Refractive Eye Surgery

Refractive Eye Surgery

Leo D. Bores MD

BORES EYE INSTITUTE

SCOTTSDALE, ARIZONA

WITH A CONTRIBUTION BY

Richard D. Smith MD

FOREWORD BY

José I. Barraquer

BOSTON

Blackwell Scientific Publications

OXFORD LONDON EDINBURGH

MELBOURNE PARIS BERLIN VIENNA

© 1993 by
Blackwell Scientific Publications, Inc.
Editorial offices:
238 Main Street, Cambridge
  Massachusetts 02142, USA
Osney Mead, Oxford OX2 0EL, England
25 John Street, London WC1N 2BL
  England
23 Ainslie Place, Edinburgh EH3 6AJ
  Scotland
54 University Street, Carlton
  Victoria 3053, Australia

Other editorial offices:
Librairie Arnette SA
2, rue Casimir-Delavigne
75006 Paris
France

Blackwell Wissenschafts-Verlag
Meinekestrasse 4
D-1000 Berlin 15
Germany

Blackwell MZV
Feldgasse 13
A-1238 Wien
Austria

First published 1993

Set by Excel Typesetters, Hong Kong
Printed in Italy by Vincenzo Bona srl, Turin
and bound in France by SIRC, Marigny-le-Châtel

93 94 95 96 5 4 3 2 1

DISTRIBUTORS

USA
  Blackwell Scientific Publications, Inc.
  238 Main Street
  Cambridge, Massachusetts 02142
  (*Orders*: Tel: 617 876-7000
            800 759-6102)

Canada
  Times Mirror Professional Publishing, Ltd
  5240 Finch Avenue East
  Scarborough, Ontario MlS 5A2
  (*Orders*: Tel: 416 298-1588
            800 268-4178)

Australia
  Blackwell Scientific Publications
  (Australia) Pty Ltd
  54 University Street
  Carlton, Victoria 3053
  (*Orders*: Tel: 03 347-0300)

Outside North America and Australia
  Marston Book Services Ltd
  PO Box 87
  Oxford OX2 0DT
  (*Orders*: Tel: 0865 791155
            Fax: 0865 791927
            Telex: 837515)

Library of Congress
Cataloguing-in-Publication Data

Bores, Leo D.
    Refractive eye surgery / by Leo D. Bores.
        p.   cm.
    Includes bibliographical references and index.
    ISBN 0–86542–152–8
    1. Refractive keratoplasty—Atlases.   I. Title.
    [DNLM.   1. Cornea—surgery—atlases.
    2. Refractive Errors—surgery—atlases.
    WW 17 B731r]
    617.7′1—dc20

Contents

Foreword

The author of this magnificent book, Dr Leo Bores, was the one to introduce radial keratotomy to the western world for the correction of myopic ametropia, a technique originally developeed by Sato in 1951 and later perfected by Fyodorov in 1977, using incisions only in the anterior face of the cornea and reducing the size of the optical zone.

Dr Bores has developed instruments and technical features to improve refractive interventions on the cornea, among them the design of diamond and sapphire blades, a corneal topographer model, an adjustable progressive increment cut turbine engine microkeratotome, keratotomy instruments, the use of centrifugal incisions, etc., instruments and techniques widely publicized in multiple journals and lectures, and which now have been gathered in this book where his experience is presented in full detail.

He puts special emphasis on the specific aspects that, if overlooked, lead to adverse results. His entire book is a paradigm of Lister's statement: "Success depends on the attention paid to details," details that the attentive reader will find in every chapter and sometimes in each paragraph.

Refractive corneal surgery has been in the past decades and is still one of the new frontiers of ophthalmology. Its basis has been well established both for lamellar and relaxation techniques. For the latter since the end of the nineteenth century and for the former since 1964, where we demonstrated that, to correct myopia, thickness must be substracted from the center of the cornea or increased in its periphery, and that to correct hyperopia, thickness must be added to the center of the cornea or substracted from its periphery. Procedures involving substraction were called keratomileusis and those involving addition received the name of keratophakia.

Procedures without freezing and laser exeresis are some recent examples of surface and intrastromal keratomileusis, without requiring a change in the procedure's name. This has been done in some cases giving the impression that the procedure in question is somehow new.

Keratotomies remain keratotomies be they straight, centrifugal or centripetal, curved, transversal, etc.; be they performed with steel, diamond, sapphire, or ruby blades; and keratomileusis remains keratomileusis, be it performed with a lathe, a microkeratome, a laser, or other exeresis procedures.

Perhaps, in the near future, and in order to avoid surgery altogether, it will be possible to soften the cornea, modify its shape, and harden it again so as to maintain its new form, thus correcting the refractive, spherical, and meridional errors in a non-surgical way.

My warmests congratulations to Dr Bores, promotor of these techniques and author of this book.

José I. Barraquer

Preface

This textbook has its beginning in the first moments of a meeting which took place almost 14 years ago on a cold, bleak, February morning between two men—one Russian, one American. The decision that led to that meeting had been taken approximately 6 months previously and seemingly by accident. Yet that decision and what came out of that meeting seems almost to have been fated.

During the spring of 1975 I had reached a crisis in my life which necessitated a change in direction. Many choices presented themselves but the one path I chose was to completely narrow my focus to two things—my family and my profession. I began to cast about for interesting things to get involved with. I was quite facile in the anterior segment and I liked the idea and potential of intraocular lens implants. So, I arranged to borrow two Copeland lenses from Henry Hirschman, a fellow Kresge Eye Alumnus, with some vague promises about "paying him back." He parted with them quite easily, which on reflection should have made me nervous. These I implanted without much difficulty but not without some reservations about their design. These lenses were the first ever implanted in Detroit and occasioned some comment, much of which was negative. Additionally, I had had no formal instruction in implantation techniques, having "learned" by attending a few presentations elsewhere (not a process generally to be recommended), so I decided to seek out an education, preferably abroad.

Since the pioneering work in intra-ocular lenses had been done mostly in England and Holland, it was there that I intended to go. Having made plans to visit Jan Worst in Gronigen in February, I chanced to mention my proposed excursion to Jo Isaacson, a colleague and former mentor. He considered what I had said and then uttered the fateful words: "Why not visit Fyodorov? No one's seen him for about 5 years—might be interesting." I was somewhat aghast; a trip to a place Winston Churchill had so aptly described as a "riddle wrapped in a mystery inside an enigma" was not quite what I had originally planned. Yet the thought piqued me. I did, after all, need to get away from everything as much as I wanted to learn new things and where better to "get away," to get shut of the world, but in Russia? "But," said I "How do I find this Fyodorov?", half hoping that there would be no answer. "Call Miles Galin," said Jo writing down the number, "he should know."

Miles Galin, as I subsequently learned, is not all that easy to reach but through some "miracle" he happened to be in his "snuggery" that day and less acerbic than usual. He took my call. "Why do you want to see Fyodorov?" he demanded in that slightly nasal and imperious tone that is so Miles. "To learn how to implant lenses," said I, unabashed. "Here's his phone number," said he. "Tell him that I recommended you. Goodbye." So I called immediately, getting Fyodorov himself on the phone. At that time his English was what can only be described as scanty, whereas my Russian was worse, consisting of "Da" and "Nyet." "Yes," he exclaimed, "you will come visit me for two weeks. We will show you all. I will send you invitation for your visa. Christmoose merry!" and he hung up.

There were still some minor details to settle before going, however. Firstly, I had no passport but luckily the US Passport Office had just streamlined their operation and I got one in 10 days. I submitted a photocopy of it and my completed visa application along with Fyodorov's cable to the Soviet Embassy in Washington. Now, never let it be said that naivety is all bad. Had I been more worldly or knowledgeable I would have *known* that there was no way that the visa would be ready in time. After all, it was only 6 weeks before I was due to leave and we're talking the Russians here. The travel agent, whose trepidations were echoed by my friends, was not hopeful and even the Soviet embassy suggested that I might reconsider my travel timetable. But again some "miracle" intervened and the visa arrived, again in 10 days. Three miracles in a row . . . I was beginning to get a little nervous. However, I had said that I was going, so armed with my *Berlitz Guide to Russian for Travelers* and some Kaopectate, I went off to visit Fyodorov at #10 Lobninskaya Ulitza, Moscow, USSR in February, 1976.

I landed at Sherymetevo Airport Number 2 on a Sunday afternoon. It was snowing and the sky was grey. Of course it was snowing, of course the sky was grey! It was February! This was Russia! Didn't the song say something about "more clouds of grey than any Russian play," etc? We debarked from the plane under brooding clouds into odorous yellow buses which took us to the old terminal, a dark concrete building of indeterminate age. "Bleaker and bleaker," said Alice. We unloaded and passed within, traversing some invisible threshold from bleakness into chaos. Therein I had my first taste of the real Russia—I got into a line. The border guards (passport control) were very solemn and very young. By the way they stared at the arrivees I half expected to be arrested and carted away to Lubyanka at any second. So far, Russia was living up to its advance billing.

Suitcase inspection was next but I had been primed by my travel agent and had placed a pack of cigarettes on top of my clothes. The pack vanished instantly and I was waved through—another miracle—everyone else was being "sifted." I passed on through the gate into still more chaos. Now what was I supposed to do? Fortunately, the professor had sent someone to meet me, Doctor Topolovna. Somehow she had found

me amongst the throng but it turned out that she had even less English than the professor and my Russian had not improved in the interim. So we stared helplessly at each other for a time until I heard my name called. I looked toward the sound, which was coming from a row of tables at which a woman was looking in my direction expectantly. When I looked back to my new acquaintance she had vanished.

The woman who had called out for me was with Intourist and spoke passable English. She handed me a fistful of vouchers and rattled off some instructions before passing me off to a rather disreputable looking specimen who turned out to be my driver to the hotel. Between he and I and a *nisilchik* (porter) we managed to get my baggage into his black Volga (for a time I thought Volga meant *black*, because I didn't see one in any other color until years later). After a mildly harrowing ride into the city I was deposited at the Gastanyeetza Nationale (National Hotel) right across from the Kremlin. I turned over my passport and vouchers to the reception desk and was taken upstairs where I was introduced to the floor lady—the Cerebrus of the Room Keys. She unlocked the 9 foot tall, etched glass fronted door and ushered me into a baroque room right out of Doctor Zhivago. I set my bag down, and closed the door behind me—I had arrived in Moscow.

The next morning, Dima, the professor's personal driver, collected me at the hotel and rocketed me to the clinic. Dima was a Tartar and his car had two speeds—stop and go-like-blazes. The clinic was a rather decrepit looking building set amongst an apartment complex and surrounded by a drunkenly leaning concrete fence. I found out later that the building was actually an annex to a gynecologic hospital nearby and that Fyodorov had it "on loan." I walked up the brick steps, through the double-doored entry and into a time warp.

My first impression was that I had been somehow transported back to the past into a hospital existing in the States some 50 or 60 years earlier. All the equipment and furnishings, the rooms, everything, seemed like photos of some by gone age come suddenly alive. I followed my driver up the stairs to the second floor, down the hall to a solitary door on the left, opened it and stepped into an adventure that changed my life and the lives of countless thousands, forever.

I wasn't sure what I expected but what I got was the greeting "Aha! Louva Boris!" and a bear hug. I gasped "Professor Fyodorov?" in that wheezy, throaty style that comes either from nervousness or from having one's breath squeezed out, or both. He looked a little like Kruschev but with hair cut to a flattopped brush. He had an enormous chest and wide shoulders with large hands and fingers (I was to find out a little later just how skilled those hands and fingers were). His eyes were bright and he had an engaging smile that lit his entire face as well as most of the room. He offered me tea, which I accepted. He was gruff. He was direct. I liked him instantly.

He was also very gracious and open and true to his word. In the next few days he "showed me all," as he had said he would. I had been there but 2 days when he announced that he wanted to show me something else. He then introduced me to a procedure involving making radiating incisions in the corneal stroma which he said was "against *blizarukist*" (nearsightedness). My initial reaction was one of disbelief, a reaction that I'm sure everyone experiences when first exposed to this procedure. After all, it seemed rather a bizarre solution to the "spectacle problem." In addition, I knew something of Sato's work. It hadn't worked for Sato, why should it work for Fyodorov? Could this perhaps be another Russian "re-invention" of previous technology? He sensed my hesitation because he said "No, it is not Sato procedure. We do incisions only from outside." Still, I would have left it at that had it not been for one thing: Slava and I had become fast friends in those past 2 days.

Everyone who meets Svyataslav Nicholævich Fyodorov is struck by the charisma of the man—I was no exception. However, there seemed to be something deeper between us, almost as though we had known each other for a thousand years. It was a mutual connection that had manifested itself the very first instant we met. We soon began to communicate "*dusha-a-dusha*" or soul to soul. We quickly found that we thought very much alike and there was understanding and absolute candor between us. In some instances we would finish each others sentences, at other times no sentences at all were necessary. Somehow, despite the barrier of language, we understood and trusted one another, completely. Therefore, when he explained this procedure to me, I was disposed to believe him, despite my initial reservations.

I was allowed to examine, without interference, all of the available patients who had had the surgery to that point; there were 135 in all and it took several days to round them up. Each had unaided visual acuity ranging from 6/5 to 6/9 (20/15 to 20/30) with a follow-up period ranging from 2 weeks to 2 years. An examination of their records showed that preoperatively they all had unaided vision of 20/100 or less (Cyrillic numerals are the same as ours). If the records were correct, and there was no reason to believe that they were not, then there was no question that the corneas of these patients had become flatter as a consequence of this "bizarre" surgery "against *blizarukist*."

I suggested that I would like to check the next group of pre-operative patients personally. I carefully recorded the examinations and matched them with the names both on the chart and their wristbands. I also followed them into the operating room and observed their surgery. Post-operatively I found that their corneas had become flatter and that the myopia had disappeared. In some cases the refractions were on the plus side. It being Friday and since I was going by train to Leningrad that evening, I would have the weekend to ponder this phenomenon and to offer comment. Upon my return to Moscow early Monday morning, I found Slava there to greet me at the train station. He asked if I felt like doing a "little surgery." When I replied positively he said "good!" because he had eight cases lined up for me, four of which were keratotomy cases. I broke out in a sweat despite the temperature being 20 below zero.

We were whisked to the hospital where we exchanged mufti for hospital attire. After scrubbing up, I was led into the operating theater where I was gowned and then seated, gloveless, at the operating microscope, an Opton (which is a Zeiss in disguise). My assistant was Boris Feldman, the "interpreter" who had been with me most of the previous week. His English was terrible and I didn't know a "*britva*" from a "*nosh*". I looked around for Slava but he had unaccountedly vanished! Then I looked through the scope at the case before me. "Ye merciful Gods!" I thought. (That is *not* what I *actually* thought but it's close.) It was a hypermature membranous cataract! The eye was already open, and Boris handed me two hooks! "*Jehosophat!*" thought I (which is *not* what I thought but . . . well, you get the picture). Here I was, a stranger in a strange land trying to perform eye surgery with strange tools and not a familiar face in sight! The feeling was right up there with the sensation of falling off a building.

So I did what I always did in situations like this— put myself on automatic pilot. Upon closing the eye after having lost only a small bit of vitreous and implanting my very first Sputnik intra-ocular lens, a disembodied voice said: "Very nice, Louva! You may operate in my clinic any time you want." I looked around and then it hit me—Slava had been watching the whole thing via television! But I wasn't thinking about the joke he had just played on me (he confessed later) but about what he had just said. I have never told him just how much that simple statement meant to me at that time or since but I would not trade that moment for any other in the world.

Within a few minutes, Slava rejoined me in the operating theater and we began my first "dosaged dissection of the circumferential ligament of Kokott" (which was what Fyodorov called the surgery; a somewhat droll name which I subsequently changed to *radial keratotomy*). At that time the surgery was done "free hand" with an unguarded razor blade held in a blade breaker. Slava assisted and guided me step-by-step through each case. It was a peak experience for me, needless to say. The incisions were all made beginning outside the limbus and moving in toward the optic center, a nerve wracking proposition I can assure you. After each stroke of the knife, a "dipstick" gauge was used to check the depth of the incision. Thirty-two incisions were each made in that manner. One week later we did the other eye of each patient. In each case, corneal flattening occurred and the myopia vanished. Furthermore, the fellow corneas were still flat.

Needless to say I was thrilled. I was also apprehensive because if this operation really worked, and it certainly seemed that it did, it should be introduced into the United States. The potential of this procedure for doing great good was enormous. Considering the temperament of my colleagues, however, there was also an enormous potential for personal disaster. After all, who the devil was this upstart Leo Bores? Supposing that it did not work after all? *Chort voz me*, the devil take me!

When I returned to the United States I tested the waters. I conferred with some of the other physicians who had visited Fyodorov but had not known about this operation. They all gave me the same answer: "too risky," "too variable," "too unpredictable," "won't last," etc. Others mentioned Sato. So I decided to lay low. Also, the follow-up in the Russian series had only been 2 years, hardly enough time to decide if the method really effected a permanent corneal change.

Nevertheless, I mentioned it, almost in jest, to a couple of problem patients of mine. They weren't very happy with their glasses and were having difficulties with their contact lenses as well. I must confess that I was not prepared for their reaction. They practically exploded. They demanded the procedure on the spot. "Never mind the follow-up, just get me out of these damned glasses!" was one of the milder retorts. That was my initiation into the world of myopes. I had not realized until that moment just how trapped and helpless many of these people felt, how dependent they were on a simple visual aid. I began to realize that myopia was a very real problem, a congenital anomaly that we were "treating" with crutches.

In the fall of 1976, Slava came to the United States as my guest and stayed at my home in Detroit, Michigan. I arranged for him to give a lecture at the Kresge Eye Institute on the topic of "dosaged dissection". The response was polite but indifferent.

In May 1977, I returned to Moscow, bringing with me a retinue of well-known eye surgeons from the States including the late Bill Valloton, then director of the Storm Eye Institute at the University of South Carolina in Charleston. My Chief Resident, Steve Gianarelli, accompanied us as well. The others were shown the procedure and again the response was one of indifference. Steve and I examined the patients that I had operated on the year before. Very little change had taken place in the shape of their corneas and they were still seeing well. I also examined the records of some of the earlier cases, as well as more of the previous patients themselves. They were all doing well. There were no regressions (beyond that expected in the first 3 months), no infections, and no decompensatory changes in the cornea. "Now," said Slava, "You will do in the United States!"

However, the possibility of being "burned at the stake" still loomed before me. If I did do it, while I may be thought of as some sort of god by the patients, I felt that I was bound to be "God something else" to my colleagues. Steve opined that that sort of possibility had never stopped me before this and suggested that I purchase a pair of asbestos BVDs and a flak jacket and get on with it.

Considerable dialog followed between Slava and myself *vis-à-vis* this procedure in the insuing months. Finally, in the early spring of 1978, he showed me the records of the patients that I had operated 2 years previously. That, coupled with the good results and 4 years of follow-up on almost 200 other Soviet patients, was sufficient—I had to get off dead center. Therefore, in November of 1978, when Bob Jampel (my Department Chief) was out of town, I "sneaked" a patient into the hospital and did the case under general anesthesia (the Russians at that time were doing the surgery under topical anesthesia, consisting of 1% tetracaine). That first patient was a young black woman in her thirties who had bilateral myopia of −3.25 D, and a long history of contact lens intolerance with skin irritation from her spectacles. She had been a patient of mine for years and had begun nursing school with my wife.

I must tell you that doing the first eye, all alone, was the most trying and difficult experience in my entire life. It was worse than doing that first case in Russia. Unless you have been there it is impossible to appreciate the degree of stress such a situation can engender. Your whole life passes in front of your eyes like an old-time movie. I was "assisted" by an ignorant first year eye resident who, mercifully, shall remain anonymous and who bombarded me with incessant and inane questions and who, I'm sure, ran off bleating to the Chief as soon as he was able. Sweat poured from my body in torrents. I wanted to be elsewhere. A voice within me kept crying out "What the hell are you doing here, Bores?". "Everything is cool," thought I. After all, 4 years of experience were in the can. This procedure worked! "Oh yeah?" said the voice, "Suppose you blow it?" Meanwhile I was filming it, and as I worked away the room began to fill up with spectators. Through the whispering I caught words like "What is it *this* time?", "crazy bastard," "Fantastic!" "He's gone bonkers," "never a dull moment with Bores around!" etc. But I didn't "blow it," it was fantastic, and 2 weeks later I operated her other eye. Her uncorrected visual acuity was 20/25 (where it has remained to this day). The operation worked, as it was supposed to, and as I really knew it would deep down.

In January, I proudly presented my patient at Grand Rounds and showed the film that I had made. I also presented some of the Russian data—zero response! Correction, there was *one* question: "Isn't this the Sato procedure?" and that from one of the most learned of the group. Apparently no one had been listening. By that time, however, I was totally convinced that any attempt by me to communicate this idea to my esteemed local colleagues was an exercise in futility. It was obvious that I was hearing different music than they were and marching to a different drummer altogether.

I therefore decided that the best course of action was to proceed according to my convictions. The Chief, bless him, looked the other way while I did two more cases before he "asked" that I submit a proper research protocol to the university human research committee, which I did. It was a carefully constructed protocol which met all of the requirements of the NIH, the Hague Convention, and the University Safety in Human Research guidelines. It passed with flying colors and was pronounced by the chairman of the Human Research Committee, Dr Prasad, as the best example of such a protocol he had ever seen, and well it should be having been modeled on the one devised for intra-ocular lenses written by Miles Galin. It later became the basis of other such protocols throughout the world including the PERK study.

I also decided that this procedure was too big for just one man. Accordingly, I set up the framework for the National Radial Keratotomy Study Group and went about selecting individuals whom I felt were "team players" and not afraid to stick with a program. Thus the stage was set for what followed, the start of a new era in the annals of eye surgery and the birth of a new sub-specialty, refractive eye surgery. The stage was also set for a fire storm of criticism and rebuke hardly to be imagined. I did expect *some* controversy based on the response to the surgery by my local colleagues. It was still a shock and trial though when it really "hit the fan."

The mildest criticism offered was that radial keratotomy was not new, that it had been done before and that it didn't work (referring to the Sato operation). Of course, the wheel is not new either; it had been done before as well—lo these many years ago. However, no one confuses the earlier product with our new and modern wheel and I doubt that anyone would care to return to that older design.

Worse was the accusation that we were irresponsibly endangering vision by incising normal corneal tissue in an effort to cure something that was not even a disease. We were branded as "buccaneers" capitalizing on peoples' fears and misinformation (a sword, as later shown, that cuts both ways, see Chapter 11). But we knew that we were not the monsters we had been painted to be. We also knew that the critics were wrong. Myopia *is* a congenital "disease." It is every bit as disabling and as disheartening a handicap as a withered arm or leg or a cleft palate. It meets the conventional definition of a handicap in that it requires an external or artifical appliance for the afflicted to function normally. It interferes with normal functions as much as deformed limbs. It can be life-threatening as well. Furthermore, visual appliances are a hoax and a cruel joke on the patient. Their presence engenders false hope and breeds dependence. Patients are fooled into thinking that they can see, but when the appliances are lost, the patient is lost.

This disease causes discrimination both consciously and subconsciously. "Men don't make passes at girls who wear glasses" is not just a clever jingle, it is an insight into a strong social prejudice. Manufacturers recognize this and "fancy up" spectacles to make the wearer "more attractive." But in truth, the wearer is isolated, behind a window, peering out at the world —*ænigmatate*—through a glass, darkly.

Contact lenses are also an attempt to remove the stigma. There is no denying that, for some, contact lenses provide the only hope of usable vision. But there is also no question that this type of wearer is in the minority. Most people wear contacts because "they look terrible in glasses." They may not admit this. Their usual explanation is that they "see better." Anyone who has fitted more than two pairs of contact lenses will recognize the contact lens "failures" who insist that they won't give up the lenses because they "see better" (even when the patient's best corrected vision with contacts may be 20/30 as opposed to 20/15 with spectacles).

Yet, who is to say that they don't see better? What do we mean by "see better" anyway? There is ample evidence to show that vision is more than reading the small print on an eye chart—witness the small success of the Bates Method. Yet for lack of the ability to read that chart without a visual aid, doors are closed to the afflicted. How many potential Neil Armstrongs or Amelia Earharts are sitting out their lives on the side lines, not even getting a chance to participate?

Anyone can visualize a small child with a leg brace, a victim of a congenital defect. Everyone can see that the child's progress is impaired. Who would deny the right to discard that brace, that crutch, that dependence? It would take an insensitive person indeed not to picture his joy at running and climbing unencumbered. It would take a granite heart to state, "he gets along well enough with his braces; he can survive and function well enough." However, only a champion of mediocrity and the status quo would opt for that kind of choice. Why should a visual handicap not entitle that individual to relief? Why should he be doomed to the status quo? Why cannot he partake of the "forbidden fruit"? Who gave *us* the mandate to make that judgement anyway?

Still, someone will invariably say: "Surely this argument is all nonsense. What has the patient's sense of well being got to do with it? What does 'quality of life' have to do with the 'sacred' art and science of medicine? The patient has no choice. He's incapable of choice. How could anyone be so irresponsible as to propose to actually cut into a normal cornea, just to do away with glasses? That's utter foolishness! Why, any fool can see that it's dangerous. It exposes the eye to infection! The whole idea is utter nonsense!" However, like the measurement of time and space, the concept of nonsense is relative, and we can always be sure when we use it, that from some frame of reference, it applies to us. Reality is never as we suppose it to be or wish it to be. Experience is the only reality. What is—is. There is no "supposed to be." The only "truth" is what is there. Perishing few of the frightful things that were "supposed" to happen with this surgery have ever happened!

I had hoped that recognition of this Zen-like concept of reality on the part of detractors, well meaning and otherwise, would have ended the discussion and let us get back to the task at hand, namely refining the "wheel." Unfortunately, that hope was not to be realized for some years. It is a sad commentary on our human species that the NIH ("Not Invented Here") syndrome is so pervasive. It seems that there is a tendency for those of the species *Homo sapiens* to look with suspicion upon anything not personally created. While in the past this had great survival value, its usefulness has diminished in a cooperative society. Some have developed this tendency to a fine art, and have carried it to the extreme of telling others how to order their lives (witness the "Carrie Nations" of the world). This propensity is defended under the guise of teaching the "great unwashed" the error of their ways. The common denominator here is the belief that others are incapable of thought and that only the "professor" possesses the qualities of honesty, knowledge, and forthrightness. Do I hear an "amen," brothers and sisters?

This phenomenon was not confined to just my situation, Trokel and Munnerlyn encountered the same problem early in the history of excimer laser surgery of the eye. Which prompts the author to cry: "Ye merciful gods, will there be no respite!?" Where, pray, do these "seers" and keepers of ultimate "wisdom," who have, unfortunately, elbowed their way into controlling positions, come from? "History does not repeat itself, only man does." So goes the saying and how true it is. After having been thrashed completely over their opposition to penetrating keratoplasty, vitrectomy, α-chymotrypsin, intraocular lenses, and radial keratotomy, the "nay-sayers" persist in saying nay. How quaint. How old. How utterly boring—perhaps they're betting on being "right" one of these times. Considering their dismal track record, my advice would be to stay away from Las Vegas—the disease of *chronic recurring wrongness* is obviously incurable. Many of these down-putters are, no doubt, puffing up about their current acceptance of radial keratotomy and many have wriggled their way into the forefront of the excimer laser arena. It has been said that the essence of humankind is intelligence and that the essence of intelligence is learning from one's mistakes. This does not speak well of the nay-sayers. In scientific and medical endeavors there will always be disagreement, this is healthy. Discourse and open-mindedness are the key to medical progress—suppression and censorship are its death. Oliver Wendell Holmes, Jr, said it quite well:

> When men have realized that time has upset many fighting faiths, they may come to believe even more than they believe the very foundations of their own conduct that the ultimate good desired is better reached by free trade in ideas—that the best test of truth is the power of the thought to get itself accepted in the competition of the market, and that truth is the only ground upon which their wishes safely can be carried out.

The author addresses this additional thought to the young reader who is both new upon this scene and who is experiencing his/her greening within the profession: Study and heed the lessons of medical history, recent and remote, so that you will not be included amongst those mean spirited of your colleages to whom nothing is sacred but their own petrified opinion. Admit to yourself the possibility, nay the probability, that you will often be mistaken in your views. And have a care to husband your opinion and remember that: "It is better to keep silent and be thought a fool than to speak and remove all doubt." [Abraham Lincoln]

It hardly seems possible that almost 16 years have passed since that first visit to Hospital #81, 10 Lobninskaya Street. When it all began, much of what has transpired since was then only a dream. When the contents of my first radial keratotomy syllabus were transcribed, a battle was raging over what had begun as a simple and earnest desire to improve the lives of an unrecognized group of sufferers—the myopes. Since then the storm of that war has passed by leaving only sporadic "guerrilla" action. Energy has been turned to the more important task of furthering the art of refractive surgery. During these past 16-plus years there has been born a new sub-speciality, refractive eye surgery. To be sure, such surgery had been done before (*c.* 1713?) but quietly and by very few. Not until I performed that first case of radial keratotomy in 1978 did that interest change from a tiny spark into a raging fire. The knowledge that I have been instrumental in igniting and fanning those flames has sustained me through some very dark times. All in all, I think that I acted wisely, time will tell. I must confess, though, that during the early part of this adventure I became quite empathetic with the frontiersmen's penchant for lynching rustlers and claim jumpers. That, however, is a story best left for another time and another place.

Leo D. Bores MD
Scottsdale, Arizona

Acknowledgments

No one can be the sole author of a work of this magnitude—no matter how fervently they may wish it or how hard they may try to accomplish it. The ghosts of authors past are forever peering over the writer's shoulder, whispering criticism and advice. At times the murmuring can become so insistant and strident as to cause the writer to temporarily lose his identity. Sometimes the "conversation" takes on the flavor of a fireside chat with friends:

Whate'er I feel I cannot feel alone.
When I am happiest or most forlorn,
Uncounted friends, whom I have never known
Rejoicing stand or grieving by my side,
These nameless, faceless friends of mine who died
A thousand years or more e'er I was born.
[Rosalind Murray]

In fact, the very process of such an undertaking triggers a metamorphosis in thought and being. It is not possible to come away from such an experience with a whole skin. Had I realized this potential hazard at the outset, perhaps I would have declined the challenge. Perhaps, but not likely. Such an opportunity is not proferred to all who seek it—thus one must grasp the nettle. Carpe diem. Kismet.

Fortunately I had help. Firstly, from Richard Smith who initially had to be bludgeoned into acquiescence. To him was assigned the task of writing the chapter on corneal anatomy and the pathology of corneal wound healing. Heavy stuff, that. To his credit he did admirably. Frank Thompson was next on my "hit list." My man Vito convinced Frank to supply materials for the chapter on scleral reinforcement. This contribution is, in fact, fitting. It is not possible to do justice to that subject without incorporating the important work of this distinguished pioneer.

To my good friend and fellow adventurer Akira Momose, go the laurels for shedding light on the early days of refractive surgery in Japan—*á la* Sato. His own work on posterior scleral support is not without merit. It would have been difficult, to say the least, to write the ametropia chapter without the help and encouragement of "Doctor Myopia" Brian Curtin. His monumental work *The Myopias* is recommended reading for all refractive surgeons, aspiring or otherwise. And if the text of the current treatise sometimes transcends the usual pedantic style expected of a work of this type, thank Guido Majno. His wonderful book *The Healing Hand: Man and Wound in the Ancient World* proved to me that it is possible to be scholarly without being stuffy. I am indebted, as well, to Professor Gabriel van Rij of the Academisch Ziekenhuis, Gronigen, Netherlands, for the history of Lans and other Dutch investigators. The "Learned Man", Houdijn Beekhuis, kept me in stitches if nothing else.

His droll perspective on certain aspects of medicine was enlightening to say the least.

To all the ghosts—Imhotep, Hippocrates, Aristotle, Galen, Al Hazen, Keppler, Tadini, Boerhaave, Young, to name but a few—my profound and humble thanks. Take a break.

My earnest and heartfelt good wishes to those others of my colleagues (cited throughout the text) without whose support much of this treatise would be figureless. Without the able assistance of Dick Wolf, curator of Harvard's Countway Library, and Reva Hurtes, librarian and rare book guru at the Bascom Palmer Eye Institute, we would be without many of our historic illustrations. My profound thanks to Karla VanderSypen, Head of the Rare Book Room at the library of the University of Michigan, and especially to Mary Lou Goldstein, Chief Librarian at Scottsdale Memorial Hospital-North and her able assistant Deborah LaBarbera, who provided assistance above and beyond their requirement to do so. Kudos as well to the charming May Cheney, whose beautiful artwork graces many of these pages.

I am particularly indebted to my professional critics who continually provided me with stimulation and helped me to remember exactly what it was that I was trying to accomplish with refractive surgery. This kept me from becoming lazy and complacent and forced me to weigh everything that I said carefully and to be prepared to back it up—it still does.

I have enjoyed the support and encouragement of my many friends as well as my family from the very beginning of this medical adventure. Much of what lies within these pages was stimulated both by experience and in intimate discussion with these friends, but of course, none of this was accomplished without episodes of depression and self-doubt. The example of Slava Fyodorov, as he struggled to build his dream, was a constant inspiration to me. The numerous "skull sessions" with him were always sure to strike sparks of inspiration in us both. I am grateful to my long-suffering wife Leara who gave back as good as she got and then some. She has provided insight into areas of which I was untutored and used her "sharp stick" when I became down and feeling sorry for myself. To her and to Molly, my secretary at the Kresge Eye Institute; to Ella, Karen, Kathy, and Laura, my tough assistants; and to Bob, Jane, Carlo, Mahmud, and the other patients too numerous to name who played a part, my undying gratitude—I hope that I have not let you down. To Mother Nature, I got the message and thanks.

Finally, to the late Professor A.D. Ruedeman, Sr, my first *sensei*, whose gruff model of bulldog determination and no nonsense approach to medicine has served me well; to my gentlemanly chief, the late Windsor S. Davies, who inherited the rough beginnings and put the final polish on a brash young eye resident; to my mentor and friend, José Ignacio Barraquer, whose paradigm of diligence and rectitude is always before me; and of course to my dear friend Slava, I dedicate this text.

Leo D. Bores MD
Scottsdale, Arizona

Refractive
Eye
Surgery

1
Introduction

It has long been an axiom of mine that the little things are infinitely the most important. [Sir Arthur Conan Doyle]

This work is about a new type of eye surgery—refractive eye surgery—designed primarily to remove the visual handicap of ametropia, chiefly myopia. To be sure, hyperopia and astigmatism take their toll in diminished vision. However, it is myopia that is, by far, the greatest scourge and toward which the majority of our energies have been focused. This treatise is designed to prepare the beginning refractive surgeon for this adventure by providing a firm grounding in basic fundamentals and techniques and to assist the general ophthalmologist in understanding these methodologies. The experienced refractive surgeon will find much that is of value within these pages as well. All aspects of the problem including hyperopia and astigmatism are included and practical tips and methods of surgical treatment are detailed.

This work is not, however, encyclopedic nor does it attempt to be. The author has found through experience that eclecticism has no place in refractive surgery. If ever the old saw, too many cooks spoil the broth, were true it is surely here. All too often instruction courses are given in which many guest speakers present so many differing points of view, undoubtedly in the spirit of non-bias, that the erstwhile refractive surgeon goes away more confused and bewildered than before. It is just not possible, however, to "mix-and-match" with this surgery. Beginning refractive surgeons cannot be eclectic in their surgical approach and expect it to be effective. Nor are they in any position to decide what to choose and what to discard. They must first adopt the surgical method of a particular, experienced, surgeon and follow his or her method assiduously until such time that they have become absolutely confident in their understanding of all the nuances of the surgery. Then and only then will it be possible for the surgeon to "vary the theme" and strike off on his or her own. Thus this present work emerges as the point of view of one individual—with a little help from friends—admixed with a tincture of philosophy to give it some spice.

Refractive eye surgery is defined as that surgery upon the eye which acts to change the light-bending characteristics of that eye. This definition would include such things as cataract surgery, with or without the implantation of an intra-ocular lens. This discussion will, however, confine itself to surgery performed upon the cornea, sclera, or lens of the eye specifically for modifying its refractive characteristics.

In 1708, Hermann Boerhaave suggested that high myopia could perhaps be treated by couching the clear lens in such patients. Von Haller, in 1746, may well have tried it but it was not until 1894 that Fukala published his first reports on the technique of clear lens extraction for myopia. In 1869, Snellen, in an article published in the German literature, discussed the possibilities of correcting corneal astigmatism, possibly drawing on the attempts of Von Galezowski to achieve the same purpose through resection of a crescentic piece from the cornea. Bates, in 1894, described a surgical technique for such modification and reported a number of cases, as did Lans in 1898. Thus the search for effective surgical means to modify ametropia began.

The evolution of such surgical techniques resembles, in many ways, the development of manned flight. As experience and technical skills improve, early and more primitive efforts give way to more advanced ideas and methods. Sometimes ideas that were previously discarded or not implemented because of technical deficiencies are revived at a later time when they are capable of being used or their worth fully recognized.

Parallel to these and other technological advances have come changes in the psycho-social makeup of human society. In the early days, the battle against disease was black and white. Disease was once thought of as God's punishment to the ungodly and meddling with its progress sinful. As medicine advanced, the subject of preventive medicine began to play a more important role. Today there is more emphasis on the quality of life and the human condition than ever before and procedures designed to modify human existence, such as genetic engineering, plastic reconstructive surgery, and refractive surgery of the eye, are being employed.

Throughout such evolution, however, the innovator must battle not only with those specific problems that accompany the treatment itself, but must also confront and surmount those generated by the actions and attitudes of contemporaries and colleagues. Such circumstances are, of course, not new and given human nature, are very likely to continue.

There are currently five methods of surgically modifying the corneal curvature presently in general usage. These are:

1 Mechanical modulation of corneal shape—keratomileusis.
2 Relaxing incisions—radial keratotomy.
3 Corneal onlays—epikeratophakia.
4 Corneal inlays—keratophakia.
5 Tissue replacement—keratoplasty.

Of these five, keratoplasty does not always have as its primary goal (except in cases of keratoconus) the modification of the corneal curvature and so will be discussed only incidentally. Additionally, clear lens extraction or intra-ocular lens implantation can be employed to reduce high myopia and scleral reinforcement can shorten axial length and prevent further elongation of the globe. Such approaches to the problem, once considered bizarre and risky, are now being more seriously entertained as primary or alternative treatments of ametropia.

To be successful as a refractive surgeon, the ophthalmologist must develop a special mind-set. He or she must come to terms with the fact that refractive surgery is truly micro-surgery and that micro-meters count. He or she must not be swayed by the argument that because biological systems are variable in nature, precision is unnecessary in the performance of this surgery. It is vital that the surgeon should make precise those things that he or she can control and minimize the imprecision of those things that he or she cannot. The surgeon must also avoid the tendency to simplify the surgical decision-making process *ad absurdum*.

There is a strong tendency by the neophyte to take short cuts and because of inexperience to overlook data deemed insignificant. However, as in no other aspect of ophthalmology, the careful gathering and integration of numerous parameters to affect a desirable end result are paramount. As never before, beginning surgeons cannot rely upon common sense to guide them through the learning experience. They cannot "wing it." They must instead rely upon the hard-won experience of fellow surgeons who have gone before. As John Dickinson said: "Experience must be our only guide. Reason may mislead us." Because of this fact, this surgery finds no place for instant experts and incisional configurations of the month. Good ideas will still be good ideas 6 months or a year from now. Sudden flashes of inspiration are too often found to be mere glints of the egoist's eye which pale when exposed to the harsh light of time and reality. Small changes in technique, often made for no other reason than that "it seemed right," can produce a domino effect not apparent for some time, perhaps years.

Radial keratotomy is a case in point. This surgery is said to be simple and that it is not necessary to do "all those measurements." If it were possible to perform this surgery optimally through the consideration of only a few parameters or by consultation of rigid tables, then those who have labored long and hard to bring this surgery about would be doing it the simple way.

Such simplifications have led, for example, to overcorrections and progression of effect after radial keratotomy. It was such innovation that produced circular-radial keratotomy in some 30 patients with resultant increased myopia, and non-healing and marsupialization of the wounds. This was done by an "expert" some 7 days after taking his first course in radial keratotomy. It was another "expert" who kept his patients on topical steroids four times daily for more than 6 months to "enhance the effect" of his ineffective surgical technique and induced cataracts. It was another "expert" who over-extended his blade in the presence of a flat chamber and incised the anterior capsule of the lens. It was still another "expert" who neglected to cover his patient with antibiotics after a microperforation; the eye then went on to develop endophthalmitis.

It is simple to watch this surgery being done by an expert who often makes it look so easy. After all, how could it be hard to make a cut on the eye? It's done all of the time. But the incision made for a cataract extraction is not expected to produce a precisely modulated change of corneal curvature—it's expected only to provide access to the anterior chamber. This surgery is only simple to "screw up." There are too many factors involved, all supported by clinical results over time, to take the casual approach. It is possible to guide an aircraft to a landing or simply to "arrive." One can also "arrive" on the first floor by leaping from the 10th, but the results would not be as satisfactory as taking the elevator. Some surgeons find the elevator too slow for their tastes and insist upon leaping—taking the patient with them.

All of these surgeries continue to evoke controversy despite successful application of the basic principles and techniques. Some of the cautious statements that were made in the beginning were valid then but not today. Moreover, some problems previously trumpeted have resulted from inappropriate application or execution of these procedures and are not inherent, as once believed.

These cases have served to emphasize a point often overlooked: this surgery is micro-surgery in its strictest sense. It requires of the surgeon a particular mind-set. He or she must convert from "macro" to "micro" thinking. He or she must think in terms of micrometers instead of millimeters. He or she must pay attention to pre-operative testing as never before. He or she must consider, and weigh as significant, parameters which heretofore seemed "not to matter." It should not be surprising that some surgeons fail in

this conversion. A gifted cataract surgeon may not make a gifted micro-refractive surgeon. If it happens to you, don't blame the surgery; some of us can't ride skateboards very well either. Kismet.

This is no place for the casual or occasional surgeon. This is no province for the surgical dilettante. None of these techniques are simple despite their appearance and some are on a par with open-heart surgery in their complexity. No general surgeon would dream of performing open-heart surgery, leaving that to specialists. So too refractive surgery. There are a myriad of small details that must be constantly considered and concentration on the case at hand is essential to success. Such necessity does not fit in well with the general practice of ophthalmology. The proper performance of this surgery is best left to specialists who have dedicated themselves to it and are prepared to continue to dedicate themselves to it. Teaching of these techniques should not be done as a matter of course in a residency program but afterwards in a program devoted to refractive surgery alone. This represents a shift in my previous position on this subject. However, continued misapplication of these techniques by general ophthalmic surgeons has made this shift in opinion necessary.

This is not a definitive text—no text on this subject could ever be—rather consider it a primer on refractive eye surgery. The type of surgery we are describing is undergoing an evolution of impressive dimension. Still the basics have not changed. The rationale behind each technique remains. It is hoped that the refractive surgeon, beginner and shellback, will find within these pages those tools necessary to take the next step, whenever or where ever that might be. Thus the thrust of this text is as a foundation, a sheet-anchor from whence one can cast off on the great adventure that is refractive surgery.

2
The Nature of Ametropia

The newly invented optick glasses are immoral since they pervert the natural sight, and make things appear in an unnatural and false light. [Mr Cross, Vicar of Chew Magna, Somersetshire, England (13th century)]

Introduction and historical background

Near-sighted people have sought ways to get rid of their glasses for centuries. Tradition says the ancient (presumably myopic) Chinese slept with sandbags on their eyes to flatten their corneas. It is certain Purkinje tried the same thing in the 1820s with only temporary improvement of his 5 D of myopia. In the mid 1800s, a Dr J Ball advertised a small mallet mounted on a spring in an eye cup that struck the cornea through the closed eyelid, pounding it flat. "It restores your eyesight and renders spectacles useless," he claimed. "Professor" Charles Tyrell claimed a similar effect from the use of his Ideal Sight Restorer at the turn of the century (Figures 2.1 and 2.2) [1]. Ridiculous perhaps, ineffectual certainly, but not all such notions were either ridiculous or ineffectual—they may have just been untimely. Timing, as someone once said, is everything. This is especially true in medicine. Methods considered bizarre, far-fetched, impractical, or fantastical in some yesteryear, are not so seen today. That being true, who can say what the verdict of tomorrow will be?

It is not possible to say with assurance just who it was that first conceived of treating ametropia or altering the refractive power of the eye surgically. Perhaps some long-forgotten troglodyte had his myopic vision restored after an injury—before his visual handicap led to his demise—and may have wondered over it. It is not clear that the ancients (before Aristotle) even recognized ametropia as such. Nevertheless, many of these early physicians were astute observers, and many of their medical techniques made sense even if they seemed to have ascribed the cure to supernatural intervention. Certainly visual problems other than that due to disease were observed and treated from the earliest of times, but we lack direct and pertinent documentation of such treatments.

The Egyptians had a long and apparently deserved reputation as physicians *swnw* (sounou). Homer speaks of Egypt in Book IV of the *Odyssey*:

> In that country the fertile soil produces all kinds of juices which may have a good or bad effect. There everybody is a physician and surpasses in experience all other men; because verily they are from the family of Paeon.

That Egyptian medicine was apparently sacerdotal does not mean that superstition held sway over common sense, despite some modern views to the contrary. Their knowledge of treatment of trauma was quite advanced and thorough, as evidenced by the Edwin Smith surgical and Ebers papyri [2–4]. Figure 2.3 shows the Stele of Iry (2400 BC), the earliest known ophthalmologist, while Figure 2.4 shows a physician treating an eye.

However, except for some references to weak vision

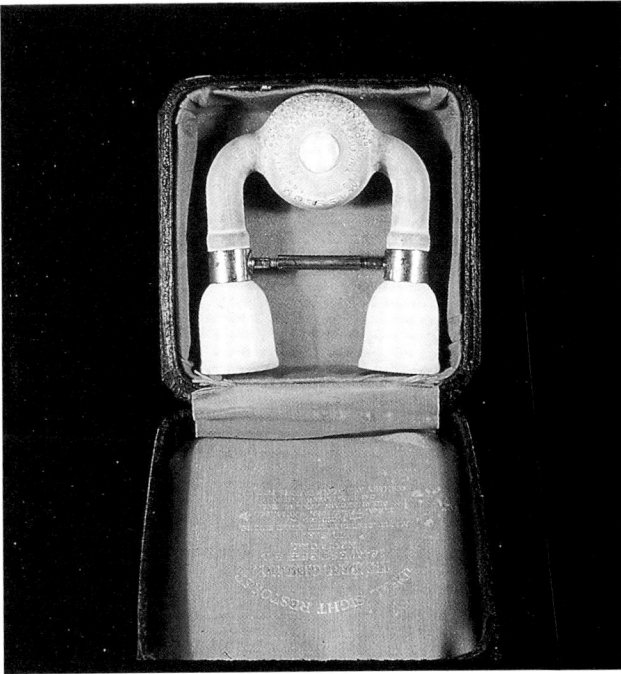

Fig. 2.1 The Ideal Sight Restorer of "Professor" Tyrell, circa 1909 (Andrew Ferry, MD).

NEVER DID A POET SING OF THE BEAUTY OF A SPECTACLED EYE OR INDITE A SONNET TO "MY ADORABLE LADY WITH THE EYEGLASSES."

SIGHT RESTORED
Spectacles Useless
AVOID HEADACHE OR SURGICAL OPERATION. READ "ILLUSTRATED TREATISE ON THE EYE. IMPAIRED VISION, WEAK, WATERY, SORE OR INFLAMED EYES, ASTIGMATISM, PRESBYOPIA, MYOPIA, CATARACT, AND THE WORST DISORDERS OF THE EYE." MAILED FREE. SAVE YOUR EYES.
THE IDEAL COMPANY, 239 BROADWAY, NEW YORK.

Fig. 2.2 Advertisement extolling the virtues of the Sight Restorer (Andrew Ferry, MD).

Fig. 2.3 The Stele of Iry (2400 BC)—the first ophthalmologist (Kunsthistorisches Museum, Vienna).

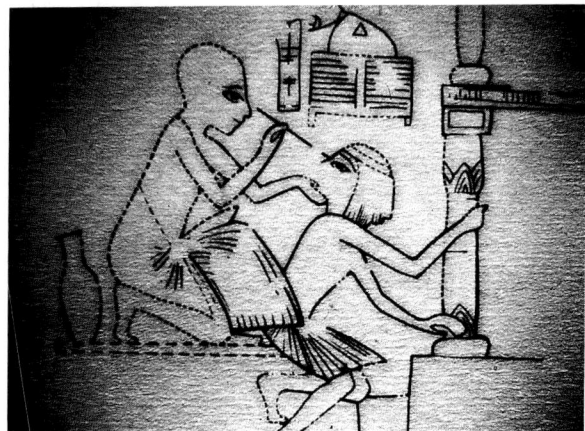

Fig. 2.4 An inscription from the temple of Ipuy showing a physician or his assistant probably removing an ocular foreign body at a construction site.

and remedies for this and other problems which could have been cataract, there is no indication that the Egyptians (or for that matter, the Sumerians) knew anything about myopia, hyperopia or presbyopia. Likewise, while there is evidence of the use of magnifying lenses by lapidaries in Nineveh, such usage is not described in extant Egyptian writings but may have been known and kept as a guild secret (Figure 2.5). Nothing resembling spectacles has been found either in inscriptions or with any mummies. While early Greeks borrowed much from the Egyptians and were familiar both with the magnifying as well as the heating potential of a water-filled glass globe, it is not clear whether such knowledge came from other cultures or originated with the Greeks themselves.

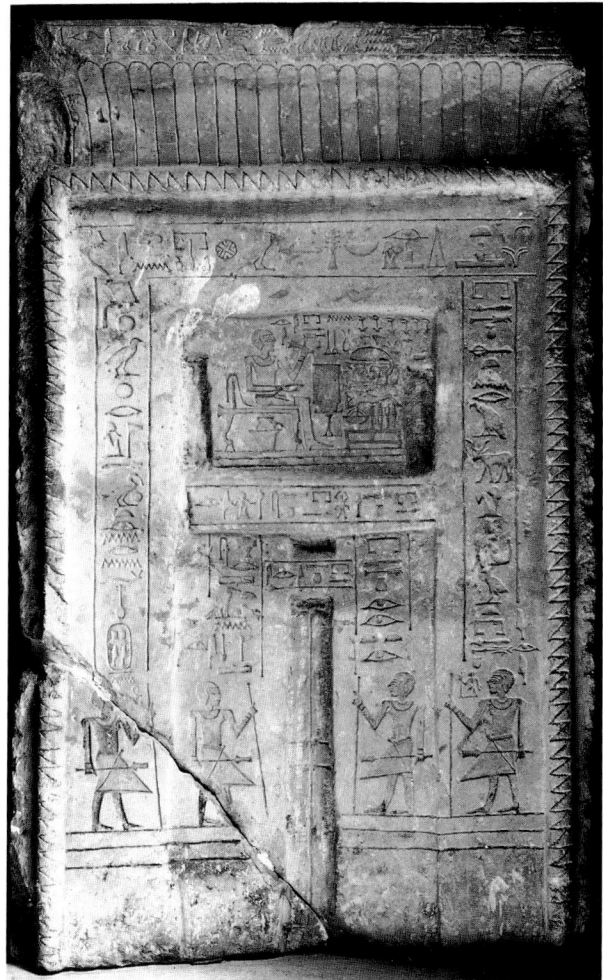

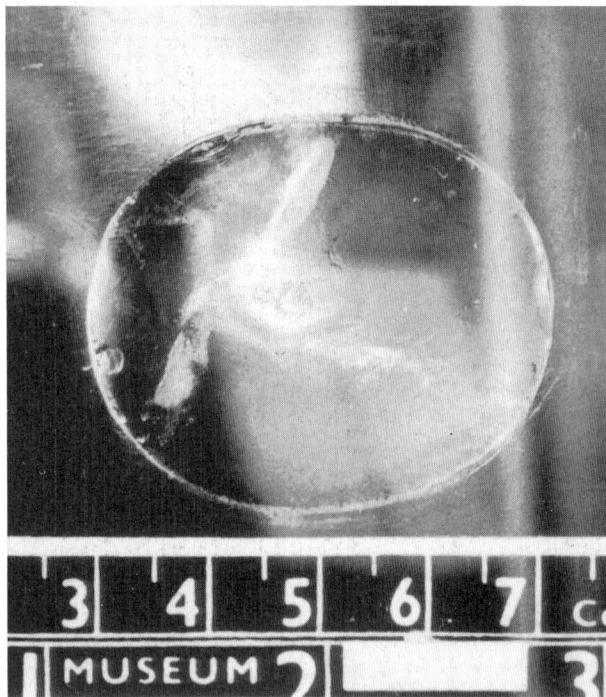

Fig. 2.5 A polished crystal excavated at Nineveh that might have been used as a magnifying lens (British Museum, London).

Aristotle and myopia

The first real discussion or mention of refractive errors came later in the works of Aristotle who lived about 100 years after Hippocrates and therefore before the collection of Hippocratic books was completed. These books by Aristotle should be able to show us what the Greeks of the classical period and shortly after it knew about this topic. Unfortunately, those works which would primarily be concerned with this field, the so-called *Problems* of Aristotle, do not belong to the authenticated works by the famous philosopher [5–6]. Nevertheless, these quotations are of interest. They are probably the oldest citations which explain the name and the concept of myopia and the first ones which allude to presbyopia:

> There are two kinds of weak eyes. The one is the myope and the other one occurs in old people. The first one will hold objects close in order to see sharply while the other one will hold them far away.

> The vision of old people is opposite to that of myopes: the first do not see clearly what is close, but see well at distance.

> Why does the myope hold everything close and the old man everything far away?

Some hints about myopia and hyperopia can be found in the authentic works by Aristotle, however. We find an allusion to presbyopia there as well. He says that old people do not see sharply because the transparent membrane in front of the pupil becomes wrinkled and casts a shadow. He had apparently already observed an elongation of the visual axis in myopic eyes (*Origin of Animals*) [7]. In these works he also asks:

> Why do myopes write in such small letters?

> Why do the myopes [those who squint their eyes] have a tendency to squint their lids?

This is the first time the word *myops* is encountered in the literature: a word which even today, 2000 years later, is used in the same sense. *Myein* means to close, especially the eye or the mouth; *myops* means to close or blink the eye. The same word also signifies the condition of myopia; only the later authors substitute for this term myopia. Before that the term *myopiasis* was used [8]. It aptly describes the facial expression of the uncorrected myope trying desperately to clarify the world. Until the general introduction of spectacles for the myope, squinting the lids, with the resultant production of a horizontal stenopeic slit, was the only practical means whereby clear distance vision could be achieved.

According to Hirschberg:

> *Presbys* means the old man or venerable man; *presbytes* is the senile man. This is also the meaning of the word in the original Greek quotation above; the meaning is obvious because in general old people will hold a book farther away, though exceptions exist. The meaning of this word as "poor vision in old age" was only acquired in modern times [6].

As to vision itself, the emanation hypothesis of vision, propounded by Pythagoras, held sway [9]. Accepted in one form or another with its many obscurities by such philosophers as Epicuros (341–270 BC), Euclid, Hipparchos (second century BC), and eventually by Ptolemy (AD second century) in Alexandria, and propagated to Arabic and thence to western medicine by the writings of Galen (AD 130–200), it claimed that vision was accomplished by the emission of a subtle "visual spirit" or "pneuma". This originated in the brain, the center of sensation and the seat of the ruling soul (probably located in the ventricles), circulated constantly through the hollow optic nerves (which were considered to be extensions of the brain itself) into the eye, and filled the crystalline lens from which it emanated in linear rays resembling sunlight (in the form of a cone) into space. In this view the lens was the essential organ of vision, and the retina, a thinned expansion of the optic nerve, acted as a guide to enable

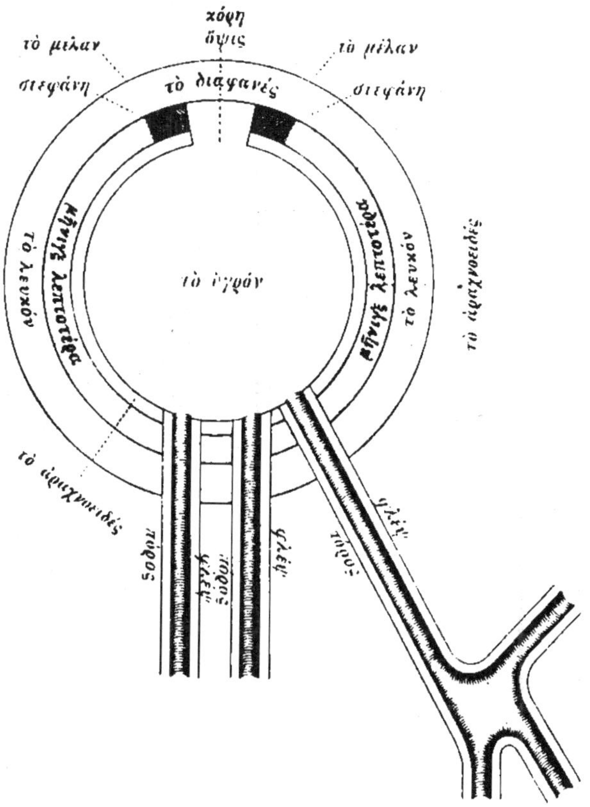

Fig. 2.6 The eye as understood in Hippocrates' time.

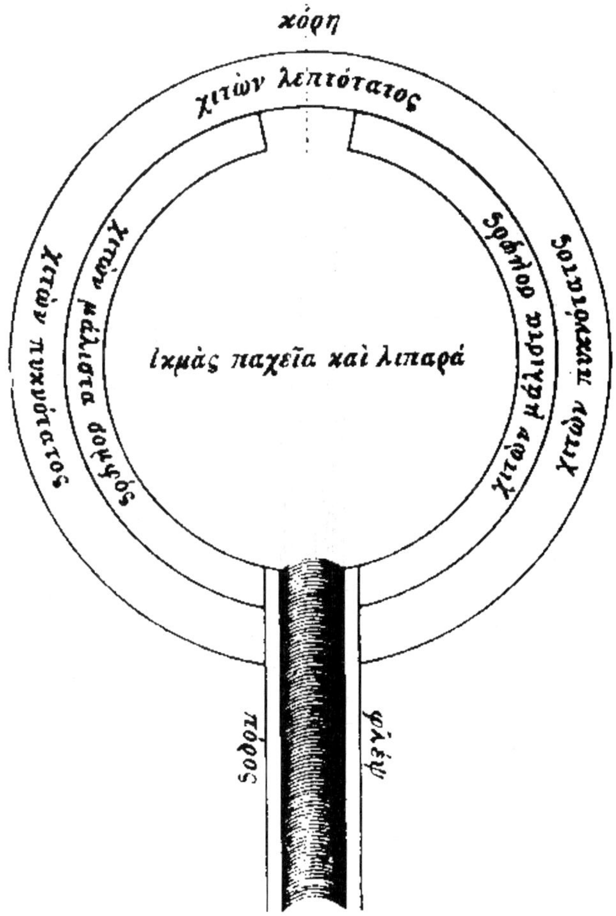

Fig. 2.7 The eye according to Democrites and as understood by Aristotle.

the visual spirit to reach this vital organ and with its blood vessels also served as a means of nourishment to the vitreous and thus to the lens (Figure 2.6).

The alternative and rival view of Democrites (500 BC), accepted and elaborated by Aristotle, that light was an activity of an external ethereal substance originating from luminous or illuminated bodies, was largely ignored, although an attempt was made by Plato (429–327 BC) to combine the two opposing views in his somewhat vague concept that the rays of "inner light" emanating from the eye united with the rays of "outer light" emitted by the luminous object to accomplish the visual act. In this theory, if the corpuscles of inner light were sufficiently large to split up the outer light, the eye saw black; if they were small enough to be split up themselves, the eye saw white; colors emerged by different reactions of the two streams, and dazzling when the process of splitting occurred close to the eye. In either case vision centered upon the lens which acted as the essential organ of photoreception, a function conferred upon it by the circulating visual spirits (Figure 2.7).

Regardless that they may have differed in their opinions as to the nature of vision, the Alexandrian scholars seem to have agreed that light traveled in a straight line and at high speed. The major part of their knowledge of optics, however, concerned itself with catoptrics—the optics of mirrors or reflection (see also Chapter 4). It will suffice at present to say that the ancient scholars were hampered in their understanding of optics by their almost complete misunderstanding of vision and refraction, not to mention anatomy. Consequently, spectacles were also unknown to the Greeks.

The Roman period

In 30 BC, upon the death of the last of the Ptolemaic rulers—Cleopatra—Rome took over control of Egypt and the curtain fell on one of the glorious periods of medicine's history. Very little of Roman medicine was indigenous or original. All that was worthy of the name was Greek, practiced only by slaves, recently emancipated slaves or foreigners (Greeks or Egyptians), until the time of Julius Caesar. It was he who conferred Roman citizenship upon physicians resident in the Imperial City.

There were public lectures about medicine, but medical education was not regulated. There were no examinations, nor were the practicing physicians burdened with heavy responsibilities. Therefore many untrained and unskilled tried to practice the art. The income of well-known physicians was rather high. Not everything was always ethical. However, one should not believe everything that Pliny wrote—he hated *medici*.

It was Pliny who started the rumor that "the Emperor Nero used to observe the fights of the gladiators in an emerald." The much discussed paragraph in Pliny discusses only reflection, however. Nevertheless, emeralds are transparent and while some authors would have us believe that Nero viewed a reflection of the fights in the emerald with his back turned, as paranoid as he seemed to be, it is highly unlikely that he would sit with his back to armed men. The jury is still out on this but the emeralds were cut concave so that they acted like a mirror and produced an erect image—just what myopes need. If it was used in this dubious way then the episode represents the first known use of an optical aid to improve distance vision.

The most influential practitioner and writer of the Roman period was Claudius Galenus (Galen) of Pergamon (AD 130–200). Though the importance of his contribution to medicine can hardly be exaggerated, unfortunately it was not all to the good. His system was based on anatomic–physiologic foundations, but permeated with the Hippocratic dogmas—especially those of humoral pathology—freely leavened with sophistry. To Hippocrates medicine was factual and what was unknown to him was freely acknowledged. Galen had no use for doubt and, where knowledge

was lacking, metaphysics was called in as substitute. Everything was imbued with a divine purpose and each experimental observation had to be submitted to teleological analysis. This may seem naive but this view is still held subconsciously today. As von Bruecke put it: "teleology is a lady without whom no biologist can live; yet he is ashamed to show himself in public with her." Whereas Hippocrates had freed medicine from religious superstition, Galen, solving all problems and answering all questions, left it bound to dogma.

In Galen's view the retina was an expansion of the optic nerve which nourished the vitreous which in turn nourished the lens (Figure 2.8) [8]. This last—a tissue considered to be divine (*divinum oculi*)—was the essential organ of vision. From it visual emanations were emitted into outer space in the form of a cone to touch the objects seen; and from it also visual sensations were dispatched up the optic nerves to the mysterious third ventricle of the brain, the abode of the soul. To Galen the myope possessed a clear visual spirit but in too small a quantity to reach a distant object.

These two misconceptions—the sensory function of the lens and the emission hypothesis of vision dating from Pythagoras—although denied by Aristotle in the classical Greek period and later by Al-Hazen in the Middle Ages, dominated ophthalmological thought and retarded the progress of the subject up to the time of Johannes Kepler in the 17th century [10]. Just as Galen himself idolized Hippocrates, so also was his system accepted throughout the medical world with-

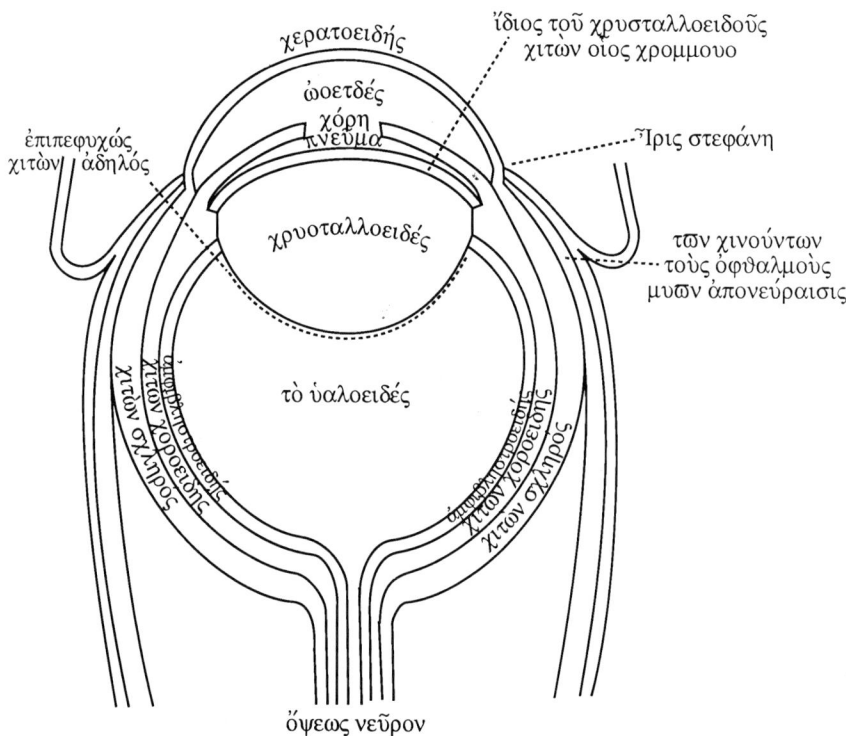

Fig. 2.8 The eye in the time of Galen.

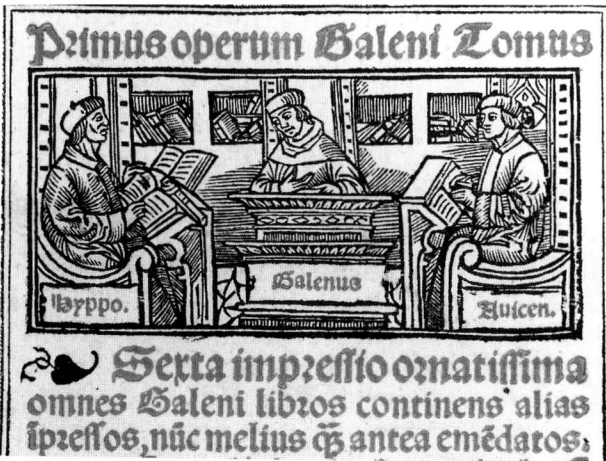

Fig. 2.9 Manuscript illustration showing Galen flanked by Hippocrates and Avicenna from an edition of the works of Galen published in 1528 (National Library of Medicine, Washington).

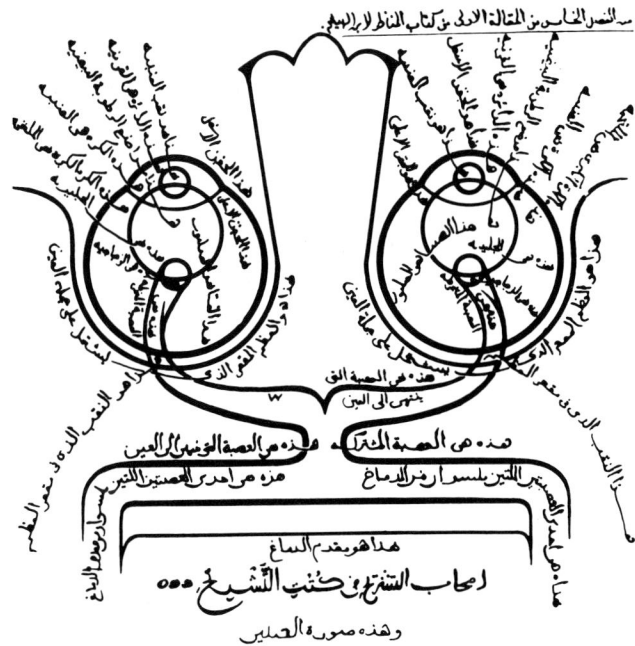

Fig. 2.10 The eye, from Al-Hazen's *Opticae Thesaurus*—AD 1038.

out question for nearly 15 centuries, partly because its theistic implications suited both Islam and Christendom and partly because his comprehensive works were available at a time when books were scarce. Of the 500 or so known works of Galen, 83 medical treatises have survived to this day (Figure 2.9). The unsettled conditions of the Middle Ages provided a fertile ground for his concepts to thrive. Unrest produced a longing for certainty and authority—an attitude especially prevalent in the Muslim East and the Christian West. Galen's dogmatic style, leaving no question unanswered, satisfied the desire for absolutes and his teleologic reasoning made his ideas easy for the Christian Church to embrace.

In the paralyzing atmosphere of clerical obscurantism which pervaded the Eastern Empire, all scientific investigation ceased. Little was added to ophthalmology and nothing at all to ocular anatomy. Finally, with the moral, economic and physical decay of Rome and its fall to the barbarians in AD 455, the Dark Ages engulfed the west, lasting from the 5th to the 10th centuries.

It is possible, indeed, that much which had been gained to that point would have been lost had not the fanatical followers of Mohammed embraced science with the same enthusiasm with which they waged their religious wars. However, this Arabian renaissance of learning was preservative rather than creative, revering authority rather than observing and experimenting. Had not the Koran prohibited dissection, Mohammedan medicine might have been very different. Nevertheless, though largely borrowed from Greek sources, these Arabic writings were not by any means always uncritical and several new observations were made in that period.

Al-Hazen (Ibn Al-Hytham Al Basri), among his many varied writings, transformed this science in *The Book of Optics (Opticae Thesaurus)* and *De Luce*. The oldest

extant diagram illustrating the eye and its central nervous connections is found in the latter book. Adopted by Al-Hazen's Persian commentator Kamal al-Din al-Farisi in 1316, it received wide publicity. In Al-Hazen's diagram the lens is more or less central and since it was considered the essential organ of vision the optic nerves ran directly to it (Figure 2.10).

Al-Hazen conducted experiments with plane, spherical, cylindrical and parabolic mirrors. Additionally, his studies of magnifying glasses brought him close to a rational theory of convex lenses. Of more importance, however, was the philosophical theory he presented on the nature of light; he discarded the emanation hypothesis and adopted the Aristotelian view that rays of light traveled from external objects into the eye (although Al-Razi had rejected the Pythagorian theory 100 years earlier) [11]:

> However, those who are convinced that vision consists in the formation of an image of the object which is produced within the eye have to assume that rays are propogated on a straight line from the object toward the center of the eye . . . The straight lines which extend from the center of the eye toward the viewed object are those which are used by the light beam. [12]

However, he still placed the formation of the image on the anterior surface of the lens.

As to glasses and the treatment of refractive disorders, they had nothing to add. Even within the complete textbook of ophthalmology by Ali Bin Isa there is not the slightest mention of any concave or convex lenses but of ametropia there is a hint:

A patient who sees well at distance but not at near (an affection which usually occurs in old patients) should keep a healthy lifestyle and should put styptic medication into his eye. A patient who sees well at near but not at distance should take liquid food and should sometimes use a salving medication into his eye. [11]

Neither mirrors nor specially cut gemstones or glass are mentioned in the Arabic literature for the treatment of refractive disorders—certainly spectacles are not described.

The best that can be said for that period in medical history from the fall of the Byzantine Empire to the Renaissance is that it was a holy mess, quite literally. The traditional seat and focus of learning—the clergy (priests)—were caught up in ecclesiastical pursuits of relics of the true cross or fragments of a saint's bones. The philosophical discussions, if any, concerned the pressing question of whether angels were male or female and how many could stand on the head of a pin. The medieval Christian God was portrayed as a rigid, non-philosophic, gloomy, and intolerant God. The body was looked upon not as a temple for the soul and a manifestation of God's grace—it was rather an object of scorn not worth knowing nor saving. Disease was once again a punishment for sin, real or imaginary. Nature was overwhelmed by a supernaturalism which had in it no place for scientific observation; miracles were expected rather than reasoned therapeutics, fables credited before facts. Thus Galen fit right in—the main reason for his influence over the centuries: his was "right" thinking.

Physicians of the time were forced to rely on works which were poor copies of the Arabic references. Typically slavishly copied by ignorant and probably lazy scribes working under conditions of poor lighting and poorer health, they abounded in mistakes. The crude drawings of the Arabic literature—transliterated from

Greek texts—were reduced to meaningless circles and lines (Figure 2.11). Knowledge of the function of the eye was stagnated by the persistent belief that the lens was the visual receptor and by the Pythagorean concept that visual rays emanated from the eye itself. Anatomic studies which would eventually lead to decipherment of this mysterious organ were stymied by the interdiction of dissection. In an age which featured the Inquisition and encouraged death and torture in God's name, there was an absolute horror of the anatomist's knife.

The church was not totally successful in stamping out the rational spirit however. Within the maelstrom there appeared, over time, small islands of enlightenment and reason which withstood the assault of conformity. Ironically, but not surprisingly, some of the first chinks in the wall were created by members of the establishment itself—the clergy—representing as they typically do the most educated of the prevailing society. Through these cracks began a trickle of rationality which enlarged into a torrent and which eventually led to that second golden period of human existence—the Renaissance.

Roger Bacon

Roger Bacon (1214–1294)—*doctor mirabilis*—a Franciscan friar and philosopher at Oxford was one of the most notable of the early writers who swam against the main stream. A product of an aristocratic family, he studied philosophy and science at the University at Oxford and then in Paris, joining the Franciscan order where in 1250 he became a monk. That was bad judgment for he was temperamentally unsuited for the contemplative life of a friar. His fractiousness, particularly with respect to educational reform within the Franciscan order, led to his censure and eventual incarceration where he was provided with ample time to contemplate his sins. He took advantage of the opportunity to compile a reference work on scientific knowledge. Upon his release by Pope Clemens in 1267, he dedicated his *Opus Majus* (as well as his *Minus* and *Tertium*) to his benefactor. In this work he commented upon the phenomenon of magnification as gleaned from the writings of Al-Hazen. He suggested that the difficulty experienced by the aged in seeing near objects was due to an increase of moisture in the eye and a wrinkling of the cornea resembling the wrinkling in the aged skin. He suggested as a remedy the magnification given by a segment of a sphere of glass or crystal when laid upon the letters to be read; by such means, he said, the "smallest particles of sand or dust could be seen."

> If anyone examine letters or other minute objects through the medium of crystal or glass or other transparent substance, if it be shaped like the

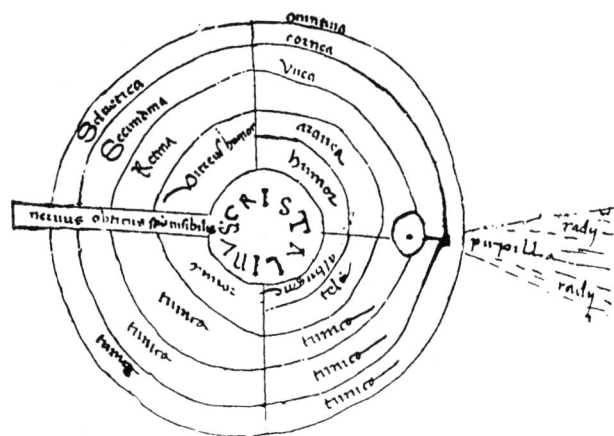

Fig. 2.11 The eye at the beginning of the Renaissance. Redrawn from the *Codex Trivultanius* (14th century).

lesser segment of a sphere, with the convex side towards the eye, and the eye being in the air, he will see the letters far better, and they will seem larger to him. For according to our canon concerning a spherical medium beneath which the object is placed, the centre being beyond the object, the convexity being towards the eye, all causes agree to increase the size, for the angle in which it is seen in greater, the image is greater, and the position of the image is nearer, because the object is between the eye and the centre. For this reason such an instrument is useful to old persons and to those with weak eyes, for they can see any letter, however small, if magnified enough.

For we can so form glasses and so arrange them with regard to our sight and to objects that the rays are refracted and deflected to any place we wish, so that we see the object near at hand or far away beneath whatever angle we desire. And so we can read the smallest letters or count grains of sand or dust from an incredible distance owing to the magnitude of the angle beneath which we see them, and again the largest objects close at hand might be scarcely visible owing to the smallness of the angle beneath which we see them; for it is on the size of the angle on which this kind of vision depends, and it is independent of distance save per accidens. So a boy can appear a giant, a man seem a mountain, and in any size of angle whatever, for we can see a man under as large an angle as though he were a mountain and make him appear as near as we desire. So a small army might seem very large, and though far away appear near, and conversely: so, too, we could make sun, moon and stars apparently descend here below, and similarly appear above the heads of our enemies, and many other similar marvels could be brought to pass, that the ignorant mortal mind could not endure the truth (*Opus Majus*, Part V).

Bacon's idea of a "glass" was a handled, segmented sphere to be used as a reading aid. He sent such a glass to Pope Clemens in 1267. This does not make Bacon the inventor of spectacles as some claim, however, because other than the reading glass mentioned (which does not qualify as a spectacle) he apparently never carried out any practical experiments of his ideas (Figure 2.12).

Spectacles

Spectacles as we know them did not make an appearance until sometime around 1276 in Venice, Italy. It is possible that Bacon's idea made its way to the glass capital of Europe but the exact inventor is not known

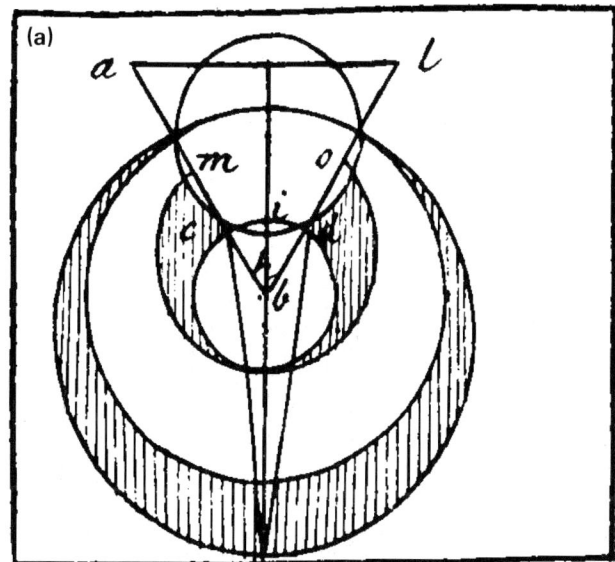

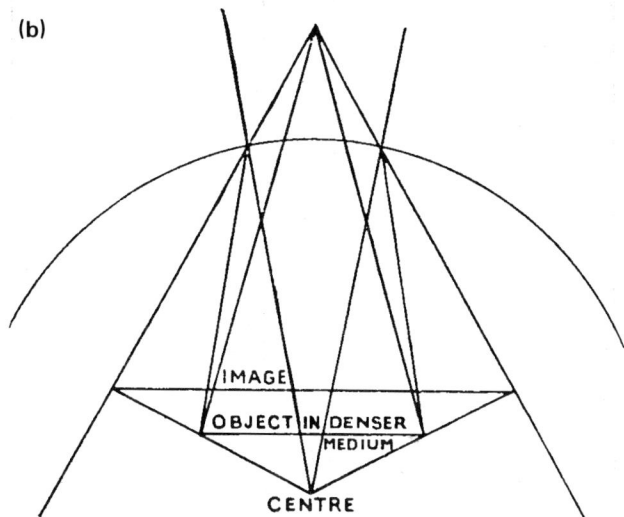

Fig. 2.12 (a) Roger Bacon's drawing of the eye from his *Opus Majus*, 1268. (b) Roger Bacon's diagram of a plano-convex lens. The diagram is wrong but the idea is there.

with certainty. The premise that Europeans learned of spectacles from the Chinese, however, is not tenable even though they are supposed to have been mentioned in the memoirs of Marco Polo. Polo's ventures lasted from 1271 to 1295 but the *Travels* were not dictated until 3 years later and were revised 9 years after that; by that time spectacles had been in use in Europe for several years [11]. In any case, nowhere in Polo's original writings are spectacles mentioned [13].

The first authenticated mention of spectacles is in a collection of minstrel's ballads dating from 1280. In 1305, according to Francesco Redi, Brother Giordano da Rivalto, of the Order of St Dominic stated in a sermon: "Not even 20 years have passed since the art to make spectacles has been invented. These help us to

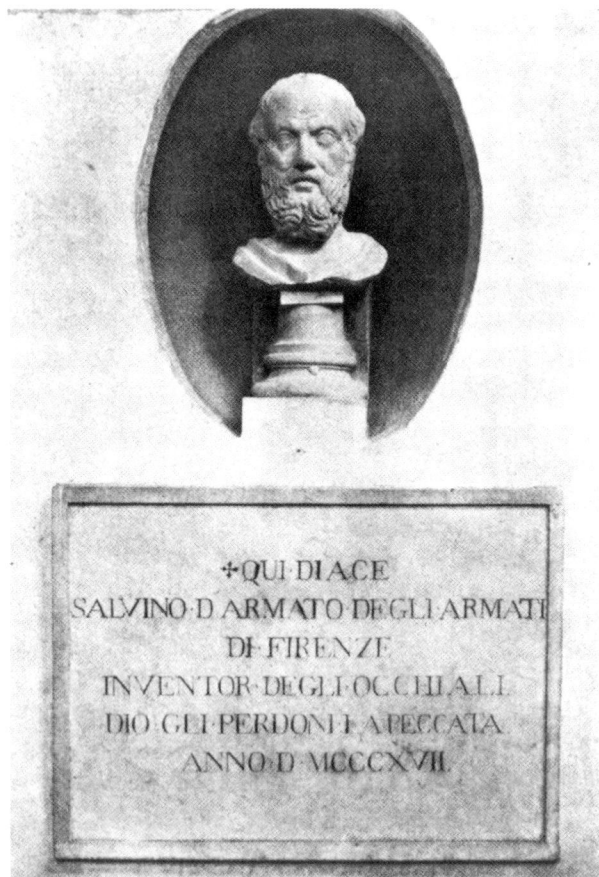

Fig. 2.13 Tombstone of Salvino d'Armato, inventor of spectacles—1317.

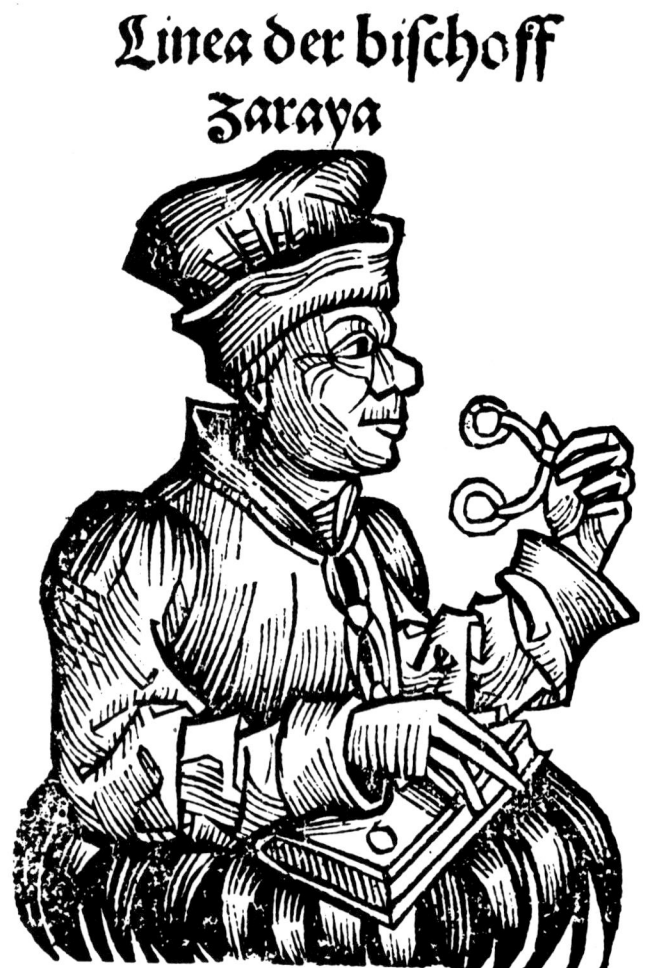

Fig. 2.14 The first printed illustration of spectacles—Schedel, *Liber Chronicarum*—Nürnburg, 1493 (Countway Library, Harvard School of Medicine).

see and this is one of the greatest and most necessary inventions the world has seen." [14] Redi also mentions in one of his letters not the inventor, but the re-inventor of spectacles:

> In the library of the Dominican Monastery of Santa Caterina in Pisa there is an old manuscript which represents the chronicle of this monastery. Within this manuscript, the following comments are found: "Brother Alexander de Spina of Pisa could make with his hands whatever he wanted to. He preached charity to others. When somebody invented the glasses and it was proven to be a useful invention nobody could make other spectacles. Then our good brother started making spectacles without a teacher and taught this procedure to others who wanted to learn it" [11,14].

Whoever the inventor may really have been, the following interesting inscription is found on a grave stone from the churchyard of Santa Maria Maggiore (Figure 2.13):

> Here lies Salvino d'Armato of the Armati of Florence
> Inventor of the spectacles.

God pardon him for his sins.
AD 1317

Certainly spectacles were well known by 1300 although still expensive and somewhat of a novelty, not becoming popular until the 15th century—the advent of printing. Medical manuscripts mention spectacles only from this time on (Figure 2.14). Even then they were not widely prescribed by physicians. In the *Lilium Medicinae* (1305) of Bernard of Gordon, he described the use of a collyrium of such strength "that it makes old people read the smallest print again without that they need to use spectacles (*oculus berrelerius*)" [15]. Guy de Chauliac (1300–1368) of Lyons mentions in his *Chirurgie* of 1363 first some good medications against poor vision and then adds, less cynically: "If this does not work one has to turn to the spectacles." [16,17]

Furthermore, such spectacles as existed were only available for presbyopia (hyperopia was confused with presbyopia and thought only to occur in the aged)—the myope was doomed to suffer for some 200–300 years more (Figure 2.15). They were also prescribed for

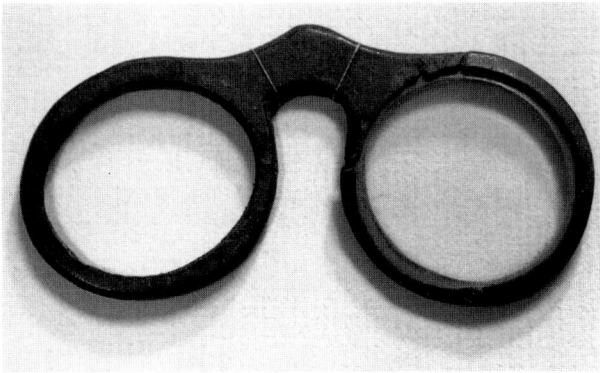

Fig. 2.15 Leather spectacle frames, circa 1400 (American Academy of Ophthalmology).

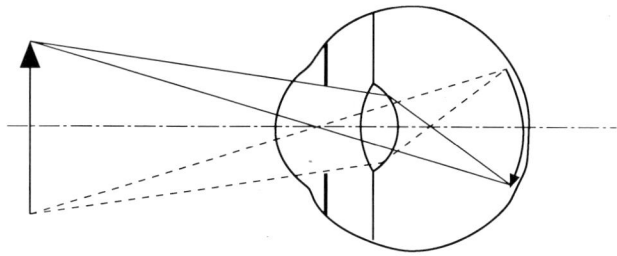

Fig. 2.16 Kepler's refraction of the eye—from his *Ad Vitellionem Paralipomena*, 1604.

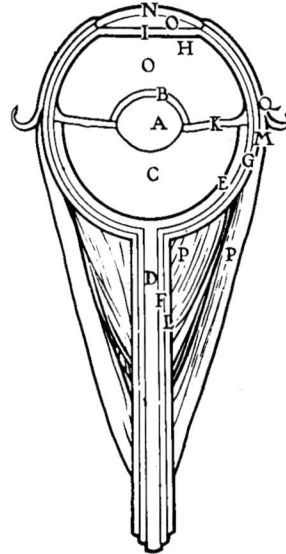

Fig. 2.17 The eye at the time of Kepler. From Vesalius' *De humani Corpus Fabrica*, 1543, Basel.

aphakic patients but the problem was still considered to be presbyopia. Hollerius, the famous French professor (1553), was supposedly the first physician who prescribed them for myopes [11]. However, it has only been since the middle of the 19th century that ophthalmologists have seriously involved themselves in the selection and calculation of lenses. Moreover, cylindric lenses were only produced in the 19th century—probably because of an incomplete understanding of the optics of the eye which still prevailed.

Felix Platter

Felix Platter (1539–1614) altered the whole of the theory of ophthalmic optics by advancing the revolutionary view, already suggested four centuries previously by Ibn Rushd, that the retina and not the lens was the visual receptor. Platter proved his thesis by showing that vision was still possible after severing the zonule through which the visual impulses were supposed to pass from the lens to the retina and optic nerve [18]. For the first time the lens was thus accurately described as the dioptric mechanism and the retina as the photoreceptor. This view was proved by Christopher Scheiner, by the simple expedient of observing an image formation after the sclera and choroid had been removed from an eye. Descartes repeated this experiment by cutting off the back of an ox eye and observing the image on a piece of paper [19].

Johannes Kepler

The optics of myopia, however, were not clearly explained until the 17th century by Johannes Kepler (the founder of dioptrics) in his classical works, *Ad Vitellionem Paralipomena* (A Supplement to Vitello, 1604) and *Dioptrice* (1611) [20–23]. In the first treatise, Kepler applied his vast optical and mathematical skills to the problem, demonstrating the role of both the lens and the cornea in vision and again placing the inverted image on to the retina where it belonged (Figure 2.16). Kepler's anatomy of the eye, however, was drawn

from Platter and Aquapendente and is quite similar to that of Vesalius and thus adheres to the Galenic view (Figure 2.17). He described the curvature of an image cast by a lens secondary to the stronger refractive power of its periphery than its center—220 years before Airy. He defined the action of concave and convex lens upon this system, although he only approximated the laws of refraction which were finally codified by Snell.

In the second treatise—a mere 80 pages in length—he revolutionized contemporary thinking on optics. In his initial clarification of ophthalmic dioptrics he correctly assumed that in myopia, the incident light was brought to a focus in front of the retina, a view subsequently accepted by Isaac Newton 100 years later. Both of these pioneers in optics also considered myopia and presbyopia to be antitheses.

> Those who see clearly at distance but indistinctly at near are helped by convex spectacles, and those who see poorly at distance but well at near are helped by concave spectacles. How amazing that while the practical use of this fact is so widespread, its scientific cause remained obscure.

Kepler, himself myopic, also wrote about accommodation but did not identify it as such. In this area of his writings there is a considerable degree of confusion as a result of his inability to appreciate the fact that presbyopia occurred in both myopia and hyperopia. Kepler attributed the ability to see clearly at both distance and near to alterations in the shape of the eye, proposing that the lens moved backwards and forwards (through changes in the length of the eye) to provide clear near and far vision.

> It is impossible for the retina, which is fixed within the eye, to perceive clear images simultaneously from near and far. Some see well at distance, some at near. Those who see everything confused have imperfect eyes due to faulty structure. In those who see everything distinctly, either the retina or the lens must change its position relative to one another.

> It is probable that in young and healthy eyes the globe is alternately compressed and dilated at the equator when vision shifts to different distances.

Kepler attributed this action to the ciliary processes which act like a muscle. When they contract the equator is pulled inward and the eye becomes elongated, as happens in encirclage for retinal detachments. In this case Kepler deduced that the retina had to be moved back in order for a near object to be seen clearly. Kepler made all his observations through deduction only—as he told a friend: "I am no empiricist concerned with the accumulation of observed data" [20]. Hence he could probably never get his work published in today's journals which require original data and documented facts. But as Dewey wrote: "Every great advance in science has issued from a new audacity of imagination" (John Dewey—*The Quest for Certainty*).

He went on to propound the "near-work" hypothesis for myopia by stating that study and fine work in childhood rapidly accustom the eye to near objects. According to Kepler, with advancing years this adaptive mechanism produces a permanent, finite far point such that distant objects are seen poorly:

> It is false that only old people see poorly at near and the young at distance. Both conditions may occur at all ages [here is an important observation and a clue to hyperopia—which he missed]. With age, however, the power of changing the view from distance to near weakens, and hence those with healthy eyes at youth see well only at distance. Furthermore, it is more natural and less tiring to hold the eyes parallel rather than converged on near objects. Therefore, too, tired old eyes remain focused for distance. Those who do much close work in their youth become myopic.

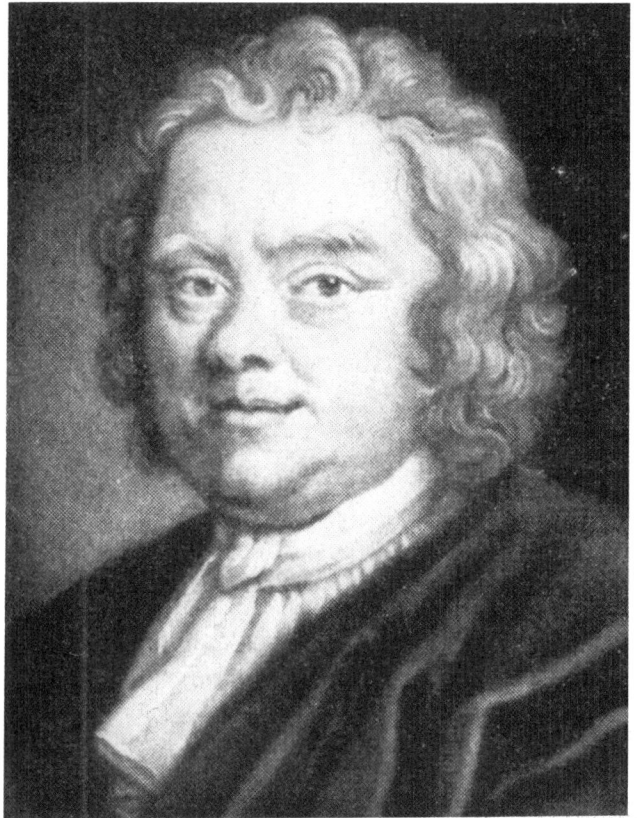

Fig. 2.18 Hermann Boerhaave (1708)—the first to suggest clear lens extraction for myopia (Mary & Edward Norton Library, Bascom Palmer Eye Institute).

This theory led to the formation of "myopia schools" in later years and is still very much in evidence today.

Plempius

Vopiscus Fortunatus Plempius, professor of therapeutics at Loewen in Holland, described anatomically the unusual distance between the lens and the retina in myopic eyes [24]. This view was confirmed by Georg Albert Hamberger, professor of mathematics at Jena who also correctly described the phenomenon of "second sight" in the aged with an early cataract—100 years before it was rediscovered by Demours and others [25].

Boerhaave

Hermann Boerhaave of Leyden, who was the first university professor to teach the correct concept of vision as well as Kepler's explanation of myopia and hyperopia, attributed the defect of myopia to either an increased convexity of the cornea or the undue length of the globe. This latter cause was factually confirmed by Morgagni and Scarpa among others [26,27]. Still other causes that were postulated were an increase in

V S O

DE LOS ANTOIOS

PARA TODO GENERO DE VISTAS:
En que fe enfeña a conocer los grados que a cada vno le
faltan de fu vifta, y los que tienen qualef-
quier antojos.

Y ASSI MISMO A QVE TIEMPO SE AN
de vfar, y como fe pediran en aufencia, con otros avifos impor-
tantes, a la vtilidad y confervacion de la vifta.

POR EL L. BENITO DAÇA DE VALDES,
Notario de el Santo Oficio de la Ciudad de Sevilla.

DEDICADO A NVESTRA SEÑORA
de la Fuenfanta de la Ciudad del cordoua.

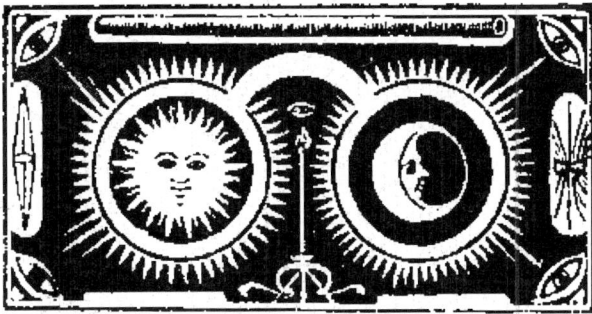

CON PRIVILEGIO
Impreffo en Seuilla, por Diego Perez Año de · 5 1 1.

Fig. 2.19 Title page of Valdes' book on the use of spectacles to treat far-sight (1623).

the thickness of the lens, an increase in its refractive index, and a change in its position. Boerhaave's picture is shown here (Figure 2.18), though for quite another reason. In 1708 he made the observation that since after cataract surgery, myopes see quite clearly without lenses, it seemed reasonable to treat myopia by extracting the clear lens: "This will allow the eye to focus the rays onto the retina, whereas before the operation the focus was in front of the retina." [28] This is the earliest reference to this technique that the author could find. Clearly, Fukala did not invent this technique—of which we will have more to say in Chapter 13.

Hyperopia

Since the refractive power of the cornea is largely abolished when it is immersed in water, divers become so hyperopic that clear vision is impossible. This is, in fact, the method whereby Young discovered his

astigmatism. Benito Daza de Valdes prescribed convex lenses for distant as well as for near vision in the aged—in fact, such use was described in his book *Uso de los Antojos y Comentarios a Propósito del Mismo* (Figure 2.19) [29]. The first optical explanation of the anomaly, however, was not made until 1696 by Hamberger who described the phenomenon as occurring sometimes in the young as well as congenitally [30]. However, long-sight was still considered identical with presbyopia. The latter was thus explained by Newton:

> If the Humours of the eye by old age decay, so as by shrinking to make the Cornea and the Coat of the Crystalline Humour grow flatter than before, the Light will not be refracted enough, and for want of a sufficient Refraction will not converge to the bottom of the Eye but to some place beyond it . . . This is the reason for the decay of sight in old Men and shews why their Sight is mended by Spectacles. For their Convex glasses supply the defect of plumpness in the Eye, and by increasing the Refraction make the Rays converge sooner, so as to convene at the bottom of the Eye if the Glass have a due degree of convexity. And the contrary happens in short-sighted Men whose Eyes are too plump. For the Refraction being now too great, the Rays converge and convene in the eyes before they come to the bottom . . . unless the Object be brought so near to the Eye as that the place where the converging Rays convene may be removed to the bottom . . . or the Refraction is diminished by a Concave-glass of a due degree of concavity [31].

With Newton's concept of hyperopia as a condition due to parallel rays of light converging *behind* the retina, the stage was set for the acceptance of the axial length of the eye as the sole determinant of refraction, thereby opening a floodgate of speculation.

The same theme was described and illustrated by the great mathematician of Cambridge, Robert Smith [32]. Kastner, professor of mathematics at Leipzig, in his annotated translation of Smith's book, called the optical state in long-sighted individuals *hyperpresbytas* [33]. The general outline of the optics of long-sight, still described as presbyopia, was also understood by Thomas Young, who stated clearly:

> A convex lens is necessary for far-sighted or presbyopic eyes. And it often happens that the rays must be made not only to diverge less than before, but even to converge towards a focus behind such an eye, in order to make its vision distinct.

This is probably the first unequivocal description of hyperopia. From the clinical point of view Janin distinguished three types of sight—normal, short-sight and long-sight, "the first two occurring naturally and the third fortuitous and occurring only in old people" [34].

Many investigators conducted studies on the axial length during that period. Morgagni [26], Guerin, Geudron, and Pichter [35] and some—Scarpa [27] and von Ammon [36]—noted posterior staphylomas but did not associate them particularly with myopia. It wasn't until 1856, in an excellent monograph by von Arlt [37], that a convincing association was made, though it had been suggested 2 years before by von Graefe [38] in a combined ophthalmoscopic and ana-tomical study of two eyes measuring 29 mm and 30.5 mm in length.

As a consequence of these studies the greatest efforts of the ophthalmologic community were concentrated on a search for the causes of the increased axial length of the eye. That this search became indiscriminate and almost absurd can be appreciated by a review of the early theories of the etiology of myopia. It is interest-ing to read the medical papers of that era and note the plethora of treatises on the causes and nature of myopia. It resembles, in some ways, the feeding frenzy of sharks in its irrationality, ferocity, and redun-dancy of attack. It has its parallels even today, in a more "enlightened" time.

In 1793, Young had described the mechanism of accommodation in which he posited that the lens was a muscular organ. In this same paper, while discussing the fibers within an ox lens, he declared that sclerosis of these fibers with age explains, at least partially, presbyopia [39]. Young retracted his muscular lens theory in his next publication but stated that the lens did have the ability to change its shape [40]. He proved this by using his optometer with aphakic patients, finding that the refractive power remained absolutely stationary.

In 1813, Ware made it clear that long-sight was not necessarily associated with presbyopia. He described "young persons who have so disproportionate a con-vexity of the cornea or crystalline, or of both, to the distance of these parts of the retina, that a glass of considerable convexity is required to enable them to see distinctly, not only near objects, but also those that are distant" [41]. Such an idea, however, was not well-understood and some ascribed such a visual defect to asthenopia until Stellwag von Carion gave a relatively clear account along with an optical explanation in 1855 [42,43]. Nevertheless, it was left to Franz Donders to establish the optical nature and frequent occurrence of hyperopia and point out its differentiation from pre-sbyopia [44].

Astigmatism

While the optics of astigmatism were briefly described by Kepler in 1604, the first clinical description of this problem was made by Young in 1801 (Figure 2.20), by practicing Scheiner's experiment (see below) and find-

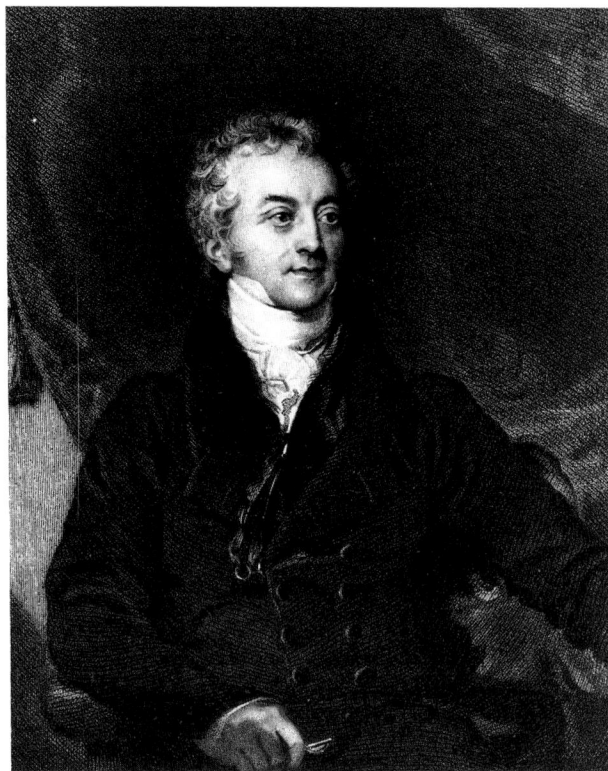

Fig. 2.20 Thomas Young, ophthalmologist and natural philosopher (Countway Library, Harvard School of Medicine).

ing that he had 3.94 D of myopia in the vertical meridian and 5.62 D in the horizontal [19,40]. Curiously, he did nothing to follow up his discovery. Young, a Quaker, was one of those singular human phenomena that occur sporadically through time. After qualifying in medicine, he went on to make major contributions in physiologic optics, the theory of light and the deci-phering of Egyptian hieroglyphics and the Rosetta Stone. At the age of 19 he read his first paper, on the accommodation of the eye, to the Royal Society [39]. In a course of lectures given while professor of natural philosophy at the Royal Institution, the definition of the familiar Young's modulus of elasticity was given as well as the wave theory of light.

The introduction of astigmatic lenses, however, had to wait until Sir George Biddell Airy. Airy, 24 years after Young, described the astigmatic change that had occurred in his own eyes, and to correct it designed and had made an astigmatic spectacle lens [45]. The name astigmatism itself was suggested to Airy in 1849 by the Reverend Whewall, who was then professor of mathematics and philosophy at Cambridge.

In those days, astigmatism was considered an oddity and worthy of notice and report. Several such cases were reported in 1847 by Sir William Hamilton of Dublin, visually characterized by the distinctness of horizontal and the indistinctness of vertical lines, and also by Henry Goode the same year. One case was reported from Europe by Schnyder [46] in 1849, who corrected the error in his own eyes by astigmatic lenses, and three by Isaac Hays in the American edition of *Lawrence's: A Treatise On Diseases of the Eye* [47]. One of the cases described by Hays is of particular interest because it represents the first instance of astigmatism treated by spectacles in the New World. A Reverend Goodrich managed to figure out the cause of his weakened sight and had lenses ground to correct it [48].

The optics and the importance of the defect were clearly defined by Donders in 1864 [44]. Generally speaking, very little was done to deal with the problem until the beginning of the 20th century when Jackson fitted the first sphero-cylinder spectacles. Prior to these attempts, astigmatism was compensated for by fitting spherical spectacles alone—a compromise at best. In 1869, Snellen, in an article published in the German literature, discussed the possibilities of surgically correcting corneal astigmatism. Bates, in 1894 [49], detailed a surgical technique for such modification and reported a number of cases, as did Lans in 1898 [50]. We will have more to say about these gentlemen when we examine more thoroughly the subject of the surgical correction of astigmatism in Chapter 9.

Ametropia

The nature of ametropia is an extensive subject, and complete coverage would require an entire book—something not in our mandate. The reader is referred to the section on further reading for assistance in that regard. It is within our mandate, however, to discuss ametropia in some detail in order to more completely understand attempts to correct it. Thus we will hit the high points, defining ametropia as well as presenting a sketch of its prevalence and development and how it impacts on the human condition. An understanding of the nature of ametropia is an essential precursor to any attempt to correct it, be it by surgery or any other method.

In the physiologically normal eye parallel light rays converge to form a principal focus upon the retina; when these ideal optical conditions occur with the eye in a state of rest the condition is termed emmetropia. Since the principal focus is of a size approximating a point and lies in one plane, such a system is also called stigmatic (from the Greek meaning point or mark). Since this requires a rather precise correspondence of all the optical components of the eye it would, as so aptly expressed by Duke-Elder,

> . . . be strange indeed if this were a common state of affairs, for its attainment depends on an almost perfect correlation of such measurements as the length of the eye and the shape of the cornea and the lens. Such regularity and conformity to optical perfection necessitates a mathematical accuracy which is nowhere realized in the constitution of living organisms. Emmetropia may be optically normal, but it is no more biologically normal than would be the universal attainment of a uniform height of 5 feet 6 inches [51].

In fact, its opposite condition, ametropia, wherein light rays are not focused exactly on to a single point at rest, is by far the more common. With more exact means of measuring, emmetropia is found to be very rare indeed. However, if small errors in refraction are neglected (up to 0.25 D), most people are emmetropic or very nearly so. An examination of a large series of

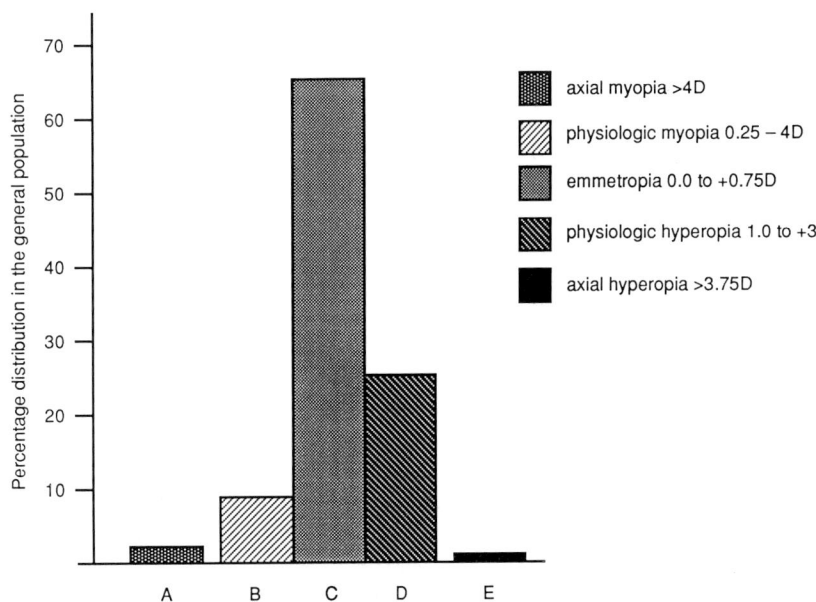

Fig. 2.21 Percentage incidence of ametropia in the general population (from Stromberg. Refraction and axial length of human eyes. Acta Ophthalmol, 1936).

patients reveals that emmetropic cases are more prevalent than would be predicted and that the incidence of myopia is disproportionately excessive. The relative incidence of refractive errors is shown in Figure 2.21.

Complicating this picture is the fact that the refracting components of the eye are not symmetrically arranged around a common axis and even if a reasonable facsimile of one could be constructed, the fovea would not be on it. Furthermore, the refracting surfaces are highly aspheric. In any event, even in the best of circumstances, the focus of the eye is not a discrete point but rather a diffusion circle of measurable diameter. Considering the imperfections that exist within the optical components of the eye it is no wonder that von Helmholtz stated:

> If an optician should try to sell me an instrument possessing the faults mentioned above, it seems to me—without overstressing the matter—that I should think myself wholly justified in using the most severe language with regard to the carelessness of his work and returning the instrument under protest [52].

Classification of ametropia

Ametropia has three main sub-divisions or types: hyperopia, myopia, and astigmatism. In hyperopia (or hypermetropia), the rays of light come to a focus behind the retina. The eye is said to be relatively too short (see section on hyperopia, below). In the opposite case, the eye is relatively too long and the focus occurs in front of the retina. Such a condition is termed myopia and is by far the greatest part of ametropia (see section on myopia, below). In the event that conditions are such that the rays of light converge to not one but several foci, such a condition is nonstigmatic or, as commonly termed, astigmatic. The various foci may, in turn, lie entirely before the retina —compound myopic astigmatism; wholly behind the retina—compound hyperopic astigmatism; or partly before and partly behind—mixed astigmatism (see section on astigmatism, below). There can be a number of different causes for any one of these conditions to exist or in some instances all three may occur in a single eye. The following classification is after Duke-Elder and will serve to introduce the reader to the subject [51]. It will be expanded upon in the individual sections that follow.

Ametropia due to positional anomalies

The eye may be of a length which does not correlate with the corneal curvature or the lens may be malpositioned.

1 If the axial length of the eye is too long relative to the power of the cornea and lens, the resultant myopia is said to be of the axial type. In this case the corneal curvature is relatively too steep.
2 Conversely, if the eye is too short, the corneal curvature is said to be relatively too flat and axial hyperopia exists.
3 If the lens is dislocated forward, the principal focus is also moved forward of the retina, and myopia will result; if backward, hyperopia results. This can occur in a traumatic recessed angle.

Anomalies of the refractive surfaces

The curvature of the cornea or of the lens may be too steep, giving a curvature myopia; or too flat, giving a curvature hyperopia; or be toroidal (toric surfaces are discussed more thoroughly in Chapter 3), varying in different meridians, giving astigmatism. Typically, a greater and (relatively) lesser curvature of the surface can be identified (major and minor meridians) simultaneously (see section on astigmatism, below).
1 If the major and minor meridians are at right angles to one another, the condition is called regular astigmatism and the refractive surface has the properties of a regular toroidal lens.
2 If they are not so related, the astigmatism may be called bi-oblique [53]. The author terms this condition asymmetrical astigmatism, preferring to confine the term oblique to describe astigmatic axes other than at 90 or 180°.
3 In some cases there may be no symmetry whatsoever in the system. In these instances the rays may form foci at different positions which may not be aligned on the optic axis nor lie in a single plane. This occurs, for example, in the cornea after corneal ulceration or in the lens in developing cataract. The astigmatism is termed irregular, and the surface possesses the characteristics of an irregular toroidal lens.

Since the latter two are asymmetrical toroidal surfaces not easily corrected by spectacle lenses, they are usually grouped together as irregular astigmatism.

Obliquity of the system elements

The refractive elements may not be aligned with the optic center or may be rotated.

Lenticular obliquity. If the lens is placed obliquely or subluxated, astigmatism will result.

Retinal obliquity. The posterior pole of the eye may be placed obliquely, as when it bulges backwards in a staphyloma in high myopia, and if the summit of the staphyloma does not correspond to the fovea the rays do not fall upon this region perpendicularly.

If the focus were a point this would be without effect, but since it is a diffusion circle the obliquity will deform and increase it, thus diminishing visual acuity.

It is likely, as well, that the latter two conditions will produce astigmatism of the irregular variety. In these cases, compensation by either spectacles or contact lenses may not be possible.

Anomalies of the refractive index

The refractive index of the transparent media may be abnormal.

1 If the refractive index of the aqueous humor is too low, or that of the vitreous humor is too high, there will be an index hyperopia. This can happen when silicone oil is used to replace vitreous during retinal detachment surgery. Conversely, if the refractive index of the aqueous is too high, as in certain types of iridocyclitis (this has also been postulated as one of the reasons for induced myopia in the uncontrolled diabetic) or that of the vitreous too low (gas replacement in retinal detachment surgery or liquefaction of the vitreous gel), there will be an index myopia.

2 If the refractive index of the lens as a whole is too low, the light is bent less, and there will be index hyperopia. If the index of the cortex increases relatively and approximates that of the nucleus, as it does normally with age, the lens tends to act as a single refractive element with flatter refractive surfaces, and consequently has less converging power than normal; the eye therefore becomes hyperopic. Conversely, if the refractive power of the nucleus increases, as frequently occurs in early cataract, index myopia is produced. Such induced myopia offsets the normal presbyopia and produces the phenomenon called in the laity "second sight." In this case the patient finds that he or she is able to read much better without spectacles than before—in fact, may be able to dispense with them entirely. If the increase in the refractive index of the nucleus is very marked a false lenticonus may be produced wherein the central part of the pupil is myopic and the periphery hyperopic. In these cases the patient may find that both near and distant vision is relatively clear and may be able to function—for a time at least—without bifocals.

Absence of system element

The absence of the lens produces extreme hyperopia. Astigmatism of the against-the-rule variety is almost always present following wide incision cataract surgery as well but is reported less and less as the incisions have become smaller [54,55].

Many of the definitions just given in this classification of refractive anomalies are much too simplistic and require qualification. The concept of an eye which is too long or too curved or has any other physical or geometric abnormality of optical significance leads by implication to the notion that normal values can be established. This is not the case. The range of variability of the optical components of the eye can be considerable. Small errors of total refraction can be associated with extreme variation of the refractive constituents. In fact these deviations can be much greater than those occurring in conditions considered pathologic.

The axial length of an eye with emmetropia can, in some instances, be found to be greater than that of one with progressive myopia. A typical case showing progressive changes in the fundus may have an axial length shorter than normal (mean 22.39 mm). Nevertheless, it is useful to retain the distinction between axial ametropia wherein an alteration in axial length is the main factor, and refractive ametropia wherein the anomaly lies principally in the curvature or indices of the refracting media.

Myopia

In myopia, parallel rays of light entering the eye are brought to a focus anterior to the retina (Figure 2.22). That is, the total refraction is greater than that required for emmetropia. If they are to be brought to a focus upon the retina, parallel rays coming from distant objects must be rendered more divergent at the cornea, and this can only be done by placing a concave lens in front of the eye (Figure 2.23). It follows that distant objects cannot be seen clearly without artificial aid; only divergent rays will meet at the retina, and thus, in order to be seen clearly, an object must be brought close to the eye, so that the rays coming from it are rendered sufficiently divergent. This point, the furthest at which objects can be seen distinctly, is called the far

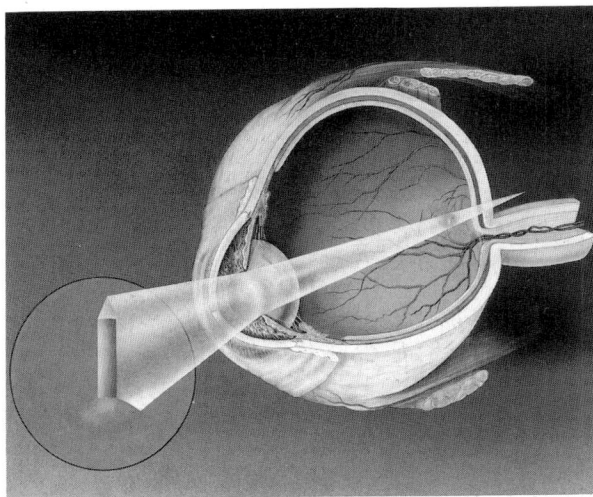

Fig. 2.22 The myopic eye.

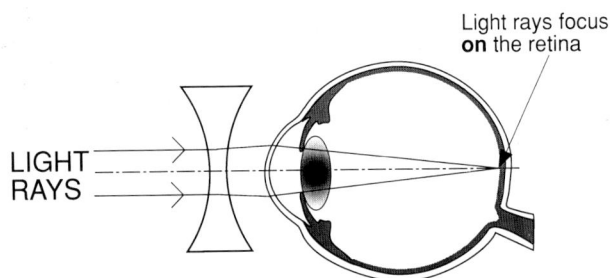

Fig. 2.23 A corrected myopic eye.

point (*punctum remotum*). In the emmetrope it is at infinity; in the hyperope it is behind the eye and therefore virtual; in the myope it is a finite distance in front of the eye and therefore real, and the higher the myopia, the shorter is this distance.

It is important, at this point, to note that the symptom of blurred distance vision and the diagnosis of myopia are common denominators of what have been described as two different clinical entities: physiologic myopia and pathologic myopia.

Physiologic myopia

Physiologic (simple, school, low, benign) myopia is an optical condition of the eye in which a chance combination of normal refractive components renders the eye near-sighted. An increase in curvature of the surfaces of the cornea or lens (decrease in radius of curvature) and an increased axial diameter of the eye attained by normal growth are factors which are both capable of producing myopia unless proportional compensatory changes are present in the other components. The axial length of the eye as well as the corneal and lens power are within the normal limits for the population, but are mismatched, so the image does not fall on the fovea.

Pathologic myopia

Pathologic (degenerative, progressive, malignant) myopia is a direct consequence of an abnormal component of refraction. In its general usage and as a strict diagnostic term, it indicates those cases associated with an abnormal lengthening of the eye. The condition may be generalized and involve the entire posterior sclera as far forward as the insertions of the recti muscles. This diffuse process is usually associated with a herniation of an area of the posterior pole, which yields the dramatic picture of a posterior staphyloma (Figure 2.24). This is generally attributed to the stretching of the scleral wall. In pathologic myopia, the total refraction of the cornea and lens falls within normal limits and the myopia state is produced by excessive axial elongation; the axial diameter of the eye lies outside the normal binomial curve [56]. Ectatic and degenerative changes are often present in the posterior globe (Figure 2.25).

The differential diagnosis between physiologic and pathologic myopia is not discrete [57]. As a general rule, we separate the two by:

Degree of myopia. Pathologic myopia usually has −6 D or more of refractive error.

The axial diameter of the eye. Adult eyes of more than 26.5 mm show an increased incidence of degenerative fundus changes.

History. Pathologic myopia is a congenital (or neonatal) disease, whereas physiologic myopia has its onset anywhere from 5 to 12 years of age.

Ophthalmoscopic findings. This is by far the best differential point. The posterior fundus of the physiologic myopia eye has a normal appearance, although a small temporal crescent (0.3 disk diameter or less) is compatible with this diagnosis. Pathologic myopia, on the other hand, almost always has changes in the retinal pigment epithelium that are present at the

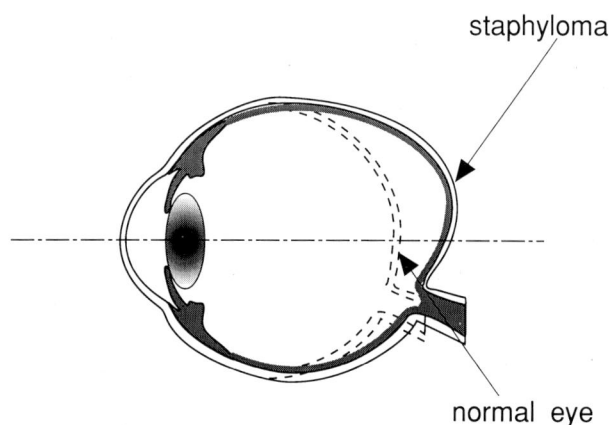

Fig. 2.24 Staphyloma in pathologic myopia.

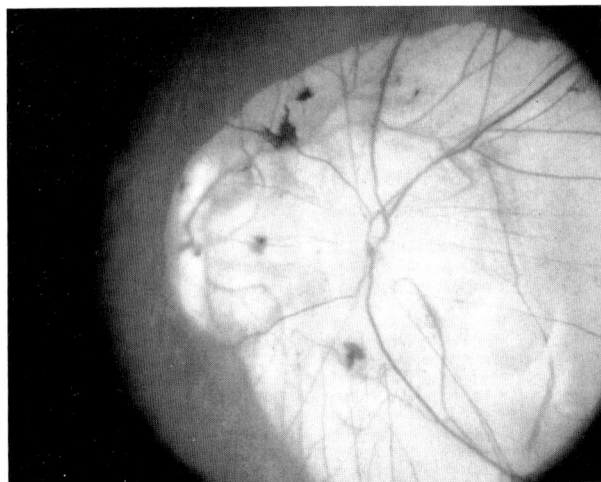

Fig. 2.25 The fundus in pathologic myopia.

earliest age and appear as a localized or generalized pallor and tessellation of the posterior fundus. Stereoscopic fundus examination will reveal an ectasia of the posterior globe that begins in the second decade and expands in the third. The scleral crescent is also present at earliest examination, is usually large (greater than 0.5 disk diameter), and often encircles the disk. The degenerative changes of small punched-out areas of focal chorioretinal atrophy within the staphyloma confirm the pathologic nature of the myopia (see Chapter 14 for a classification of pathologic myopia fundi).

Progression. Physiologic myopia progresses during childhood, slows during the second decade and is stable by the third decade, whereas pathologic myopia usually becomes worse during the second decade and may progress in the fifth decade.

Technically, the term pathologic myopia, in its broadest sense, can be applied to such myopias as those found in keratoconus and spherophakia. To avoid confusion these entities are probably best termed curvature myopias. In this textbook the term pathologic myopia will be used only in the strict sense to mean a myopia due to abnormal axial lengthening of the eye accompanied by staphyloma formation. There is clearly, however, a large group of myopic eyes that cannot be classified as physiologic because they show evidence of abnormally increased axial lengths. On the other hand, they should not be classified as pathologic since they do not display the classic degenerative fundus changes of this disease. These eyes should be classified as intermediate in type, as suggested by Curtin [35].

Hyperopia

We have said that in the emmetropic eye parallel rays of light are brought to a focus upon the retina; but with hyperopia (hypermetropia or far-sight), parallel rays come to a focus behind the retina, and the diffusion circles which are formed result in a blurred and indistinct image (Figure 2.26). It follows that with the emmetropic eye objects theoretically at infinity are seen distinctly when the eye is at rest, while in hyperopia the formation of a clear image of any kind is impossible unless the converging power of the optical system is increased either by placing a convex lens in front of the eye or by an effort of accommodation (Figure 2.27).

This condition is the normal state in the newborn and persists in 50% of the population in most of the countries of the world. The normally 2–3 D of hyperopia present at birth usually decreases rapidly in the early years and is all but gone by the age of puberty. In some hyperopes it may actually increase between the ages of 5 and 14 years [58]. Any residual hyperopia will tend to remain stable until middle life where it

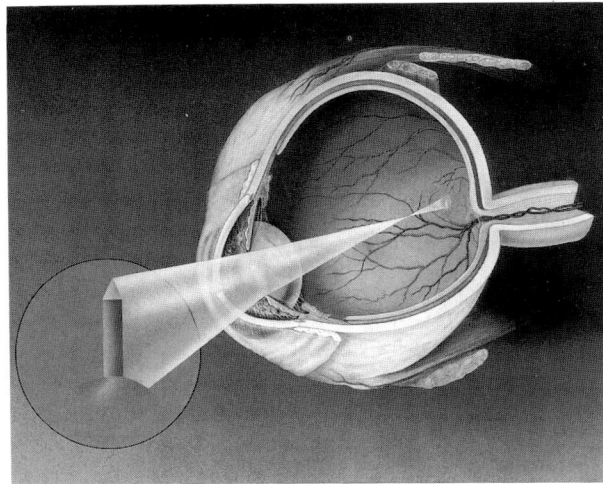

Fig. 2.26 The hyperopic eye.

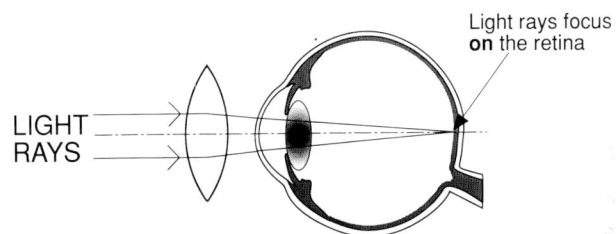

Fig. 2.27 The corrected hyperopic eye.

again re-appears due to lens changes (so-called senile hypermetropia of Straub). The vast majority of simple hyperopia is under 3 D but in the presence of ocular malformations or pathology can reach 20 D or more.

The structure of the hyperopic eye

These eyes are typically small, not just axially, but in all dimensions. The cornea is small as well. Since the human lens appears to vary little, if any, in size—it is relatively large leading to a shallowed anterior chamber—this carries with it the increased likelihood of angle closure glaucoma. Additionally, the macula is situated farther from the disk than in emmetropes and the cornea is likewise decentered, typically showing a large angle α (see Chapter 3).

Axial hyperopia is due to abnormal shortening of the globe; each millimeter of change is equal to 3 D. This condition is typically developmental, as in microphthalmos (where in some cases the refraction may even be normal). Progressive hyperopia can be seen in certain diseases such as orbital tumors or retinal exudates. Rarely the cornea can be found to be markedly flattened—as flat as 29 D—cornea plana. In some of these cases the total hyperopia may not be high at all

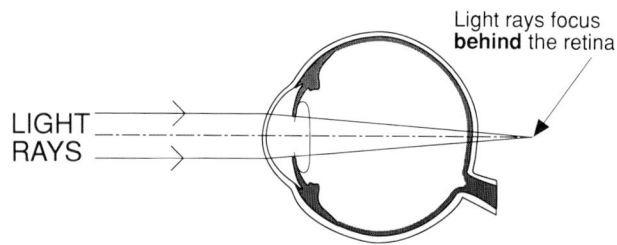

Fig. 2.28 The aphakic eye.

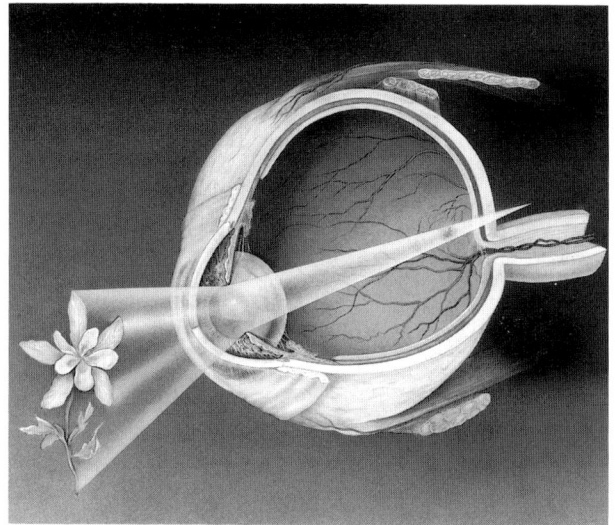

Fig. 2.29 Presbyopia.

(2–3 D) whereas in others it could be considerable. The latter are usually associated with high degrees of astigmatism as well.

The best-known form of acquired hyperopia is, of course, aphakia (Figure 2.28). Here the absence of nearly +19 D of refractive power pushes the focal point as far back as 31 mm behind the retina. This necessitates strong convex lenses being placed before the eye to compensate—typically +10 to +11 D in power. Such lenses were supposedly first advocated by Benito Daza de Valdes, though the first mention of such usage is to be found in the writings of Nicholas Cusanus (1401–1464) in his work, *De Beryllo* (Spectacles) [59,60]. Writing one of the earliest works on spectacles, not only did Valdes suggest such use in aphakes but recommended concave spectacles for myopes and convex lenses for hyperopes. In that period such lenses were only prescribed for presbyopes (Figure 2.29) and it wasn't until 1725 that their use in aphakia was finally put into practice by Heister. It was to be another 225 years before the suggestion of Tadini to replace the cataractous lens was successfully carried out by Ridley [61] (see also Chapter 13).

Characteristics of hyperopia

Hyperopia is called far-sight because the near point is at a considerable distance in front of the eye, making far vision more comfortable and clearer than near vision. In some cases, this deficit can be overcome by the act of accommodation. However, while this might suffice to clarify objects at a distance, sufficient accommodative amplitude may not exist to produce clear images at near.

The amount of hyperopia compensated for by normal tonus of the ciliary muscle is called latent while any remaining is termed manifest. Taken together the two constitute total hyperopia. It follows that the amount of latent hyperopia decreases over time as the lens becomes less flexible until presbyopia results, at which time all the hyperopia becomes manifest. Manifest hyperopia is further made up of facultative hyperopia, which is that amount that can be compensated for by the act of accommodating. That remaining uncompensated is termed absolute hyperopia.

Since accommodative amplitude varies from individual to individual as well as by age, it follows that cycloplegic examination of the hyperope (occasionally into the 50s) is necessary to uncover the total hyperopia present.

Frequently, fogging techniques are insufficient to uncover the latent and/or facultative hyperopia. In fact, the amount of unsuspected facultative hyperopia can be astonishing. The author once examined a 36-year-old naval supply officer who was complaining of asthenopia (his commanding officer was also complaining about this man's surly disposition). Uncorrected, and with no obvious effort, his visual acuity was 20/20 on the Snellen chart, both for near and far. On manifest examination his refraction was +1 D OU, while on cycloplegic his refraction was +4.00 D! He was unable to tolerate any plus correction until we adopted the expedient of administering cycloplegia and ordering him to wear his glasses while the drop was wearing off. That ploy worked and he was finally able to wear +3 D comfortably, banishing his asthenopic complaints. Interestingly, his disposition improved markedly as well.

The neglected hyperope

In the literature concerning ametropia, myopia has received most of the attention, and hyperopia has been all but ignored. In a review of references listed in the huge database compiled by the National Medical Library (from 1966 to the present), 3411 articles exist dealing with myopia and only 773 with hyperopia (4:1). Within that enduring "bible" of ophthalmology, *System of Ophthalmology* by Sir Stewart Duke-Elder, 72 pages are devoted to myopia and only 14 to hyperopia (5:1). Refractive surgery too is about myopia and astigmatism, or so it seems. In a review of extant literature, less than 10% of the articles dealing with the surgical treatment of ametropia, excluding aphakia, are about hyperopia. Yet hyperopia appears to be more prevalent than myopia by at least 2:1. Thus hyperopia would seem to be a poor relative indeed. Why should this be? After all, the first spectacles were prescribed—in 1290—for hyperopia (actually for presbyopia), not myopia. It wasn't until almost 300 years later than myopes had some relief from their affliction.

Perhaps it's because myopes need a correction most of the time or perhaps it's because myopia is perceived as more threatening [62–64]. Probably the main reason for this emphasis is that being associated with poor vision, myopia alone seems to hold the threat of blindness. In fact, throughout the world myopia is listed as one of the leading causes of visual loss—hyperopia is not on that list. Interestingly, the first schools for partially sighted children, established in London, were called myopia schools and designed for the express purpose of enabling high myopes to avoid eyestrain and thereby prevent further progression of the myopia. Whatever the reason, myopia has received the lion's share of attention. Many methods have been devised for the prevention or control of myopia but little or no effort has been expended for a like process with hyperopia.

Yet a significant number of the world's population (almost 50% in most countries) are hyperopic *de novo*, not to mention those cases iatrogenically produced through one means or another. If Grosvenor is correct, hyperopia *per se* represents a significant impediment to the learning process [65]. Evidence exists connecting it with behavioral problems as well as low academic standing amongst elementary school children (see section on ametropia, intelligence, and scholastic standing, below). Still and all, hyperopia does not seem to be regarded as a problem of pressing proportions. In fact, hyperopia amongst adults is not often discussed, perhaps because the malady is dealt with (most of the time) behind closed doors where the afflicted can wear their "grannies" or bifocals in secret. Also most hyperopes are of such degree that they can "muddle through" the day without exposing their "weakness." Broekema showed that normal visual acuity occurred in 82% of the hyperopes in his study whose refractive error was 1–2 D; in 64% from 3 to 4 D; in 44% from 5 to 6 D; and in only about 15% from 7 to 10 D [66].

Many vision practitioners, as well as the general public, still consider myopia a weakness and all the more so because the myope displays his or her weakness in public by wearing spectacles. For despite efforts at destigmatization, the wearing of spectacles still carries with it significant social penalty. Even in this age of "enlightenment" the wearing of glasses, especially by a child, tends to set one apart. In contrast, many

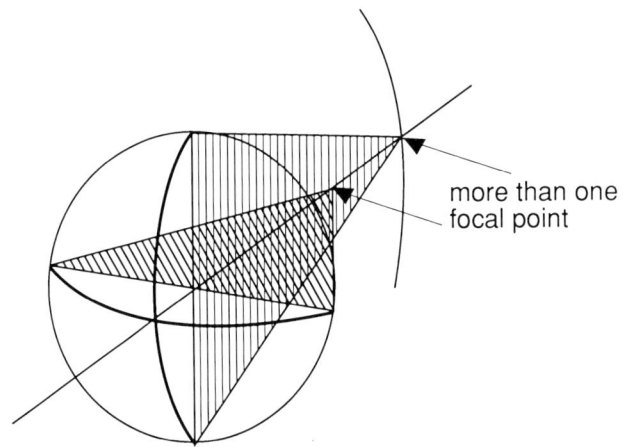

Fig. 2.30 The astigmatic eye.

hyperopes find that they can conceal their anomaly by only wearing glasses in the privacy of their homes or offices—at least for a while—for close work. The wearing of glasses is also perceived as being a sign of intelligence—a paradox to be sure. It's very likely that we are more concerned about the appearance of weakness than in the malady itself, however. This is underscored by the fact that optometrists, once heavily involved in attempts to control or prevent myopia by visual training, under-correction, or plus lenses for reading, have almost completely abandoned these attempts and have turned instead to the fitting of contact lenses. Of course some of the impetus to this trend may stem from the demonstrated failure of these methodologies to make more than a token dent in the problem.

Whatever may be the *casus omissus* of the situation, considerable evidence exists in the literature pointing to the relationship of ametropia to intelligence test scores, reading ability and school achievement. It is apparent that at least some hyperopes are having problems in that regard. Grosvenor reviewed the situation and suggested that more attention be paid to this sector of the population [65]. He presents some compelling arguments to support his thesis.

Astigmatism

We have said previously that in the eye when light rays converge upon, behind, or in front of the retina, and the principal focus approximates a point lying in one plane, such a system is termed stigmatic (pointlike). This condition can also be termed anastigmatic (without astigmatism). When the principal focus lies not within one plane but in many planes no one principal focus is formed, and the condition is termed astigmatic (Figure 2.30). Ocular astigmatism is physiologic and almost invariable, but usually small in degree and of little visual effect (Figure 2.31).

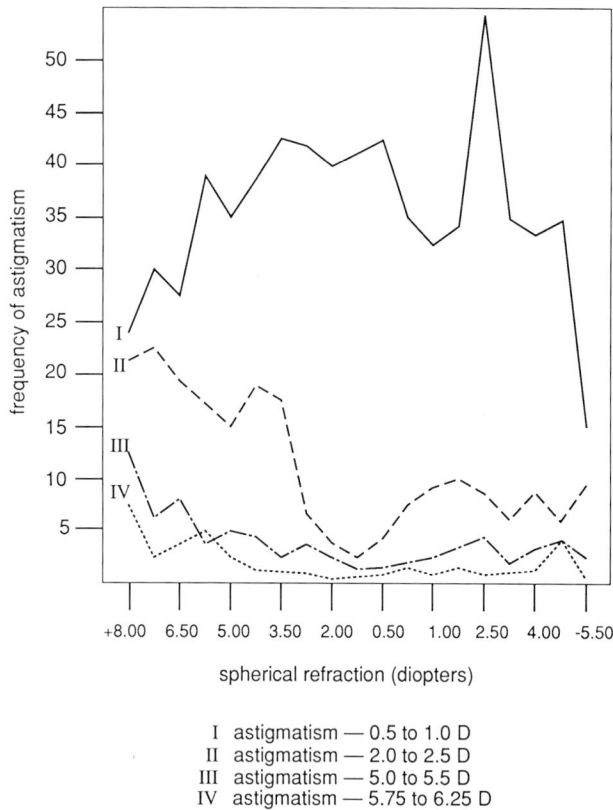

I   astigmatism — 0.5 to 1.0 D
II astigmatism — 2.0 to 2.5 D
III astigmatism — 5.0 to 5.5 D
IV astigmatism — 5.75 to 6.25 D

Fig. 2.31 The variation in frequency of various degrees of corneal astigmatism associated with different refractive states (from Kronfeld and Devney. The frequency of astigmatism. Arch Ophthalmol, 1930).

Astigmatism ordinarily depends on the presence of toroidal instead of spherical curvatures of the refracting surfaces of the eye. The refractive power as a whole, therefore, instead of being equal in all meridians, changes gradually from one meridian to the next by uniform increments, and each meridian generally has

a uniform type of curve. If the axes showing the greatest difference in curvature are at right angles to one another, the condition is called regular astigmatism and is correctable by a cylindrical lens. If they are not so related, the astigmatism may be called bi-oblique and can be treated by a cross cylinder. Typically the major and minor axes are oriented such that one of them is at or near 90°. If they are not so oriented, the astigmatism is said to be oblique. When, however, as in cases of corneal disease such as keratoconus or in lenticular sclerosis, there are irregularities in the curvature of the meridians, the condition is called irregular astigmatism. Unless such a defect is corneal, it cannot be compensated for by spectacle lenses, but sometimes can be by contact lenses (Figure 2.32).

Types of astigmatism

We have already noted that astigmatism can be regular or irregular; oblique or bi-oblique. Additionally, the curvatures producing the astigmatism can cause the foci to vary in their antero-posterior relationship to the fovea. Thus, in hyperopic astigmatism, for example, the curvatures of both axes are unequal and too flat (large radii). In myopic astigmatism they are both unequal and too steep (small radii). If both foci lie either before or behind the retina, the condition is termed compound astigmatism (Figures 2.33 and 2.34). When the two conditions are combined so that one axis is hypermetropic and the other myopic—that is, the principal foci lie both before and behind the retina —the condition is termed mixed astigmatism (Figure 2.35). If one focus lies upon the retina and the other before or behind it, the astigmatism is considered simple astigmatism (Figures 2.36 and 2.37).

Regardless of whether the astigmatism is simple,

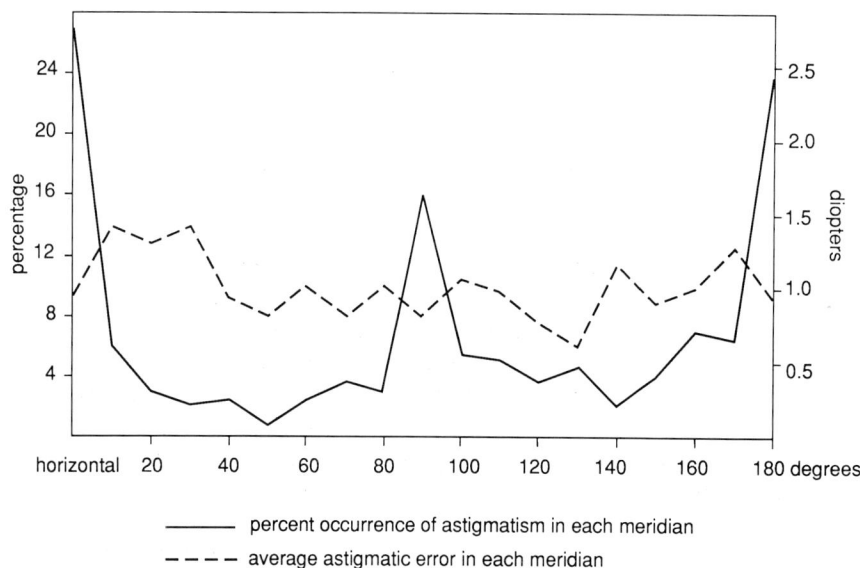

——— percent occurrence of astigmatism in each meridian

- - - - average astigmatic error in each meridian

Fig. 2.32 The percentage incidence of the direction of the axis of astigmatism. (from Lang, Br J Ophthalmol, 1920).

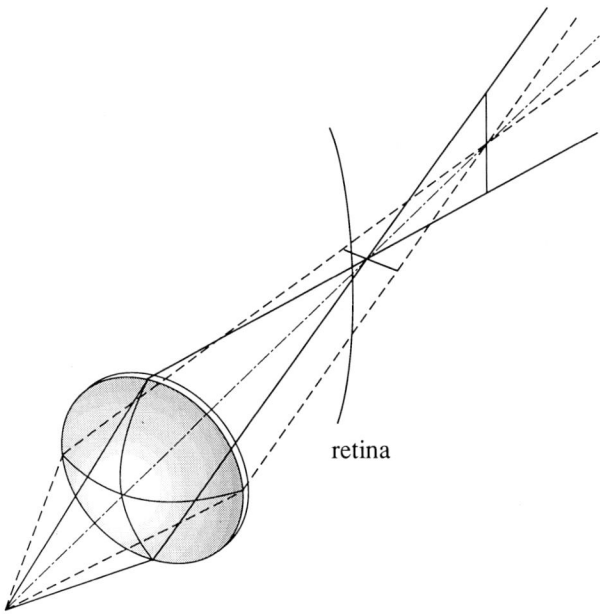

Fig. 2.33 Compound hyperopic astigmatism.

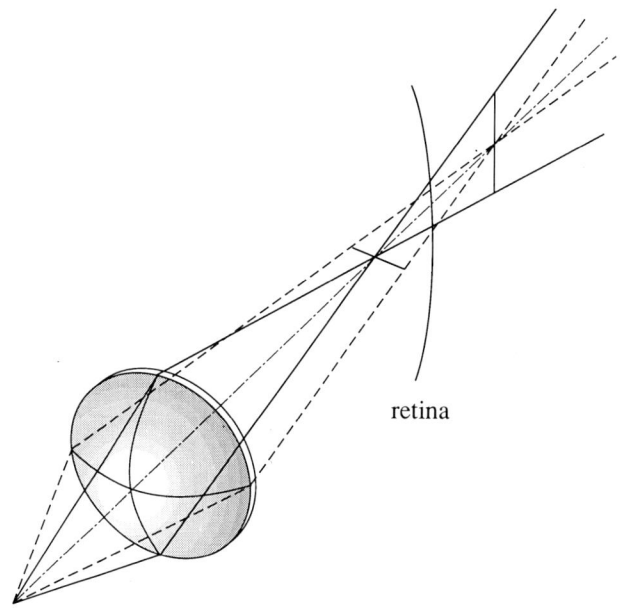

Fig. 2.35 Mixed astigmatism.

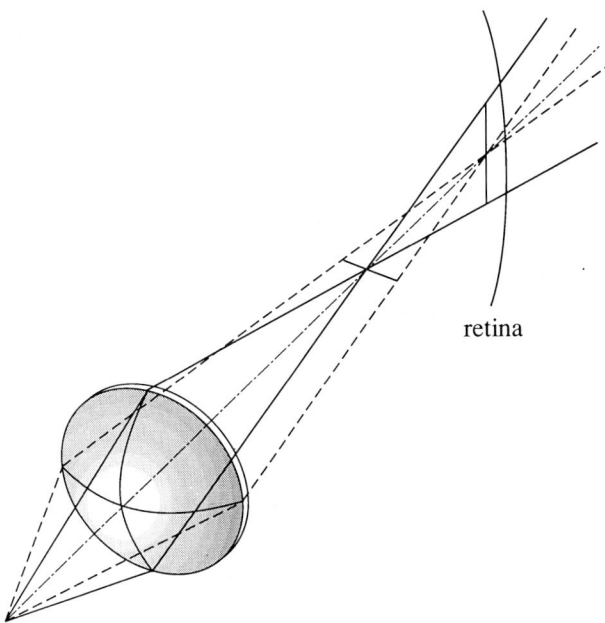

Fig. 2.34 Compound myopic astigmatism.

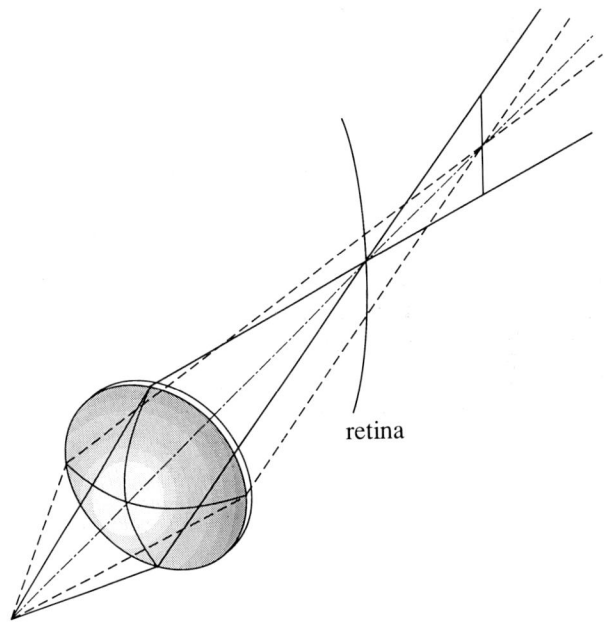

Fig. 2.36 Simple hyperopic astigmatism.

mixed, or compound, there is more than one focal point strung out along the visual axis. The interval between the anterior and posterior focus is called the interval of Sturm and varies in its extent depending upon the amount of astigmatism present in the optical system (Figure 2.38). The diffusion "circles" formed at these points are typically elliptical in shape. There is one point between the most anterior and the most posterior focus where the focal spot is circular, however. This circle is called the circle of least confusion

and is located approximately one third of the way from the anterior-most focus. At this point in space, in the absence of any optical correction, the image formed by the system is the best possible. Before the advent of sphero-cylindric spectacle lenses, physicians compensated for astigmatism by choosing a spherical lens which basically moved the circle of least confusion on to the retina. Typically this power corresponds to the so-called spherical equivalent of the refractive system; that is, a spherical lens of that power will produce a

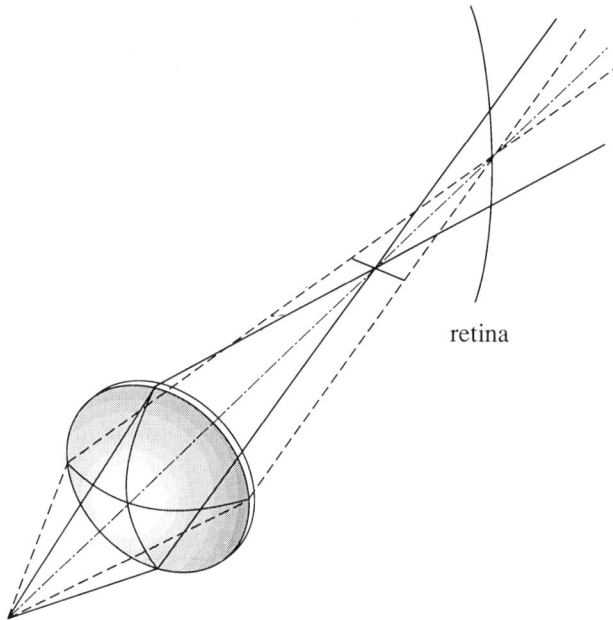

Fig. 2.37 Simple myopic astigmatism.

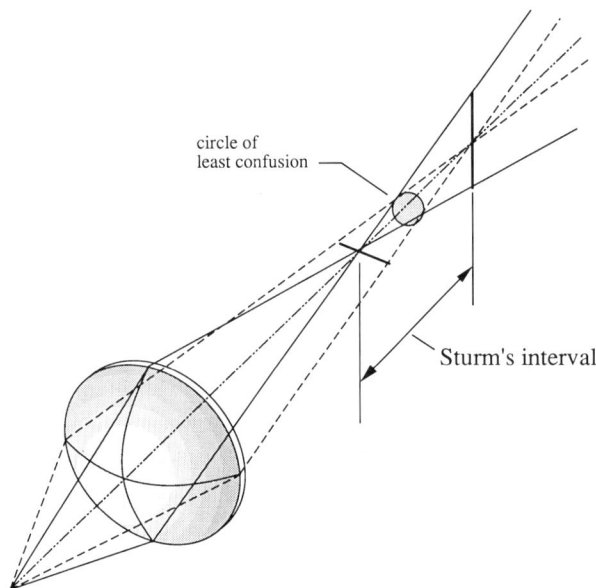

Fig. 2.39 Astigmatism axes.

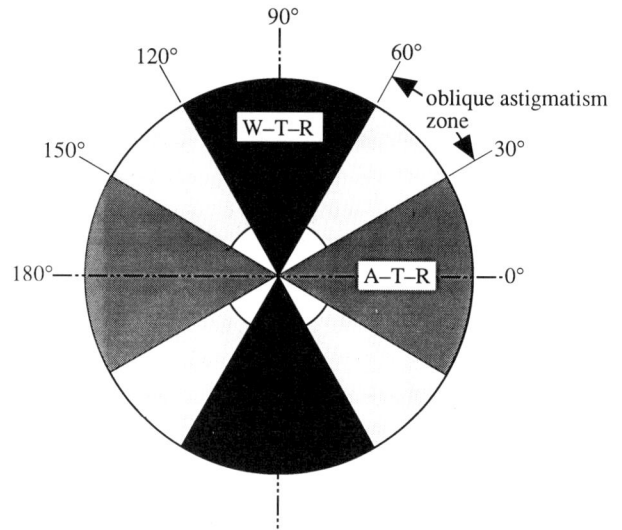

Fig. 2.38 Astigmatism and the interval of Sturm.

circle of least confusion on the retina similar to that of the astigmatic system alone.

The components of total astigmatism

Curvature variation of the anterior surface of the cornea occurs physiologically and is thus responsible for the majority of cases of astigmatism. The average difference between the refractive powers of the two corneal meridians lies between 0.5 and 0.75 D. Donders [44] gave a mean value of 1 D, Pfalz [67] of 0.75 D, Sørensen [68] of 0.75 to 0.5 D, Steiger [69] and Gullstrand [70] of 0.5 D, while Kronfeld and Devney [71] suggested that any value over 1 D should be regarded as pathologic. The author prefers to consider any astigmatism over 1 D as significant and any over 4 D as pathologic. Furthermore, the author considers any astigmatism that equals or exceeds 20% of the associated spherical component as significant and an indication for surgical intervention. In about 90% of these cases the meridian of least curvature (flattest) is horizontal (Figure 2.39). If that meridian lies within 30° of the horizontal plane, the astigmatism is said to be direct or with the rule (W-T-R). If it makes such an angle with the vertical plane so that the horizontal curvature is greater, it is said to be inverse or against the rule (A-T-R).

This tendency toward W-T-R astigmatism has never been adequately explained although Snellen associated it with pressure on the globe from the eyelids [72]. This view has had considerable support from other investigators and may be true to some degree. In keratoconus, where the cornea is extremely malleable, W-T-R astigmatism is quite frequent. This also occurs if external ocular pressure is increased by forceful lid closure or by increased weight of the eyelid as with lid tumors. It may be thought that increased intra-ocular pressure alone, as in glaucoma, may have the effect of producing inverse astigmatism. However, while this may occur in experimental animal models, it does not seem to be of clinical significance. It seems more likely that, since the corneal curvature is an extension of the same general curvature as the sclera, the cause is more a defect in growth of the eye. This view is substantiated by the common occurrence of high astigmatism in deformities of the globe—even of the posterior segment. Inverse astigmatism often follows the healing of a large horizontal scar such as is seen in large-incision cataract surgery (see also Chapter 13).

The posterior surface of the cornea also shows an astigmatic curvature which typically ranges from 0.25 to 0.5 D, sometimes reaching 1.0 D [73]. It is usually inverse in type neutralizing that of the external surface. In some cases, it may be the cause of so-called residual astigmatism encountered in contact lens fitting and can also account for that seen after refractive surgery in the presence of a spherical anterior surface.

Curvature astigmatism of both lens surfaces is also a normal occurrence and is typically less than that of the cornea and in the opposite direction. For example, Tscherning's measurements for the radii of the anterior lens surface were 10.2 mm horizontal and 10.1 mm vertical, and of the posterior surface 6.17 and 6.13 mm respectively [74]. Typically, such asphericity is small in degree—0.50 D. In an otherwise normal eye, it is assumed that most, if not all, astigmatism is corneal in origin. However, many patients do, in fact, possess considerable degrees of lenticular astigmatism. This is of particular importance in refractive surgery. It is essential to compare the net refractive error with that of the corneal curvature when evaluating a patient for this type of surgery. The presence of A-T-R astigmatism in a young individual should alert the examiner to the possibility of significant lenticular astigmatism. Only occasionally will the cornea be steeper horizontally; it typically shows direct or vertical astigmatism.

Astigmatism from decentration of the optical system is also physiologic and invariable since the refracting surfaces are neither geometrically centered nor concentric to the anatomic axis. Thus, the optic axis intersects the cornea as much as 0.25 mm below and nasal to the corneal apex. This is a small deviation and tends to neutralize physiologic direct astigmatism. Additionally, the fovea is not on the optic axis but some 1.25 mm down and temporal. The pupillary axis is somewhat eccentric as well, lying to the nasal side of the corneal center. Thus, if we accept Gullstrand's usual 5° angle between the pupillary and optic axes, the resultant astigmatism is 0.1 D for a pupil of 2.0 mm [74].

The total astigmatism of the ocular system is made up primarily by that of the corneal surface with the rest (the residual astigmatism contributed by the surfaces of the posterior cornea, lens, and component decentration) tending to neutralize this effect. This residual astigmatism, while usually of small degree, cannot be totally ignored. Jackson examined a large number of young adults and found the average corneal astigmatism to be 1.04 D while the residual averaged 0.61 D —a not inconsiderable amount [75]. The extremes were 8.0 D of corneal, 4.25 D of lenticular, and 6.0 D of total astigmatism. It seems evident from these figures that it is not possible nor rational to attempt to correct astigmatism through keratometry readings alone. Thus, it would be unwise to rely on Javal's rule [51], especially in refractive surgery. Javal's rule gives an empirical relationship between total or subjective astigmatism (AST) and the keratometric (corneal) astigmatism (ASC) but is prone to too many exceptions:

$$AST = k + 1.25\,ASC$$

where $k = 0.25\,D$ against the rule. It is interesting to note that while the total astigmatism of one eye may be quite different from its fellow, the residual astigmatism is similar [76].

Astigmatism and age

Regular astigmatism is age-variable with a small degree of W-T-R astigmatism occurring early in life. This astigmatism may not be present at birth, however— the neonate cornea is usually spherical—but develops somewhat later in life and changes little during the school years. During early adulthood on, there is a slight tendency for the W-T-R astigmatism to decrease or even reverse, with changes occurring more usually in men than women [77,78]. Jackson's figures [75] are illustrated in Table 2.1.

Accommodation

Accommodation is not ametropia *per se*, but this would appear to be the most appropriate place to discuss it, particularly as it applies to the post-operative course in refractive surgery. The existence of accommodation was proved by the classic but little appreciated experiment of Scheiner in 1619 (Figure 2.40) [19]. Alteration of ocular length was, for 150 years, the most popular theory by which this phenomenon occurred. Kepler described accommodation as occurring through elongation and shortening of the globe through the action of the ciliary processes [22,23]. This mechanism was elegantly disproved by Young in 1801 [40]. Having prominent eyes, he was able to place, after strong convergence, a ring, both at the inner orbital angle and at the outer, which pressed against the eye, the latter

Table 2.1 Astigmatism and age. From Jackson E, Norms of refraction. JAMA 1932; 98:132

	Nil	Horizontal	Vertical	Oblique
Corneal astigmatism				
Before 25 years	52	24	910	32
After 50 years	84	118	737	86
Residual astigmatism				
Before 25 years	62	817	61	52
After 50 years	72	726	63	163

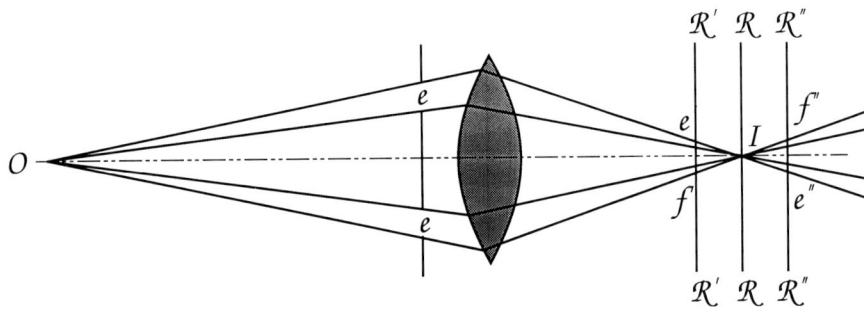

Fig. 2.40 Scheiner's classic experiment. If two holes are made in a card (e–e'), the object O is brought to a focus on the screen R where one image, I, will appear. If the screen is held at R' or R'', two images will appear ($e'f'$ and $e''f''$). The experiment proves that there is a focusing mechanism within the eye (from Scheiner C. *Occulus Hoc est: Fundamentum Opticum*. Innsbruck, 1619).

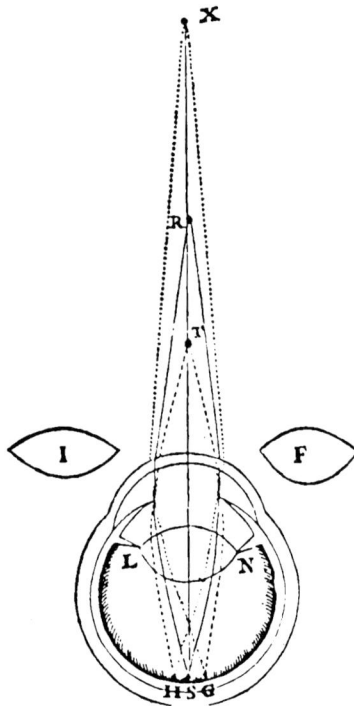

Fig. 2.41 Descartes' theory of accommodation. "In order to represent the point X distinctly it is necessary that the whole shape of the humor NL be changed and that it becomes a little flatter as that which is marked I, and to represent the point T it is necessary to become a little more convex like that which is marked F" (from Descartes R. *Traité de l'Homme*. Paris, 1677).

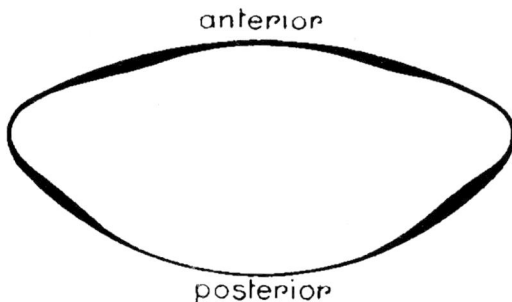

Fig. 2.42 Fincham's diagram of the lens capsule (from Fincham EF. The changes in the form of the crystalline lens in accommodation. Trans Opt Soc Lond 1925; 26:239–269).

over the macula. Pressure on the rings produced bright circular spots in the field of vision called phosphenes. On strong accommodation, neither of the images was displaced nor altered, thus showing that elongation of the eye did not occur in accommodation. In the same paper he dispelled the theory of Lobé that changes in the corneal curvature occurred to produce clear near vision. This was accomplished by showing that accommodation was unimpaired if corneal refraction was eliminated by attaching a glass lens to his cornea (one of the first, if not the first, examples of a contact lens) and filling the space between with water. Interestingly, it was while conducting this experiment that he discovered that he had astigmatism (see also section on astigmatism, above).

It is also interesting to note that corneal curvature changes actually do occur during accommodation, but not the radius change from 8.0 to 6.8 mm needed to accomplish clear near vision in the normal eye [52]. These changes in the normal have been attributed to convergence by some investigators [79,80]. That the accommodative mechanism is capable of altering corneal shape was demonstrated in a study of post-radial keratotomy patients with mild presbyopia [81].

This left only the lens which, it was suggested, moved backward and forward during accommodation [23]. However, it would require a total movement of 10 mm to produce the effects seen. Thus it remained that perhaps accommodation did occur—in the manner originally suggested by Descartes [82] (Figure 2.41), demonstrated by Porterfield and corroborated by Young—due to a change in lens shape [83]. Helmholtz demonstrated that accommodation resulted from increased curvature of both the anterior and posterior capsules of the lens, commenting on the conoidal shape of the postero-central part of the lens when accommodated [52]. Fincham explained this singular shape change by the molding capacity of the peculiar configuration of the lens capsule (Figure 2.42) [84]. In this he was in opposition to the view of Helmholtz who suggested that this shape was due to some elasticity of the lens itself which opposed that of the capsule. This latter view was shown to have some validity in the work of Kikawa and Sato [85] as well as Fisher [86]. Despite this hard evidence, Bates insisted that the lens was unnecessary in accommodation and persisted in his teaching that he, and he alone, was correct [87]. We will have more to say about William Bates in Chapter 10.

The significance of accommodation

The farthest point at which an object can be seen clearly is called the far point. When maximum accommodative effort is exercised, the closest point at which an object can be seen clearly is the near point. Range of accommodation is defined as the distance from the far point to the near point and represents the distance over which the near focus is effective. Amplitude of accommodation is defined as the difference in the refraction of the eye between these two values expressed in diopters, thus it is an expression of work done or to be done. Typically, the range of accommodation for an uncorrected myope decreases in nonlinear proportion to the degree of myopia, whereas the reverse is true in the hyperope (Figure 2.43). In the myope, full spectacle correction increases the accommodative demand, that is, the fully corrected eye must exert more accommodative effort to discern near objects clearly—the reverse is true for the hyperope. The demand is more for a myope than for a hyperope due to the relative inefficency of spectacle lens for divergent as opposed to parallel light rays. This difference is typically on the order of 0.9 D and depends upon the vertex distance. This is especially evident in contact lens wearers who may find that their demand increases as much as 50% [88]. This explains the middle-aged myopic contact lens wearer who finds that in giving up his spectacles he has attained the dubious advantage of having clear vision for distance but now requires spectacles with which to read. This fact may also mean the necessity of prescribing reading correction for presbyopia sooner than in the hyperope.

This phenomenon is especially evident after refractive surgery, even in young individuals, who often complain of difficulty with reading which was never experienced before. In some cases this is also seen in contact lens wearers who had not experienced this problem while wearing contacts prior to surgery. The fact of increased demand has encouraged some clinicians to advocate the under-correction of the myope or even to prescribe plus lenses for near to offset the need for increased accommodation. Articles advocating such an approach were prevalent in the literature (including in the USA) from the middle 19th century through the early 20th [89,90]. Today, most advocacy seems to be centered in the Japanese and Russian literature [91,92]. It is of interest that the wearing of contacts to increase accommodative demand is advocated to reduce progression of myopia by the most ardent proponents of the theory of environmental myopigenesis, particularly the role played by the malignant effects of accommodation and convergence.

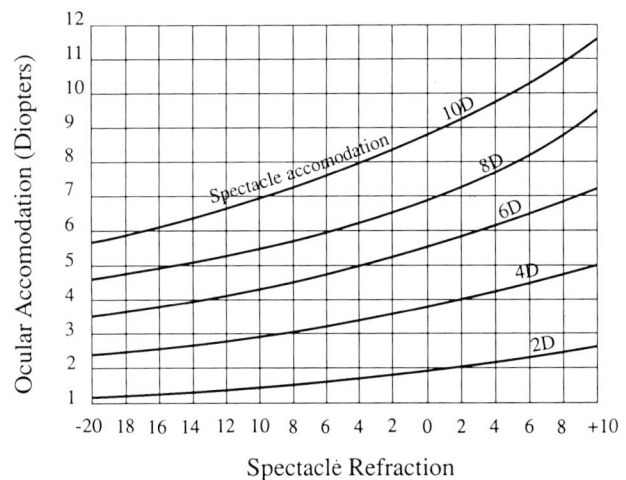

Fig. 2.43 Spectacle accommodation (from Bennett. *Optics of Contact Lenses*. 4th edn. Association of Dispensing Opticians, 1966).

The natural history of ametropia

Our discussion will begin by considering the condition (for want of a better, more universal description) of myopia—by far the greater portion of the problem of ametropia.

Ametropia—affliction or disease?

It seems somehow ironic that a condition, considered by many authorities [35,44] to be one of the leading causes of visual impairment in this country (as well as in others), is described by some others not even as a disease [93,94]. Yet myopia meets the definition of a disease in *Webster's International Dictionary*, namely: "an impairment of the normal state of the living animal or plant body or any of its components that interrupts or modifies the performance of the vital functions." Would anyone argue that vision is not one of the vital functions? Not to put too fine a point on it, but the author submits that vision has survival value and that any impairment of it reduces one's chances in an increasingly hostile world.

The evolution of our knowledge of myopia has been marked by occasional giant strides based on careful investigations and their impartial analysis. All too often, however, the contributions to this subject have been bewildering in their protocols, their results, and their conclusions. A tendency toward advocacy rather than investigatory curiosity can especially be seen to permeate the early literature.

Regardless of the somewhat blurred data representing the prevalence of myopia among the world's population, there is no doubt that myopia (except in its milder forms) and, to a lesser extent hyperopia, inflict a grave socio-economic burden upon the individual. This burden has not been truly appreciated by some and has been deprecated by many. We can make a beginning in our assessment of the question by considering that the cost of optical aids amounts to something in excess of $4 billion annually in the USA alone! This burden starts early and continues for a lifetime. In a survey conducted by the Department of Health, Education, and Welfare in 1974, it was found that 34% of individuals between ages 12 and 17 years were wearing correcting lenses. Myopic corrections accounted for an increasing proportion of these wearers —72% at age 12 to 87% at age 17 [95].

If myopia only caused a significant reliance upon optical corrections, it would be a problem of major proportions. Unfortunately it has been found to be the fifth most frequent specific cause of impaired vision in the USA; the seventh most frequent cause of legal blindness and the eighth most frequent cause of severe visual impairment (Table 2.2).

Curtin feels that these data may be somewhat misleading, however. He points out that pathologic myopia is a single disease entity, and in these tabulations it is ranked behind such disease groupings as cornea or sclera, uveitis, optic nerve disease, prenatal, vascular, and the like [35]. It is apparent that as a single cause of visual loss, pathologic myopia is under-estimated to a significant extent by some of these surveys. An equally important aspect in the consideration of the visual loss produced by myopia is its relatively early onset.

A recent investigation in the USA attributes 5.6% of blindness among school children to myopia, mak-

ing it the fifth most frequent cause of blindness after retrolental fibroplasia, cataract, optic nerve atrophy, and the combined category of anophthalmia–microphthalmia [96]. The prevalence of world blindness in general and myopic blindness in particular varies widely with the parameters used in different surveys (Table 2.3).

The Model Reporting Area studies on blindness conducted by the US Department of Health, Education, and Welfare indicate that, in addition to ranking seventh as a cause of blindness (1969–1970), the incidence of myopic blindness increased from 0.1% in children under 5 years of age to 0.6% in the aged [97]. The sharpest increase was noted to occur in the middle of the fifth decade. This, unfortunately, coincides with that period of life in which the talents and productivity of those affected are at a maximum, as well as with that time at which there is a peak in financial respon-

Table 2.3 The world's major blinding conditions. From Lim AS, Jones BR. World's major blinding conditions. Vision 1981; 1:101

Country or territory	Ranking as cause of blindness	Percentage of population affected
USA	7th	3
Hong Kong	5th	8
Japan	5th	8.4
Sri Lanka	5th	Not reported
Denmark	3rd	Not reported
German Democratic Republic	1st or 3rd	14.7 or 13.9
German Federal Republic	7th	6.6
Malta	1st	19.4
Poland	3rd	11
USSR	2nd	Not reported

Table 2.2 Estimates of prevalence of impairment from vision disorders, in thousands. From *Support for Vision Research*. Publication no. [NIM] 76–1098. Department of Health, Education and Welfare, Washington, DC, 1976

Type of eye affection	Impaired vision	Severe visual impairment	Legal blindness
Glaucoma	1070	207	56
Cataract (prenatal, other)	1711	217	64
Retinal disorder (prenatal, diabetic, other)	815	392	118
Retrolental fibroplasia	19	19	10
Myopia	715	36	14
Cornea or sclera	294	67	22
Uveitis	285	67	23
Optic nerve disease	121	107	41
Multiple affections	90	90	23
Refractive errors with lesser disability	1662	0	0
Other affections	3656	103	45
Unknown	221	179	53
Total (all affections)	10 699	1483	468

sibility; thus, the impact of this blindness upon the family is particularly severe (Figure 2.44).

In Europe a large number of such studies have been conducted. The data from the UK are of particular note because of Sorsby's interest in myopia [98]. In an early survey of blindness in England and Wales, he found myopia to be the second most frequent cause of blindness in persons between the ages of 30 and 49 years. In the next age group (50–69 years) it ranked second only to cataract. Overall, myopia was ranked as the third most prevalent cause behind cataract and glaucoma. In a more recent study of the same population, Sorsby found myopic atrophy and retinal detachment to be the cause of 14% of blindness in all age-groups behind diabetic retinopathy and cataract. It would appear that in Scotland the problem of myopic blindness is even more grave. Here it has been found as the single greatest cause in persons in the fifth decade of life. According to surveys conducted in 1942 and 1946, it was ranked second only to cataract among all age-groups. The combination of these data revealed a significantly earlier onset of blindness among myopic persons (mean 52.1 years) as compared with persons with blindness due to other causes.

Unfortunately, there has been wide variance in the definition of blindness and, specifically, myopic blindness. In some surveys, the blindness of a myopic eye due to glaucoma, for example, may be reported as myopic in nature. Conversely, blindness due to retinal detachment in eyes with substantial degrees of myopia is reported as due to retinal and not myopic causes. In some surveys blindness secondary to cataract as well as retinal detachment in myopic eyes was reported as myopic in nature. The inclusion of the former is of questionable validity however, and a somewhat exaggerated picture of the importance of myopia emerges from this review.

The development of ametropia

It is apparent, in retrospect, that this central canon of the old school would eventually be challenged. That axial length was not the sole determinant of refrac-

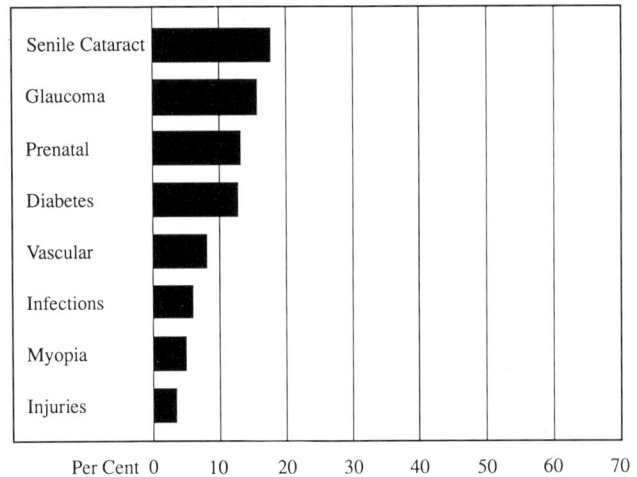

Fig. 2.44 The eight major causes of blindness in the USA: population 20 years of age and above (from *Estimated Statistics on Blindness and Visual Problems*. National Society for the Prevention of Blindness, New York, 1966).

tion was appreciated by Donders [44]. Schnabel and Herrnheiser [99] had found axial diameters varying from 22.25 to 26.24 mm in 23 emmetropic eyes and postulated that emmetropia was determined by the relation between axial length and total refraction. It was, however, Steiger's work in 1913 [69] on 5000 juvenile eyes that finally de-emphasized the role of axial length as the sole contributor to the myopic condition. Despite defects in his methodology, especially in assuming lens power as a constant, his work ushered in a new era in the study of myopia. The variability of lens power had been alluded to as early as 1575 by Maurolycus [100], and variations in lens thickness, refractive index, and position had been enumerated as possible causes of myopia prior to Donder's time. Furthermore, actual lens power measurements, albeit in small samples, had been demonstrated by von Reuss [101,102] and Awerbach [103] as showing considerable variations (Table 2.4).

Tron confirmed most of Steiger's earlier work (avoiding its pitfalls) and in addition showed that axial length was a determinant in ametropia only in ranges beyond

Table 2.4 Range and mean values of the four components of refraction obtained by three major studies. From Curtin BJ. *The Myopias. Basic Science and Clinical Management*. Harper & Row, New York, 1985

	Tron		Stenstrom		Sorsby	
	Range	Mean	Range	Mean	Range	Mean
Corneal power (D)	37–49	43.41	39.2–48.5	42.84	39–47	43.14
Anterior chamber depth (mm)	2.16–5.05	3.27	2.8–4.55	3.68	2.6–4.4	3.47
Lens power (D)	15–29	20.44	12.5–22	17.35	17–26	20.71
Axial diameter (mm)	21–38	25.14	20–29.5	24.00	21–37	23.94

See text for details.

+4 and −6 D [104,105]. Stenstrom [64] elaborated on some earlier work by Rushton [106] on determining the axial length using X-rays. In a series of 1000 eyes he confirmed Tron's earlier data showing essentially normal distribution curves for corneal power, depth of anterior chamber, lens power, and total refraction. It was also noted by Stenstrom that the distribution curve of refraction had basically the same pattern as that of axial length, featuring both a positive excess at emmetropia and a skewness toward myopia. This deviation in the population refraction curve had been noted previously by Scheerer [107,108] and Betsch [109] (Figure 2.45), who had attributed this to the incorporation of eyes with crescent formation at the optic nerve.

When these eyes were deleted from the data, a symmetric curve was obtained for the distribution of refraction. In the analysis of these data it was pointed out that a positive excess still persisted in the corrected curve. Stenstrom's refractive curve after the removal of eyes with crescents also demonstrated an excess. This central peaking was attributed to two factors: the first was the effect of component correlation in the emmetropic range as postulated by Wibaut [110] and Berg [111] and the second was the direct effect of axial length distribution upon the curve of refraction.

Sorsby's work in 1957 and again in 1961 [112,113] stands as the model and framework for our current understanding of the evolution of ametropia, particularly myopia. Sorsby and co-workers demonstrated conclusively in their study of 341 eyes that an "emmetropization" effect was noted in distribution curves of refraction as a result of a correlation of corneal power and axial length. In ametropias of ±4 D and above, this correlation appeared to break down, however. Their study also indicated that neither the lens nor the anterior chamber depth was an effective emmetropizing factor. In all of their investigations, the dominant finding was the high correlation of total refraction with axial length. This is true especially in the emmetropic range of refraction (−0.75 to +1.50 D) in which the correlation of corneal power diminishes the impact of axial length upon the refraction. The latter remains, for the most part, as the primary determinant even in this range of refraction. The question then arises, what is the natural history of physiologic myopia?

By and large myopia illustrates marked changes at three periods of development: newborn, childhood, and adult. From premature infant to about 6 months of age, the trend in myopia is downward, showing a marked rise from age 5 to 13 years. Following this period, until age 20, a gradual decline in the degree of myopia is seen.

In a classic paper, Brown performed atropine refractions at least 1 year apart on 1203 eyes, from birth to age 51, for a total of 8820 comparative measurements (Figure 2.46) [114]. He concluded that:

> myopia increases and hyperopia decreases rapidly from age 8 to 13 years. From 14 to 20 years, this increase in myopia continues each year, but at a rate barely half that of the previous period. Puberty possibly tends to bring about an *emmetropization*. [This concept makes some investigators uncomfortable. Acceptance of the fact of this mechanism, however, does not mean the phenomenon is teleologic in nature.] Increase of myopia after the age of 20 is practically negligible . . . between 20 and 33 years the increase continues at a very low average yearly rate (0.04 diopter). Between 34 and 42 years, the refraction shifts to the low yearly decrease in each successive year, averaging only 0.03 diopter.

Lepard [115] performed 797 examinations on 55 patients aged 1–28 years and found that his "data indicate that eyes with normal visual acuity become progressively more myopic with growth and development until 25 years of age, and are in excellent agreement with the data of Brown." On the basis of these studies, we can conclude that changes in refraction after radial keratotomy in individuals aged 21 or older are most likely due to the surgery, since spontaneous regression of myopia is virtually unheard of and since the progression of myopia after this age is very small compared to the effect induced by the surgery.

Ocular growth manifests in two distinct phases: the first or rapid phase occurs from birth to 3 years and the second or slow phase is from age 3 to 13. The different refractions and axial lengths are not related to bodily

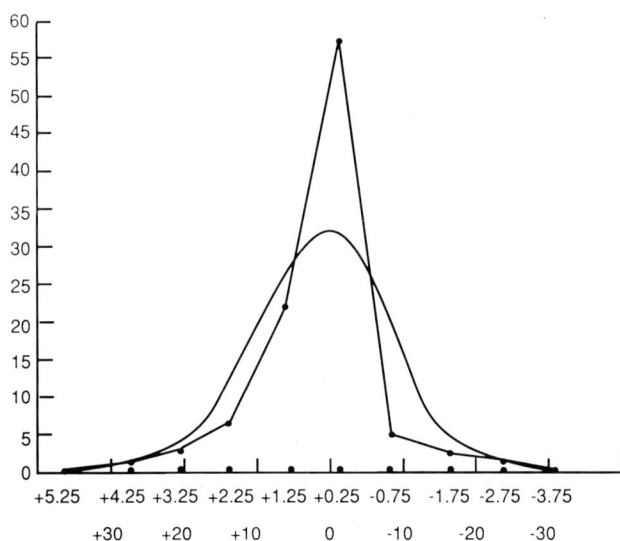

Fig. 2.45 Refraction curves of Scheerer and Betsch compared with a theoretical binomial curve.

stature and weight, nor does there appear to be a spurt in growth at puberty. Furthermore there is no sexual predilection—the growth of the eye appears to be completed by the age of 13 or 14 in both boys and girls [112]. This latter observation is in line with the growth pattern of the central nervous system in general, of which the eye is, of course, an integral part.

The corneal diameter attains its full adult size (mean 11.7 mm) by 5 years of age, and may possibly reach it by age 1 year. This was well demonstrated in Priestley Smith's classic study [116] and substantiated by others [117]. The remainder of the eye does not show the same degree of stability—particularly the weight and axial length [118]. In the full-term infant, ocular length ranges from 17.5 to 18.5 mm. Since the mean adult length lies between 23 and 25 mm, 6 mm would seem to be the usual increase in ocular size during childhood. This growth is neither uniform nor marked but still necessitates considerable change in the dioptric powers of the lens and cornea (to a lesser extent the anterior chamber depth) in order to compensate.

The eye grows most of the remaining 6 mm (an additional 5 mm) between birth and age 3 years [113]. The lens and/or the cornea must therefore undergo almost 20 D of compensatory change during this period, for there is no drastic change in the refraction of the eye during this time. Whether the cornea and lens are equally concerned in this compensation is uncertain; it has been shown that changes in corneal power in the order of 20 D do occur in the rabbit but comparable changes have not been satisfactorily demonstrated in humans. It follows that the changes must therefore occur mostly in the lens during infancy but evidence for these changes is not clear-cut.

During the next 10 years there is a gradual elongation of the eye by approximately 1.0 mm. Consequently, less change is required of either the cornea or the lens. The increase in axial length represents a potential reduction of some 3 D of hyperopia, but the actual reduction is less since flattening of the lens reduces its power by about 1.5 D, and there is also some flattening of the cornea. It is apparently the shortfall of such changes that results in ametropia. That is, it is the failure to compensate for axial growth that produces myopia and it is the failure of ocular growth itself that produces hyperopia. That these changes do occur is evident by the fact that the percentage of eyes showing axial elongation is greater than those eventually showing myopia. This correlation of increasing ocular elongation and decreasing power of the lens and cornea is the normal pattern in childhood. Sorsby [79] was able to demonstrate flattening of the corneal curvature

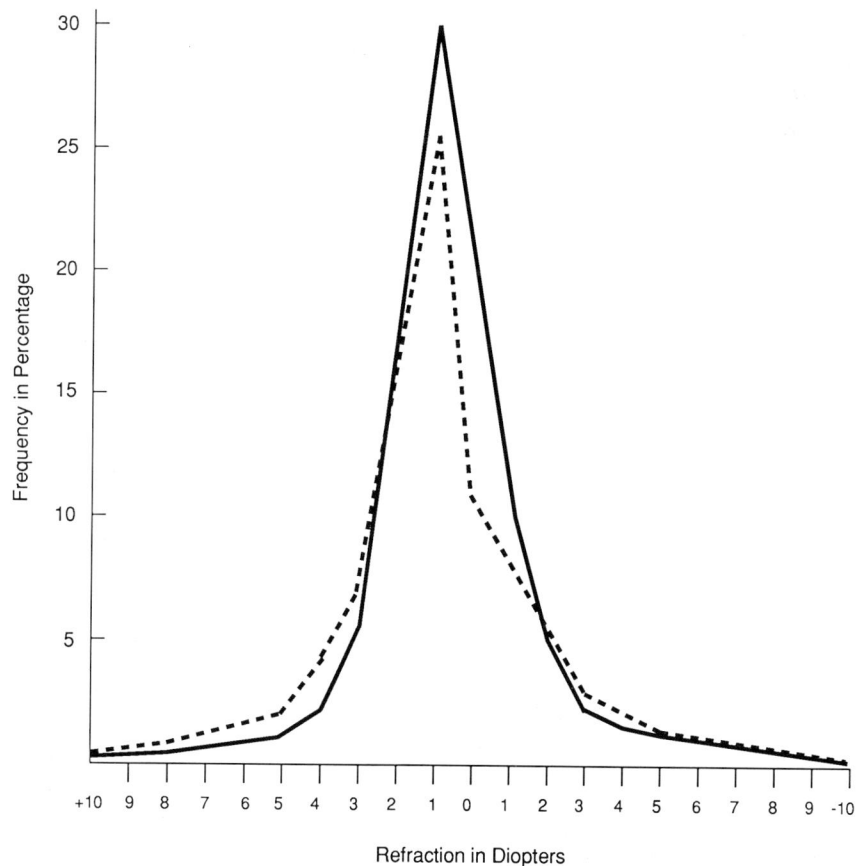

Fig. 2.46 Relative incidence of refractive errors in adolescents under 25 (from Brown Kronfeld. The refraction curve in the U.S. with special reference to the first two decades. Thirteenth Council Ophthalmol 1929; 1:86.

Frequency in Percentage

+10 9 8 7 6 5 4 3 2 1 0 1 2 3 4 5 6 7 8 9 -10

Refraction in Diopters

associated with increasing ocular elongation. There-fore, the main trend is toward emmetropia; marked reduction in hyperopia or the breakdown of this cor-relation leading to myopia is uncommon.

That a slight increase in hyperopia was the rule during the first 7 years of life was found by Brown in his study [119]. This rather surprising finding was con-firmed by Slataper, but his figures for refraction in the early years of life were restricted and he included Brown's figures in his own series [120]. On the other hand, the longitudinal studies of Hirsch and Wey-mouth on a slightly older age-group appear to indicate that, while an increase of hyperopia is found in a small proportion of children, a decrease is the rule [121].

The more rapid changes in axial length as well as the capacity to compensate are greater in the younger age-groups. The slower rate of growth as seen in the older age-groups along with a diminished capacity to com-pensate correlates well with the greater incidence of myopia in those older age-groups. This phenomenon must be kept in mind when evaluating studies that purport to show that myopia increases during later school and college years and that therefore near-work produces the impetus for such change. The temptation to conclude that *post hoc, ergo propter hoc*, while tempt-ing, must be resisted.

Component coordination

How this coordinated growth is achieved is uncertain. In an earlier study it has been shown that the eye is a coordinated organ and not a haphazard association of optical components [112]. It was therefore suggested that the axial length is the determining factor in the dioptric architecture of the globe, and that normally the curvatures of the cornea and of the lens are deter-mined by axial length. In the case of the cornea this followed from the fact that a larger globe had flatter surfaces; in the case of the lens the physical basis was not so obvious. Full coordination and automatic adjust-ment gave emmetropic eyes, and less full coordination resulted in errors falling within the range of ±4.0 D. It appears that all but some 3–4% of eyes in the general population have full or fairly full coordination.

Sorsby and his associates amplified these findings in showing that the process of coordination is active throughout childhood (Figure 2.47). Here the adap-tation of the cornea and of the lens to axial elongation is seen in operation. It was also shown that compen-sation by flattening of the cornea and lens tends to lag behind the axial elongation, so that during growth the optical components are not only coordinated, but so keyed that some reduction in refraction follows: this is the process of emmetropization in action. Since growth of the eye implies increase in axial length and decrease of the curvature of the lens—and to a lesser extent of

the cornea—it follows not only that the child's eye is smaller but that the quotient of axial length to the curvature of the lens is lower than in the adult.

Sorsby and his group invoked embryonic organiz-ation as the factor responsible for the negative cor-relation between the power of the lens and the axial length. Simple mechanical factors, however, may pro-vide a partial explanation as well. As an example, the ring into which the outer extremity of the suspensory ligament is inserted increases in diameter with the growth of the globe and so will tend to flatten the lens, and it has been suggested that the tone of the ciliary muscle may itself affect the axial length of the globe [56,122,123].

This latter concept has led to an exploration of the role accommodation may have in promoting the pro-gression of myopia [124]. Various authors have advo-cated the use of atropine drops to suspend accom-modation, claiming a slowing or arresting of the growth of the eye [125–128]. Atropine is a dangerous drug, however, and its potential side-effects must be weighed against its potential benefits, because the evidence of its efficacy is not clear-cut. However, Curtin feels that the possible risk of atropine therapy in intermediate myopia is outweighed by the real morbidity of an increase in myopia from 3 to 5 D, for example, which might otherwise occur [35].

Ocular development between the ages of 3 and 14 years is both slow and slight compared with the rapid and marked changes that occur in the infant under 3 years of age. Of this infantile phase we know little beyond the fact that it does occur. It is tempting to postulate that just as there are individual variations in development after the age of 3, so there are individual variations before that age. It is possible that in some eyes axial elongation falls short of the usual 5 mm or so, and that in consequence the infants enter on the second phase of ocular growth—the definitive phase—with globes considerably shorter than normal. Such adjustments that take place during the definitive stage would not be enough to carry these eyes into the normal range, and thus it is these that remain markedly hyperopic. Such a hypothesis recalls the older view that the hyperopic eye is an undeveloped one and it is probably true that the highly hyperopic eye is struc-turally abnormal. Similarly, while low degrees of myopia can be precipitated by the breakdown of co-ordination of the ocular components at the end of the definitive phase of growth, the highly myopic eyes, like the highly hypermetropic ones, fall outside the range of the changes that are part of normal growth.

The individual variations in axial elongation and in reduction of corneal and lens powers are such that it is impossible to forecast the refraction of a child who is, for example, emmetropic at the age of 8. The axial length may remain stationary and the refraction un-

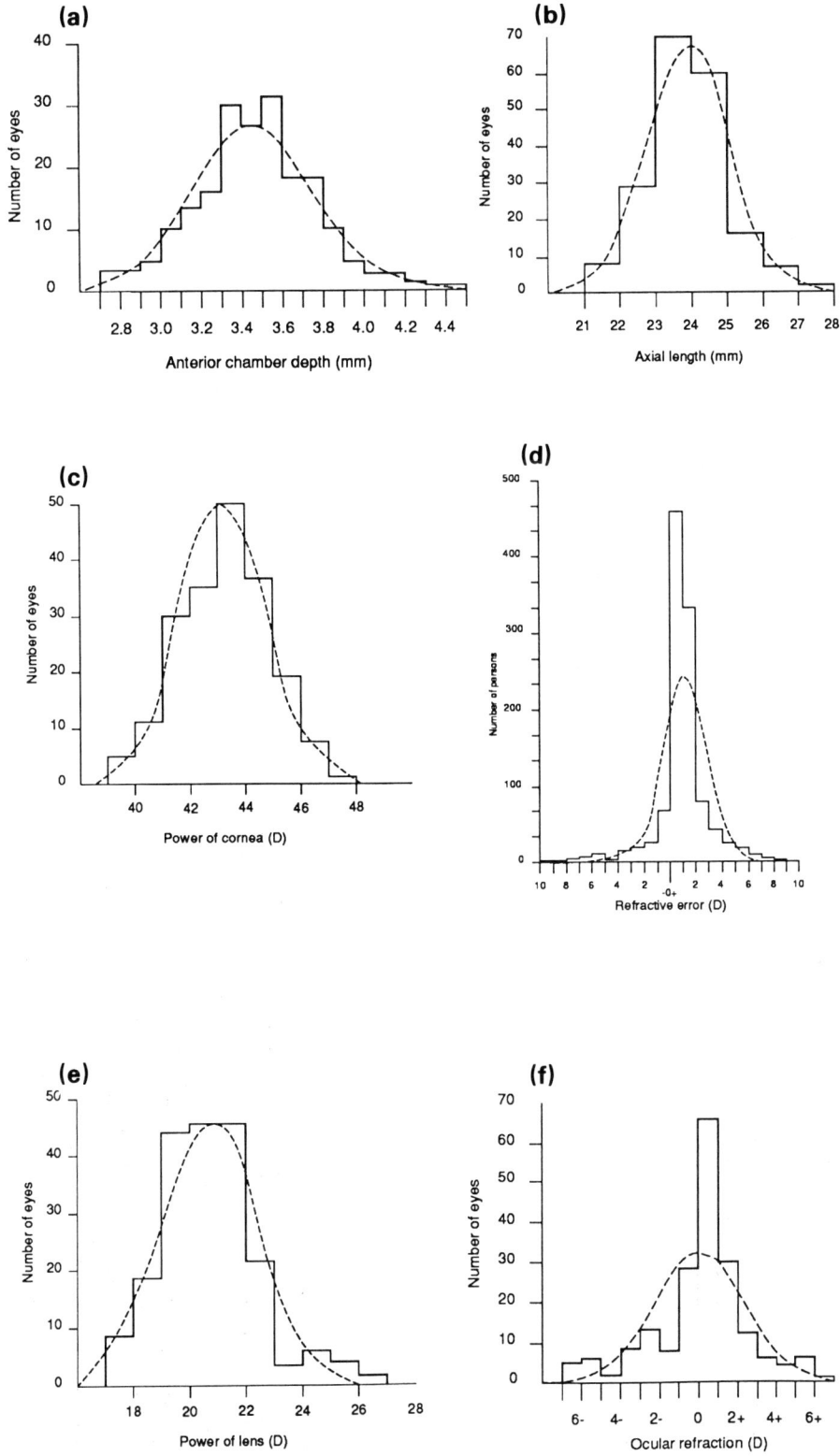

Fig. 2.47 (a,b) Ocular component dimensions in children: AC depth/axial length. (c,d) Corneal power/distribution of refractive error. (e,f) Lens power/total refraction (from Sorsby A, Benjamin B, Davey J. Tanner *Emmetropia and its Aberrations*. Medical Research Council, London, 1937.

changed; there may be axial elongation which will be fully compensated for and so leave emmetropia, or there may be axial elongation only partially compensated for, giving myopia. Each of these three patterns was observed by Sorsby in his short follow-up study, as were similar patterns for hyperopic eyes. It seems clear that there is much to be learned from an adequate follow-up study of a substantial number of children throughout growth (Figures 2.48 to 2.50, Tables 2.5 and 2.6).

Changes in the refractive state in the adult

We have seen that it is probable that significant growth of the eye proceeds only until early puberty; thereafter in the majority of subjects the axial length of the globe remains practically unaltered. Nevertheless, after ocular growth has ceased, the evidence indicates that refractive changes still occur with age. Thus Slataper found that there was a slight but steady increase in hyperopia from the third to the seventh decade, and it is generally recognized that this process, although mild in degree, is the rule after the age of 40 [58,77]. Thus an eye which was emmetropic at 30 years of age will show 0.25 D of hyperopia at 55, an addition of 0.75 D may be evident at 60, of 1 D at 70, and at 80 years this may increase to about 2.5 D. Hyperopia of this origin is frequently designated as acquired hyperopia (senile hypermetropia of Straub). On the other hand, in extreme old age, a trend toward myopia

may develop but this change is probably due to the presence of nuclear sclerosis. Slataper, in an examination of 1404 subjects in the eighth decade, found that only 18% had clear lenses [120].

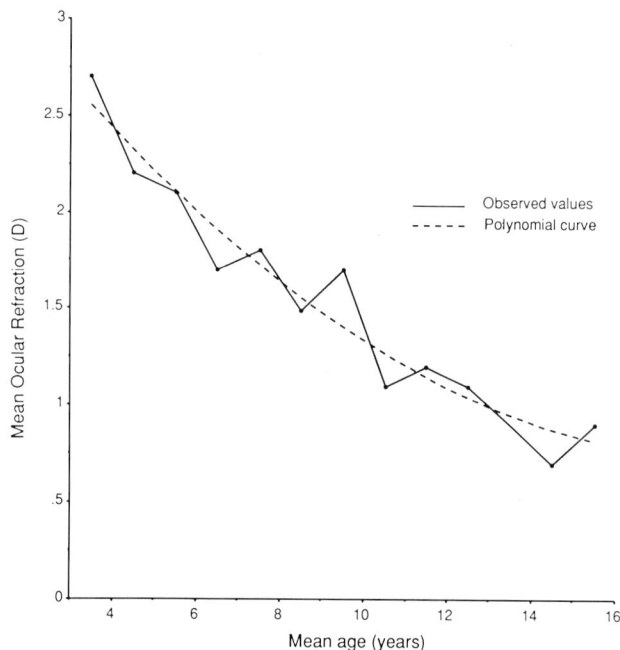

Fig. 2.49 Mean axial length in millimeters (from Sorsby M, Benjamin B, Sheridan M. *Refraction and its Components During the Growth of the Eye from the Age of Three.* Medical Council Special Report series no. 301. Her Majesty's Stationery Office, London, 1961).

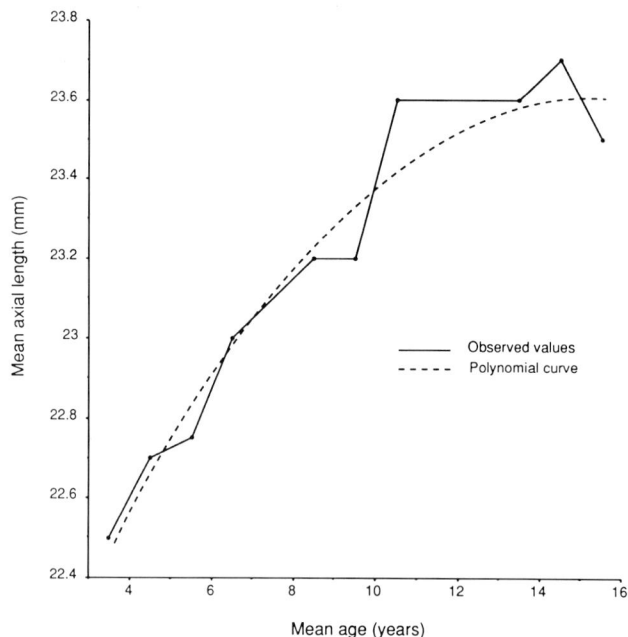

Fig. 2.48 Mean ocular refraction in diopters (from *Refraction and its Components During the Growth of the Eye From the Age of Three.* Medical Research Council Special Report series no. 301. Her Majesty's Stationery Office, London, 1961).

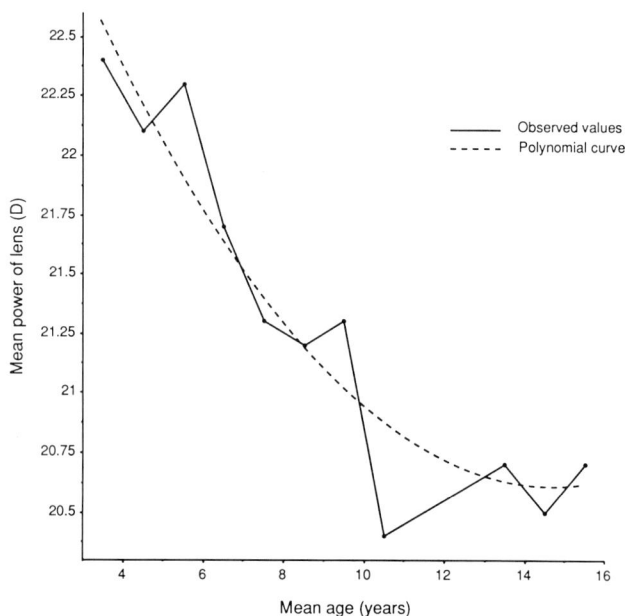

Fig. 2.50 Mean power of lens in D (from Sorsby M, Benjamin B, Sheridan M. *Refraction and its Components During the Growth of the Eye from the Age of Three.* Medical Council Special Report series no. 301. Her Majesty's Stationery Office, London, 1961).

Table 2.5 Mean values of ocular refraction during growth in 1432 children. From Sorsby A, Benjamin B, Sheridan M. *Refraction and its Components during the Growth of the Eye from the Age of Three.* Medical Council Special Report series no. 301. Her Majesty's Stationery Office, London, 1961

		Boys			Girls	
Age (years)	No.	Mean ocular refraction (D)	Standard error of mean	No.	Mean ocular refraction (D)	Standard error of mean
3	56	+2.33	±0.24	39	+2.96	±0.19
4	54	+2.24	±0.12	51	+2.33	±0.15
5	56	+2.21	±0.16	58	+2.20	±0.17
6	56	+1.71	±0.16	54	+1.83	±0.19
7	64	+1.92	±0.20	57	+1.98	±0.20
8	60	+1.76	±0.19	60	+1.63	±0.15
9	50	+1.52	±0.24	56	+2.03	±0.24
10	51	+1.43	±0.22	63	+1.33	±0.20
11	57	+1.63	±0.23	85	+1.50	±0.20
12	67	+1.19	±0.23	60	+1.04	±0.19
13	58	+1.38	±0.20	61	+0.96	±0.13
14	42	+0.93	±0.38	80	+0.62	±0.26
15				37	+0.64	±0.18
	671			761		

Table 2.6 Comparison of correlation coefficients for five refraction variables. From van Alphen GWHM: On emmetropia and ametropia. Ophthalmologica 1961; 142 (suppl):7

For refractions between column	Stenstrom ±10 D I	British ±8 D II	Stenstrom ±3 D III	British ±3 D IV
12	−0.75	−0.77	−0.45	−0.59
13	−0.34	−0.46	−0.40	−0.50
14	−0.19	−0.30	−0.21	−0.26
15	−0.02	+0.28	+0.13	+0.42
23	+0.44	+0.46	+0.45	+0.39
24	−0.31	−0.28	−0.52	−0.51
25	−0.39	−0.49	−0.60	−0.60
34	+0.09	+0.19	+0.09	+0.14
35	−0.26	−0.46	−0.32	−0.44
45	−0.10	−0.10	−0.09	−0.09
Number of right eyes	1000	96	886	78

The cause of these variations in refraction originates from changes in the lens. The decreasing curvature of its surfaces as it continues to grow throughout life is probably of importance, while it has been suggested that changes in the refractive index involving an increase in optical density of the cortex, thus making the lens more uniformly refractive, could also contribute to a decrease of its optical power [129]. However, it is by no means certain that the refractive index of the nucleus of the normal lens or cortex alters with age. Possibly the relative or absolute size of the nucleus may decrease with advancing years, thereby reducing the lenticular power.

Prevalence of ametropia

The question that invariably arises during the course of any discussion of refractive surgery is: just how prevalent is ametropia anyway? Figure 2.51 shows a combined graph for the prevalence of myopia as reported by several authors [62,75,130].

There are any number of monographs and treatises dealing with this subject which have been printed over the years. The problem lies in separating the wheat from the chaff, as it were. Authors have faulted their own studies by poor sampling or restricted or too broad interpretation of the term ametropia. In some studies of myopia, cases with astigmatism were eliminated, in others such cases were retained. In others such cases were included but only the spherical equivalents recorded. In still others cycloplegia was used in the examinations, in others not.

Coupled with those variants is the apparent inherent variable incidence of myopia among certain racial and ethnic groups associated with the influence of the

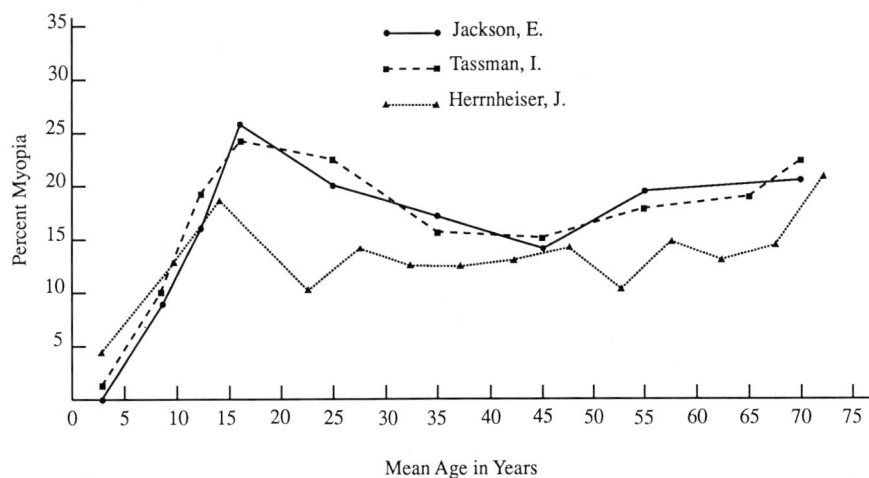

Fig. 2.51 Prevalence of myopia (derived from Jackson, Herrnheiser and Tassman).

environment. For example, a study of 120 000 rural Chinese undertaken in 1912 has no real bearing on the incidence of myopia amongst urban Britons nor, for that matter, on contemporary rural Chinese. The prevalence of myopia demonstrates considerable changes with age as well. Then too, some studies examine a specific population in cross-section while others examine a smaller group at regular intervals over time.

The classic example of this variability is the relatively homogeneous population of Germany. Reports from the Federal Republic of Germany find myopia to be the seventh most frequent cause of blindness (6.6% of cases) [131]. The neighboring Democratic Republic to the east finds myopia to be either the first or second most frequent cause in two surveys (14.7 and 13.9% of cases respectively) [131]. More reliable data will be forthcoming when international health agencies can standardize such reportage. In spite of the obvious shortcomings of these surveys at the present, the prevalence of myopia as a blinding disease is most impressive.

There is evidence that the incidence of myopia may be even higher in Orientals. Blacks seem to show a lower incidence of myopia than do non-blacks and there is a slight skewing toward a higher incidence amongst urban populations. Some studies show as much as a 2:1 ratio of occurrences in Jews as opposed to non-Jews; others show it to be 33% more amongst persons of Jewish extraction. This was not shown in Sorsby's work, however (Figure 2.52).

The prevalence of ametropia also varies with age. The typical incidence of myopia at age 6 months is 4–6%. The overall incidence of myopia amongst school children ranges from 4% in ages 4–14 in England to 25% in the same age group in Japan. In the USA, the large HANES study examined the incidence of myopia among youths aged 12–17 and found that the incidence rose from 29.3% at age 12 to 33.2% at age 17 [132]. Curtin's study, conducted during the early part of this century, aptly demonstrates the changes in myopia during rapid childhood development. Among children in the 1st through 4th grades, the frequency of myopia was 10%; in grades 5 through 8, 14%; and in grades 9 through 12, 16.35%. Sorsby found a gradual decrease in hyperopia for the same age groups: +2.65 D at age 3, +1.77 D at age 6 [133]. Later he demonstrated a change from +2.33 D to +0.93 D in males aged 3–14 years. Girls showed a similar, slightly larger change in the same age group. In a group of 231 hyperopic school children followed over a 3–8-year period, Sorsby showed that 6% had an increase in their hyperopia, 60% were stable and the remainder became less hyperopic. In a parallel study of 130 myopic school children, 65% showed an increase in their myopia from −0.75 D to more than −4.00 D [134]. Most showed an increase in the range of −1.25 to −2.00 D. A somewhat later study demonstrated a change of −1.00 to −2.00 D in 72% of the students [135]. This gradual reduction in hyperopia during childhood has also been found in the studies of Herrnheiser [130],

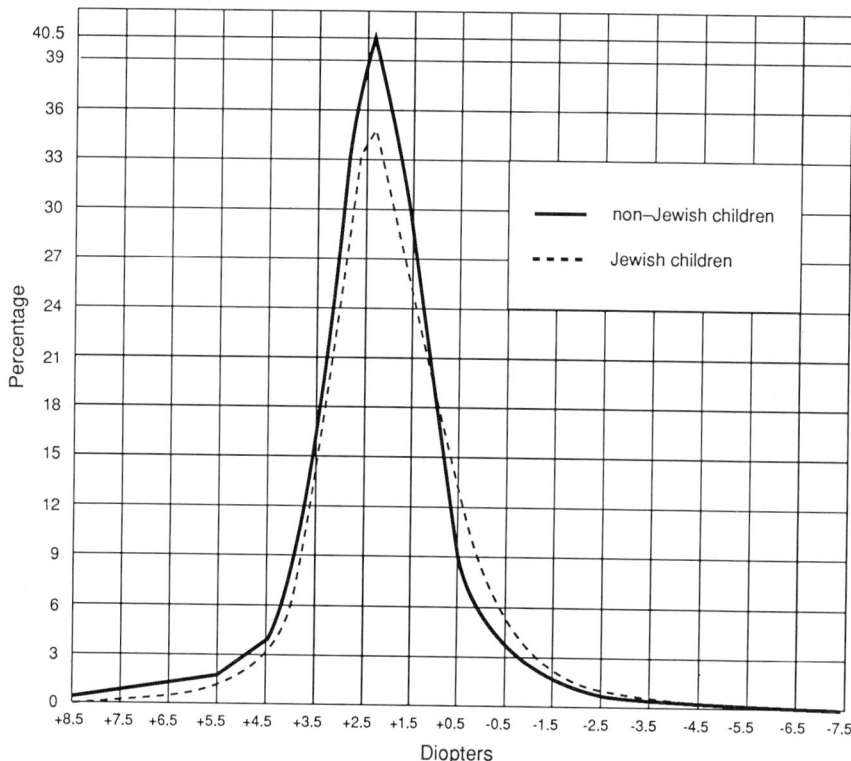

Fig. 2.52 Relative incidence of refractive errors in children age 4–8 (Sorsby, op cit)

and Hirsch [136,137]. Cross-sectional studies will occasionally show an increase in average hyperopia during an isolated 1-year interval depending on how the sample is obtained. Three such shifts are exhibited for both boys and girls in Sorsby's data [113] and one at age 6 (male), is demonstrated in Hirsch's data [121], but these changes can be attributed to the nature of cross-sectional sampling rather than to actual longitudinal increases in hyperopic refractions. In view of the general agreement regarding the behavior of refraction during childhood, the data of Brown and Slataper (see above), for example, must be taken with reservations. Their data showed an increase in mean hyperopic refraction through the 7th year, then a gradual decrease in hyperopia was found. This variation can probably be attributed to the population sampled since, of those children below age 8 in Brown's population sample, over 50% had strabismus. Because Slataper incorporated Brown's population in his study, the unusual incidence of high hyperopia in this group could affect the findings of both studies. This shows the importance of longitudinal studies in interpreting data gleaned from cross-sectional investigations.

Ametropia and personality

Much has been written about the personality characteristics of the myope, less about the hyperope. Schapero and Hirsch refer to the inhibited disposition and over-controlling nature of the myope as opposed to the happy-go-lucky, carefree affect of hyperopic brethren [138]. Other studies have reported similar findings.

The psychologic effects of myopia are operative, for the most part, during the crucial periods in the development of personality. The gradual loss of efficient distance vision tends to concentrate the interest and energies of these patients more and more on near tasks. This obligatory shift to near is capable of producing subtle as well as striking changes in the attitudes and aptitudes of the individual. Justly or not, the myope has always been considered the introverted, bookish, non-athlete who is the academic bane of more outgoing emmetropic and hyperopic fellows. Rice stressed the tendency of the myope to become finicky, painstaking, and scrupulous. These characterizations were more the impressions of the author and were unsupported by scientific data, however. There is, nevertheless, more than fragmentary evidence that this impression is true, at least to a limited extent. Rice also observed that the use of correcting lenses, as in the case of Theodore Roosevelt, could prevent the development of such an intolerant personality (how much that helped in this case is debatable) [139].

In an early study of college students, it was found that myopes did indeed show a slight but consistent tendency toward introversion when compared with normally sighted colleagues [140]. The average difference as measured by the Bernreuter Personality Inventory was not statistically significant and, in addition, was unaffected by the degree of myopia and the duration of the use of corrective lenses. A number of other tests consistently show differences in the mental make-up and attitudes of the myope. Schapero and Hirsch [138], using the Guilford–Martin Temperament Test, found myopes to be more prone to emotional inhibition and disinclined toward motor activity. These authors noted that the myope was inclined toward social leadership—somewhat at odds with introverted personality traits, one would think.

A later study by Stevens and Wolff using a test for the evaluation of leveling–sharpening mentation, showed a significant correlation with refraction [141]. Myopia was associated with highly differentiated memories as a result of minimal perceptual interaction. In 1967 Young used the Edwards Personal Preference Schedule and found that myopes scored higher than non-myopes in achievement, introspection, abasement, heterosexuality, and aggression needs [142]. Non-myopes scored higher in deference, order, exhibitionism, dominance, and change. Statistical significance was achieved only in abasement (guilt feelings, willingness to accept blame), exhibitionism (need to be noticed), and change (the desire to vary or avoid routine).

Using the Rorschach test, Rosanes compared the myope with the emmetrope and hyperope and presented the hypothesis that myopia might be a protective or adaptive mechanism, a reaction pattern to anxiety [143]. She theorized that myopia might be one of a series or constellation of tendencies or reactions to stress by a certain type of personality configuration—a somewhat teleological explanation of myopia. The cock crows and the sun rises, therefore it is the crowing of the cock that causes the sun to rise. To propose that myopia is a *result* of a personality disorder is a novel concept indeed. This study concluded that myopes have a statistically significant increase in covert anxiety, with a decrease in motor activity compared with other refractive groups ($P < 0.01$). Rosanes also noted the fact that both hyperopes and myopes demonstrate less variability in exhibiting anxiety than do emmetropes ($P < 0.01$). These two groups also showed less variability in exhibiting hostility compared with those who were emmetropic ($P < 0.01$). She further concluded that myopes have a high tolerance for anxiety and exhibit excessive control. They are less likely to place themselves in a situation where they can be attacked. They are innately cautious and use compromise generously. She found that the typical attitude of the hyperope could be characterized as "fight" and that of the myopes as "fright"—understandable in any sentient who finds him- or herself "hemmed in" by a blurred and uncertain environment.

An earlier Rorschach test survey conducted by van Alphen had found that myopes demonstrated a unique system of abstract thinking but had a deep-seated anxiety pattern [56]. From these results it would appear that myopia is associated with certain differences in cerebration that are accompanied by distinguishing personality traits. Guilt feelings, anxiety, and introversion are frequently cited in this regard, and these emotions may have much to do with the greater achievements of the myope.

Ametropia, intelligence, and scholastic standing

The earliest and most extensive reports on this subject were those of Cohn in Germany [144]. He found 1.4% of children in the primary grades to be near-sighted. This increased to 26.2% at the university level. Cohn compiled an extensive, international survey of the relationship between myopia and academic achievement. In Japan this same phenomenon has been seen. A very large 1937 study found that myopia increased in the school population from 27% in the elementary grades to about 46% in middle grades to a high of 67% in high schools [145,146]. Myopes seem to cluster amongst the high achievers as well, whereas hyperopes seem to be scattered through the ability groups at random. Goldschmidt made a careful survey of school children in the Danish population in 1968 [147]. He noted a significant plurality of myopes in the academic groups as compared with the other two, intellectually less rigorous, comprehensive and general groups. He also noted that whereas the frequency of this condition was about the same in the normal school populations and in schools for emotionally disturbed children and those for the deaf, the frequency of myopia was significantly less among retarded children.

The remarkable academic success of the myopic population has naturally raised questions regarding the association of myopia and intelligence. Various studies relating ametropia to intelligence scores have been reported in the literature [80,148–150]. A variety of tests have demonstrated a measurable difference in the intelligence quotient (IQ) of persons with various refractive states. The myope usually scores perceptibly higher than the emmetrope and hyperope. All of these studies indicate that, on average, hyperopes achieve lower intelligence scores than do myopes (Table 2.7).

Although numerous studies have found the IQ of the myope to be somewhat higher than that of non-myopes, statistical significance has not been established. At this time there is no body of scientific evidence to support or refute this concept. Hirsch's

Table 2.7 Reading scores and ametropia. From Angle J, Wissmann DA. The epidemiology of myopia. Am J Epidemiol 1980; 111:220–228. Roberts J, Slaby D. Refraction Status of Youths 12–17 Years. United States Vital Health Statistics Series 11, No. 148. (HRA) 75:1630, 1974

	Myopic (%)
Reading test (deciles)	
1 (low)	19.7
2	24.9
3	27.6
4	30.9
5	31.3
6	32.4
7	31.0
8	38.1
9	37.5
10 (high)	45.3
Time spent reading in a typical day	
<1 hour	27.7
1–3 hours	32.8
>3 hours	34.6

study of 14–17-year-olds is of interest because it showed that IQ scores increased in proportion to the degree of myopia while a reverse relationship was shown in hyperopes; this was especially apparent when reading was used as a basis for the score [80]. Taken together the indicators are that hyperopes are not necessarily less intelligent than myopes but that their average reading scores on such tests are lower.

Still, there is very little unequivocal evidence that overall, hyperopes have a greater reading disability than do myopes. Most studies purporting to show this relationship often neglect to indicate the spread of refractive error and frequently neglect to use cycloplegia. One of the most widely quoted studies on this subject is the one by Eames [151]. In this study, refraction without cycloplegia was done in 1000 children who were judged reading failures. Of this group 43% were found to be hyperopic as opposed to only 13% in a group selected at random. Unfortunately, no distribution of the hyperopia is given. Thus the 30% differential between the two groups is meaningless. It is likely that these data are skewed by the high incidence of hyperopia in the general school population.

In the USA, Dunphy *et al.* in 1968, found a disproportionately high frequency of myopia in 200 graduate students attending the Harvard schools of business and law [152]. The implication is that the level of education affected the degree of myopia. This study is flawed, however, in the manner of establishing the cohort and many students failed to return for follow-up examinations.

Nadell *et al.*, administering the California Test of

Mental Maturity (CTMM) to 414 students, demonstrated a data trend that indicated that myopes were generally more intelligent, but not to a significant degree [148]. One year later Hirsch published the results of another study in which he administered the Stanford–Binet test to children 6–7 years of age and the CTMM to older pupils: 544 students were tested in all [80]. He found no statistical difference in scores among youngsters 6–9 years of age, but among those aged 10–13, myopes scored higher ($P < 0.001$). In these data there was an almost linear increase in IQ from students with hyperopia of greater than $+2\,D$ to myopic students of greater than $-2\,D$. These results were seen as being the result of several possible mechanisms: an over-developed eye associated with greater cerebral development; the effect on test scores of reading experience and proficiency; the tendency of intelligent children to read more and thereby become myopic; and the superior reading ability of myopes leading to an increase in their scores.

Young later studied 251 students using both the Stanford–Binet and the CTMM. All correlations were low and negative. The larger differences favoring myopes were contained in the results of the CTMM, which requires greater reading ability. Young then tested the reading ability of 117 students and found that myopes were significantly better readers than the emmetropes [149].

In summary it may be said that myopes generally score higher on intelligence tests, although not to a significant degree. Part of this, but not all, can be attributed to their demonstrably superior reading ability and their personality traits. Given the hereditary background of myopia, scholarship re-inforcement is also more likely to be present at home. The myopic student more often has a similarly affected parent, often of academic achievement, who would stress intellectual pursuits and academic hobbies. Even the very wearing of spectacles may play a small part in the tendency to regard myopes as more intelligent.

Thornton found that merely wearing glasses can give the impression of intelligence [118]. Additional observations of those with short-sight have included the allegation that they are essentially night people who like to stay up late. This is said to be related possibly to the greater security felt by the myopic child at night, at which time the darkness neutralizes the handicap to some degree. If dimness of the external world of the myope retards the development of an extroverted, gregarious personality, it appears to be a superb catalyst for the development of artistic skills. Or as Curtin put it:

> It has been said that "success dwells in the silences". It is conceivable that myopia provides just such a "silence" for the young it afflicts [35].

References

1 Ferry AP. "Professor" Charles Tyrell and His Ideal Sight Restorer. Ophthalmology 1986; 93(9):1246–1257.
2 Breasted J. *The Edwin Smith Surgical Papyrus.* University of Chicago Press, Chicago, 1930.
3 Ebers G. *Papyrus Ebers, das hermetische Buch über die Arzeneimittel der alten Ägypter in hieratischer Schrift.* Leipzig, 1875.
4 Bryan CP. *The Papyrus Ebers.* Geoffrey Bles, London, 1930.
5 Aristotle. *Problems,* 2 volumes. WS Hett (transl). Harvard University Press, Cambridge, Mass, 1961.
6 Hirschberg J. *Antiquity, vol. 1. The History of Ophthalmology,* FC Blodi (ed). Wayenborgh Verlag, Bonn, 1982.
7 Aristotle. *Parts of Animals,* 1 volume. WS Hett (transl). Harvard University Press, Cambridge, Mass, 1961.
8 Galen C. *On the Use of the Parts of the Body,* 2 volumes. MT May (transl). Ithaca, 1968.
9 Moon RO. The influence of Pythagoras on Greek medicine. In Proceedings of the Seventeenth International Congress of Medicine, Sect 23, London, 1913.
10 Duke-Elder S, Abrams D. Historical development. In: *System of Ophthalmology. II. The Anatomy of the Visual System,* SS Duke-Elder (ed). C.V. Mosby, St. Louis, 1970.
11 Hirschberg J. *The Middle Ages, vol 2. The History of Ophthalmology,* F Blodi (ed). Wayenborgh Verlag, Bonn, 1982.
12 Al-Haytham I. *Opticae Thesaurus Alhezeni libri VII.* Risner, F., Basel, 1572.
13 Polo M. *The Travels of Marco Polo.* Yule, London, 1875.
14 Manni D. Lettera intorno all'invenzione degli occhiali. In: *Degli occhiali da naso inventati da salvino Armatis, Gentiluomo Florentino.* Accademico Florentino, Florence, 1738.
15 Gordon B. *Practica su Lilium Medicinae, Particula III: De passionibus oculorum.* J. & G. DeGregoriis, Venice, 1496.
16 Cooper S. The Medical School of Montpellier in the fourteenth century. Ann Med Hist 1930; 2:163.
17 Chauliac G. *Chirurgia magna.* Venice, 1553.
18 Platter F. *De corporis humani structura et usu.* Officinia Ionnis Oporinus, Basel, 1583.
19 Scheiner C. *Occulus Hoc est: fundamentum opticum.* Daniel Agricolam, Innsbruck, 1619.
20 Mark HH. Johannes Kepler on the eye and vision. Am J Ophthalmol 1971; 72:869–878.
21 Nutton V. *From Democedes to Harvey: Studies in the History of Medicine.* Variorum Reprints, London, 1988.
22 Pliny the Elder. *Natural History,* 10 volumes. H Rackham, WHS Jones and DE Eicholz (transl). Loeb Classic Library, Harvard University Press, Cambridge, Mass, 1942.
23 Rogers S. *Primitive Surgery: Skills Before Science.* Thomas, Springfield, 1985.
24 Plempius V. *Ophthalmologica.* Henrici Laurentii, Amsterdam, 1632.
25 Hamberger G. *Optica Oculorum.* Literis Gollnerianis, Jena, 1696.
26 Morgagni GB. *De Sedibus et Causis Morborum per Anatomen Indiaatis.* Remenainiana, Venice, 1761.
27 Scarpa AA. *A Treatise on the Principal Diseases of the Eye.* J. Bregg, London, 1818.
28 Boerhaave H. *Praelectiones Publicae, de Morbis Oculorum.* A. Vandenhoek, Göttingen, 1746.
29 Valdes BD. *Uso de los ateojos y comentarios a propósito del mismo.* Diego Perez, Seville, 1623.
30 Hirschberg J. *The Renaissance of Ophthalmology in the Eighteenth Century, part 2, vol 4. The History of Ophthalmology,* F Blodi (ed). Wayenborgh Verlag, Bonn, 1982.
31 Newton I. *Opticks.* Smith and Walford, London, 1704.

32 Smith R. *A Compleat System of Opticks.* Cornelius Crownfield, Cambridge, 1738.

33 Kästner AG. *Vollständiger Lehrbegriff des Optick.* Altenberg, 1755.

34 Janin de Combe-Blanche J. *Mémoires et Observations Anatomiques, Physiologiques et Physiques sur l'Oeil.* Didot, Paris, 1772.

35 Curtin BJ. *The Myopias. Basic Science and Clinical Management.* Harper & Row, New York, 1985.

36 von Ammon FA. Uber die angebornen Spaltungen in der Iris, Chorioidea und Retina des menschlichen Auges. (About congenital colobomas of the iris, choroid and retina in the human eye.) Ophthalmologie 1831; 1:55.

37 von Arlt CF. *Ueber die Ursachsen und die Entsehung der Kurzichtigkeit.* Wilhelm Braumuller, Vienna, 1856.

38 von Graefe A. Zwei Sektionbefunde von Scleratio-Chronivites posterior und Bermerbegen uber diese Krankeit. Arch Ophthalmol 1854; 1:390.

39 Young T. Observations on vision. Phil Trans R Soc Lond 1793; 83:169.

40 Young T. On the mechanism of the eye; the Bakerian lecture. Phil Trans R Soc Lond 1801; 91:23–88.

41 Ware J. Aberrations relative to the near and distant sight of different persons. Phil Trans Lond 1813; 1:31.

42 MacKenzie W. *A Practical Treatise on the Diseases of the Eye.* Longman, London, 1830.

43 Stellwag von Carion K. Refractive anomalies. S B Akad Wiss Wein, Math Klasse 1855; 16:187.

44 Donders FC. On *the Anomalies of Accommodation and Refraction of the Eye.* WD Moore (transl). The Hatton Press, London, 1864.

45 Airy G. On a peculiar defect in the eye, and a mode of correcting it. Trans Camb Phil Soc 1827; 2:267–273.

46 Schnyder. Ann Oculist (Paris) 1849;21:222.

47 Hays I. Ocular Astigmatism. In: *Lawrence's: A Treatise On Diseases of the Eye,* I Hays (ed). Lea & Blanchard, Philadelphia, 1854.

48 Noyes HD. Cylindrical glasses in astigmatism. Am J Med Sci 1872; 63:355–359.

49 Bates WH. A suggestion of an operation to correct astigmatism. Arch Ophthalmol 1894; 23:9–13.

50 Lans L. Experimentelle Untersuchungen uber die Entstehung von Astigmatismus durch nicht Perforirende Cornea-wunden. (Experimental studies of the treatment of astigmatism with non-perforating corneal incisions.) Albrecht von Graefes Arch Klin Exp Ophthalmol 1898; 45:117–152.

51 Duke-Elder S, Abrams D. Anomalies of the optical system. Types of ametropia. In: *System of Ophthalmology. V. Ophthalmic Optics and Refraction,* SS Duke-Elder (ed). C.V. Mosby, St. Louis, 1970.

52 Helmholtz H. *Treatise on Physiological Optics,* vol. 1. J Southall (transl). Opt Soc Amer, New York, 1924.

53 Roure MF. Deux problèmes sur la correction de l'astigmatisme cornéen par les verres cylindriques. Ann Oculist (Paris) 1896; 115:99–107.

54 Brint S, Ostrick D, Bryan J. Keratometric cylinder and visual performance following phacoemulsification and implantation with silicone small-incision or poly (methyl methacrylate) intraocular lenses. J Cataract Refract Surg 1991; 17:32–36.

55 Parker W, Clorfeine G. Long-term evolution of astigmatism following planned extracapsular cataract extraction. Arch Ophthalmol 1989; 107:353–357.

56 van Alphen G. On emmetropia and ametropia. Ophthalmologica 1961; 142:33.

57 Curtin BJ. Physiopathology and therapy of the myopias. Trans Can Ophthalmol Otolaryngol 1966; 5:331–339.

58 Hirsch MJ. The longitudinal study of refraction. Am J Optom 1964; 41:137.

59 Cusanus N. *Opscula, Part II: De Beryllo.* Nuremberg, 1441.

60 Duke-Elder S, Abrams D. Spectacles. In: *System of Ophthalmology. V. Ophthalmic Optics and Refraction.,* SS Duke-Elder (ed). C.V. Mosby, St. Louis, 1970.

61 Ridley H. Intraocular acrylic lenses. Trans Ophthalmol Soc UK 1951; 71:617.

62 Tassman I. Frequency of the various kinds of refractive errors. Am J Ophthalmol 1932; 15:1044.

63 Tenner AS. Refraction in school children: 4800 refractions tabulated according to age, sex and nationality. NY Med J 1915; 102:611.

64 Stenstrom S. Untersuchungen uber die Variation und Kovariation der optischen Elemente des menschlichen Auges. Acta Ophthalmol (suppl) 1946; 26:7.

65 Grosvenor T. The neglected hyperope. Am J Optom 1971; 48:376–382.

66 Broekema O. Bijdrage tot de kennis der hypermetropie. Thesis. Amsterdam, 1909.

67 Pfalz G. Ophthalmometrische untersuchungen uber cornealastigmatismus; mit dem ophthalmometer von Javal und Sciötz. Graefes Arch Klin Exp Ophthalmol 1885; 31:201.

68 Sørensen SK. L'astigmatisme du cristallin, déterminé comme la différence entre l'astigmatisme cornéen et l'astigmatisme total, illustré par l'examen de ses variations d'après l'âge. Acta Ophthalmol (Kbh) 1944; 22:341.

69 Steiger A. Die Entstehung der Sparischen Refraktionen des menschlichen Auges. Karger, Berlin, 1913.

70 Gullstrand A. Beitrag zur Theorie des Astigmatismus. Scand Arch Ophthalmol 1890; 2:269–359.

71 Kronfeld PC, Devney C. The frequency of astigmatism. Arch Ophthalmol 1930; 4:873–884.

72 Snellen H. Die Richtunge des Hauptmeridiane des Astigmatischen Auges. (The axis of the major meridians of the astigmatic eye.) Albrecht von Graefes Arch Klin Ophthalmol 1869; 15:199–207.

73 Tscherning M. Physiological optics. Encycl Franc Ophthalmol (Paris) 1904; 3:105.

74 Gullstrand A. *Einfuhrung in die Methoden die Dioptrik des Auges.* Leipzig, 1911.

75 Jackson E. Norms of refraction. JAMA 1932; 98:132.

76 Hofstetter HW, Baldwin W. Bilateral correlation of residual astigmatism. Am J Optom 1957; 34:388–391.

77 Exford J. A longitudinal study of refractive trends after age forty. Am J Optom 1965; 42:685–692.

78 Forsius H, Eriksson AW, Fellman J. Corneal refraction according to age and sex in an isolated population and the heredity of the trait. Acta Ophthalmol (Kbh) 1964; 42:224.

79 Steiger A. Beitrage zur Physiologie und Pathologie der Hornhautrefraction. Arch Augenheilkd 1894; 29:98.

80 Hirsch M. The relationship between refractive state and intelligence test scores. Am J Optom Arch Am Acad Optom 1959; 36:12–21.

81 Bores L. *Pseudo-accommodation Following Radial Keratotomy.* Quintum Forum, Bogota, Columbia, 1987.

82 Descartes R. *Tractatus de Homine.* Elsevier, Amsterdam, 1977.

83 Porterfield W. *Treatise on the Eye, the Manner and Phenomena of Vision.* Hamilton & Balfour, Edinburgh, 1759.

84 Fincham EF. The changes in the form of the crystalline lens in accommodation. Trans Opt Soc Lond 1925; 26:239–269.

85 Kikawa N, Sato T. Lenticular elasticity. Exp Eye Res 1963; 2:210.

86 Fisher RF. The significance of the shape of the lens and capsular energy changes in accommodation. J Physiol 1969; 201:21–47.

87 Bates WH. *Cure of Imperfect Sight by Treatment Without Glasses.*

Central Fixation, New York, 1920.

88 Kuster A. Myopieprogression bei Kontaktlinsen und bei Brillentragern in 400 Fallen. [The progression of myopia in wearers of contact lenses and spectacles. 400 cases.] Klin Monatsbl Augenheilkd 1971; 159:213–219.

89 Warren GT. Myopia control and abatement. Opt J Rev Optom 1955; 92:33.

90 Takemura T. The influence of the use of glasses on the progress of myopia. Acta Ophthalmol (Jpn) 1943; 47:906.

91 Savolyuk MM. Optical correction and progressive myopia. Vestn Oftalmol 1968, 1:82.

92 Takamaya H. The effects of glass correcting corneal astigmatism on refractive components. Acta Soc Ophthalmol (Jpn) 1974; 78:220.

93 Rubin ML, Milder B. Myopia—a treatable "disease"? Surv Ophthalmol 1976; 21:65–69.

94 Safir A. Orthokeratology. II. A risky and unpredictable "treatment" for a benign condition. Surv Ophthalmol 1980; 24:291, 298–302.

95 Roberts J, Slaby D. Refraction status of youths 12–17 years. United States Vital Health Statistics Series 11, No. 148 (HRA) 75:1630, 1974.

96 Hatfield E. Why are they blind? Sight Sav Rev 1975; 45:3.

97 Kahn H, Moorhead U. Statistics on blindness in the model reporting area. (NIM) 73–427 1970.

98 Sorsby A. The incidence and causes of blindness: an international survey. Br J Ophthalmol 1950, 34 (suppl):13–14.

99 Schnabel I, Herrnheiser J. Uber Staphyloma posticum, Conus und Myopie. Z Augenheilkd 1895; 16:1.

100 Maurolycus F. *Photismi de lumine et umbra.*Venice, 1597.

101 von Reuss A. Augen-Untersuchungen an zwei Weiner Volksschulen. (Eye examinations in two Viennese public schools.) 1881; 22:200.

102 von Reuss A. Untersuchungen uber die optischen Constanten ametropischer Augen. Albrecht Von Graefes Arch Ophthalmol 1880; 23:183.

103 Awerbach M. The dioptrics of refraction (in Russian). Thesis, Moscow, 1900.

104 Tron E. Variationsstatistiche untersuchungen uber Refraction. Graefes Arch Ophthalmol 1929; 122:1–34.

105 Tron E. Ein Beitrage zur Kenntnis der Refractionskurve. Graefes Arch Ophthalmol 1930; 124:544–565.

106 Rushton RH. The clinical measurement of the axial length of the living eye. Applied Optics 1938; 58:136–142.

107 Scheerer R. Zur entwicklungsgeschlechtlichen Auffassung der Brechzustande des Auges. Ber Zusammenkunft. Dtsch Ophthalmol Ges 1928; 47:118.

108 Scheerer R, Seitzer A. Ueber das Auftreten von sogenannten myopischen Veranderungen am Augenhintergrund bei den verscheidenen Brechungzustanden des Auges. Klin Monatsbl Augenheilkd 1929; 82:511.

109 Betsch A. Ueber die menschliche Refraktionskurve. [Regarding the human refraction curve.] Klin Monatsbl Augenheilkd 1929; 82:365.

110 Wibaut F. Uber die Emmetropisation und den Ursprung der Spharischen Refraktionsanomalien. Albrecht von Graefes Arch Ophthalmol 1925; 116:596.

111 Berg F. Uber Variabilitat und Korrelation bei den verscheidenen Abmessungen des Auges. Albrecht von Graefes Arch Ophthalmol 1931; 127:606.

112 Sorsby A, Benjamin B, Davey J, Tanner JM. Emmetropia and its aberrations. Med Res Counc Spec Rep Ser (London) 1957; 293.

113 Sorsby A, Benjamin B, Sheridan M. Refraction and its Components during the Growth of the Eye from the Age of Three. Medical Research Council Special Report Series No. 301. Medical Research Council, London, 1961.

114 Brown EVL. Net average yearly changes in refraction in atropinized eyes from birth to beyond middle life. Arch Ophthalmol 1938; 19:719.

115 Lepard C. Comparative changes in the error of refraction between fixing and amblyopic eyes during growth and development. Am J Ophthalmol 1975; 80:485–490.

116 Smith P. On the size of the cornea in relation to age, sex, refraction, and primary glaucoma. Trans Ophthalmol Soc UK 1890; 10:68.

117 Peter R. Ueber die Corneagrosse und ihre Vererbung. Albrecht von Graefes Arch Ophthalmol 1924; 115:29.

118 Thornton G. The effect of judgment of personality traits of varying a simple factor in a photograph. J Appl Psychol 1944; 28:203.

119 Brown EVL, Kronfeld PC. The refraction curve in the US with special reference to the first two decades. Thirteenth Council of Ophthalmology 1929; 1:86.

120 Slataper F. Age norms of refraction and vision. Arch Ophthalmol 1950; 43:466.

121 Hirsch M, Weymouth F. A longitudinal study of refractive state of children during the first six years of school. Am J Optom Arch Am Acad Optom 1961; 38:564.

122 Collins ET. Lectures on the anatomy of the eye. Lancet 1890; 2:1329.

123 Weale RA. *The Aging Eye.* Harper & Row, London, 1963.

124 Armaly M, Burian H. Changes in the tonogram during accommodation. Arch Ophthalmol 1958; 60:60.

125 Kelly TS, Chatfield C, Tustin G. Clinical assessment of the arrest of myopia. Br J Ophthalmol 1975; 59:529–538.

126 Young F. The nature and control of myopia. J Am Optom Assoc 1977; 48:451–457.

127 Dyer J. Role of cycloplegics in progressive myopia. Ophthalmology 1979; 86:692–694.

128 Bedrossian RH. The treatment of myopia with atropine and bifocals: a long-term prospective study. Ophthalmology 1985; 92:716.

129 Parsons JH. The pathology of the eye. Br J Ophthalmol 1906; 3:929.

130 Herrnheiser J. Die Refraktionsentwicklung des menschlichen Auges. (The refraction development of the human eye.) Z Augenheilkd 1892; 13:342.

131 Lim A, Jones B. World's major blinding conditions. Vision 1981; 1:101.

132 Sperduto R, Seigel D, Roberts J, Rowland M. Prevalence of myopia in the United States. Arch Ophthalmol 1983; 101:405–407.

133 Sorsby A. Normal refraction in infants and its bearing on development of myopia. London Co Council Rep 1933; 4(3):55.

134 Sorsby A, Leary GA. A longitudinal study of refraction and its components during growth. Med Res Counc Spec Rep Ser (London) 1969; 309:1–41.

135 Sorsby A. *Epidemiology of Refraction. Historical: a Qualitative Approach.* Little, Brown, Boston, 1971.

136 Hirsch MJ. The changes in refraction between the ages of five and fourteen: Theoretical and practical considerations. Am J Optom 1952; 29:445.

137 Hirsch ND. Sex differences in the incidence of various grades of myopia. Am J Optom 1953; 30:135.

138 Schapero M, Hirsch M. The relationship of refractive error and Guilford-Martin temperament test scores. Am J Optom 1952; 29:32.

139 Rice T. Physical defects and character: II. Nearsightedness and astigmatism. Hygeia 1930; 8:644.

140 Mull H. Myopia and introversion. Am J Psychol 1948; 61:575.

141 Stevens D, Wolff H. The relationship of myopia to performance on a test of leveling-sharpening. Percept Motor

Skills 1965; 21:399–403.

142 Young F. Myopia and personality. Am J Optom 1967; 44: 192–201.

143 Rosanes M. Psychological correlates to myopia compared to hyperopia and emmetropia. J Proj Tech Pers Assess 1967; 31:31–35.

144 Cohn H. *Hygiene of the Eye in Schools*. Simpkin, Marshall, London, 1886.

145 Sato T. *The Causes and Prevention of Acquired Myopia*. 1957.

146 Otsuka J. Research on the etiology and treatment of myopia. Nippon Ganka Gakki Zasshi 1967; 71:1–212.

147 Goldschmidt E. On the etiology of myopia. An epidemiological study. Acta Ophthalmol (Copenh) 1968; 98:1.

148 Nadell M, Hirsch M. The relationship between intelligence and the refractive state in a selected high school sample. Am J Optom 1958; 35:321–326.

149 Young E. Reading, measures of intelligence and refractive errors. Am J Optom 1963; 47:257.

150 Grosvenor T. Refractive state, intelligence test scores, and academic ability. Am J Optom 1970; 47:355–361.

151 Eames T. Visual problems of poor readers. In *Clinical Studies in Reading*, H Robinson (ed). University of Chicago Press, Chicago, 1953.

152 Dunphy E, Stoll M, King S. Myopia among American male graduate students. Am J Ophthalmol 1968; 65:518–521.

Further reading

Badawi A. Kom-Ombo sanctuaries. Inst Fr d'Arch Or, XXXII, Cairo, 1921.

Biedermann H. *Medicina Magica: Metaphysical Healing Methods in Late-antique and Medieval Manuscripts with Thirty Facsimile Plates*. Classics of Medicine Library, Birmingham, 1986.

Biggs R. Medicine in Ancient Mesopotamia. In *History of Science*, A Crombie and M Hoskins (eds). Heffer, Cambridge, 1969.

Breasted J. *The Edwin Smith Surgical Papyrus*. University of Chicago Press, Chicago, 1930.

Breasted J. *A History of Egypt*. 2nd edn. Hodder and Stoughton, London, 1950.

Castiglioni A. *A History of Medicine*. New York, 1958.

Celsus. *De Medicina*, 3 vols. W Spencer (transl). Loeb Classic Library, London, 1935.

Cockburn A, Cockburn E. *Mummies, Disease and Ancient Cultures*. Cambridge University Press, Cambridge, 1968.

Davis A. *Medicine and its Technology*. Greenwood Press, Wesport, 1981.

Dawson WR. The Egyptian medical papyri. In *Science, Medicine and History*, EA Underwood (ed). Oxford University Press, London, 1953.

Estes JW. *The Medical Skills of Ancient Egypt*. Science History Publications, Canton, 1989.

Galen C. *On the Use of the Parts of the Body*, 2 vols. MT May (transl). Ithaca, 1968.

Garrison F, Morton L. *A Medical Bibliography*. J.B. Lippincott, New York, 1970.

Harper R. *The Code of Hammurabi King of Babylon about 2200 BC*. University of Chicago Press, Chicago, 1904.

Hippocrates. *The Genuine Works of Hippocrates*, 2 vols. F Adams (transl). Sydenham Society, London, 1849.

Jackson R. *Doctors and Disease in the Roman Empire*. University of Oklahoma Press, Norman, 1988.

Jastrow M Jr. Babylonian-Assyrian medicine. Ann Med Hist 1917; 1:231–257.

Kramer SN. *History Begins at Sumer*. The Falcon's Wing Press, Garden City, 1959.

Levey M. Some objective factors of Babylonian medi-cine in the light of new evidence. Bull Hist Med 1961; 35:61–70.

Lyons AS, Petrucelli RJ. *Medicine: An Illustrated History*. Harry N. Abrams, New York, 1987.

Nutton V. *From Democedes to Harvey: Studies in the History of Medicine*. Variorum Reprints, London, 1988.

Pliny the Elder. *Natural History*, 10 vols. H Rackham, WHS Jones and DE Eicholz (transl). Loeb Classic Library, Harvard University Press, Cambridge, 1942.

Rogers S. *Primitive Surgery: Skills Before Science*. Thomas, Springfield, 1985.

Sandison AT. Diseases of the eyes. In *Diseases in Antiquity*, D Bothwell and AT Sandison (eds). Thomas, Springfield, 1967.

Saunders JB. *The Transitions from Ancient Egyptian to Greek Medicine*. University of Kansas Press, Lawrence, 1963.

Scarborough J. *Roman Medicine*. Cornell University Press, Ithaca, 1969.

Sigerist HE. *A History of Medicine*. Oxford University Press, London, 1951.

Waterman L. *Royal Correspondence of the Assyrian Empire*. University of Michigan, Ann Arbor, 1930.

Wells C. *Bones, Bodies and Disease*. Thames & Hudson, London, 1964.

Whipple AO. Role of the Nestorians as the connecting link between Greek and Arabic medicine. Ann Med Hist 1936; 8:313–323.

3

Light, Optics, and Refractive Surgery

He who does not imagine in stronger and better lineaments and in stronger and better light than his perishing mortal eye can see, does not imagine at all. [William Blake]

While complete elucidation of the subject of light and optics lies beyond the scope of this work, some elaboration on the topic is in order. The author is keenly aware of the anathema with which the subject of optics is greeted by most ophthalmologists—still, we must acknowledge that optics plays a vital role in our specialty. To paraphrase a familiar expression: without optics, the eye is nothing. That's because the eye serves to focus light on to the prime receptor organ of the brain—the retina—via its optical properties. That's what optics do—focus that light. Of course we all know what light is, or at least we think we do. Actually, no one knows for certain what light is—not really. It seems to be two things, or at least acts as though it were two things, or one thing with two properties. Whatever, nobody really knows, although we can make some reasonable assumptions based upon its properties and its actions. Nevertheless, despite our relative ignorance, let us review what we think we know about light and then move on.

The nature of light

Light is a form of energy. Not to put too fine a point on it, light is therefore us: we too are energy, as are all things in the universe. It's just that we are more sedate than other forms of energy—except for rocks. Some energy forms move along in a more sprightly manner. Light moves very snappily indeed—some 186 000 miles per second—which makes light the fastest thing in the universe. Light is, furthermore, a special kind of energy—electromagnetic energy. That is, it possesses both electric and magnetic characteristics. More specifically, light is only a small portion of the total spectrum of electromagnetic energy. This portion is the relatively narrow band from 400 to 700 nm (a nanometer equals 10^{-9} m or 10^{-6} mm), and is called the visual spectrum because these wavelengths can be perceived by the human retina (Figure 3.1).

Sources of light

Before we can talk more about what light is, it will probably be a good idea to discuss from whence light comes. Basically it comes from hot matter—so-called thermal and spectral emitters. Thermal emitters are characterized by producing light as a portion of the continuous electromagnetic spectrum; an example is a light bulb. In classic pre-Planckian physics, electromagnetic waves are said to be induced by vibrating charged particles whose frequency of vibration decreases as their energy is removed by the induced electromagnetic waves; this results in a continuous energy spectrum. Max Planck forever modified this view by demonstrating that electromagnetic energy could be emitted only in discrete amounts or packets

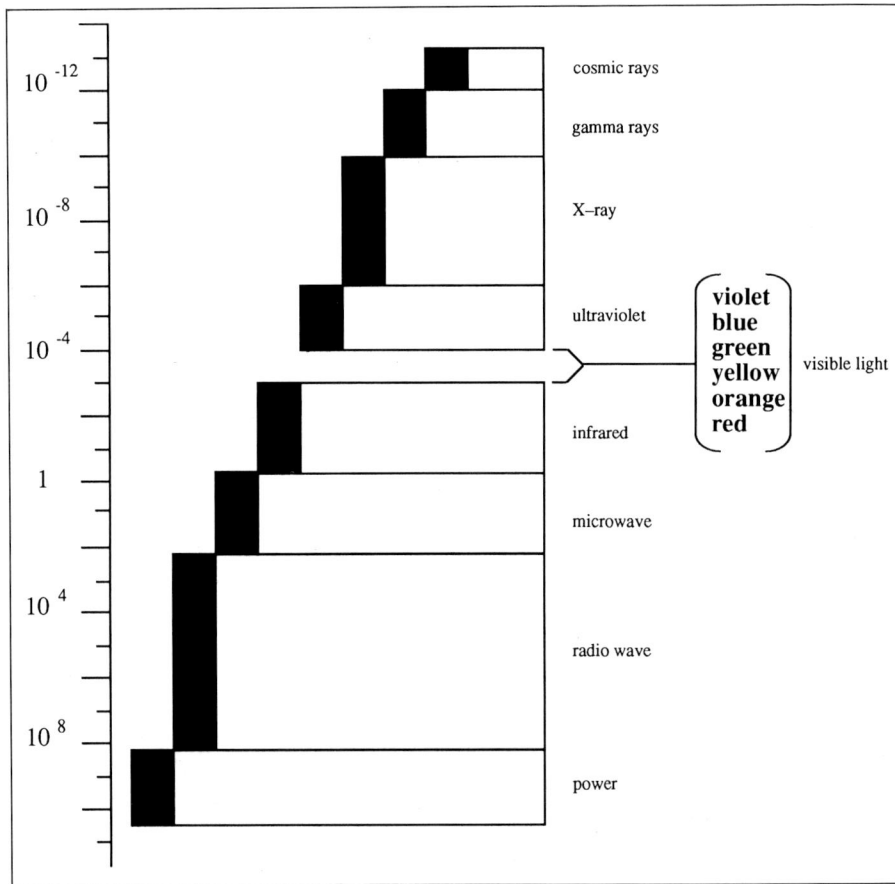

Fig. 3.1 The electromagnetic spectrum.

which he termed quanta. The energy of these quanta is proportional to a fundamental constant and the frequency of the light:

$$E = \hbar f$$

where E is the energy of the electromagnetic wave, $\hbar$ is Planck's constant, and f is the frequency of the emitted wave and therefore of the vibrating charged particle.

Prior to Planck, classic theory predicted that every object with a temperature above absolute zero continuously emitted an infinite amount of very high-frequency energy, which was decidedly contrary to experience—after all, the stars still shone. This prediction was called the ultraviolet catastrophe, and was obviously erroneous because any object that radiates an infinite amount of energy would destroy the universe in short order (Figure 3.2). However, Planck's theorem, which led to the creation of quantum mechanics and modern physics, correctly predicted the emission spectrum of hot objects. So the classic viewpoint gave way, grudgingly, to the new.

The laws of physics for hot objects were derived originally for so-called black bodies. A black body absorbs all energy striking it and re-radiates that absorbed energy until it goes into thermal equilibrium with its surroundings. Under a steady-state condition

it would be the same temperature as its surroundings. At room temperature, a lump of charcoal (or other black object) is a reasonably good example of this. At higher temperatures, the same charcoal lump heated to glowing is another. Figure 3.3 represents the various spectra of black bodies at different temperatures. Note that the higher the temperature the higher the frequency (shorter wavelength) at which the maximum energy is radiated. This explains why objects at higher temperatures feel hotter (they radiate more energy)

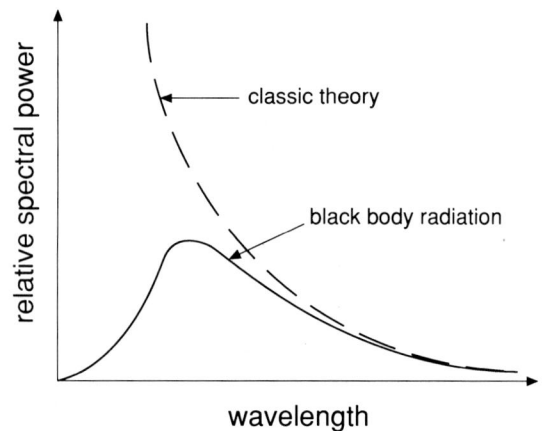

Fig. 3.2 The emission spectrum of black bodies.

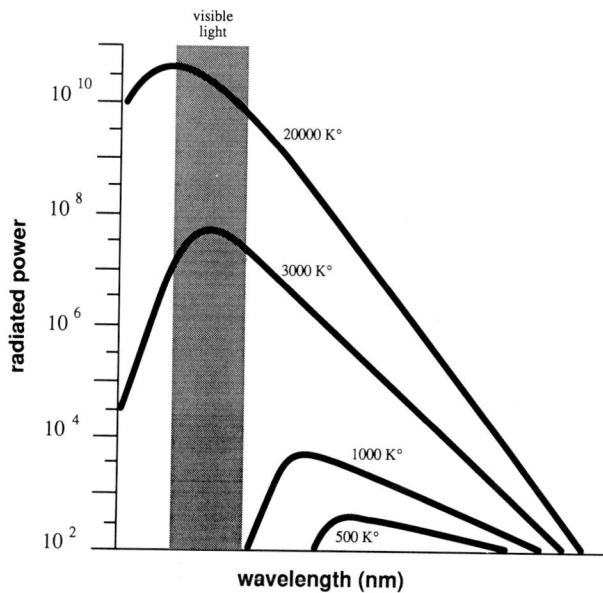

Fig. 3.3 Radiation power curves of black bodies.

and are therefore bluer in color (more of their radiation is at higher frequencies or the blue end of the spectrum). Wien's displacement law, which predicts the wavelength at which the black body emits at maximum power, is:

$$\lambda_m T = 0.2867 \text{ cm deg}$$

where λ_m is the wavelength of maximum emission in centimeters and T is the temperature of the black body in degrees Kelvin; thus the emission of a black body depends only upon its temperature.

The energy radiated per unit area of a black body is proportional to the fourth power of its temperature. Raising an object to twice its original temperature will cause it to radiate 16 times as much energy ($2^4 = 16$). This is the reason why it is difficult to get objects to very high temperatures. The hotter an object gets, the more efficiently it radiates its energy and the harder it is to get it hotter.

The other most common source of light is the discrete spectral emitter, which emits light at discrete frequencies rather than as a continuous spectrum. The spectrum of a black body (thermal emitter) in a spectrograph is a continuous blur between red and blue, whereas the spectrum of a discrete emitter consists of numerous distinctly colored lines, called a line spectrum. A line spectrum can also be produced through dispersion (see below). These discrete lines derive from the fact that the electrons which create the light are restricted to certain orbits in their atoms according to the rules of quantum mechanics. The orbit depends upon the angular momentum of the electron—thus its energy. The orbital angular momentum can only be an integer multiple of $\hbar$, Planck's constant, that is:

orbital angular momentum $= n\hbar$

where $n = 1, 2, 3, \ldots$, and so on. Because of various angular momenta and spins there may be no more than $2n^2$ electrons in any orbit; therefore two electrons for $n = 1$, eight for $n = 2$, etc. The lower the orbit the less energetic an electron is in the orbit. If all of the electrons in the atom are in their lowest possible orbits, the atom is said to be in a ground state. If one of the electrons somehow absorbs energy, it can be pushed into a higher orbit but it may not stay there. According to quantum theory, the electron can give its energy away in the form of an electromagnetic wave or photon. Since the energy of the orbits is quantized, when an electron drops into a lower orbit the energy it gives off to the photon is equal to the energy difference of the two orbits. The various transitions between different orbits therefore result in different and discrete wavelengths of light. In general, the more complex an atom, the more possible are transitions and the more allowable are frequencies (or colors or lines) in the spectrum. Hydrogen, for example, has only four lines in the visible spectrum while iron has thousands.

According to the laws of quantum mechanics, there are some transitions that an electron is likely to undergo—the so-called allowed transitions—and some transitions that are unlikely—the so-called forbidden transitions. Einstein's transition probability states that there are two ways in which an electron can drop from a higher to a lower state. The first is by spontaneous emission, that is, the electron in an excited state has a certain probability to drop into a particular lower level just by chance. The probability of a particular transition occurring depends upon the similarity of the various separate quantum numbers of the upper and lower levels. The second way for a transition to occur is by induced emission. If an electron is in an upper state and is hit by a photon of exactly the energy difference of a given transition to a lower orbit, the photon will induce the electron to make the transition, thus radiating a photon of exactly the same frequency and polarization of the original photon. Because of this interaction there are now two identical photons and one atom in the ground state, where there were originally one photon and one atom in the excited state. This phenomenon is important and will be discussed in Chapter 11—which is the whole point of the preceding discussion.

Wave property of light

As stated in the beginning of this chapter, light has a dual nature, acting both as a particle and as a wave. When discussing its creation or destruction, the particle nature fits best. When discussing the propagation of light through space, the wave model, as enunciated by Thomas Young in 1801, is more apt [1]. This theory was probably first proposed by Aristotle around 360 BC. Actually all matter can be described in terms of waves and particles, although the wave-like nature of matter is more significant for particles the size of electrons or smaller. All wave motion consists of a disturbance moving through a medium. The medium itself does not move along with the wave (this is easily demonstrated by floating a cork on water). In the case of a water wave, the surface of the water moves up and down as the wave passes. The same thing happens with a wave propagating along a rope. This wave motion is usually described as a relatively small back-and-forth, or up-and-down, motion of the particles of the medium, as the wave passes through the medium.

Two types of waves can be described: longitudinal and transverse. Longitudinal waves—such as sound makes—require a medium through which to travel. In this case condensation and rarefaction of the particles of the medium occur. Transverse waves need no medium in order to propagate. The disturbance caused by the wave is perpendicular to the direction of the wave. Thus light takes the form of a transverse wave. Furthermore, for the purposes of our discussion on optics, we will agree that a light wave has the properties of a simple vertical sine wave, even if it doesn't.

A light wave actually is two waves having two different properties. The electronic portion of light moves along the direction of travel or propagation and is our simple vertical sine wave. At the same time, the magnetic portion of the light vibrates at right angles to the line of propagation, again in the form of a sine wave (Figure 3.4). Light tends to move along in a straight line unless acted upon by an external force. One of the forces that acts on light is gravity, but since it is a relatively weak force we mere mortals do not notice its effect upon light here on Earth. We have, however, observed the effect of gravity upon light in space in the form of a galactic lens and the displacement of star images near the sun.

The maximum displacement of a particular wave (crest-to-midpoint) is termed amplitude (Figure 3.5).

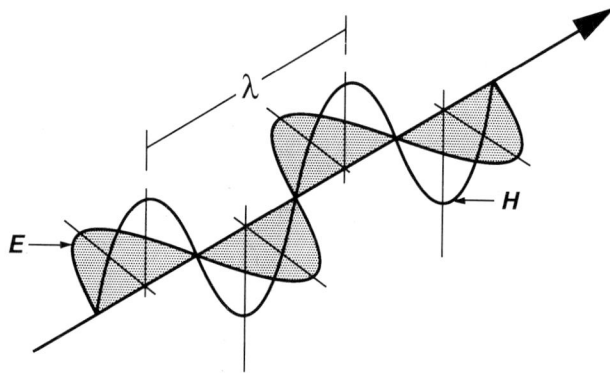

Fig. 3.4 Schematic of an electromagnetic wave—light. A light wave has a magnetic as well as an electronic part.

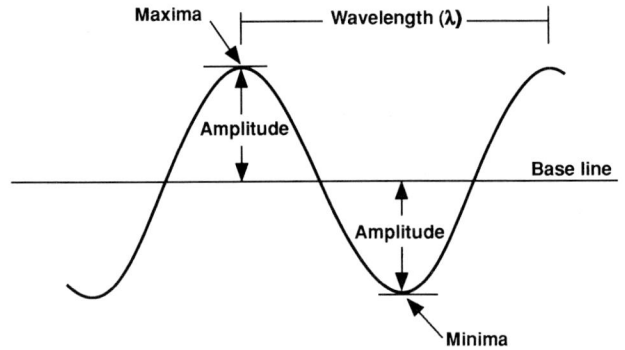

Fig. 3.5 The anatomy of a light wave.

The crest of any such wave is called the maxima, and the trough, the minima. The distance between two successive maxima or any other two successive corresponding points describes one cycle of the wave and is called the wavelength. A fraction of a complete cycle is called the phase. The phase difference between two waves traveling in the same direction is the fraction of a wavelength by which one wave leads the other. If an imaginary particle passes through a complete cycle, it is conventionally denoted as having a phase change of 360°. The period of the wave is the time necessary for an imaginary particle to travel one complete cycle. Distances along a wave may be measured in units of length, such as meters, or in units of angle, such that one cycle is equal to 2π rad, or 360°.

The length of any given wave of light is inversely related to just how energetic the photons are in the wave. That is, the more energetic, the shorter the wavelength. This relationship is classically described in terms of a weight attached to a spring which is set into oscillation—ignoring the effects of friction. The number of complete excursions (maxima-to-maxima) within a given time period is the frequency of oscillation of the weight—the number of vibrations per unit time. If one were to attach a pen to the weight such that it could inscribe a mark upon a moving piece of paper, the line drawn would be in the shape of the sine wave previously described. If the paper were to be moved at a constant rate, it follows that the peak-to-peak dimension of a wave (the wavelength) would depend upon the speed with which the weight is oscillating. Since (as far as we know) the speed of light is constant, wavelength is therefore inversely related to frequency.

Both the electric and magnetic portions of the light wave are related to each other in time and share the energy of the wave, which is proportional to the square of its amplitude. Physically, electric and magnetic fields are force fields that act upon charged particles. An electric field pulls in a positively charged particle and repels a negatively charged particle. A magnetic field acts only upon moving charges, which are deflected at right angles to both the direction of motion of the charge and the direction of the magnetic field. Being force fields, they are described by vectors—that is, with magnitude and direction—and can be resolved into perpendicular components. This property will be important later in the discussion of polarization.

Color of light

Color is determined by the frequency of the light wave. Red light falls at the low-frequency or long wavelength end of the spectrum while blue light falls at the high-frequency or short wavelength end of the spectrum. All other colors occur in between these limits. The visual spectrum is bordered on the long wavelength side by infrared and on the short wavelength side by ultraviolet. By convention, infrared and ultraviolet are called light, although, strictly speaking, since they are not visible to the human eye, they are not light.

Refractive index

We have said that light moves along at 186 000 miles per second and so it does—in a vacuum, at least. However, when light travels through another transparent medium it interacts with the atoms of that medium and slows up, just a little. The slowing occurs because the photons produce an oscillation in the electrons of the medium. The energy produced is released in the form of heat. Since heat is also a form of electromagnetic energy it would seem that if the induced oscillations were of sufficient frequency the energy released could reach the visual spectrum or higher. That is, in fact, similar to what happens in a laser (see Chapter 11). This property of light was first postulated by Pierre Fermat in his "principle of natural economy" and confirmed by Roemer (who had also established that light moved at a constant and finite velocity) in 1676 [2,3].

If the light enters such a medium at an angle, its path is changed, sometimes profoundly (Figure 3.6). We can express the ratio of that slowing and hence the bending by dividing the speed of light (c) in a vacuum, or in air, by its speed within the medium, c_m. This ratio is always larger than 1 and is called the index of refraction. The index of refraction of the human cornea is approximately 1.3776. The importance of this index will be discussed more thoroughly in the section on geometric optics, below.

Dispersion

The actual amount of deflection that occurs is related to the wavelength or frequency of the light itself for any given medium. That is, the shorter, more energetic

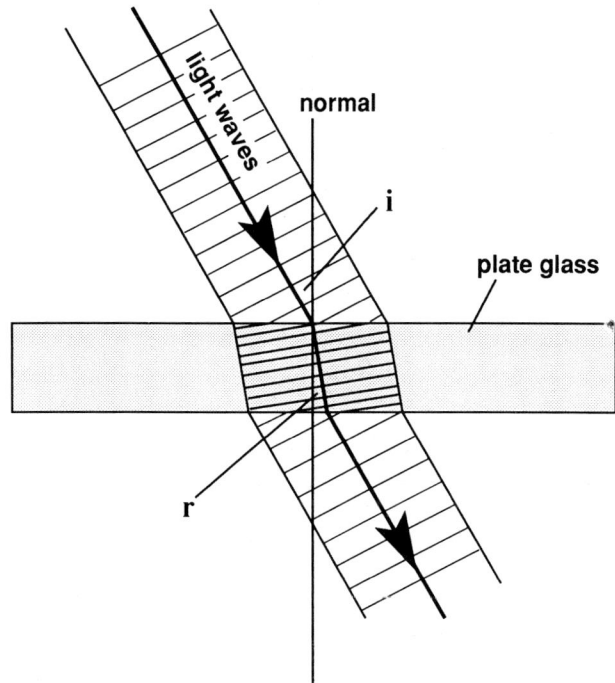

Fig. 3.6 Path of light from one medium to another.

wavelengths are slowed more than the longer, less energetic waves. This phenomenon is termed dispersion. Dispersion is related to index of refraction in that the higher the index, the greater the dispersion of the light. It is dispersion that produces chromatic aberration in uncorrected lens systems. The spectrograph uses the property of dispersion to separate light into its various wavelengths. Combining a prism with a slit aperture, this device breaks a light source down into discrete bands of color called a line spectrum. Various elements produce different kinds of light when heated, thus a spectrograph can be used to analyze the content of unknown substances or even to detect such substances in outer space. The relative intensity of the lines can also be used to determine the temperature of an object.

Interference

Because of the wave nature of light, it seems logical that it might be possible for two or more light waves to collide or otherwise interfere with one another, and so they can, if the light is coherent. That is, if the waves have the same polarization and wavelength and are of constant phase difference, then the resultant amplitudes at that point remain constant and a pattern of light and dark bands will be produced. However, if the two waves are not coherent, the resultant amplitudes change from one instant to the next, depending upon the differences in the relative phases, no collisions occur and thus no pattern emerges. This is

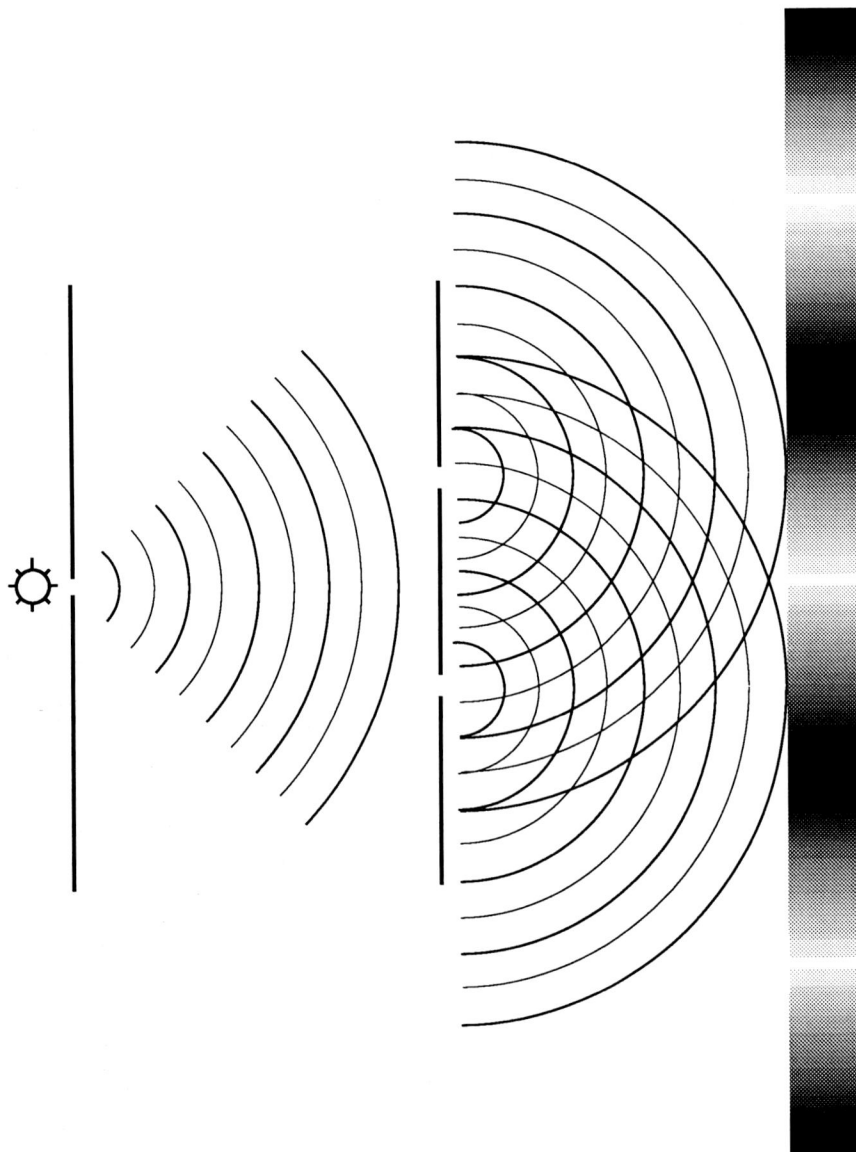

Fig. 3.7 Thomas Young's experiment showing the interference phenomenon.

the principle of Young's classic experiment, which was one of the first to prove that light acts as a wave [4]. In Young's experiment, light from a small source is filtered to make it monochromatic and is then allowed to pass through two narrow slits separated by a few tenths of a millimeter. When the light waves that have passed through the two slits illuminate a screen, a pattern of light spots and dark spots is seen (Figure 3.7). The light spots correspond to places where the waves arrive with the same phase, and the dark spots are places where the waves from the two slits have opposite phases and so cancel each other.

The results of Young's experiment follow directly from the wave nature of light. Nevertheless, it is quite contrary to all our ordinary experience for two light waves to combine and produce darkness. This is because ordinary light sources are not coherent and there is no fixed relationship between the phases of waves from different places on the source. Since so many different, independent atoms are involved, the relative phases fluctuate rapidly and the intensity at places on the illuminated screen is some average value. Interference is therefore a phenomenon associated with coherent light except in certain circumstances when it

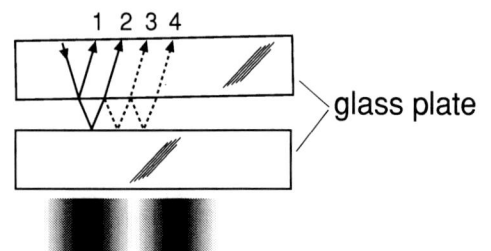

Fig. 3.8 Rays reflecting from two almost parallel glass surfaces. When the optical path traversed by ray 2 is one-half wavelength greater than the path for ray 1, destructive interference occurs. A dark band (fringe) is seen at that point.

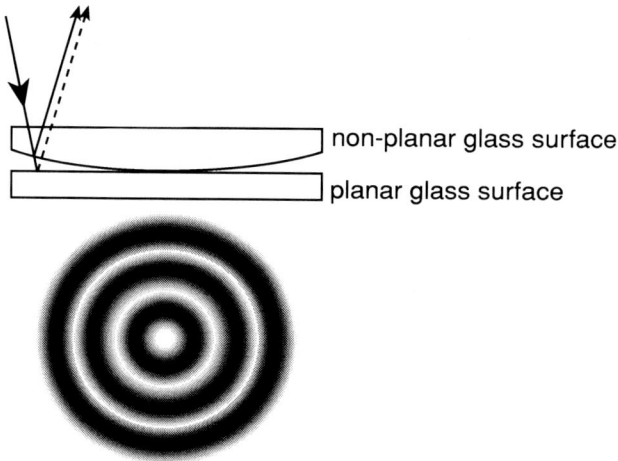

Fig. 3.9 Newton's rings.

reflections from each of the two surfaces determines the phase difference between the waves, which in turn determines the final fringe pattern. The fringe pattern is thus an indication of the physical distance between the two surfaces. When a spherical transparent surface is in contact with a plane reflecting surface, a phenomenon called Newton's rings occurs which is a bullseye-shaped pattern of alternating white and dark rings (Figure 3.9). Finally the rainbow colors seen in the surface of a soap bubble or in a thin oil film on water are interference patterns. In each of the preceding three cases, reflections from the interfaces partially polarize the light rays which in turn produce the phase differences resulting in interference patterns.

The result of such interference depends on whether the waves are in or out of phase—that is, whether the troughs and crests correspond or overlap. If the troughs and crests exactly overlap—their phase difference is zero—then the maxima will add to maxima and minima to minima. The intensity of the light therefore increases. Since the intensity of light is proportional to the square of the amplitude, if two waves are in phase the intensity will increase fourfold. This is called constructive interference (Figure 3.10).

If the waves are 180° out of phase so that troughs match crests, then the maxima add to minima and the sum is zero—no light is present; that is, the intensity is zero (Figure 3.11). In between these two conditions the light intensity will vary (Figure 3.12). This is destructive interference. Thus there will be seen an alternating series of bright and dark lines; the bright areas cor-

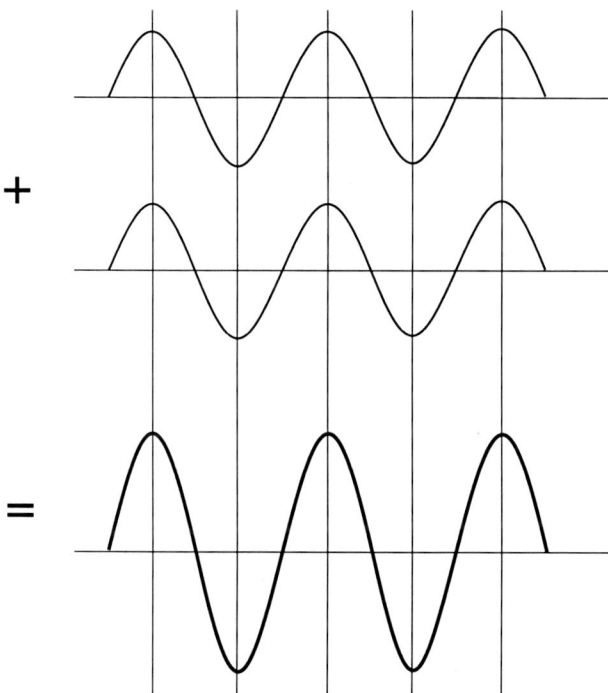

Fig. 3.10 The interaction of coherent light. Constructive interference.

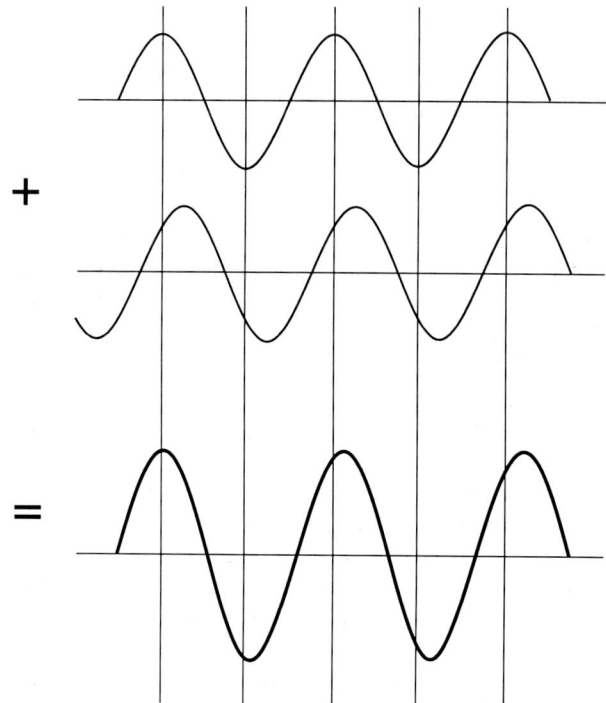

Fig. 3.11 Waves slightly out of phase.

can occur in white light. They may be observed when two nearly parallel glass surfaces are in close proximity (Figure 3.8). This is the problem sometimes encountered in microscopy when there is air between a slide and its cover glass. Waves are partially reflected from the glass–air surface and from the air–glass surface. Interference occurs between these two waves of light and the result is a fringe pattern. In this illustration, light is depicted as rays so that the sites of reflection may be more clearly indicated. The optical path between the

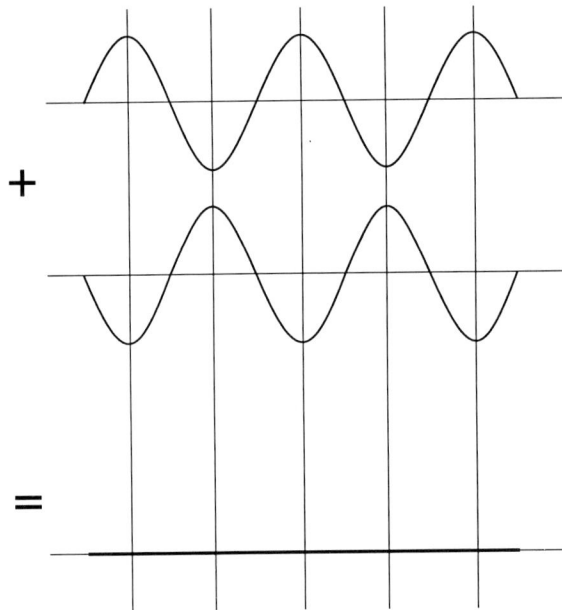

Fig. 3.12 Destructive interference.

respond to superimposition of two maxima or two minima and the dark areas to the superimposition of waves 180° out of phase with each other. The alternating bright and dark lines obtained on a screen are known as an interference fringe pattern (Figure 3.13).

Just because there is no light does not mean that the light was destroyed, however. In coherent light, the energy gained at the interference maxima because of constructive interference is exactly matched by the energy lost elsewhere as a result of destructive interference. The same total amount of energy is present whether or not the waves are coherent, but the energy falls into a sort of large blur.

The distance traveled by the light going between two points is called the optical path; in the illustration in Figure 3.13, this is the distance from the source of light to the screen. If the optical path from one source were changed slightly, as by a curved reflecting surface, the result would be a change in the location of the maxima from that source. This in turn would alter the location of the bright and dark fringes, since the intersection site of the maxima and the minima would be similarly altered. The change in optical path would be manifested as a shift in the interference pattern. The extent of this shift can be used to gain information about the reflecting surface.

If the location of the sources of light in Figure 3.13 is unchanged but the color of light (that is, the wavelength) is changed, the fringe pattern would also be altered. Shortening the wavelength causes the maxima to be closer together, and in the resultant fringe pattern the bright and dark fringes are also closer together.

Longer wavelengths would produce a fringe pattern in which the bright and dark fringes are separated by a greater distance.

The phenomenon of interference is used to design lens coatings to reduce unwanted reflections. These coatings are typically made from dielectric (non-conductive) materials that have been vacuum-deposited on to a lens surface to a thickness of one-fourth wave. Some of the light striking the surface will be reflected at the air–material interface and some at the material–glass interface while the rest will be transmitted. If the index of refraction of the coating has been chosen to equal that of the lens material, exactly the same amount of light will be reflected from each interface. Since the light from the second reflection has to pass through the coating twice, it will be 180° out of phase with that of the first reflection, hence each cancels the other out. The result is 0% reflection and 100% transmission. The rub is that the coating can only be made to match one-fourth of one particular wavelength—which is not too effective in white light. Also, no one material has been found that is equal in refractive index to that of spectacle crown glass. The problem can be partially solved by depositing multiple coating layers, each one of which is tuned to a different frequency and related to one another with respect to their indices of refraction.

The phenomenon of interference has become of increasing importance, especially as regards refractive surgery. This special property of electromagnetic radiation provides us with an extremely sensitive tool to measure with. This property is also important in measuring the efficiency of an optical system by means of the modulation transfer function. This function is discussed under the section on geometric optics, below. The most familiar form of such a device is the laser visual acuity tester. In this device two pinpoint beams of a low-wattage laser are directed into the eye. As the light waves traverse the eye they interfere with one another producing alternating light and dark bands which can be perceived by the patient. It is possible to adjust the separation of these bands so as to correspond to dimensions equal to that of a standard vision chart letter form. In practice, the beams are adjusted until the banding can no longer be detected. The acuity is taken as the next highest setting. As long as the medium has some ability to transmit light, the use of this device can give both the surgeon and the patient some practical assessment of the vision to be expected after cataract extraction.

Another application, of more immediate concern in refractive surgery, is holography. Anyone who has visited Disneyland has been exposed to one or more holograms, particularly some of the ghost-like images in the Haunted Mansion. A hologram is made using

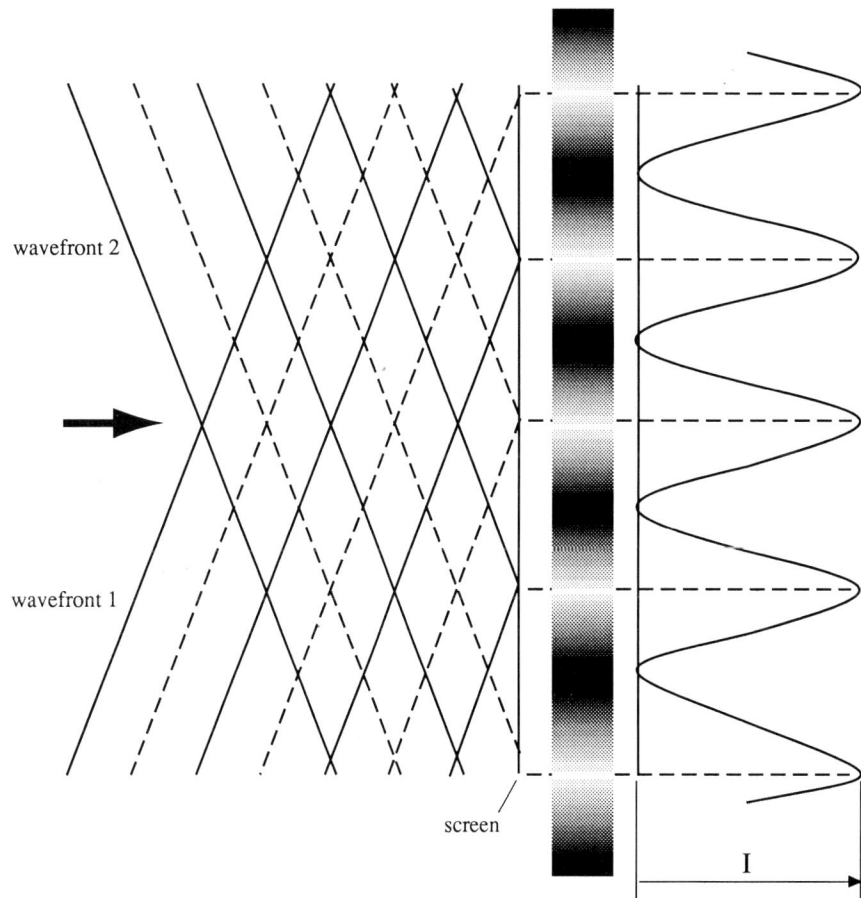

Fig. 3.13 Interference produced by two intersecting waves.

laser light that has been split into two beams, a reference beam and an object beam (Figure 3.14). The reference beam is directed on to the photographic (or other) recording medium without being focused. The object beam is directed on to the subject and the reflected light allowed to strike the recording media, again without being focused.

Since the two beams of light are coherent and parts of the object beam will be out of phase with the reference, an interference pattern will be produced on the recording medium. When the film is developed, no recognizable image will be seen. However, if the negative is illuminated with the reference beam and then viewed, that light will react with the pattern to form an exact replica of the object beam and hence an image of the object will be clearly visible. Since all the data present in the original object have been duplicated by the object beam, the image will appear to be fully dimensional.

Outside of its amusement value, the same principle can be used to construct a two-dimensional image of the corneal surface which can then be manipulated and its curvature measured. Because we know the exact wavelength of the light used to construct the image,

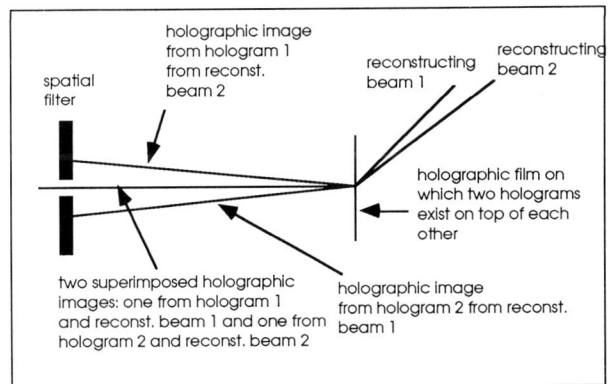

Fig. 3.14 Schematic of two-beam holographic system.

we can reproduce the corneal elevations exactly as well (see also Chapter 6).

Scattering

We have described how light is slowed when it passes through a medium other than a vacuum by interacting with the atoms within that medium. If those particles are larger than atoms—perhaps molecules—the light will be reflected and diffused. If the particles are even larger, such as large dust grains or ice crystals in the sky, all wavelengths of light will be affected. In this case the intensity of the light will be less and more diffuse, causing grey skies and soft shadows. If, however, the particles are smaller than the wavelength of light, the proportion of the light scattered will be inversely related to the fourth power of the wavelength. Thus blue light, whose wavelength is approximately $4/7$ that of red, is scattered $(4/7)^4$ or 10 times as much, which gives the sky its blue color and makes the sun appear much redder than it actually is. In the evening, when the low level of the sun causes light to travel a much greater distance, the sun appears redder still.

Diffraction

When light is projected through an aperture, secondary wavelengths will be formed at the edge of the aperture which interfere with the main wave front. This phenomenon is called diffraction. As the aperture is made smaller the more important this edge effect becomes and the larger the bullseye-like diffraction pattern which results. The size of the "x-ring" of the bullseye—the central bright spot—is called the Airy disk and is given by the formula:

$$R = \frac{1.22\lambda F}{d}$$

where R is the radius of the disk, F the distance from the aperture to the screen, λ the wavelength, and d the diameter of the aperture. About 83% of the energy of the point source will be found within the Airy disk (Figure 3.15). Since this disk is an image of the source, the smaller this disk the sharper the image and therefore the greater the resolving power of the system. The resolution of a lens is the smallest possible distance between two point sources at which their images can be recognized as distinct. This distance is typically the point where the minimum of the Airy pattern of one source falls upon the maximum of the second source, thus the absolute limit to resolving power is set by the laws of diffraction (see the section on resolving power, below).

Since diffraction occurs at every obstacle to a wave motion or aperture, the effect is always present in optical systems, including the eye. An ideal lens with no aberrations when imaging a point source will still form a diffraction pattern instead of a point image as predicted by the theory of geometric optics. An image can be improved by reducing the size of the aperture which reduces or eliminates aberrations in the system. The size of the imaging aperture is limiting, however. There is a size aperture beyond which the edge effects become dominant and the image becomes

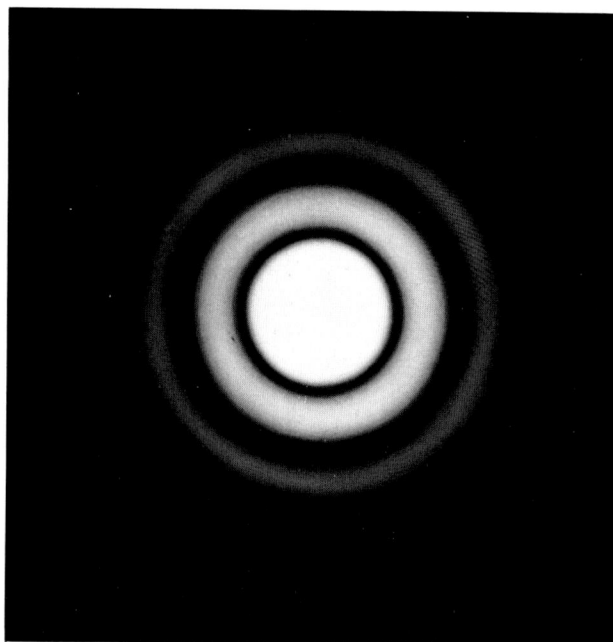

Fig. 3.15 An Airy disk at the limit of resolution.

degraded or blurred. Such a system is described as diffraction-limited.

If one considers the human eye, the most efficient diameter of the pupil is 2.5 mm. Above that various refractive aberrations limit the resolution and below that diffraction effects limit the resolution. Because of these diffraction effects, the typical pinhole used to estimate latent visual acuity will not improve that acuity to better than 20/25. We will have more to say about this phenomenon when we discuss the optics of the human eye in the following section on geometric optics.

Polarization

If light waves are traveling in the same direction, their electric fields may or may not be parallel to one another but will instead be randomly related. Such light is said to be non-polarized (unpolarized)—the condition of almost all light sources. Polarized light can be created from unpolarized light by one of three methods—transmission, reflection, or scattering.

If unpolarized light passes through a medium containing asymmetrically charged molecules that are oriented in the same direction, these molecules will absorb the electric field of the light in the same direction—thus causing the wavefront to collapse—and transmit the remainder. This phenomenon is typically described by using the analogy of a rope being wriggled through a picket fence, the idea being that only when the waves (wriggles) are parallel to the pickets will they be passed through. That's a lovely

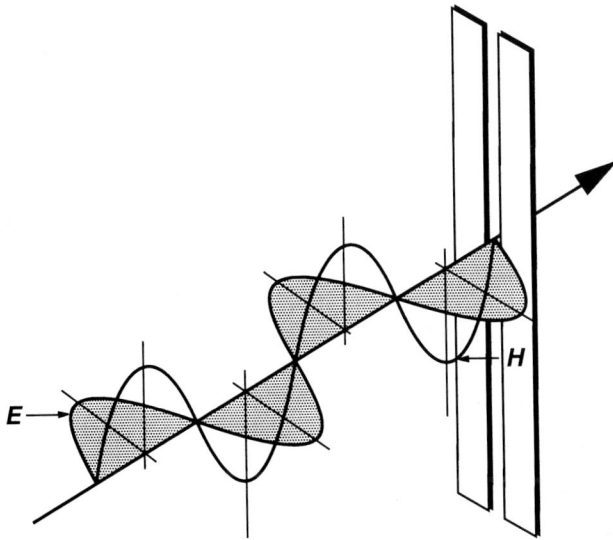

Fig. 3.16 Polarization of light. Note that the electrical portion of the light wave (E) is perpendicular to the pickets, hence this light wave is not passed through.

analogy but for the fact that reality is exactly the reverse of that picture. The electrical component is $\perp$ to the magnetic portion (Figure 3.16). Since the molecules within the polarizing material absorb the electrical portion, they only pass the light that is $\perp$ to their arrangement. This is the type of polarization that exists naturally in crystals.

Artificial polarizing materials were created 40 years ago by spraying iodide crystals on plastic and then stretching the plastic so that all the crystals would line up in the same direction. Since then, more sophisticated techniques have been found, but the basic principle remains the same.

An interesting experiment that shows some of the physical properties of polarized light consists of taking a linear polarizer and putting it in the path of a white light source. A second linear polarizer is placed perpendicular to the first, also in the path of the light. This is known as crossed polaroids. Light that passes through the first polarizer is polarized 90° to the plane of the other polarizer so that no light will get through the combination of crossed polaroids. However, if we interject yet a third polarizer between the first two at 45°, some light will get through. This happens because light is a vector. When the unpolarized light reaches the first polaroid it is oriented parallel to this polaroid. When it strikes the second polaroid it is at 45° to the plane of that polaroid, which means it can be resolved into components perpendicular and parallel to the second polaroid. The perpendicular component is absorbed but the parallel component is transmitted, which then strikes the third polaroid, which is now 45° to the plane of polarization of the light. This can then be resolved once more into light polarized perpendicu-

lar to the polaroid. Again, the parallel light will get through. Only about an eighth of the light actually gets through the system, as half was absorbed at the first polaroid and half again was absorbed at the second polaroid.

Polarization can also be created if the light falls on a partially transmitting material at an oblique angle. Some of the light will be reflected and some will be transmitted. The light will be bent according to Snell's law:

$$n_1 \sin a_1 = n_2 \sin a_2$$

where n_1 is the index of refraction of the first medium and n_2 is the index of refraction of the second medium. The two angles, a_1 and a_2, are the angles that the light makes with the component perpendicular to the surface of the interface of the first and second media, respectively. The law of reflection says that the angle of incidence is equal to the angle of reflection. As the light strikes the interface at an oblique angle, it is bent by the medium to a new angle, as given by Snell's law. In general, it bends toward the normal (a normal in optics is a line drawn perpendicular to a surface) in going from a less dense to a more dense medium. Likewise, some of the light is reflected by the molecules of the second medium at an angle, as given by the law of reflection. The reflected angle cannot be perpendicular to the angle of refraction, however, because then the electric field of the light in the molecules would be parallel to the direction of the propagation of the reflected light. This is impossible because light is a transverse wave. Therefore, at this angle only light with an electric field parallel to the direction of propagation may be reflected, thus the light is polarized (Figure 3.17). This is important because glare is reflected light and therefore polarized to some extent, thus polarized sunglasses reduce reflected glare more than the background illumination, which is unpolarized light.

Light is polarized by scattering molecules in the atmosphere in a very similar way. This scattering of

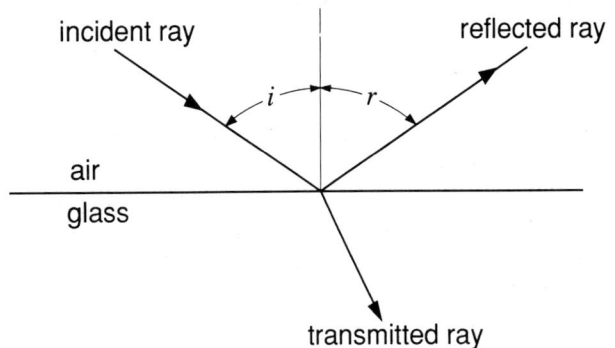

Fig. 3.17 Polarizing angle. The reflected light is polarized.

sky light can be easily verified by looking at a clear sky 90° to the direction of the sun while wearing polarized sun glasses. If one's head is rotated somewhat while looking in this direction, the light of the sky will be diminished considerably, but any clouds in that area will remain fairly constant in brightness. This is because the light from the atmosphere reaches the eye exclusively from scattering by relatively few air molecules and is thus polarized. Light from the clouds reaches the eye from scattering by many, much larger water droplets in the cloud, which destroys the polarization.

Fluorescence

Light may be absorbed by an electron in the ground state, raising the electron into an excited state. The excited electron may then decay to a lower level. If the electron decays to a state higher than the ground state, it will emit a photon that is less energetic than the absorbed photon, and therefore of a longer wavelength. This process is called fluorescence. A commonly used dye in ophthalmology, fluorescein, absorbs light at 490 nm in the blue and re-radiates it at 530 nm in the green when stimulated by white light.

Absorbance

When light falls upon an object it may be transmitted, reflected, absorbed, or, more usually, undergo some combination of the aforementioned. A number of optical devices such as light filters and sunglasses make use of absorption. If light of intensity I_0 falls upon a partially transparent plate, the intensity of the transmitted light would be $I = TI_0$ where T, called the transmittance, is a unitless number between 0 and 1. If several plates are stacked, the total transmittance of the stack is the product of the individual transmittances. It is sometimes more useful to add terms than to multiply them, so another term, called the density, was invented.

$$D = \frac{\log I}{T} = 10^{-D}$$

where D is the density. Since numbers can be multiplied by adding their logarithms, the density of a series of plates is the sum of the densities of the individual plates. Absorbed light is usually converted into heat by the absorbing electrons, but it may be used to excite an electron into a higher level and be re-radiated, as in the case of fluorescence.

Photometry

Photometry is concerned with the measurement of light in a system and the effect that the light has upon the visual sensation. Light that differs only in wavelength can be distinguished by the eye because of two properties—color and apparent intensity. The eye is more sensitive to some parts of the spectrum than to others, so that the apparent intensities of the different parts of the spectrum will be different, even if the incident light intensity is the same at all wavelengths. There are four characteristics of the eye that determine its response to light.

Spectral sensitivity. From an inspection of the luminosity curve, one can see that an eye is very sensitive to green light and rather insensitive to red and violet light. If violet illumination is to give the same sensation of brightness as a green source, much more power is needed.

Range of sensitivity. The human eye can detect energies of a few photons per second up to bright sunlight, a difference in sensitivity of 10^{15}.

Fechner's law. The relative sensation of an increase in sensitivity is proportional to the log of the change, so that by increasing the intensity of a lamp from 1 to 10 foot-candles, the same sensation of change as from 10 to 100 foot-candles is given. This law applies for four orders of magnitude.

Weber's law. The change of brightness necessary to be noticed is proportional to the original brightness, that is, $DL = KL$, where DL is the least amount of change of intensity noticeable, K is a constant, and L is the brightness of the light. Therefore, the change necessary before a difference is noticed in a bright light source is larger than in a dim one.

Geometric optics

The process of discovery and furtherance of knowledge is often a painful process, resembling the ebb and flow of the tides. Low water alternates with high, with the occasional neap or excessively high tidal flow. So it was with the optics of the eye. While myopia and hyperopia were recognized and described in Aristotle's time, the possibility of definite treatment beyond medicinal awaited the more complete understanding of the optical nature of the human eye. Much of the progress in this was stymied by the prevailing notions of the time regarding sight itself.

The manner in which vision works has been the subject of much philosophic discussion down through the ages. Nothing, however, exists in the extant ancient Egyptian or Sumerian writings alluding to vision or the phenomenon of sight, though a practical knowledge of refraction existed among the Assyrians (see also Chapter 2). The first such writing comes from the time of Pythagoras, in 600 BC, referring to his "emanation theory" of vision. Vision was supposed to result from the emission of a subtle "visual spirit" or pneuma originating in the brain, traveling down the hollow optic nerves and filling the lens from whence it emanated in rays similar to those of sunlight. How this concept persisted in the face of the fact that vision is impaired in the absence of light is a mystery.

This thesis was denied by Aristotle (360 BC) who adopted and expanded on an original proposal of Democrites (500 BC). Sixty years later, Plato tried without success to reconcile both views. The Arabic writers al Hazen and Ibn Rushd also supported this concept of Aristotle, expanding it to include the retina as the seat of visual reception, to no avail. Leonardo Da Vinci attempted and failed to combine both views as well. The "consecration" of the Pythagorean view by Galen centuries before had insured its acceptance for 2500 years, practically unchallenged. This hypothesis held sway until the time of Felix Platter in 1583, when it was finally put to rest.

The durability of this thesis is surprising in view of the knowledge of optics possessed by the Greeks. Although something of optics must have been known to the Babylonians and Egyptians before then, it would seem likely that it was limited to deductions from ordinary observable phenomena. The first optical treatise (*Optics*) was written by Euclid in 300 BC. This work was followed shortly thereafter by that of Aristarchus; next by the *Catoptrics* of Heron in the first century AD and finally the *Optics Thesaurus* of Claudius Ptolemeus (Ptolemy) in AD 100; Ptolemy was described as the father of optical science and his work remained the essential source of knowledge until the 1600s. The sum of this knowledge concerned itself with catoptrics or the optics of reflecting surfaces, however; of dioptrics little was known. Ptolemy's construction of an object AB, as seen under water, is shown in Figure 3.18. The rays from the eye, OM and ON, are refracted at the surface and reach the object along paths MA and NB. Ptolemy knew that a normal ray was not refracted and concluded that the virtual image, A'B' is located by protracting the rays, OM and ON until they reach the perpendiculars, AK and BL. He postulated that the image was magnified because the visual angle, A'OB', was greater than the angle AOB, through which it would be seen if in air.

The ancients had observed the magnifying qualities of a water-filled flask, as well as its ability to concentrate the sun's rays. Though the Roman physician Heliodorus described this as a refractive phenomenon, its nature was apparently not understood. Ptolemy's construction remained the standard explanation for centuries—it was even copied by Roger Bacon—and remained so until corrected by Barrow in 1674. This understanding was undoubtedly hampered by the inability of such philosophers to break the bonds of dogma and theocratic meddling. It takes great moral courage and not a little chutzpah to fly in the face of established precedent—it is safer to "go along." It

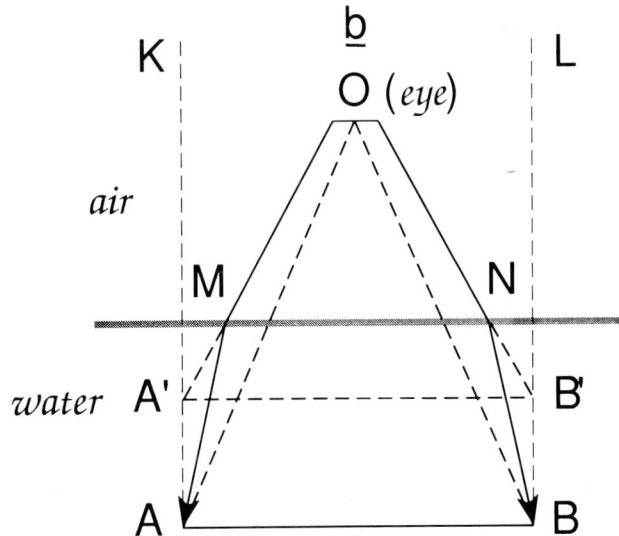

Fig. 3.18 Refractive concepts of Ptolemy.

would have helped had not the authorities stymied the science of anatomy by interdicting human dissection. Nevertheless, even when dissection was allowed, the study of the eye continued to be hampered by the difficulty in preserving it intact for study.

Newton (Figure 3.19), in his *Opticks* (Figure 3.20), consolidated the entire system of optics, reflection, refraction, image formation, and dioptric system of the eye and included the rudiments of color theory. He did it so thoroughly that nothing more was added for nearly a century. In 1841 Gauss (a prodigy ranked with Archimedes and Newton) produced the elegant mathematic construction that solved the problem of complex optical systems, which essentials are still accepted today. Listing, Gauss' student, devised a very accurate theoretical schematic eye which culminated in the simplified, but still elegant, schematic eye of Allvar Gullstrand [5].

Geometric optics deals with light as rays and the formation of images using optical devices such as lenses, prisms, and mirrors and the physical laws governing the characteristics of such images. It concerns itself with three aspects:

1 The size of the image.
2 The distance of the image from the optical surface.
3 The characteristics of the image: inverted or erect; real or vitual.

We are interested in such things because we are choosing to meddle with the mechanism by which we see—the eye—and the eye is, of course, an optical device. Our discussion will touch upon some aspects of the science of optics. The reader is referred to the section on further reading for more detailed coverage.

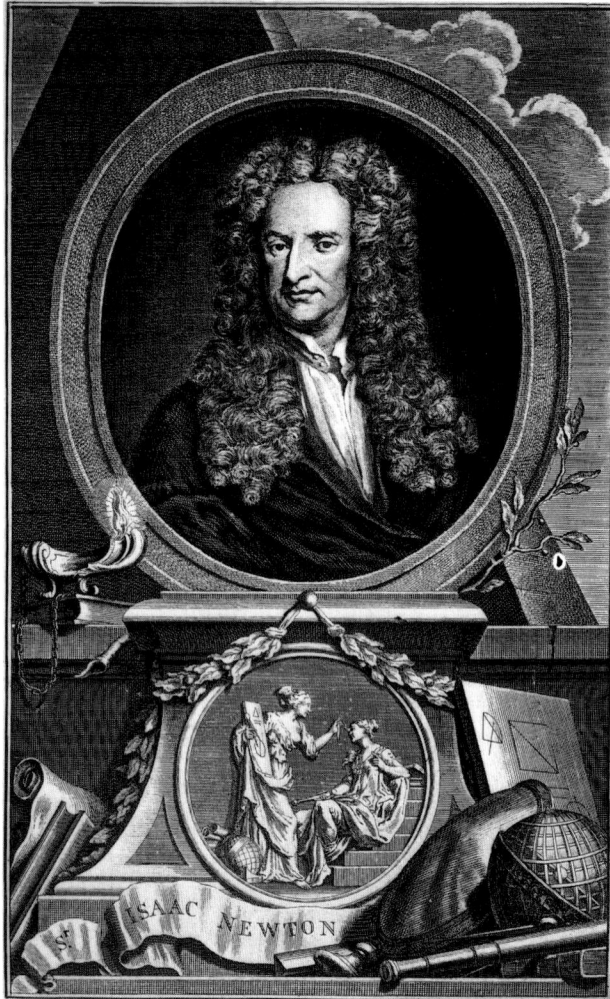

Fig. 3.19 Sir Isaac Newton.

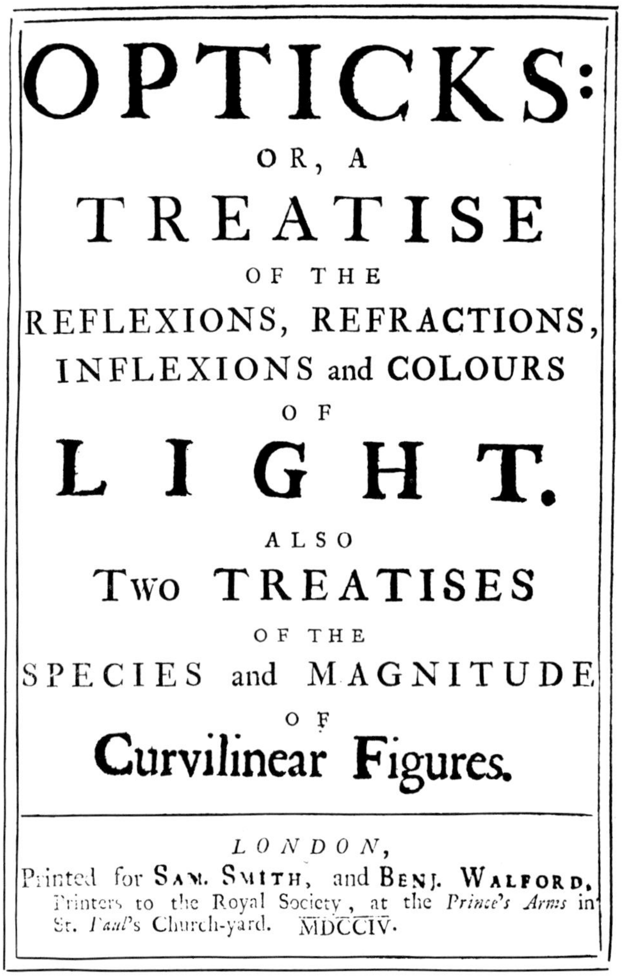

Fig. 3.20 The title page of Newton's *Opticks*.

To deal more adequately with this subject, however, we must define some terms of usage.

Object. This is a source of light or the origin of rays directed toward an optical system. An object may be real or tangible or it may be virtual or intangible, formed by projection of the rays through an optical system to a location where it cannot be imaged on to a screen.

Image. An image is a concentration of rays from an object by an optical system to produce a likeness of the object. As in the case of an object, the image may be virtual or real.

Optical axis. This is an imaginary line, about which the components of an optical system are centered.

Infinity. In the classic sense this term has no dimension and refers to the location of an object or image. In the sense in which we will use it in our discussion, this distance refers to that which is greater than that of the optical system itself.

Focal length. This is the distance between a lens or mirror and the image of an object located at infinity and is abbreviated *f*. The position of the image is the point at which the parallel rays from an object are brought to a focus by the optic. The designation of this point is *F*. Focal length is commonly employed as an expression of optical power.

Diopter. This term is also used to express optical power. It is expressed in this manner:

$$D = \frac{1}{f \text{ (in meters)}}$$

Thus, a 1D lens would deviate a ray 1 cm at a distance of 1 m. If such a lens (or mirror) causes a ray to be deviated toward the optic axis of the system (converge), that lens is said to have plus power. In this case the lens would be described as $+1\,D$. If the lens (or mirror) were to cause the ray to deviate away from the optic center (diverge), it is said to have minus power. By convention, an unsigned diopter is considered to be of plus power.

Magnification. The relationship between the size of the object and is the size of the image expressed thus:

$$M = \frac{\text{image size}}{\text{object size}}$$

Transparent. This is an optical medium that transmits light with minimal attenuation. These substances (or media) are typically clear, such as glass, water, and air.

Opaque. Opaque is the opposite of transparent and either reflects or absorbs the light.

Incident. In the discussion the term is used to describe a ray of light striking a surface. Thus the ray was incident to the surface of the mirror. Dropping the mirror would also be an incident but of a different category and consequence.

Interface phenomenon

An interface is the junction of two optical media. For a lens in air, the interface is located at the surface of the lens. This interface is thus an optical surface. Three things can happen to a ray of light when it strikes such a surface:

Reflection. The light is bounced back into the initial medium. Depending upon the quality of the surface the reflection can be specular (from a mirror-like surface) or diffuse (as from a flat painted surface) or a combination of both.

Absorption. The light is so attenuated by the medium that it is converted to heat. Sometimes the absorption is not obvious, as in a shallow pan of clear water which becomes heated if left in sunlight.

Refraction or transmission. Refraction is the bending of a ray as it passes (is transmitted) from one medium to another.

Optical surfaces

The optical interface or surface can take many shapes. It can be flat or plano. It may also be convex, in which case the surface is curved toward the object (or thicker at the optic axis) or it may be concave, the opposite condition. If the surface has an even curvature overall as if sliced from a round ball, such a surface is said to be spherical. If the curvature is not so shaped it is called aspherical. A regular aspherical surface has a curvature which deviates from a single radius of curvature from center to the periphery in the same manner in all meridians. It should be obvious that such a surface would not have a single point of focus, although the defocus spot would be a circle.

The corneal surface is highly aspherical and cannot be described in simple geometric terms. This fact has serious implications when attempts are made to measure the curvature of this surface. These implications will be discussed more thoroughly in the sec-

tion on corneal topography (see Chapter 6). Wavefront analysis techniques are more appropriate for the study of surfaces of this nature.

An aspherical surface can have other properties. In Chapter 2 we discussed how such a surface can have astigmatism. In an astigmatic system the surface curvature can vary in a regular fashion from one meridian to another such that the extreme deviations lie at 90° to one another. Such a condition is termed regular astigmatism. Astigmatism is usually considered to be a deviation from the underlying spherical surface, hence the surface is termed sphero-cylindric—a cylinder lens superimposed on to a spherical lens. A cylinder lens is one in which the refracting power is directed along one axis only, as if the lens were a slice from a glass rod or cylinder, hence its name. Such a surface would not have a single point of focus either but in contradistinction to a regular asphere, the focal spot would be an ellipsoid (oval).

Astigmatism can also result from misalignment of an optic. Thus if a lens deviates from the vertical (or horizontal) plane, if it is tilted, astigmatism due to tilt results. If the lens is not so tilted but is slightly off-center, a type of astigmatism results called coma (pronounced comma). The eye encompasses all of these aberrations within its optical system, some of which tend to cancel or neutralize each other. Tilt and coma are not usually considered in corneal surface analysis using current techniques (since they are not easily measured with photokeratoscopic methods) but are important when dealing with the corneal surface, particularly when attempting ray tracing (see also Chapter 6).

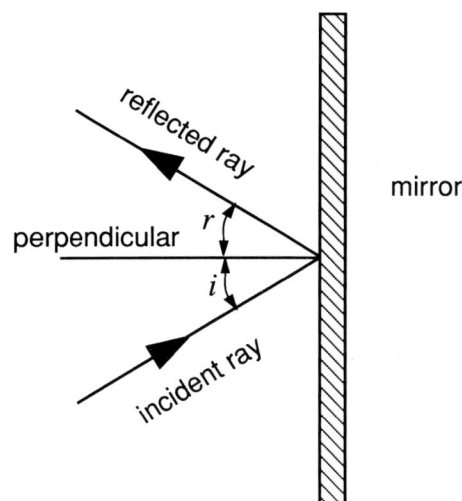

Fig. 3.21 The law of reflection applied to a plane surface.

Index of refraction

This is one of the most important characteristics of an optical medium. It is expressed mathematically as follows:

$$n = \frac{c}{c_m}$$

where c is the speed of light in a vacuum (or air) and c_m is the speed of light in the medium. The indices for some ocular media media are:

Saline   1.33
Cornea   1.3775
Air   1.0003

Certain laws govern the behavior of single rays at an optical surface. These are the law of reflection, and the law of refraction (Snell's law).

The law of reflection

This rule or law applies when a ray is reflected back into the initial medium after striking an optical surface. It basically states that the angle of reflection is equal to the angle of incidence and is expressed thus (Figure 3.21 and 3.22):

angle i = angle r

It is true for all optical surfaces.

The law of refraction (Snell's law)

When a ray is transmitted rather than reflected, Snell's law (derived in 1621) applies (Figure 3.23). This rule states that the angle of refraction at an optical surface is proportional to the sine of the angle of incidence and the ratio of the refractive indices. It is written algebraically as follows (Figure 3.24):

n sine $I = n'$ sine I'

In small angles of incidence (under 6°) the sine of the angle is almost equal to the angle, thus Snell's law is greatly simplified:

$$I' = \frac{n}{n'} I$$

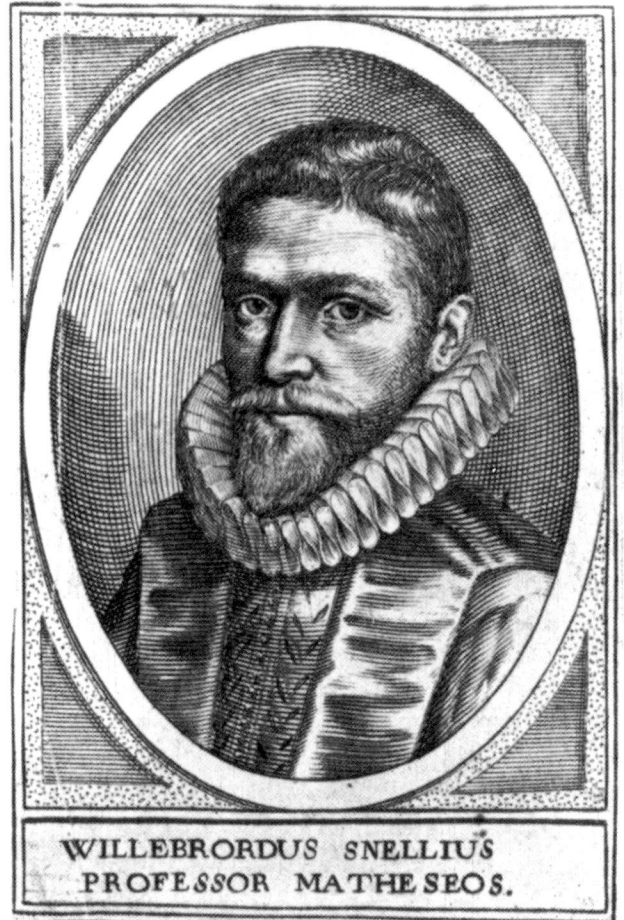

Fig. 3.23 Willebrord Snell.

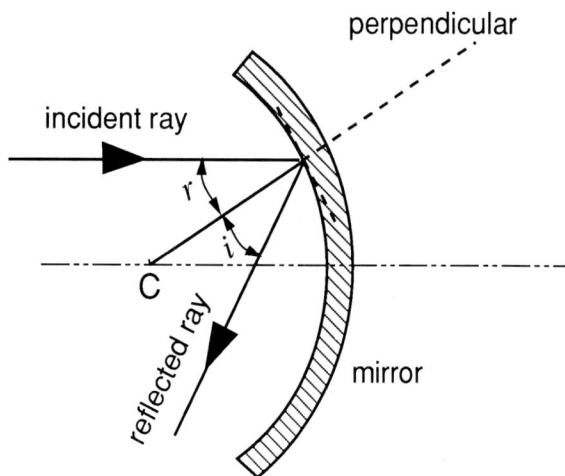

Fig. 3.22 The law of reflection applied to a curved surface.

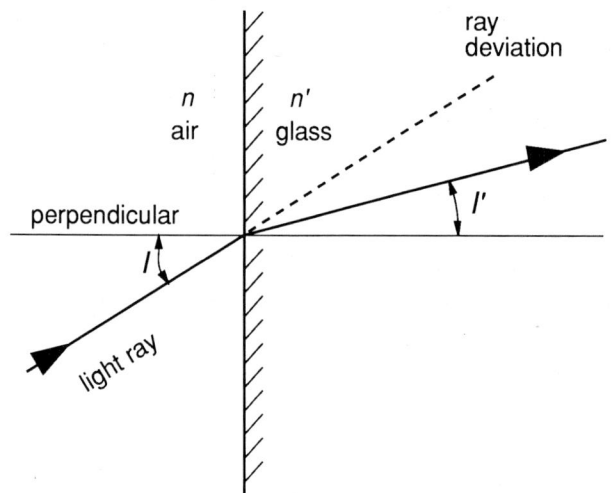

Fig. 3.24 Basic principle of Snell's law of refraction.

Selected ray imaging is another technique for determining the size, location, and characteristics of an image in any optical system. This technique employs only two rays. To use this technique we must assume that no aberrations exist in the optical system—all rays emanating from a single object will converge at a single point. The two rays selected for this purpose are these:

1 Any incident ray parallel to the optic axis must pass through the focal point after refraction or reflection.

2 A ray passing through the center of rotation of the surface is not refracted or is reflected back on itself. Thus the angle of incidence is zero. In a lens this would only be true if it were infinitely thin but is close enough when dealing with the cornea.

The reflecting characteristics of the cornea are of special interest to us when measuring its curvature. The refracting characteristics must also be understood when calculating the effect that any surgical procedure on this surface has on total refraction of the eye. In the latter case the cornea is treated like a thin meniscus lens.

Cardinal points and planes

Cardinal points and planes are constructions located to permit the use of two-ray procedures in thick lenses. The use of these constructs will result in greater precision but the thin-lens alternative is adequate for most ophthalmic purposes. There are three pairs of cardinal points on the optic axis. The cardinal planes, which correspond to these points, are planes perpendicular to these points. The points and planes commonly encountered are the principal planes, nodal points, and focal points.

Principal plane

The formal definition of this plane is that it is a plane of unit magnification (see Figure 3.25).

Focal point

The focal point is located on the optic axis at the point where rays from an object at infinity cross (are focused). The focal length is that distance from the principal plane to the focal point (Figures 3.26 and 3.27).

Nodal point

The nodal point of a thin lens is characterized by no deviation from the initial to the final media of a refracted ray passing through the point (Figure 3.28). The angle of incidence of the ray passing through the nodal point is therefore equal to the angle of refraction. Thick lenses have two nodal points. A ray of light directed toward the first nodal point will appear to be

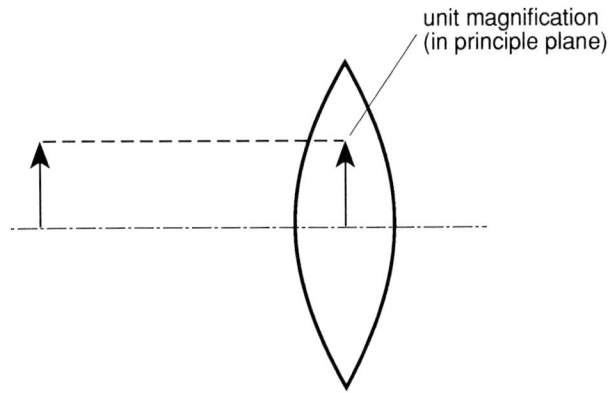

Fig. 3.25 Definition of principal plane.

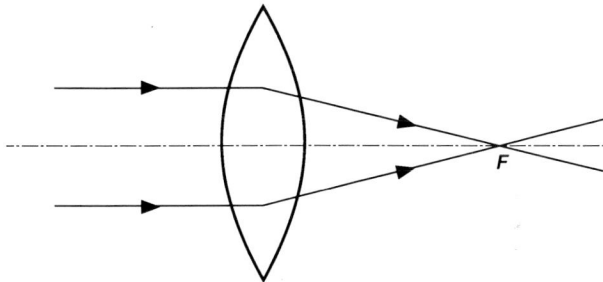

Fig. 3.26 The focal point.

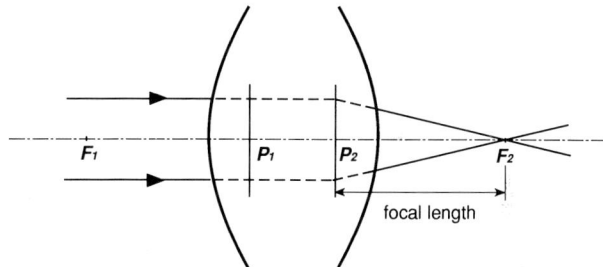

Fig. 3.27 The focal length of a lens defined.

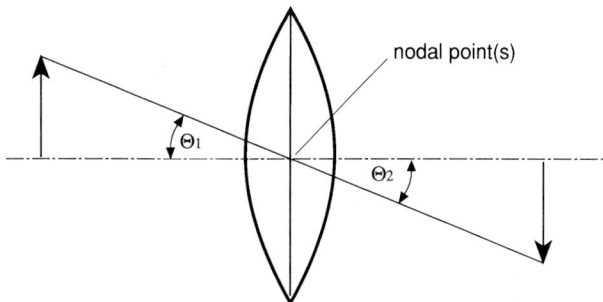

Fig. 3.28 Nodal points—thin lens.

coming from the second (Figure 3.29). In most situations the indices of refraction of the media in which both the object and image are located are equal. In the case where this medium is air, the nodal points are superimposed on the principal planes (Figure 3.30).

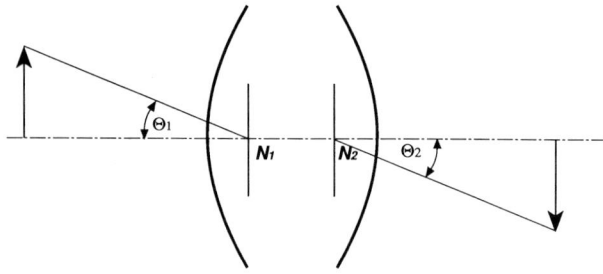

Fig. 3.29 Nodal points—thick lens.

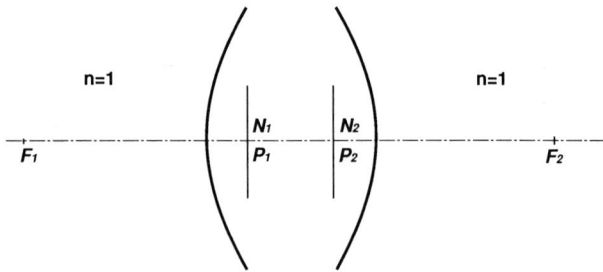

Fig. 3.30 In air, the nodal points and principal planes coincide.

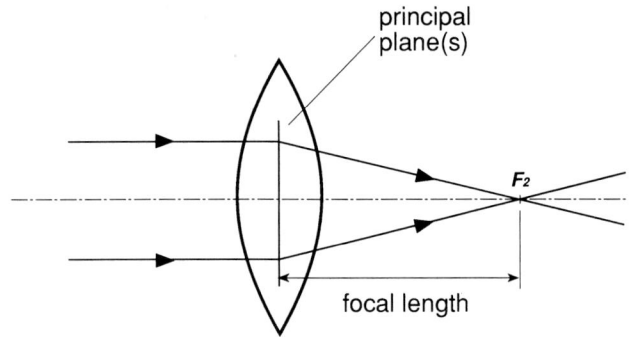

Fig. 3.31 Single refracting surface. There is only one principal plane and one focal point.

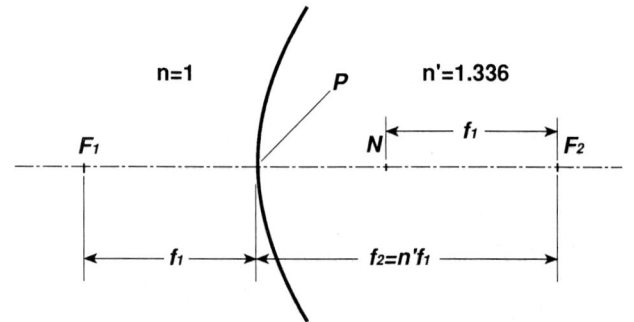

Fig. 3.32 In a single refracting surface, the focal length is proportional to the index of refraction.

Single refracting surfaces

A single refracting surface is one in which refraction occurs at one surface with the image located in a medium whose index of refraction differs from that in which the object is located. The behavior of cardinal points is as follows:

1 There is only one nodal point, one principal plane, and one focal point (Figure 3.31).
2 The principal point is located at the refracting surface.
3 The focal length is proportional to the index of refraction (Figure 3.32), therefore:

$$F_2 = n'F_1$$

4 The nodal point is not located at the principal plane. It is shifted toward the second focal point at the center of curvature of the surface (Figure 3.32). Thus the distance from the first focal point to the principal plane is equal to the distance from the nodal point to the second focal point.

Vergence

One other method employed to determine image characteristics is vergence, used with the two-ray trace procedure (Figure 3.33). Most problems should be solved using both methods. The application of vergence requires the use of five rules:

1 Distances of the object and image have dioptric value. This is expressed as the reciprocal of those dimensions, in meters.
2 Divergent beams have minus power.
3 Convergent beams have plus power.
4 The power of each element is expressed in diopters.
5 The ray, mirror, and lens powers are added algebraically.
Figure 3.34 shows a reduced eye using this method.

Magnification

Magnification refers only to the relationship between the image and object size, as expressed by:

$$M = I/O$$

It is evident that magnification can also be expressed in terms of object and image distance (Figure 3.35):

$$M = \frac{\text{image distance}}{\text{object distance}} = \frac{D'}{D}$$

Greatest magnification occurs when the object is located at the first focal point of the lens. Changing the distance from the lens to the eye only alters the size of the field of view through the magnifying lens, not the size of the resultant image. Telescopes are two-stage

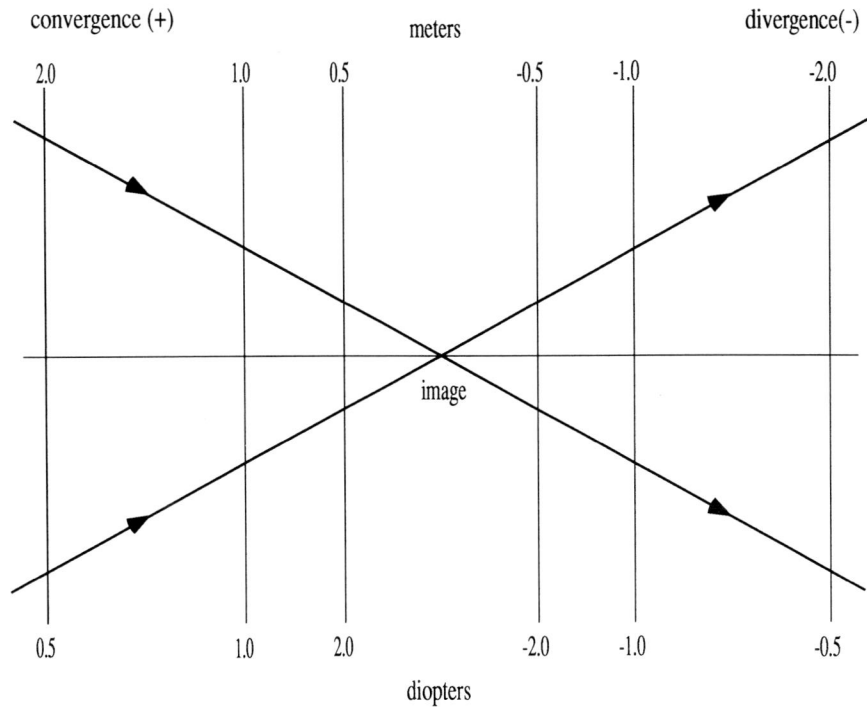

Fig. 3.33 Vergence of light rays. Converging light rays are plus and diverging beams are minus. The power of the ray is determined by its distance from the image.

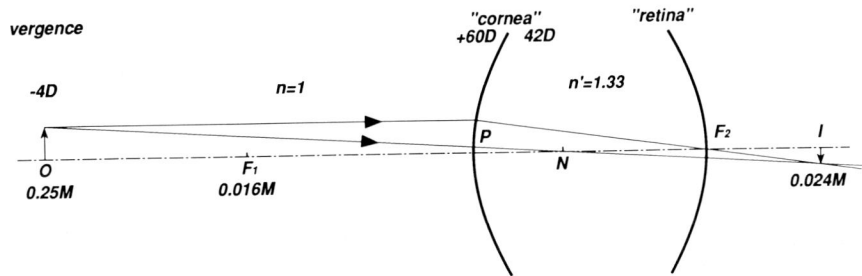

Fig. 3.34 A single-surface schematic eye demonstrating the use of vergence.

magnifiers in which the object lens (objective) forms an image of the object. This image is further imaged by the much stronger magnifying power of the second lens, the ocular (Figure 3.36).

Optical aberrations

In all the foregoing, we have assumed a perfect optical system—that is, every ray of light passing through the system must converge to or diverge from a single point on the image. The image must also lie in a plane perpendicular to the optic axis and must be a symmetric copy of the object whether erect, inverted, larger, or smaller. However, no optical system is ever perfect nor are all the light rays identical. If Snellen's law is applied to various parts of a spherical lens, it will be discovered that greater refraction occurs at the periphery than at the center. Unless incoming rays are paraxial, the rays of light will not come to a point focus;

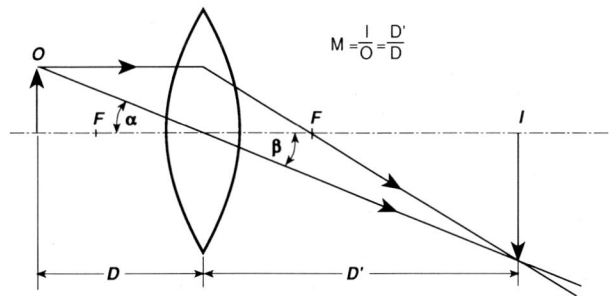

Fig. 3.35 Magnification.

instead the image will take the shape of a blurred circle (Figures 3.37 and 3.38). Lord Rayleigh suggested that the image does not deteriorate appreciably as long as the maximum difference in equivalent optical path at best focus does not exceed a quarter wavelength of light—the Rayleigh limit. Thus it can be expected that some abnormalities will exist in the image formed by

(a)

(b)

(c)

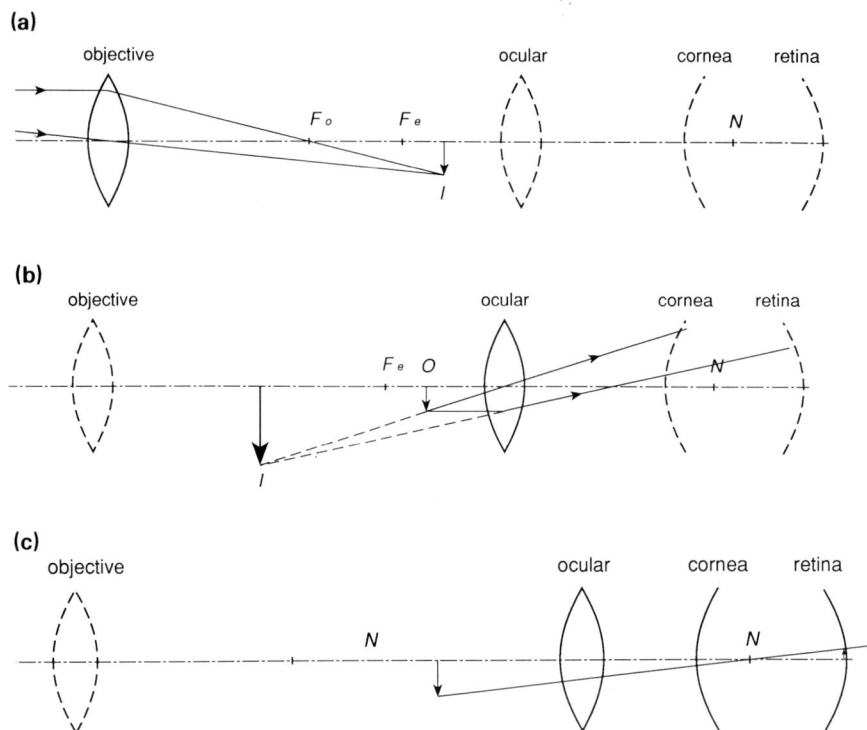

Fig. 3.36 (a–c) Telescopic magnification.

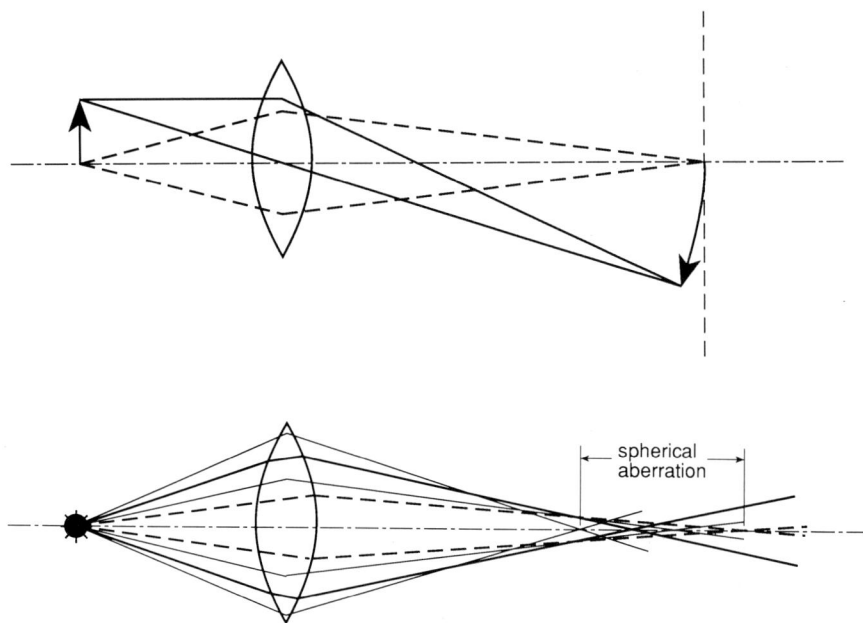

Fig. 3.37 Field curvature from a thick lens. Note that rays striking the periphery of the lens undergo more refraction.

Fig. 3.38 Spherical aberration showing the resultant caustic or shape of the bundle at the putative focal point.

any system. These deviations or aberrations are divided into two main groups.

1 Aberrations due to the multi-wavelength nature of light—chromatic aberrations.

2 System aberrations:

    (a) occurring on the optic axis—spherical aberrations.

    (b) occurring off axis—astigmatism, coma, distortion, field curvature, tilt.

Chromatic aberration

Chromatic aberration is not negligible, but neither is it considerable. The eye is not achromatic, as once believed (Figure 3.39). The magnitude of this phenomenon was first measured by the Astronomer Royal, Nevil Maskelyne, in 1789. He found a difference in focal length of the eye for red and violet light of 0.535 mm—quite close to more modern averages. While

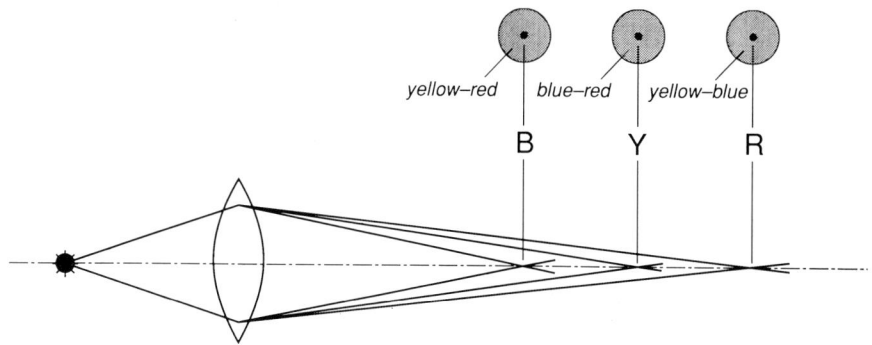

Fig. 3.39 Chromatic aberration.

there is some variability, it is low and the average amount of this difference is 0.9 D. With a 2 mm diameter pupil, 70% of the light falls on an area 0.005 mm in diameter and thus the effects of chromatic aberration fall within the same magnitude as diffraction. As the pupil widens, the effects of increased chromatic aberration are offset by increasing diffractive effects. The net result is that image definition is practically unchanged.

Spherical aberration

The effects of spherical aberration in the eye are small (Figure 3.40). This is partly due to the relative flatness of the cornea in the periphery. However most of the correction occurs because the lens nucleus is more dense than the periphery, refracting the axial rays more strongly than the marginal ones. It might be expected that the act of accommodation would affect the aberration present. It can be seen that during accommodation, the aberration becomes over-corrected and is least when 1–2 D of accommodation is exerted (Figure 3.41).

Other types of aberrations typically found in optical systems are negligibly small in the eye. Thus, although some obliquity of the light rays striking the retina occurs (because the optics are not coincident with the visual axis), the angle is usually very small. Therefore, as far as central vision is concerned, the effects of oblique astigmatism, lateral spherical aberration, tilt,

and coma are not operative to any significant degree. However, any or all of these factors can take on more significance after the corneal surface shape has been altered through surgical, or other means.

Image curvature

One of the factors affecting image quality is image curvature. This occurs because the periphery of any lens has greater refracting power resulting from the greater obliquity of its surface there; thus peripheral

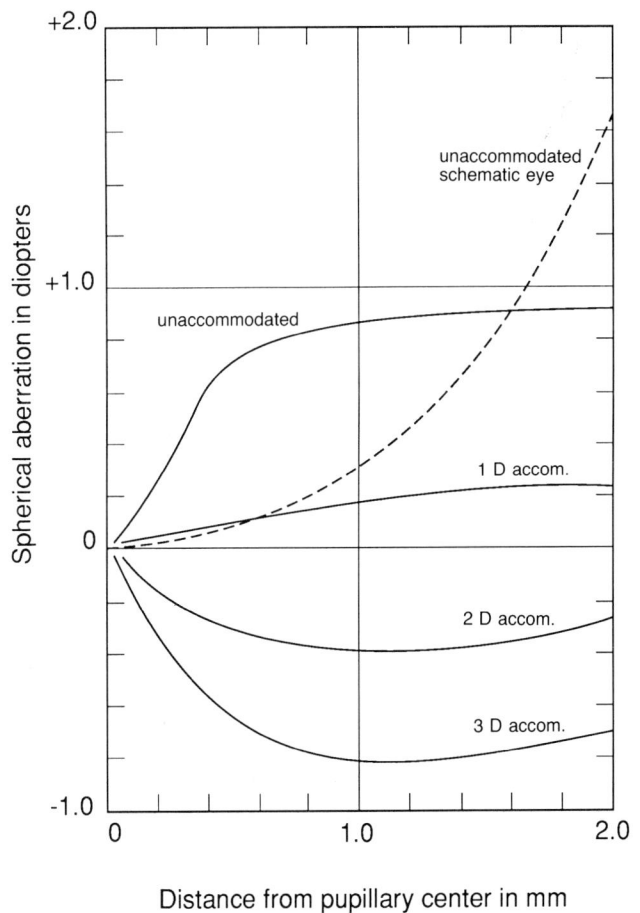

Fig. 3.40 Aberration in the human eye is small.

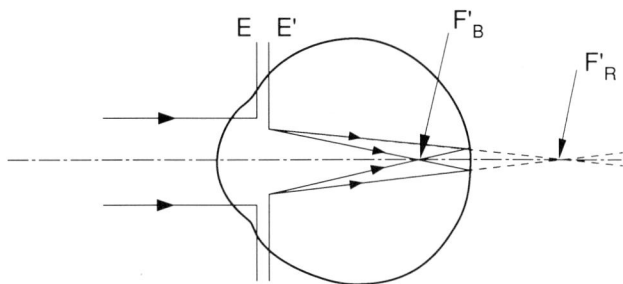

Fig. 3.41 Spherical aberration in the human eye is modified by accommodation.

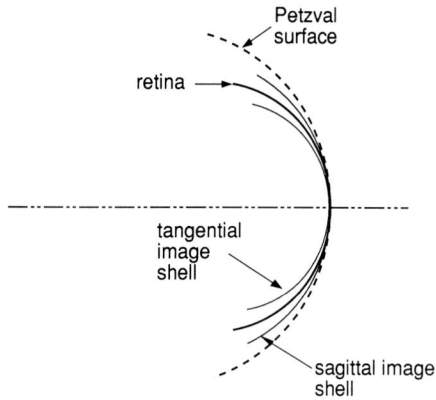

Fig. 3.42 Petzval's curvature or natural plane of focus for a thick lens, as in the human eye. Note that the image shells approximate the curve of the retina.

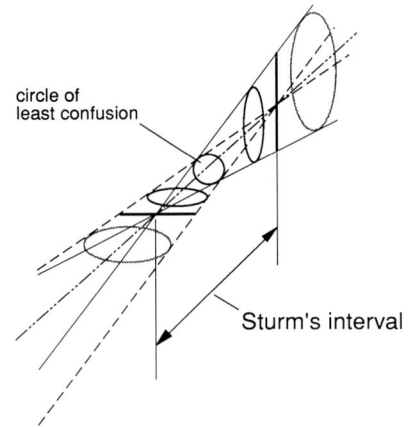

Fig. 3.43 An astigmatic system showing the shape of the light bundle making up Sturm's conoid.

rays are brought to a focus sooner (Figure 3.37). This phenomenon was clearly described by Kepler in 1604 [6,7]. Although first elucidated mathematically by George Biddle Airy in 1827, this curvature is generally known as Petzval's curvature or surface. Airy's formula for the curvature is:

$$\frac{1}{r} = -\frac{1}{n_1 f'_1}$$

Two factors lessen the effect of such aberrations in the periphery. The first of these is the fact that the back-surface of the eye is curved. Thus the image shells approximate the true shape of the retina (Figure 3.42). The second point is that the resolving power of the peripheral retina is much less than that of the center, therefore more aberration can be tolerated without notice.

Astigmatism

Astigmatism is a characteristic of spherical surfaces in that the aberration results in more than one point of focus along the optic axis. This is true only in the sense that, typically, the major and minor meridians are spheres whose radius of curvature differ. However, astigmatism can also occur in surfaces that are regular aspheres (such as the cornea). The interval between the anterior and posterior focus is called the interval of Sturm and varies in its extent depending upon the amount of astigmatism present in the optical system (Figure 3.43). Anterior to the first focal plane, the vertical rays converge more rapidly than the horizontal, and consequently the bundle's cross-section will be that of a horizontal ellipse. At the first focal plane, all the vertical rays have come to a focus and the bundle now takes the shape of a horizontal line. Beyond this point the vertical rays begin to diverge while the horizontal rays are still converging and the ellipse begins to

shorten. At the posterior (second) focal plane, the condition is such that the horizontal rays have all come to a focus as a vertical line. Beyond that point the bundle again takes on the appearance of a vertical ellipse. There is one point between the anterior and posterior focus where the bundle's cross-section is circular, however. This circle is called the circle of least confusion and is located approximately one-third of the way from the anterior-most focus (Figure 3.43). At this point is space, in the absence of any optical correction, the image formed by the system is the best possible. Typically this power corresponds to the so-called spherical equivalent of the refractive system; that is, a spherical lens of that power will produce a circle of least confusion on the retina similar to that of the astigmatic system alone.

The simplest form of astigmatic system is one in

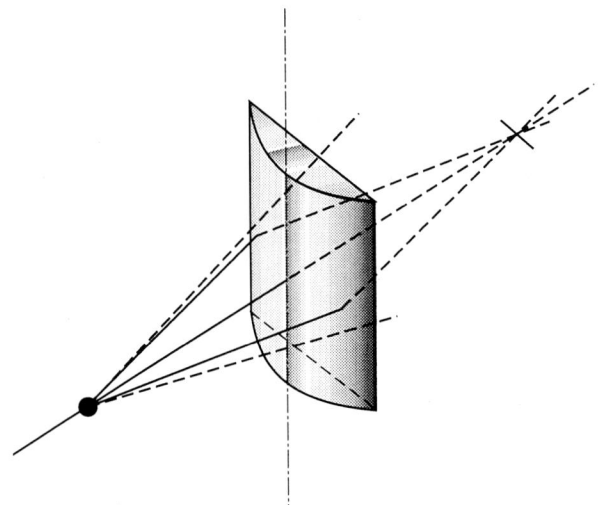

Fig. 3.44 A cylindric lens. Note that the image is a line perpendicular to the long axis of the lens.

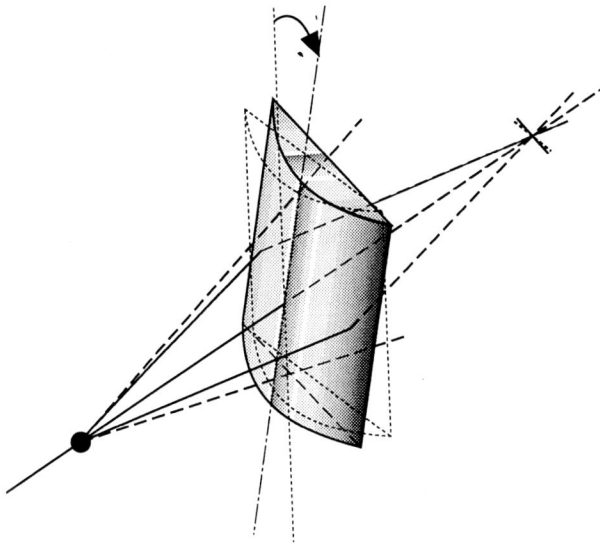

Fig. 3.45 When a cylinder lens is rotated, the image also rotates. Thus a cylinder lens has direction.

which the curvature exists in only one direction (Figure 3.44). In this event the image of a circle would be a straight line whose direction would depend upon the angle of rotation of the surface (Figure 3.45). Thus we see that astigmatic lenses possess a direction or axis. An astigmatism occurring in a spherical system could be thought of as a cylinder lens superimposed on a spherical lens (Figure 3.46). Such a surface would be called sphero-cylindric or toroidal. An example of an extreme toroid would be a doughnut.

Coma and tilt

Coma and tilt are special forms of astigmatism. Coma occurs in images of objects located off the optic axis (Figure 3.47). The resultant image is characteristic, having a bright center with a less bright tail, hence its name. Less discrete objects will appear to be smeared. Tilt occurs when an element is rotated around a plane perpendicular to the axis (Figure 3.48). The resultant image is also smeared but in two or more directions. Such aberrations have less effect in the eye due to the fact that the asymmetry of the ocular system corrects part of these aberrations and also because the image falls on to a curved surface (the retina).

Resolving power

To distinguish two luminous points, two cones must be stimulated with the one between unstimulated. The smallest resolvable image therefore has a diameter just slightly larger than a macular cone cell. This distance has been shown to be around 0.002 mm. Therefore, the

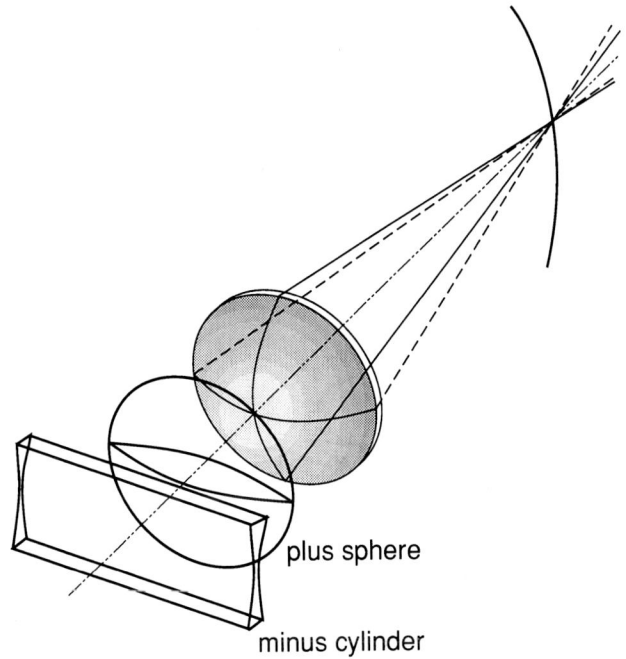

Fig. 3.46 A regular toroidal astigmatic refracting surface is corrected by applying both spherical and cylindric lenses of appropriate power.

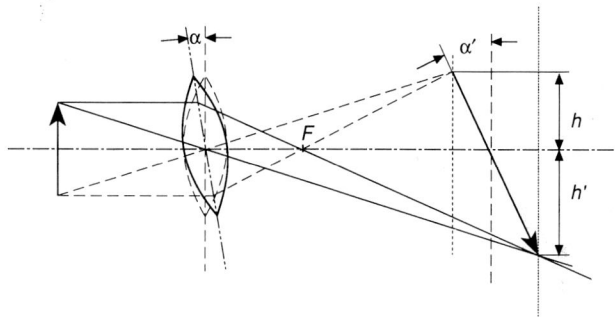

Fig. 3.47 Tilt in an optical system. Tilt is axisymmetric whereas coma is not.

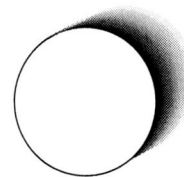

Fig. 3.48 Characteristic appearance of coma.

minimal visual angle possible is:

$$\tan aNb = \frac{ab}{bN} = \frac{0.002}{17.054} = \tan 24.14\,\text{s}$$

However, the ultimate resolving power of the eye is really determined by Rayleigh criterion. Here we must

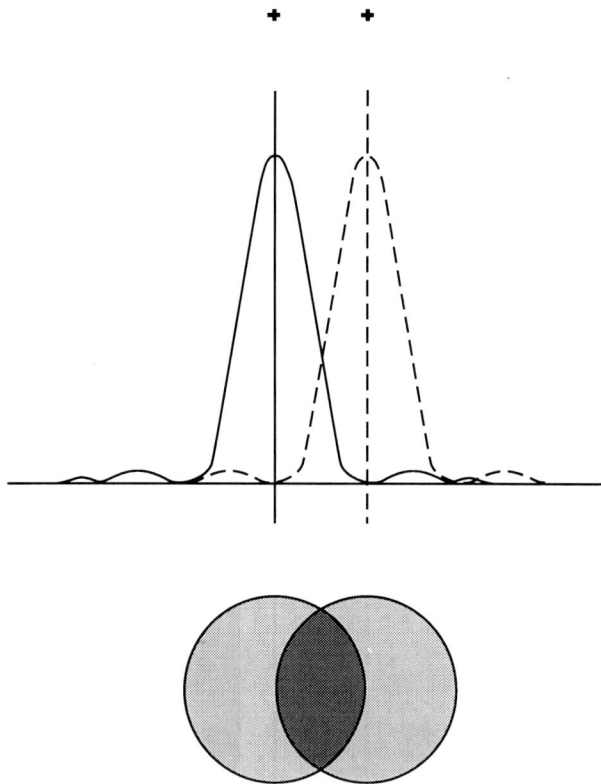

Fig. 3.49 Superimposed Airy disks demonstrating the principle of Rayleigh's criterion for resolving discrete objects. Only the central, bright spot is represented.

return to the wave nature of light and the subject of wavefronts. It must be remembered that a circular aperture such as the iris produces a diffraction effect resulting in an image that is made up of alternate dark and light rings surrounding a bright central disk (see Figure 3.15). The size of this disk is usually expressed as the angular radius of the first dark ring. In order to distinguish (resolve) two points, Lord Rayleigh suggested that a separation of the Airy disks by this magnitude is necessary (Figure 3.49). Thus the resolving power of the eye can be measured by calculating the size of the Airy disk using the formula:

$$\phi = \frac{1.22\lambda}{d}$$

where λ is the wavelength and d is the diameter of the pupil. Thus for yellow light and a pupillary diameter of 6.0 mm, the visual efficiency would be 0.3 min of arc; for a 2.0 mm pupil, 1.22 min (in blue light, 1.05 min).

We are used to estimating the efficiency of an optical system such as the eye by its resolving power. Today, however, we are hearing about a more sophisticated methodology of measurement—the modulation transfer function—applied to optics and the eye. This concept is borrowed from the study of electricity and

works because of the similarity of optical and electric systems. It is important for the reader to grasp this concept since it applies not only to light transmitted through the optical system of the eye but also to that reflected from its surface. Since it is the reflecting (or catadioptric) nature of the cornea which allows us to study its surface changes, a working knowledge of the concept of modulation transfer functions will assist in the interpretation and understanding of modern topographic mapping devices.

Any signal entering an electric system can be considered as a series of sinusoidal waveforms by means of Fourier analysis. According to Fourier's theorem, any wave, regardless of its complexity, can be reproduced by combining a number of waves of different amplitudes, frequencies, and phases. The emerging signal can be treated in the same manner, but the waves will differ among themselves depending upon how they have been attenuated by the system through which they have passed. The curve of attenuation against frequency is called the frequency response function.

The optical analog to this system lies in considering the light as a series of spatial frequencies, each representing an imaginary grating. The curve of amplitude against the spatial frequency is the optical transfer function. In both cases we are concerned with the change in frequency or phase; in other words, the modulation of the signal. Hence the term, modulation transfer function. Above a certain critical frequency, the "noise" from diffraction cancels out the response, thus the frequency is dependent upon the aperture. For 100% modulation, the absolute sensitivity of the eye with a 2.0 mm pupil is 0.5 min of arc.

It is possible to use this method to measure the contrast sensitivity of the retina alone since the production of interference fringes is largely unaffected by the focusing mechanism of the eye (we will have more to say about interference fringes in our discussion on corneal topography in Chapter 6). The relationship of this measurement and that of the visual apparatus as a whole is the transfer function of the dioptric apparatus.

The optics of the eye

It should be evident by now (see also Chapter 2), that the optics of the eye is a complex subject. It is made more so by the fact that a large part of the refraction occurs at a single surface, yet the eye must be considered as a thick-lens system. Despite the confusing behavior of the cardinal and nodal points of the eye their locations are the result of a logical application of the optical rules discussed in the previous section. Thus:

1 The eye cannot be considered a thin-lens system.

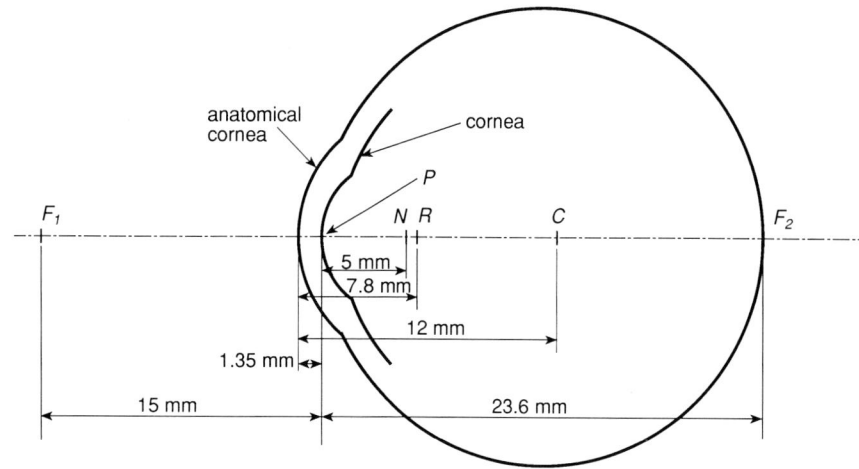

Fig. 3.50 The schematic eye of Listing.

Thus P_1, P_2, N_1, and N_2 are not superimposed in one position.

2 The eye has characteristics of a single refracting surface. Thus the anterior focal length is shorter than the posterior focal length. This means that the nodal points are shifted posteriorly. The distance between the first nodal point and the first principal point is equal to the distance between the second nodal point and the second focal point.

3 The eye is not optically homogeneous—there are several surfaces where refraction occurs because the eye is made up of various structures all having different indices of refraction. This fact also separates each of the principal and nodal points.

4 The eye is a variable optic. That is, accommodation can shift the overall refractive power of the eye toward the center of the lens.

Optical constants

Because of the complexity of the human optical system, ray tracing using the two-ray method becomes tedious. It has proved useful, therefore, to employ a schematic representation of the eye taking into account the various factors and replacing them with approximations. Several such schematic eyes have been devised. Listing was one of the first to do so, but most students of the human eye use the reduced eye of Gullstrand.

Table 3.1 Power of optical elements. Adapted from Helmholtz H. *Treatise on Physiological Optics*. JPC Southall (transl). Optical Society of America, New York, 1924

	Far	Near
Cornea	43	43
Lens	20	33
Total	60	71

Table 3.2 Indices of refraction. Adapted from Helmholtz H. *Treatise on Physiological Optics*. JPC Southall (transl). Optical Society of America, New York, 1924

Air	1.00
Cornea	1.37
Aqueous	1.33
Lens cortex	1.38
Lens nucleus	1.40
Vitreous	1.33

Table 3.3 Refracting surfaces. Adapted from Helmholtz H. *Treatise on Physiological Optics*. JPC Southall (transl). Optical Society of America, New York, 1924

	Radius (mm)	
	Far	Near
Anterior cornea	7.8	7.8
Anterior lens	10.0	5.3
Posterior lens	6.0	5.3

Table 3.4 Cardinal points. Adapted from Helmholtz H. *Treatise on Physiological Optics*. JPC Southall (transl). Optical Society of America, New York, 1924

	Distance from vertex of cornea (mm)	
	Far	Near
First principal point, P_1	1.5	1.8
Second principal point, P_2	1.6	2.0
First focal point, F_1	15.2	12.3
Second focal point, F_2	22.3	18.9
First nodal point, N_1	6.9	6.5
Second focal point, N_2	7.3	6.9
First focal length	16.7	14.1
Second focal length	22.3	18.9
Position of near point		100.8

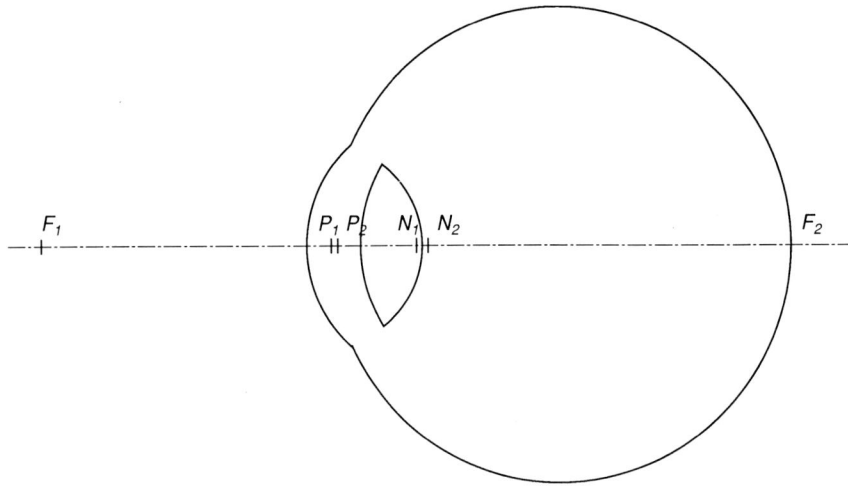

Fig. 3.51 The schematic eye of Gullstrand.

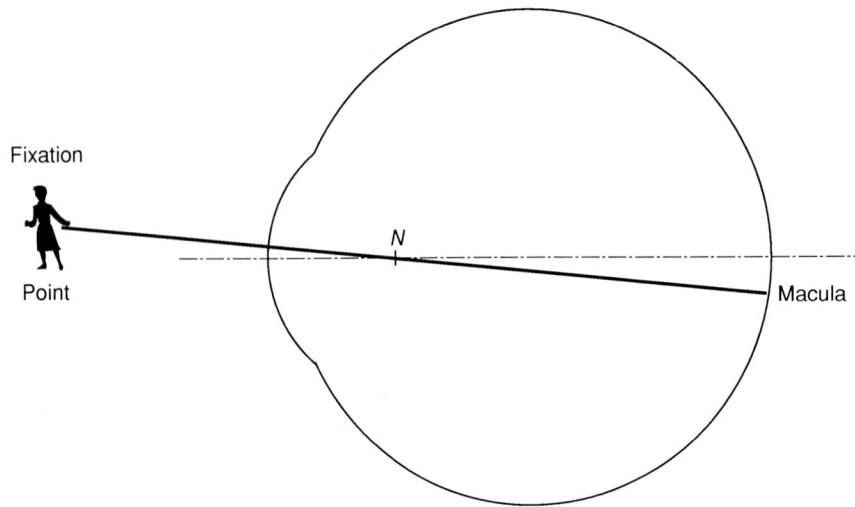

Fig. 3.52 The visual axis. It does not correspond to the geometric axis.

Reduced eye of Listing

This is somewhat more complex than that of Gullstrand. Figure 3.50 is derived from the modification by Donders.

Gullstrand's eye

The groups of ocular constants in Tables 3.1–3.4 are derived from Helmholtz and refer to Figure 3.51, the schematic eye of Gullstrand.

Those of particular concern to us are the anterior and posterior surfaces of the cornea and lens. Pertinent indices of refraction are those of the cornea, aqueous, lens, and vitreous. The axial length is also important in ray tracing and determines, many times, the optical state of the eye [8]. This schema can be even further simplified but the constants given will provide sufficient information and accuracy to use with any ray tracing computer program; among these the author

recommends BEAM4. The methods by which these constants were, are, or can be derived are many but are not germane to our discussion. The reader is referred to the appropriate literature for that information.

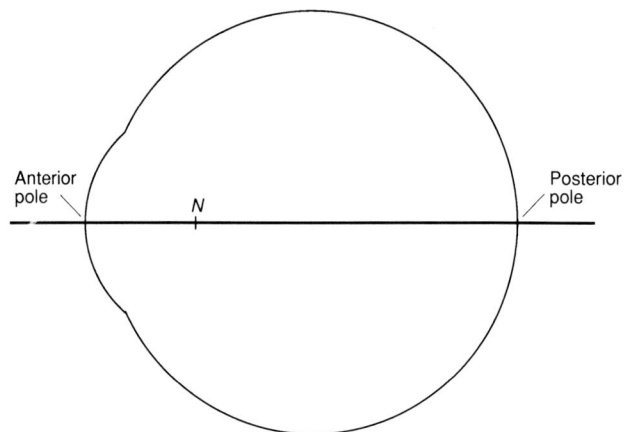

Fig. 3.53 Optic or geometric axis.

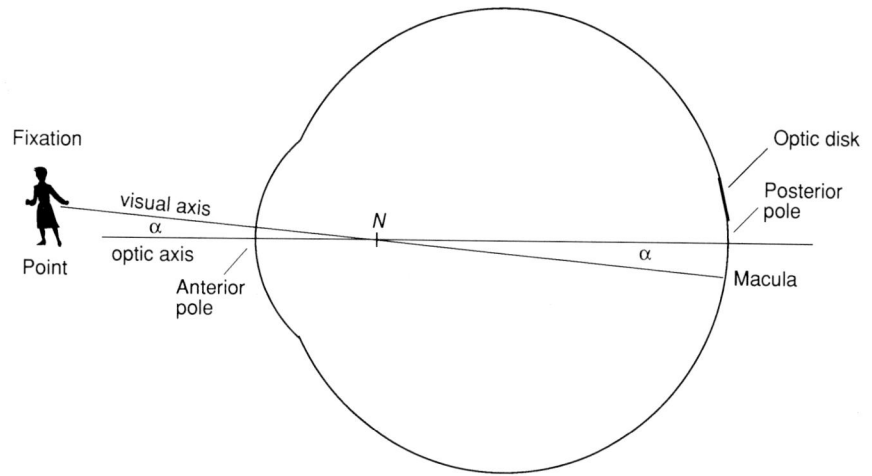

Fig. 3.54 Angle alpha.

Angles and axes of the eye

As we have already pointed out in Chapter 2, the optical complexity of the eye is compounded by the fact that the ocular components are not symmetrically aligned along a common axis. This fact has led to a veritable stew of angles and axes which are defined as follows:

1 The visual axis is an imaginary line passing through the macula, the nodal point and the object (fixation) point (Figure 3.52).

2 The optic axis (a real imaginary line—the stuff of fantasy) passes through the anterior and posterior poles of the eye and through the nodal point (Figure 3.53). As in any optic system it is the line along which

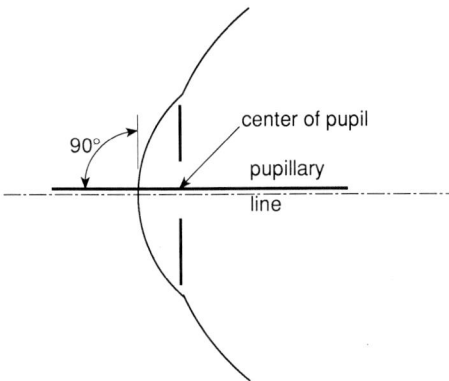

Fig. 3.55 Pupillary line.

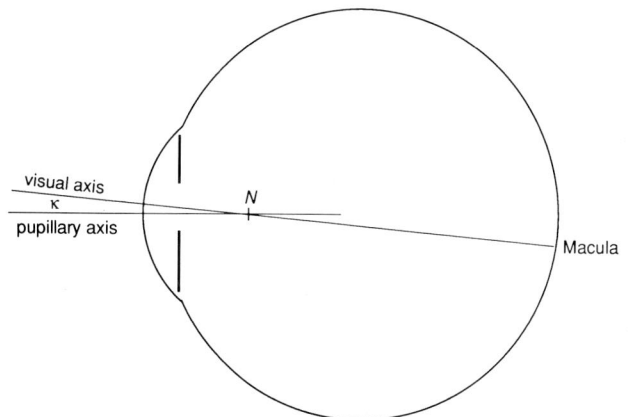

Fig. 3.57 Angle kappa—defined as the angle between the visual and pupillary axis at the nodal point.

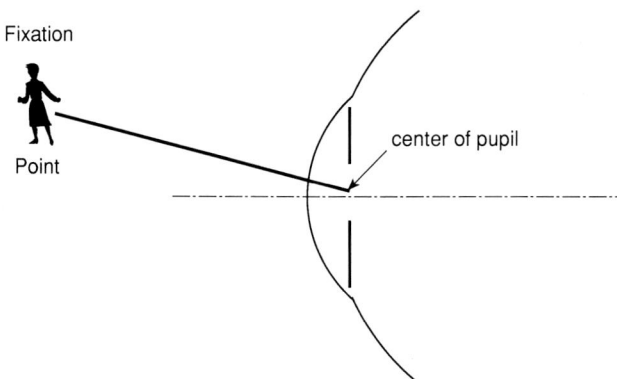

Fig. 3.56 The principal line of vision.

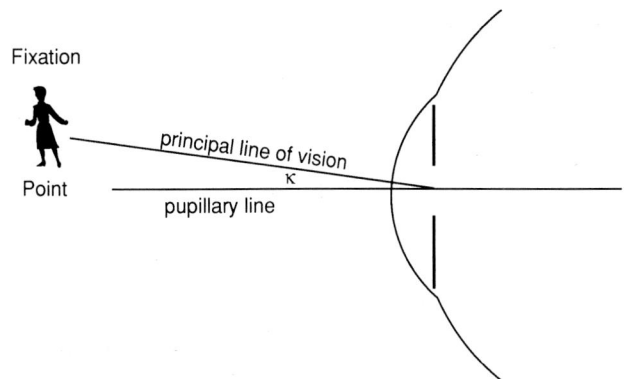

Fig. 3.58 Angle kappa—defined as the angle between the visual axis and the principal line of vision.

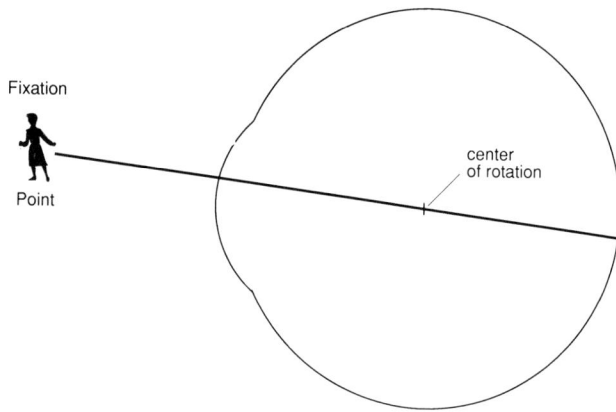

Fig. 3.59 The fixation axis passes through the center of rotation of the eye.

all the optical components of the eye are, theoretically, aligned. The operative word here is theoretically.

3 Angle α, typically 5°, is formed between the optic and visual axes at the nodal point (Figure 3.54).

4 The pupillary line (or axis) is drawn through the apparent center of the pupil, perpendicular to the corneal surface (Figure 3.55). It is not symmetric to the remainder of the optic system because the pupil is usually displaced nasally.

5 The principal line of vision is the axis from the apparent center of the pupil to the object (Figure 3.56). Note that this is not the same as the pupillary axis.

6 Angle κ is the angle formed between the visual and the pupillary axis (extended posteriorly) at the nodal point (Figure 3.57). It has also been defined as the angle between the pupillary axis and the principal line of vision (Figure 3.58). The difference between the two definitions is very small and can be ignored.

7 The fixation axis is the line joining the object with the center of rotation of the eye. The rotation point is usually located on the optic axis 13 mm posterior to the corneal surface (Figure 3.59).

8 Angle γ is the angle formed by the fixation and optic axes at the center of rotation (Figure 3.60).

Visual acuity

The current method of deriving the visual acuity uses various-size letters (called optotypes) printed or projected in a high-contrast setting (Figure 3.61). The acuity is recorded in terms of Snellen's fraction where the numerator is the distance (typically 20 ft or 6 m) at which the letter is viewed and the denominator is the relative distance (also in feet or meters) at which the letter will subtend an angle of 1 min on the retina. Other ways of expressing the fraction are in decimal notation or as a percentage. Thus 20/20 = 1.0 (or 100%),

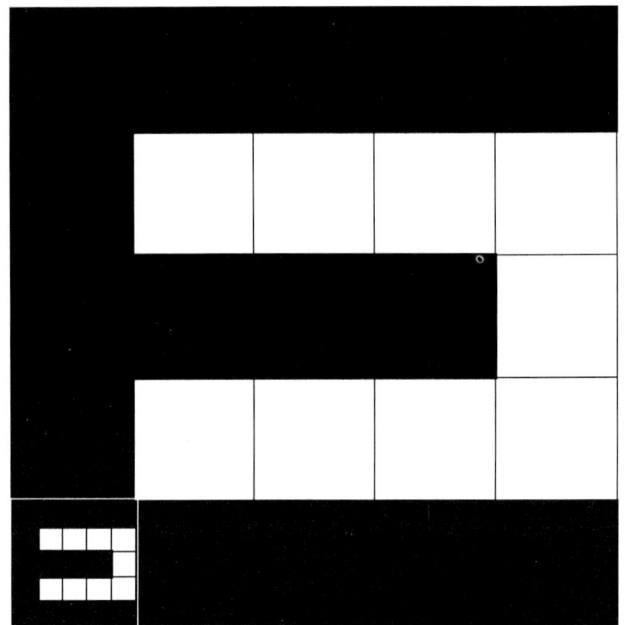

Fig. 3.61 The Snellen optotype showing the relationship between a 20/20 and a 20/200 letter.

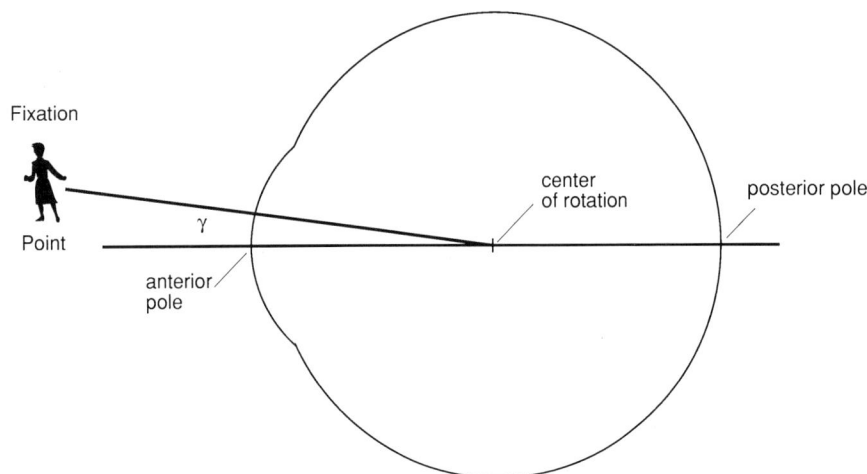

Fig. 3.60 Angle gamma.

20/40 = 0.5 (50%), 20/200 = 0.1 (10%), and so on. This method, in use for around 125 years, is a way to record ocular resolution in an artificial environment. The acuity measurement very much depends upon the contrast of the letter with the background. Unfortunately, the technique has few counterparts in the real world and equally unfortunate is the fact that it is firmly entrenched in society. It is well-known in clinical practice that the visual acuity as measured by the Snellen chart is often in no way indicative of the existence of a visual handicap. Many individuals with increased lenticular turbidity can discern 20/40 or better and yet are unable to recognize a face in normal lighting or drive safely at night. Contrast sensitivity methods are probably a more realistic test of visual efficiency but a standard has not yet been established for their use.

In any event this subject completes our brief discussion of light and optics, for the moment. Do not despair, however; we will encounter certain of the principles reviewed here from time to time in other parts of this treatise.

References

1 Young T. *A Course of Lectures on Natural Philosophy and the Mechanical Arts*. Royal Society, London, 1807.
2 Taton R. Roemer et la vitesse de la lumiere. In *Proceedings of the Centre National Reserche Scientifique*, Paris, 1976.
3 Fermat P. *Varia Opera Mathematica*. Joannem Pech, Tolosa, 1679.
4 Young T. On the theory of light and colours. Phil Trans R Soc Lond 1802; 92.
5 Gullstrand A. *Einfuhrung in die Methoden die Dioptrik des Auges*. Leipzig, 1911.
6 Kepler J. *Ad Vitellionem Paraliponema*. Frankfurt, 1604.
7 Kepler J. *Dioptrice*. Frankfurt, 1611.
8 Helmholtz H. *Treatise on Physiological Optics*, vol 1. J Southall (transl). Optical Society of America, New York, 1924.

Further reading

Born M, Wolf E. *Principles of Optics*. Macmillan & Co., New York, 1964.
Donders FC. *On the Anomalies of Accommodation and Refraction of the Eye*. WD Moore (transl). The Hatton Press, London, 1864.
Hardy AC, Perrin FH. *The Principles of Optics*. McGraw-Hill, New York, 1982.
von Helmholtz H. *Treatise on Physiological Optics*, vol 1. J Southall (transl). Optical Society of America, New York, 1924.
Jenkins F, White H. *Fundamentals of Optics* 3rd edn. McGraw-Hill, New York, 1957.
Ogle K. *Optics: An Introduction for Ophthalmologists*. Charles C. Thomas, Springfield, 1961.
Sears FW. Optics. In: *Principles of Physics*, vol III, 3rd edn. Addison-Wesley, Cambridge, 1948.
Tscherning M. *Physiological Optics*. C Weiland (transl). Philadelphia, 1904.

4

Anatomy and Physiology of Corneal Wound Healing

Iago: How poor are they that have not patience!
What wound didst ever heal but by degrees?
Thou knowest we work by wit and not by witchcraft?
And wit depends on dilitory time.
[Othello, Act II, Scene iii]

Corneal anatomy and physiology

The healing of corneal wounds is of vital concern to all ophthalmic surgeons. Recent years have seen the advent of many refractive surgical procedures. Such surgery has created entirely new wounding patterns and post-surgical stresses and tissue repair play a pivotal role in the end results of such procedures. It is appropriate, therefore, to consider the complex processes which take place during healing of the cornea. An understanding of the unique anatomic features of this structure also deserves review as a preface to a discussion of wound healing.

The constituents of the cornea are few, comprising only three distinctive cell types—epithelium, keratocytes, and endothelium—and an extracellular matrix made up of collagen and glycosaminoglycans (GAGs). The corneal structure includes five layers, the epithelium, Bowman's membrane, the stroma, Descemet's membrane and the endothelium (Figure 4.1).

Corneal epithelium

The corneal epithelium (Figure 4.2) is composed of five to eight layers of cells and is the most regularly arranged of all such squamous epithelia in the body. The nuclei of the basal layer are aligned with their long axes perpendicular to the corneal surface. Mitotic activity takes place in this basal layer. As new cells are produced, they gradually move to the surface. During this process, they become more flattened and are eventually cast off in the tear film, much like the epidermis. Unlike the skin, however, the normal cornea lacks a protective layer of keratin.

The epithelial cell membranes have complex interdigitations or folds which serve to hold them together along with fine filaments—tonofibrils (Figure 4.3). On the surface, these cell membrane folds take the form of microplicae and microvilli. This plication (folding) increases the effective epithelial surface and plays a key role in adhesion of the tear film. The basal cells secrete a basal lamina, which is intimately associated with Bowman's membrane. These basal cells are firmly attached to the basement lamina by hemidesmosomes, which are cytoplasmic/cell membrane modifications. Multiple fine, unmyelinated branches of the trigeminal nerve insinuate themselves between the cells of the basal layer to provide corneal sensation.

Although the term Bowman's membrane is in common use, it is not a true membrane—the preferable term is Bowman's layer. The thickness of this layer varies between 8 and 14 μm and is composed almost entirely of collagen with small amounts of GAGs interspersed, as a filler. Posteriorly, it blends imperceptibly with the corneal stroma.

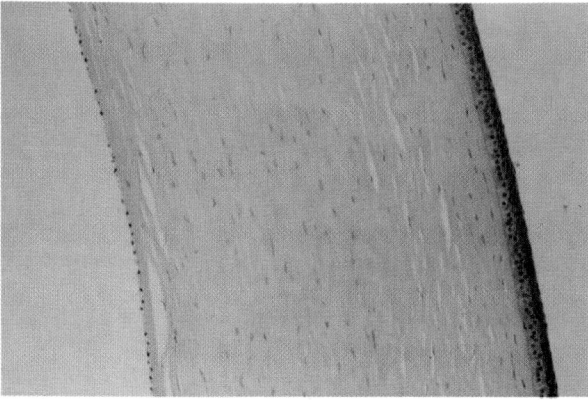

Fig. 4.1 Normal cornea. Hematoxylin & eosin, original magnification × 10.

Glycosaminoglycans

GAGs are macromolecules of the class proteoglycans (in the past called mucopolysaccharides). The bulk of corneal GAGs (65%) is made up of keratin sulfate and 30% is chondroitin-4 sulfate; the remainder is other types of chondroitin-GAGs. The role of GAG seems to be as a filler between collagen fibers and between the stromal keratocytes (see below). This filler role binds and separates the collagen fibers, this process maintains the transparency of the corneal stroma. It is remarkable that the cornea is as clear as it is, consider-

ing that it is made up of layers of fiber bundles all of which can produce diffraction and scattering of light [1]. There are, after all, some small variations in refractive index of the fibers and surrounding matrix. However, as discussed in Chapter 3, if such differences in indices are distanced less than half the wavelength of light apart (or about 200 nm), transparency is preserved. If that distance increases—such as from interstitial edema—the corneal fibers begin to act as a sinusoidal grating, the modulation transfer function of the stroma is altered and scattering is increased, as happens in a sunset on a dusty day [2,3]. GAGs also seem to be responsible for the imbibition (swelling) pressure drawing water into the cornea [4].

Collagen

Collagen is made up of another group of macromolecules termed glycoproteins (which also includes mucins). Collagen makes up approximately 71% of the dry corneal weight, and is the most abundant protein in the body [5]. In the cornea, collagen is present as the sub-epithelial basement membrane, the fibrils of Bowman's layer, the stromal lamellae, and Descemet's membrane.

Production of collagen begins intracellularly with the synthesis of recursor forms in the rough endoplasmic reticulum, followed by secretion, probably through the

(a)

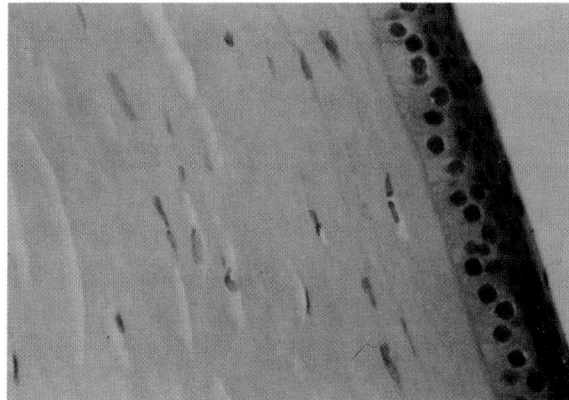

(b)

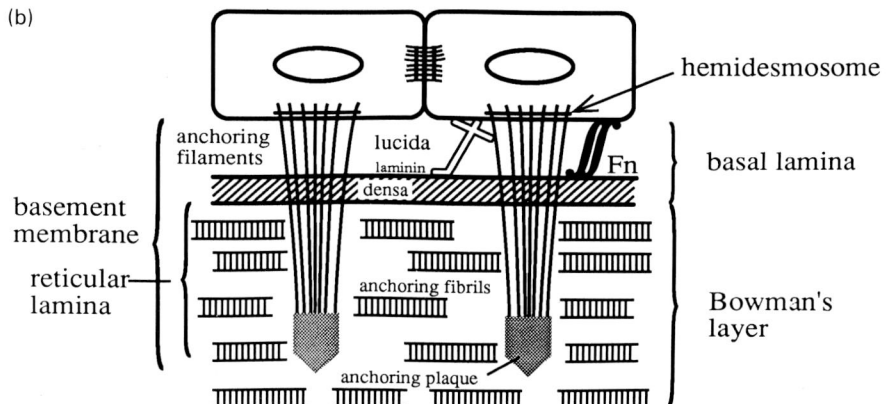

Fig. 4.2 (a) Corneal epithelium, Bowman's membrane and anterior stroma. Hematoxylin & eosin, original magnification × 80. (b) Schematic of the relationship of the basal columnar cells to Bowman's layer (from Beuerman RW, Crosson CE, Kaufman HE. *Healing Processes in the Cornea*, vol 1. Gulf, Houston, p 243, 1989).

(a)

(c)

(b)

(d)

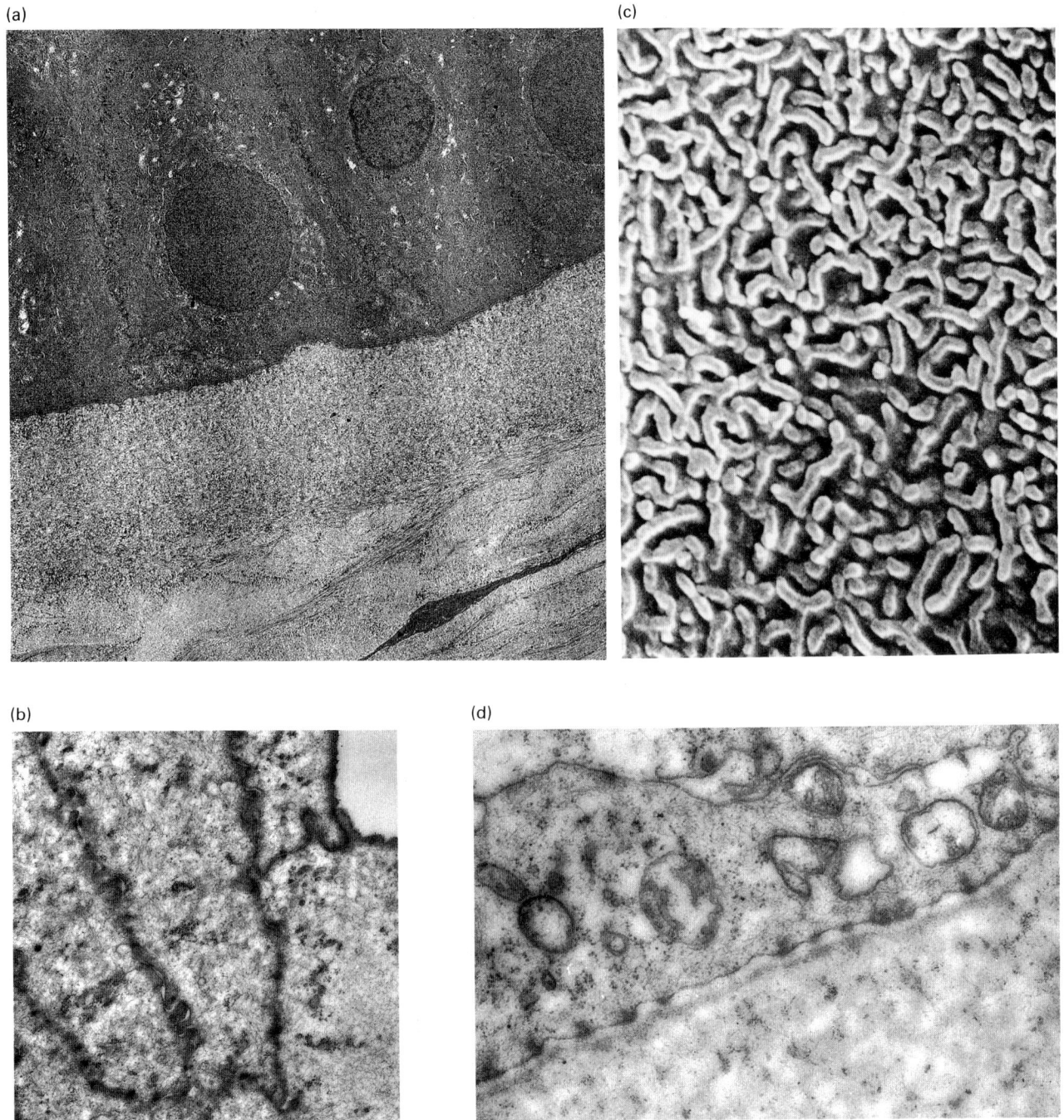

Fig. 4.3 (a) Corneal section at Bowman's layer showing columnar basal cells, and basal lamella. Note how Bowman's blends into the underlying stroma. Original magnification × 15 200. (b) Corneal epithelium, showing the numerous sites of attachment along adjacent cell membranes. Original magnification × 27 400.

(c) Microvilli. Original magnification × 15 000. (d) Basal layer of corneal epithelium. Numerous hemidesmosomes attach to a thin basal lamina which merges with Bowman's membrane. Original magnification × 31 800.

Golgi apparatus. Production of sub-units called pro-α chains comes first with linking of amino acid chains. Hydroxylation of these chains then takes place along with some glycosylation. This process causes the maturing pro-α chains to twist into individual helices which then ravel together with two others, to form procollagen. Looking for all the world like loosely twisted yarn with fuzzy ends—one end twisted and one straight—they are then excreted from the cell. Further development continues extra-cellularly where the non-helical peptide ends are trimmed off enzymatically leaving the finished basic unit of collagen—

chain and is designated as $\alpha 1(I)_2\alpha(2)$. Type II collagen, found in cartilage, is designated as $\alpha 1(II)_3$. Type III, which is frequently found in association with type I in skin, blood vessels, and smooth muscle, is designated as $\alpha 1(III)_3$. There is also basement membrane collagen (type IV) whose exact α chain composition has not been completely worked out and type AB (type V) probably consisting of two αB and one αA chains [6,7].

Corneal stroma

The corneal stroma comprises over 90% of the normal corneal thickness. The major component of the stroma consists of mainly types I and V collagen arranged in a lamellar array (Figure 4.5). The corneal lamellae have an average thickness of 2 μm and each extends across the entire breadth of the cornea. These lamellae are arranged in a highly regular fashion, as are the collagen fibers, of which they are composed. This regular arrangement plays a central role in corneal transparency, as noted above. Small amounts of GAGs are also present and constitute about 1% of the cornea's wet weight. The keratocytes are modified fibroblasts which are few in number and show little activity in the normal cornea.

Descemet's membrane

Descemet's membrane is the acellular basal lamina of the corneal endothelium. Compared with other basal laminae, it is unusually thick, reaching 10–12 μm by adult life (Figure 4.6). It is composed of fine filaments of collagen—probably type IV in large part—which merge with the corneal stroma. It is highly unusual in that it has a high carbohydrate content and is amor-

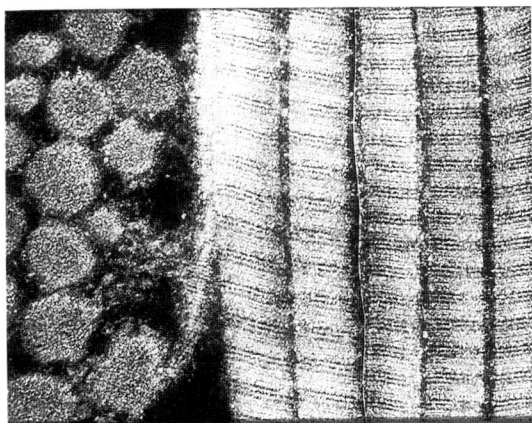

Fig. 4.4 Characteristic banding seen in collagen fibrils. Original magnification × 50 000.

tropocollagen. Collagen fibrils in their native state are made up of these tropocollagen molecules (approximately 300 nm in length) arranged in a staggered manner with about a 25% overlap. It is this overlapping that produces the characteristic banding pattern seen in electron micrographs, at approximately 67 nm (Figure 4.4).

There are five collagen types which are defined by the kinds of α chains present, of which there are four. These four α chains are $\alpha 1$, $\alpha 2$, αA and αB, among which there is some heterogeneity depending upon the location of certain amino acids within these chains. Thus there is a type I $\alpha 1$ chain (denoted as $\alpha 1(I)$) found primarily in skin, for example. Of the five collagen types there is type I found in bone tendon and skin—Bowman's layer probably contains type I collagen. Type I collagen consists of two $\alpha 1(I)$ chains and one $\alpha 2$

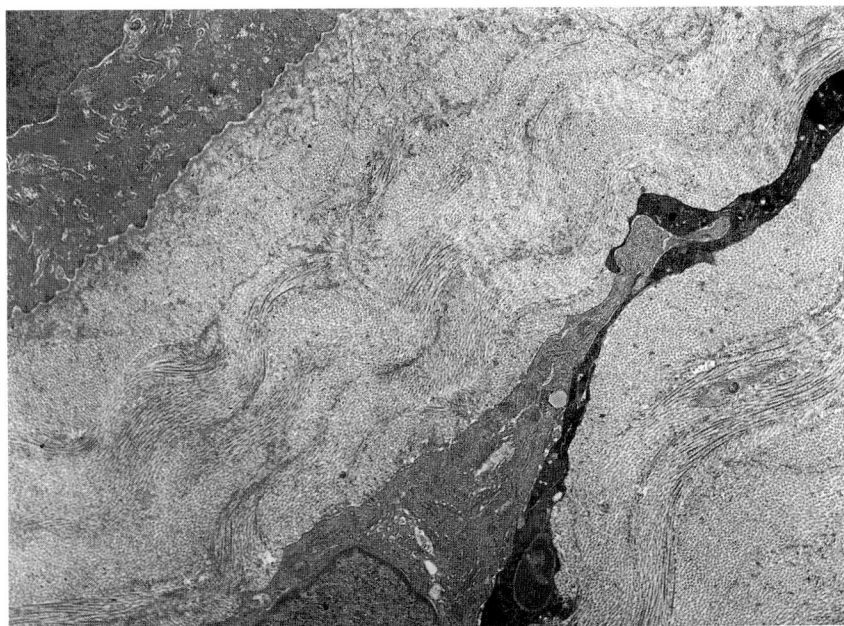

Fig. 4.5 Corneal stroma demonstrating the interlacing of collagen fibers surrounding a keratocyte. Note the layered nature of the stroma. Original magnification × 10 500.

(a)

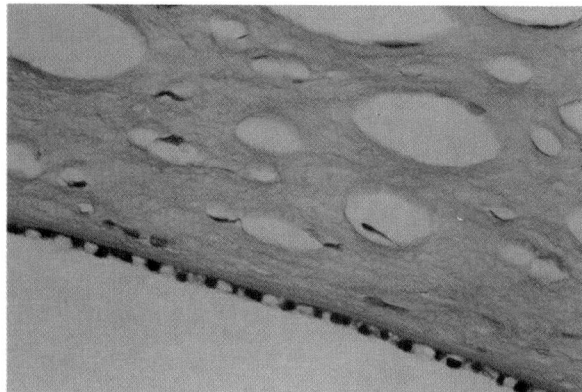

(b)

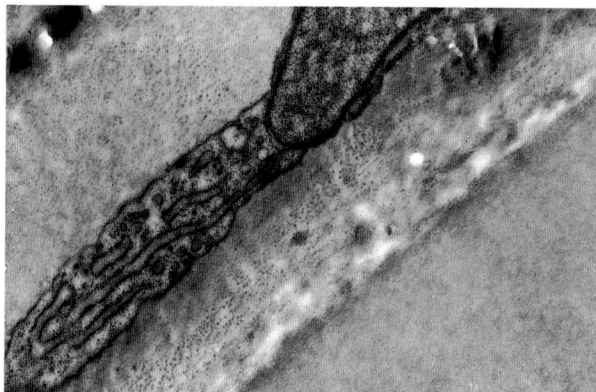

Fig. 4.6 (a) Corneal endothelium, Descemet's membrane and the posterior corneal stroma. Hematoxylin & eosin, original magnification × 100. (b) Next to the stroma, Descemet's membrane is a heterogeneous layer of larger collagen filaments. Original magnification × 16600.

phous. Although Bowman's layer does not undergo repair if interrupted, small gaps in Descemet's membrane may be healed by overlying endothelial cells. Descemet's membrane undergoes a variety of pathologic changes during life and in various disease states. The most common of these changes is diffuse or focal thickening—corneal gutta.

Corneal endothelium

The corneal endothelium (Figure 4.7) is a monolayer of cells which, in humans, does not proliferate during adult life. Because of this, there is a progressive decline in cell density with age. Focal defects in the endothelial sheet are covered by spreading of adjacent cells; individual cells become larger and the cell count drops. Accidental or surgical trauma may produce a precipitous decline in the endothelial cell population. Because the endothelium is responsible for normal corneal detumescence, a significant loss of endothelial cells may be associated with corneal decompensation and edema (see also Chapter 7). The intercellular space between adjacent cells is closed at the apex (facing the anterior chamber) by gap junctions and tight junctions which impede the flow of some substances. Many mitochondria are found in the endothelial cells, reflecting their vigorous metabolic activity [8]. Most of this activity appears to involve the active transport of bicarbonate and is capable of moving fluid at 6.5 ml/cm² per hour against normal hydrostatic pressure [9–11].

Corneal hydration

We have already alluded to corneal transparency and the role that GAGs play in it. It should be apparent that the hydration of the cornea is crucial to the maintenance of this transparency. Corneal stroma ordinarily has a higher water content than most connective tissue elsewhere in the body. The presence of this water is due to the water-binding capacity of GAG. This affinity for water tends to swell the cornea producing stromal swelling pressure (SP) (Figure 4.8). This pressure is considerable—amounting to 40–50 mmHg at normal corneal thickness—thus variations in intra-ocular pressure up to 50 mmHg will have virtually no effect on corneal thickness [12,13]. However, this pressure decreases as the cornea swells such that when it is twice its normal thickness, the SP has dropped to about one-third (Figure 4.9). This mechanism also works in the opposite direction. Thus if the cornea becomes dehydrated, the tendency to swell (by imbibition) is greatly increased, and an equilibrium is therefore maintained, normally.

Both the epithelium and endothelium act as barriers to the rapid influx of water into the stroma—some leakage occurs. Epithelium is 2000 times more resistant to fluid transfer than the stroma and 200 times more than the endothelium. This osmotic gradient tends to retain fluid within the stroma and requires an active pumping mechanism to remove it [14]. The epithelium is, therefore, an almost perfect semi-permeable membrane but it is highly vulnerable to damage.

Evaporation of water from the corneal surface is a constant process between blinks. This results in hypertonicity of the tear film layer which produces an osmotic gradient causing fluid to be pulled out of the cornea. In the normal cornea this results in a slight thinning of the cornea during the day, increasing in the afternoon when the blink rate decreases [15]. This mechanism has more effect on epithelial edema and accounts for the fact that many patients with mild or early epithelial edema experience poor vision immediately upon awakening which gradually clears as the day goes on. Sometimes edema will persist in the upper part of the cornea hidden by the upper lid, which is not exposed to the effects of evaporation. As the epithelial gets

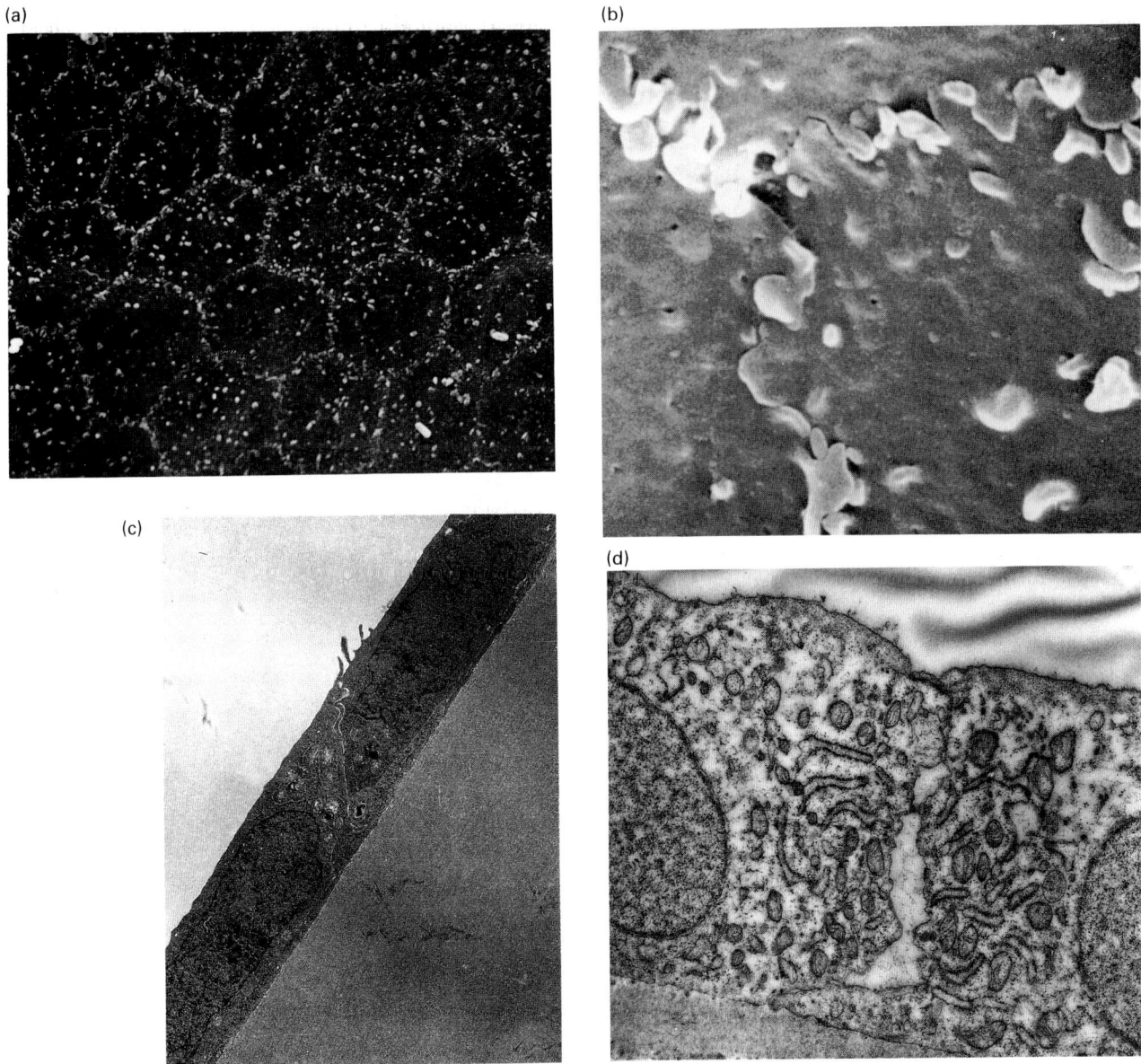

Fig. 4.7 (a) Scanning electron micrograph of corneal endothelium, showing the hexagonal pattern of the cells and their complex interdigitations. Original magnification × 2250. (b) Higher-power view of the endothelium. Original magnification × 30 000. (c) Side view of the endothelium showing how the interdigitation lies in two planes. Original magnification × 10 250. (d) The corneal endothelium lies on Descemet's membrane. The cells are joined on the anterior chamber side by short flap junctions. Original magnification × 26 100.

"sicker," edema becomes so severe that evaporation cannot keep up with the influx of fluid.

It is surprising just how thick the cornea can become as a result of edema before it produces a noticeable effect on vision. For example, in bovine cornea, a transparency equivalent of 20/30 was maintained with up to a 60% increase in thickness [16]. This swelling is an almost universal finding after radial keratotomy. Simple incisions through Bowman's layer deep into the stroma are always accompanied by an increase in corneal thickness without noticeable changes in corneal clarity. This swelling begins immediately and is prob-

ably responsible for the incision depth irregularity seen in early cases (see also Chapter 8). It is also persistent. The author has recorded significant increases in corneal thickness (20–30μm) for periods in excess of 22 months; this has also been reported elsewhere [17]. In a cornea whose pre-operative central thickness is 500 μm, such an increase would amount to 6% of the total. This is a significant amount and must be considered in any repeat incisional refractive surgery (see also Chapter 8).

On the other hand, epithelial edema affects vision much sooner and to a greater extent, even when the

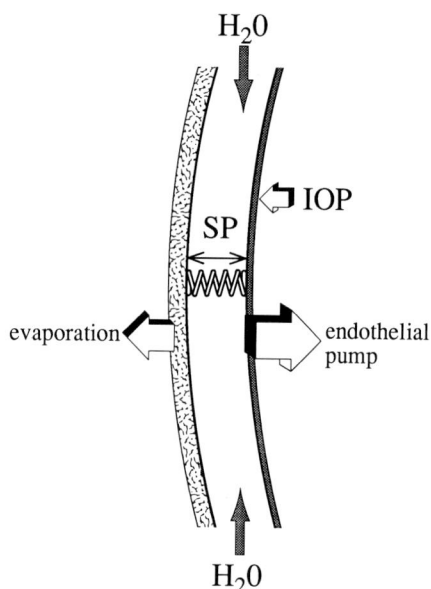

Fig. 4.8 Factors affecting hydration of the cornea. The tendency of the stroma to swell (swelling pressure (SP)) is balanced by the barriers imposed by the epithelium and endothelium, as well as by the endothelial pump. Evaporation plays a minor role, and intra-ocular pressure has almost no effect over a wide range of pressures.

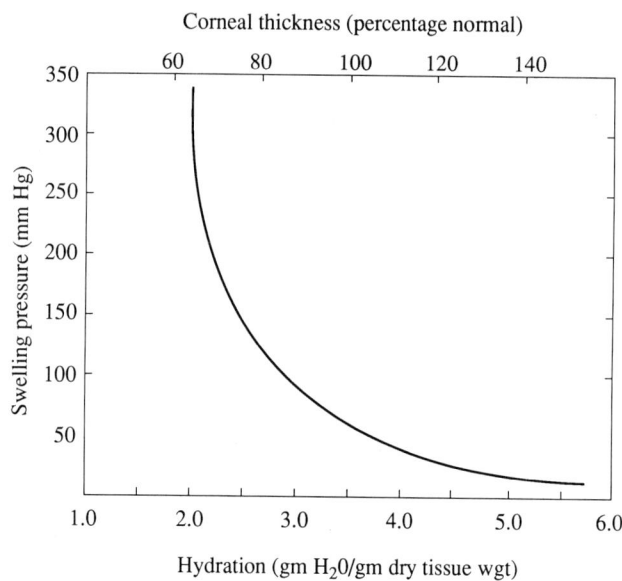

Fig. 4.9 Swelling pressure, hydration, and thickness of the cornea. As corneal thickness and hydration increase, the tendency to swell decreases (from Dohlman CH. Physiology of the cornea: corneal edema. In: *The Cornea. Scientific Foundations and Clinical Practice*, G Smolin and RA Thoft (eds). Little, Brown, Boston, 1983).

swelling can only be seen at the slit-lamp. This is probably due to the scattering of light within and between the cells themselves but also due to the increased microscopic irregularity of the surface, as in a poorly glued tile floor whose edges are beginning to curl up.

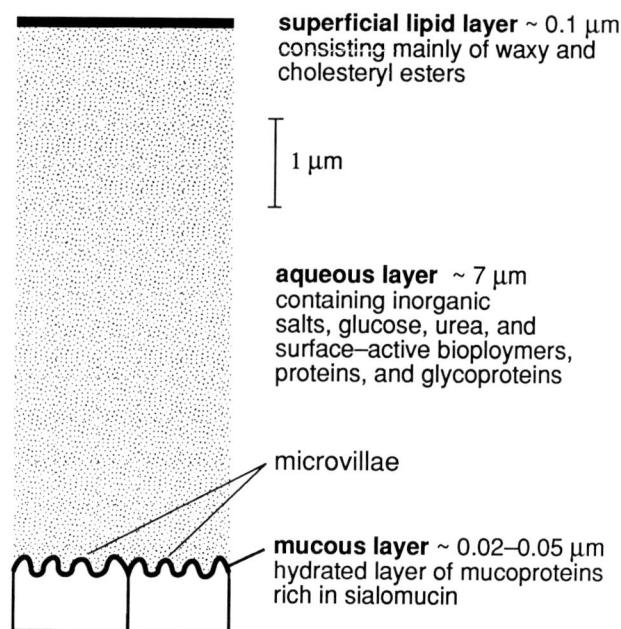

Fig. 4.10 The three layers of the tear film (from Holly FJ, Lemp MA. Tear physiology and dry eyes. Surv Ophthalmol 1977; 22:69–87).

The tear film

Of the layers of the cornea, the tear film can be thought of as the sixth since the cornea does not function well without it and because it is more complex than a mere aqueous layer (Figure 4.10). Classically, the tear film has been considered a three-tiered structure composed of lipid, aqueous, and mucous layers from top to bottom. It is probably better thought of as a two-layer structure—a thin lipid layer (0.1 μm) overlying a thick aqueous lake—because the mucous layer belongs to the epithelial cells to which it is intimately attached [18,19]. This tear film, including the mucous layer, is about 7 μm in thickness.

The lipid layer is secreted by the meibomian glands and is always fluid in the living eye. It should be considered as independent of the underlying aqueous layer. Anchored as it is to the orifices of the meibomian glands, it does not take part in tear flow. It is compressed on a blink and rapidly spreads over the corneal surface upon opening of the lids. Its purpose is to retard evaporation of the aqueous layer and to prevent overflow of tears. As the lipid spreads over the aqueous layer it drags liquid with it, thickening the tear film—the Marangoni effect (Figure 4.11). This of course presupposes a relatively smooth corneal surface—something which may not be present immediately following corneal refractive surgery.

Table 4.1 represents a composite of studies on the content of the aqueous layer [19]. At one time it was thought that the cornea obtained its nutrients from the

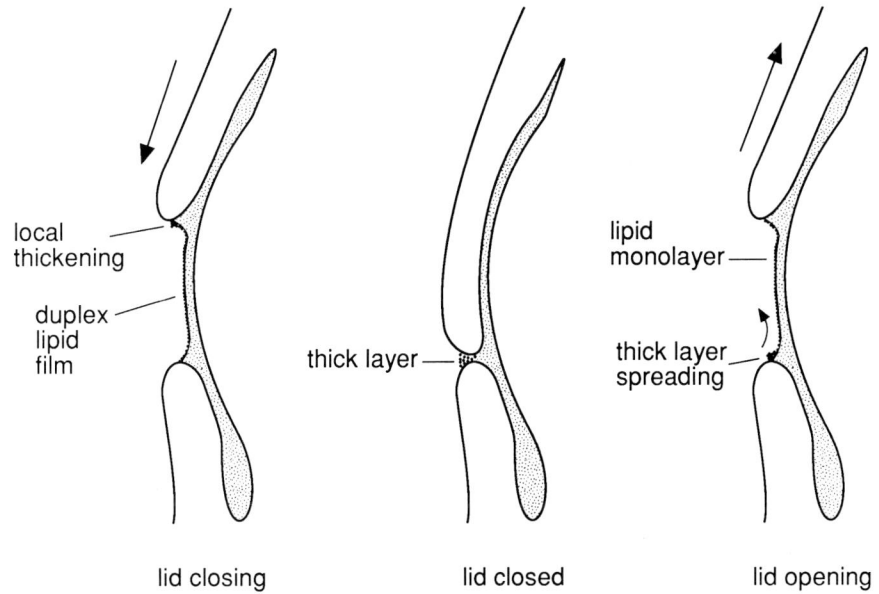

Fig. 4.11 The dynamics of the tear film during a blink.

lid closing   lid closed   lid opening

Table 4.1 Composition of tears. From Lamberts DW. Physiology of the cornea: physiology of the tear film. In: *The Cornea. Scientific Foundations and Clinical Practice*, G Smolin and RA Thoft (eds). Little, Brown, Boston, 1983

Component	Concentration
Water	98.2%
Sodium	145 mmol/l
Potassium	20 mmol/l
Chloride	128 mmol/l
Bicarbonate	26 mmol/l
Calcium	2.11 mg/dl
Magnesium	Trace
Zinc	Trace
Glucose	3 mg/100 ml
Amino acids	8 mg/100 ml
Urea	7–20 mg urea N/100 ml
Oxygen	155 mmHg (eyes open)
Total protein	$0.9 \pm 0.1\%$
Lysozyme	1.3 ± 0.6 mg/ml
Complement	Present
Mucus secretory substance	Present
Lysosomal hydrolases	Present
Lysosomal enzymes	Present
Lactate and pyruvate	Present

tear layer. This has been shown not to be true [20]. However, the cornea does receive the major portion of its oxygen supply from the tear layer. Another important component within the tear film is lysozyme, which is secreted by the lacrimal gland [21]. Lysozyme destroys bacterial cell wall integrity and thus aids in keeping the corneal surface relatively sterile. Other enzymes are also said to be present.

The entire immunoglobulin complement pathway is also present within the tears as well as specific antibodies against such things as herpes simplex, trachoma, and influenza viruses [19].

The mucous layer

The hydrophilic mucous layer serves to make the hydrophobic epithelial cells wettable both by coating the surface and resisting lipid contamination. This layer is secreted by the goblet cells of the conjunctiva and serves also to stabilize the tear film. This stabilization is assisted by the second role of the mucus, as a surfactant. Sufficient mucus dissolves within the aqueous layer to lower its surface tension, thus making it a better wetting agent.

Tear film dynamics

An understanding of the tear film dynamics can be useful. The process proceeds as follows: after a blink, the upper lid wipes the cornea and resurfaces it with a fresh, clean layer of mucus. At rest, the mucous layer is separated from the lipid layer by the aqueous phase of the tear film. After a blink, however, the lipid becomes admixed somewhat with the aqueous layer, eventually reaching the mucus. The lipid adheres to the mucus and eventually this lipid contamination can reach such a level that the mucus becomes hydrophobic. The tear film then ruptures, and a dry spot forms on the cornea (Figure 4.12). Enough mucus must be present to resist the lipid contamination until the next blink occurs—which is what happens in a normal eye—a blink occurs before a dry spot appears [22].

Rose Bengal dye is a useful tool that does not see sufficient application, in this author's opinion. However, it is a beneficial adjunct to the surgeon's "tool-

evaporation

superficial lipid layer
aqueous
adsorbed mucin layer
corneal epithelium

flow   diffusion   flow

tear breakup

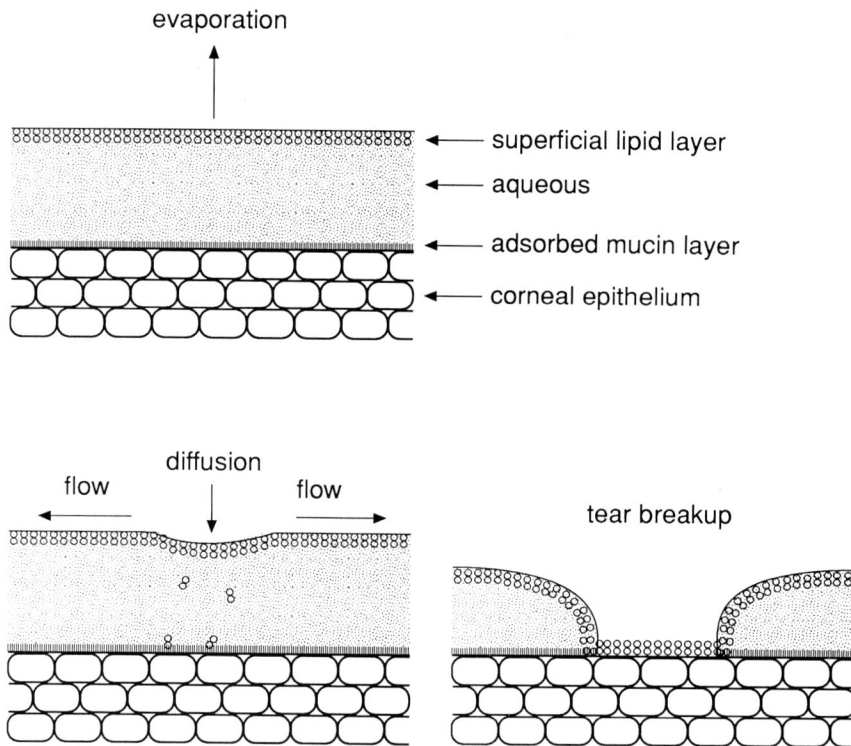

Fig. 4.12 The mechanism of tear breakup. Lipid contaminates the mucin layer from the mixing that occurs during the blink. Eventually the hydrophilic mucin layer becomes hydrophobic.

box." It is a vital stain that marks not only injured epithelium but also lipid-contaminated mucus and corneal filaments—which fluorescein will not.

Tear breakup time

Another useful tool is the tear breakup time (BUT), a measure of the stability of the tear film and thus indirectly the health of the goblet cells as well as the lacrimal apparatus (although there can be many causes for a shortened BUT). The test is conducted by placing a drop or two of fluorescein dye on the eye and having the patient blink several times. Without touching the lids, the time in seconds from the blink to the appearance of a dark spot on the surface (where there is no wetting) is measured. This event should be recorded several times and averaged. The dark spots should appear in random areas for the test to be accurate. While the test itself has been subjected to criticism for several shortcomings, it does, withal, provide useful information on the state of the tear film and is easily done. It is recommended in all cases of corneal refractive surgery as part of the pre-surgical workup. A subnormal BUT, while not contraindicating surgery, can serve as a harbinger of possible problems in the postoperative period. To be forewarned is to be forearmed —sufficient irregularity may exist in the corneal surface following refractive surgery to make a marginal case of inadequate tearing pre-operatively take on the proportions of a major problem post-operatively.

Corneal wound healing

Our understanding of corneal wound healing is enhanced by comparing it with events in other tissues. Wound healing throughout the body is the end result of a sequence of events, controlled and modulated by many factors. Briefly, when a wound occurs, there is bleeding, the clotting cascade is activated, and bleeding ceases. Concurrently, proteolytic enzymes digest the injured tissues, local cells become active and proliferate, and there is an acute inflammatory response. Phagocytosis of devitalized tissue is followed by fibroblastic and vascular proliferation. Collagen synthesis is succeeded by contraction and remodeling of the scar which closes off the process. It is pertinent to note that while much attention has been paid to the processes which initiate healing, little is known about how it ceases. In the cornea, for example, vessels will grow in response to a stimulus, but stop when the stimulus is removed. The control mechanism for this phenomenon is unknown. Elements of the clotting cascade, growth factors, and angiogenic factors may all prove pivotal in the control of wound healing and vascularization.

Compared to cutaneous healing, corneal wound repair is more complex. The cornea has a higher degree of differentiation and organization than does the dermis. Bowman's and Descemet's membranes and their healing patterns are unique. The vital role played by the corneal endothelium has no exact parallel elsewhere in the body. The absence of a vascular system in the normal cornea leaves the immune system out of the healing loop in many instances, which results in a slower rate of healing.

It would be easy to conclude that the hemostatic system plays no role in corneal wound healing. However, plasminogen activator has been detected in clear cornea [23] and free fibrin is found in the tissues during the critical period of endothelial mitosis, when corneal vascularization is induced [24]. Indeed, fibrin appears at the earliest stages of neovascularization and then disappears when new vessel growth is complete. This suggests a relationship of this clotting product to the process of new vessel formation, a hypothesis which deserves additional study.

Formation and contraction of scar tissue, which usually signals a successful conclusion to wound healing elsewhere, can be a functional disaster in the cornea, leading to loss of vision, irregular astigmatism, or corneal ectasia. Control of scar tissue formation and vascularization is essential for proper healing of corneal wounds. The purpose of this first section is to review the pathophysiology of corneal wound healing and to provide a basis for the following section which deals with histology and wound healing in refractive surgery.

Epithelial healing

When an epithelial wound is made without damage to other corneal structures, the physical process of healing is relatively simple. Two steps are involved: migration of existing cells and proliferation of those cells to restore the normal thickness of the epithelial sheet. Shortly after the occurrence of an epithelial defect, the basal epithelial cells at the wound margin become flatter and begin to slide across the defect (Figure 4.13) [25,26]. The movement is mediated by intercellular actin filament formation and contraction. The process is inhibited by exposure to cytochalasin B which is known to block the assembly of actin filaments within the cytoplasm of epithelial cells. In contrast, colchicine, which inhibits microtubule formation, has no effect on epithelial migration [27].

A second essential component for epithelial migration is fibronectin. Both in tissue culture and in living animals, fibronectin has a role in epithelial resurfacing. Cell surface receptors for fibronectin have been identified. These receptors help the corneal epithelial cell bind to fibronectin by way of the intercellular actin filaments. Contraction of the actin filaments helps the cell move across the epithelial defect. When corneal healing is complete, the fibronectin disappears [28].

The next steps in healing of an epithelial defect are mitosis and proliferation of the epithelial cells which serve to return the epithelium to its original thick-

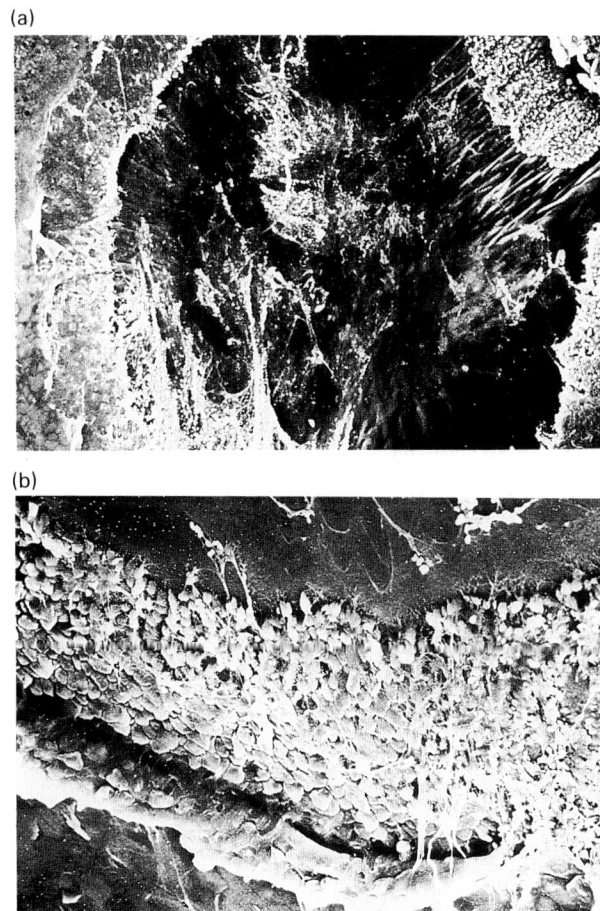

Fig. 4.13 (a) Scanning electron micrograph of healing corneal abrasion. Original magnification × 1000. (b) Epithelium sliding covers bare stroma. Original magnification × 4000.

ness [29]. There is increasing evidence that these changes are mediated by growth factors. In 1953, Levi-Montalcini and Hamburger discovered nerve growth factor (NGF) and demonstrated its ability to cause nerve cells to grow [30]. In 1962, Cohen isolated epidermal growth factor (EGF) from the submaxillary glands of mice [31]. Subsequently, a host of other growth factors have been isolated and characterized. Many of these factors may exert an influence on corneal wound healing.

EGF is a strong mitogen for corneal epithelium in the presence of stroma, but does not have this effect on isolated epithelial cells in tissue culture. This is a good example of the interaction of different corneal tissues, discussed later in this chapter. The effect is so strong that in some experimental situations the epithelium becomes hyperplastic and thicker than normal [32,33]. In contrast, the use of EGF in clinical situations is disappointing. It is hypothesized that this may be due to saturation of the system. In other words, all receptor sites are occupied by naturally occurring EGF and the system is being driven at maximum speed [34]. Fibroblast growth factor (FGF) is also a mitogen for corneal epithelium. Its effect varies with the dosage, unlike EGF. Its role in normal healing remains to be defined [35]. It is highly likely that other growth factors may also modulate wound healing. There has been some discussion about the possible use of FGF or other growth factor to accelerate healing in radial keratotomy, for example. If such an application succeeded in stabilizing the normally seen curvature fluctuations, that would be good. If, instead, it stimulated the progression of the scarring mechanism that would be bad—some radial keratotomy patients have already demonstrated spontaneous and progressive corneal flattening. Additionally, some of the effect of radial keratotomy is seen over time, thus timing of the application of growth factor would be critical. Some mechanism to turn off the action and thus prevent progression of the scarring complex would be handy to have.

The normal corneal epithelium becomes attached to its basement membrane and to Bowman's layer by the hemidesmosomes. These filamentous microstructures join the basal cells to their basal lamina. These attachment bodies are absent in epithelium migrating over a debrided surface and during the proliferative phase of healing. When healing is complete, they reform, at which point the corneal epithelium returns to a resting state.

The situation is more complex if a wound extends into Bowman's layer or the stroma. With a small wound in Bowman's, the defect is filled by epithelium to form an epithelial facet (Figure 4.14). Bowman's layer does not regenerate. If the damage to Bowman's layer and the basement membrane of the epithelium is severe, epithelial healing may be slowed. The absence of a basement membrane often interferes with the formation of hemidesmosomes by the basal cells. The lack of attachment of the basal cells can lead to repeated epithelial breakdown—a finding characteristic of a number of corneal problems, such as recurrent erosion, Cogan's microcystic dystrophy, and other anterior membrane dystrophies [36,37]. The loss of Bowman's layer in laser ablative techniques suggests that there may be a risk of recurrent corneal erosions, if there is interference with hemidesmosome formation.

In a deep stromal wound, the healing process shows interaction between the epithelium and stroma. Inflammatory cells from the tear film are attracted to the injured tissue. The tendency of epithelium to cover bare surfaces results in a migration of epithelial cells into the stromal wound. Epithelial proliferation fills the gap and forms an epithelial plug (Figure 4.15). This chain of events is typical of an early radial keratotomy wound. In the normal course of events, stromal healing occurs. Formation of new collagen and scar tissue pushes the epithelial plug out with a return to a more normal appearance (Figure 4.16). With broad, irregular stromal wounds, this may be a prolonged process.

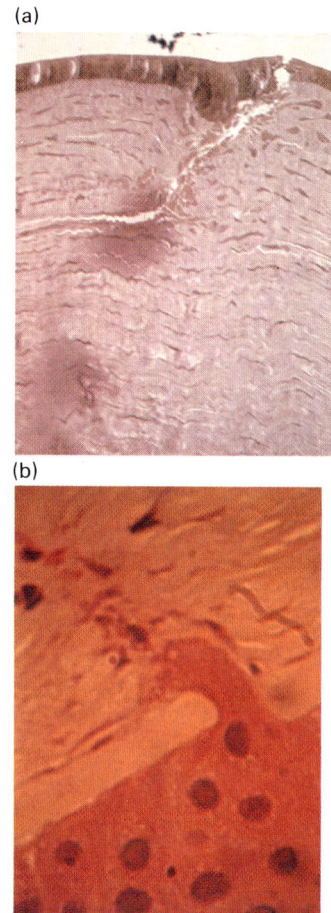

Fig. 4.14 (a) Epithelial facet formation following experimental stromal incision. Paraphenylene-diamine, original magnification × 80. (b) Break in Bowman's layer. Hematoxylin & eosin, original magnification × 80.

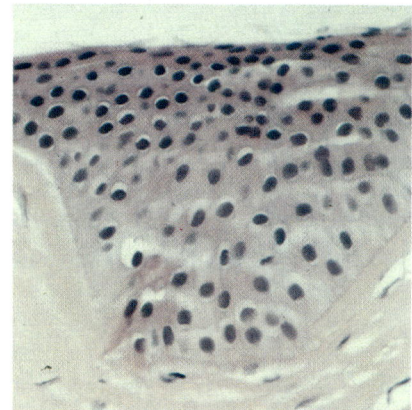

Fig. 4.15 Epithelial plug, filling wound after radial keratotomy. Hematoxylin & eosin, original magnification × 80.

Persistence of the epithelial plug for a year or more has been documented in radial keratotomy patients. A wound bridged by epithelium is obviously not as strong as one closed by collagen. Fibroblast [35] and mesodermal growth factors can accelerate stromal healing [38] and may have therapeutic value.

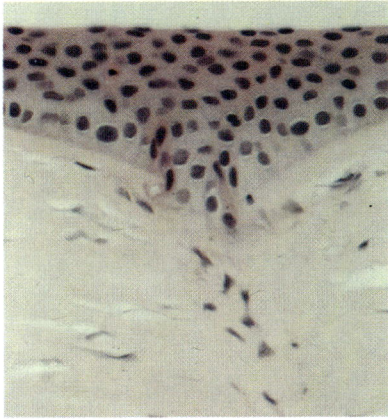

Fig. 4.16 Regressing epithelium and stromal scar following radial keratotomy. Hematoxylin & eosin, original magnification × 80.

(a)

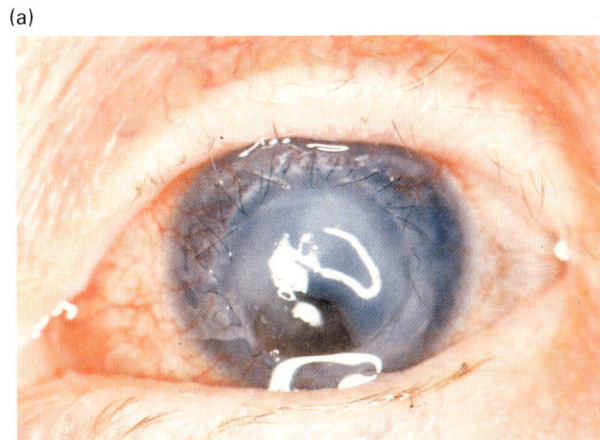

(b)

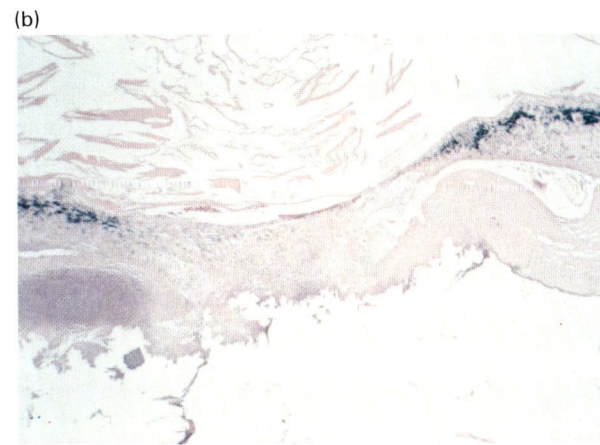

Fig. 4.17 (a) Corneal melting at graft margin with descemetocele formation. (b) Marked stromal loss from corneal melting. Hematoxylin & eosin, original magnification × 10.

It is important to consider both physical and bio-chemical factors that affect wound healing. Without a doubt, the most important physical factor in epithelial healing is the quality and integrity of the tear film. The corneal epithelium is the major barrier to infection. When there is a tear deficiency, the ability of the epithelium to cover a defect is compromised and the possibility of invasion by micro-organisms is enhanced [39]. Tear deficiency can lead to chronic epithelial defects which may be associated with stromal inflammation and scarring. Chronic epithelial defects are often associated with production of collagenase which can cause stromal melting and necrosis [40]. This melting process, which can be rapid or slow, can eventually lead to corneal perforation. A failure of proper epithelialization can lead to stromal melting in epikeratophakia (Figure 4.17). In addition, the tears carry a variety of substances such as lysozyme, which inhibits bacterial growth.

Abnormal corneal wound healing

In the context of refractive surgery, it is important to review abnormalities of corneal wound healing, as they may play a significant role in post-operative problems. The importance of an intact tear film and epithelial surface has been noted from the point of view of resistance to infection. Of even greater importance in refractive surgery, the epithelial sheet must be smooth and regular for best-quality vision.

Pharmaceutical agents

Many commonly used ophthalmic pharmaceutical agents interfere with epithelial healing. These include topical anesthetics, antivirals, corticosteroids, and aminoglycoside antibiotics [41]. Excessive use of any of these drugs leads to superficial punctate keratitis (Figures 4.18 and 4.19). Breakdown of the epithelial

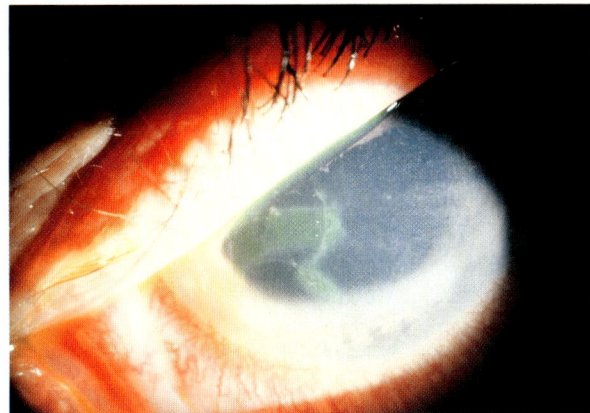

Fig. 4.18 Persistent epithelial defect in an anesthetic abuser.

barrier increases the risk of secondary infection with bacteria or fungi. While this most often occurs as a consequence of non-surgical treatment, it may also occur in refractive surgery patients. There is a particular risk with the lamellar procedures, since the tear film is disturbed at the same time that drug therapy may be intense (see section on the tear film, above). The super-

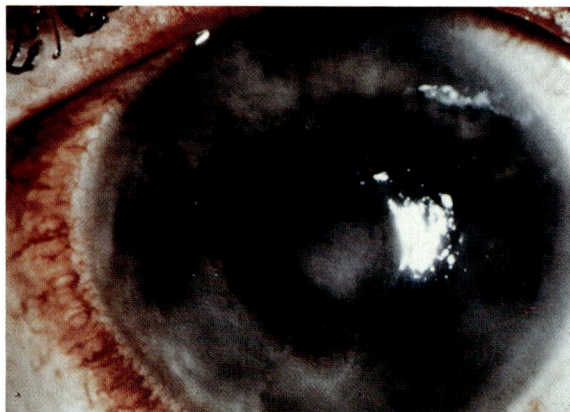

Fig. 4.19 Indolent ulcer in a patient with chronic stromal herpes keratitis.

ficial punctate keratitis, always present initially, may progress to persistent epithelial defects, which could lead to eventual corneal melting.

Anterior membrane dystrophies

Abnormal epithelial healing is a hallmark of the anterior membrane dystrophies. These include microcystic dystrophy, Meeseman's dystrophy, macular dystrophy, and lattice dystrophy [36]. All of these conditions are characterized by abnormalities of the epithelial basement membrane and all may be associated with a recurrent erosion syndrome. The mechanism is the same as that following a traumatic corneal abrasion in that the hemidesmosomes of the basal epithelium do not form properly and fail to attach the epithelium to the basement membrane. The presence of any of these conditions may be a contraindication to refractive surgery.

Epithelial downgrowth

Another example of abnormal epithelial wound healing is epithelial downgrowth (Figures 4.20–4.22). This problem has been reported after penetrating keratoplasty, cataract, and glaucoma filtration surgery as well as after trauma [42]. While the risk of this complication is low in refractive surgery, an inadvertent perforation during radial keratotomy or epikeratophakia could provide an avenue for classic epithelial downgrowth (see Chapter 15).

Although unlikely to occur in refractive surgery, epithelial downgrowth is a major clinical disaster. Any wound that remains open for a period of time provides a pathway for epithelium to grow through the wound and into the eye [43]. The epithelium continues to grow and may eventually totally cover the endothelial surface of the cornea as well as the iris and other intraocular structures. This leads to endothelial death and

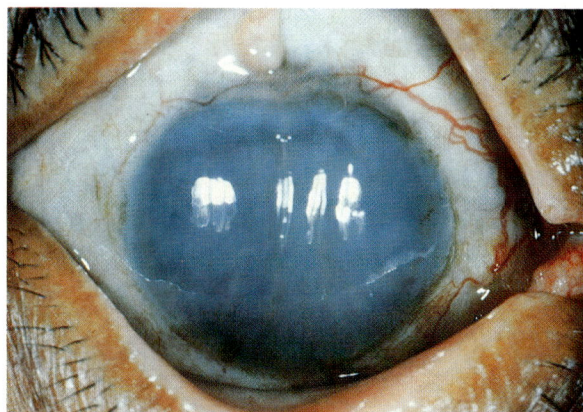

Fig. 4.20 Epithelial downgrowth following cataract surgery. A small filtering bleb above indicates the point of entry. Note the scalloped white border inferiorly, marking the advancing epithelium. The overlying cornea shows marked edema.

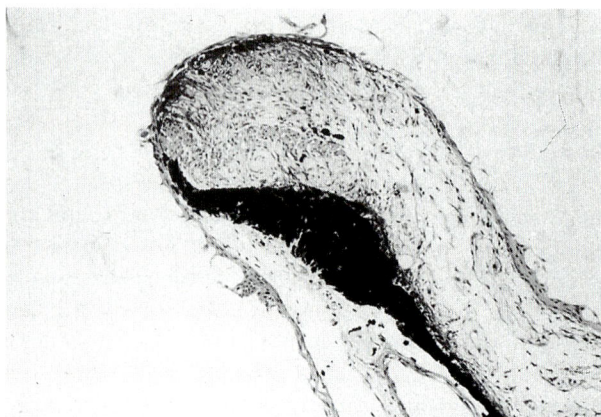

Fig. 4.21 Epithelium growing on the anterior iris surface has produced a prominent ectopion uvea. Hematoxylin & eosin, original magnification × 60.

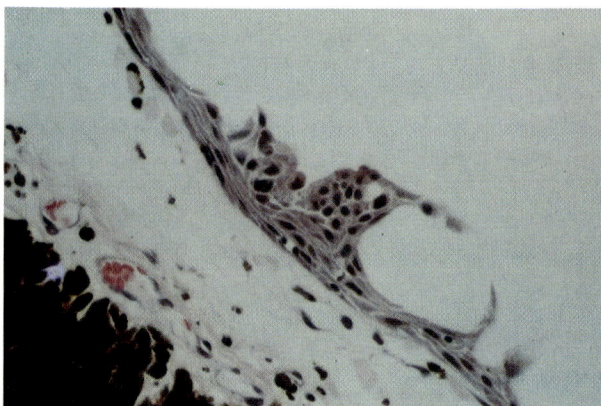

Fig. 4.22 High-power view of Figure 4.21, showing a part of the epithelial sheet from the iris surface. Hematoxylin & eosin, original magnification × 100.

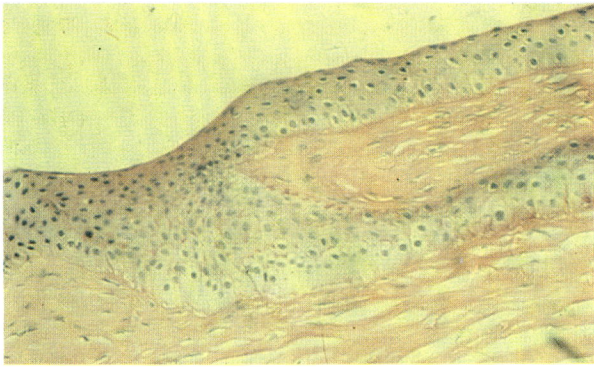

Fig. 4.23 Epithelium infiltrated beneath an epikeratophakia lenticule. Hematoxylin & eosin, original magnification × 100.

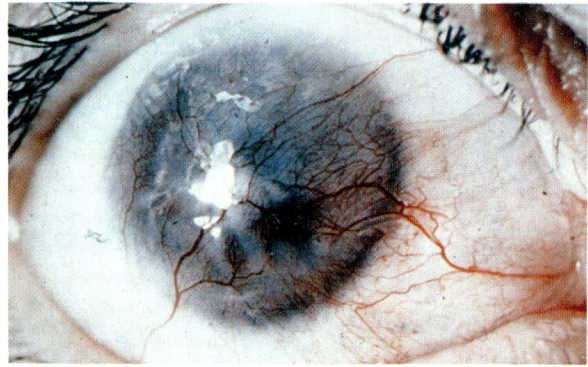

Fig. 4.24 Corneal vascularization in a patient with chronic aphakic bullous keratopathy.

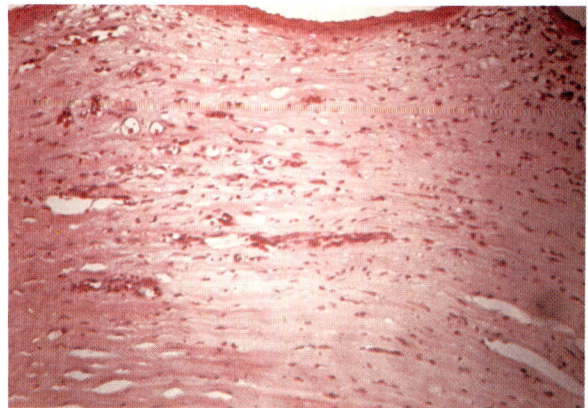

Fig. 4.25 Anterior and mid stromal corneal vascularization in a corneal button from a patient with bullous keratopathy. Hematoxylin & eosin, original magnification × 80.

corneal decompensation and often produces and intractable glaucoma [42]. If caught at an early stage, a 50% cure rate has been reported. The treatment is drastic, requiring double freezing of the involved cornea, excision of all affected intra-ocular tissue and extensive vitrectomy [44]. More advanced cases may lead to loss of all useful vision. It is appropriate to emphasize that while the corneal epithelium is only fulfilling its role of covering bare surfaces, the results are destructive.

Ingrowth of epithelium beneath donor lenticules has been reported in epikeratophakia (Figure 4.23) and could well occur with intra-stromal alloplastic implants. In both instances the mechanism is similar. The natural tendency of epithelium to cover a bare surface—which works to our advantage in corneal abrasions—can cause serious problems in refractive surgery. Ingrowth of epithelium beneath a homologous or heterologous lenticule may lead to opacification of the lenticule/recipient interface [45]. In the case of epikeratoplasty, such ingrowth might result in unsatisfactory wound healing at the interface with loss of the lenticule.

The interaction of the corneal epithelium with the rest of the cornea is well-illustrated by indolent ulcers. In patients with herpes simplex or other chronic stromal inflammation, portions of the epithelium may slough off and resist efforts at healing for many weeks (Figure 4.19). The chronic inflammation, combined with damage to Bowman's layer and the epithelial basement membrane, prevents reformation of the epithelial sheet [46]. Tear film abnormalities potentiate this problem.

In patients with repeated episodes of epithelial disruption, as seen in bullous keratopathy, inflammation can stimulate growth of fibrovascular tissue from the limbus (Figures 4.24 and 4.25). This degenerative pannus contributes to loss of vision [47]. The potential for a similar occurrence is present with refractive surgery in the presence of chronic and recurrent epithelial defects.

Stromal healing

Although epithelial wound healing seems much faster than stromal healing, laboratory research has shown that within a few hours of stromal wounding, there is activation of keratocytes. This change is characterized by the development of phagocytic activity in the keratocytes as well as by proliferation of cytoplasmic organelles. DNA synthesis and mitotic activity are seen by 24 hours. In addition, macrophages enter the stromal wound from the tear film and undergo fibroblastic transformation [48]. Initially there is a breakdown of damaged collagen. Within a few days, the wound shows uptake of radio-labeled hydroxylysine, hydroxyproline, and sulfur, which leads to the formation of new collagen and GAGs [49]. Over a period of several weeks, collagen synthesis occurs and amino acid uptake ceases.

In excimer laser keratectomy, the epithelium must grow and heal over bare corneal stroma in the absence of Bowman's layer. This is exactly the situation in

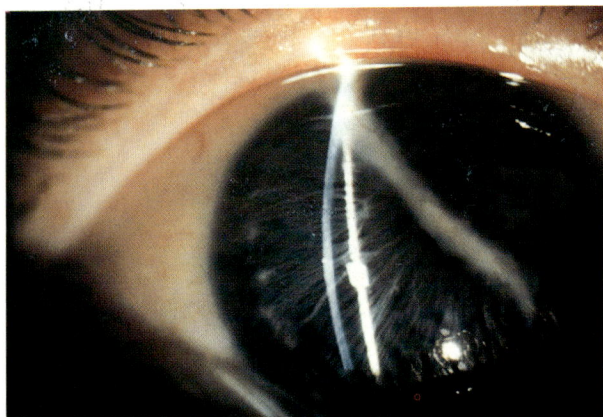

Fig. 4.26 Corneal scar following accidental penetrating wound.

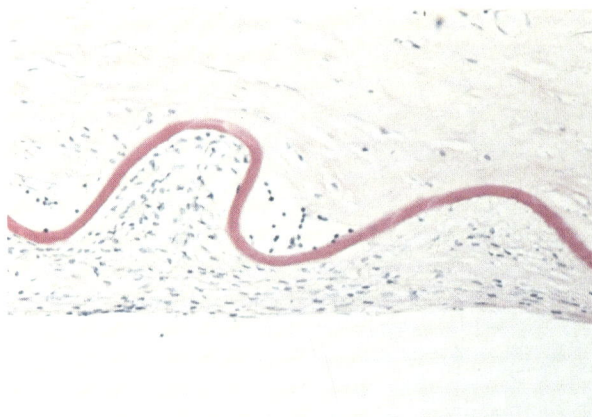

Fig. 4.28 Retrocorneal membrane after failed keratoplasty. Note the fixed folds in Descemet's membrane. Periodic acid Schiff, original magnification × 60.

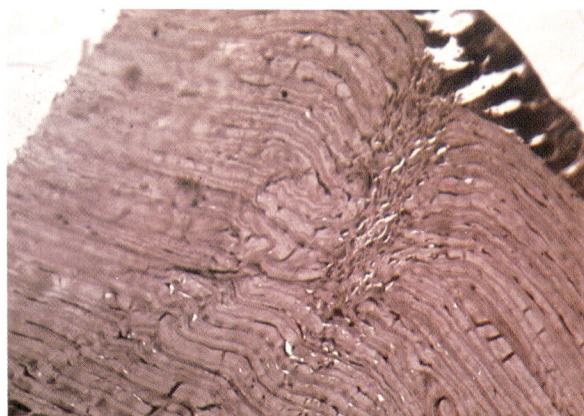

Fig. 4.27 Irregular stromal scar following a penetrating corneal wound. Paraphenylene-diamine, original magnification × 60.

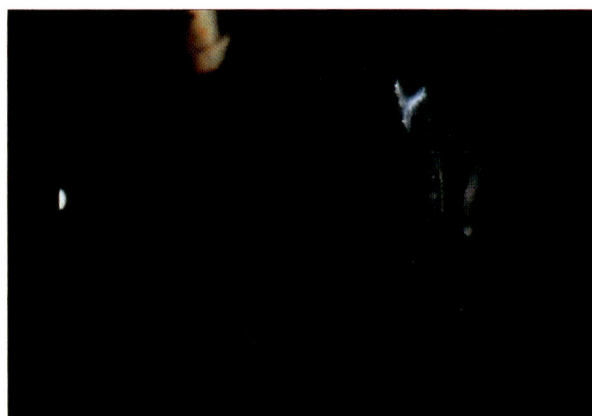

Fig. 4.29 Sub-endothelial fibrous proliferation following a micro-perforation.

which recurrent erosions and indolent ulcers occur. Early studies of excimer keratectomy suggest this is not a problem [50]. Injury to Bowman's layer and epithelial healing problems may relate to the problem of prolonged corneal haze, which has been observed in animals and humans after laser keratectomy, however.

In a dermal wound, the final change in the sequence of wound healing is contraction of the scar tissue. Fibroblasts develop actin filaments and are transformed into myofibroblasts. It is the contraction of these cells associated with collagen bundles that produces the shrinkage of the wound [51]. The role of this process in the cornea is less clear. Nevertheless, the opacity of corneal scars is clear evidence that the normal orderly array of stromal collagen has been lost (Figures 4.26 and 4.27).

Scarring with proliferation is more likely to occur with penetrating wounds, although degenerative pannus is a similar phenomenon. Retrocorneal membranes after keratoplasty and stromal ingrowth after cataract surgery are examples of proliferative scarring (Figure 4.28). Similar problems might potentially occur with perforations during refractive surgery (Figure 4.29). When Descemet's membrane is covered by a retrocorneal membrane, the endothelium is destroyed. The loss of this fluid barrier results in corneal edema and further visual loss.

This visual loss can occur in several ways. One of these is through surface irregularity to such an extent that irregular astigmatism results. Another is through light scattering by the scar tissue. Recall that corneal transparency depends upon uniform collagen fiber diameters and spacing. This spacing should be less than half the wavelength of light or about 200 nm. Unfortunately, the response to wounding produces collagen fibers that vary in diameter considerably, from 20 to 120 nm. Because the response is hasty and chaotic, these fibers never become organized into the normal lamellar arrangement with elements less than 200 nm apart. Some of this spacing differential is, of course, due to the edema that inevitably follows wounding. Additionally, the collagen fibers themselves differ in GAG content from that of the normal and hence have different indices of refraction.

Corneal vascularization

Because of the primary involvement of the stroma, it is appropriate to consider corneal vascularization in a discussion of stromal healing. This process has fascinated researchers for many years. Cogan was the first to suggest that corneal vascularization was related to a loss of stromal compactness. He demonstrated that stromal swelling always preceded the ingrowth of new vessels [52]. That this is not the sole factor in vascularization is shown by the avascularity of many eyes with severe stromal edema in bullous keratopathy.

More popular theories have suggested that vascularization is due to loss of an inhibitor of vascularization or to the release of an angiogenic substance [53,54]. The latter theory has received strong support from the work of Folkman with tumor angiogenesis factor. Tumor cells injected into the anterior chamber will proliferate to form a clump of cells about 1 mm in diameter. Growth then ceases, unless the cell mass settles on the iris and establishes a blood supply. When this occurs, there is accelerated growth of the tumor. Tumor extract or a tiny piece of tumor tissue implanted in the cornea causes the ingrowth of vessels from the limbus. Tumor angiogenic factor is now established as another growth factor [55]. While this probably does not play a role in the normal cornea, there may be naturally occurring angiogenic substances which take part in wound healing.

Descemet's membrane and the endothelial cell layer

Changes in Descemet's membrane and the corneal endothelium may occur with refractive surgery, but the need for primary healing of these structures is present only when there is a full-thickness corneal wound. The endothelium is able to regenerate short stretches of Descemet's membrane, although there are limits to this ability (Figure 4.30). Regeneration of the endothelium by mitosis does not occur to an appreciable degree in the human eye [56]. Defects in the endothelial layer are covered by the spreading of adjacent cells, which results in lower endothelial cell counts. Both migration and spreading are mediated by changes in intracellular actin filament organization [57].

Accidental perforation of the cornea in refractive surgery, such as radial keratotomy, causes a focal injury to Descemet's and the endothelium which is not functionally significant. It has been shown that the endothelial cell loss which occurs following radial keratotomy is acute, non-progressive, and limited to between 5 and 7% [58]. Others have shown a net cell gain, which just goes to point out the margin of error present in endothelial cell counting methodology [59]. On the other hand, an unhealthy endothelium may

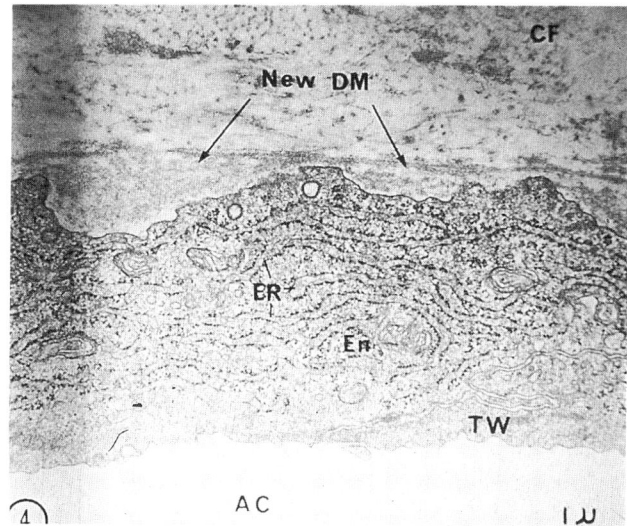

Fig. 4.30 Healed Descemet's membrane following injury. Original magnification × 22 500.

respond with greater cell loss resulting in corneal decompensation after refractive surgery.

Corneal wound healing and its sequelae are complex processes which may result in an uneventful recovery of visual function or which may lead to a permanent loss of vision. While much remains to be learned about the events which occur in this process, it is important for the refractive surgeon to understand the known mechanisms and use them to achieve a successful surgical result. The next section will deal with the specific problems of healing as related to refractive surgery.

Healing of the cornea in refractive surgery

The previous section emphasized the interaction of the various layers of the cornea during the healing process. In all refractive surgery, a successful result depends on proper healing of the corneal surface and control of stromal scarring. Defects in either process may result in serious complications such as infection or stromal melting.

The intact corneal epithelium, and more specifically, the overlying tear film provide the primary refractive interface of the cornea and also present a major barrier to invasion by micro-organisms. Most of the refractive surgical procedures discussed in this chapter cause an initial loss of some or nearly all of the surface epithelium. The epithelium which remains must slide over the bare surface of the cornea, attach to the basement membrane, and then proliferate to return to normal. Damage to the basement membrane of the basal epithelial cells retards effective healing, since hemidesmosomes may fail to reform. Inadequate development of hemidesmosomes is associated with re-

Table 4.2 Radial keratotomy. From Binder PS. What we have learned about corneal wound healing from refractive surgery (Barraquer lecture). Refract Corneal Surg 1989; 5:98–120

Acute surface features

Rupture/loss of cells within 50–100 μm of either side of wound

Debridement of epithelium in a triangular pattern with apex toward optical clear zone (concordes)

Inadvertent epithelial implantation into wounds

Focal fractures in Bowman's layer and basement membrane when grasped with forceps or with attempted re-entry of wounds with the blade

Blade entry site smaller and more sharply demarcated than blade exit

---

Acute stromal and endothelial features

Loss of keratocytes within 200–300 μm of wound

Jagged wound edge with fragmented collagen fibers

Posterior bowing of Descemet's membrane toward anterior chamber

Ruptured endothelial cells along posterior Descemet's folds

Table 4.3 Radial keratotomy. From Binder PS. What we have learned about corneal wound healing from refractive surgery (Barraquer lecture). Refract Corneal Surg 1989; 5:98–120

Chronic features

Epithelium
Abnormal surface cells over wounds

Epithelial ridges over wounds

Map-dot-fingerprint dystrophy changes affecting basal lamina

Iron deposition

Bowman's layer
Focal fractures

Inward bowing at incision sites

Stroma
Viable epithelium in wounds (cysts, plugs)

Epithelial degenerative products in wounds

Neovascularization proximal to limbus

Non-aligned collagen lamellae/fibers

Activated keratocytes under incisions

Bowing of lamellae toward anterior chamber

Variable incision depths within the same wounds and between wounds in the same specimen

Non-perpendicular incisions in the same corneal specimen

Descemet's membrane
Bowing of Descemet's membrane toward anterior chamber

Normal endothelial morphology over incisions except at micro-perforation sites

---

current erosions and persistent epithelial defects. The repercussions of a failure of epithelial resurfacing may also include infection, increased stromal scarring and corneal melting.

The transparency of the cornea depends on the highly regular arrangement of the collagen fibers which form the stromal lamellae. An opaque scar may lead to a visual failure of the refractive surgery. In some procedures, such as radial keratotomy, the scarring plays a role in production of the optical effect of the procedure. However, scarring in the visual axis leads inevitably to a variable and permanent loss in visual acuity.

Aberrant healing of the epithelium interacts in a negative way with stromal healing, either contributing to a failure of stromal healing or resulting in enhanced stromal scarring. Following incisional types of refractive surgery, the epithelium may invade the incision and persist for long periods. Because the epithelium has little tensile strength, these areas of the cornea are severely weakened. Epithelial cysts migrate beneath the stroma in the lamellar procedures and cause an interface opacity. Finally, if there is an accidental corneal perforation during surgery, epithelium may migrate through the perforation and produce epithelial downgrowth. The serious consequences to the eye

(a) 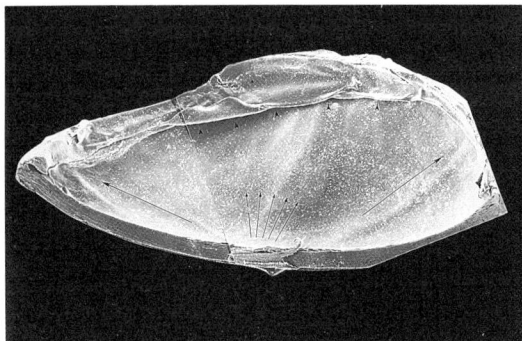   (b)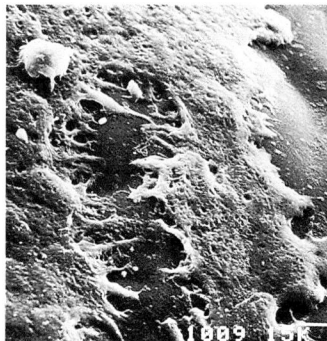

Fig. 4.31 (a) Scanning electron micrograph of a trephined section showing the "log under a rug" effect beneath radial keratotomy incisions. (b) Endothelial damage following radial keratotomy in a rabbit. Original magnification × 15 000. (Figure 4.31 b from Yamaguchi T, Polack FM, Valenti J, Kaufman HE. Endothelial damage after anterior radial keratotomy. An electron microscopic study of rabbit cornea. Arch Ophthalmol 1981; 99:2151–2158.)

caused by this downgrowth were outlined in the previous section.

Failure of the epithelium to re-establish its integrity may produce corneal melting. It is well established that such a failure may encourage the production of collagenase from invading neutrophils or from the injured epithelium itself [40]. Persistence of collagenase then leads to liquefaction of the stroma. In some instances, the melting may progress to perforation and loss of the eye.

The normal eye with intact corneal epithelium is highly resistant to micro-organisms. An epithelial defect is a potential portal of entry for bacteria, fungi, viruses and *Acanthamoeba*. Corneal ulcers from these pathogens often occur in contact lens wearers and may also follow refractive surgical procedures. The end result of a corneal ulcer is stromal scarring and loss of vision [60,61].

Incisional procedures

Radial keratotomy

Wound healing problems in radial keratotomy take two forms: those related to faulty production of the incisions at the time of surgery and those related to abnormal wound healing (Tables 4.2 and 4.3). Accurate knowledge of corneal thickness and precise calibration of the cutting instrument are critical factors in all forms of keratotomy surgery. Effectiveness of the surgery is directly related to the depth of cut. An incision that is too deep will result in a micro- or macro-perforation. After healing of a micro-perforation there is a focal loss of endothelial cells from direct trauma as well as localized proliferation of fibrous tissue. A micro-perforation also presents the possibility of invasion by micro-organisms or by epithelium to cause a downgrowth.

A macro-perforation usually causes termination of the procedure and may require suturing of the wound to maintain the anterior chamber. All of the possible complications of micro-perforations must be entertained in this event. Additionally, the full-thickness wound and its repair may cause irregular stromal scarring which may then interfere with visual rehabilitation. Deep wounds also tend to push on Descemet's, causing focal raised surfaces seen in some sections—"log under a rug" (Figure 4.31). In some cases, endothelial cells can be destroyed. Severe regular or irregular astigmatism may result, as with any healed corneal scar. This is more likely with wounds made with steel blades which typically show more jagged wound edges.

Nearly all radial keratotomy patients report glare after surgery, which may last from 1 to 3 months. The glare results from the scattering of light by incisional

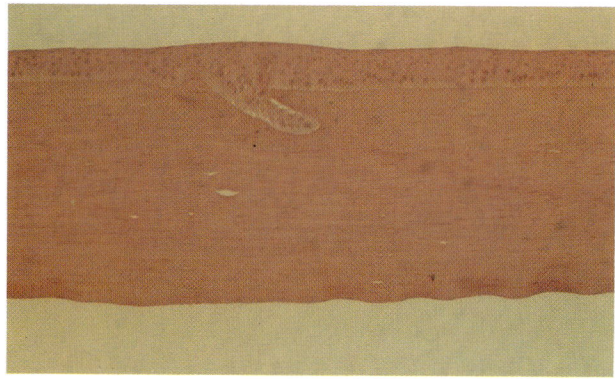

Fig. 4.32 A healed radial keratotomy scar is marked by a small epithelial plug, which extends obliquely across the cornea for two-thirds the stromal thickness. Such a scar is associated with severe and persistent glare. Hematoxylin & eosin, original magnification × 50.

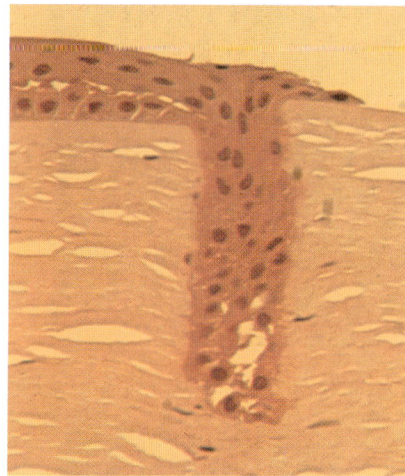

Fig. 4.33 An early radial keratotomy incision is filled by an epithelial plug. Hematoxylin & eosin, original magnification × 100.

edema and scar tissue. The ideal incision should be made perpendicular to a tangent to the cornea. An oblique incision (Figure 4.32) produces a broader base for light scattering and aggravates the glare. If scarring is sufficiently severe, disabling glare may be present—permanently.

As previously noted, the stromal wound is usually sealed with an epithelial plug which disappears as the wound heals. The way in which the wound is produced may alter the sequence of events. For example, radial keratotomy wounds show a relatively simple form of healing. Following the acute surgical incision, the corneal epithelium migrates (Figure 4.33) down the lateral walls of the incision and then proliferates, forming an epithelial plug [62]. In the normal sequence of events, fibroblastic repair and proliferation gradually push the plug out of the wound with formation of an

(a)

(b)

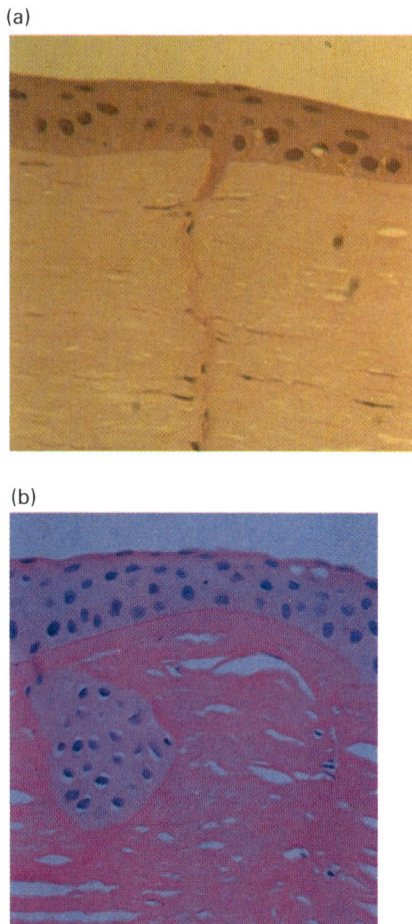

Fig. 4.34 (a) A late radial keratotomy scar. The incision is marked by a break in Bowman's membrane and a well-healed stromal scar. Hematoxylin & eosin, original magnification × 100. (b) Epithelial island or cord trapped within corneal stroma. Hematoxylin & eosin, original magnification × 100.

avascular scar (Figure 4.34). Unlike a single isolated stromal wound, final healing of a radial keratotomy wound and expulsion of epithelium may be prolonged in some patients. In some cases, the epithelial plug persists for many months or years [63]. In fact, small inclusions of epithelium can become implanted within the scar; these can lead to incomplete or prolonged healing. It has been suggested that this prolonged healing phase is also due to flexure of the multiple stromal wounds, which prevents normal healing, although there has not been good correlation with pathology [64]. The situation is different in epikeratophakia where healing must take place between the stroma of the lenticule and the host Bowman's layer, in addition to epithelial healing.

Marsupialization can also occur, especially if the wounds gape too much [65]. If epithelial cells are implanted within the incision, these can proliferate to form cystic structures, sometimes of considerable size. Talcum from incompletely washed gloves can find its way into these incisions, as can other foreign bodies. Red blood cells, if not irrigated from the wound, can be converted by the keratocytes into lipid deposits—sometimes of impressive dimensions (see also Chapter 15) [66].

There also may be something different about the corneas of myopes of differing degrees. Kurasova has noted that wound appearance correlates with result and has defined four different types of wounds seen post-radial keratotomy [67]. This "feathering" of the wound margins has been described by the author and others [68] but the clinical appearance has not been correlated histologically [69]. It is possible that we are dealing with a different type of collagen in these cases; certainly there is something different about the healing processes in radial keratotomy [70,71].

Map-dot changes have been reported following radial keratotomy (see also Chapter 15) [72]. Binder attributes these to improper handling of the cornea—these are less likely to occur when the sclera and not the wound is grasped during surgery [71]. Handling the wound edge is a violation of Bores' Second Rule—"Thou shalt not twiddle with the incision;" see also Chapter 8.

Astigmatic keratotomy

In addition to all of the above problems, astigmatic keratotomy has other complications. At one time, it was customary to connect the transverse cuts with the radial cuts performed in a Ruiz procedure. Many patients were found to have one or more V-shaped corneal flaps at the incisional crossings after this procedure. The flaps (Figure 4.35) became edematous and elevated above the surface of the remainder of the

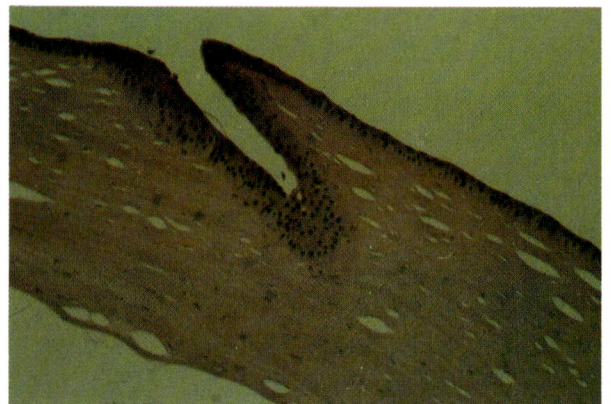

Fig. 4.35 A persistent stromal defect lined by epithelium is seen after a Ruiz procedure with intersecting incisions. An elevated stromal flap has resulted from the improper healing. Hematoxylin & eosin, original magnification × 50.

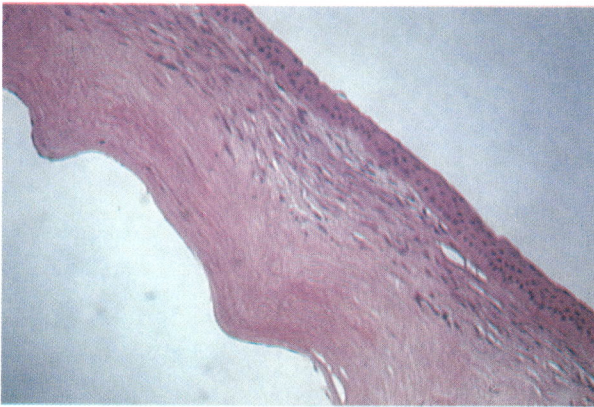

Fig. 4.36 Cornea following thermokeratoplasty. Bowman's membrane is absent and there is irregular anterior stromal scarring. Hematoxylin & eosin, original magnification × 50.

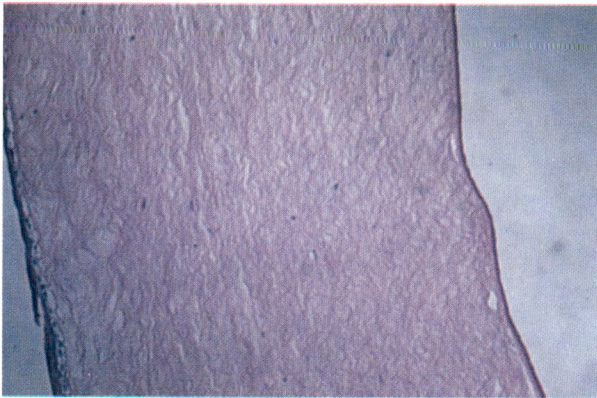

Fig. 4.37 Cornea following thermokeratoplasty. Basilar epithelial edema is present and there is epithelial thinning related to poor healing. Corneal edema is prominent and there is a marked decrease in the number of keratocytes. Hematoxylin & eosin, original magnification × 100.

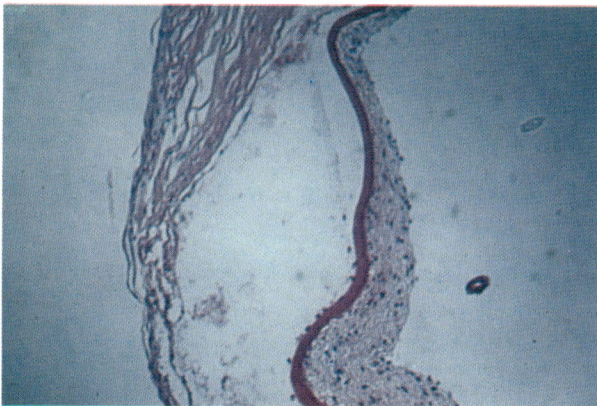

Fig. 4.38 The corneal epithelium is absent following thermokeratoplasty. There is marked central stromal melting resulting in a descemetocele. A fibrin plaque is present on the posterior surface of Descemet's membrane. Hematoxylin & eosin, original magnification × 50.

cornea. Chronic epithelial defects, corneal melting and irregular scarring are possible complications, which cannot be completely avoided even in the best of hands [73].

Thermal procedures

Thermal (planiform) keratoplasty

Collagen undergoes shrinkage when heated, a fact which suggested a potential application in refractive surgery (see also Chapters 8 and 14). At one time it was felt that thermal shrinkage could be used in patients with keratoconus to alter corneal curvature, improve contact lens fitting, and avoid the need for keratoplasty. Thermokeratoplasty was thus attempted with a number of instruments, all of which cause similar complications. Whatever the mode of heat production, the procedure damages Bowman's layer which in turn interferes with re-establishment of the epithelial sheet, leading to stromal scarring (Figure 4.36). The heat often destroys stromal keratocytes as well (Figure 4.37) which may lead to additional stromal scarring. The persistent epithelial defect can potentiate production of collagenase, leading to corneal necrosis and melting (Figure 4.38). These problems have been observed in a number of patients [74]. Binder [71] has observed that severe corneal damage can occur with as few as four burns. Hyperopic thermokeratoplasty employs 12–96 deep stromal burns.

Hyperopic (punctiform) thermal keratotomy

Fyodorov in Russia and Neumann in the USA have proposed a radial thermal pattern for the treatment of hyperopia (see also Chapter 14). No animal studies have been published, but one might predict irregular astigmatism, persistent epithelial defects, and perhaps

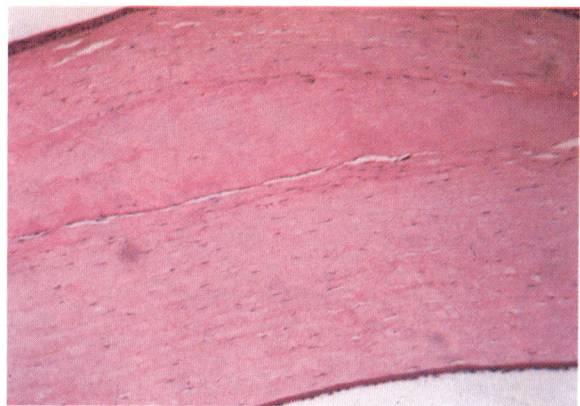

Fig. 4.39 In keratophakia, keratocytes are absent in the lenticular stroma. Hematoxylin & eosin, original magnification × 100.

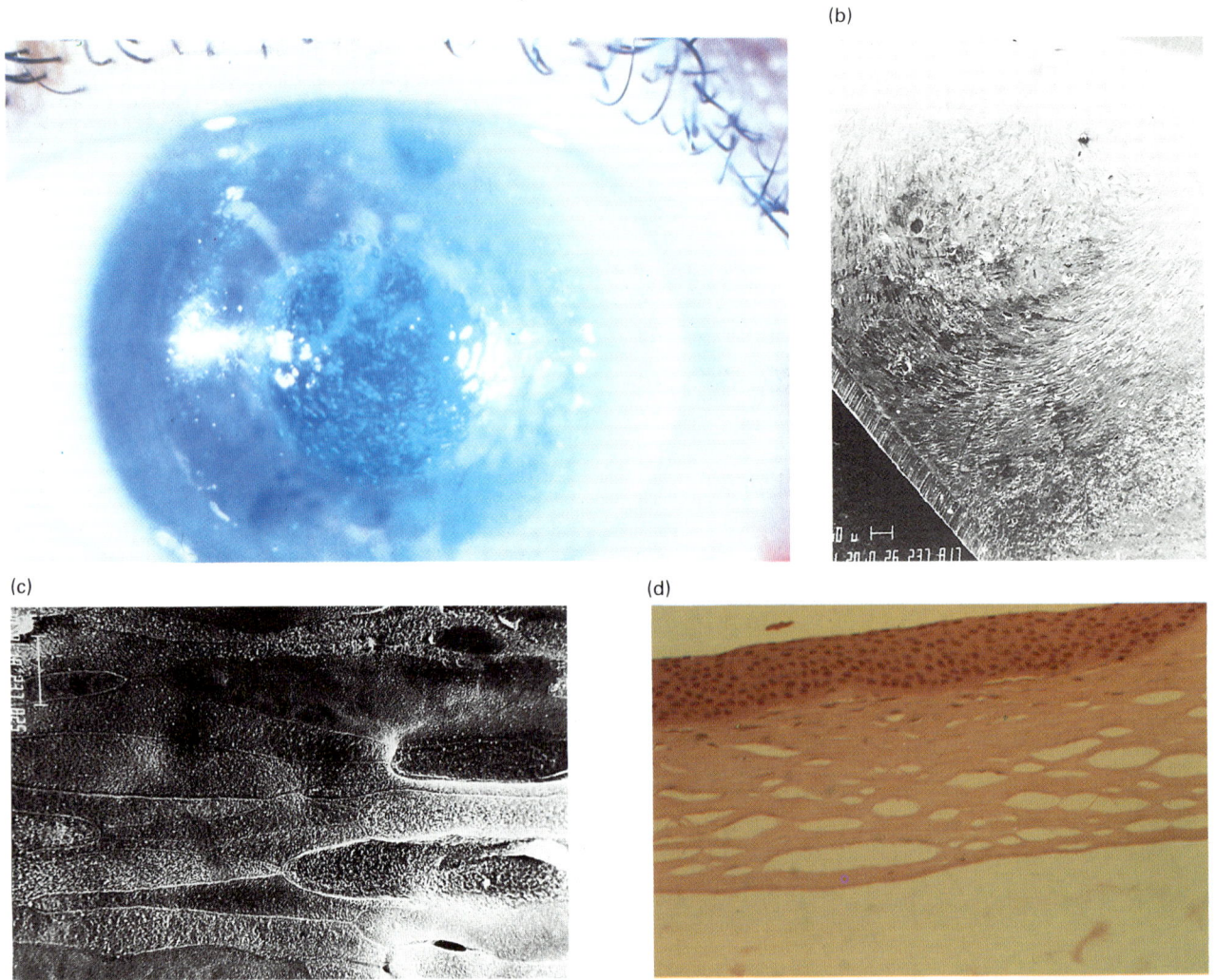

Fig. 4.40 (a) Spiral epithelialopathy following MKM. (b) Scanning electron micrograph of the surface of the failed lenticule. Original magnification × 2250. (c) Higher-power view showing the peculiar nature of the epithelium. Original magnification × 10 500. (d) Bowman's membrane is absent and there is anterior stromal scarring following failed myopic keratomileusis. Hematoxylin & eosin, original magnification × 100.

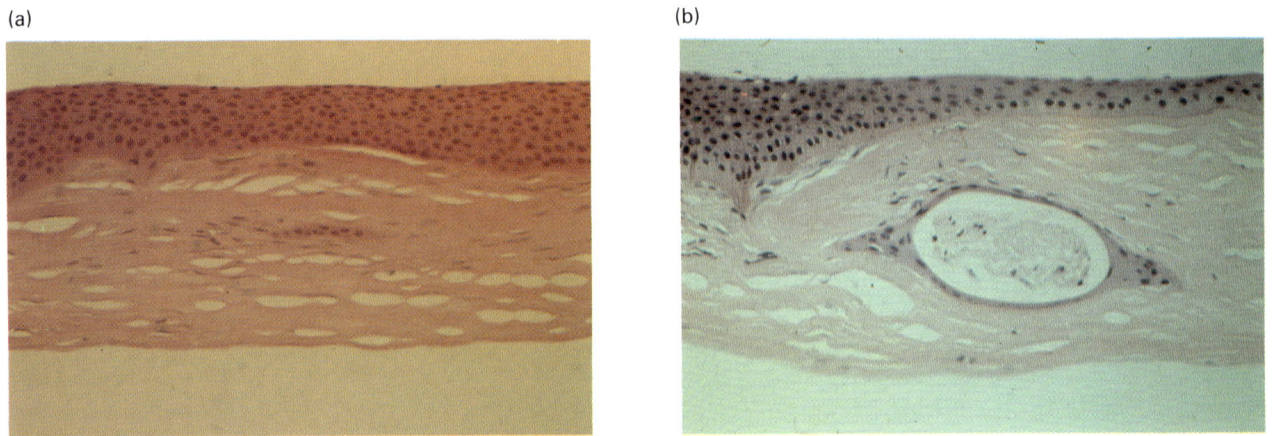

Fig. 4.41 (a) Epithelial inclusion at the interface between lathed tissue and deep stroma following myopic keratomileusis. Superficial stromal irregularity and thickened epithelium is also evident. Hematoxylin & eosin, original magnification × 100. (b) Epithelial cyst following MKM. Note bulging of Descemet's membrane. Hematoxylin & eosin, original magnification × 100.

some of the problems associated with planiform thermokeratoplasty.

Lathed tissue procedures

Barraquer is the father of corneal lathing as a method of altering the anterior curvature of the cornea. Kerato-phakia, keratomileusis, and epikeratophakia all make use of this general concept. Because the operative techniques vary, there are specific abnormalities of wound healing associated with each procedure. For example, epikeratophakia uses a lathed donor button of either frozen or fresh tissue which is placed directly on the recipient Bowman's layer.

Keratophakia

In keratophakia, a donor lamellar disk is cryolathed and then placed within the patient's cornea in a pre-viously prepared lamellar bed. Since the donor lenticule is frozen prior to being implanted, there are no viable keratocytes within it. Collagen and GAGs by light microscopy are apparently undisturbed by the freeze-processing other than distortion of the lamellae. Unlike keratomileusis, the donor button shows little repopu-lation by keratocytes, even up to a year after surgery (Figure 4.39) [75,76]. Electron microscopy, however, demonstrates distorted and occasionally fractured col-lagen along with reduced ground substance. It has been suggested that this failure of keratocyte invasion is due to interface pressure or lack of horizontal edge alignment. Irregular healing in this and the other lathed tissue procedures often results in irregular astigmatism. The most frequent reason for removal of a kerato-phakia lenticule, however, is inappropriate optical correction.

Keratomileusis

In keratomileusis, a lamellar button from the patient's own cornea is frozen, lathed to a new shape, and placed back into the bed. Both hyperopic and myopic correction may be achieved by this procedure. Epithel-ial vacuolization and intra-epithelial cyst formation may occur, perhaps related to freezing damage (see also Chapters 11 and 15). In some cases, the epithelium is separated from Bowman's layer by fibrocellular pro-liferation. Despite the fact that the lenticule was frozen, it is rapidly repopulated by keratocytes [75,76]. The lamellar arrangement of collagen is undisturbed. Frac-tures of Bowman's layer, however, are particularly likely to occur in myopic keratomileusis (Figure 4.40) [76]. This is due to physical distortion of the very thin central portion of the lenticule during surgical mani-pulation. Damage of the epithelial basement mem-brane results in fewer hemidesmosomes which can

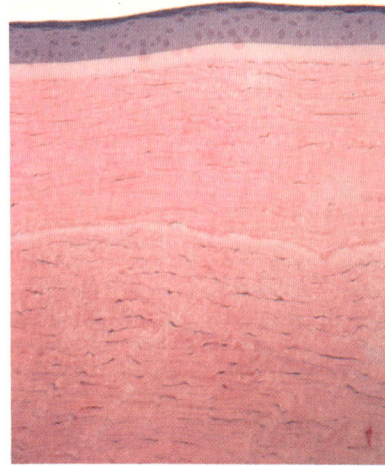

Fig. 4.42 Penetrating keratoplasty button after epikeratoplasty. The interface between the epikeratoplasty lenticule and the recipient is shown. Hematoxylin & eosin, original magnification × 50.

lead to persistent epithelial defects, as well as the potential risk of infection and scarring. To avoid this, the central lenticular thickness is held to a minimum of 0.015 mm. When this is done, cracking of Bowman's layer and scarring, in the author's experience, rarely occur.

Additional interference with vision may result from epithelial invasion of the interface between the lenti-cule and the underlying stroma (Figures 4.41 and 4.42). This can also occur in the non-freeze forms of kerato-mileusis but the incidence is low. This is probably related to the fact that the donor epithelium is un-damaged in the non-freeze method, thus the area to be covered by epithelial cells is less and consequently, so is the collagenase activity (L.D. Bores, 1991, unpub-lished data). Table 4.4 summarizes the histologic fea-tures of keratophakia and both freeze and non-freeze keratomileusis.

Epikeratophakia

The original epikeratophakia buttons were prepared by cryolathing eye bank donor tissue designed to pro-duce the desired refractive effect. Both hyperopic and myopic lenticules can be produced and, in the com-mercial lenticules, are lyophilized for storage. The pa-tient's epithelium is removed prior to placement of the donor tissue on to the recipient's Bowman's layer. The prepared lenticule is sewn into a circular keratotomy of varying diameter. The practice of annular keratectomy —removal of a ring of corneal tissue—the source of irregular healing and astigmatism, has been aban-doned. Although little histopathology is available, there has been a recent interest in lathing fresh, unfrozen tissue, a technique which avoids death of the donor

Table 4.4 Histologic features of lamellar surgery. From Binder PS. What we have learned about corneal wound healing from refractive surgery (Barraquer lecture). Refract Corneal Surg 1989; 5:98–120

Keratophakia	Keratomileusis	Non-freeze keratomileusis
Acute features		
Killed keratocytes	Killed keratocytes	Viable keratocytes
Distorted lamellae	Normal lamellae	Normal lamellae
Stromal edema	Minimal edema	No edema
—	Dead epithelium	Normal epithelium
—	Bowman's fractures	Bowman's fractures —peripheral
Chronic features		
Stromal edema	Bowman's fractures	Intact Bowman's
—	Normal epithelium	Normal epithelium
Distorted lamellae	Thin central stroma	Normal thickness
Interface epithelium	Interface epithelium	Interface collagen
Anterior cap pannus	Normal keratocytes	Interface keratocytes
Neovascularization	Interface keratocytes	—

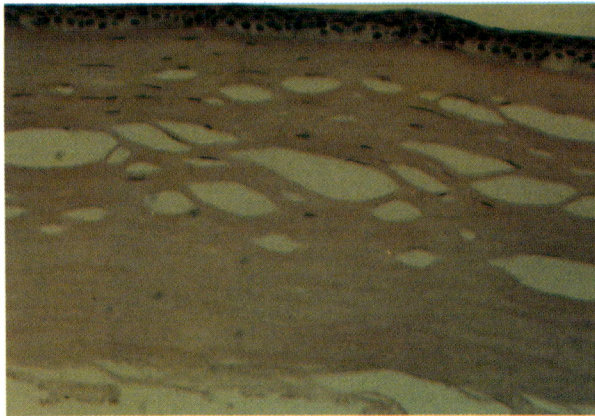

Fig. 4.44 Failed epikeratoplasty. The corneal epithelium is absent. The artifactual clefting of the stroma suggests edema. Keratocytes are absent. Hematoxylin & eosin, original magnification × 50.

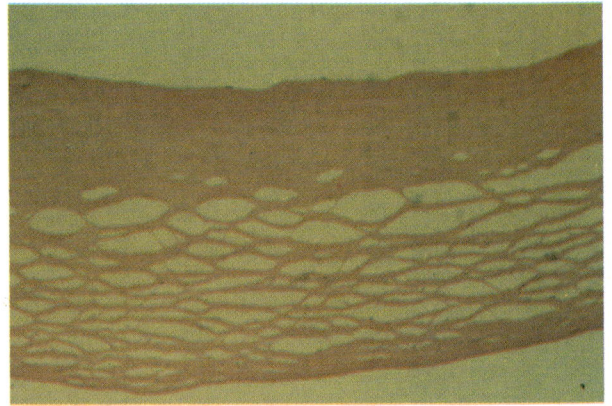

Fig. 4.45 At the edge of a failed epikeratoplasty, epithelium is growing around the edge of the lenticule. This resulted in improper healing and ectasia of the lenticule. Hematoxylin & eosin, original magnification × 100.

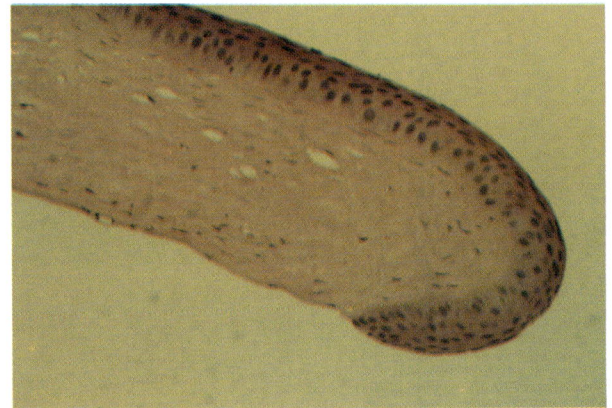

Fig. 4.43 Failed epikeratoplasty. Keratocytes are absent. Hematoxylin & eosin, original magnification × 100.

keratocytes (see also Chapter 11) [77–85]. In the frozen lenticules, the keratocytes are destroyed as they are in keratophakia and keratomileusis. In lenticules which have been studied some time after surgery, keratocytes are usually present anteriorly and peripherally, but are sparse or absent in the posterior aspects of the lenticule (Figure 4.43). Some have ascribed this irregular keratocyte re-population to interference with diffusion of nutrients by the host Bowman's layer [86].

A major problem in epikeratophakia relates to resurfacing of the donor lenticule with host epithelium [87]. Re-epithelialization plays a role in lenticular clarity— the faster this occurs, the clearer the final result. Persistent epithelial defects are common in epikerato-

phakia (Figure 4.44)—the epithelial basement membrane may be abnormal in some cases; fractures and folds can occur [88]. As in other procedures, such defects may provide an entry for infectious agents or may be associated with corneal melting of both host and donor cornea at the interface, forcing removal of the lenticule. Subsequent scarring may interfere with visual function and necessitate a penetrating keratoplasty [89,90]. Epithelial cells pile up at the host–graft edge. While this tends to smooth out the change in corneal curvature, thickened epithelium may prove to be unstable in the long run.

The edge of the lenticule may provide a route for epithelium to grow downward and between the lenticule and donor cornea (Figures 4.45–4.50), although this is more likely in keratomileusis. This will produce an interface opacity if not removed, and sometimes even if it is. Such opacities may also result from scar-

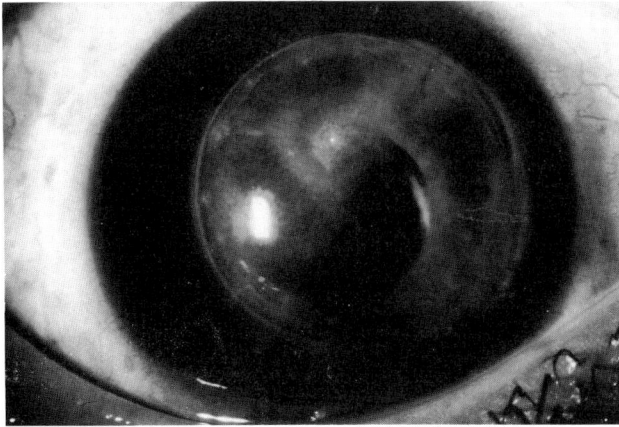

Fig. 4.46 Patient received lyophilized (AMO) lenticule but had persistent epithelial defect not responsive to therapy. Clinical appearance 4 months after surgery with scarring of the epikeratoplasty lenticule (from Grossniklaus HE, Lass JH, Jacobs G, Margo CE, McAuliffe AM. Light microscopic and ultrastructural findings in failed epikeratoplasty. Refract Corneal Surg 1989; 5:296–301).

(a)

(b)

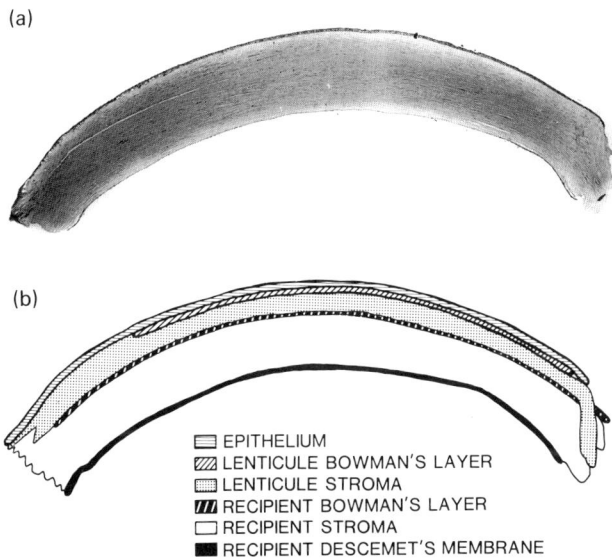

☐ EPITHELIUM
▨ LENTICULE BOWMAN'S LAYER
▦ LENTICULE STROMA
▥ RECIPIENT BOWMAN'S LAYER
☐ RECIPIENT STROMA
■ RECIPIENT DESCEMET'S MEMBRANE

Fig. 4.47 (a) Corneal button. Masson's trichrome, original magnification × 4. (b) Corresponding diagram (from Grossniklaus HE, Lass JH, Jacobs G, Margo CE, McAuliffe AM. Light microscopic and ultrastructural findings in failed epikeratoplasty. Refract Corneal Surg 1989; 5:296–301).

(a)

(b)

(c)

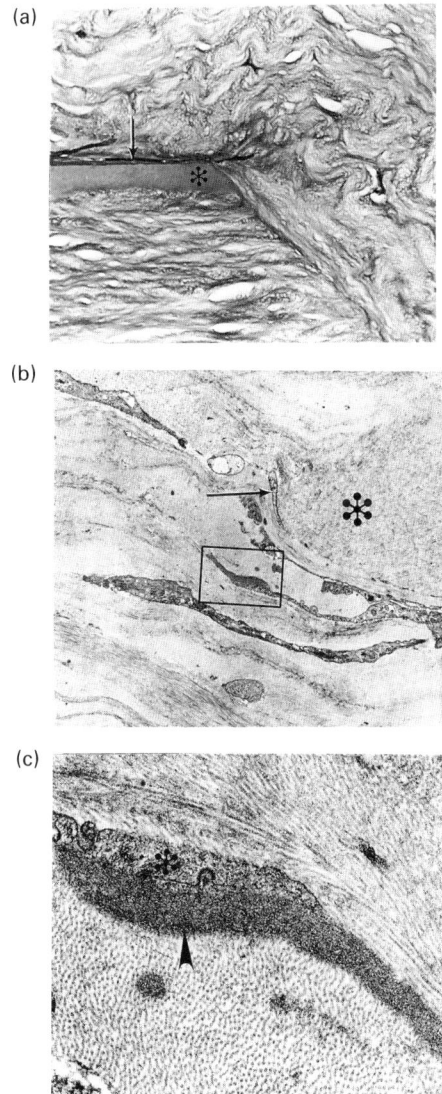

Fig. 4.48 (a) Keratocytes (arrow) are present anterior to cut margin of recipient Bowman's layer (arrowhead). Lenticule stroma contains relatively more keratocytes than recipient in this particular field; however there was an overall decrease in the number of keratocytes in the lenticule, as compared to the recipient stroma. Periodic acid Schiff, original magnification × 700. (b) Electron micrograph of cut edge of recipient Bowman's layer (asterisk) corresponding with (a). Lenticular keratocytes (arrow) are draped over the edge of Bowman's layer. Electron-dense material is associated with a lenticule keratocyte (bracketed area). Original magnification × 1700. (c) Higher magnification of bracketed area shown in (b) demonstrates fibrillogranular material (arrowhead) associated with a lenticule keratocyte (asterisk) in surrounding collagen matrix. Original magnification × 35 000 (from Grossniklaus HE, Lass JH, Jacobs G, Margo CE, McAuliffe AM. Light microscopic and ultrastructural findings in failed epikeratoplasty. Refract Corneal Surg 1989; 5:296–301).

ring (see also Chapter 15). An additional cause of interface opacification is seen in keratoconus patients. Epikeratophakia has been used in keratoconus to flatten the cone and to provide an improved optical surface (see also Chapter 11) [91]. If central scarring is present in the host, vision is not improved by the clear epikeratophakia button (Figure 4.51). The tension exerted by the tightly sewn epikeratophakia button can also produce wrinkling of Bowman's layer (Figure 4.52) which

may also contribute to a reduction in visual acuity. Tables 4.5 and 4.6 summarize problems leading to lenticule removal in epikeratophakia and their histologic features.

(a)

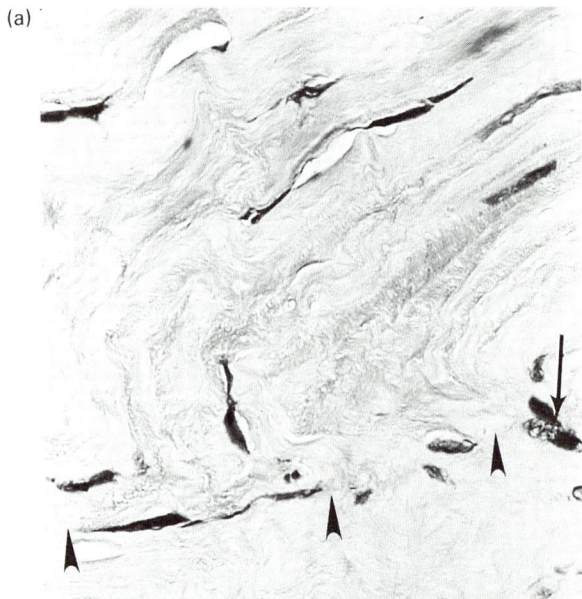

(c)

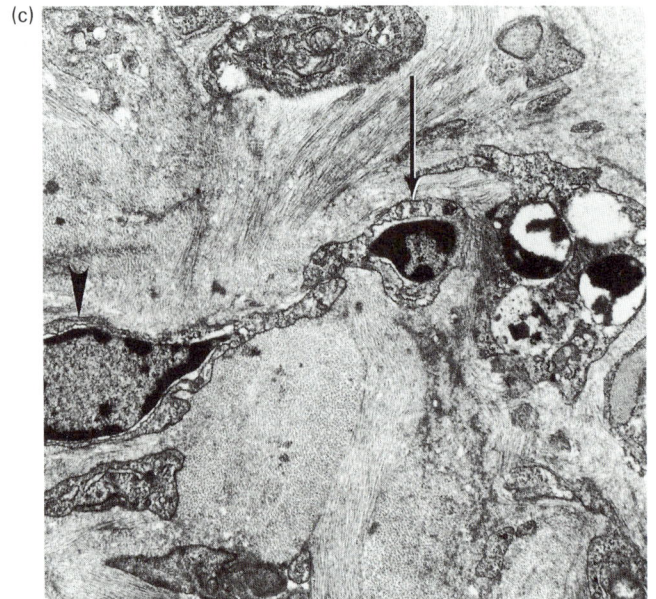

(b)

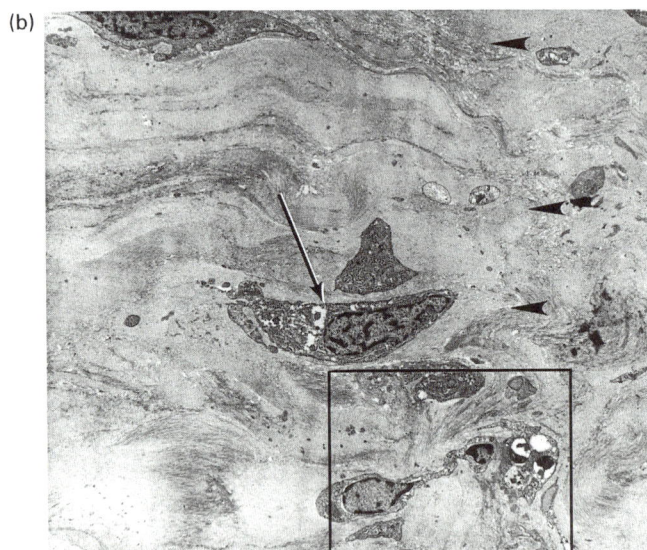

Fig. 4.49 (a) Trephination wound (arrowheads) interface of recipient stroma on left and donor stroma on right. Note apparent migration of plump keratocytes (arrow) between recipient and lenticule. Masson's trichrome, original magnification × 700. (b) Electron micrograph of recipient–lenticule interface (arrowheads corresponding to area shown in (a). Note plump keratocyte (arrow) and apparent migration between recipient keratocyte on left and lenticule keratocyte on right (bracketed area). Original magnification × 7500. (c) Higher magnification of bracketed area shown in (b) shows keratocyte in recipient (arrowhead) is in contact with a keratocyte in the lenticule (arrow) via an opening in the collagen lamellae. Original magnification × 24 000 (from Grossniklaus HE, Lass JH, Jacobs G, Margo CE, McAuliffe AM. Light microscopic and ultrastructural findings in failed epikeratoplasty. Refract Corneal Surg 1989; 5:296–301).

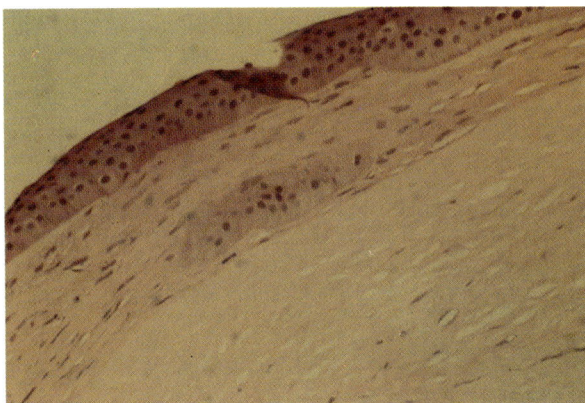

Fig. 4.50 An isolated island of epithelium is present centrally at the interface between the epikeratoplasty lenticule and the host. This produces a local opacification which interferes with vision. Hematoxylin & eosin, original magnification × 100.

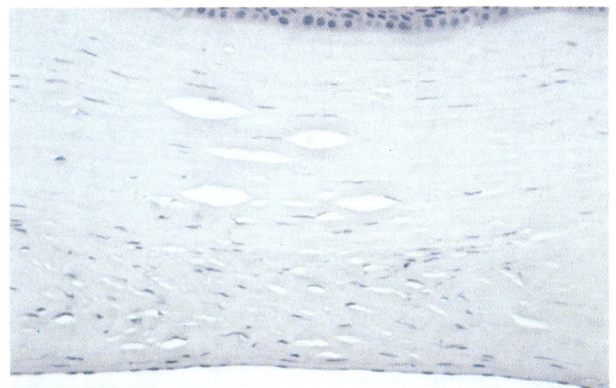

Fig. 4.51 Although the epikeratoplasty lenticule is clear, host stromal scarring persists in this keratoconus patient. Hematoxylin & eosin, original magnification × 100.

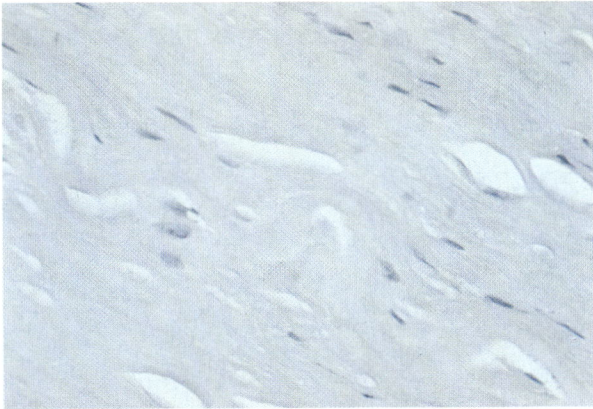

Fig. 4.52 There is marked wrinkling of the host Bowman's membrane in this keratoconic epikeratoplasty. Hematoxylin & eosin, original magnification × 200.

Table 4.5 Epikeratophakia. Indications for lenticule removal. From Binder PS. What we have learned about corneal wound healing from refractive surgery (Barraquer lecture). Refract Corneal Surg 1989; 5:98–120

Loss of best corrected acuity for no apparent reason
Loss of best acuity due to irregular astigmatism, epithelial ingrowth, Bowman's scarring or particulate material
Significant under- or over-correction
Lack of lenticular clarity in the absence of an infective process
Chronic non-healing epithelial defect with or without stromal melting
Infection within cornea or lenticule
Progression of keratoconus under lenticule

Implantation procedures

Intrastromal lenses

Another approach to refractive surgery is to implant a plastic material of appropriate refractive index to alter the patient's underlying refractive error (see Chapter 11). Early experience with methylmethacrylate and other water-impermeable substances failed because nutrients were blocked from the portions of the cornea anterior to the implant. This often resulted in necrosis, melting, and extrusion of the implant. Subsequently, water- and oxygen-permeable plastics such as HEMA and polysulfone have been somewhat more successful [71].

Polysulfone lenses

These lenses are inserted through a superior corneal incision to a pocket created by an intra-stromal dissection, sometimes aided by sodium hyaluronic acid. As

Table 4.6 Epikeratophakia. Histologic features from failed specimens. From Binder PS. What we have learned about corneal wound healing from refractive surgery (Barraquer lecture). Refract Corneal Surg 1989; 5:98–120

Epithelial ulceration
Stromal tissue loss (melting)
Increased collagen interfibrillar distance
Loss of ground substance GAGs with stromal edema
Abnormal epithelium covering lenticule (too thin or too thick)
Focal epithelial cyst formation within stromal wounds
Scars in recipient Bowman's layer
Absent to decreased keratocyte re-population of lenticule
Neovascularization and/or epithelium, collagen, keratocytes in interface
Frank bacterial ulceration

with the lamellar procedures, debris and epithelial cells may be accidentally implanted into the pocket along with the lens. Opacities similar to those seen with epikeratophakia may result. Animal studies have shown that the epithelium and endothelium generally remain intact over these lenses [71].

These lenses are able to correct large refractive errors, but acute failures occur because of edema and severe stromal inflammation. Late effects include epithelial thinning, anterior stromal melting with implant extrusion, gray anterior interface deposits, and neovascularization. Evidence of chronic keratocyte damage, such as vacuolization and lipid degeneration, is also seen. The anterior stroma typically shows a significant decrease in keratocytes. These changes seem to indicate interference with normal corneal nutrition [92] and to avoid this possibility, lenses were fenestrated (Figure 4.53) [93]. This procedure decreases the severe complications, but collagen invades the fenestrations with localized opacification. Lipid deposits have also been reported beneath the unfenestrated areas [71]. Although these lenses are easy to insert, it seems apparent that new materials must be developed before this class of plastic shows clinical usefulness.

Hydrogel lenses

These lenses are inserted either into a free-hand stromal pocket or preferably into a space created by a microkeratome. As with all lamellar procedures, the implantation of epithelial cells and debris can cause problems because of localized opacification. In contrast to the polysulfone lenses, hydrogel lenses are well-tolerated. The typical cornea is optically clear both in front of and behind the lens (Figure 4.54). The corneal endothelium is normal. There is a remarkable absence

(a)

(c)

(a)

(b)

Fig. 4.54 (a) Intra-stromal hydrophilic (KeratoGel) implant. (b) Intra-stromal alloplastic implant. Inflammation and stromal scarring are absent. Toluidine blue, original magnification × 100 (courtesy Bernard McCarey, PhD).

(b)

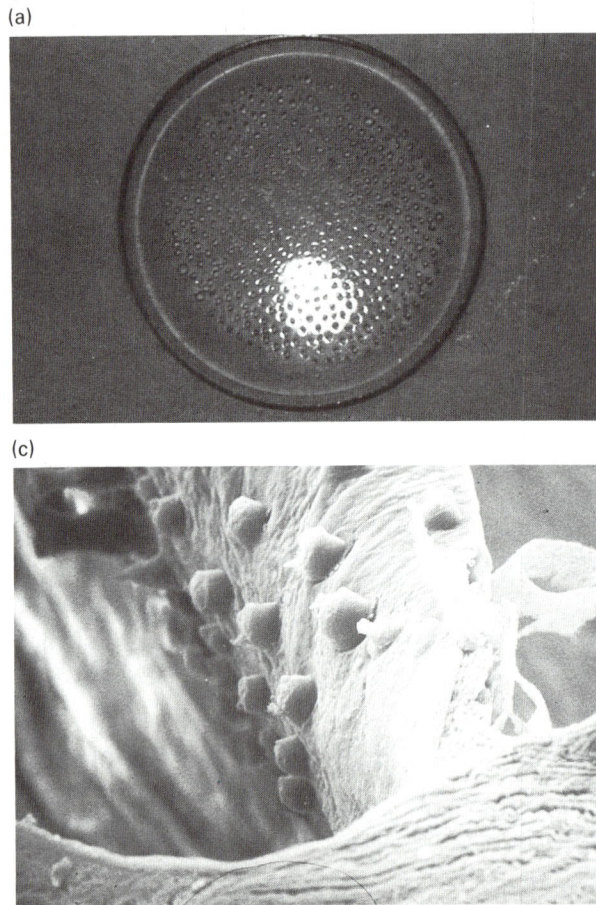

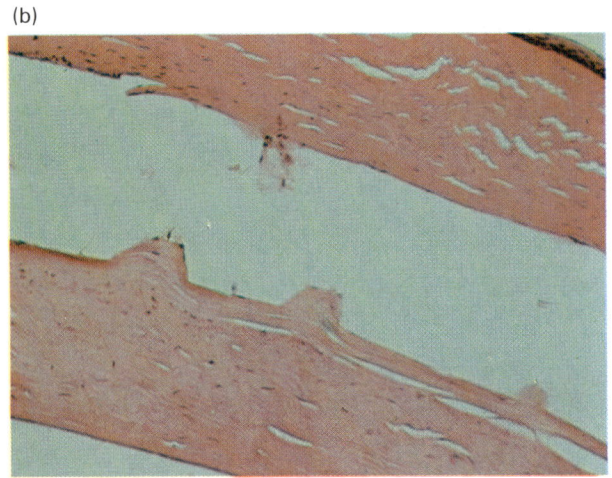

Fig. 4.53 (a) Fenestrated polysulfone lenticule. (b) Histologic section of intralamellar pocket following removal of a fenestrated lens. Note normal keratocytes within pegs of corneal stroma growing through the fenestrations. Hematoxylin & eosin, original magnification × 10. (c) Scanning electron micrograph demonstrating corneal stromal pegs and smooth intralamellar pocket. Original magnification × 22 (from Lane SS, Lindstrom RL. Polysulfone intracorneal lenses. Int Ophthalmol Clin 1991; 31:37–46.

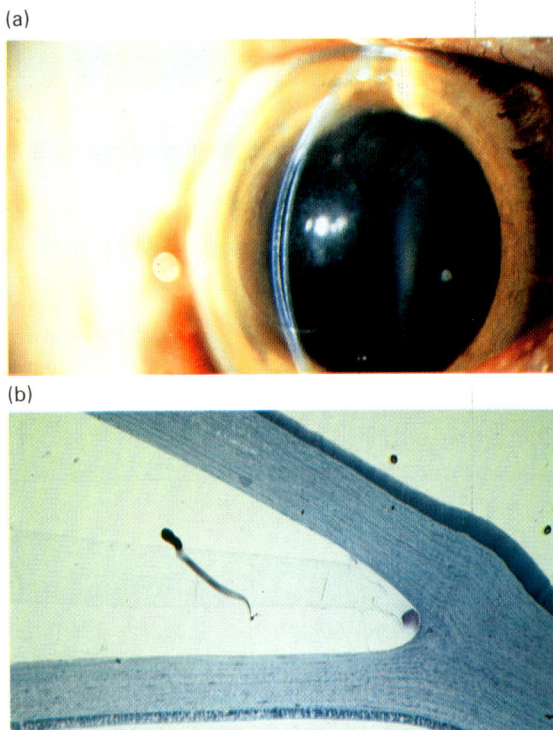

of inflammation and stromal scarring. In a few eyes there has been anterior stromal melting, but the majority of cases show a healthy Bowman's layer and corneal epithelium [71,94]. In those lenses inserted into freehand pockets, there may be consequent wrinkling of Bowman's and Descemet's membranes which can cause interference with visual acuity; this is avoided by removing the upper layer with a microkeratome. Fibrosis may also occur around the implant because of faulty edge design which leaves an unfilled space.

With all lamellar procedures, there is always a risk of infection in the post-operative period or if there is erosion of the anterior stroma and epithelium. The results are predictably disastrous with peri-implant abscess formation and permanent loss of vision. Table 4.7 lists the acute and chronic histologic changes with allopathic stromal implants.

Laser ablative procedures

Laser radiation in the far ultraviolet (150–200 nm) can be produced by a number of different lasers using halogens or noble gases. Extensive animal studies have shown that the argon fluoride excimer laser, operating at 193 nm, has the optimal effect on corneal tissue. The effect of these lasers is produced by ablative photodecomposition in which the irradiated tissue is broken down into volatile fragments without heat effects in the adjacent tissues [95].

The excimer laser may be used for refractive surgery

Table 4.7 Histologic features of alloplastic stromal implants. From Binder PS. What we have learned about corneal wound healing from refractive surgery (Barraquer lecture). Refract Corneal Surg 1989; 5:98–120

Hydrogel implants	Polysulfone implants
Acute features	
Lamellar separation	Lamellar separation
Interface epithelium	Interface epithelium
Microkeratome damage to Bowman's	Descemet's perforation
Chronic features	
Thinned epithelium	Thinned epithelium
Interface collagen	Absent/decreased keratocytes
Interface keratocytes	Interface keratocytes, epithelium
	Anterior lipoid degeneration
	Epithelial ulceration
	Anterior stromal melting
	Descemet's scarring

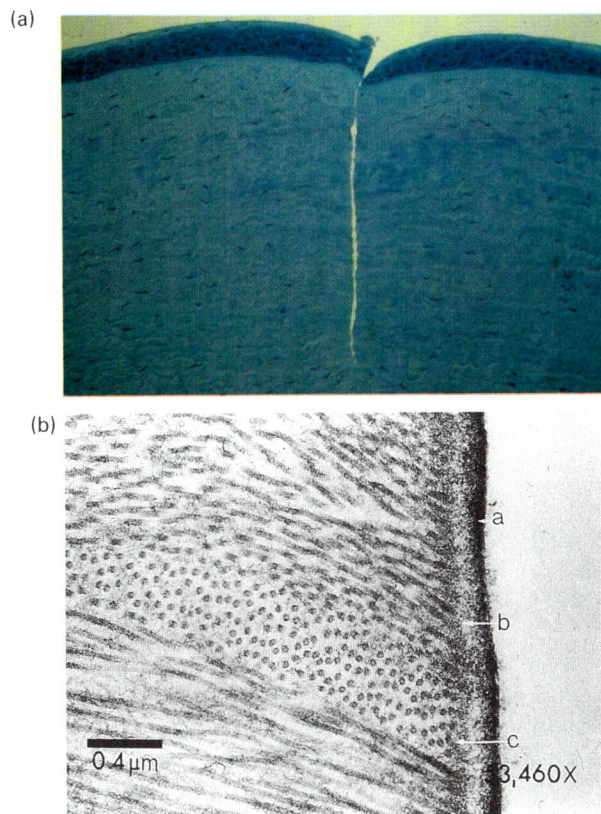

Fig. 4.55 (a) Incision made in rabbit cornea using 193 nm ultraviolet laser (excimer). (b) Edges are smooth and the typical stromal edema and destruction seen in thermal burns are absent. The zone of abnormality consists of an outer densely staining region (a), middle lightly staining region (b), and an inner region (c) showing some increased staining in an area where the fine collagen structure is partially preserved (from Ophthalmology 92:6, 741–748, 1985).

either in a cutting mode, to produce a radial keratotomy wound, or in a broad ablative mode to alter the curvature of a central optical zone. Most of the radial keratotomy studies have been limited to the laboratory. In experimental animals, the excimer laser can make a sharp vertical cut with good depth control. Light microscopic studies show no damage to the adjacent tissues and no inflammatory reaction other than a thin pseudomembrane on the stromal edge (Figure 4.55) [95]. Incisions which approach Descemet's show endothelial cell rupture immediately over the excision site [96]. These wide excision sites (wherein the beam acts like a trenching tool, or "ditch witch") provide a formidable obstacle for the epithelium to cross. These sites accumulate a large epithelial plug similar to that seen in wide gaping radial keratotomy incisions or where such incisions cross. Marsupialization of such wounds is a distinct possibility but has not been reported to date (R.E. Fenzl, 1991, personal communication).

Clinical studies of excimer laser photorefractive keratectomy have been reported [97]. Animal studies in rhesus monkeys demonstrate that corneal changes are limited to the area of laser treatment [98,99]. Immediately after ablation, a marked reduction in the numbers of keratocytes in the anterior stroma was seen. Damaged keratocytes were present within a week of treatment, epithelium had grown over the bare stroma and was thicker than normal. Focal production of basement membrane and hemidesmosomes was seen (see also Chapter 11). Marshall and co-workers hypothesize that a pseudo-Bowman's layer is created by the ablation process, supporting the establishment of a normal epithelial layer [100]. Fibroblasts were present in the anterior stroma.

By 3 weeks, there was a further increase in the number of fibroblasts in the anterior stroma. Electron microscopy of these cells showed intense metabolic activity, suggesting protein synthesis. The anterior stromal lamellae were irregular. Clumps of extracellular matrix were present adjacent to the fibroblasts [98,99]. Because ultraviolet light is known to be mutagenic concern has been raised over the effect on tissue from far-ultraviolet exposure. Nuss and colleagues demonstrated unscheduled DNA synthesis (a marker indicating chromosome damage) in corneal tissue subjected to both 193 nm and 248 nm radiation. The rate was much higher for 248 nm laser light [101]. Trentacoste *et al.* found no increased incidence of anaplastic changes in fibroblast cell culture after exposure to 193 nm radiation [102].

Some of these animals showed a dense anterior stromal haze at 3 months. Microscopic study revealed dark basal cells with vacuolization at the stromal–epithelial junction. The basement membrane remained fragmented in these animals. Numerous fibroblasts and abundant extra-cellular matrix persisted. However, these features were absent in the animals which showed only minimal or absent corneal haze [98,99].

At 6 and 9 months after surgery, the severe changes had disappeared in most animals. Those with persistent haze continued to show some fragmentation of the basement membrane as well as a few active fibroblasts. Throughout the time periods, the posterior stroma, Descemet's membrane, and the corneal endothelium appeared within normal limits. Despite the changes noted in the basement membrane, recurrent epithelial erosions were not observed. The lack of uniformity in histopathology and clinical appearance was felt to be due to individual variation in response to the phototic injury [98,99].

Intra-ocular procedures

The effects upon the cornea by the implantation of an intra-ocular lens have been well-documented [103–106]. Certain of these have been reduced by the advent of folding lens technology and small incisions but they have not been completely eliminated. The possibility of corneal decompensation, while less, is still there. Thus the concern with the implantation of IOLs into phakic eyes. The poor results obtained by Strampelli [107,108] and Barraquer [109] cannot be ignored. Some of these newer lenses are similar to the design of Kelman and rely upon scleral angle fixation, with all that implies. Baikoff has reported endothelial cell loss in some of his cases—two severely [110, 111]. At least one case of cataract formation has been reported with the angle-supported myopic lens [111]. While mild uveitis has also been reported, no cases of the UGH (uveitis–glaucoma–hyphema) syndrome have been documented to date. No clinical reports of the "collar button" lens advocated and implanted by Fyodorov's group is, as yet, available. It remains to be seen how well the crystalline lens tolerates these types of implanted lenses. We will have somewhat more to say on these implants in Chapter 13.

Scleral procedures

The reader is referred to standard texts on ophthalmic pathology and retinal detachment surgery for a thorough discussion of the histology of these procedures (see also Chapter 14).

Principles of wound healing as applied to refractive surgery

The following is excerpted from Binder's excellent work [71] on healing in refractive surgery:

1 Permanent corneal curvature changes occur when Bowman's layer is severed.

2 Fewer radial incisions and a standard surgical approach to radial keratotomy may improve the safety, predictability, and stability of the procedure.

3 Optical interfaces tend to degrade the visual image. The potential space that is created can serve as a location for foreign material, keratocytes, and epithelium, which collectively have the potential further to degrade the visual image.

4 Freezing and lyophilization produce severe morphologic changes in the cornea. Refractive procedures that utilize fresh tissue appear safer.

5 Water-impermeable (bioincompatible) intra-stromal implants cannot be used for refractive surgery.

6 All thermal collagen shrinkage procedures produce severe and permanent stromal damage and only temporarily produce collagen shrinkage.

7 The wound healing response of the cornea needs to be controlled if photorefractive keratectomy is to be successful.

The above pretty much encapsulates the current thinking in refractive surgery. The reader is advised to take note and heed these observations.

References

1 Miller D, Benedek G. *Intraocular Light Scattering*. Thomas, Springfield, 1973.
2 Goldman J, Benedek G, Dohlman C, Kravitt B. Structural alterations affecting transparency in swollen human corneas. Invest Ophthalmol 1968; 7:501–519.
3 Farrell RA, McCalley RL, Tatham PER. Wavelength dependencies of light scattering in normal and cold swollen corneas and their structural implications. J Physiol (Lond) 1976; 233:589.
4 Hedbys BO. The role of polysaccharides in corneal swelling. Exp Eye Res 1961; 1:81.
5 Newsome DA, Gross J, Hassell JR. Human corneal stroma contains three distinct collagens. Invest Ophthalmol Visual Sci 1981; 22:376.
6 Miller EJ, Gay S. Collagen: an overview. Methods Enzymol 1982; 82:3.
7 Piez KA, Miller A. The structure of collagen fibrils. J Supramol Struct 1974; 2:121.
8 Hogan MI, Alvarado JA, Weddell JE. *Histology of the Human Eye*. W.B. Saunders, Philadelphia, 1971.
9 Baum JP, Maurice DM, McCarey BE. The active and passive transport of water across the corneal endothelium. Exp Eye Res 1984; 39:335–342.
10 Hodson S, Miller S. The bicarbonate ion pump in the endothelium which regulates the hydration of the rabbit cornea. J Physiol (Lond) 1977; 203:563.
11 Hull DS. Corneal endothelial bicarbonate transport and the effect of carbonic anhydrase inhibitors on endothelial permeability and fluxes and corneal thickness. Invest Ophthalmol 1977; 16:883.
12 Dohlman CH, Wortman B, Hedbys BO, Mishima S. The swelling pressure of the corneal stroma. Invest Ophthalmol Visual Sci 1963; 1:158.
13 Dohlman CH. Physiology of the cornea: corneal edema. In: *The Cornea. Scientific Foundations and Clinical Practice*, G Smolin and RA Thoft (eds). Little, Brown, Boston, 1983.
14 Klyce SD. Electric profiles in the corneal epithelium. J Phy-

siol (Lond) 1972; 226:407.

15 Manchester PT. Hydration of the cornea. Trans Am Ophthalmol Soc 1970; 68:425.

16 Zucker B. Hydration and transparency of the cornea. Arch Ophthalmol 1966; 75:228.

17 Fyodorov SN, Agronovsky A. Long term results of anterior radial keratotomy. J Ocul Ther Surg 1982; 1:217.

18 Holly FJ. Formation and rupture of the tear film. Exp Eye Res 1973; 15:515.

19 Lamberts DW. Physiology of the cornea: physiology of the tear film. In: *The Cornea. Scientific Foundations and Clinical Practice*, G Smolin and RA Thoft (eds). Little, Brown, Boston, 1983.

20 Thoft RA, Friend J. Corneal epithelial glucose utilization. Arch Ophthalmol 1972; 88:58.

21 Gillette TE, Greiner JV, Allansmith MR. Immunochemical localization of human tear lysozyme. Arch Ophthalmol 1981; 99:298.

22 Holly FJ. The precorneal tear film. Contact Intraocular Lens Med J 1978; 4:134.

23 Geanon JD, Tripathi BJ, Tripathi RC, Barlow GH. Tissue plasminogen activator in avascular tissues of the eye: a quantitative study of its activity in the cornea, lens, and aqueous and vitreous humors of dog, calf, and monkey. Exp Eye Res 1987; 44:55–63.

24 McCracken JS, Burger PC, Klintworth GK. Morphologic observations on experimental corneal vascularization in the rat. Lab Invest 1979; 41:519–530.

25 Crosson CE, Klyce SD, Beuerman RW. Epithelial wound closure in the rabbit cornea. Invest Ophthalmol Visual Sci 1986; 27:464–473.

26 Buck RC. Cell migration in repair of corneal epithelium. Invest Ophthalmol Visual Sci 1979; 18:767–784.

27 Soong H, McClenic B. EGF does not enhance corneal epithelial cell motility. Invest Ophthalmol Visual Sci 1989; 30: 1808–1812.

28 Ding M, Burstein NL. Review: Fibronectin in corneal wound healing. J Ocular Pharmacol 1988; 4:75–91.

29 Jumblatt MM, Neufeld AH. A tissue culture assay of corneal epithelial wound closure. Invest Ophthalmol Visual Sci 1986; 27:8–13.

30 Levi-Montalcini R, Hamburger V. A diffusable agent of mouse sarcoma producing hyperplasia of sympathetic ganglia and hyperneurotization of viscera in the chick embryo. J Exp Zool 1953; 123:233–288.

31 Cohen S. Isolation of a mouse submaxillary gland protein accelerating incisor eruption and eyelid opening in the newborn animal. J Biol Chem 1962; 237:1555–1562.

32 Kitizawa T, Kinoshita S, Fujita K. The mechanism of accelerated corneal epithelial healing by human epidermal growth factor. Invest Ophthalmol Visual Sci 1990; 31:1773–1778.

33 Baudouin C, Fredj-Reygrobellet D, Caruelle J. Acidic fibroblast growth factor distribution in normal human eye and possible implications in ocular pathogenesis. Ophthalmic Res 1990; 22:73–81.

34 Leibowitz HM, Morello S, Stern M, Kupferman A. Effect of topically administered epidermal growth factor on corneal wound strength. Arch Ophthalmol 1990; 108:734–737.

35 Soubrane G, Jerdoin J, Karpouzis I. Binding of basic fibroblast growth factor to normal and neovascularized cornea. Invest Ophthalmol Visual Sci 1990; 31:323–333.

36 Fogle JA, Kenyon KR, Stark WJ, Green WR. Defective epithelial adhesion in anterior corneal dystrophies. Am J Ophthalmol 1975; 79:925–940.

37 Werblin TP, Hirst LW, Stark WJ, Maumenee I. Prevalence of map–dot–fingerprint changes in the cornea. Br J Ophthalmol 1981; 79:925–940.

38 Smith RS, Smith LA, Rich LF, Weimar V. Effects of growth factors on corneal wound healing. Invest Ophthalmol Visual Sci 1981; 20:222–229.

39 Musch DC, Sugar A, Meyer RF. Demographic and predisposing factors in corneal ulceration. Arch Ophthalmol 1983; 101:1545–1548.

40 Berman M, Dohlman CH, Gnadinger M, Davison P. Characterization of collagenolytic activity in the ulcerating cornea. Exp Eye Res 1971; 11:255–257.

41 Fraunfelder FT, Meyer SM. *Drug Induced Ocular Side Effects and Drug Interactions*. Lea and Febiger, Philadelphia, 1989.

42 Smith RS. Clinical diagnosis and management. In *Corneal Disorders*, HM Leibowitz (ed). W.B. Saunders, Philadelphia, 1984.

43 Claoue C, Lewkowicz-Moss S, Easty D. Epithelial cyst in the anterior chamber after penetrating keratoplasty: a rare complication. Br J Ophthalmol 1988; 72:36–40.

44 Stark WJ, Michels RG, Maumenee A, Cuppless H. Surgical management of epithelial ingrowth. Am J Ophthalmol 1970; 85:772–780.

45 Yee RD, Pettit TH. Corneal intrastromal cyst following lamellar keratoplasty. Ann Ophthalmol 1975; 7:644–646.

46 Kenyon KR. Decision-making in the therapy of external disease: non-infected corneal ulcers. Ophthalmology 1982; 89:44–51.

47 Waring GO, Rodrigues MM, Laibson PA. Corneal dystrophies. II. Endothelial dystrophies. Surv Ophthalmol 1978; 23:147–168.

48 Weimar V, Fellman M. Connective tissue cell mobilization and migration following wounding. I. Inhibition of mobilization by chloroquine and inhibition of migration by colchicine. Exp Eye Res 1970; 9:12.

49 Cintron AC, Schneider H, Kublin C. Corneal scar formation. Exp Eye Res 1973; 17:251–259.

50 McDonald MB, Frantz JM, Klyce SD et al. One-year refractive results of central photorefractive keratectomy for myopia in the nonhuman primate cornea. Arch Ophthalmol 1990; 108: 40–47.

51 Welch MP, Odland GF, Clark RA. Temporal relationships of F-actin bundle formation, collagen and fibronectin matrix assembly, and fibronectin receptor expression to wound contraction. J Cell Biol 1990; 110:133–145.

52 Cogan DG. Vascularization of the cornea. Its functional induction by small lesions and a new theory of its pathogenesis. Arch Ophthalmol 1949; 41:406–416.

53 Klintworth GK. The contribution of morphology to our understanding of the pathogenesis of experimentally produced corneal vascularization. Invest Ophthalmol Visual Sci 1977; 16:281–284.

54 Furcht LT. Editorial: Critical factors controlling angiogenesis: cell products, cell matrix and growth factors. Lab Invest 1986; 55:505–509.

55 Folkman J, Klagsbrun M. Angiogenic factors. Science 1987; 235:442–447.

56 Laing RA, Neubauer L, Oak SS. Evidence for mitosis in the adult corneal endothelium. Ophthalmology 1984; 91:1129–1134.

57 Joyce NC, Meklir B, Neufeld AH. In vitro pharmacologic separation of corneal endothelial migration and spreading responses. Invest Ophthalmol Visual Sci 1990; 31:1816–1826.

58 MacRae SM, Matsuda M, Rich LF. The effect of radial keratotomy on the corneal endothelium. Am J Ophthalmol 1985; 100:538–542.

59 Smith RS, Cutro J. Computer analysis of radial keratotomy. CLAO J 1984; 10:241–248.

60 Ormerod LD, Smith RE. Contact lens-associated microbial keratitis. Arch Ophthalmol 1986; 104:79–83.

61 Schein OD, Glynn RJ, Poggio EC. The relative risk of ulcerative keratitis among users of daily-wear and extended-wear soft contact lenses. N Engl J Med 1989; 321:773–778.

62 Ingraham HJ, Guber D, Green WR. Radial keratotomy. Clinicopathologic case report. Arch Ophthalmol 1985; 103: 683–688.

63 Binder PS, Nayak SD, Deg JK. An ultrastructural and histochemical study of long-term wound healing after radial keratotomy. Am J Ophthalmol 1987; 103:432–440.

64 Yamaguchi T, Kaufman H, Fukushima A, Safir A, Asbell P. Histologic and electron microscopic assessment of endothelial damage produced by anterior radial keratotomy in the monkey cornea. Am J Ophthalmol 1981; 92:313–327.

65 Jester JV, Villasenor RA, Miyashiro J. Epithelial inclusion cysts following radial keratotomy. Arch Ophthalmol 1983; 101:611–615.

66 Roth AM, Ekins MB, Waring GO, Gupta LM, Rosenblatt LS. Oval corneal opacities in beagles. III. Histochemical demonstration of stromal lipids without hyperlipidemia. Invest Ophthalmol Visual Sci 1981; 21:95–106.

67 Kurasova TP. Klinicheskoe techenie posleoperatzionnovo perioda pri keratotomii. (Clinical course of the postoperative period following keratotomy.) In: Surgery of Refractive Anomalies of the Eye, AI Ivashina and SA Kolmanovskii (eds). Moscow Scientific Research Institute for Eye Microsurgery, Moscow, pp 27–32, 1981.

68 Waring GO, Steinberg EB, Wilson LA. Slit lamp microscopic appearance of corneal wound healing after radial keratotomy. Am J Ophthalmol 1985; 100:218–224.

69 Coalwell K, Binder PS. High voltage electron microscopic evaluation of human radial keratotomy. Invest Ophthalmol Visual Sci (AMA Abstract) 1988; 29:280.

70 Davison PS, Galbavy EJ. Connective tissue remodeling in corneal and scleral wounds. Invest Ophthalmol Visual Sci 1986; 27:1478–1484.

71 Binder PS. What we have learned about corneal wound healing from refractive surgery (Barraquer lecture). Refractive Corneal Surg 1989; 5:98–120.

72 Nelson JD, Williams P, Lindstrom RL, Doughman DJ. Map-fingerprint-dot changes in the corneal epithelial basement membrane following radial keratotomy. Ophthalmology 1985; 92:199–205.

73 Deg JK, Binder PS. Wound healing after astigmatic keratotomy in human eyes. Ophthalmology 1987; 94:1290–1298.

74 Aquavella JV, Smith RS, Shaw EL. Alteration in corneal morphology following thermokeratoplasty. Arch Ophthalmol 1976; 94:2082–2085.

75 Barraquer JI. Queratofaquia. In: Cirugia Refractiva de la Cornea. Instituto Barraquer de America, Bogota, Colombia, 1989.

76 Pokorny KS, Kenyon KR, Swinger C et al. Histopathology of human keratorefractive lenticules. Cornea 1990; 9:223–233.

77 Bores LD. Mechanical modulation of the corneal surface. Int Clin Ophthalmol 1991; 31:25–36.

78 Krumeich JH, Swinger CA. Nonfreeze epikeratophakia for the correction of myopia. Am J Ophthalmol 1987; 103:397–403.

79 Krumeich JH, Knuelle A. Non-freeze epikeratophakia (live epikeratophakia). Fortschr Ophthalmol 1990; 87:20–24.

80 Rostron CK, Brittain GP, Morton DB, Rees JE. Experimental epikeratophakia with biological adhesive. Arch Ophthalmol 1988; 106:1103–1106.

81 Binder PS, Krumeich JH, Zavala EV. Laboratory evaluation of freeze vs non-freeze lamellar refractive keratoplasty. Arch Ophthalmol 1987; 105:1125–1128.

82 Zavala EY, Krumeich JH, Binder PS. Clinical pathology of non-freeze lamellar refractive keratoplasty. Cornea 1988; 7: 223–230.

83 Lieurance RC, Patel AC, Wan WL, Beatty RF, Kash RL, Schanzlin DJ. Excimer laser cut lenticules for epikeratophakia. Am J Ophthalmol 1987; 103:475–476.

84 Maguen K, Pinhas S, Verity SM. Keratophakia with lyophilized cornea lathed at room temperature: new techniques and experimental surgical results. Ophthalmic Surg 1983; 14: 759–762.

85 El-Maghraby MA, Vitero E, Ruiz L. Keratomileusis in situ to correct high myopia. Ophthalmology 1988; 95(Suppl):145.

86 Jaeger MJ, Berson P, Kaufman HE, Green WR. Epikeratoplasty for keratoconus. A clinicopathologic case report. Cornea 1987; 6:131–139.

87 Steinert RF, Grene RB. Postoperative management of epikeratoplasty. J Cataract Refract Surg 1986; 14:255–264.

88 Binder PS, Zavala EY, Baumgartner SD, Nayak SK. Combined morphologic effects of cryolathing and lyophilization on epikeratoplasty lenticules. Arch Ophthalmol 1986; 104: 671–679.

89 Binder PS, Baumgartner SD, Fogle JA. Histopathology of a case of epikeratophakia (aphakic epikeratoplasty). Arch Ophthalmol 1985; 103:1357–1363.

90 Binder PS, Beal JPJ, Zavala EY. The histopathology of a case of keratophakia. Arch Ophthalmol 1982; 100:101–105.

91 Dietze TR, Durrie DS. Indications and treatment of keratoconus using epikeratophakia. Ophthalmology 1988; 95:236–246.

92 Climenhaga H, Macdonald JM, McCarey BE, Waring GO. Effect of diameter and depth on the response to solid polysulfone intracorneal lenses in cats. Arch Ophthalmol 1988; 106:818–824.

93 Lane SS, Lindstrom RL, Cameron JD. Fenestrated intracorneal lenses. Ophthalmology 1987; 94(Suppl):125.

94 Beekhuis WH, McCarey BE, van Rij G, Waring GO. Complications of hydrogel intracorneal lenses in monkeys. Arch Ophthalmol 1987; 105:116–122.

95 Trokel SL, Srinivasan R, Braren B. Excimer laser surgery of the cornea. Am J Ophthalmol 1983; 96:710–715.

96 Dehm EJ, Puliafito CA, Adler CM. Endothelial injury in rabbits following excimer laser ablation at 193 and 248 nm. Arch Ophthalmol 1986; 104:1364–1368.

97 Taylor DM, L'Esperance FAJ, Del Pero RA et al. Human excimer laser lamellar keratectomy. A clinical study. Ophthalmology 1989; 96:654–664.

98 Fantes F, Hanna KD, Waring GO et al. Wound healing after excimer laser keratomileusis (photorefractive keratectomy) in monkeys. Arch Ophthalmol 1990; 108:665–675.

99 SundarRaj N, Geiss MJ, Fantes F et al. Healing of excimer laser ablated monkey corneas. An immunohistochemical evaluation. Arch Ophthalmol 1990; 108:1604–1610.

100 Marshall WJ, Trokel SL, Rothery S. Photoablation reprofiling of the cornea using an excimer laser photorefractive keratectomy. Lasers Ophthalmol 1986; 1:21–48.

101 Nuss RC, Puliafito CA, Dehm E. Unscheduled DNA synthesis following excimer laser ablation of the cornea in vivo. Invest Ophthalmol Visual Sci 1987; 28:287–294.

102 Trentacoste J, Thompson K, Parrish RK, Hajek A, Berman MR, Ganjei P. Mutagenic potential of a 193-nm excimer laser on fibroblasts in tissue culture. Ophthalmol 1987; 94: 125–129.

103 Castroviejo R. Comments on cataract surgery. Usual and unusual procedures including an evaluation of cryoextraction. Am J Ophthalmol 1966; 61:1063–1077.

104 Charlin R. Peripheral corneal edema after cataract extraction. Am J Ophthalmol 1985; 99:298–303.

105 Cotlier E, Rose M. Cataract extraction by the intracapsular methods and by phacoemulsification: the results of surgeons in training. Trans Am Acad Ophthalmol Otolaryngol 1976; 81:163–182.

106 Panariello GF, Cooper J. Complications in cataract surgery. J Am Optom Assoc 1983; 54:713–718.

107 Strampelli B. Lentilles camerulaires après 6 années d'experiences. Acta Conc Ophtal Belgica (Brussels) 1958; 11:1692–1698.

108 Strampelli B. Sopportabilita di lenti acriliche in camera anteriore nella afachia e nei vizi di refrazione. Atti Soc Oftal Lomb 1953; 8:292.

109 Barraquer J. Anterior chamber plastic lenses. Results and conclusions from 5 years' experience. Trans Ophthalmol Soc (UK) 1959; 79:393–424.

110 Baikoff G, Colin J. Damage to the corneal endothelium using anterior chamber intraocular lenses for myopia: letter. Refract Corneal Surg 1990; 6:383.

111 Baikoff G. The refractive IOL in a phakic eye. Ophthalmic Pract 1991; 9:58–61.

5
Patient Workup

Science is facts, just as houses are made of stones, so is science made of facts; but a pile of stones is not a house and a collection of facts is not necessarily science.
[Henri Poincaré]

The proper evaluation of a candidate for refractive surgery includes a number of considerations. The following criteria are those currently utilized to screen candidates for refractive surgery within my clinic. These are subject to modification by circumstances which may from time to time arise.

1 Any patient whose age is 18 or more and whose myopia is greater than 1.00 D and who has shown no progression of the myopia for the last 18 months is a good candidate for surgery. This does not preclude anisometropic children. However, no protocol for children has, as yet, been evolved. A change of ±0.50 D within a year is considered normal. A change of 1.0 D within a year is considered significant. In addition, any patient (as above), whose hyperopia is greater than 1.50 D would be suitable for refractive surgery.

2 Patients with astigmatism >1.00 D (or 20% of the spherical component) are also candidates but may require special procedures (see also Chapter 9).

3 Patients with corneal curvatures less than 40 D are not considered good candidates unless they have low to moderate myopia.

4 No evidence of corneal disease and/or dystrophic changes can be present.

5 Any patient with an external ocular disease process should be off medication and clear for 3 months before scheduling surgery. Surgery on patients with a past history of actual or suspected herpes simplex keratitis is contraindicated at this time.

Patient evaluation

The following workup procedure is offered as a guide to establishing your own specific schedule. Recommendations will be made as appropriate within this outline in order to establish those points the author deems important. The general outline of the workup process will be followed by a more detailed description of the examination procedures.

Preliminary screening and intake

Patients will inquire of your receptionist to find out if indeed you do perform refractive surgery. The receptionist should be prepared to answer that question and also those of a more general nature, briefly. It is suggested that patients be offered information about the surgery either by mail or by pickup. This information can take many forms.

To determine whether a patient is a possible candidate prior to making an appointment, the receptionist should request that the patient bring or mail in copies of his or her most current eyeglass and contact lens prescriptions (if available). This is particularly important for patients intending to travel long distances for this service. In these cases this information is vitally important and may save the patient considerable time and expense.

Dealing with contact lenses

When making an appointment for a patient, the receptionist should ascertain if the caller is a contact lens wearer and what type lens is being worn. The patient is requested to remove any contact lenses for the period of time that you have determined adequate (Table 5.1). For example, hard contacts should be out for a minimum of 7 days—longer if possible. The length of time can be adjusted depending upon the time duration of spectacle blur. At my clinic, we add 3 days for each 30 min of spectacle blur. As an example, a patient experiences 45 min of blur from the time he or she removes the contacts until he or she can see clearly with current spectacles. The length of time the patient should have the lenses out would be: 7 + 4 = 11 days minimum. Patients like this should be routed to your nurse or assistant to insure that the response obtained is correct. Soft contacts should be removed for a minimum of 48 hours. On the other hand, if the patient is wearing "retainer lenses" for orthokeratology, these lenses must be out a minimum of *6 months!* These lenses are known to produce long-standing corneal distortion [1–3].

An occasional patient will state that he or she does not have "fall-back" spectacles. Here the nurse or assistant should become involved. The patient is requested to remove the lens from the non-dominant eye for the duration specified. If coming from a distance, he or she should be advised to obtain an inexpensive pair of spectacles (or find an old pair) to wear for the interim.

The patient should bring any old optical aids that he or she has retained and may have worn in the last few years. These will be useful during the initial visit to determine how stable the patient's refraction and keratometry readings are. Old prescriptions are also requested to be brought.

The initial visit

Workup outline

1 Complete ocular history.
2 Visual acuity—corrected/uncorrected (near and far).
3 Refraction—cycloplegic as warranted.
4 Intra-ocular pressure.
5 Keratometry.
6 Slit-lamp examination.
7 Measurement of corneal diameter.
8 Determination of dominant eye/handedness.
9 Fundoscopic examination.
10 Viewing of informed consent tape.

Table 5.1 Length of time contact lenses should be removed before the initial visit

Lens type	Minimum time*
Hard	1 week
Soft	48 hours
Ortho-K	6 months

* See text.

11 Patient questions to be answered.
12 Patient expectations to be recorded on chart.

A patient intake form is to be supplemented through careful history-taking by your nurse or assistant (Figure 5.1). Reading over this form and your nurse's notes is helpful prior to examining the patient yourself and may suggest some important avenues to explore further. After this form is filled out, it should be checked by the receptionist and any blanks filled in or marked NA by inquiry. Sometimes patients will prefer not to reveal some history to the receptionist. In this event that fact should be noted or flagged to the attention of the doctor and/or nurse, to be followed up. The receptionist should photocopy all submitted prescriptions, referral letters etc. during this period and attach them to the chart. Any spectacles should be neutralized, the age of each noted and that information affixed to the record as well.

The patient is placed in an examination room where preliminary information is obtained. A careful recording of the patient's visual acuity both with and without correction is vital. If the patient is a contact lens wearer, these lenses should be removed before the initial visit and must be kept out for a period of time corresponding to the type of lens and amount of spectacle blur being experienced after removal (see above). In these cases, we recommend a pre-examination or acuity screening visit prior to the workup if possible.

Contrast sensitivity and glare testing should also be performed, especially in contact lens wearers. There has been some discussion about the validity of devices such as the Miller–Nadler Glare Tester (marketed by the Titmus Company). It has been said that devices such as these do not truly measure glare, but rather flare. Since there is no general agreement as to the definition of glare or flare, it is difficult to decide this question unequivocally. Test results from these instruments do not correlate well with so-called contrast sensitivity testers—each appears to be measuring something different. Still, the results of such tests seem to relate to the real world much more closely than do high-contrast Snellen letter charts. Furthermore, the results of such tests may bear on the experience of the patient post-operatively.

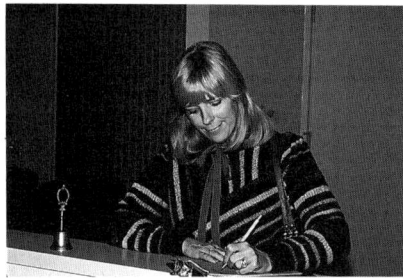

(a)

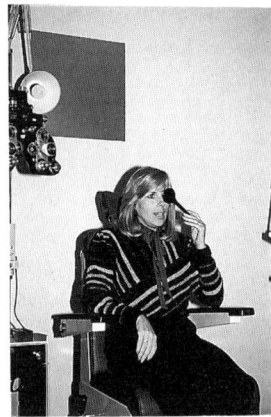

(b)

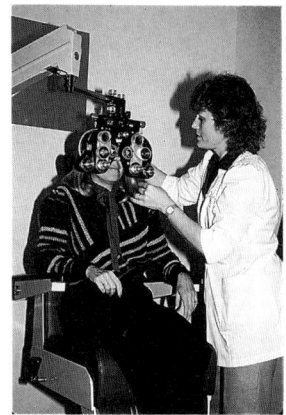

(c)

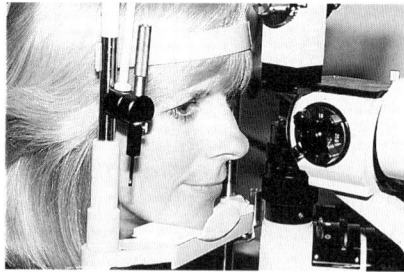

(d)

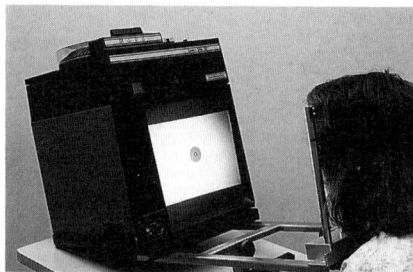

(e)

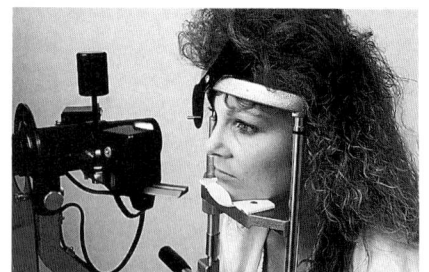

(f)

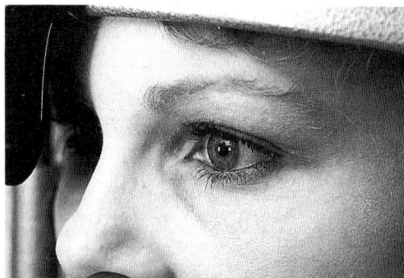

(g)

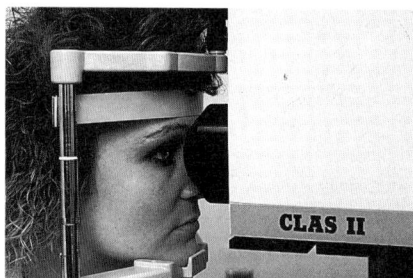

(h)

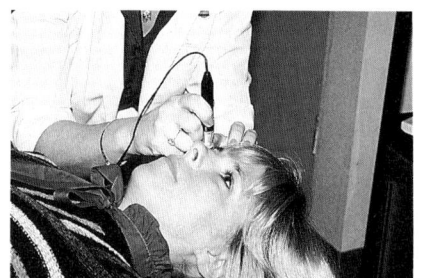

(i)

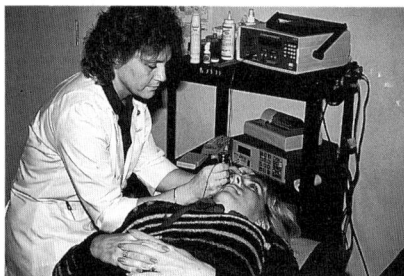

(j)

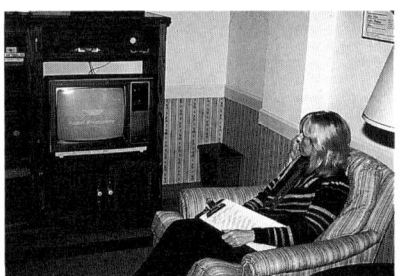

(k)

Fig. 5.1 Patient intake: (a) get information; (b) check vision; (c) refract with phoropter—not with computer; (d) examine cornea with slit-lamp; (e) do glare or contrast sensitivity testing; (f,g) record Ks; (h) do topography; (i) A-scan; (j) measure thickness over entire cornea; (k) watch informed consent tape.

The acuity measurement very much depends upon the contrast of the letter with the background. Unfortunately, the technique has few counterparts in the real world and equally unfortunate is the fact that it is firmly entrenched in society. It is well-known in clinical practice that the visual acuity as measured by the Snellen chart is often in no way indicative of the existence of an actual visual handicap. Many individuals with increased lenticular turbidity can discern 20/40 or better and yet be unable to recognize a face in normal lighting or drive safely at night. Contrast sensitivity methods are probably a more realistic test of visual efficiency but a standard has not yet been established for their use.

It would be well to consider that the Snellen optotypes were invented 125 years ago. They have been used universally and religiously ever since to record the visual acuity. Religiously is not too strong a word to use in connection with the Snellen vision chart—mainly because its employment is almost a matter of canonical law. To suggest that it is time it was supplanted by a modern method which has more relevance to the real world is to commit an act of heresy. Yet the Snellen chart measures only the ability of an eye to discern the shapes of high-contrast objects—not the efficiency of the visual system in a normal environment. It is not unusual for an individual to score 20/40 vision on a Snellen chart and yet be unable to recognize a familiar face at arm's length. That same individual may be found to fail a contrast sensitivity test altogether. Regardless, such a Snellen visual acuity score permits that individual to drive an automobile— day or night—regardless that the visual efficiency may be below par. However, until such time as these contrast sensitivity measuring devices are standardized their results will not be universally accepted. That's the nice thing about glare "standards"—there are so many to choose from. None the less, their employment in the evaluation of pre- and post-operative refractive surgery patients is highly recommended.

Glare testing generally follows the recording of the visual acuity, after which are also recorded the keratometry readings. The sequence of events is arranged so as to produce the least possible alteration in the results of the following examination. In any case, pachymetry and the intra-ocular pressure are the last measurements to be taken, after the informed consent.

The informed consent

The patient is then removed to the secondary waiting area where, alone or with others, an informed consent video tape presentation is viewed. A short written examination follows this video presentation and is so arranged as to insure that the essential material is understood by the viewer. The patient is then returned to the examination room and awaits refraction, slit-lamp examination, fundoscopy etc.

When the examination is completed, any questions that the patient may have are answered at that time. Patients are then asked if there are any more questions that they would like answered; if the answer is yes, these additional questions are answered. If no other questions are pending, then the informed consent portion of the exam is ended. However, the patient is encouraged to write down any questions that inevitably come up after leaving the office and have them answered at a later time. Complete candor is essential at this point. If the patient is a candidate for surgery, his or her expectations are recorded, in the patient's own words, into the record. If they agree to have surgery performed, they are required to sign both the video test and the informed consent, even though surgery may not actually be scheduled. Patients are assured that they are under no obligation when they do this and may change their minds at any time. It is important to get the consent signed while everything is fresh in the patient's mind and more importantly, to avoid the possibility of the patient reaching the operating room with an unsigned consent form. Once the patient is pre-medicated, it's too late to get the consent signed—postponing the case to a later day (at least a week hence) is the only alternative. In any case the patient is now ready for the pre-operative testing and is placed into the surgical workup queue. Photokeratometry and/or corneal surface topography needs to be done and lastly pachymetry, axial length and the intra-ocular pressure are recorded.

One of the questions frequently asked by patients is their chance for success. The answer should be based upon your percentage of success in cases similar to their own. Success is described as the achievement of 20/40 unaided visual acuity post-operatively. You can demonstrate varying degrees of refractive error reduction for patients by adjusting their correction within the phoropter or trial frame and allowing them to observe their surroundings with and without this correction. You may find that, in some cases, uncorrected vision less than 20/20 is acceptable to patients. In that event patients will express themselves and this should also be recorded in the record. This process can help patients decide whether or not the surgery meets their needs. If patients' expectations seem unreasonable or they insist that they want or expect "perfect" vision after surgery, gently but firmly suggest that they reconsider having any such surgery performed on their eyes and dismiss them.

Gathering pre-operative data

It should be evident by now that, although the outcome of radial keratotomy surgery (for example) is

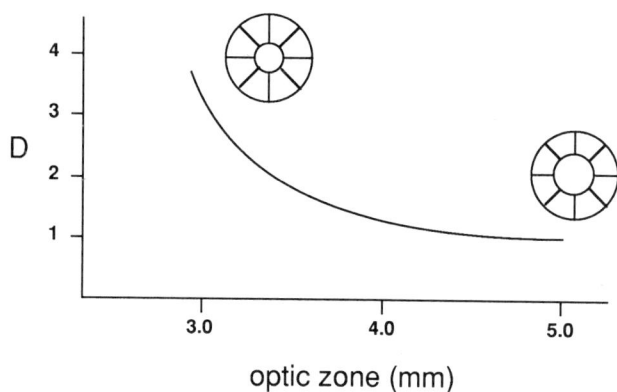

Fig. 5.2 Effect of optic zone size on surgical outcome.

Table 5.2 Comparison of methods of Snellen visual acuity notation with logarithm of the minimal angle of resolution (LogMAR) values. From Ferris FL, Kassoff A, Bresnick AH. New visual acuity charts for clinical research. Am J Ophthalmol 1982; 94:91–96

6 m	20 ft	Decimal equivalent	LogMAR
6/60	20/200	0.10	+1.0
6/48	20/160	0.125	+0.9
6/38	20/125	0.16	+0.8
6/30	20/100	0.20	+0.7
6/24	20/80	0.25	+0.6
6/20	20/63	0.32	+0.5
6/15	20/50	0.40	+0.4
6/12	20/40	0.50	+0.3
6/10	20/32	0.63	+0.2
6/7.5	20/25	0.80	+0.1
6/6	20/20	1.00	0.0
6/5	20/16	1.25	−0.1
6/3.75	20/12.5	1.60	−0.2
6/3	20/10	2.00	−0.3

inversely related to the size of the surgical optic zone (Figure 5.2), there are other factors that have been shown to modify this outcome as well. The "trick" in all this is to combine these factors into a surgical plan that will result in a satisfactory result—satisfactory to the patient and surgeon alike. This is also true of any of the various refractive surgical procedures. During the workup of the patient, you will be gathering the raw materials to determine the surgical parameters you will use. It will behoove you to make sure that the information obtained is as accurate and complete as possible and that no short-cuts are taken, either in the gathering of the data or, ultimately, in the performance of the surgery.

Some of the tests suggested, such as A-scan, endothelial studies, AC depth etc. may not seem to be strictly required for evaluation from a surgical standpoint. However, some of these measurements are essential in high myopia and it is recommended that you make them, especially if you hope to obtain accurate predictions with the computer programs.

Visual acuity

Any method of taking the visual acuity is acceptable as long as the method is standardized for all patients. If you have more than one refraction lane, make sure that the projectors used are the same, as well as the room lengths. If this cannot be done, perform the acuity testing in one specific room. Try to keep the room lighting at the same level for each examination and the methodology of testing the same as well. Record the acuity for each eye separately with and without correction both for near and distance, and then test binocular acuity as well. The recommended acuity chart is that promulgated by the National Eye Institute (NEI). A separate chart is used for each eye (to minimize chances of a patient memorizing the letters). It is possible to use the logarithm of the minimal angle of resolution (LogMAR), which for the NEI chart

changes 0.1 unit for each line. Each line has five letters, thus each letter can be assigned a value (0.02 LogMAR) and the total of all the letters read correctly results in a visual acuity score. The 20/200 equivalent line is assigned a LogMAR value of +1.0 while 20/20 is valued at 0.0 units. If an individual read down to the 20/50 line (value +0.4) plus two letters from the 20/40 line ($0.02 \times 2 = 0.04$), the score would be: $0.4 - 0.04 = 0.36$. The lower the score, the better the vision (Table 5.2).

Ocular dominance

An attempt should be made to determine which of the eyes is dominant. Typically this will correspond to the handedness of the patient, but not in all cases. It is crucial that surgical planning should take into account this factor. The rationale for determining the ocular dominance is simply to indicate which eye will have the surgery first. Experience has shown that the postoperative course of patients is much smoother when the non-dominant eye is operated first. There are compelling reasons for this approach—not the least of these is the relative unpredictability of the current surgical techniques. Since the two eyes can be assumed to have the same physical and healing characteristics (except in unusual cases of anisometropia), the first eye acts as the bellwether for the other or "work horse" eye.

Allowing sufficient time for the eye to react to surgery points up any potential over- or under-shoot in the results of the first procedure; this knowledge can then be applied to the second. This is of special significance if one is planning "mono-vision." It is simply not possible to know in advance the exact results of your surgical plan. Thus if you are attempting to under-correct one eye, it makes more sense to operate on the reading eye for the lesser amount first and find out where it ends up. Hence, if the patient is very under-corrected, allowances can be made for this in the other eye and the first eye can be corrected further later. If there is an over-correction (unlikely but possible), an unpleasant surprise is avoided. This is because it can be used as a control for the fellow or dominant eye. Thus any "misses" can be corrected for in the dominant eye. In case of over- or under-correction, the non-dominant eye will cause less post-operative problems to the patient. In addition, the side-effects of the surgery are better tolerated in this eye. By the time the patient is ready to have the other eye done he or she will be better equipped to handle any post-operative sequelae.

Generally speaking, do not schedule surgery upon the fellow eye until the first eye has achieved a vision of at least 20/40—with or without correction—or is at a level, at 1 week, that experience leads you to believe will come up to 20/40 or better within a reasonable period of time. This has been standard procedure at my clinic from the beginning and we have never had cause to regret it. However, if the correction has been sufficiently successful so as to produce some degree of symptomatic anisometropia, it is better to continue with the second eye as soon as possible. This is true even if an over-correction has occurred with the first surgery. It is unlikely that a similar over-correction will occur in the second eye, but even if it does, the patient will be much better served by that condition than one of major anisometropia which would result if the second eye is left untouched.

Regardless of any normal, high score on the pre-surgical testing for glare, some patients may experience incapacitating glare post-operatively. This problem proves to be easier to cope with when it is the non-dominant eye that is affected. A legitimate question then is: What happens when it's the other eye's turn? The answer is that patients seem to cope with the glare much more easily after they have experienced it and single vision the first time in the non-dominant eye.

Many tests for determining ocular dominance depend upon correspondence to handedness. A more objective method, proposed by Milder and Rubin, is recommended to be used [4]. A 1 in (2.5 cm) diameter circular hole is cut in the center of an 8½ × 11 in (21.5 × 28 cm) white piece of cardboard. The patient, seated in the examining chair, is instructed to hold the paper in his/her lap with both hands, and to observe a 20/100 letter on the screen. The following instruction is then given: "Keep both eyes on the letter, quickly lift the paper up with your arms extended in front of you, and observe the letter through the hole with both eyes. Keep the letter in view and slowly bring the card toward your face." The hole will be in front of the dominant eye. This procedure is repeated five times and the eye that is dominant three or more times is recorded as the dominant eye. The number of times this eye appeared to be dominant out of five is recorded for future reference.

Near point of accommodation

Mount a Prince rule on a phoropter and place either a Rosenbaum pocket vision screener card or the standard Prince rule reading card in the clip. Place the patient's manifest refraction in the phoropter before each eye. Slide the test card toward the patient and have him/her read the 6 point (20/40) print. If the patient can see the print at 40 cm, continue to slide the test card toward the patient, instructing him or her to identify the point at which the print begins to blur. If it is difficult to tell this end point, and the patient has 6/6 visual acuity, try the small 5 or 4 point print, which may detect the point of blur more precisely. If the patient cannot see the print at 40 cm, place a +1.50 D lens in front of each eye and increase the power of the lens until the patient can see the print at 40 cm. Then slide the test card toward the patient and detect the first point of blur. If the patient's best corrected visual acuity is worse than 6/6 (20/20), use a test type that is big enough so the patient can see it at 40 cm.

Record the results as follows:
1 Print size (in point notation).
2 Power of the additional plus lens in the phoropter.
3 The location on the Prince rule where the first blur occurred, in both centimeters and diopters.

Corneal diameter (Figure 5.3)

Note that there is space provided for corneal diameter on the biometry form as well as the evaluation form. While this is important in the final outcome (see Chapter 7) no one has, as yet, suggested a foolproof

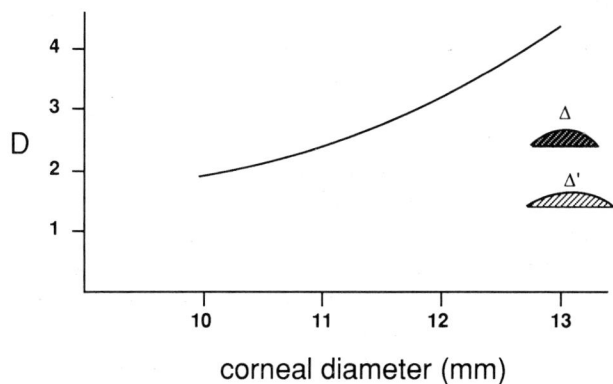

Fig. 5.3 Effect of corneal diameter on surgical outcome.

method of determining the exact diameter of the cornea—as those of you who have implanted anterior chamber lenses can attest. The use of a Castroviejo muscle caliper is recommended for this purpose. The cornea is measured from "white-to-white" at 90, 180, 45 and 135° and each measurement is recorded. The average of these four readings is taken as the nominal corneal diameter.

Scleral rigidity

Scleral rigidity is an important measurement and must be derived using either the Maklakov tonometer, or by allowing the computer to calculate the statistical mean for you.

For years physicians in the former Soviet Union have been taking measurements of intra-ocular pressure using the Maklakov tonometer. This instrument, which consists of several dumb-bell-shaped weights, is held in a wire holder that allows the weight to slide freely. Argyrol (or similar silver solution) is applied in a thin coating to each of the ends of the weight via a pad similar to a rubber stamp inkpad. The weights are applied to the anesthetized cornea of the supine patient in ascending order with two applications made for each weight, one for each end. The imprint is then either transferred to paper using alcohol as a mordant or better, the footplate is examined directly—a method utilized at the Bores Eye Institute. In either case, the small white center section is measured across its smaller diameter with the plastic nomogram supplied with the instrument. A deviation of 0.1 mm between successive readings (of the same weight) is cause for a remeasurement.

It is a characteristic of this device that as the weights increase so does the measured intra-ocular pressure. Since this results in a false-positive reading, tables have been constructed to compensate for this induced error. If the pressures are plotted on a graph against the weights, a straight line can be drawn between these points. The angle of the resultant slope gives a fair indication of the resistance of the cornea to flattening and thereby an indication of its rigidity. The tangent of this angle is the coefficient of corneal rigidity (Figure 5.4). Such a coefficient is typically 0.95 for the average myope and gets smaller as the myopia increases and larger as it decreases. It also increases with the age of the patient and is somewhat less for females of the same age up to approximately 45 years of age (Figure 5.5) [5].

The Maklakov tonometer, however, has been difficult to obtain in the USA and requires a fair amount of expertise to produce repeatable readings. Consequently, few individuals have utilized this measurement in the calculations required to determine the surgical parameters for an individual case. Many have

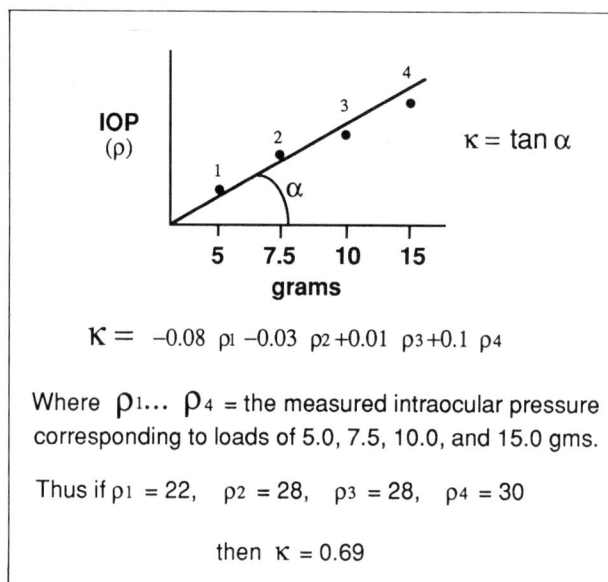

$$\kappa = \tan \alpha$$

$$\kappa = -0.08\ \rho_1 - 0.03\ \rho_2 + 0.01\ \rho_3 + 0.1\ \rho_4$$

Where $\rho_1 \ldots \rho_4$ = the measured intraocular pressure corresponding to loads of 5.0, 7.5, 10.0, and 15.0 gms.

Thus if $\rho_1 = 22$, $\rho_2 = 28$, $\rho_3 = 28$, $\rho_4 = 30$

then $\kappa = 0.69$

Fig. 5.4 Derivation of the rigidity coefficient.

derived empiric age or age/sex factors to account for the relationship between rigidity and age, sex, and surgical outcome. Recently, the instrument has become available through Meditech (Bausch & Lomb). The Differential Tonomat, manufactured by Ocular Instruments of Redmond, Washington, is no longer available. It uses the same principles but requires that only two measurements be taken. It still has some of the disadvantages of the other instrument, however.

It is impossible to state with assurance that such a factor represents the true corneal rigidity: other factors could be acting. The observer must make the assumption that the intra-ocular pressure remains constant during the measurement and that the sclera has the same factor of rigidity as the cornea. Regardless of the exact nature of this factor, there is a positive correlation between it and the outcome of the surgery. Therefore, until a better instrument is evolved, one of these devices will have to be used or some other means employed to account for this factor. The radial ketatotomy Datamaster computer program utilizes a statistically derived table built into the main calculation module to arrive at this factor. Other programs, such as the Deitz–Retzlaff–Sanders (DRS) use built-in factors based on the patient's age and are essentially accounting for the same thing (Figure 5.6).

Table 5.3 shows the average scleral rigidity for the various parameters illustrated. These figures were obtained through measurement of over 560 patients in six groups divided equally between males and females. The sex of the patient is also important and must be taken into account. There is sufficient evidence to show that women get significantly less result for a given set of parameters than do men. Since both age

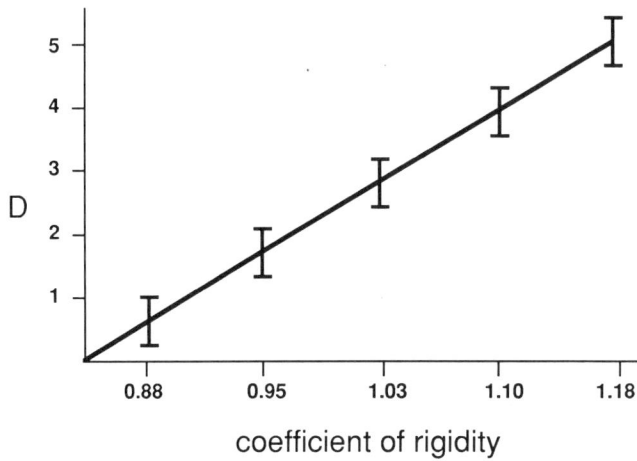

Fig. 5.5 Effect of corneal rigidity on surgical outcome.

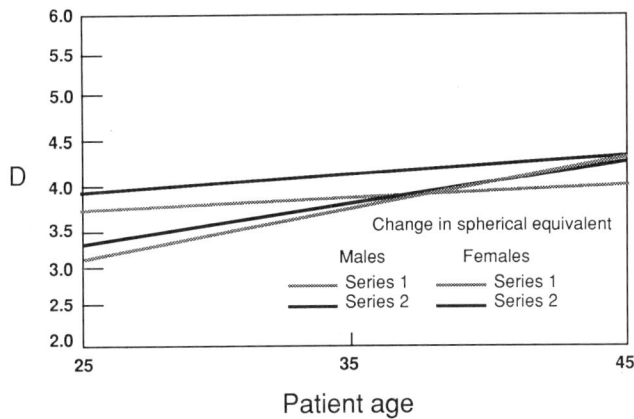

Fig. 5.6 Effect of age and sex (from Deitz M, Sanders D, Marks R. Radial keratotomy: an overview of the Kansas City study. Ophthalmology 1984; 91:467–478).

Table 5.3 Mean corneal rigidity

Myopia	Sex	Age (years) 25	35	45
1.5 D	Male	0.95	1.02	1.12
	Female	0.92	1.00	1.11
3.0 D	Male	0.90	0.95	1.04
	Female	0.88	0.90	1.03
5.0 D	Male	0.86	0.90	0.99
	Female	0.81	0.87	0.98
7.0 D	Male	0.80	0.82	0.96
	Female	0.70	0.78	0.95

and sex play a role in the outcome of the surgery they have been integrated into this table. Besides helping select the size of the optical zone this table can help weed out those patients who have an abnormally low rigidity and who do not seem to do well, statistically, with radial keratotomy surgery.

Axial length

Axial length is not currently used in the computer programs to predict the outcome of refractive surgery. The omission of this reading will not significantly reduce the accuracy of the predictions for radial keratotomy but you are encouraged to obtain these measurements whenever possible. They are, of course, essential in clear lens extraction and in scleral re-inforcement procedures.

Refraction

A careful manifest and/or cycloplegic refraction must be done. Auto-refractor data should not be relied upon. Do a manifest in addition if you are using this type of equipment. Cycloplegic refractions are routinely performed in the initial examination of all hyperopic patients and in the presence of mixed astigmatism. It is suggested that the duochrome (red–green) test be performed to avoid over-minusing the myopic patient during the manifest refraction. In this test the patient is shown a screen of grouped letters of varying size over which is superimposed a vertically split red–green screen. Spherical lenses are added and subtracted in 0.25 D increments until the patient's response to the question: "Which color makes the letters darker? Red or green?" is answered "about the same" or the patient indicates a slight preference for the red. This will insure that the image is focused upon the retina without undue accommodative influence. The cylinder should be measured and recorded in plus cylinders (see also Chapter 10).

Ophthalmometry (keratometry)

Keratometry is, in the author's view, the single most important pre-operative measurement that must be obtained in refractive surgery. There has been some controversy over the exact role this factor plays in radial keratotomy surgery in the past, as far as surgical outcome is concerned. Some authors have suggested that the pre-operative K-readings are not relevant to the result and need not be accounted for in the surgical plan [6]. Since the study referred to was done on cadaver eyes, it is difficult to take its conclusions seriously, especially in view of the published experience of other investigators, including this author [5,7–9]. However, Barraquer's calculations for lathing procedures are dependent upon these values, as are those for stromal implants and epikeratophakia [10–14]. Hence it is essential that this measurement be done. At the same time, the surgeon should be aware of the major short-comings of this method of corneal curvature measurement (see Chapter 7).

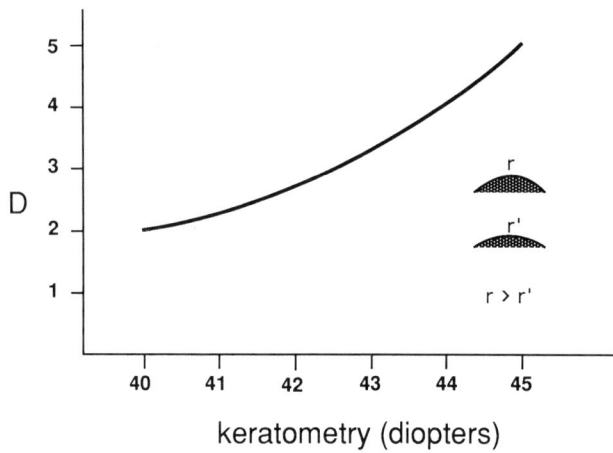

Fig. 5.7 The effect of preoperative K on surgical outcome (from Deitz M, Sanders D, Marks R. Radial keratotomy: an overview of the Kansas City study. Ophthalmology 1984; 91:467–478).

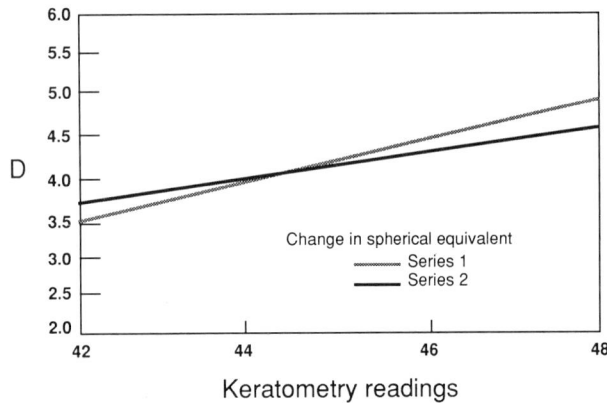

Fig. 5.8 The effect of pre-operative K on surgical outcome.

Figure 5.7 is from Deitz *et al.* and represents the findings of a study of two groups of patients undergoing radial keratotomy [15]. The influence of pre-operative keratotomy on the post-operative spherical equivalent is very evident. This relationship was noted early on in the history of radial keratotomy surgery and, while remarked upon frequently, was not given sufficient weight by many investigators. From the very beginning of this surgery, Fyodorov and the author have taken the pre-operative K-readings into account in establishing the surgical parameters (Figure 5.8) [5,16,17]. Figure 5.9 illustrates the results of surgery in a series of patients in whom the K-readings were integrated into the pre-operative calculations used to establish the surgical optical (or free) zone size. The trend of this plot shows a definite slope upward to above the emmetropia line. If the K-readings did not have any appreciable effect on the surgical outcome, then the results of surgery in those groups whose corneal curvatures are the steepest should have had less effect from

the surgery than those with flatter corneas. This should occur because the optical zones in the steeper cases were made larger to account for the increased corneal power and to prevent over-correction. It is evident, in examining the plot, that the steeper cases are showing a slight tendency toward over-correction, leading one to the conclusion that not enough weight has been given to those K-readings. If the K-reading is not taken into consideration, as some have recommended, over-corrections are likely to occur. This could account for the cases of progressive corneal flattening which were reported in the prospective evaluation of radial keratotomy (PERK) study [18].

These measurements are taken with a calibrated keratometer and for best results should be taken by the same person each time. The axis, while not needed in the calculations, should be recorded as well (see Chapter 9 for a discussion on the significance of the axis of K). Be aware that routine measurements represent only the central 4.00 mm of the corneal surface and that keratometers are designed to be most accurate when measuring spherical surfaces. Furthermore, the keratometer assumes an average index of refraction for the cornea as a whole. The limitations of the keratometer are discussed further in Chapter 6.

The refractive power of the cornea, which is a curved surface, depends upon a number of factors, some of which are constant and some variable. The ability of a curved surface to bend or refract light when situated between media of differing refractive indices is well known in optical physics.

The refractive power (D) of such a surface is given by the formula:

(a)

$$D = \frac{n' - n}{r} \times 1000$$

(b)

$$D = \frac{n' - n}{r} \times 1000$$

(c)

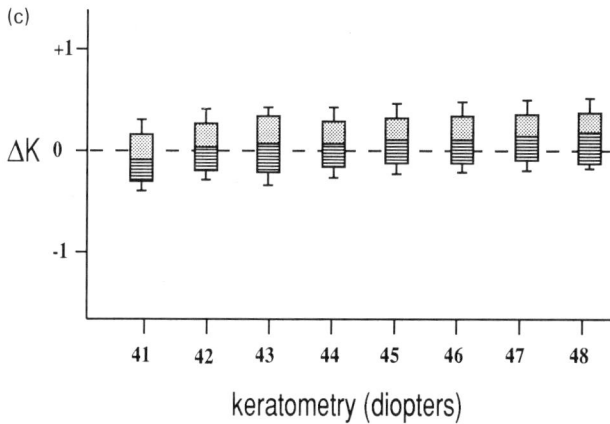

where D = dioptric power; n' = index of refraction of the second medium; n = index of refraction of the first medium, and r = radius of the refractive surface in millimeters.

Constants

Index of refraction of air	1.000
Index of refraction of cornea	1.376
Index of refraction of aqueous	1.336

If for the cornea, the variables are:

Radius of anterior cornea	7.70 mm
Radius of posterior cornea	6.80 mm
Corneal thickness	0.50 mm

Then the refractive power at the anterior surface is:

$$D = \frac{1.374 - 1.000}{7.70} \times 1000 = 48.83\,D$$

and the refractive power at the posterior surface is:

$$D = \frac{1.334 - 1.376}{6.80} \times 1000 = -5.882\,D$$

The resultant corneal power is thus:

$$D = 48.83 + (-5.882) = 42.95\,D$$

Because the cornea is composed not merely of two surfaces but has a definite thickness, there is a small refractive power (0.1 D) due to this factor. Therefore we can consider the dioptric power of the cornea as arising from three factors:

1 Anterior surface	=	48.83
2 Posterior surface	=	−5.88
3 Corneal thickness	=	0.10
		43.05 D

The readings displayed by the typical keratometer are in diopters and represent the effective corneal power. This value for corneal power is derived by taking an arbitrarily low value for the corneal refractive index—1.3375—which takes into account the front and back surface powers of the cornea and its thick-

ness. That this is effective corneal refractive power must be kept in mind when evaluating the output of some corneal topographers. These instruments typically give the actual corneal curvature and not the effective refracting power of the cornea. Hence a conversion must be made when trying to equate the resultant values with those of standard keratometers. Some instruments, such as the CLAS II, display the effective total corneal power—the front surface corneal power as well as the true external corneal curvature.

It should be apparent that attempts to modify the refractive power of the eye would most effectively be applied to the anterior corneal surface where there exists a variable factor of considerable magnitude. It is important to remember always that the keratometer is an instrument for directly measuring radius of curvature, not refractive power. Furthermore, certain assumptions are made about conditions which may not exist in a given eye. The power reading given by the keratometer assumes a given value for n' such that for a given radius of anterior corneal curvature, the net power displayed approximates that which would be obtained if one calculated the net power from both the anterior and posterior surfaces (as illustrated above). This assumption is reasonably valid over the range of curvatures normally found clinically—at least for the central 4.00 mm of the cornea.

However, a problem arises once we have modified the corneal thickness by the Barraquer procedures (MKM, KP, and HLK) or by epikeratophakia because now the anterior and posterior surfaces deviate considerably from parallel. For this reason one must calculate the net corneal power by solving for both surfaces. In short, K-readings taken after such procedures will not represent the true corneal net power. No current topographer units, except the CLAS II laser holographic topographer, are capable of rendering both the anterior and posterior corneal curvatures to facilitate these types of measurements. Useful, if inaccurate, expressions of corneal power can still be obtained with standard keratometers, though, so don't get rid of your instrument yet. These devices come in handy for "quick and dirty" measurements when extreme accuracy is neither needed nor warranted—such as in current methods of contact lens fitting. Furthermore, until additional investigation and standardization of topography nomenclature and displays are effected—not to mention clinical work to establish the relationship between the shape of the cornea pre- and post-operatively—the K-readings will continue to be important (see also Chapter 7).

Central keratometry

The standard clinical method to measure corneal shape is central keratometry. Accurate keratometric measure-

ments are important in this surgery for three reasons:
1 The pre-operative keratometry readings have an effect on the amount of correction achieved with these techniques—the flatter the cornea, the less effect.
2 The change in central keratometry after surgery is a major response variable that indicates not only how flat the cornea has become, but also whether the surgery has induced astigmatism, either regular or irregular.
3 Although the keratometer measures the curvature of only the central 3.4–4.2 mm, the keratometric readings are analyzed and communicated easily.

To insure that your results are in line with those of other surgeons, use instruments that are optically interchangeable, i.e. the Bausch & Lomb, the Topcon, and the Haag–Streit devices. This uniformity is desirable, since different types of keratometers assume different indices of refraction for the cornea to convert the radius of curvature measurements, which the keratometer reads directly, to power measurements in diopters. For example, the Haag–Streit and Bausch & Lomb instruments use an index of 1.3375, whereas the American Optical instrument uses 1.336, and the Gambs instrument uses 1.332—the true refractive index of the cornea is 1.376. In these three examples, a radius of 7.8 mm will read 43.27 D, 43.08 D, and 42.56 D, respectively.

Basic principles of keratometry are discussed in standard textbooks and the procedures specified here for using the Bausch & Lomb instrument are modified from their instruction manual [19–22].

Keratometer set-up

To calibrate the instrument, secure a steel test ball of known curvature (usually 45.00 D and supplied with the device) on the concave end of a magnetic rod that can be attached to the frame of the instrument. Position the steel ball in the optical axis of the keratometer, set both drums to 45.00 D, adjust the eyepiece (described below), and superimpose the crosses of the focusing circle and horizontal drum. If the reading on the horizontal drum is 45.00 D, the instrument is properly calibrated. If the reading differs from 45.00 D, re-adjust the eyepiece. If the reading is still inaccurate, the instrument must be properly calibrated by the manufacturer. Repeat this calibration check annually.

Eyepiece calibration

Particular attention must be given to adjustment of the eyepiece of the keratometer each time the instrument is used in order to assure accuracy of readings for each patient. The first time the operator uses this instrument, he/she must adjust the eyepiece for his or her

eye, otherwise the readings taken will be erroneous. To adjust the eyepiece, proceed as follows:
1 Position the white-backed occluder in the optical axis of the instrument (unless the steel calibration ball is used).
2 Turn the eyepiece cap counterclockwise as far as possible.
3 Turn the instrument lamp on and look through the eyepiece—a blurred cross will be seen.
4 Continue looking through the eyepiece and slowly turn the eyepiece in a clockwise direction, to come from the plus side and which avoids accommodation, to that position where the cross is in the sharpest focus. (*Note*: Do not turn the eyecap back and forth to focus the cross. This tends to stimulate accommodation and will result in erroneous readings.)
5 When the cross is in the sharpest focus, note the reading on the outer periphery of the eyecap.
6 Repeat the previous three steps at least three times. If the results are approximately the same each time, the eyepiece is adjusted for your eye. Make sure that this setting is recorded somewhere for each person designated to perform this examination. If possible, assign one person to do all these readings.

The calibrated scale on the outer periphery of the eyecap is for the operator's convenience. Once the operator has assured that the eyepiece is adjusted for his or her eye, he or she should note and remember or record the setting. The next time the instrument is used, the eyecap is turned to this setting and it will be in adjustment for the operator's eye. However, this setting should be verified occasionally.

The patient's chin should fit snugly into the chin rest. For accurate results, it is necessary for the patient to hold his or her head firmly against the head rest during the complete keratometer examination. For the patient with an extremely receding forehead or with deep-set eyes and a protruding forehead, it may be necessary to adjust the forehead or chin rest.

Grasp the grip that rotates the keratometer drum and rotate the instrument so that the axial scale reads exactly 90° and 180° at the axis marks. Release the set screw so the tube of the instrument can be moved to one side. Raise or lower the instrument until the pin on the side of the lamphousing and the white axis marker are aligned, like gunsights, with the patient's pupil or outer canthus. Cover the eye not under examination with the occluding shield.

After the patient's head has been accurately lined up and leveled, turn the instrument so that it points directly at the eye to be examined. Looking from the side, the observer will then see a tiny, bright ring in the center of the cornea (the corneal image of the circular mire). When the correct position has been found, the patient will see a reflection of his or her own eye in the tube of the instrument with an image of the mire

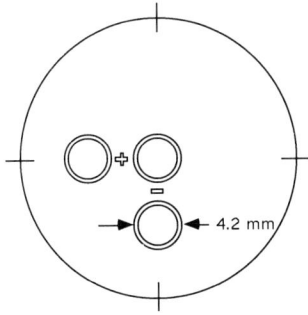

Fig. 5.10 Typical keratometry mires of Bausch and Lomb keratometer.

in the center of the pupil. The patient should fixate on this image. If there is difficulty with this procedure, shine a penlight through the eyepiece to assist with alignment.

Technique of measurement

Looking through the eyepiece, the operator will see images of the target mire, perhaps very blurred (Figure 5.10). These may be cleared with the focusing knob. By swiveling the instrument slightly and by making fine adjustments of the elevator knob, the black cross-hairs may be put near the center of the double circle. This doubled circle is called the focusing circle. When this is done, tighten the locking screw and measure the corneal surfaces.

It is important that the cross-hairs be near the center of the focusing circle, for when this condition is attained, the optic axis of the instrument will coincide with the visual axis of the patient's eye, as it should for accuracy. At the same time, the image of the patient's eye will be directly in front of the operator. These conditions constitute the triple alignment so necessary to precision measurements. When the instrument is out of focus, the central focusing circle and the plus and minus signs are doubled, but when the exact focus is located by turning the focusing knob, the focusing circle will appear single and sharp.

In an astigmatic cornea, all of the central focusing circle will not appear exactly in focus at the same time. Therefore, for greater accuracy the operator may direct attention to the doubled plus sign and focus it sharply. The focus of the minus sign can be disregarded until a later step.

Locating the cylinder axis

Two plus signs will be seen between the left-hand and the central focusing circles within the telescope. The axis of the cylinder can be found most easily when the tips of these plus signs just touch. Turn the horizontal measuring drum until the plus signs are barely separ-

ated. If the horizontal lines of the plus sign appear to be continuous and unbroken, the instrument is already set at the position of the axis of the astigmatism. If the horizontal lines appear discontinuous, the keratometer is not at the cylinder axis.

Grasp the keratometer at the rotating grip and rotate the entire tube while looking into the eyepiece. At some position, which can readily be found by watching closely, the horizontal lines of the plus signs will appear continuous and unbroken. A further check on the accurate location of the axis may be obtained by throwing the instrument slightly out of focus. Then the plus sign of the central focusing circle will be doubled. If the axis is correct, the horizontal line in the plus sign of the left circle will be exactly midway between the double horizontal line of the other plus sign.

If it is not at the midpoint, a slight rotation of the instrument one way or another will move the line to the midpoint. The double cross should next be focused, so that it becomes single. The two horizontal lines will then become continuous. This extra check on the corneal axis is particularly valuable in low astigmatic errors. When these horizontal white lines of the plus signs appear tip to tip and continuous, the keratometer is set so as to indicate the axis of the astigmatism.

Measuring the horizontal principal meridian

After the axis has been found, turn the horizontal measuring drum knob and the left-hand plus sign will move to the right or left. Move this plus sign until it is exactly superimposed on the plus sign of the central focusing circle. This completes the setting for the rear horizontal meridian. The scale of the left-hand or horizontal measuring drum indicates the actual diopter power of the cornea in the horizontal or near horizontal meridian.

Measuring the vertical meridian

You should use the crosses to measure the vertical meridian, since they are more accurate than the minus signs described by the manufacturer. To measure the curvature in the vertical meridian, rotate the drum so that the plus sign of the central focusing circle is vertical, and repeat the procedure followed for the horizontal meridian.

While measuring, one hand should be constantly on the focusing screw to keep the meridian being measured in sharp focus. The operator's judgment of focus in this instrument is very keen, thanks to the coincident method of focusing. This permits him or her to keep the mire, whose image in the cornea he or she measures, a constant distance from the eye in spite of the small movements which every eye constantly makes. Unless the object distance is a fixed one, the measurements of the image size will be erroneous.

Reading the amount of astigmatism

On the left, or horizontal, measuring drum, the power of the cornea in the meridians nearest to 0–180° is read. When the drum is rotated vertically, the difference between these two readings is the amount of corneal astigmatism. If the two readings are the same, there is no measurable corneal astigmatism.

Axis of astigmatism

The meridian indicators of the keratometer tube are engraved white lines on the body bearing facing the operator. The horizontal marks on each side indicate the meridian measured on the horizontal drum, and the vertical mark on top indicates the meridian measured when the drum is turned vertically. If the astigmatism is to be measured in a minus cylinder form, take for its axis that mark representing the drum having the lower dioptric reading. If the astigmatism is to be measured in a plus cylinder form, take for its axis the mark representing the drum having the higher dioptric reading. The two curvatures in diopters and the axis of each are recorded on the data forms.

Extended range for flat corneas

A loose trial frame lens may be used with the Bausch & Lomb keratometer to extend the range to read flatter corneas. If the keratometer drum is turned to its flattest extent, and still cannot accurately read the corneal curvature, a −1.25 lens is taped, convex side out, over the front aperture of the keratometer, the drum reading is obtained, and the supplied nomogram chart is used to determine the true keratometric reading.

Determining degree of corneal asphericity

There is a relationship between the successful outcome of radial keratotomy surgery and the relative

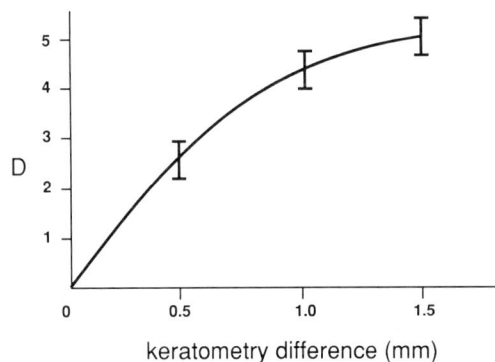

Fig. 5.11 Effect of corneal asphericity (Fyodorov).

asphericity of the cornea (Figure 5.11). If the cornea is too spherical, that is the peripheral corneal curvature approaches in degree that of the center, very little, if any, effect will result from the surgery. At first the myopia will be reduced, but within a short period of time the curvature will return to the same (or very nearly) as that of the pre-operative state. For this reason the peripheral corneal curvature should be measured in the horizontal and vertical meridians and compared with those of the center. In the author's experience, if the difference between the two readings is equal to the degree of myopia present, the result will be that predicted by the calculations. If the difference is equal to or less than half the myopia, it is very likely that no lasting change will occur in the corneal shape as a result of the surgery. It can be argued that, given the nature of keratometers, measurement of the peripheral cornea with these instruments is completely inaccurate. While this is true, peripheral K-readings are of sufficient clinical reliability to recommend their use—as opposed to nothing—until something better comes along.

Take the measurements as in central K-readings except that the patient is directed to fixate eccentrically. The patient should be encouraged to move the eyes sufficiently off axis so as to cast the mires on to the limbal zone. The mires will inevitably be distorted when this occurs. To reduce this distortion and to obtain a reading, have the patient blink several times in succession and rotate the eyes medially so as to move the mire somewhat closer to center. Use only one drum to make the measurement (preferably the plus) and rotate the tube as necessary to clarify the mire. Record both the horizontal (temporal) and vertical (6 o'clock) readings.

Glare testing

There are three ways in which a retinal image may be degraded:
1 It may be out of focus, as in uncorrected ammetropia.
2 It may be degraded by light scatter from opacities in the ocular media.
3 It may be affected by a combination of both factors. In patients having refractive surgery both ammetropia and glare from surgical scars may degrade the retinal image.

The standard visual acuity test projects a high-contrast black letter or number on a white background. The patient with glare may read all letters correctly but fail to comment that the letters appear as a washed-out faded gray. In the world outside the examining room, the person observes that delicate shades of gray and subtle color tones may be lost in a non-descript hazy fusion and that image outlines are blurred. Thus, the standard visual acuity chart gives no information about the quality of contrast, and may be dangerously misleading regarding visual function under real-life conditions, particularly in bright light and night time.

Many researchers have sought ways to evaluate glare sensitivity by way of contrast measurements [23–29]. The Miller–Nadler Glare Tester (Titmus) is one of several such instruments available, enabling the clinician to quantify glare sensitivity. The instrument consists of a constant bright rectangular glare source that surrounds a series of randomly oriented, constant-sized, black Landolt rings positioned on a background that is progressively darkened until a contrast threshold is reached. The apparatus consists of a desktop slide projector which provides the constant glare source and a series of specially made 35 mm slides.

Nadler [30] and LeClaire et al. [31] have proposed that glare sensitivity be graded by using a comparison method, as occurs in determination of Snellen acuity. By this method, most normal individuals in the first three decades of life can see to a contrast level of 5%. This means that there is only 5% contrast between the Landolt ring and its immediate background. If a patient's glare contrast sensitivity is such that a 10% contrast between the Landolt ring and its surround is required before the Landolt ring can be seen, the increase in contrast compared to normal is 2×, still an excellent score.

Wolf found a clear division of glare sensitivity between patients below and above age 50 [26]. An increase in contrast of 3× or 4× (10–20% contrast) may be normal for patients above age 50 who have no obvious opacities in the ocular media. A glare contrast sensitivity of 11–15× (55–75% contrast) or more may indicate severe visual disability under bright light conditions, even though a good Snellen acuity may be obtained in the refracting lane. Such patients can be visually crippled with an effective acuity as low as 20/800 outside on a bright day.

LeClaire et al. performed glare and visual acuity tests on 161 normal eyes, 144 eyes with cataracts, 100 eyes with intra-ocular lenses, and 26 eyes wearing aphakic spectacles. They found that the normal patients averaged 6% contrast level, those with Copeland intra-ocular lenses 15% contrast, those with Lynell intra-ocular lenses 20% contrast, and those with aphakic spectacles 18% contrast. The glare readings of normal patients were significantly different from the corrected aphakic patients, regardless of the method of correction ($P < 0.001$). For management of glare see Chapter 16.

Description of the Miller–Nadler Glare Tester

The glare tester described consists of a Fairchild desktop sound/slide projector, Model 3501, Type SS-35, which is used under low lamp illumination. Newer models use a Kodak Ektagraphic Model 260 or similar.

The bulb used is a projection lamp, 19 V and 80 W (must be purchased with part no. PN9–1251 or specify type DDM #34–100, available through Fairchild Industrial Products, or through the Titmus Company). The projector is mounted on an adjustable instrument support pan that has a frame protruding in front of the screen for positioning the patient's head. A set of test slides calibrated specifically for the illumination and optics of this model projector consists of a dark Landolt ring against a 30 mm round background created by the use of gelatin neutral density filters. The Landolt rings are all the same size—20/400 Snellen equivalent—and are randomly oriented for patient testing. For optical reasons, accurate positioning of the patient directly in front and perpendicular to the center of the screen is important.

The percentage contrast is defined as:

$$C = \frac{L_{max} - L_{min} \times 100}{L_{max} + L_{min}}$$

where L_{max} = maximal luminance in the surround; and L_{min} = minimal luminance in the target.

Glare testing technique

Preparation of slides

Position a Carousel 80 slide tray (or preferably Carousel Diamagazin Cat# 700–1266 or Universal 80 with the full Plexiglas cover to keep out dust) on to the projector. Face the screen of the projector and hold the slides so that the numbers on the white side of the plastic mounts are in the upper right-hand corner facing you. Insert the slides so that their numbers match the tray slots 1–17. Secure the slides in the tray with the locking ring cap (or clear cover). Use the adhesive strip which comes with the slides to label each slide position by peeling off the protective backing and attaching it to the side of the carousel tray so that the slide orientation letters are precisely centered over the slot numbers 1–17.

Assembly of the projector and frame

Place the projector on the support pan with the screen facing the chin rest and head support assembly. Verify that the screen is 14 in (35 cm) from the eye. An elevating device on the front end of the pan has a height adjustment knob to help make the patient comfortable. The chin cup assembly and forehead rest at the front part of the frame have marks on the vertical posts indicating the level to which the eye should be adjusted. This is done by elevating or dropping the chin cup. The cup should always be locked into position once the eyes are brought to the level of the post marker. The chin cup assembly should be moved laterally and locked in position to center the eye being tested in front of the screen. Slide it to the right for testing the left eye and to the left for testing the right eye.

Procedures for patient testing

Glare testing should be done in a darkened room. If the subject wears glasses or contact lenses, be sure they are clean and lack surface defects, so they do not induce glare themselves. If the patient wears bifocals, raise the frames so that he or she can read the target through the bifocal segment. Pre-operatively test with spectacles or contact lenses *on*. Post-operatively test without correction and with *best* spectacle correction if one is needed.

Seat the patient in front of the glare tester and adjust and secure the height of the chin cup so that the eyes are level with the marker on the vertical post of the forehead rest. Move and secure the chin cup so the eye to be tested is aligned directly with the center of the screen. Tilt the whole instrument support pan up or down for patient comfort.

Explain the test to the patient. Use a Landolt C on a demonstration card to show how the opening is oriented in one of four directions. Explain that the C will become increasingly difficult to see, but that the patient is to indicate its orientation—even if he/she must guess—until it simply cannot be perceived. Begin the test with the right eye.

Darken the room to simulate scotopic conditions, place the patient's head in the chin rest, turn on the projector, and use a Rosenbaum pocket vision screener to estimate the pupil size.

Have the patient occlude the eye not being tested with a hand-held occluder, but warn not to press it tight enough on the glasses to be distracting.

Advance the slides as rapidly as the patient can make an accurate response, but not fast enough to generate a sense of haste. As the Landolt ring orientations become difficult to identify, allow additional time for recognition. When the subject indicates that no further recognition seems possible, wait a full 20 seconds before going to the next slide. Record on the data sheet the number of the final slide which is correctly identified. Repeat the procedure on the other eye.

Optional testing

Darken the room to simulate scotopic conditions and measure the physiologically dilated pupil with the subject fixating at the end of the room. Shine a penlight obliquely across the eye and measure the pupil size with a ruler in millimeters. This will estimate pupil size under dark ambulatory conditions. Dilate

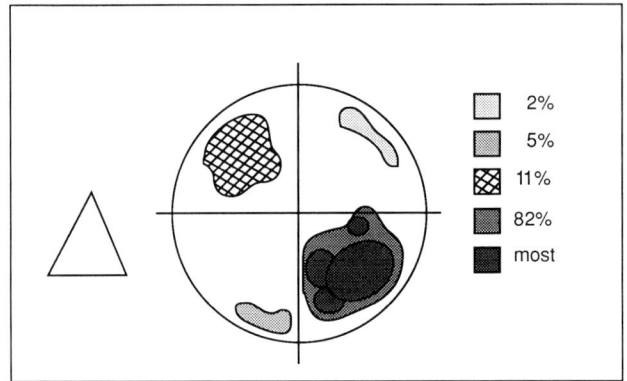

Fig. 5.12 Distribution of thin areas.

the pupil with 2% cyclopentolate and measure the pupillary diameter again with the patient looking at the glare tester light 20–30 min later. When the dilatation attains and holds the approximate size measured under the scotopic conditions, repeat the glare test first on the right eye and then on the left, documenting the results along with the last measurement of pupil size in millimeters.

Pachymetry

Until the advent of radial keratotomy it was assumed that the corneal thickness varied smoothly from a relatively thinner central portion to a relatively thicker peripheral portion. However, the occurrence of microperforations in areas of the cornea in which these were not anticipated spurred a search for the cause. These perforations generally occurred in the mid-periphery and, for the most part, non-uniformly. In other words they were happening where the cornea was supposed to be thicker and sometimes when incisions had already been made across this same mid-zone in other parts of the cornea with the same blade. This stimulated the author to begin mapping out the corneal thickness over its entire surface. This study was facilitated by the use of ultrasonic pachymetry. It was found that in approximately 11% of the cases, small isolated areas of abrupt corneal thinning—dubbed corneal dimples—were found. While these initially appeared to occur at random, a pattern soon emerged such that they seemed to group primarily in the infero-temporal part of the cornea at the mid-periphery (Figure 5.12). In addition, some older patients exhibited rather large areas of pre-limbal corneal thinning—again mostly in the infero-temporal quadrant.

From this work certain corneal thickness patterns have been recognized:

Type 1

Type 1 is the most common: corneal thickness proceeds in a smooth, even transition from a thinner

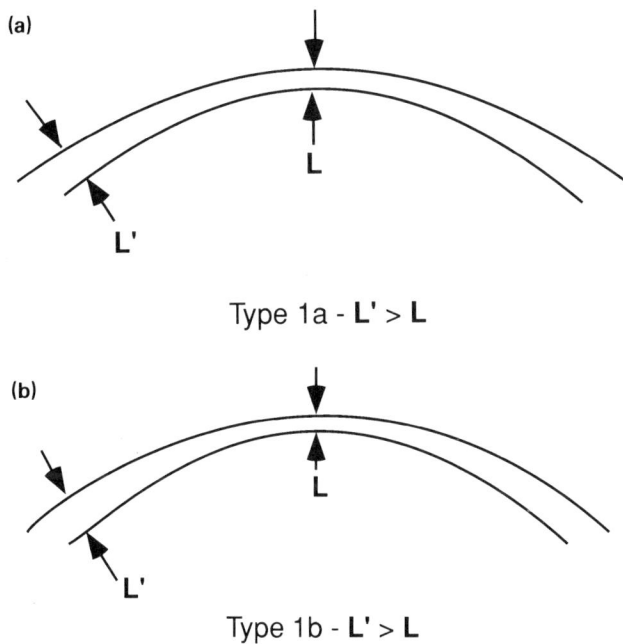

Fig. 5.13 Corneal thickness types: type 1 (most common)—corneal thickness proceeds in a smooth, even transition from a thinner central section to a thicker peripheral section. Within this type two sub-types occur: (a) type 1a; (b) type 1b.

central section to a thicker peripheral section. Within this type two sub-types occur.

Type 1a

In this type the transition is smooth and gradual (Figure 5.13a).

Type 1b

Here the transition is smooth but the thickening occurs more rapidly than type 1a in the pre-limbal area (Figure 5.13b). The limbal cornea is typically thicker than in type 1a.

Type 2

In this type (sometimes called the plateau cornea), the corneal thickness varies very little from the central zone until somewhere near or just past the mid peripheral point where it begins to thicken rapidly. This type of cornea is seen in higher myopes and the average peripheral pachymetry is typically thinner than in type 1.

Type 3

Type 3 is, for the most part, similar to type 1, with the added feature that the cornea becomes thinner again at the periphery in the infero-temporal quadrant. This type is seen most often in eyes over 50 years of age.

Type 4

Type 4 possesses the characteristics of type 1 with the addition of having small, well-circumscribed areas of abrupt corneal thinning—corneal dimples. Most of these occur in the infero-temporal quadrant and there does not appear to be any association with age. However, no patient has been described with both type 3 and 4 in combination, either in the same eye or in opposite eyes.

Instrumentation

Ultrasonic pachymetry is the recommended method for obtaining corneal thickness measurements [32]. None of the optical methods previously in use (Haag–Streit, Zeiss, or Heyer–Schulte) have proved to be of sufficient accuracy or reproducibility for use in difficult cases or in aiding predictability. Also, as incisions have become deeper, more precise measurements are necessary to prevent or reduce the incidence of perforations.

Ultrasonic pachymetry possesses the advantages of:
1 Reproducibility.
2 Ability to take measurements anywhere on the cornea.
3 Not being dependent upon patient fixation.
4 High accuracy.
5 Ability to be used intra-operatively (not recommended).
6 Ease of use by relatively unskilled personnel.

All the available ultrasonic instruments represent a sizable investment. It is not possible, however, to perform this surgery with any degree of confidence without one. In a comparison of all the available pachymeters (done by an independent ophthalmologist) which were donated by the manufacturers, the one that tested out as the best was the DGH-1000/2000. This instrument embodies all of the design characteristics that the author desired. It has an integral printer, which not only lists out the readings but where they were taken, plus a frontal map of the reading format or mode selected as well as a profile of corneal thickness across the cornea in up to four sections. There is an internal memory allowing for editing of the recorded data prior to print-out; selection of multiple measurement modes with incremental guide map; and two self-test modes—one for the device and one for the solid probe tip. Tip coupling is provided by the standard, solid probe tip, which eliminates the usual ultrasound gel (filled once daily). Other features include a two-stage foot switch, provided for obtaining and storage of the measurements; digital read-out of data with two-tone signal; rejection of non-perpendicular readings; provision to pre-set the bias for automatic blade-setting calculations; automatic gain control; provision to re-set speed of sound (default 1640 m/s); and there is a port at the rear of the instrument to allow direct input into a computer and to allow it to interact with the other planned instruments in the series.

The 2000 series embodies all the above features with the additional ones of:
1 Automatic averaging of rings.
2 Programmable mapping.
3 Optional plug-in predictability module.

The newer Pachette has no printer or programmability, nor can a predictability module be used with it. It does, however, have a special measurement sensing probe that does away with the foot switch.

Making the measurements

The following description applies particularly to the DGH-2000 Series ultrasonic pachymeter. Some differences exist with different manufacturers.

Prepare the instrument by switching it on. Upon power up, the DGH-2000 will run through a short self-testing program to insure that all systems are nominal. Next press the CLR button followed by PQT (probe quality test). The instrument will respond by producing a reading on the screen. (i.e. PROBE EFFICIENCY = 81%). If there is not enough gel (in the older model probe), the socket is dry or the probe is not plugged in, you will get a message telling you about the problem. In this case, remove the tip and re-fill the cavity, insuring that no air bubbles are trapped in the gel. If the read-out indicates an efficiency of 75% or greater, the probe is ready for use. Newer probes have a go–no go mode, thus if the probe is defective that message will appear, otherwise the system will cycle to the next step.

Press CLR again and then press BIAS—it should be 100%. You can re-set this using the keyboard if desired. If you make a mistake in entry, repeatedly pressing the CLR key will cause the reading to march off the screen digit by digit. When you are satisfied press ENTR. Next select the mode by pressing MODE, followed by a number from 1 to 9. The number does not matter since only the central corneal measurement is important. Corneal mapping is not absolutely necessary in HLK, KMK, or KMIS. However, it is recommended that mapping be done in all refractive cases and that all 33 points on the map be recorded (Figure 5.14). The left-hand group of light-emitting diodes will light up in a pattern specific to the number entered. In addition the screen will display the characteristics of the read-out, such as what each circle represents. When you are satisfied press ENTR and you are ready to take readings.

The patient is placed supine in a well-lit room. An auxiliary floor lamp shining obliquely upon the cornea will facilitate accurate placement of the transducer probe. Under these conditions the pupil will be constricted to between 2.5 and 3.0 mm in most cases.

The operator sits at the right side of the patient's head with the foot switch so placed that the foot straddles the middle of the switch. By moving the foot slightly to the right the measurement side of the switch is depressed to the left and the reading is stored. The instrument should be placed to the patient's left so that the entire front panel can be clearly seen by the operator.

Two drops of appropriate topical anesthetic are applied to each cornea. To begin the measurements the operator depresses the right-hand foot pedal once. This will cause the light-emitting diodes to go out and be replaced by a single blinking central red light. The position of the blinking light indicates where the next reading is to be taken. The read-out on the screen will also spell out the two-letter code for that location.

The probe is now applied to the central cornea (Figure 5.15) within the pupil, slightly indenting the corneal surface. The right foot pedal is depressed once again. If the probe is perpendicular to the cornea the instrument will respond with an immediate short beep. A reading will also appear on the screen. Press the left pedal once to store the reading. Note that the flashing light has now become a steady light and the next position is flashing. If there is no immediate beep the instrument will try to take more measurements and then will give you the raspberry and print NO READING POOR APPLANATION on the screen. If that happens adjust the orientation of the probe and try again.

Next, move the probe so as to straddle the pupillary margin. Depress the right-hand foot pedal to acquire a reading. This is the para-central (PC) reading corresponding to the first or A circle (Figure 5.16).

Press the left-hand foot pedal to store the reading and move the probe tip to a point that causes the tip to butt against the edge of the epithelial imprint from the previous reading.

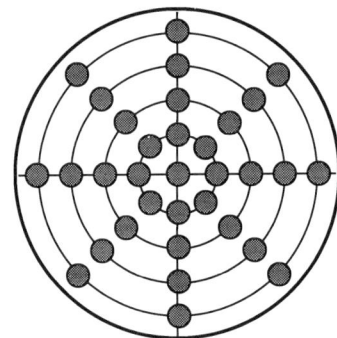

Fig. 5.14 Typical mapping pattern.

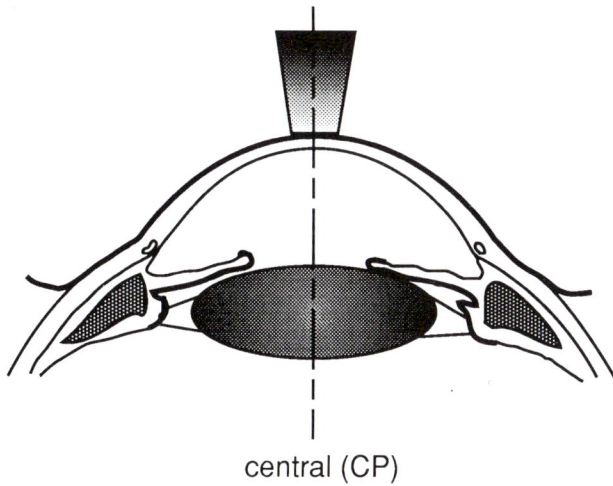

central (CP)

Fig. 5.15 Central pachymetry (CP).

(a)

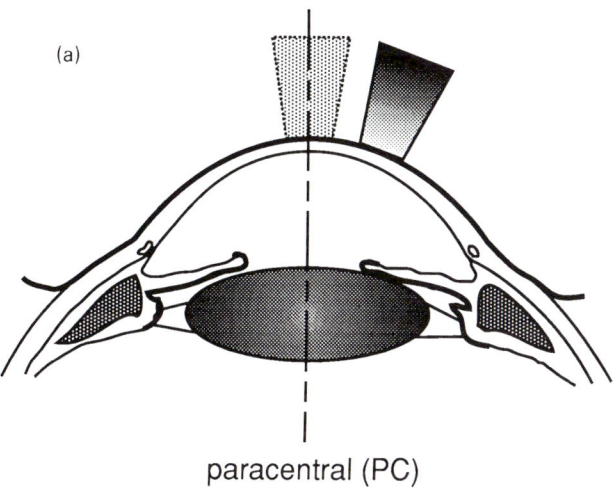

paracentral (PC)

(b)

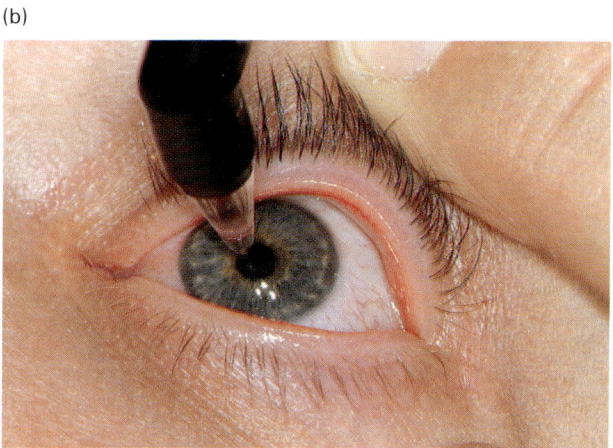

Fig. 5.16 (a,b) Para-central pachymetry (PC).

This next reading is the mid-peripheral (MP) reading and corresponds to the B ring on the map (Figure 5.17). Store the reading. Note that again the blinking light becomes steady and the next lit spot begins to blink.

The probe is now moved to a point halfway between the para-central point and the limbus (Figure 5.18). This is the para-peripheral (PP) measurement point.

Acquire and record this reading. Finally, the probe is moved so as to straddle the transition between clear cornea and the limbus. This is the far peripheral (FP) reading and corresponds to the outer or D ring on the map. Acquire and store the reading as before (Figure 5.19).

Continue in this manner until all 33 points in the map are recorded. If you have difficulty with any particular reading, depress the left-hand side of the foot pedal to store a null or blank reading. This will cause the corresponding map light to turn off. When you have completed the mapping, use the UP/DOWN (arrow) buttons to move back to this point and try again.

It helps if you seat yourself on the same side as the eye you are attempting to measure. With practice, a typical corneal mapping will take less than 5 min. It is not necessary to lift the probe between readings.

When using the Pachette to map the cornea, it is not necessary to utilize a foot pedal. The instrument will

(a)

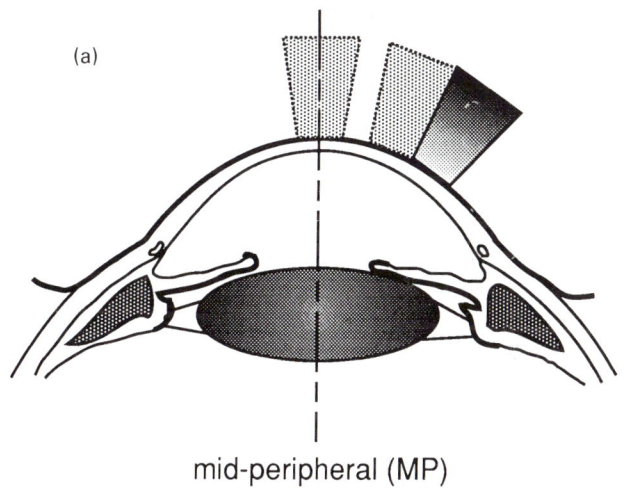

mid-peripheral (MP)

(b)

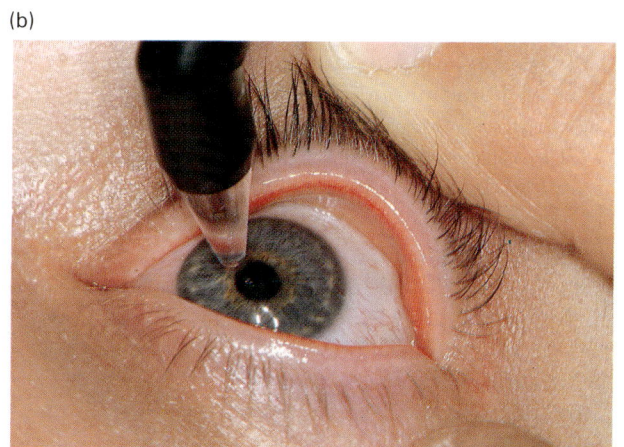

Fig. 5.17 (a,b) Mid peripheral pachymetry (MP).

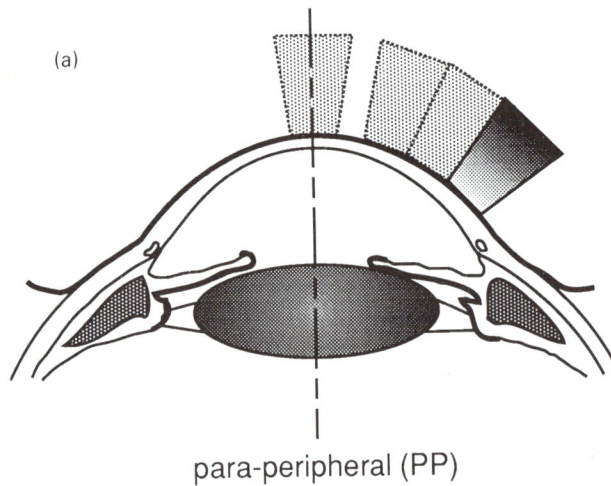

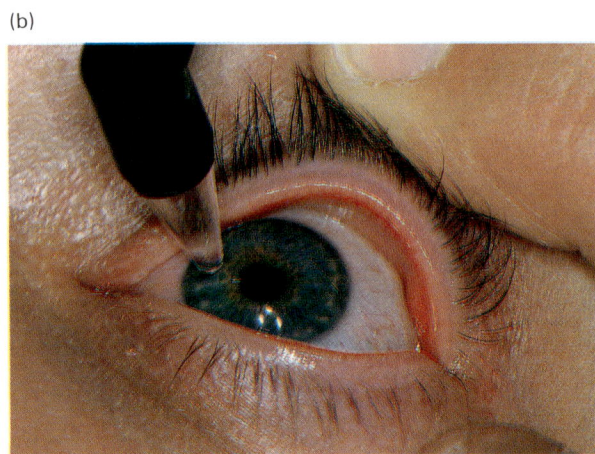

Fig. 5.18 (a) and (b) Para-peripheral pachymetry (PP).

Fig. 5.19 (a) and (b) Limbal pachymetry: far peripheral (FP).

sense when it is in contact with the corneal surface and attempt to take a reading. If it is successful, it will store the reading automatically and get ready for the next input. Simply move the probe into position and the unit will take another reading.

When you have completed the mapping process, pressing the PRINT button will cause the readings stored in memory to be printed out. When the printing is completed it is a good idea immediately to record the eye measured and write the patient's name and the date on the print-out. Press CLR and re-enter the desired mode to get ready for the left eye.

The probes can be used for intra-operative pachymetry by dry gas sterilization or by soaking in CIDEX. However, CIDEX can leave a residue and has been implicated in causing post-operative keratitis, so take care that the tip is thoroughly rinsed before use. Do not autoclave any portion of the probe and do not soak the plug portion of the probe. If soaking the older-model, fillable probes, remove the probe tip beforehand. If using the BEN-VENUE cartridge gas sterilizer be aware that the cartridges contain freon which will craze the surface of the plastic probe tip. This hazard

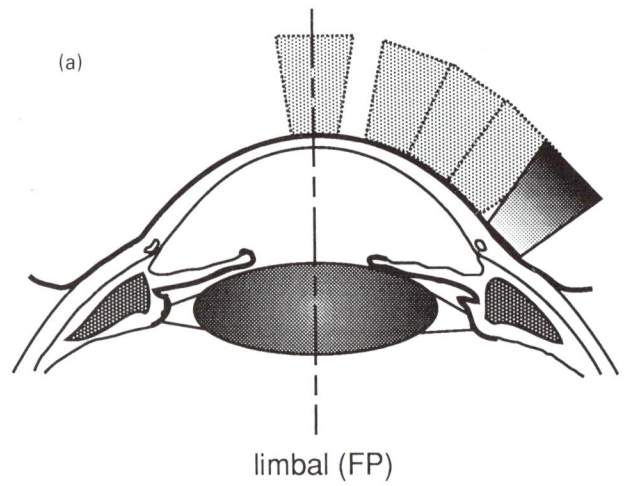

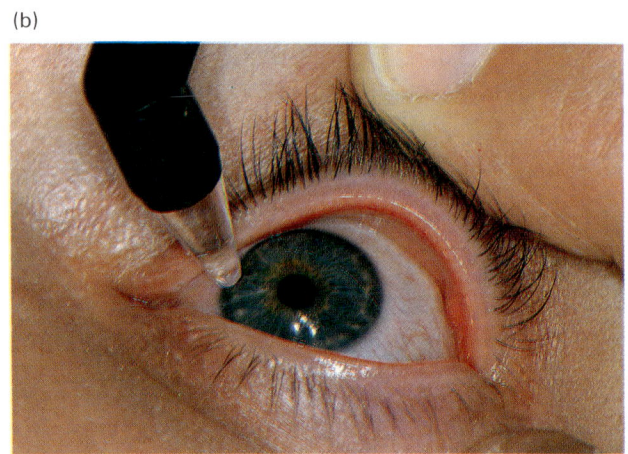

can be minimized by placing the packaged probe in several layers of cloth wrappers and supporting the probe above the bottom of the chamber on loosely packed cotton. I prefer to gas the cord and transducer and soak the probe tip. Use sterile methylcellulose or A-scan gel as a coupling medium. *Do not use saline!*

References

1 Binder PS, May CH, Grant SC. An evaluation of orthokeratology. Ophthalmology 1980; 87:729–744.
2 Levy B. Permanent corneal damage in a patient undergoing orthokeratology. Am J Optom Physiol Opt 1982; 59:697–699.
3 Polse KA, Brand RJ, Vastine DW, Schwalbe JS. Corneal change accompanying orthokeratology. Plastic or elastic? Results of a randomized controlled clinical trial. Arch Ophthalmol 1983; 101:1873–1878.
4 Milder B, Rubin ML. *Fine Art of Prescribing Glasses Without Making a Spectacle of Yourself*. Triad Scientific Publishers, Gainesville, 1978.
5 Bores L. Historical review and clinical results of radial keratotomy. Int Ophthalmol Clin 1983; 23:93–118.
6 Salz J, Lee JS, Jester JV *et al*. Radial keratotomy in fresh human cadaver eyes. Ophthalmology 1981; 88:742–746.

7 Bores LD, Myers W, Cowden J. Radial keratotomy: an analysis of the American experience. Ann Ophthalmol 1981; 13: 941–948.

8 Cowden JW, Bores LD. A clinical investigation of the surgical correction of myopia by the method of Fyodorov. Ophthalmology 1981; 88:737–741.

9 Rowsey JJ, Balyeat HD, Rabinovitch B, Burris TE, Hays JC. Predicting the results of radial keratotomy. Ophthalmology 1983; 90:642–654.

10 Barraquer JI. Terminologia y calculos basicos. In: *Cirugia Refractiva de la Cornea*, Instituto Barraquer de America, Bogota, Colombia, 1989.

11 Choyce DP. Intra-cameral and intra-corneal implants. A decade of personal experience. Trans Ophthalmol Soc UK 1966; 86:507–525.

12 Werblin TP, Blaydes JE, Fryczkowski A, Peiffer R. Refractive corneal surgery: the use of implantable alloplastic lens material. Aust J Ophthalmol 1983; 11:325–331.

13 Werblin TP, Peiffer RL, Fryczkowski A. Myopic hydrogel keratophakia: preliminary report. Cornea 1984; 3:197–204.

14 Morgan KS, Asbell PA, Kaufman HE. Cataracts in children: epikeratophakia for the correction of aphakia. J LA State Med Soc 1983; 135:23–25.

15 Deitz M, Sanders D, Marks R. Radial keratotomy: an overview of the Kansas City study. Ophthalmology 1984; 91:467–478.

16 Fyodorov SN, Durnev VV. The use of anterior keratotomy method with the purpose of surgical correction of myopia. MSIEM, 47, Moscow, 1977.

17 Fyodorov SN, Durnev VV. Operation of dosaged dissection of corneal circular ligament in cases of myopia of mild degree. Ann Ophthalmol 1979; 11:1885–1890.

18 Waring GO, Lynn MJ, Culbertson W *et al*. Three-year results of the prospective evaluation of radial keratotomy (PERK) study. Ophthalmology 1987; 94:1339–1354.

19 Duke-Elder S, Abrams D. Ophthalmic optics and refraction. In: *System of Ophthalmology*, SS Duke-Elder (ed). C.V. Mosby, St Louis, 1970.

20 Sampson WG. Keratometry. In: *Corneal Contact Lens*, LJ Girard, JW Soper and WG Sampson (eds). C.V. Mosby, St Louis, 1970.

21 Mohrman R. The keratometer. In: *Clinical Ophthalmology*, TD Duane (ed). Harper & Row, Hagerstown, 1976.

22 Ruben M. *Contact Lens Practice*. Williams & Wilkins, Baltimore, 1975.

23 Miller D, Benedek G. *Intraocular Light Scattering*. Thomas, Springfield, 1973.

24 Miller D, Jernigan MS, Molnar S. Laboratory evaluation of a clinical glare tester. Arch Ophthalmol 1972; 87:324.

25 Holladay LL. The fundamentals of glare and visibility. J Opt Soc Am 1926; 12:492.

26 Wolf E. Glare and age. Arch Ophthalmol 1960; 4:502.

27 Hess R, Woo G. Vision through cataracts. Invest Ophthalmol 1978; 17:428.

28 Arden GB, Jacobson JJ. Simple grating test for contrast sensitivity: preliminary results indicate value in screening for glaucoma. Invest Ophthalmol 1978; 17:23.

29 Paulson LE, Sjorstand J. Contrast sensitivity in the presence of a glare light. Invest Ophthalmol 1980; 19:401.

30 Nadler MP. New glare tester (letter). Arch Ophthalmol 1982; 100:1676.

31 LeClaire J, Nadler MP, Weiss S, Miller D. A new glare tester for clinical testing. Results comparing normal subjects and variously corrected aphakic patients. Arch Ophthalmol 1982; 100:153–158.

32 Villasenor RA, Santos VR, Cox KC, Harris DF, Lynn M, Waring GO. Comparison of ultrasonic corneal thickness measurements before and during surgery in the prospective evaluation of radial keratotomy (PERK) study. Ophthalmology 1986; 93:327–330.

6

Corneal Topography

Nature confuses the skeptics and reason confutes the dogmatists. [Blaise Pascal (1623–1662)]

The shape or profile of the corneal surface has always been a tantalizing and elusive mystery. True, in the past, devices have been designed and constructed which have measured something of its properties. But its exact nature, like the dark side of the moon, has, until recently, remained out of sight and out of reach and like the dark side of the moon in the past, has been described rather fancifully. Those measurements that have been taken have, unfortunately, muddied the waters by creating certain mind-sets and preconceptions that are difficult to overcome.

As our interest in refractive modulation of the corneal surface and ocular components of the eye has grown, our attention has become more focused on the actual shape of the cornea. No longer can we rely upon presumptive topography as gleaned from centuries-old technology, namely keratometry and Placido's disk. It is no secret that keratometry is only accurate for spherical surfaces—that fact has been known from the outset. Placido's disk surface representation—as manifested by photokeratoscopy—has not changed the inherent problem of that technique, despite the increased sophistication of instruments designed to that method. It is both tantalizing and frustrating to deal with such devices, all the while knowing the limitations of both.

To understand fully the shape changes the cornea undergoes following anterior segment surgery, trauma, and contact lens wear, there is a need for methods and instruments that can be used for the accurate and high-resolution mensuration of corneal shape. There can be no more compelling demonstration of this need than the cases described by Maguire and McDonnell *et al.* [1–3]. These studies add further evidence to the hypothesis that a sub-set of patients who undergo radial keratotomy are left with a post-operative topography characterized by a small central area of minimum power surrounded by concentric bands of increasingly higher power [4]. When these bands of higher power are located within or close to the entrance pupil, they have the ability to allow "good" visual acuity (as measured by standard visual acuity charts) to be maintained over a greater refractive range than is possible with normal corneal surface optics. For the radial keratotomy patient with −3.00 D of residual cycloplegic refractive error who is able to maintain good quality 20/20 to 20/40 uncorrected vision, the multifocal effect of such an extremely aspheric corneal surface could hardly be deemed a complication [5]. Unfortunately, some post-radial keratotomy patients may develop a pattern of corneal asphericity severe enough to cause a significant degradation in the quality of the visual image while still maintaining 20/20 visual acuity and a multifocal lens effect over an extended refractive range. One would be hard-pressed to convince such a patient that he or she has not had a surgical complication. These findings concerning the relationship of corneal surface topography to visual performance and the hypothesis regarding the cause of this pattern of corneal irregularity lead to the following conclusion, expressed by Leo Maguire:

> Our knowledge of the effect preoperative topography has on postoperative results following refractive surgery is less than adequate. If patients are capable of maintaining excellent Snellen visual acuity in the presence of severe corneal irregularity after such surgery, is it not possible that a subset of the "normal" population demonstrates similar degrees of variable central corneal irregularity prior to surgery? It is increasingly obvious that our understanding of the topography of the postoperative corneal surface, its relation to "multifocal effects" in particular, and visual performance in general is still in its infancy [3,6].

Today, with the increased interest in refractive eye surgery, suppositions and guesswork will no longer serve. Operations such as keratomileusis, in which the central corneal cap or apex curvature is modified through tissue ablation, depend very much upon the primary curvature of that same area. Empiric formulas have been employed to control the amount of tissue removed. While such empiricism works, predictability of the outcome is still elusive. The uncertainty of the ultimate corneal shape makes even more difficult the modification of the external corneal curvature through employment of intra-stromal allopathic lenticules such as the KeratoGel hydrophilic implant. Peripheral modification of the cornea in an effort to alter the apex —the hallmark of the radial keratotomy procedure—is also affected by the overall shape of the cornea. In this instance, the corneal surface need be moved only a few tens of micro-meters to alter the refraction significantly. Laser tissue ablation is even more problematic since reliance is made on micro-meter-level tissue layer removal. Progress in intra-ocular lens design, as well as the surgery of corneal transplantation and that of cataract, all hinge on a more enlightened understanding of the surface that produces 90% of the refractive power of the eye.

The quality of vision is greatly dependent on the topography of the cornea. The keratometer is routinely used to measure the shape of the cornea in the clinical practice of ophthalmology, but this instrument measures corneal curvature from the reflection of mires at only four positions along two meridians at right angles. While this method can achieve an accuracy of better than 0.25D in measuring steel balls, clinical keratometers cannot be used to measure irregular astigmatism or corneal asphericity. For example, the keratometer cannot be used to assess the size of the central zone of uniform power following radial keratotomy.

Thus we have employed moiré keratometry, electronic keratometry, ultrasound, photogrammetry, profile photography and interferometry to perform this task. Each has its own unique advantages and disadvantages, which will be discussed within this chapter. Underlying the eclecticism of evolving topography instrumentation lies a very real and intensive attempt to understand and codify something that has proved to be a very slippery customer over the last century or so—the corneal surface shape.

The following is a synopsis of what is fittingly called the state of the art (emphasis on the last word). The term art aptly fits the *mélange* of brightly hued and occasionally abstract images facing the ophthalmologist seeking the grail of refractive surgery. Confronted with shapes and colors reminiscent of Cézanne or Kandinsky (Figure 6.1), the refractive surgeon is also forced to cope with a new vocabulary—a techno-babble unique to this emerging field, or as George Waring phrased it, keratospeak.

The vocabulary of corneal topography

It is confusing enough to try to equate data gathered on different devices or even to try to understand what each one does—if anything—without compounding the problem by employing terms when no two are used the same way, nor can their meaning always be agreed upon. This form of technical obscurantism serves no useful purpose. In an effort to shed some light into this dark medical corner, we present this section, adapted somewhat from Waring [7].

Keratometer (ophthalmometer)

A keratometer should more rightly be called an ophthalmometer, a term coined by Helmholtz in 1853 for his device which measured the central corneal curvature [8]. Keratometer, unfortunately, is a trade name owned by the Bausch & Lomb company, but has, like Xerox and Kleenex, entered the common lexicon and is, hence, used synonymously (if incorrectly) for ophthalmometer. The act of measuring the corneal curvature can be rightly termed either keratometry or ophthalmometry without fear of trade name infringement.

Radius of curvature and refractive power of the cornea

The radius of curvature of the anterior and posterior corneal surfaces affects its refractive power. A shorter radius of curvature creates a steeper arc and greater refractive power. Conversely, a longer radius of curvature creates a flatter arc and less refractive power. The image formed by light reflected from the convex anterior corneal surface is called the first Purkinje

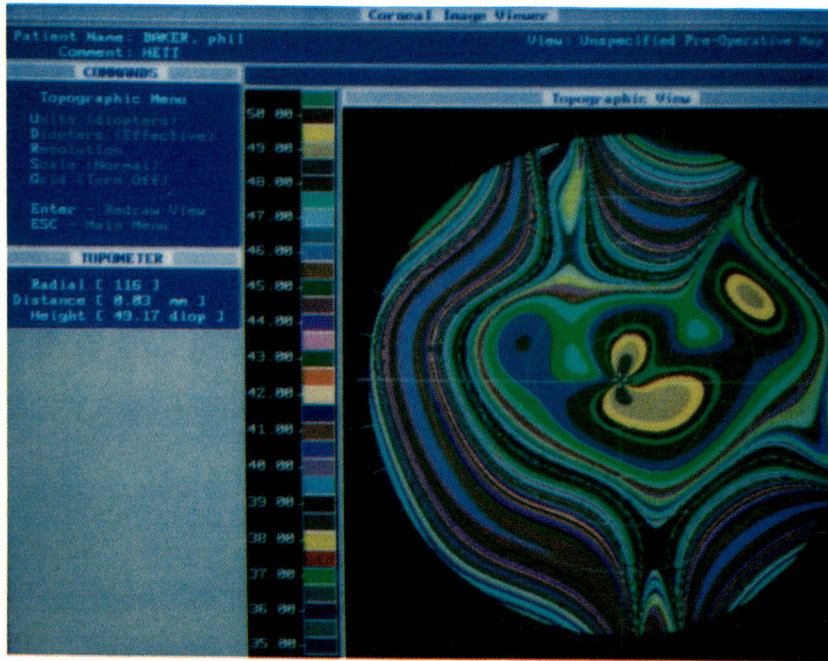

Fig. 6.1 Keratograph of post-operative radial keratotomy produced with the CLAS II holographic topographer.

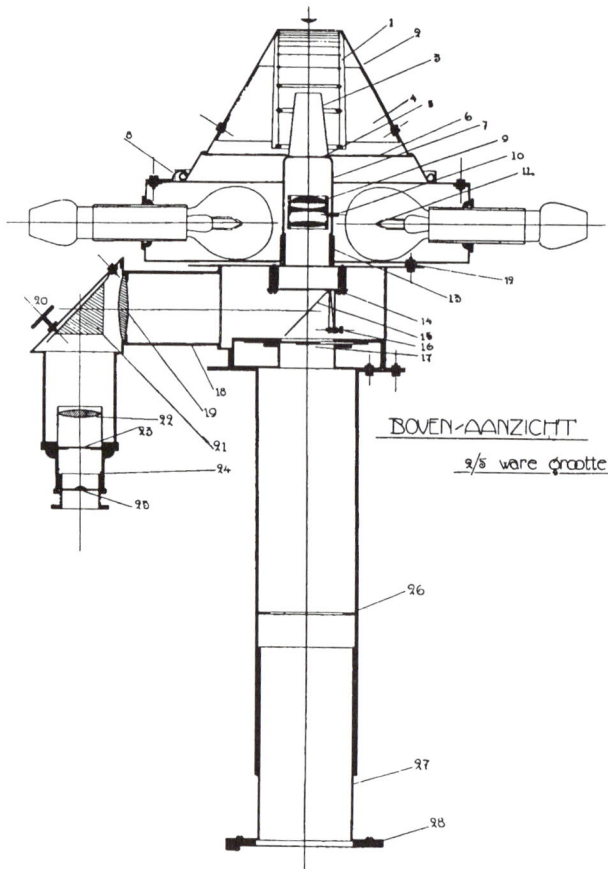

Fig. 6.2 Early model photokeratoscope (Corneoscope); from Dekking H. Fotografie der cornea, opperwlakte Assen. Groninque th. med. 1930 No. 2, Van Gorcum in Bcm, 91, 360 (1930) no. 271, 1930.

image, the corneal light reflex, or the corneal light reflection. This virtual, first-order, erect image is viewed during keratometry and keratoscopy and is located approximately 4 mm posterior to the surface of the cornea at the level of the anterior lens capsule.

Keratoscope

Fortunately no one has trade-marked the term keratoscope which describes an instrument that projects a series of mires, most commonly rings, on to the corneal surface. Keratoscopes fitted with still film cameras are called photokeratoscopes; those fitted with a video camera are called videokeratoscopes. The term Corneoscope is the trade name used by the Kera Corporation but seems headed in the same direction as keratometer. Figure 6.2 is from Dekking (1930) and represents a 50-year advance on Gullstrand's original instrument [9,10].

Keratoscopy

Direct observation of the images of mires reflected from the surface of the cornea is keratoscopy, in the same sense that examination of the ocular fundus with an ophthalmoscope is ophthalmoscopy.

Keratography

The term keratography denotes a record or portrayal of the cornea in the same sense that angiography records the pattern of vessels—the Greek word γραφειν (*graphein*) means to write. Currently, there are three methods of recording pictures (keratographs) of the mires reflected from the corneal surface:

1 With photographic film, one uses a photokeratoscope to produce a photokeratograph, a process called photokeratography (in the same sense that one uses a photomicroscope to take a photomicrograph).

2 With video recording, one uses a videokeratoscope to produce a videokeratograph, a process called videokeratography.

3 Via electronic capture one uses a video camera and a device called a frame grabber.

A keratograph can be interpreted qualitatively or quantitatively. A qualitative interpretation is done by visual inspection of the shape and spacing of the mires and has practical value in diagnosing corneal disorders such as keratoconus or in adjusting sutures after penetrating keratoplasty. Quantitative keratography is done by assigning numeric coordinate values to points on the mires and describing mathematically the curves that the points form. Complex formulas and algorithms are required for accurate quantitation of the surface topography. Quantitative analysis is usually done with the assistance of a computer that uses image analysis programs and is located in a separate instrument (as in the Kera and Nidek systems—both photokeratoscopes) or in the keratoscope itself (as in the Computed Anatomy, Visio and KeraView systems, or the CLAS II laser holographer—all computer-assisted videokeratoscopes).

Topography

Topography is the science of accurate and detailed descriptions of surface features, be they of the Earth, the moon or even the eye. The most common representation is a topographic map on which the relative elevations of the surface are delimited by contour lines. The term topology is often used to describe the study of such surfaces, typically in mathematical terms. Either word is correct but within this treatise we will use the more common one—topography.

Topographic displays

The mires used to study corneal shape have many configurations: circles, arcs, parallel lines, interference fringes, steps, etc. Those most commonly used are circular rings as in keratoscopes. The concentric ring mires are commonly called Placido rings, but strictly speaking, that designation should describe only Placido's flat disk with the equally spaced circular white rings. Modern keratoscope rings are designed differently. By convention, the rings are numbered from innermost to outermost. This can be confusing, because a specific ring (e.g. ring 3) in different instruments may cover a different location on different corneas. Therefore, it is important to designate the diameter of a projected ring and indicate the area on the cornea which it covers. There are four basic methods of displaying corneal topographic information:

1 The keratograph (Figure 6.1).

2 Representation of the radius of curvature or dioptric power at various locations on the surface of the cornea, either in a fixed pattern on a "face plate" or at any location identified by a cursor in a computer-assisted videokeratoscope (Figure 6.2).

3 Graphic three-dimensional figures often with exaggerations to show changes in curvature (Figures 6.3 and 6.4).

4 Color-coded maps using colors to designate areas of uniform radius of curvature and refractive power (Figure 6.5).

The most widely used system of color coding is reds and oranges to indicate steeper areas with greater refractive power and greens and blues to indicate flatter areas with less refractive power (LSU Topography System, Computed Anatomy Corneal Modeling System, EyeSys, KeraMetrics CLAS II) [11–13]. A quantitative scale indicates the values corresponding to each color.

Shape of the anterior cornea

Corneal asphericity

First must be understood the fact that the human cornea is a toroidal asphere—that is, its shape is neither a sphere nor a regular asphere. In fact, no human cornea is ever spherical except perhaps in that singular area called the optic or central zone—elsewhere there is always some degree of asymmetry or astigmatism. Some day our simplified conception of the cornea as a spherocylindrical lens may be replaced by more accurate "shape factors," mathematical indices or ray tracing diagrams. Until then we must muddle through with more imperfect notions.

A useful simplification to understand the topography of the cornea is to consider the corneal curvature as a section of an ellipse. In most normal corneas the central zone is steeper than the paracentral and peripheral zones, a configuration referred to as having a positive shape factor (positive because the radius of curvature becomes larger from the center to the periphery) and a prolate shape. A prolate shape is that shape taken across the narrow end of an ellipse, or better, the pointy end of an egg. The opposite topographic pattern rarely occurs in normal eyes but appears commonly after radial keratotomy: the central zone is flatter than the paracentral and peripheral zones, a configuration referred to as having a negative

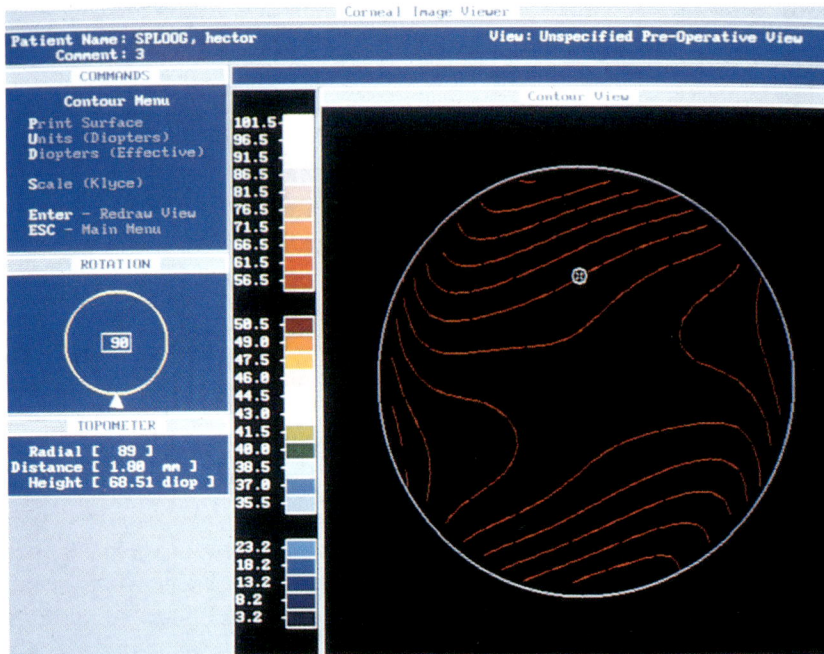

Fig. 6.3 Contour map drawn by a holographic topographer. The corneal elevation at the cursor position is indicated on the left. (Courtesy of KeraMetrics.)

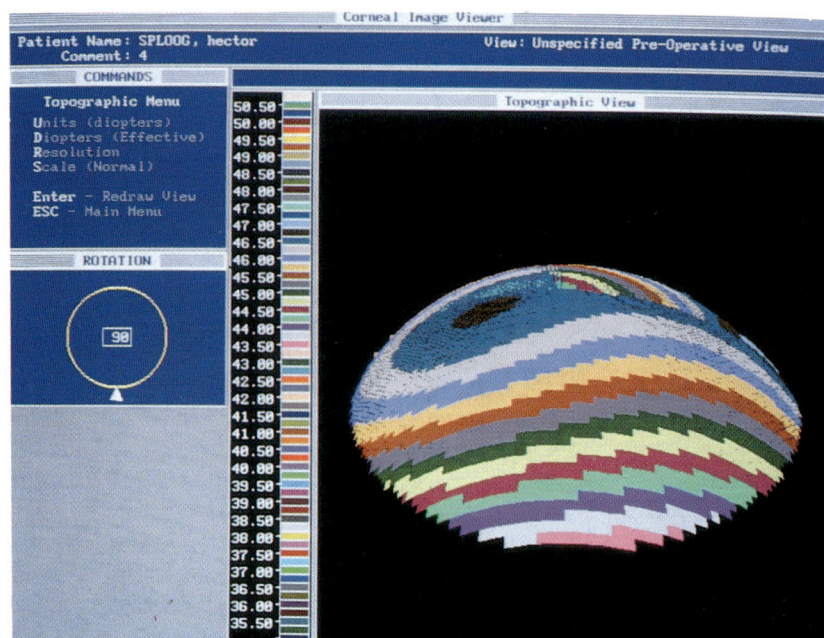

Fig. 6.4 An isometric contour map of the corneal surface. (Courtesy of KeraMetrics.)

shape factor and an oblate shape—which is the section taken across the long axis of an ellipse (Figure 6.6).

Surface zones of the cornea

A similar over-simplification takes place when the cornea is divided into surface zones (e.g. optical zone, apical zone). None of these areas is discrete, because the cornea forms continuous curves. Nevertheless, for practical optical and anatomic purposes, we can divide the surface of the cornea into two overall regions: the central optical zone and the remainder of the cornea (sometimes called the periphery) [14]. The optical zone forms the foveal image through the entrance pupil of the eye; its size, shape and curvature vary among individuals. The rest of the cornea serves as a refracting surface for peripheral vision and for the foveal image when the pupil is widely dilated, as a mechanical structure, and as a source of cells during normal turnover and repair.

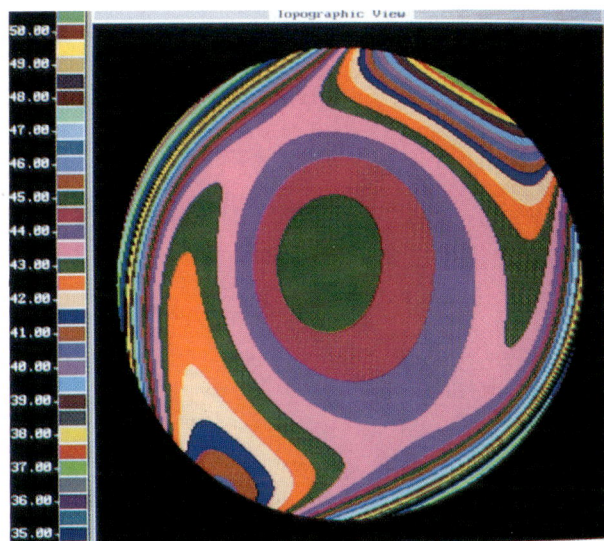

Fig. 6.5 Typical color-coded topographic map of a post-operative radial keratotomy corneal surface. (Courtesy of KeraMetrics.)

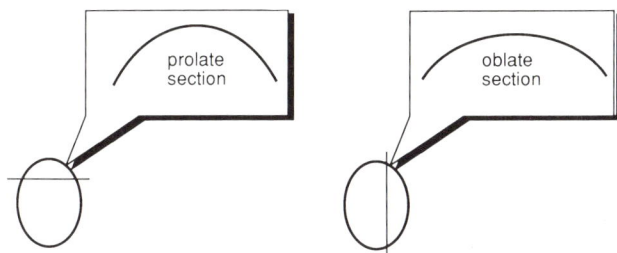

Fig. 6.6 Prolate and oblate curved sections.

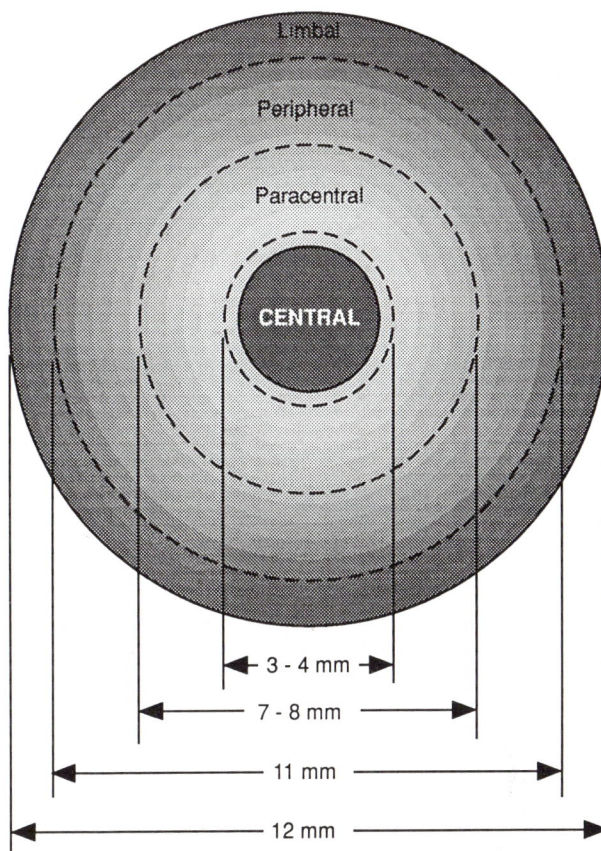

Fig. 6.7 Corneal zones.

Apex of the cornea

The apex of the cornea is the high spot of the cornea, the location of the greatest sagittal height on the surface. It is from this point that the corneal light reflection emanates and therefore it is the point around which the keratoscopy rings center. The apex or high point of the normal cornea is close to, but not coincident with, the optic axis. However, in pathologic states such as keratoconus and after corneal surgery, the apex may be so displaced that the keratoscopy rings no longer center around any clearly identifiable point or axis on the cornea, or over the entrance pupil. Thus, the patient may be looking through an area of the cornea eccentric to that portion centered within the keratoscope mires.

Conventionally, four concentric anatomic zones are recognized (Figure 6.7): central optical zone, paracentral intermediate zone, peripheral transitional zone, and limbal zone. It is important to distinguish these anatomic zones from those commonly associated with radial keratotomy so as to avoid confusion.

Central anatomic zone

The central zone is approximately 4 mm in diameter and has been called the apical zone, the corneal cap, the optical zone and the central spherical zone, all terms intended to designate this region of the cornea as the more spherical, symmetric, and optically important. The term central zone appears most apt. Now that corneal topography is requiring more careful definitions, we must distinguish among four designations:

1 The anatomic central zone, which is 3–4 mm in diameter.
2 The functional optical zone, which is the area that overlies the entrance pupil and which is smaller than the anatomic zone.
3 The spherical central part of the cornea which is present in a minority of normal corneas.
4 The apex of the cornea, which is the highest spot on the cornea (as discussed subsequently and which may not be concentric with the so-called optic axis).

The optical zone can be further defined in one of five ways, depending upon the optical circumstances (Figure 6.8):

1 The anatomic center of the cornea, equidistant from

Left eye

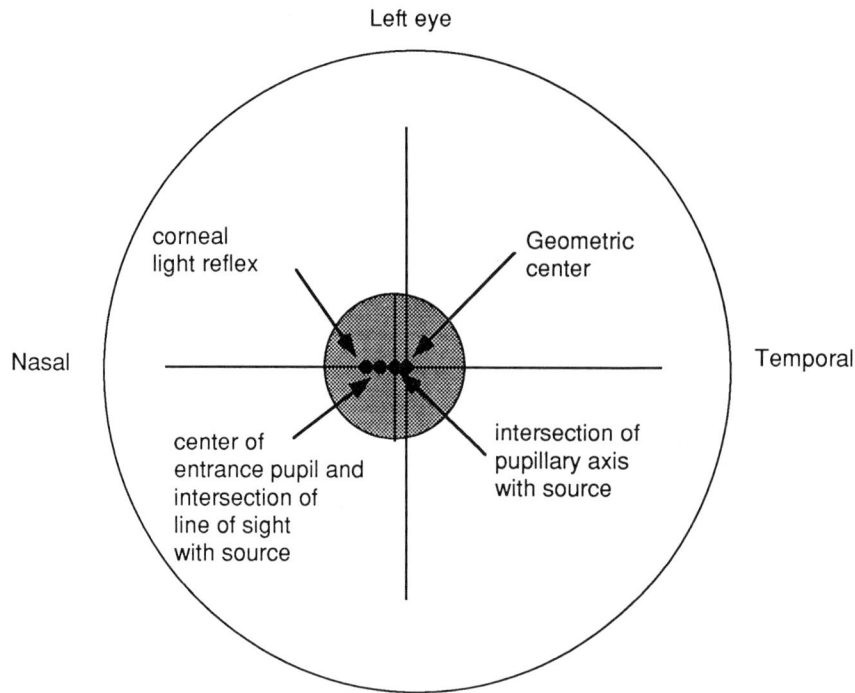

Nasal

Temporal

corneal
light reflex

Geometric
center

center of
entrance pupil and
intersection of
line of sight
with source

intersection of
pupillary axis
with source

Fig. 6.8 Pupillary axes (see also
Chapter 3).

the limbus and typically eccentric to the optic and
visual axes.

2 The optic axis that connects the center of curvature
of the cornea and centers of curvature of the crystalline
lens (which can also be slightly eccentric to the visual
axis).

3 The pupillary axis that connects the center of the
entrance pupil and the center of curvature of the
cornea.

4 The line of sight that connects the fixation point with
the center of the entrance pupil.

5 The visual axis that passes from the center of the
fovea through the nodal points of the eye.

Detailed discussion of these often confusing axes can
be found in Chapter 5. For practical purposes, the
center of the optical zone should be considered the
intersection of the pupillary axis with the cornea,
because the entrance pupil determines the image-
forming bundle of rays that reach the fovea. However
that may be, this optical zone may not be coincident
with the surgical optical or clear zone which is centered
on the visual axis.

The term optical zone is used with four different
meanings in the context of refractive surgery. The first
meaning is that just defined: the central more spherical
portion of the normal cornea overlying the entrance
pupil. The second meaning refers to the portion of a
keratomileusis or epikeratoplasty lenticule or excimer
laser surface ablation that creates the major refractive
change. The third meaning is the central uncut clear
zone in radial keratotomy; clear zone is preferred by

Waring [5] and others but with no compelling reason.
In the author's view, calling that area of the cornea
most affected by the refractive surgical technique (the
"business" part as opposed to the supportive part) the
optical zone is apt and descriptive and should cause no
confusion (except perhaps among purists). The fourth
meaning is any circular mark on the cornea used to
delineate or demarcate places where incisions begin or
end, for example, a "7 mm optical zone" used for
placement of transverse incisions. In this context,
optical zone is truly a misnomer, and should be replaced by the simple designation surgical zone or just
zone, as in "the transverse incisions were placed at the
7 mm (surgical) zone."

Paracentral anatomic zone

The paracentral anatomic zone is an annulus approximately 4–7 mm in diameter and has been called the
mid, intermediate or mid peripheral cornea. The term
mid peripheral is a misnomer because this zone
does not occupy the middle of the periphery. A transverse incision made at the 6 mm zone would be mid
peripheral because while it is still within the central
anatomic half of the cornea it is partway into the
peripheral zone and also at the midpoint of the cornea.
The paracentral surgical zone in radial keratotomy is
any zone mark from 3.0 to 5.0 mm in diameter and
refers to the first or primary surgical zone. The central
and paracentral anatomic zones together comprise
what contact lens fitters call the apical zone.

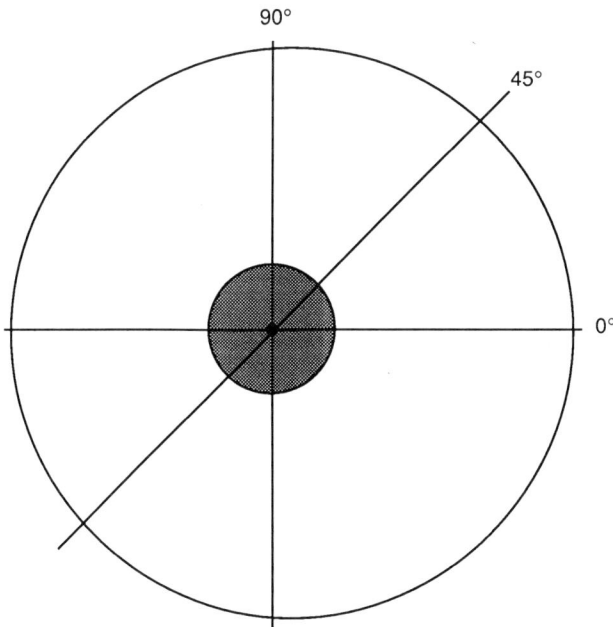

Fig. 6.9 Corneal meridians.

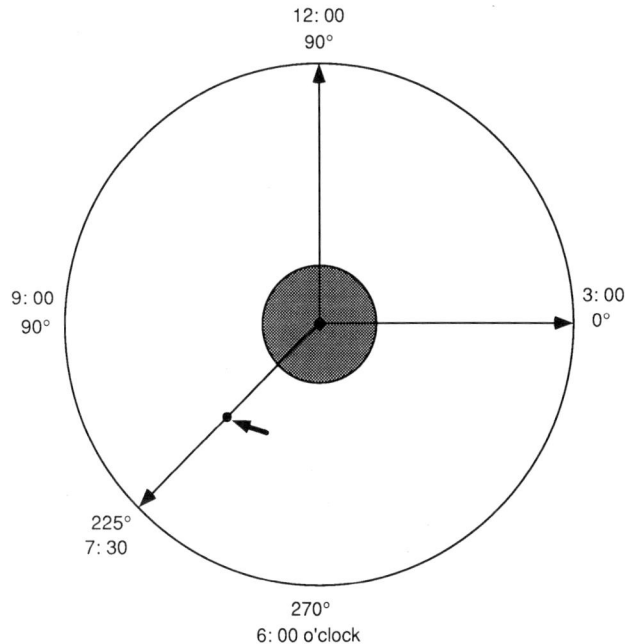

Fig. 6.10 Corneal semimeridians.

Peripheral anatomic zone

The peripheral anatomic zone is an annulus from approximately 7 to 11 mm in diameter. This is the area in which the normal cornea flattens the most and becomes more aspherical. For this reason it has been called the transitional zone. Note that this is not the same annular area described by Mandell [15]. In radial keratotomy, zones from 7 to 9 mm are called paraperipheral surgical zones.

Limbal anatomic zone

The limbal zone is the ring of cornea approximately 0.5 mm wide that abuts the sclera and contains the capillary arcade. The area from 9 mm to the limbus has been designated the far peripheral zone by radial keratotomists.

Meridians, semimeridians and axes

Locations on the surface of the cornea are designated along meridians, lines that span the diameter of the cornea from one point on the limbus to the opposite point and which have a common center. Meridians are designated from 0 to 180°, proceeding counterclockwise starting at 3 o'clock for both the right and left eyes (Figure 6.9). The term axis designates the direction in a cylindrical lens along which there is no power (see Chapter 5). Because clinicians align the axes of cylindrical lenses with meridians on the cornea, it is common practice to substitute the term axis, for

meridian, when referring to directions on the cornea. Thus, clinicians commonly refer to the steep axis of a cornea when they really mean steep meridian, a unfortunate habit that is unlikely ever to change. Thus, when clinicians refer to the steep axis or the flat axis of the cornea, the term axis is used incorrectly; the term meridian should be used when referring to the direction of corneal refractive power and axis when referring to spectacle power.

Designating meridians as 0–180° is conventional, but, unlike geographers, ophthalmologists have no north–south longitude lines to indicate a point along a meridian. Thus, if one refers to removing a tight corneal suture in the 90° meridian, it is not clear whether the activity occurs in the 12 o'clock direction or in the 6 o'clock direction. Therefore, directions from the center of the cornea are designated as semimeridians and are located around the 360° circumference of the cornea in degrees, such as "the 225° semimeridian" (Figure 6.10). The term semimeridian is preferred, since both components are derived from Latin. Another convention is to consider the cornea as the face of a clock so that 7.30 indicates the 225° semimeridian.

A specific point on the surface of the cornea is designated by indicating its location in millimeters from the center of the cornea along a semimeridian. For example: "at 3 mm from the center (6.0 mm zone) along the 225° semimeridian the corneal power may be 41.00 D." The location of a transverse incision could be described as follows: "it was placed 3 mm from the center [i.e. at the 6 mm zone], perpendicular to the 225° semimeridian" or better: "it was centered on the 225° semimeridian, transverse to a 6 mm zone." In current jargon: "A T-cut was made at the 6 mm optical zone at 7.30"—a usage to be decried and fortunately only heard among the relatively ignorant and inexperienced. This clock-hour system is too crude for refractive surgery which requires more accuracy; we can discard this designation without regret. Definitely *nekulturny* (unsophisticated).

Ophthalmometry (keratometry)

History of ophthalmometry

The concept of determining the curvature of a surface by measuring the size of the reflected image is well-established in optics. However, measuring such a reflection on the eye is made difficult by the fact that the eye is constantly in motion. At least three centuries have passed since the first attempt to measure the anterior surface curvature of the cornea was made by Scheiner, yet the exact form of this surface is still not well-understood. While the methods of measurement have been diverse, nearly all the corneal measurements realized so far have been based on one optical property of the cornea—that it is a convex reflecting surface, i.e. a mirror. In general, previous measuring devices were based on the assumption that the cornea was a conic section, i.e. a sphere, an ellipse, a parabola, or a hyperbola. In reality the living cornea is none of these but is an aspherical section with great individual variation—a toroidal asphere.

In 1619, Christoph Scheiner, a Jesuit instructor of mathematics and Hebrew, was the first to calculate the refractive properties of the various transparent media of the eye (see also Chapters 2 and 3) [16]. In one experiment, he arranged glass spheres of various known diameters next to a subject's eye and by comparing the sizes of the reflected images of a window in both, he obtained an approximation of the central spherical curvature of the cornea. This experiment naturally led many observers to assume that the cornea was a spherical surface. That assumption has handicapped ophthalmology ever since, despite evidence to the contrary.

Kohlraush measured the reflected image of an object on the cornea using a Kepler telescope [17]. Ramsden, in 1796, adopted the concept of the heliograph and visual doubling to ocular surface measurement. Helmholtz perfected this device in 1856 and his design serves as the basis for many instruments in use today. Helmholtz was the first to introduce the doubling device into an ophthalmometer. While Helmholtz's modifications made a device accurate for scientific work, some further adjustment was necessary to adapt

the instrument for use in clinical practice, particularly for the measurement of astigmatism [18]. Coccius [19], Landolt [20], Javal and Schiøtz [21], Sutcliffe [22], and Hartinger [23] followed with other measuring devices. Fincham was the first to measure directly the corneal periphery using an auto-collimation microscope [24]. The incorporation into the device of a Wollaston prism (two rectangular prisms cemented back-to-back) by Javal and Schiøtz produced a doubling refracting system which created two complete light cones rather than one [21]. Berg modified the Javal–Schiøtz ophthalmometer by placing a set of two lenses in front of it, forming an afocal system of magnification [25,26]. With this device he was able to explore a zone about 1 mm in diameter, at various points over the cornea.

Current evidence shows that the paraxial (optical) area is nearly spherical but even in this region the curvature seems to vary in different meridians. In fact, this surface astigmatism is found, at least to some degree, in such a high proportion of the population that it should be considered a normal state of affairs. Thus, by definition, the central cornea is not spherical but is more properly described as toroidal. All studies to date, based on various methodologies, have indicated that the peripheral cornea is even more irregular and cannot be described in simple geometric terms. The general shape of the peripheral cornea is flatter than is the central portion, however, and this has led to a dividing of the corneal surface into zones (see above).

As previously described, traditionally the corneal surface has been divided into two zones. The center, or corneal cap (apical zone), is the spherical or toroidal part, extending 4–5 mm in diameter. The peripheral, or annular part, extends to the limbus and is progressively flatter in contour (Figure 6.11). It is possible to define the cap as the central area having the maximum and most constant curvature. However, an annoying feature of the subject of corneal topography is the difficulty in deciding which point of the cornea to take as the apex of the cap. The center of the apical zone is not easily defined because the zone itself may be of indefinite size and extent. Defining the apex as the point of maximum curvature may find that this point does not correspond with the visual axis. Furthermore, it may be that major curvature in the toroidal form of the cornea is less marked at the apex than at the visual axis (Figure 6.12). Measurement in the latter instance may be a situation in which true toricity combines with an effect caused by tilt of an aspheric surface.

Additionally, no good data exist clearly defining either the size of the apical zone or where it ends and the peripheral zone begins. The limit or edge of this zone has been described by Mandell as the point where the radius of curvature increases by more than

optic "cap"

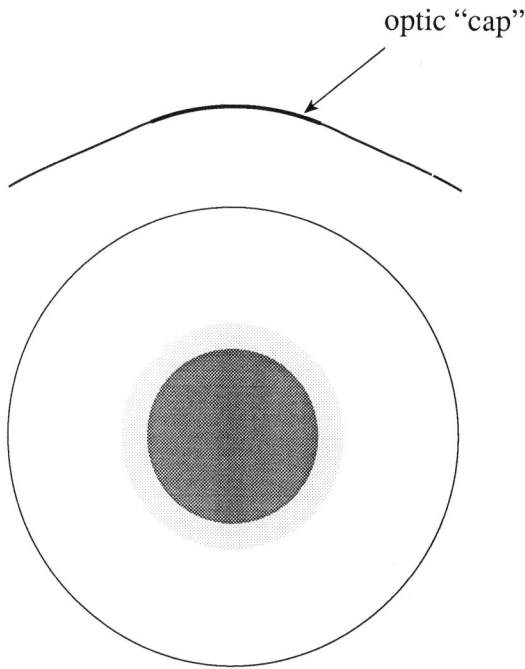

Fig. 6.11 Corneal apex or cap.

visual axis

corneal apex

note tilt of surface
(ie - intersection **is not** normal)

Fig. 6.12 The apex may not correspond with the optic axis or may be tilted.

0.05 mm (0.63 D) [11]. Thus the radius of curvature of the apex would lie between 7.2 and 8.7 mm, averaging 7.9 (46.62–38.62 and 42.50 D, respectively).

This division was originally proposed by Aubert, who described the cornea as having an optic part and a basilar part—on the basis of four measurements on six subjects—not exactly a statistically relevant sample [27]. Ericksen, using a Javal–Schiøtz type ophthalmometer, described the cap as having a diameter of 4.0 mm delineated by a change in power of 1.0 D [28]. Gullstrand supported this early work in his studies using photokeratoscopy [29]. He, too, found the central zone to be spherical. Other investigators later found the cap to be less spherical and more conical in shape with no definite boundaries—hence the borders of the so-called corneal cap are arbitrary, depending upon one's criteria.

For the purpose of our discussion, we will accept the boundary to be that place where the corneal curvature flattens by more than 1.0 D, even though this may not be entirely valid. Thus the average cap will have a diameter of 4.0 mm. If 2.0 D is used, the cap has a diameter of 6.0 mm—an interesting fact which we will touch upon later. As measuring methods have become more precise, however, it is apparent that "constant corneal curvature" is an oxymoron and that only the very central part of the cornea has an instantaneous spherical shape. The student of such things may be moved to ask: "So what?" So what, indeed; probably "so nothing" except that it is difficult to abandon the notion that there *must* exist some sort of central zone of

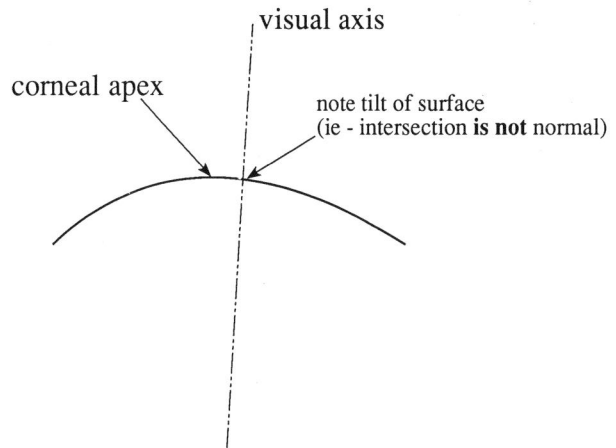

whatever stripe, else what is it that produces the reflex during skiascopy and what are we correcting with our spectacles, etc.?

Adding to the dilemma posed by such an "uncooperative" surface is the observation—reported by Reynolds and Kratt—that the cornea changes shape during the day, being flatter, and thus more hyperopic, in the morning as a rule [30]. These observations are apart from the even greater changes reported following radial keratotomy surgery [31,32]. The act of accommodation (focusing for near) itself has been shown to affect the corneal curvature by 1.5 D in the horizontal and 0.5 D in the vertical meridian in normals and by as much as 2 D in all meridians post radial keratotomy [33].

We have mentioned a visual axis as if all the optical components of the eye were somehow symmetrically aligned along a common axis. Strictly speaking such a condition does not exist. In fact, the best derived optic axis that can be conceived—assuming such an alignment—does not strike the center of vision, the fovea, at all!

Another complicating factor, which becomes more manifest as the methods of measurement become more refined, is the fact that the corneal surface is wet—a condition that has important implications as Bonnett found when he sprinkled talcum powder on the surface as a reflectant (see section on rasterstereography, below) [34].

In ophthalmometry, it is the spatial relationship between points before the cornea and the reflected image of these points that is used to calculate the average curvature between these reflected points on the cornea (Figure 6.13). To some extent, the smaller the area between these points on the cornea, the more representative of the actual surface contour the average can be.

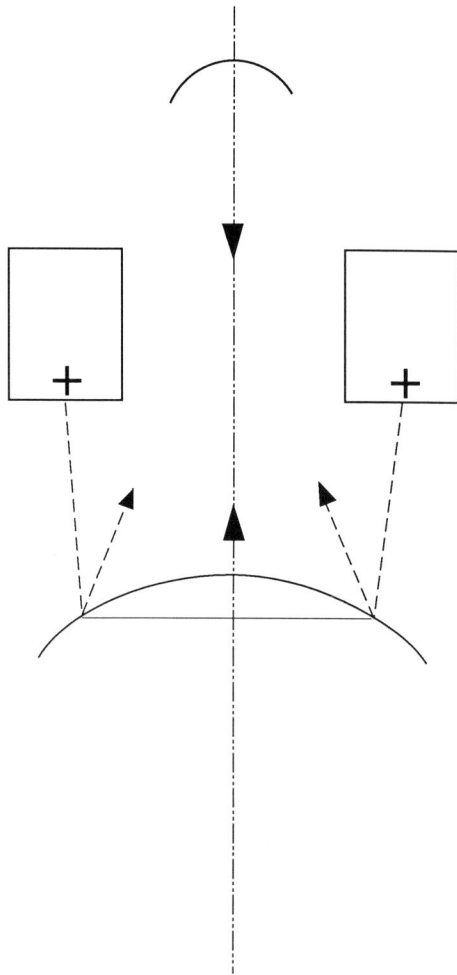

Fig. 6.13 Principle of ophthalmometry. Objects of known size are reflected by a curved surface, forming the first Purkinje image. The size of this image is related to the degree of curvature.

The mire size is fixed by the manufacturer but is generally too large to be considered to be reflecting paraxial rays from the cornea, thus optical mirror formulas cannot be used where high accuracy is needed. The keratometer does not need to measure the mire size, however. It is enough to know the relative sizes of the images for various radii—hence simple paraxial formulas can be used without concern for serious error. The derivation of this formula is based on an approximation—this is important in understanding the limitations of keratometry. Figure 6.14 illustrates the basics of keratometer optics using two-ray construction. The size of the virtual image can be found by using the relationship of similar triangles:

$$\frac{h}{h'} = \frac{f'}{x} = \frac{r/2}{x}$$

To simplify matters, the object (mire) is considered to be sufficiently far from the cornea that the virtual image is formed very near the focal point of the cornea.

Thus the distance from the mire to the focal point is very slightly different from the actual distance, d, between the mire and its image. Hence:

$$r \cong \frac{2dh'}{h}$$

The mires in the Bausch & Lomb instrument are shaped like plus and minus signs. The distance between the two plus mires represents the size of the object in the horizontal meridian while the two minus mires perform the same function for the vertical meridian. This distance is typically 64 mm. The distance from the mires to the cornea (when properly focused) is 75 mm (3 in). The circle included in the mire target is for the purpose of showing any surface irregularities or asphericity (Figure 6.15). Figure 6.16 is a cut-away drawing of the Bausch & Lomb Keratometer.

Current instruments of either the Helmholtz "variable doubling" (Bausch & Lomb Keratometer) or the Javal "fixed doubling" (Haag–Streit) type are so calibrated as to read directly the central corneal radius (in millimeters) or in diopters. This latter figure is derived through incorporation of a deliberately chosen low value for the refractive index of the cornea (1.3375) as well as an arbitrary value for the corneal back surface power—typically −5.85 D. Thus the net power of the central cornea is read out. However, the numbers obtained are really global values for the portion of the central cornea, ranging from 3.8 to 4.2 mm, and only the periphery of those areas at that. The entire center, where presumably the important part of refraction is going on, is missed. As to the peripheral cornea, the area beyond that 4.2 mm (92% of the corneal surface), out there in *terra incognita*, there, it can truly be said: "there be dragons."

Keratometry has several good points in its favor: it is easy to do; and it is a familiar methodology—beyond that it is a rubber yardstick. The measurements made with an ophthalmometer are confined to a very limited, paracentral portion of the cornea and have no relationship whatever to the rest of the cornea. Despite attempts to do so, it is not feasible to use this method for determining the curvature of the peripheral cornea (Figure 6.17). The only portions of the cornea actually measured are four in number: two vertical and two horizontal. Depending upon the design of the instrument, the mires used for this measurement are separated by a distance ranging from 3.1 (Bausch & Lomb) to 2.6 (AO) mm. Thus a spherical area having a width of at least 3.0 mm can be accurately measured. This can be verified by examining calibrated steel balls of varying radius of curvature. The degree of accuracy on such surfaces is very high indeed, probably on the order of 0.25 D or less. It is assumed, therefore, that the same accuracy can be translated to measurements

(a)

20 cm   20 cm

(b)

10 cm

(c)

11 cm

(d)

11 cm

(e)

10 cm

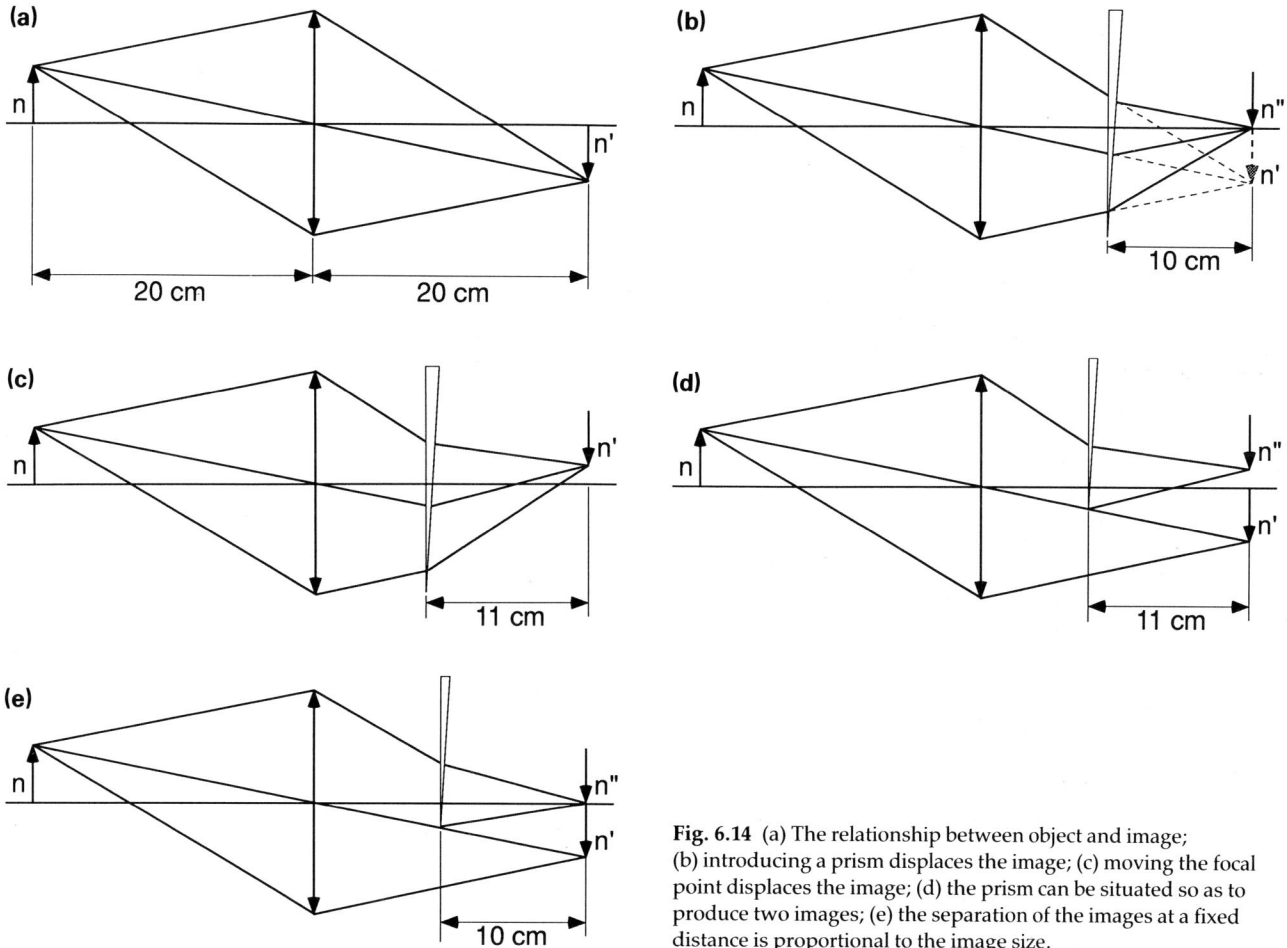

Fig. 6.14 (a) The relationship between object and image; (b) introducing a prism displaces the image; (c) moving the focal point displaces the image; (d) the prism can be situated so as to produce two images; (e) the separation of the images at a fixed distance is proportional to the image size.

of the corneal surface. Since the corneal curvature is, except in rare instances, nowhere constant, that assumption is in vain and has led to many false premises.

Photokeratoscopy

There are several technologies that might be used for the determination of corneal topography. Most current methods of topographic analysis are based on Placido's disk and Gullstrand's keratoscopic method [35]. Illuminated rings are placed in front of the eye and are reflected by the corneal surface (Figure 6.18). The position, shape, size, and spacing of the rings in the reflected image are determined by the corneal shape. This form of target has the advantage of having the same general symmetry as the cornea, guaranteeing that data points can be obtained along as many corneal meridians as desired. With reflection keratoscopes, like the Nidek PKS-1000 or the Kera Corneascope for example, a virtual image of the target is formed behind the corneal surface, and this virtual image is used in the reconstruction of corneal topography. Automated

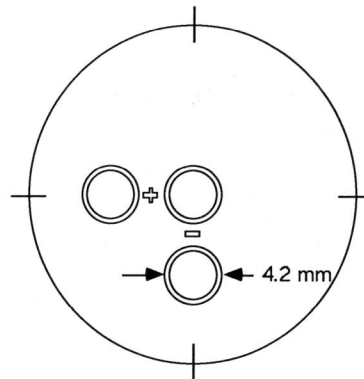

Fig. 6.15 Bausch & Lomb Keratometer mires.

photokeratography, as is used by the Corneal Modeling System (CMS) for example (Figures 6.19–6.21), is currently the most advanced technology in the field.

It is not easy (or accurate) to obtain readings sufficiently peripheral with standard keratometers nor do these instruments afford the physician any real appreciation of the corneal surface shape or topo-

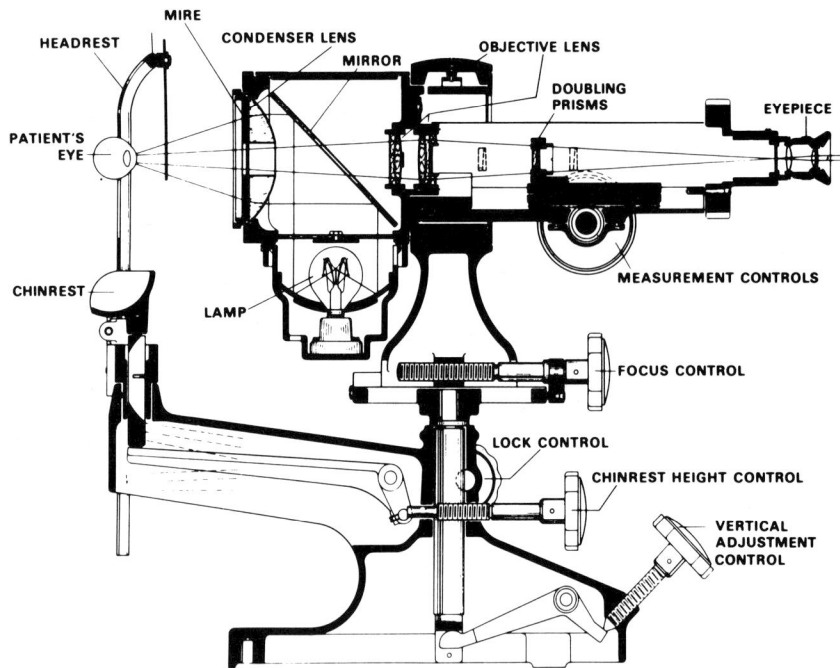

Fig. 6.16 Bausch & Lomb Keratometer.

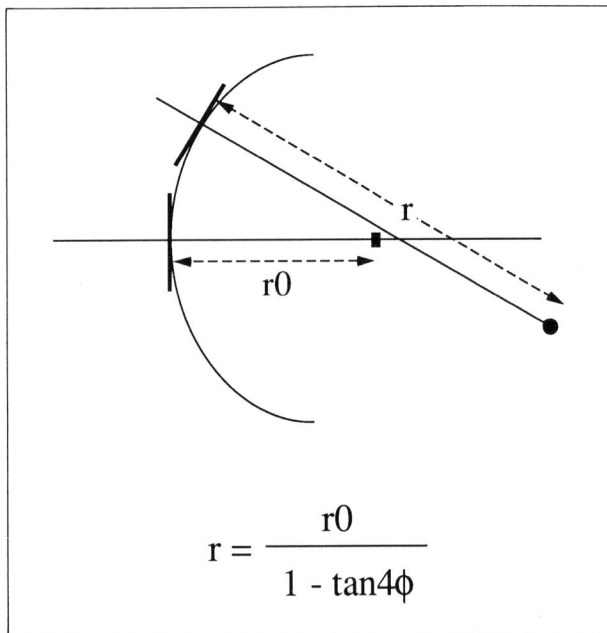

$$r = \frac{r0}{1 - \tan 4\phi}$$

Fig. 6.17 Berg's formula to calculate peripheral corneal curvature.

graphy. Furthermore, these devices are only accurate for spherical surfaces, and the human eye, most decidedly, is not spherical. It is said that Brewster, as early as 1827, suggested a practical means whereby this measurement might be accomplished [36]. Goode, in 1847, was the first to establish a method to do so

[37]. His attempts were further refined by Placido resulting in the well-known Placido's disk [38,39]. This device consists of a centrally perforated black disk upon which are painted evenly spaced, white concentric bands. When held in front of the patient's eye (while the physician looks through the hole at the reflected rings), the rings take on the shape of the cornea and reflect any aberrations thereon. If the cornea is spherical, the rings will appear round and concentric; if astigmatic, the rings will appear elliptic. The steeper the cornea in a given meridian, the closer the rings are to one another—although it takes an astute observer indeed to note all the subtleties. In fact, the instrument provides only a very crude approximation of the actual corneal distortion. Placido expanded on his original idea by devising a method of photographically recording the appearance of the rings. He was followed shortly by Javal and Schiøtz [21] and Nordensen [40]. It was Gullstrand, however, in 1896, who introduced quantitative photokeratoscopy to measure corneal contour (Figure 6.22).

Qualitative estimates of the regularity of corneal curvature can be obtained by using Placido's disk, and these can be pseudo-quantified by photographing the reflected image and measuring the distances between the concentric circles, much like one measures the distances between contour lines to determine altitudes on a topographic map. Gullstrand's original device has changed considerably over the years but still remains a useful device within its limitations (Figure 6.23).

The importance of measuring corneal contour has

(a)

(b)

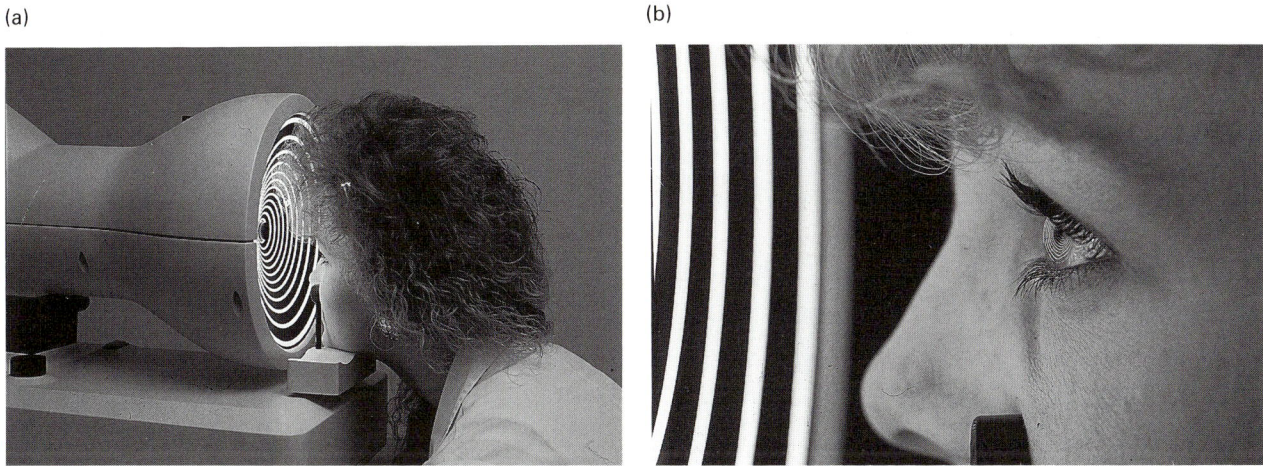

Fig. 6.18 (a) The Corneoscope; (b) note reflected rings on the subject's cornea.

(a)

(b)

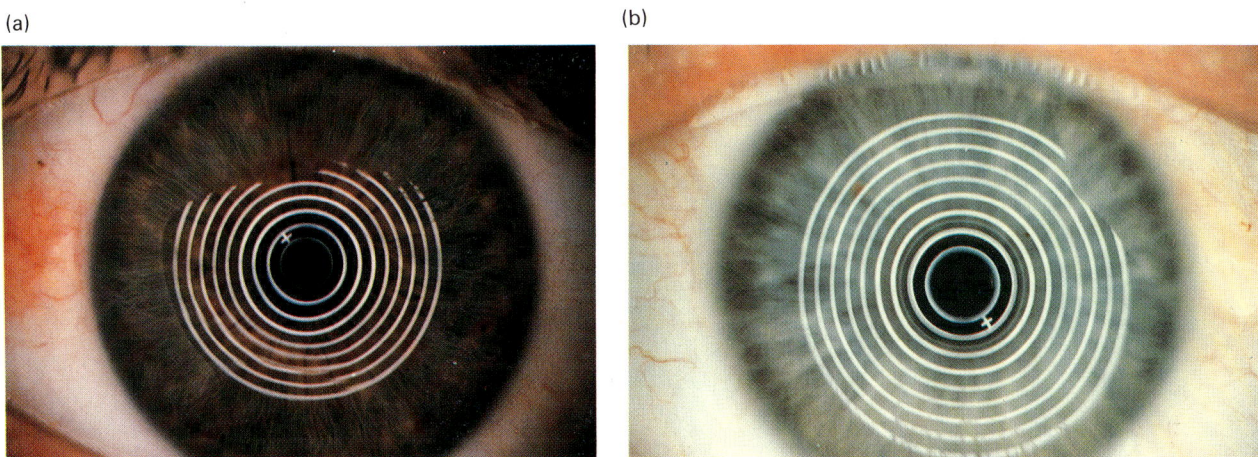

Fig. 6.19 (a) Characteristic nine-ring photokeratograph of a spherical cornea. (b) Subtle astigmatism exists on this corneal surface—against-the-rule at 15°. This cornea has low-grade keratoconus which is not demonstrated with this instrument (the patient can read 20/25 with low-power spectacles). Figure 6.20 taken with the CMS unit is more revealing. This is borne out by the color-coded surface map in Figure 6.21.

been discussed under keratometry and cannot be minimized. While the keratometer measures approximately the central 4.00 mm of the cornea (about 8% of the corneal surface), major changes in corneal shape after refractive surgery also occur in the paracentral and peripheral cornea. Measurement of the shape changes will give information about how the refractive surgical procedures work, will help document the stability of the cornea and will form a basis for future contact lens fitting, if needed. Thus these measurements must be precise.

Ophthalmometers measure an area from 2.5 to 3.5 mm in diameter around the visual axis. If the cornea was spherical, this measurement would be adequate. However, it is widely understood that the cornea is not spherical but is, rather, aspherical.

Various researchers have described it as paraboloid, ellipsoid, and conical. Regardless of which general shape one chooses to assign to it, the fact remains that up until recently the only accurate measurements of the cornea obtainable have been the sagittal height and the diameter. Between any three measurable points (Figure 6.24), the corneal surface can take any shape. It should be obvious that the keratometer cannot possibly measure such a surface.

The keratometer has a fixed focal distance between the apex of the cornea and its lens. The images of the mires are reflected off the cornea at a constant apical depth of 0.30 mm (Figure 6.25). The distance between the two reflected images is compared to the same images reflected off spheres of known radius of curvature (Figure 6.26). Since this measurement is only

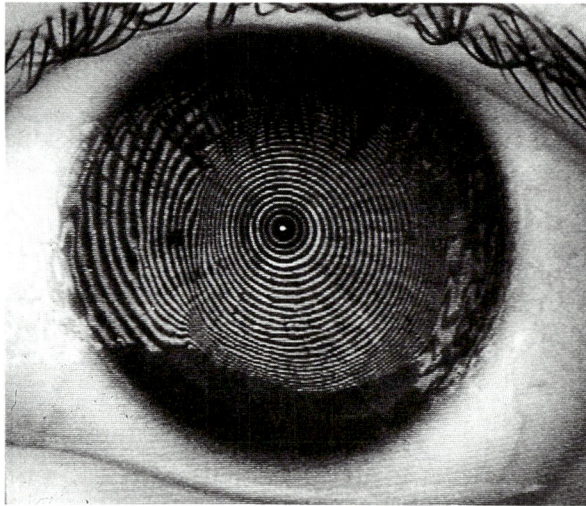

Fig. 6.20 CMS videokeratograph. (Courtesy of Computerized Anatomy.)

made in the center, K-readings give no information in the paracentral, mid peripheral or peripheral regions. A photokeratoscope attempts to solve this problem by producing successive mires which take the chord length at increasing apical depth. In the case of the Corneometer, each ring represents an increasing apical depth of 0.1 mm. The first ring is at a depth of 0.2 mm, however, because of the need to provide space for the photographic element. The second ring is therefore at 0.3 mm, the third 0.4 mm, etc.

It would be helpful to have a photokeratoscope that measured the entire corneal surface, but the anatomy of the human face, with the corneal surface recessed behind the nasal and orbital bony protuberances, makes it all but impossible to get consistent ring reflections from the peripheral cornea. The photokeratoscope most commonly being used currently has 12 rings spaced 1 mm apart. The area of the cornea covered by the rings is inversely related to the corneal

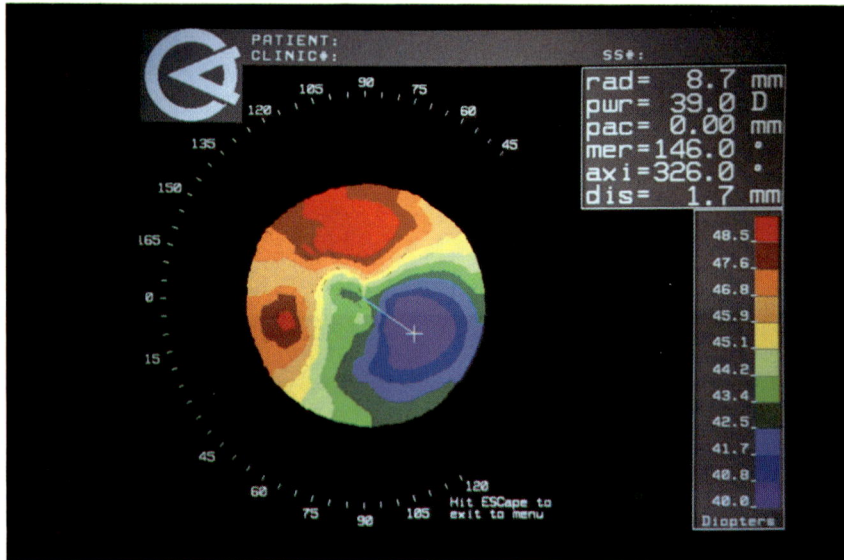

Fig. 6.21 CMS contour map of Figure 6.20. (Courtesy of Computerized Anatomy.)

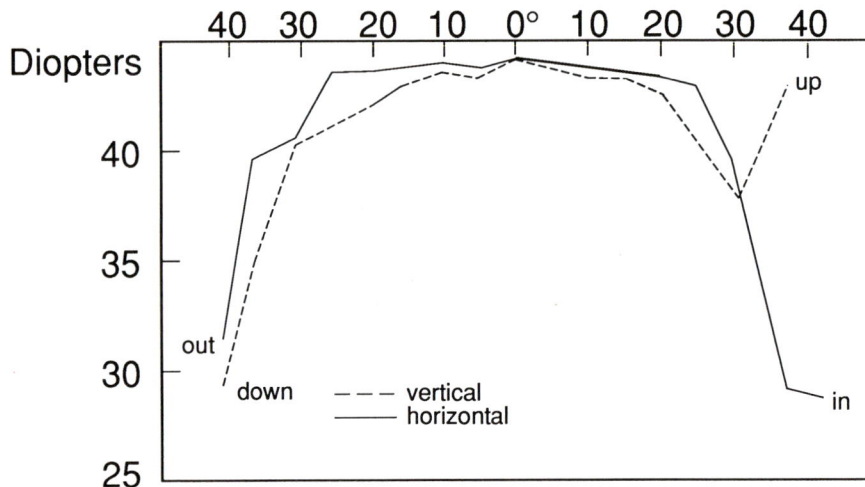

Fig. 6.22 Corneal curvature over 360° (from Gullstrand A. Photographisch-ophthalmometrische und klinishe Untersuchungen uber die Hornhautrefraktion. Kongl Svenska Vet Akad Handl 1896; 28.

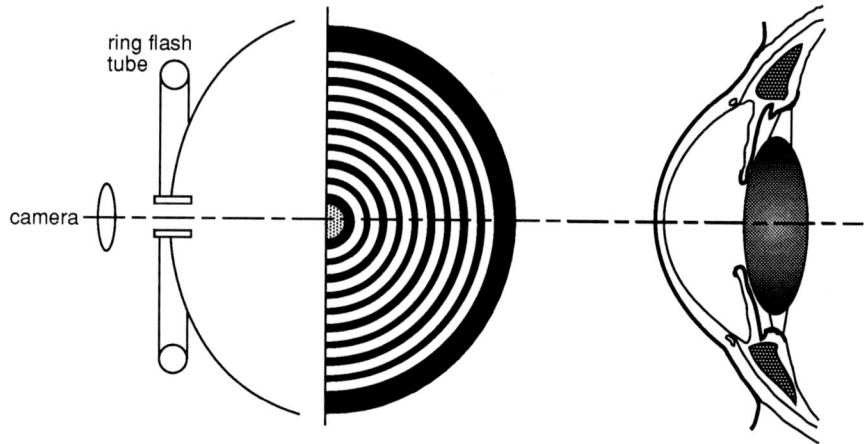

Fig. 6.23 Scheme of a typical modern photokeratoscope.

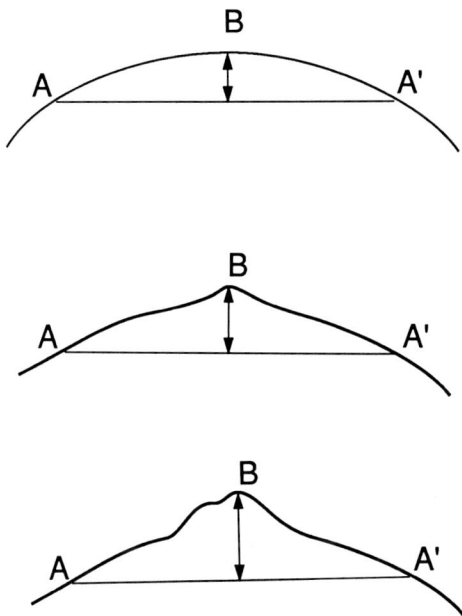

Fig. 6.24 Inherent weakness in the photokeratoscope.

power. On a 40.00 D cornea, the ninth ring has a chord length of 8.3 mm, while on a 50.00 D cornea, the ninth ring has a chord length of 6.7 mm. Using these nine rings, the Corneoscope measures the curvature of approximately 55% of the corneal surface. Twelve rings extend the range only a little more. Automated reflection keratography, as is used by the CMS, for example, using 32 rings, is currently the most advanced of this type of technology in the field.

Figure 6.27 illustrates the appearance of spherical and astigmatic corneas imaged with a nine-ring photokeratoscope. Note that the dioptric power of the cornea at any point along a ring is determined by measuring the distance from the center of the image to the middle of the ring. This becomes a problem when astigmatism is involved. The problem of imaging the cornea with this instrument is compounded by keratoconus.

Figure 6.28 shows a fairly regular form of keratoconus. Because of the limits in resolution of this type of instrument, much of the information about the cone

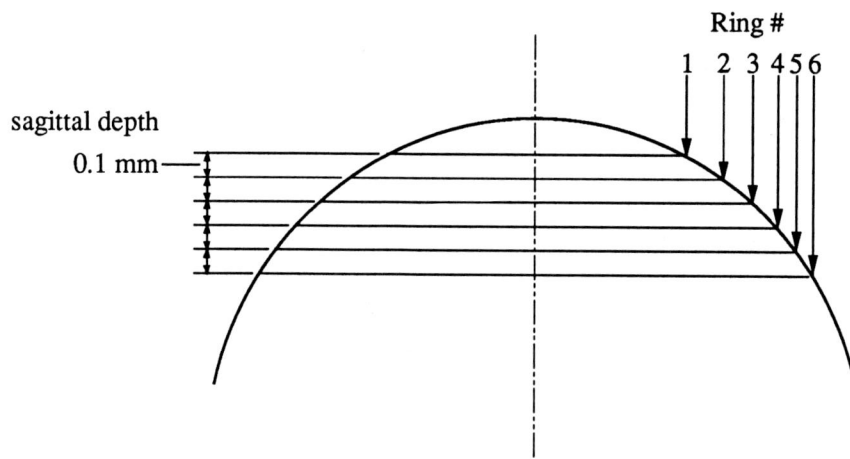

Fig. 6.25 Each ring (mire) in the photokeratoscope has a fixed sagittal depth, much like a keratoscope.

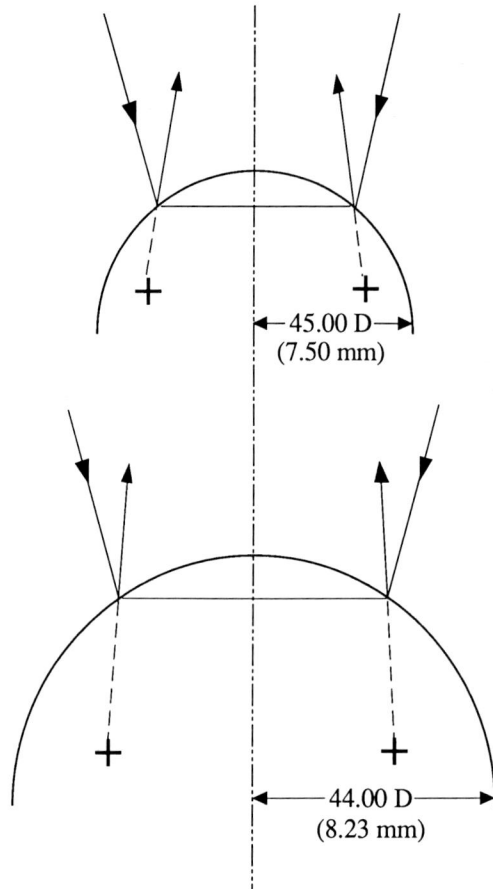

Fig. 6.26 The sagittal depth of the mires is kept constant in the keratometer.

is lost. Some increase in accuracy is obtained by using more rings. However, with present technology, the Placido's disk-type instruments have inherent limitations due not only (as noted before) to the structure of the human face and orbit but also to the increased aberration of the image as the disk becomes larger and the limits set by a Petzval's surface are exceeded. Special curved film holders (as in a Schmidt camera) have been tried but found wanting. The following illustrations demonstrate the effect of a larger number of rings on the same eyes shown previously.

The almost moiré pattern established by the rings gives a more three-dimensional appearance to the contour maps of the corneas in Figures 6.29 and 6.30.

There are only 19 rings producing this image. The Topcon unit uses 25, the CMS 32. Even with that number, the best resolution is still only about 0.5 D.

Neither the keratometer nor the photokeratoscope provides an accurate or complete measurement of the entire corneal surface. In addition, neither of these methods can determine the curvature of the inner surface of the cornea. The keratometer provides an averaged radius of curvature pericentrally and cannot be used with confidence peripherally or off-axis, even if fitted with a Soper topogonometer. The typical photokeratoscope ignores the critical central area entirely and cannot measure the peripheral 30% of the cornea. Despite the 1.0 mm ring spacing, the maximum measurement accuracy of this device is about 0.5 D in center with accuracy falling off rapidly toward the periphery. Another shortcoming of these types of instruments is in not providing a corneal profile measurement. Despite these inherent limitations, however, these devices still provide a qualitative view of the corneal surface which is not obtainable in any other way.

The CMS unit overcomes some of the difficulties with this type of imaging by utilizing monochromatic laser light. However, the problems of such optical imaging remain, even though that unit can measure all but the central 2.0 mm and the peripheral 11%.

Generally, keratoscope photographs (keratographs) have been interpreted by visual inspection of the mires [41]. With keratoscopy it is possible to detect and diagnose many forms of corneal distortion, and relatively inexpensive hand-held keratoscopes can be used intra-operatively to correct gross amounts of astigmatism. However, direct reading or visual inspection of keratographs takes a great deal of training, and even seasoned topography experts cannot detect low-amplitude or complex corneal surface distortions. Help in the form of computer transformation of the keratographs to amplify corneal distortions can be used to overcome this deficiency.

Acquisition of the corneal image

Before a three-dimensional reconstruction of the corneal surface can occur, the image must be translated from observation space into some sort of storage medium. This can take the form of a photograph (keratograph) or a video frame in computer memory. Reproducibility has been a problem with methods utilizing photographs because of the film and paper's dimensional instability. Analog video cameras built with the old-style vidicon vacuum tube detector also introduce errors because they are inherently unstable. Therefore, digital video cameras that capture their image on a semiconductor light-sensing array have been a tremendous boon to image processing because dimensional stability is guaranteed by both fixed optics and sensor.

Once the image has been captured, the next step is the digitization of the image, either manually or automatically. The LSU Corneal Topography System, for example, uses manual digitization of a photographic enlargement of the Nidek PKS-1000 photokeratoscope image [11]. Although considerable care is

(a)

Diopters = $\dfrac{2D}{f}$ (**f** = ring conversion factor)

(b)

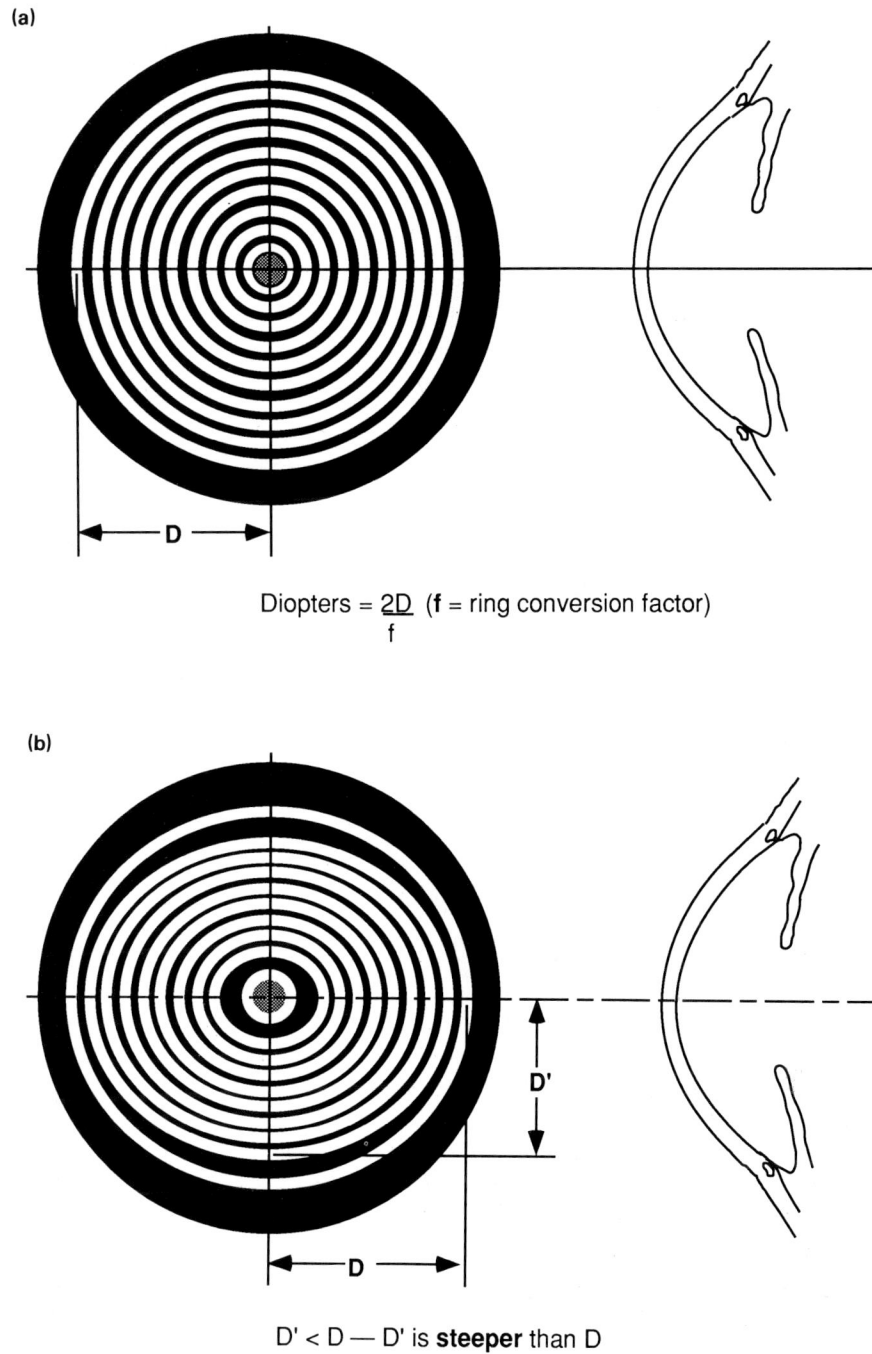

Fig. 6.27 Corneal contour map.
(a) Spherical cornea (nine-ring
instrument); (b) astigmatic cornea
(nine-ring instrument).

D' < D — D' is **steeper** than D

taken to insure accurate enlargement of the original, certain errors are inherent with dimensionally unstable photographic paper and the manual digitization process itself. Automatic densometric scanning of keratoscope photographs is used in the Kera Corporation Kerascan unit, but a limited number of semimeridians are analyzed [42]. Automatic digitization can also occur when an entire video image is digitized with a frame grabber, which permits the storage of one video frame at a time in computer memory. This is the method used by the rasterstereographic system, as well as the Computed Anatomy CMS, and the CLAS II unit [13,43,44]. The digital cameras used in these machines are able to convert images into a 512 by 512 array of numbers representing the intensity of light at corresponding points in the original image, and it is this array of pixel values which must be evaluated automatically by computer if the reconstruction of the corneal surface is also to occur automatically.

(a)

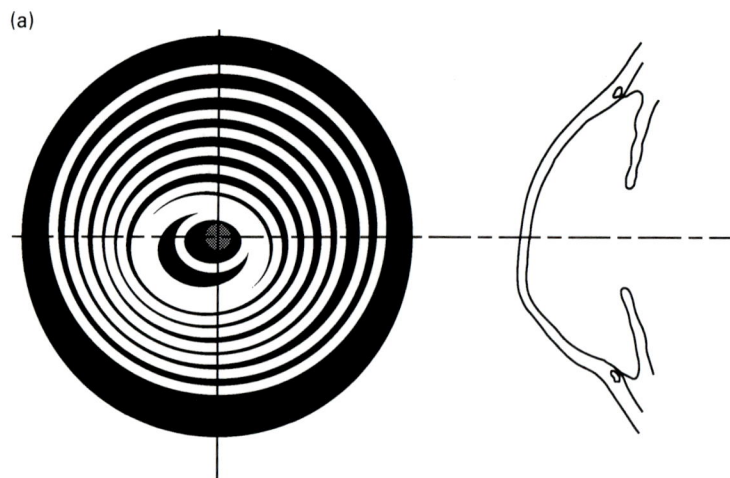

(b)

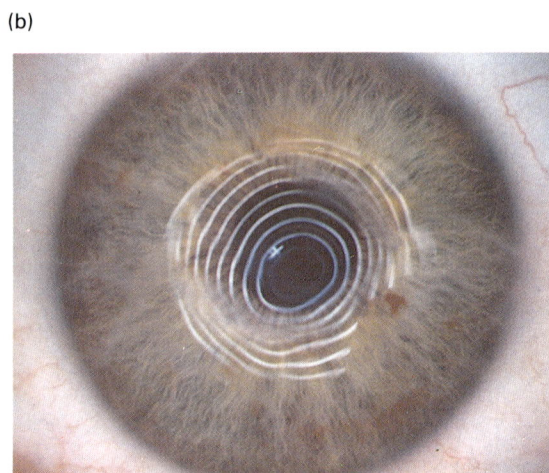

Fig. 6.28 (a) Corneal contour map—keratoconus (nine-ring instrument). This drawing is optimistic. (b) This photo demonstrates a more typical appearance of the distortion produced by an irregular corneal surface.

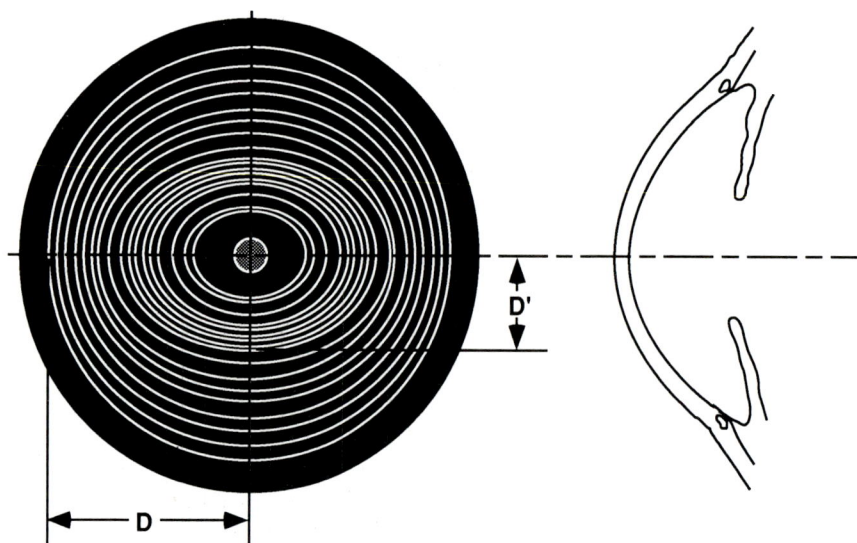

D' < D — D' is steeper than D

Fig. 6.29 Corneal contour map—astigmatic cornea (19-ring instrument).

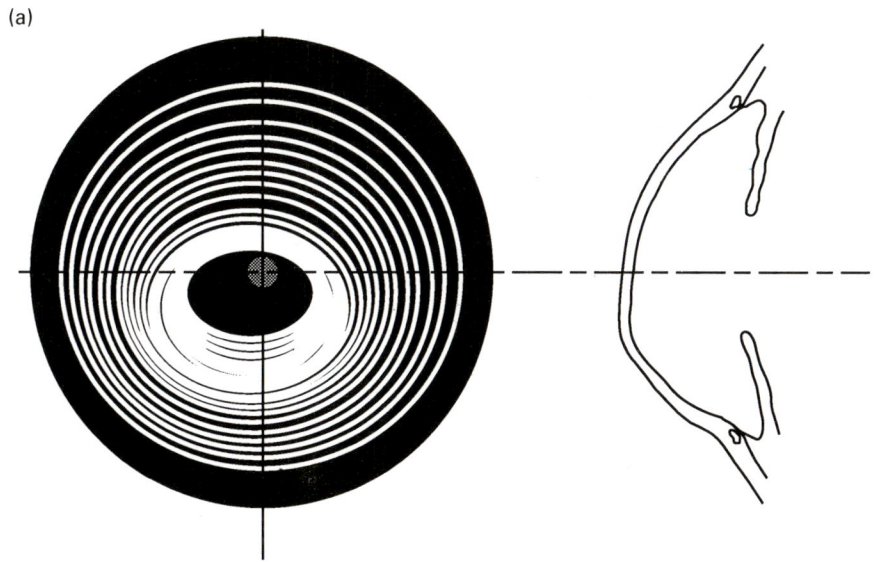

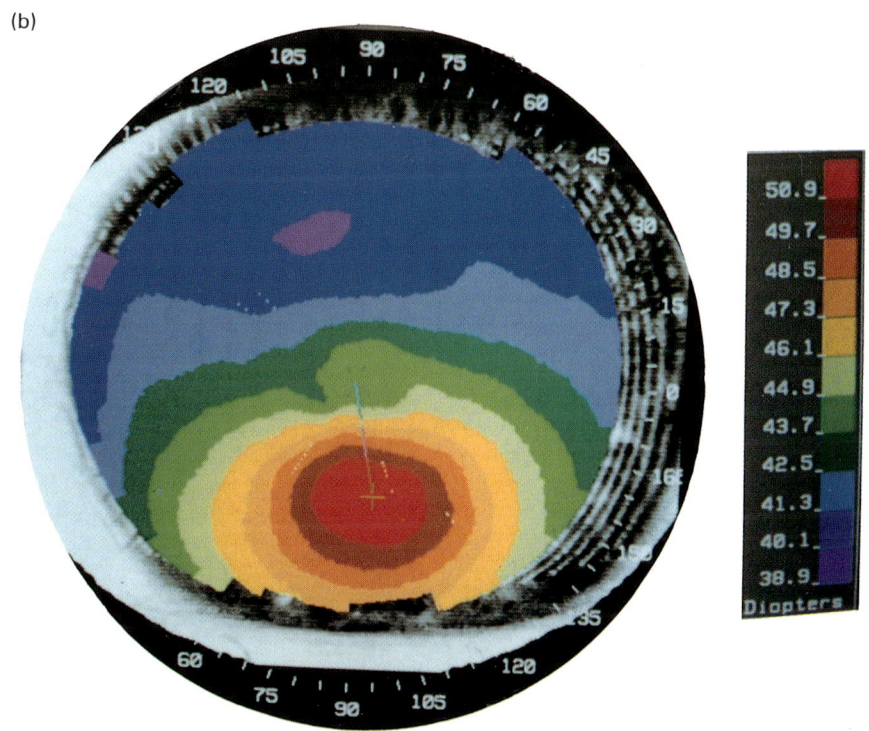

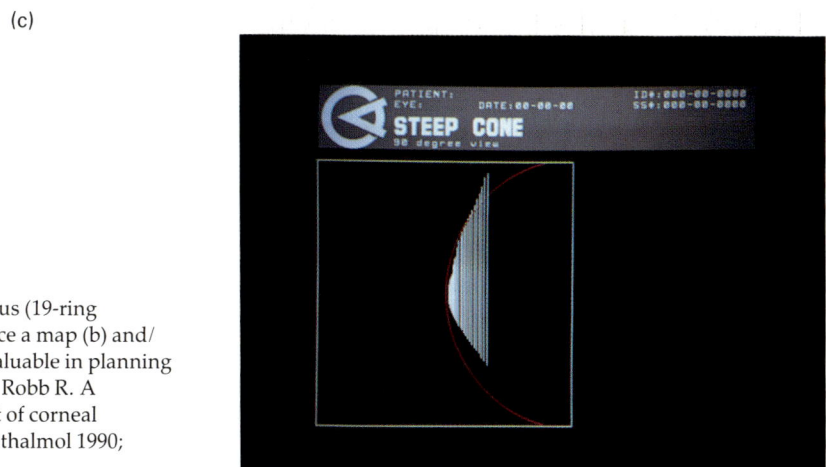

Fig. 6.30 (a) Corneal contour map—keratoconus (19-ring instrument). Computerized devices can produce a map (b) and/or a profile of the cone (c). Such maps can be valuable in planning surgery (from Camp J, Maguire L, Cameron B, Robb R. A computer model for the evaluation of the effect of corneal topography on optical performance. Am J Ophthalmol 1990; 109:379–386).

Corneal image feature extraction

With the image of the target projected on to the cornea stored in computer memory, the next task is to identify the positions of all of the projected target features, which in the case of keratographs involves finding the mires. This is the process of image feature extraction: with the LSU Corneal Topography System method the position of each of the 11 keratoscope mires is traced carefully with the digitizing pad. The mires are traced sequentially from the innermost to the outermost so that the program "knows" which set of mire image data is associated with which target mire. This is a tedious process and is prone to error.

With the rasterstereographic method, which projects a series of parallel vertical lines on the cornea, each row of the image is scanned from one side to the other in order to identify the position of each image line within the captured image. Basically, as an image is scanned from left to right, an optical density scan is obtained, with peak intensities corresponding to the presumptive position of the target image on the corneal surface. The object of the feature extraction algorithm for that methodology then becomes finding and storing the position of the brightest place in the scan, which corresponds to the assumed position of a given mire. Such positions found for 360° of all mires become the data that are used subsequently for surface reconstruction.

With the CMS, feature recognition and data capture can be thought to proceed in a fashion similar to that of the rasterstereographic method after the central fixation light in the image is automatically located. This estimated central position is used to convert the picture into polar coordinates, which has the effect of turning the nearly circular mires into nearly straight lines, which are then more easily identified and captured with image analysis technology. Some of this technology must be derived specifically for the field of corneal topography analysis to accommodate corneas with a broad range of distortions. Automatic computer recognition of image features is in its formative years—highly distorted patterns (e.g. from advanced keratoconus or from early post-operative keratoplasty) may not be correctly digitized. Hence, it is important, if not essential, that instruments that automatically identify target image features provide a means for the operator to check the accuracy of the process. The CMS, for example, displays the video image of the keratoscope frame and overlays each mire with the position determined by the computer programs; when grossly distorted corneas cause errors in identification of the mires, the analysis can be aborted. In any case, the net result is that the instrument contains the coordinates of all relevant features in the captured image for corneas that are analyzable.

The density and location of data obtained from images of the corneal surface determine the dimensions of the smallest features that can be revealed; in general the more points that are analyzed on the corneal surface, the closer they will be to each other, and the higher will be the transverse spatial resolution. For example, an instrument that collects data from several points on, for instance, eight semimeridians, would not provide enough transverse spatial resolution to depict the local circumferential corneal distortion in the vicinity of a radial keratotomy incision. There is a trade-off between the number of surface points analyzed and the speed of analysis. Obviously, a device that finds and uses 64 points on the corneal surface will calculate the data 128 times faster than a device (like the CMS) that uses 8192 points. For some applications, fewer points and faster speed may be appropriate. However, as faster computers have become available the corneal surgeon will soon be able to have the best of both worlds: high transverse resolution and real-time data acquisition and presentation.

Reconstruction of the corneal surface

So far we have covered the production and acquisition of data by corneal topography instrumentation and we have pointed out that these data, which are extracted from images, represent a translation of the actual shape of the cornea. In order to retrieve the three-dimensional original from this translation, equations unique to the optical principles employed by a given device must be derived. For the photokeratoscope class of instrument, several approaches and refinements have been reported [11,45,46]. However a major drawback to accurate corneal shape analysis by photokeratoscopy is that an exact solution is not possible from the data of the virtual image of the projected target (Figure 6.31). Hence, all of the solutions rely upon the adequacy of assumptions necessary to form a set of solvable equations. Wang et al. considered this problem and concluded that current algorithms used to reconstruct corneal topography from keratography analysis probably underestimate the magnitude of peripheral corneal asphericity such as occurs in radial keratotomy, for example [46]. The analysis of spherical calibration surfaces can be quite accurate with photokeratoscopy algorithms but few corneas requiring topographic analysis are spherical.

Despite improvements in depicting the corneal surface through photokeratoscopy, the fundamental deficiencies in that system remain. Mere ring patterns do not convey sufficient appreciation of the corneal surface shape nor do measurements of inconstant ring diameters provide an unequivocal measurement of corneal curvature. Digitization of the keratographs,

(a)

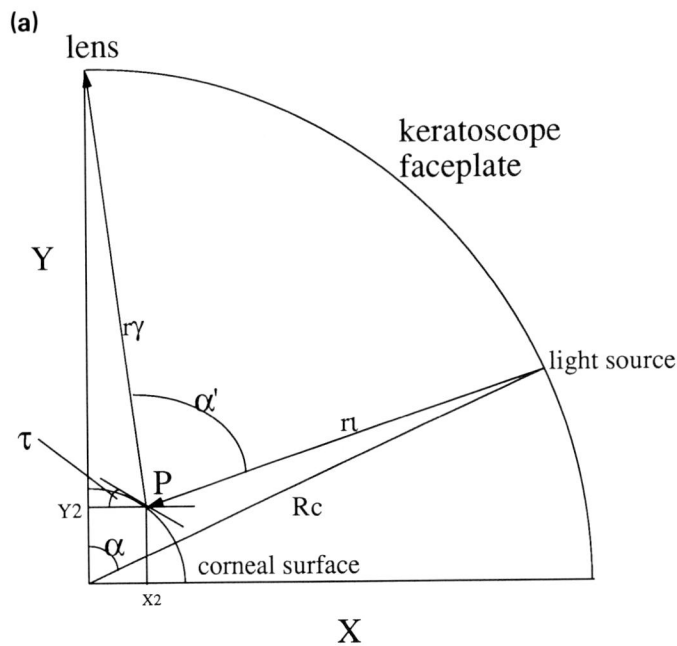

(b)

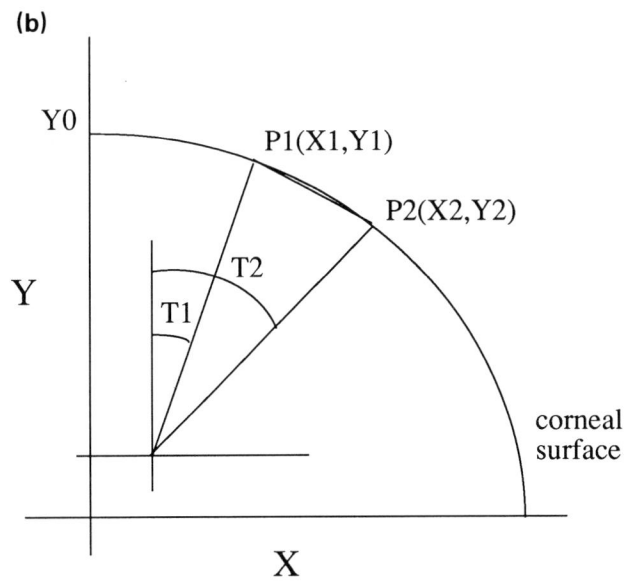

$$Y2 = Y1 - \frac{(X2 - Y2)(\cos(T1) - \cos(T2))}{\sin(T1) - \sin(T2)}$$

(c)

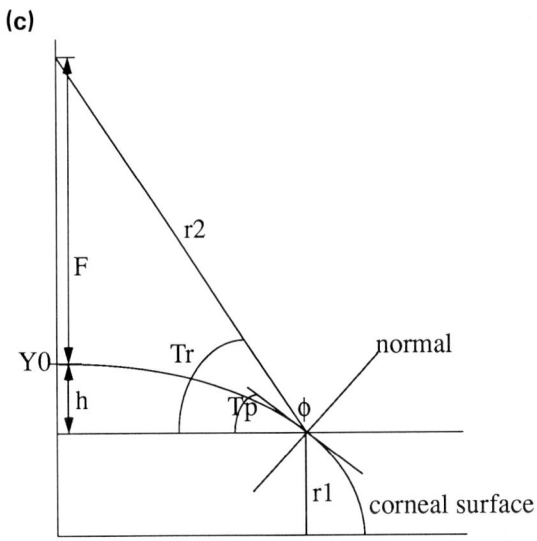

$$Tr = Tp + 90° - \sin^{-1}(1.338 \cdot \sin(Tp))$$

$$F = X2 \cdot \tan(Tr) - (Y0 - Y2)$$

Fig. 6.31 (a) General principle of establishing a datum point on the corneal surface; (b) local curvatures are established via approximation; (c) corneal Z-height is calculated from known slope angle.

either by hand or automatically through video capture with computer analysis using surface reconstruction algorithms, provides more information but no increase in accuracy. Moreover, the critical central portion and the elusive peripheral cornea remain unrecorded (Figure 6.32). Often portions of the surface are obscured by the nose, brow, or lids. Some devices employ dithering techniques to "fill in" the data gaps left by these obscurations. However, this dithering process is accomplished by making assumptions about these

gaps which may not be warranted. Moreover, since these devices depend on the reflective property of the corneal surface, any abnormality here reduces the quality of the image obtained. Epithelial defects, stromal ulcers, or scarring prevent or limit analysis. Highly irregular corneal surfaces can cause the reflected rings to run together, making it difficult or impossible to perform quantitative analysis (Figures 6.33 and 6.34). Recognizing the inherent problems in existing systems, attempts to resolve these difficulties

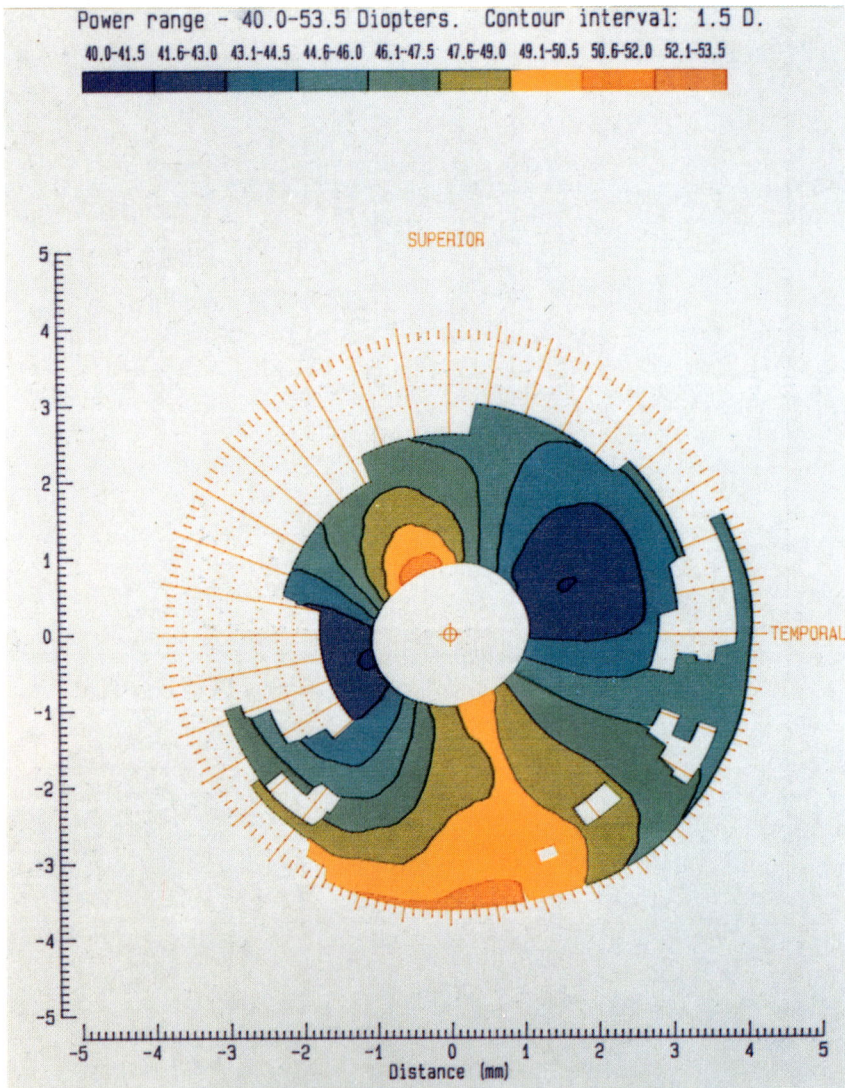

Power range - 40.0-53.5 Diopters. Contour interval: 1.5 D.

40.0-41.5 41.6-43.0 43.1-44.5 44.6-46.0 46.1-47.5 47.6-49.0 49.1-50.5 50.6-52.0 52.1-53.5

Fig. 6.32 A topographic map constructed from the LSU computer program. Note missing central data. (Courtesy of S. Klyce.)

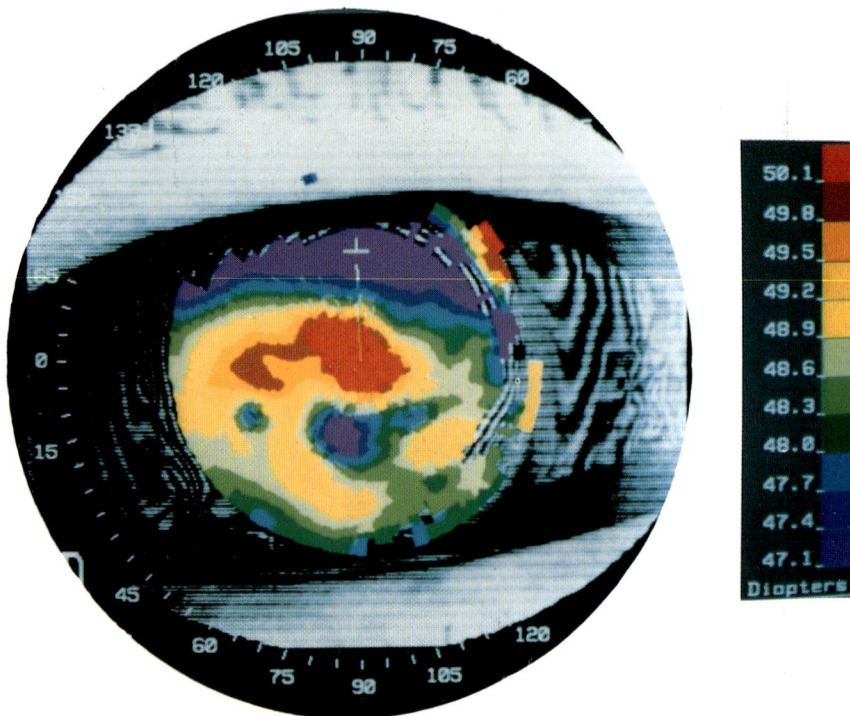

50.1
49.8
49.5
49.2
48.9
48.6
48.3
48.0
47.7
47.4
47.1
Diopters

Fig. 6.33 Contour map of a highly irregular surface from a CMS unit. Note the shape of the rings on the right. Measurements under these circumstances cannot be relied upon. As long as the surface being examined is smooth and regular, a Placido disk apparatus has no difficulty measuring the curvature changes. Surface irregularities, however, can be missed or may be unmeasurable. This fact destroys the utility of such systems in studying corneal shape post-operatively. (Courtesy of S. Klyce.)

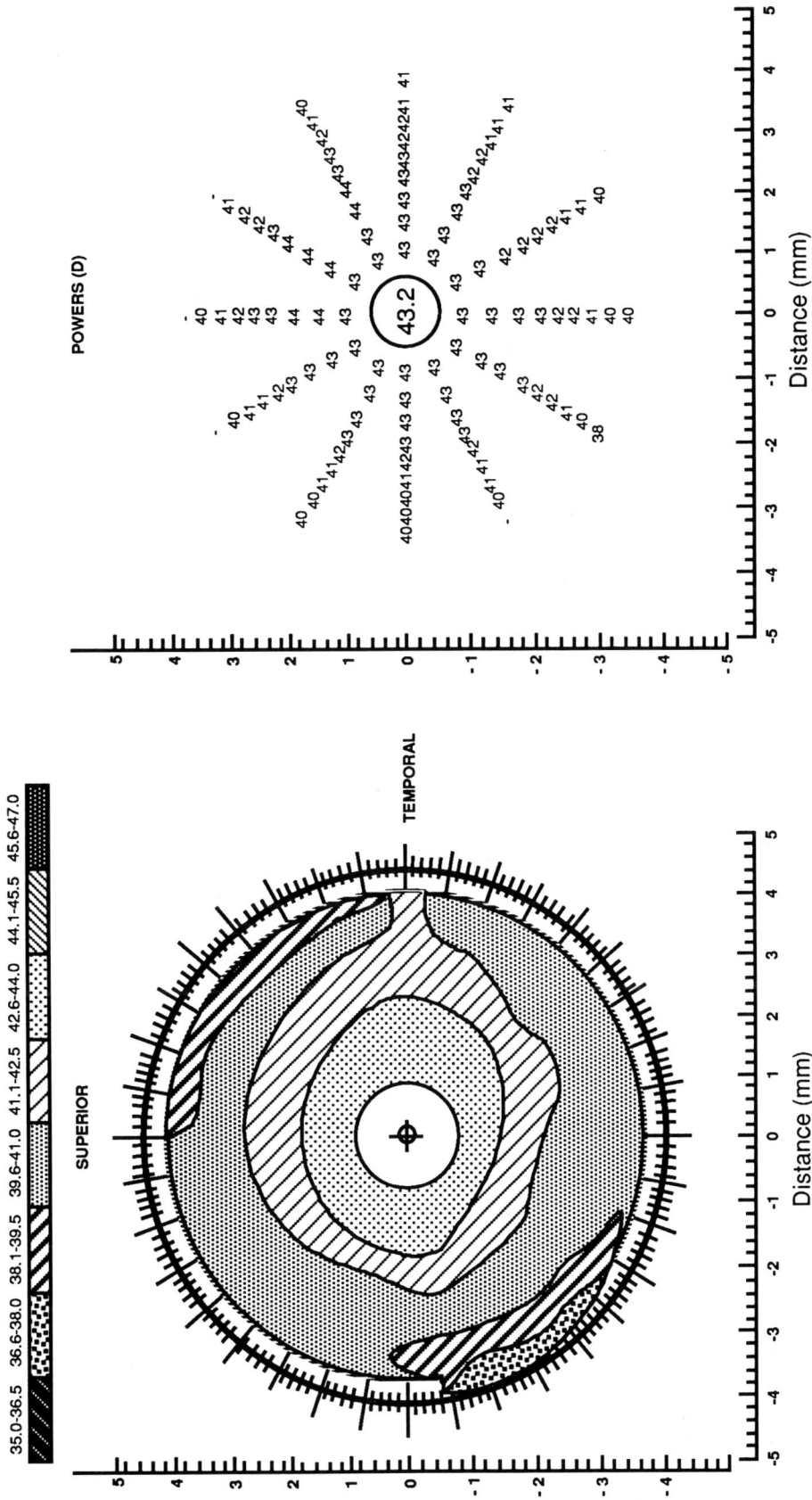

Fig. 6.34 Corneal map from conventional photokeratographic system.

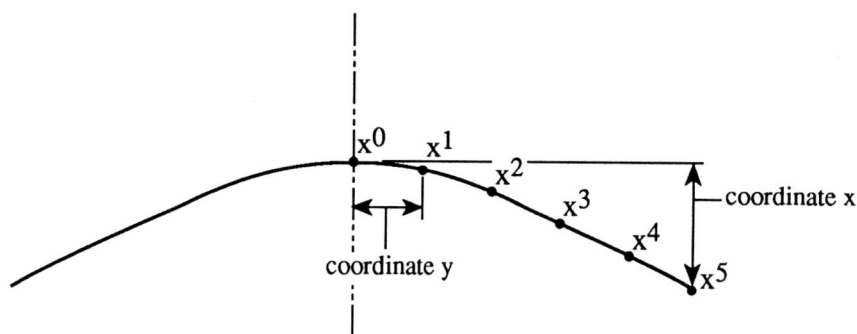

Fig. 6.35 Deriving the corneal curvature with the EyeSys system.

have been made through various other means, using the analysis of either the virtual or real image of a target projected on to the corneal surface such as in photo-contouring, rasterstereography, or by means of laser holography, or even ultrasound.

Photo-contouring

Principle of measurement

In this method of corneal analysis, the shape of the surface is dependent on the analysis of several points in a given region of the cornea. The position of these points is determined in reference to a plane tangent to the cornea and perpendicular to the optic axis of the reflected image. That is, any given point is located on this plane by its distance from the optic axis. This point is designated coordinate y in these calculations. The mathematical analysis seeks to determine the distance from the point on this plane to the reflective surface. We refer to this value as coordinate x. It is the collective values of x along a given meridian of interest that describe the shape of the reflective surface of the cornea (Figure 6.35). The apex of the cornea is located at $x = 0$ and $y = 0$. To compute corneal topography, it is essential to know the exact location of the set of object rings in space. This location is defined for each ring by its distance from the optic axis (called b) and the distance from the ring to a plane perpendicular to the optic axis through the apex (called a; Figure 6.36).

The points in object space from which the reflective image originates are formed on a cone-shaped headpiece positioned before the eye (Figure 6.37). Precisely placed on this cone are 22 transilluminated rings. The inner ring has a diameter on the cornea of 0.32 mm and the outer ring has a diameter greater than 10 mm depending on the shape of the cornea. It is important to note that the number of rings by itself has no real value. What is important to know is how many of the projected rings are really imaged, and, more importantly, with what accuracy these images are measured. The light from each of these rings is diffused in character so that some part of the emitted light

will reach the area of interest on the cornea—normal to that point.

The distance from these originating points to point 0,0 (value a), is determined by sensing devices within the apparatus and the computer. The cone is moved through commands from the computer by means of a precision stepping motor, which through a mechanical arrangement moves the entire object cone, thus changing the distance between the cone and the eye to a pre-selected value for a. Since the cone containing the object point must be centered on the optic axis of the cornea, this position is also monitored by sensing devices within the apparatus. The entire optical portion of the instrument is mounted on an $x-y$ table driven by precision stepping motors responding to commands generated by the computer. When the cone is in the proper position to satisfy the requirements of value a and is centered on the optic axis, the data are secured or "grabbed" in a few milliseconds. In the event that these automatic systems are ineffective for any reason, a manual "firing" sequence is provided. For this positioning operation to be successful, the computer and mechanical combination must be remarkably fast. The instrument is designed to be insensitive to normal saccadic movements of the eye but can be frustrated by nystagmus.

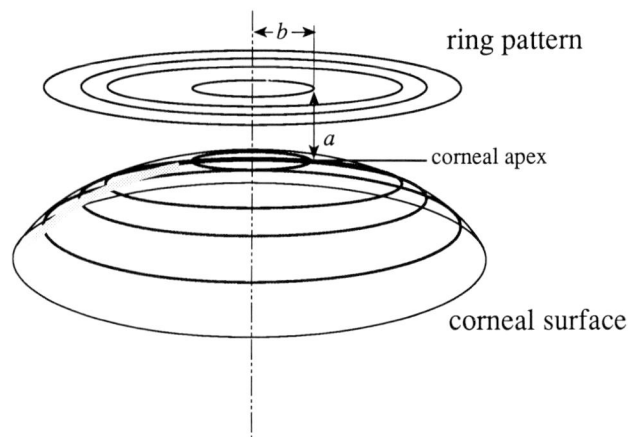

Fig. 6.36 Principle of the EyeSys photocontouring system.

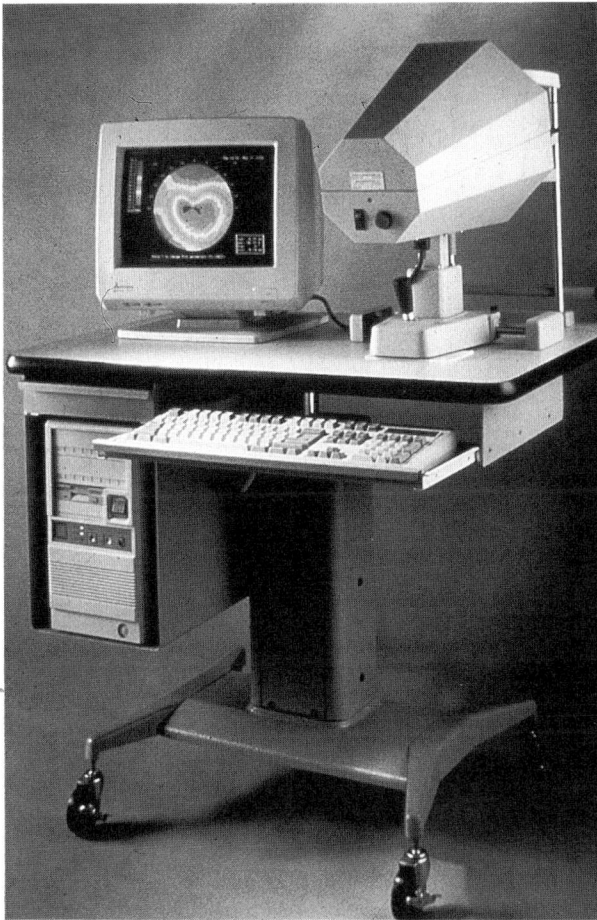

Fig. 6.37 The EyeSys system.

One of the unique optical elements of this instrument is the placement of the aperture. The stop of the objective is not near the principal plane, as is usually done, but in the back focal plane. The entrance pupil is therefore at infinity, and the chief rays reflected from the cornea are parallel to the optic axis. As it pertains to measurements of the cornea curvature this arrangement was first presented by El Hage in 1968 [47]. This arrangement has two important consequences. Normally, the aperture stop is placed at the objective so that the height (y) is not recorded directly and the angle that the chief ray forms with the optic axis is a factor in the analysis. In this instrument, y is obtained directly on the array of receptors. One advantage to this is that a slight error of focus will have negligible effect on the captured image height.

Typical measurements are done on 36 semimeridians and up to 360 semimeridians can be calculated if needed. Minimally more than 702 data points are calculated and used to describe the three-dimensional configuration of the cornea. An auto-positioning system is incorporated in the corneal topographer to improve repeatability of corneal measurements. Once

obtained, the data are fit to a high-order polynomial for each meridian. Then each datum is integrated to determine the three-dimensional configuration of the cornea along each meridian. If desired, this can be compared to a sphere for demonstration purposes. The time of the analysis is 21 seconds.

There are two functions, $a(y)$, and $b(y)$, which must be determined by the instrument. For each ring a and b, a ring image on the image receptor field is found so that the measurement gives a number of triples (a, b, y). When a and b are plotted as a function of y, two curves $a(y)$ and $b(y)$ are found, for which a polynomial interpolation within the accuracy of the measurement can give an analytic form. The two functions $a(y)$ and $b(y)$ result in a differential equation of the form:

$$x' = f(x, y)$$

Thus the instrument takes measurements only where the rings are (Figure 6.38). Since these rings are at least 1.0 mm apart and variable in number on the cornea, many areas of the cornea are not measured at all. This instrument suffers from the same restrictions as does any system employing reflected rings, although its algorithm does not need to cope with breaks in the rings, as does the CMS unit. However, it still relies upon approximations of the corneal surface which it obtains through three-point random triangulation. This method has merit in measuring large spherical surfaces but lacks the precision required for refractive surgery—small but important defects can be missed. Essentially it is a slightly more accurate keratometer and useful for contact lens fitting.

Rasterstereography

For the rasterstereographic approach to topography, a potentially more exact and efficiently calculated solution for the reconstruction of the cornea is available from the data captured [42]. This has such a great potential advantage to the various numeric solutions and approximations that have been offered for photokeratoscope analyses that additional comment is merited (see below). First, the accuracy of a given approach to measuring corneal topography is inherited from the specific methods used for imaging and reconstruction; for example, the reflection approach used in photokeratoscopy, which utilizes a virtual image, is more sensitive to corneal distortion than is the real image used by rasterstereography due to a phenomenon known as doubling. The position of the virtual image of the target reflected from the cornea is principally a function of the slope and the displacement of the cornea from the target, whereas the position of the real image is principally a function of the surface displacement alone.

Rasterstereography relies upon analysis of the real

(a)

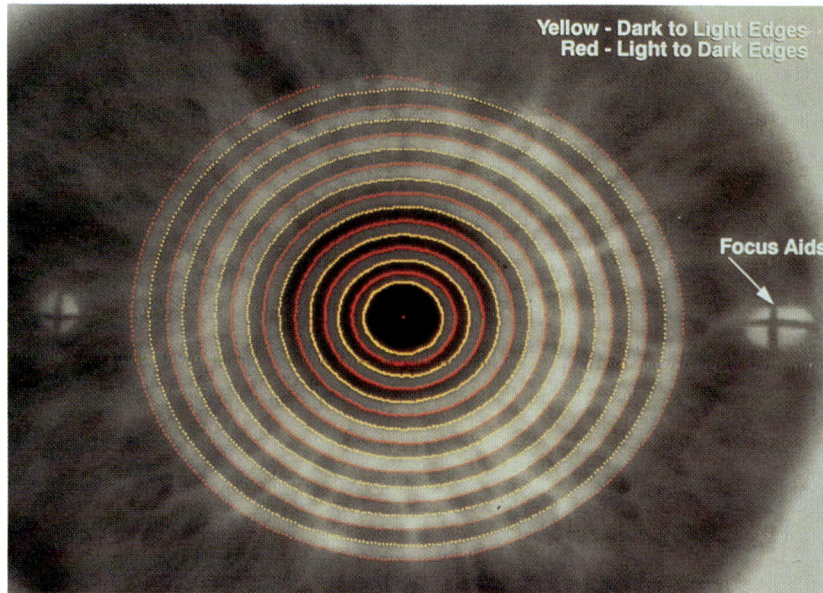

(b)

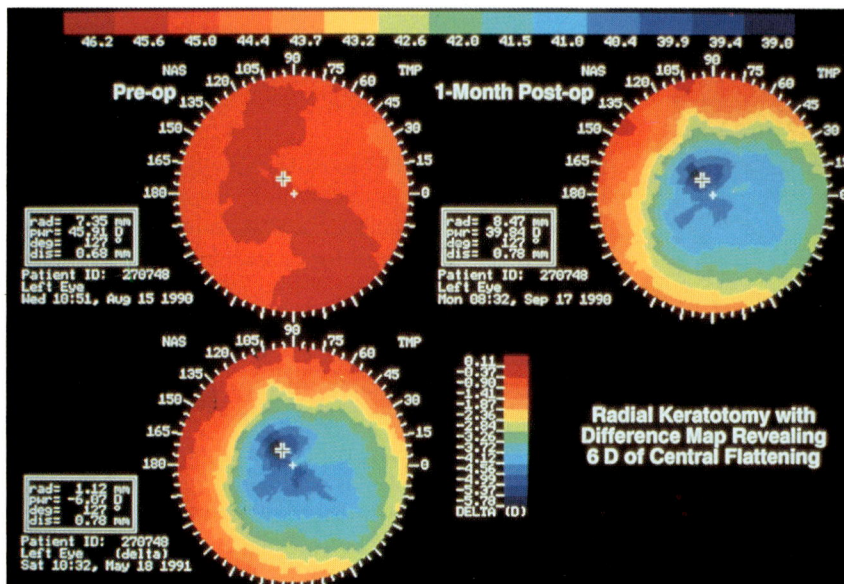

Fig. 6.38 (a) Ring pattern utilized in the EyeSys system; (b) types of topographic analyses available.

image of a target projected on to the corneal surface. This image is obtained by projecting a calibrated grid on to the fluorescein-stained tear film followed by computerized analysis [43,48]. The surface is then viewed at a pre-defined angle from the projection source, and the shape of the surface can be determined by its distortion of the projected grid. The geometry of this grid makes it possible to obtain a mesh of equally spaced data points on the corneal surface, in contrast to the circular keratoscope mires used in photokeratoscopy which provide data from corneal meridians that are equal angles apart. Typically one of the cameras of a stereo pair is replaced with a light source, which projects a grid outline on to the subject, and the other camera is used to obtain the image [49].

Rasterstereography has been used to assess spinal curvature, measure large body surfaces for reconstructive plastic surgery, size machine pads, and for depth perception in robotics [50]. This technique was adapted for corneal topography by Warnicki et al. [43]. Since a grid is projected on to the cornea surface instead of being reflected by it, a smooth intact epi-

(c)

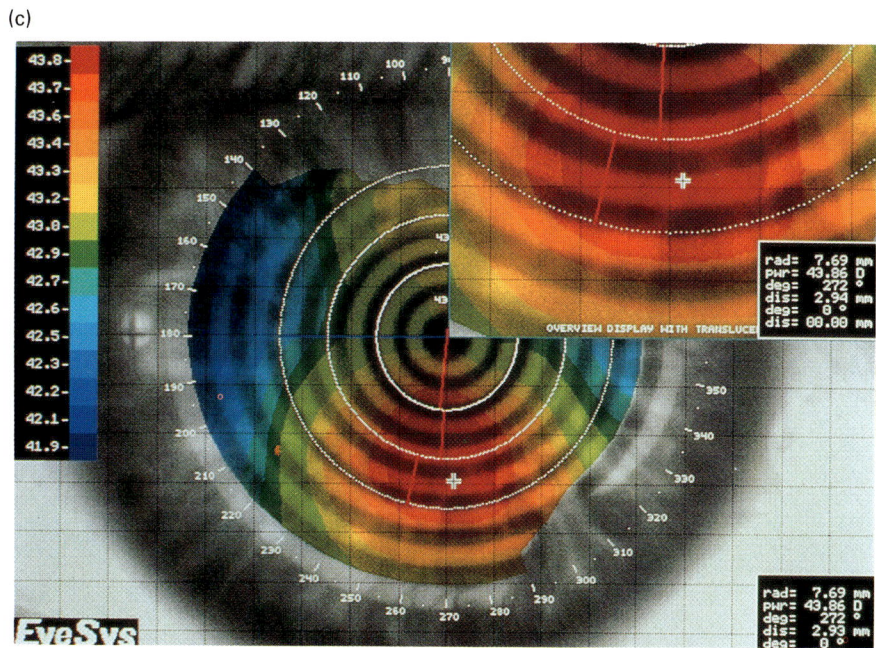

Fig. 6.38 *Continued.* (c) A nice feature of the system is the zoom mode. (Courtesy of EyeSys Laboratories.)

thelial surface is not required. Due to the narrow angle between the projection and viewing optics, shadowing is eliminated as well. Furthermore, the overall image is affected very little by highly irregular or steep corneas; small irregularities can still obscure portions of the mesh. The projected image can cover the entire cornea, including the central visual axis, far periphery and limbus, interpalpebral conjunctiva, and lid margins. The image is acquired electronically, then digitized and analyzed by a computer imaging system.

Image acquisition

A Zeiss stereophotographic slit-lamp has been adapted to acquire the corneal images (Figure 6.39). Two cine adaptors are mounted on to an accessory beam splitter: one adaptor for projection of the grid, and the other for a video camera to acquire the image. A coaxial illuminator/flash system projects through a grid mounted at the focal plane of the optical system. The grid of light is projected through the slit-lamp optics on to the corneal surface. Since a normal cornea is transparent, the projected grid· will not be visible unless a diffusing material is applied to the surface. Bonnett sprayed talcum powder on the cornea but, in the system herein described, sodium fluorescein is used [34]. A cobalt blue excitation filter is placed in the illuminating/flash pathway, making the corneal tear film fluoresce in a pattern corresponding to the grid, and a yellow barrier filter (Zeiss SB50) is placed in the viewing pathway. Previously a grid with vertical rulings was used. Recently this has been replaced with a grid with both horizontal and vertical rulings. This

improves the accuracy of measurements in the vertical meridians and helps stabilize any optical distortions which are present.

In obtaining the image, the patient is seated at the adapted slit-lamp, and fluorescein is instilled in the eye to be examined. If the fluorescein does not spread evenly over the cornea, due to tear film break-up, a fluorescein solution thickened with methylcellulose can be used. The patient looks at a fixation light on the slit-lamp, and the grid is focused on the cornea, using the slit-lamp optics. The magnification of the image can also be increased using the slit-lamp to allow more detailed examination of a localized area. The flash is fired, and the image is acquired by the black-and-white video camera.

Image processing

The image is sent from the video camera to the image processor, where it is digitized and stored. The image is displayed on a video monitor (Figure 6.40), where the operator can view it and determine whether the quality is acceptable. If it is not, the image is rejected, adjustments are made, and another image is acquired. The image processing system consists of a PC AT (MS-DOS) computer, containing a matrix-type imaging board. Operator commands can be given at the keyboard, or from a touch panel on the display screen. The position and spacing of the grid lines on the corneal image are determined by the corneal topography. The elevation of the corneal surface is calculated by comparing the horizontal and vertical positions of the grid lines projected on to the cornea

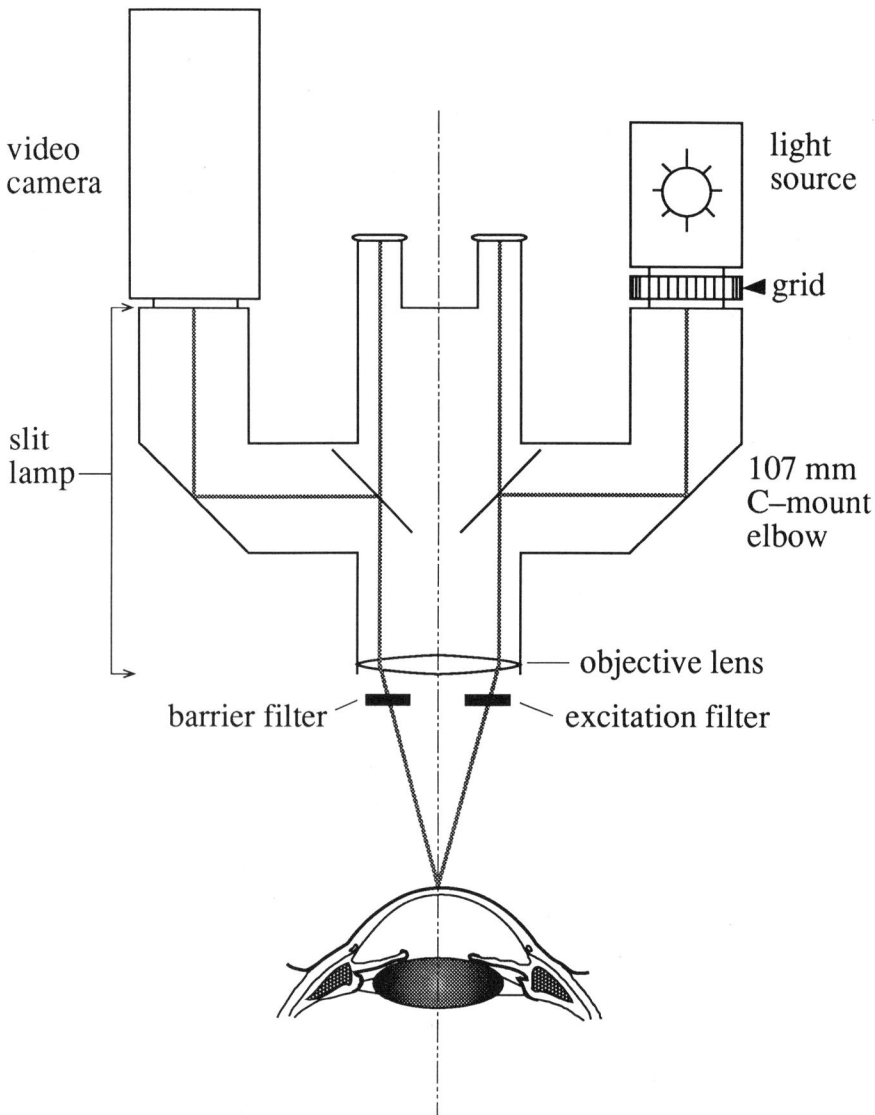

Fig. 6.39 Diagram of a rastersterographic system for measuring corneal surfaces.

with their positions when the grid is projected on to a flat plane. This requires that the computer recognize the lines, determine their center and position, and then calculate trigonometrically their displacement.

The image of the grid can vary greatly in contrast across the surface of the eye. To compensate for this the intensity is normalized across the entire image internally. The highest intensity point in each grid line is then determined, to mark the center of the line. This is done by finding the position of a sine wave which most closely matches the intensities across the grid line—this has a potential resolution greater than a single pixel, and in practice that resolution is not often obtained. The number of data points is determined by the number of grid lines, and the resolution of the video system. Approximately 3000 elevation points are currently used for analysis of the surface contour. The computer registers and displays the center points

along each grid line, in an overlay on the corneal image. It also reviews the quality of the grid points to determine the confidence of the image. The elevation of the corneal surface is then calculated at each of the center points, using the following formula:

$$\text{elevation} = \frac{\text{deviation of grid}}{\text{magnification ratio}}$$

$$= \frac{(\sin \alpha)(\cos \beta)}{\text{pixels/mm}}$$

where α = the angle between the projected grid and the viewing optics, β = half the angle of α, and the magnification ratio is the number of pixels per millimeter of the image.

The visual axis is determined by the position of the reflection of the fixation light. Since the obtained image is not coaxial with the fixation light (the light is in the

(a)

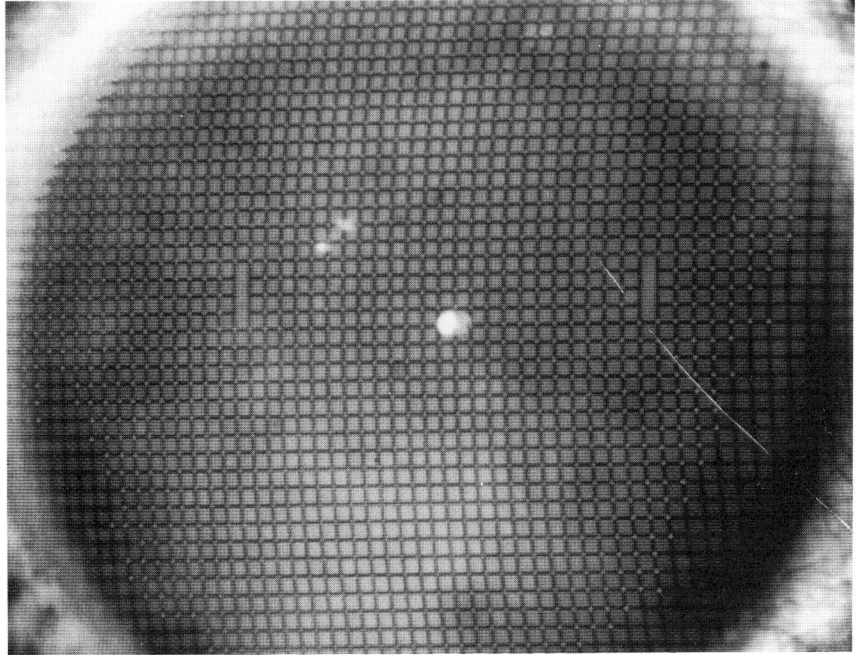

(b)

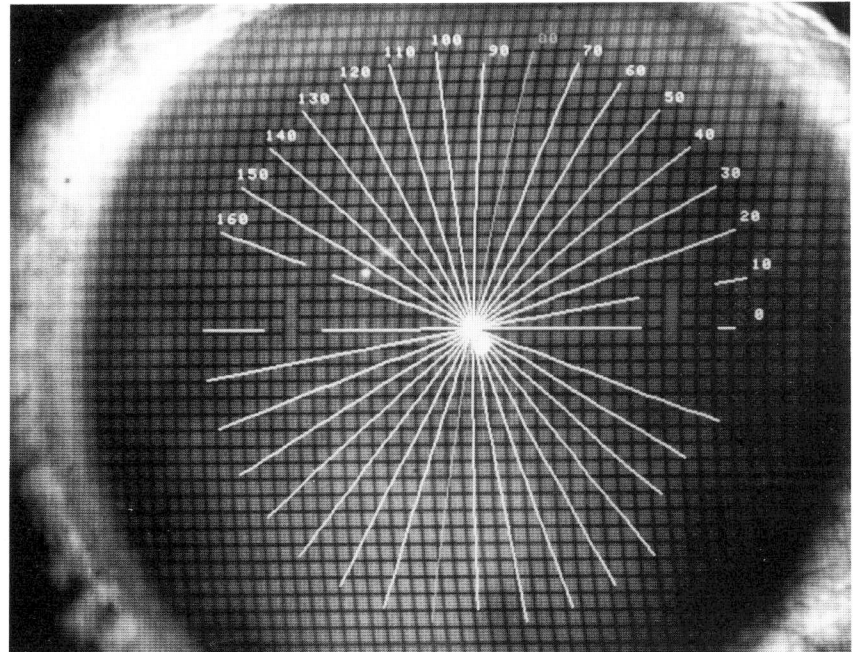

Fig. 6.40 (a) Projected grid on corneal surface; (b) vector plot of reflected grid. (Courtesy of J. Warnicki, Pittsburgh Eye and Ear Institute)

center, while the image is obtained from one of the elbows), the position of the reflection in the image is deviated from the visual axis. The amount of the deviation can be calculated, based on the curvature of the corneal surface and the angle between the fixation light and the camera. A two-dimensional matrix of the elevation points is created for each image. This matrix can then be used to create three-dimensional displays of the corneal surface, or be analyzed to determine

radius of curvature. Standard graphics-processing techniques are used to develop an orthogonal display, which can be rotated around the x or y axes [51]. The average curve of the cornea can be subtracted, to accentuate the deviations from sphericity, as described by Klyce [11]. Contour plots, based on elevation, can also be displayed (Figure 6.41). These appear like Placido disk images, but each color represents an area of equal elevation of the corneal surface, rather than

(a)

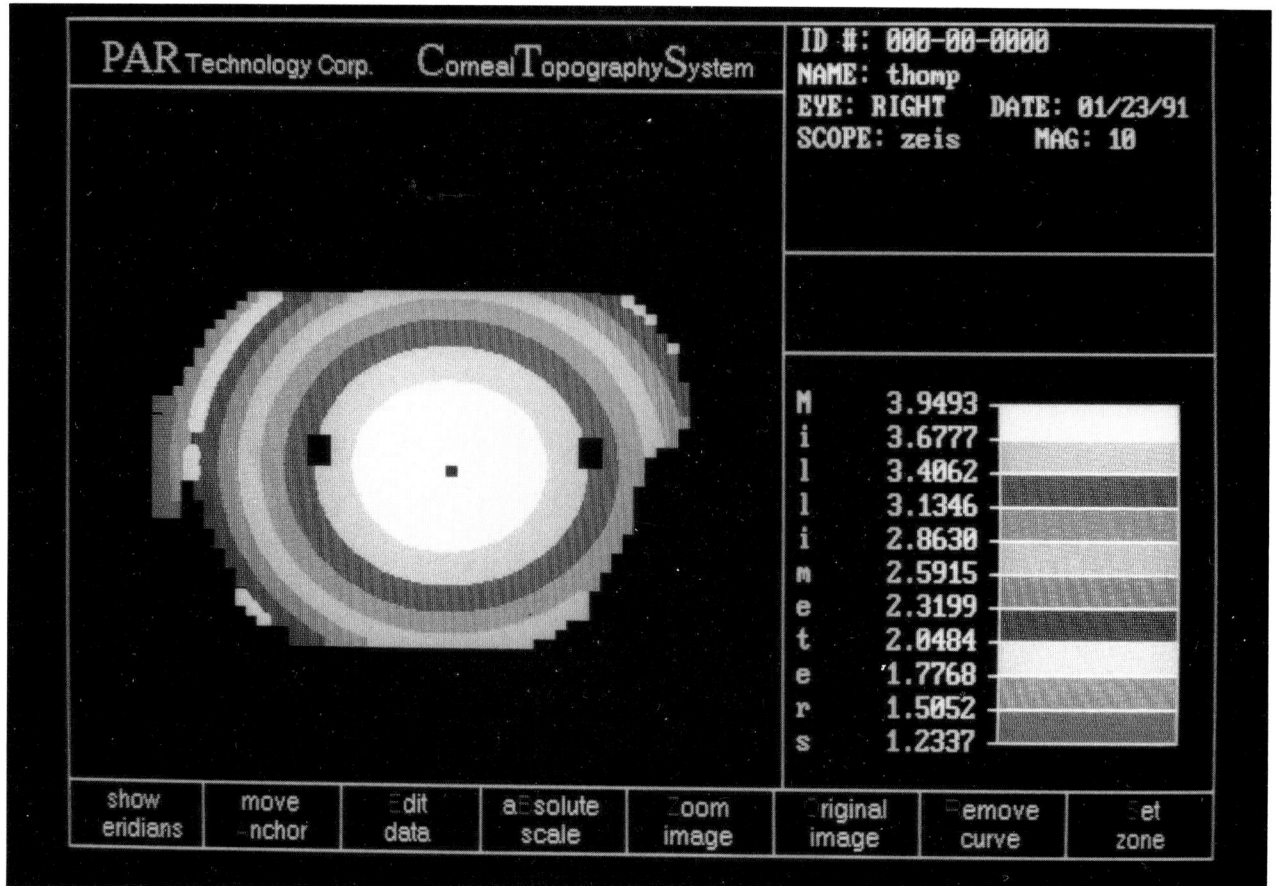

(b)

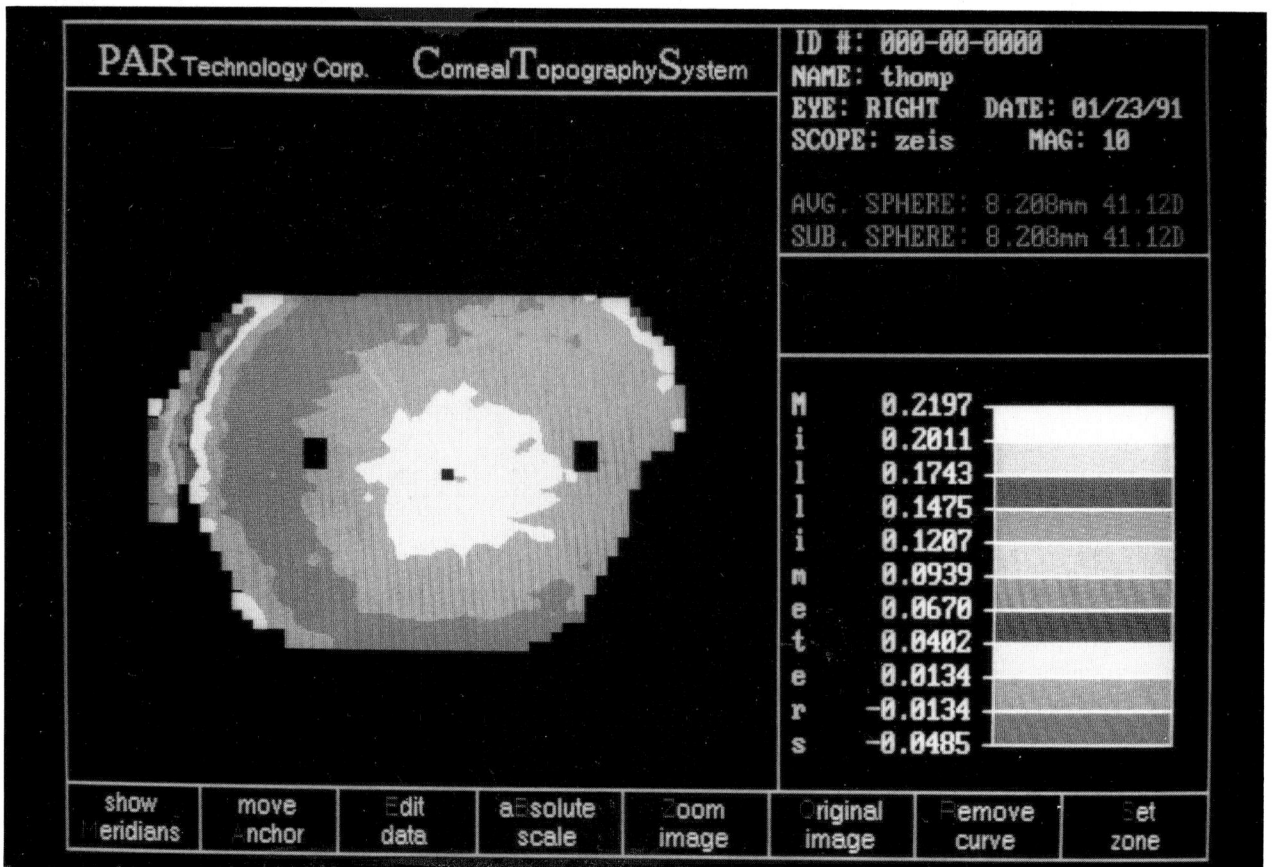

(c)

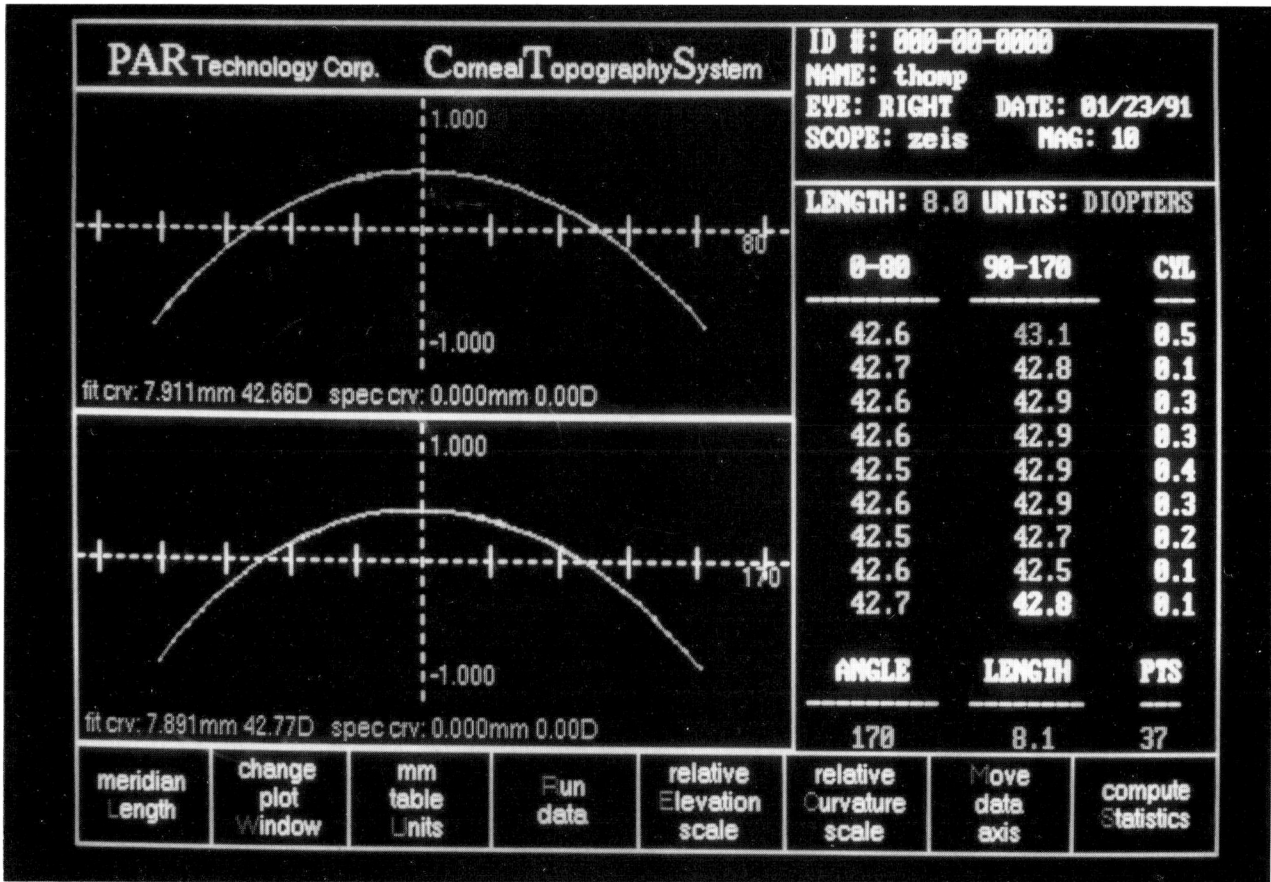

PAR Technology Corp. Corneal Topography System		

ID #: 000-00-0000
NAME: thomp
EYE: RIGHT   DATE: 01/23/91
SCOPE: zeis   MAG: 10

LENGTH: 8.0 UNITS: DIOPTERS

fit crv: 7.911mm 42.66D   spec crv: 0.000mm 0.00D

fit crv: 7.891mm 42.77D   spec crv: 0.000mm 0.00D

0-00	90-170	CYL
42.6	43.1	0.5
42.7	42.8	0.1
42.6	42.9	0.3
42.6	42.9	0.3
42.5	42.9	0.4
42.6	42.9	0.3
42.5	42.7	0.2
42.6	42.5	0.1
42.7	42.8	0.1

ANGLE	LENGTH	PTS
170	8.1	37

meridian Length	change plot Window	mm table Units	Run data	relative Elevation scale	relative Curvature scale	Move data axis	compute Statistics

Fig. 6.41 Contour map of a small cone. (a) Each ellipse represents elevations in millimeters referenced to primary focus on apex; (b) map of elevations and depressions related to reference sphere; (c) profiles of major and minor meridians. (Courtesy of J. Warnick.)

reflection of a single circle of light. Radius of curvature can be determined for any axis, and for any portion of the cornea in that axis. A problem of the corneal surface in the desired axis is displayed on the screen, and its curvature is determined using the simplex computer algorithm described by Caceci and Cacheris, which finds the radius of curvature which best fits the elevation data points [52]. The computer then displays this average curvature in an overlay on the corneal profile. Total processing time, between image acquisition and display of a contour plot, is approximately 75 seconds.

Accuracy

The accuracy of the elevation measurements depends on the magnification used. At 16×, which enables imaging of the entire cornea, the resolution of the elevation measurements is approximately 10 µm. At 40× magnification the resolution is approximately 4 µm. The accuracy depends on the number of points being used, so it varies with the length of the profile being measured. If the curvature is measured over 8 mm of a semimeridian, the accuracy is on the order of 0.11 D. However, if the curvature is calculated for only 5 mm of the semimeridian, the accuracy is reduced to 0.5 D—outside tolerable limits. Correlation of curvature measurements with this device has not yet been compared with images obtained by photokeratoscopy, or with ophthalmometry measurements.

Rasterstereography has seen its greatest value in large body imaging, where coarse measurements are tolerated. Despite its successful application in those areas this system may not have the accuracy necessary for the presentation of clinically significant corneal surface distortions. It has been said that this system does not depend upon reflection, thus irregularities of the cornea are easily measured. However, it does depend upon floating a dye on the corneal surface. While fluorescein will stain an area where epithelium is missing, the fluorescein–tear surface will be broken up and considerably distorted, both in tear film deficiencies and also in highly irregular and distorted corneas, where the dye will flow off and away from elevated areas. Thus gaps will appear within the grid. The accuracy is said to be as fine as 4 μm but this depends upon discriminating each pixel in the array. While there are edge-detection algorithms capable of detecting extremely low brightness levels, these depend upon high-density arrays as well. The brightness of the flourescein image is low and while it can be detected with a sensitive video camera, digitization of the image will inevitably result in some pixel drop-out with the current image-capturing boards commonly available. This fact coupled with the inevitable grid gaps will lower the resolution considerably. Still the potential accuracy of such a system exceeds that of photokeratography.

Holography

The use of a coherent and monochromatic light source (i.e. a laser) has extended the usefulness of different forms of interferometry, including holographic interferometry. The most fundamental of these forms are the Twyman-Green and the Fizeau interferometers. Both of these instruments are used extensively in optical surface testing. The basic configuration of these interferometers provides a foundation for other useful testing tools.

There has been interest in the utilization of wave interference techniques (e.g. laser holography) to measure corneal topography. The major advantage of such an approach is the ultrahigh precision with which such measurements can be made (less than a wavelength of the probing light). The potential for such technology is exciting, but devices using this approach have only recently been made clinically available; their resolution is very high, providing so much detail that it can become both clinically irrelevant and difficult to comprehend. They can, however, be detuned to fit the resolution to the measurement requirements. For example, replaceable modules which allow study of the tear film layer to those which can perform anterior and posterior lens surface analysis could be utilized.

The use of holographic techniques for the study of the contour of the cornea has not, however, been reported extensively in the literature. This may be due to the fact that holography requires an interferometric system that has been designed to maintain correct position of the optical components and to isolate the entire system from vibration and air movement. This has discouraged the commercial development of such a system and limited the effort of researchers.

The other reason for the lack of development of holographic contour evaluation of the cornea is the need to evaluate large disturbances on a complex surface. The imaging of the corneal contour must

provide the means to measure large-scale events without sacrificing accuracy. The requirements for precision are in the range of longer wavelength optical testing (10.6 μm source) with the ability to define the contour event to 1 μm or less. Using the interference techniques, as described in this section, accuracies of a fraction of a wavelength can be obtained. The optical path differences can be measured to less than 0.10 μm, depending on the wavelength and the analysis of the wavefront interference using an appropriate algorithm.

The surface of the cornea is measured in terms of optical path difference, with the calibration and reference being the output spherical wavefront of the optical system. The surface elevations are arrived at by summing the optical path differences with the average radius of curvature of the cornea at the center. While any point on the cornea can be referenced, the central or apical part has been chosen to relate the output to a more familiar mode of measurement, i.e. keratometry. The use of any of these techniques for the measurement of a convex aspherical surface requires auxiliary optics, commonly referred to as null optics. The purpose of these optics is to create a closely matching wavefront to impinge on the convex corneal surface and reflect the difference from the curvature of the aspheric.

A laser source that is in the visible, such as a helium–neon laser, has a sensitivity that is, at worst, sub-micron and any large mismatch between null lens optics and the aspheric that is being tested will result in a large number of interference fringes. Holographic techniques using coherent light sources (lasers) are capable of reproducing minuscule aberrations in surface contour. That sensitivity, however, is one of this method's inherent problems. Too much sensitivity produces "noise" which tends to degrade performance in the system. Besides, what constitutes practical sensitivity? That is, how accurate is accurate enough?

In the case of a cornea with moderate astigmatism—2 D of refractive power—the surface radius change would be 0.4018 mm. This would be 633.931 waves at 0.6328 μm and 1267.86 fringes at the interference plane of the interferometer. The resulting pattern on a typical video format would result in having a fringe every 0.1 mm for a 5 inch (12.5 cm) frame. The fringe pattern would also have a form that is not easily fit using standard wavefront reducing algorithms (i.e. closed-form, or circular fringes).

With that in mind, the measurement of a variable aspherical surface such as the anterior cornea requires the instrument to allow for strong irregular unknown curvatures to be imaged and to create an interference event that can be easily analyzed to produce accurate (> 1μm) surface contouring of the cornea.

The extreme amount of curvature variation on the

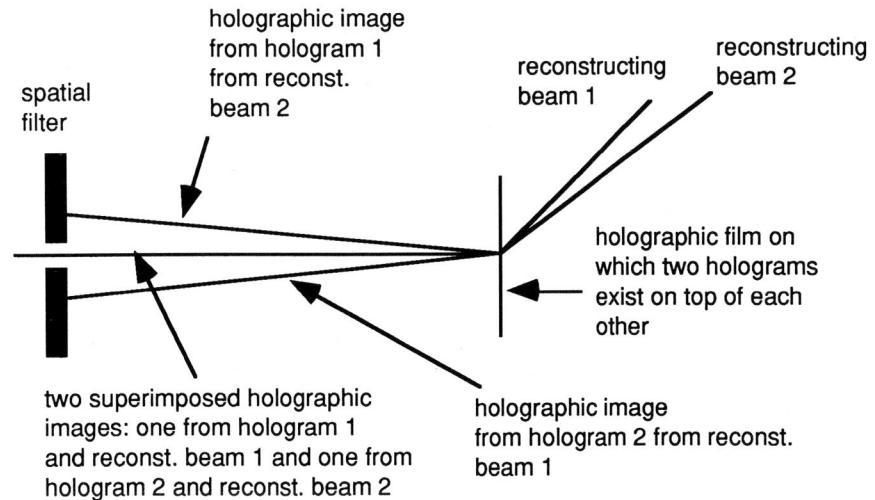

Fig. 6.42 Two-beam holographic system.

corneal surface requires the use of an extremely fast lens system in the F/0.6 to F/0.7 range. The lens system must be able to function with at least a degree of field angle to allow for off-axis events and to be able to bring enough of the direct reflection back to the imaging system [54].

The surface of the cornea is in constant movement, either from saccadic or mechanical movement, requiring fast acquisition (0.1 second) of the direct reflection to avoid loss of information and to maintain high contrast of the interference event. The returning full reflection from the corneal surface will then have its own wavefront signature from every detail that has reflected enough light to be detected by the video camera.

The author began work with this unit in 1983 when it was incarnated as a two-wavelength holographic interferometric topographer. In this device two holograms are laid one on top of the other on the same holographic film—in this case a Newport erasable media camera. Two reconstructing beams are used at one wavelength but the angle of incidence of each on the holographic recording medium is slightly different (Figure 6.42). Figures 6.43 and 6.44 show a contour map resulting from a first-generation fringe analyzer. These maps show how the shape of the corneal surface differs from the shape of the spherical wavefronts created by the focusing lens [55].

Acquisition of the corneal image

Because of the extreme changes in curvature which occur on the corneal surface, conventional holographic methods were modified to fit the peculiar requirements of this clinical modality. Happily, these requirements allowed use of a single laser beam and a much more compact, folded optical system (Figure 6.45) [14]. The current unit produces high-resolution

holographic images of the entire corneal surface (limbus to limbus) within 1/60 of a second, essentially eliminating problems associated with normal ocular movement. The working distance is quite close to the eye, necessitating a very fast lens system, but which excludes shadows created by the nose and brow which plague other methodologies. The images are captured by a high-resolution CCD array camera and relayed to a high-speed, full frame, two-page video frame grabber. The holograms in Figure 6.46 are a pair of such images of a human cornea taken with the device.

The images are then digitized and the optical path differences calculated using sophisticated Zernike polynomials. While digitization is essentially automatic, the operator, who controls all operations from the keyboard, can adjust or add data points directly on to the displayed high-contrast fringe pattern. The calculation overhead requirements are enormous requiring a central processing unit and math chip capable of operating at 25 MHz and 2 megabytes of random-access memory. The resultant topographic coordinates are displayed in false, editable colors, in high resolution on a multisync color monitor.

Corneal image feature extraction

The interference measurements used in this work are quite different to the Placido disk photographic technique. These techniques require interpretation of a complex phase and interference pattern that has been stored in a holographic medium as a diffraction pattern. The reconstruction of the complex multiple-wavelength diffraction pattern yields the phase and interference information that can be digitized to produce the wavefront of the object under test.

The digitization is illustrated in Figure 6.47. This represents the errors in the hologram shown in Figure 6.46. The contour lines are a function of the optical

(a)

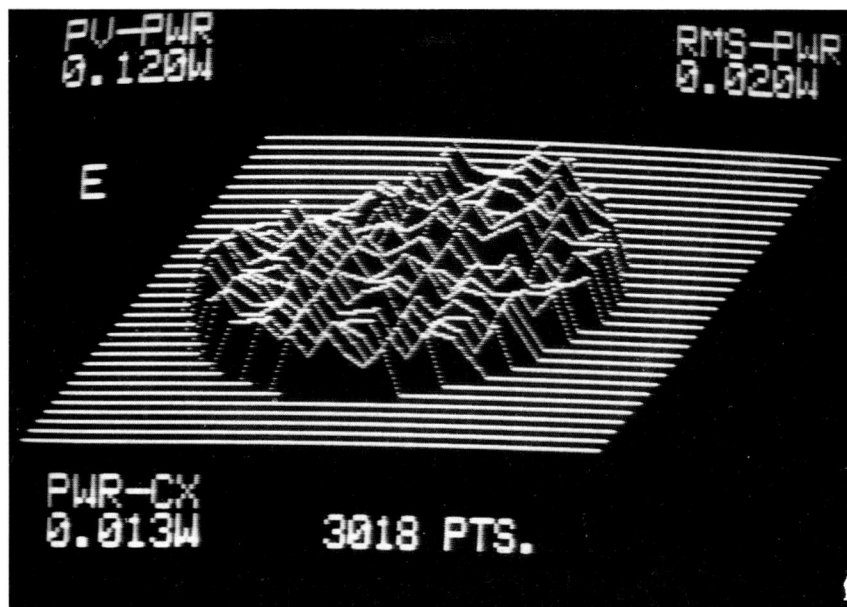

(b)

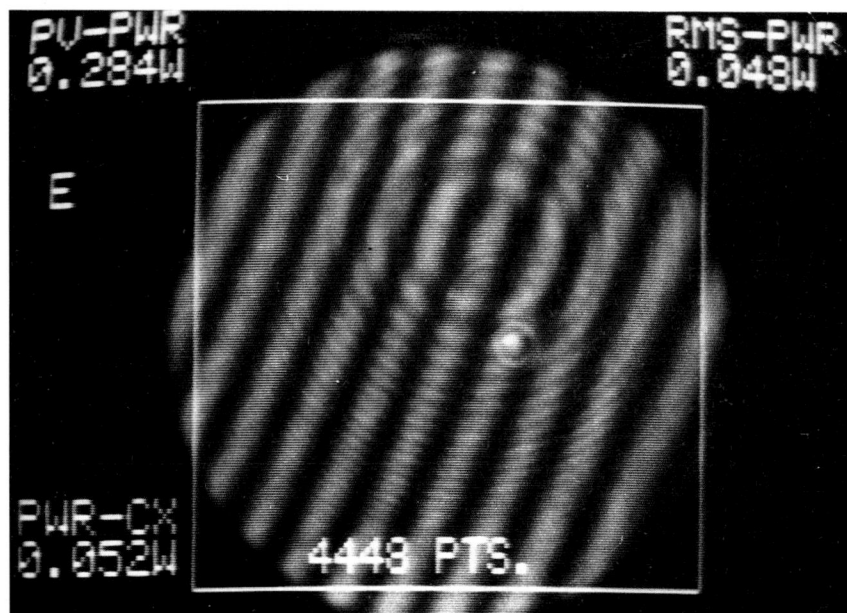

Fig. 6.43 (a) Isometric surface map and (b) the hologram from whence it was constructed. This map was made by the author in 1983 using a ZYGO unit and represents the first known curvature measurement of the human cornea holographically.

path differences recorded between the actual surface and a reference sphere. The reference sphere is obtained from an optical measurement of the corneal surface. It can also be derived from a real measurement of the limbal-to-limbal reflection of the cornea with the instrument. The value of the contour is established by the value of the equivalent wavelength. The resulting measured aberrations are in units of micro-meters which can be readily converted to dioptric equivalents.

The various aberration terms that result from the fitting of the digitized points define the optical characteristics of the measured surface. The varying degrees of astigmatism, coma, spherical, tilt, and focus that emanate from the surface being measured are converted to real surface elevations as a function of the actual value of the aberration.

The aberrations of an optical surface can be obtained from the digitized coordinates of an interference pattern that has been fit to a monomial expression:

$$W(x, y) = \sum_{i=0}^{k} \sum_{j=0}^{i} B_{ij} x^j y^{i-j} \qquad \textbf{1}$$

The polynomial is of degree k with $N = (k + 1)(k + 2)/2$ terms. The data obtained during digitization and least-squares fit to the polynomial are then transformed to a linear combination of Zernike polynomials. The angular function that has been used to convert each Zernike polynomial to its corresponding monomial form can be found by substituting this angular expression into the U_{nm} of the Zernike thus:

$$\genfrac{\{}{\}}{0pt}{}{\cos}{\sin}(n-2m)0 = p^{-(n-2m)} \sum_{j=0}^{q} (-1)^j \binom{n-2m}{2i-p} x^{2j+p} y^{n-2m-j-p} \quad \mathbf{2}$$

This is valid only for $n - 2m > 0$. The parameters for p and q are:

		n(even)	n(odd)
Sine	{p	1	1
	{q	$n - 2m/2(-1)$	$n - 2m - 1/2$
Cosine	{p	0	0
	{q	$n - 2m/2$	$n - 2m - 1/2$ $\quad\mathbf{3}$

After solving for p and substituting in terms of x and y using the following expressions:

Equation 4 determines the radial polynomials over the $n - 2m > 0$ in terms of p

$$R^{n-2m}{}_n(p) = \sum_{s=0}^{m} (-1)^s \frac{(n-s)!}{s!(m-s)!(n-m-s)!} p^{n-2s} \quad \mathbf{4}$$

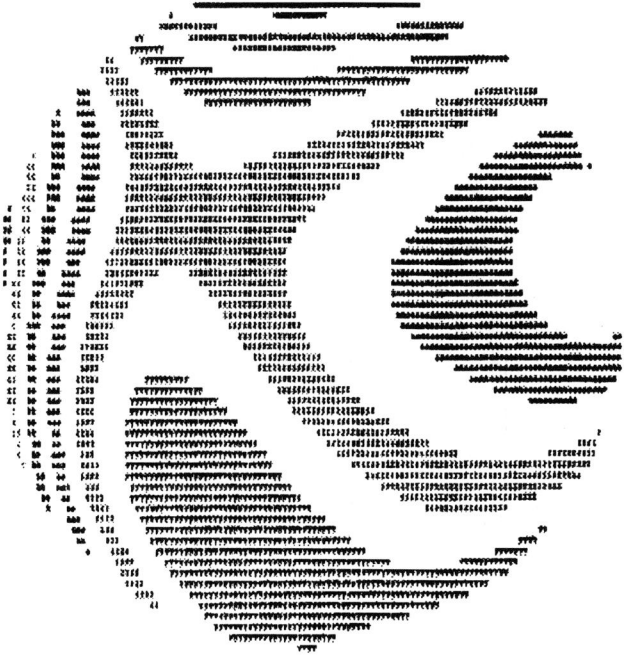

Fig. 6.44 Topographic corneal surface map derived from interference pattern data in Fig. 6.43.

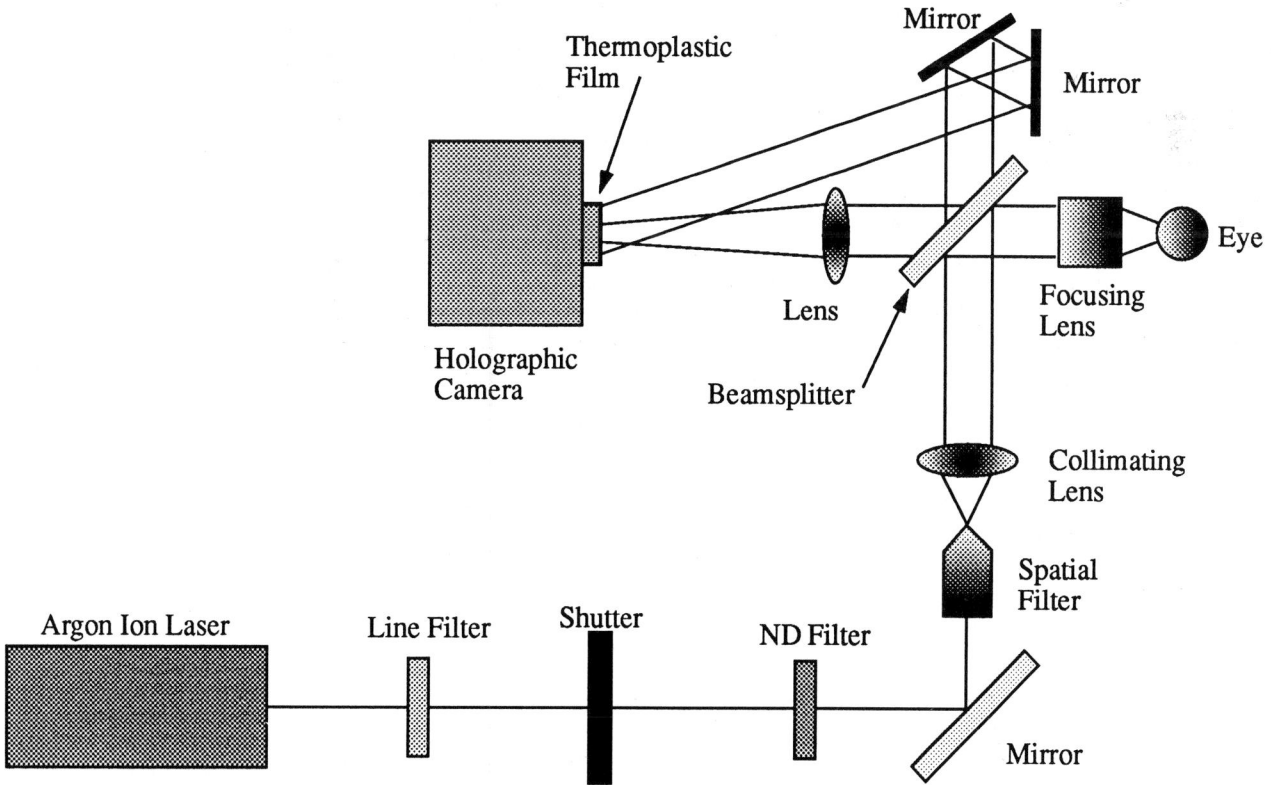

Fig. 6.45 Single side-band holographic system.

(a)

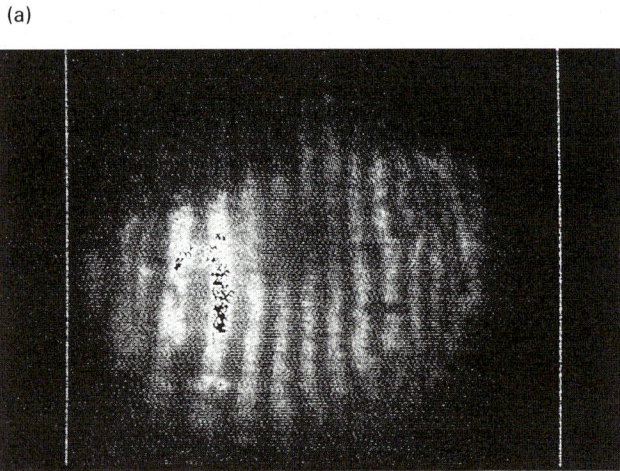

(b)

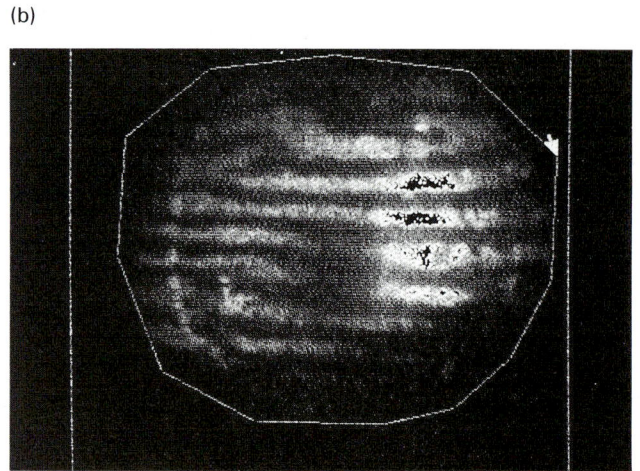

Fig. 6.46 (a and b) Typical interference pattern in x and y projection ready for digitization.

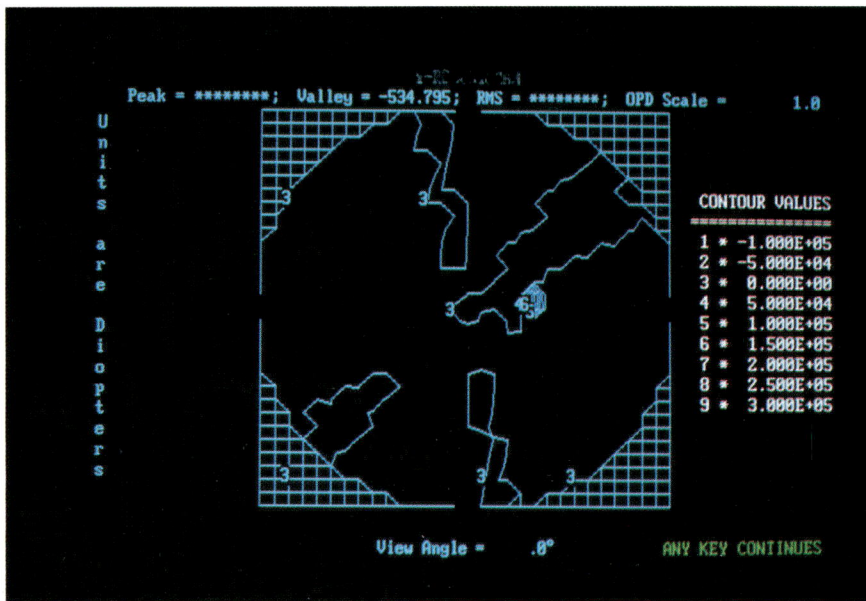

Fig. 6.47 Contour map derived from Figure 6.46. The scaling has been adjusted to show the areas of incisions. The surface distortions near four of the incisions are sufficiently great to be mapped.

$$p^{2j} = \sum_{k=0}^{q} \binom{(j)}{(k)} x^{2k} y^{2(j-k)} \qquad 5$$

The final expression for the Zernike polynomials U_{nm} in terms of powers of x and y is:

$$U_{nm} = R^{n-2m_n} \left\{ \begin{matrix} (\cos) \\ \{\sin\} \end{matrix} \right\} (n-2m)0$$

$$= \sum_{i=0}^{q} \sum_{j=0}^{m} \sum_{k=0}^{m-j} (-1)^{i+j} \binom{(n-2m)}{(2i+p)} \binom{(m-j)}{(k)}$$

$$\times \frac{(n-j)}{!(m-j)!(m-m-j)!} x^{2(i+k)+p} y^{n-2(i+j+k)-p}$$

$$6$$

The wavefront fitting that is being done is based on the fringe position caused by the reflected ray interference. This interference occurs from actual changes on the surface that perturb the return light-path from the incoming normal position. The light-path position that has been altered due to surface changes sets up interference with the reference plane, indicating a phase change in the interfering beams. The phase change is a physical difference in the distance traveled by the light reflected from the object as compared with the distance traveled by the reference beam. The total distance from the normal to the surface at any given point is the algebraic sum of the reference distance and the object distance. The path traveled by the object reflection has a value that is real with respect to the virtual image of a convex mirror or surface; this value is, however, normal to the surface and is not a value from a flat plane to a position on the corneal surface.

The surface that is constructed from the digitized points converted to wavefront monomials and then fit to circular Zernike polynomials can be treated as a real three-dimensional representation of the object with values in micro-meters, millimeters, or other units. This three-dimensional representation of the object can be operated on to present the data in required forms. The case of sagittal heights or elevations from the normals of the surface is a simple one and requires only that a perpendicular be dropped to the flat plane that has been chosen (in this case where the chord is described by the limbus), and values for the leg of the right triangle be calculated and converted to the appropriate units.

The sheared diffraction pattern produces interference fringes that could be measured as a function of the grating spacing of the holographic pattern. The shear fringes could then be analyzed for the various aberrations, i.e. spherical, focus, astigmatism, coma, etc. The use of shear fringes requires that two orthogonal patterns be analyzed in order to measure a non-symmetrical object such as the cornea. The value of astigmatism is determined from the difference in the focus of the orthogonal patterns. The amount of spherical aberration is determined by the non-linear shape of the shear fringe with the order of the fringes (number of fringes).

By adjusting the working distance and/or the lens system, measurements of the inside curvature of the cornea can and have been made. Further modifications have produced images of both the front and back lens surfaces. The most exciting aspect of this state-of-the-art technology is the ability to manipulate the laser light beam. By polarizing the beam in a certain way, corneal surface stress patterns can be seen. This ability opens the door to a whole new way of looking at post-operative results and will inevitably lead to changes in the way that all anterior segment ocular surgery is performed and complications, such as post-PKP astigmatism, are treated.

Interpreting the reconstruction of the corneal surface

The use of any new measuring system brings with it problems—we've just described some. One other is over-coming the hurdle of interpreting the data. This is especially apt in the case of holography—the output is not in a form that encourages intuitive interpretation. The interference fringes look like nothing the average ophthalmologist has seen before (Figure 6.48). However, if we are to describe the "dark side of the moon" (corneal topography) correctly, we needs must do so from a fresh perspective. Just as we cannot see the

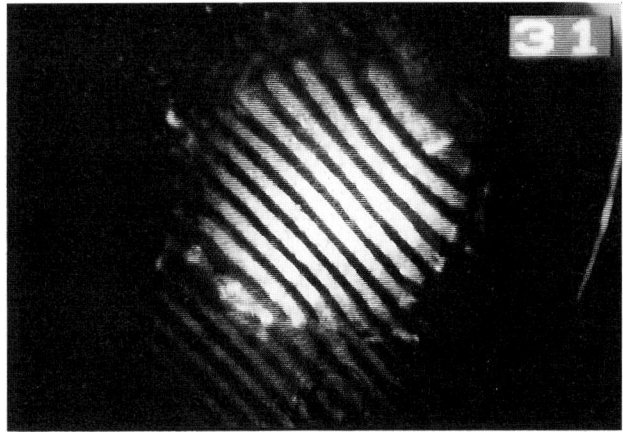

Fig. 6.48 Hologram of surface freshly ablated with the excimer laser. Photokeratoscopy is not useful in these cases. (Courtesy of M. Friedlander.)

dark side of the moon from our current point of view, so it is that our traditional viewpoint must be altered to discover and examine the true shape of the cornea. We had to leave our comfortable, familiar, and solid observation platform—the Earth—and move out into the unknown, unfamiliar, and unsteady platform of space to see the far side of the moon. So it is that we must abandon our outmoded, comfortable, and treasured—albeit erroneous—notions of the shape of the cornea we've held dear for more than 200 years. Therein lies the rub: we have relied on keratometry and its ilk for too long to discard that methodology out of hand.

While it is difficult to decipher a photo- or video-keratograph, with practice an astute observer can glean considerable information about the quality of the corneal surface as well as its shape from such an image. Not so with images produced by holographic surface measuring devices such as the CLAS II. Here the physician is confronted by a keratograph that more closely resembles a picket fence than an eye (Figure 6.46). Making sense of the image is all but impossible except for some optical engineers. The translation of image to a three-dimensional shape is not intuitive. Compounding that problem is the way in which these devices measure surfaces. Whereas in the Placido disk-type devices, the local corneal curvature is related to the diameter of the reflected ring—the chord of the arc—holograms record images through light wave interference, hence such images are often called interferograms and the dark bands produced by this interference, fringes. The image seen represents the pattern of that interference, not the shape of the cornea. In fact, except in extreme cases, the pattern may not even seem to be perturbed. Although the intervals between the dark–dark (or light–light) bands are important, they are not critical to the measurement of the surface shape because of the nature of the hologram. The corneal curve or Z-height at any point is not derived from the spacing of these bands even though the number of such bands may vary somewhat from one patient to another and one meridian to another. The number of bands is more a function of the deviation of the measured surface from the control or reference shape (sphere) and does not represent "tick" marks on a ruler. With practice, a trained and experienced observer can make reasonable assumptions about the surface by virtue of the shape of the bands and whether they are straight, curved or sinusoidal—but the actual surface profile has to be derived mathematically.

The average ophthalmologist, used to a slit-lamp, keratometer and Placido's disk, finds him- or herself at sea when viewing such a keratograph. There is nothing intuitive about such an image, no clue to aid the brain in visualizing the cornea, nothing there that resembles an eye. What must be realized is that these bands are merely addresses or locations along which are an infinite number of points holding information about the corneal profile. Selecting any point along either a dark or light band and applying sophisticated polynomial expressions to it provides the information about the corneal shape at that specific point. It is as if each band represents a road along which are erected vertical poles of varying height corresponding to the corneal profile. An observer could be dispatched down this road to pole 15. Knowing the angle of the sun the observer finds the height of the pole by measuring the shadow cast by the pole. This can be done for any number of poles along that road. The observer could then reconstruct a scale model of the poles using the data acquired and by laying a spline across the tops of the poles obtain the curvature along that road (band). The accuracy of that profile could be enhanced by increasing the number of poles measured but it is obvious that as the density of the poles increases, the height difference between adjacent poles would become less and therefore less significant. Thus having too many data points would increase only the complexity of the calculations and not the accuracy of the profile representation.

In reconstructing a holographic surface image, we can decide how many data points (poles) we wish to measure along each band as well as how many fringes we wish to use as reference points. By acquiring two images, each at right angles to the other, we can provide a grid or x–y coordinate system, at the intersection of which we can measure the "pole." By "ordering" the fringes, that is, numbering them from right to left or vice versa and down to up or reverse, we know where to apply the polynomial expression, i.e. which pole we will measure.

It is possible to automate the process to a certain extent by "grabbing" or storing each image on to a special video capture board within either the computer or the holographer. There the alternating black and white fringes are represented by individual pixels of varying intensity. By adjusting the relative brightness and contrast logarithmically the ambiguity between the black and white bands is reduced. This differentiation is further enhanced by filtering the input to reduce electronic noise. Special edge detection algorithms are used to define clearly the boundaries and path along which our observer (the computer) will travel in its measuring duties. The pole height at each intersection is duly recorded and the observer passes on to the next one. So it goes—at least in theory. Sometimes, however, the computer cannot make up its mind which direction to take and may wander down an alley and get lost. Therefore, automatic digitization of the fringes may break down partially or fail utterly. It is at this point that the eye–brain–hand "device" must be brought into play to pinpoint the missing data and it is at this point that the observer gets even more confused and skeptical—crying foul! Placing data points with a cursor device (mouse), however, is not cheating. Hand digitization is not supplying artificial or spurious data—the examiner is merely telling the computer where the next point is by taking the "lost waif" by the hand, leading it to the next pole and saying "measure here." It is, in fact, possible to do this for any number of points along any fringe without sacrificing accuracy. The whole measurement could be done in this manner but it is time-consuming and subject to human error.

Another concept used in making holographic surface measurements is that of the reference sphere—this troubles some people. They are concerned that relating the actual surface to such an artificial construct might somehow distort the rendering of that surface. This does not happen. It is in fact exactly what cartographers do when measuring elevations on the Earth's surface—they do so by relating such measurements to sea level. Despite the fact that sea level is inconstant, they can obtain sufficiently accurate elevations to serve most purposes. The reference sphere is our sea level and we can use the central corneal K-reading as the reference against which the optical path differences detected by the holographer are plotted. Thus the elevations displayed are related to some measurement in which we have inherent faith—keratometry—because we know that that measurement is accurately representative of some particular portion of the cornea (Figure 6.49). This should not be troubling either since the K-reading is only a reference value. Deviations from this reference (in terms of corneal curvature) are plotted in relationship to this known. Thus steeper points will appear above this surface and flatter points below (Figure 6.50).

The advent of holographic techniques has ushered

actual corneal surface

corneal
radius – r1

corneal
radius – r2

reference
radius

note that r1 is flatter than the reference radius
and that r2 is steeper, yet their relative positions
are such that they could be assigned a power
which is greater and lesser respectively.
Note the Z heights.

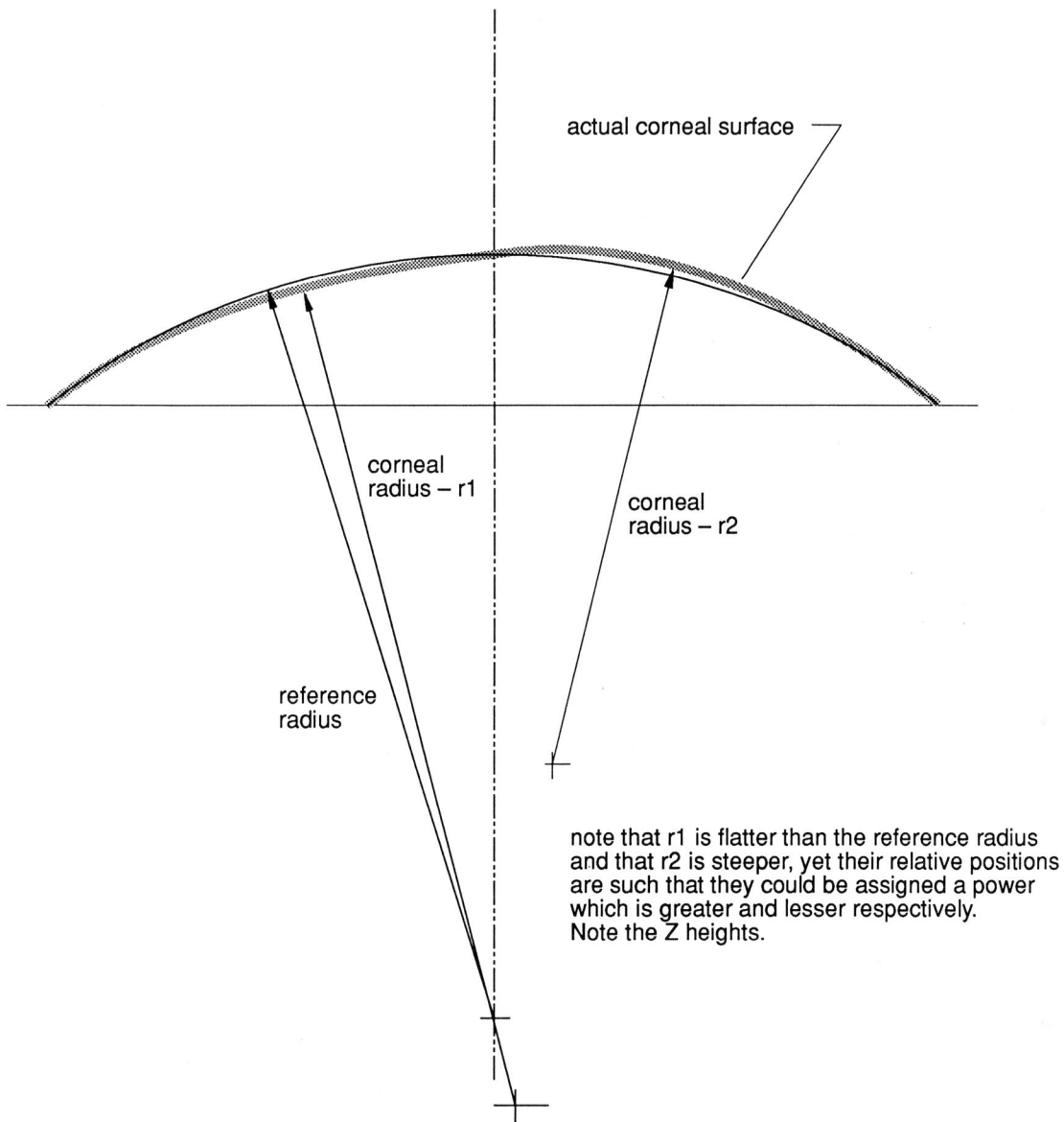

Fig. 6.49 Reference sphere/surface contour relationship.

in the use of more sophisticated and technical ways of examining not only the surface contour of the cornea, but also its effect on the light bundle traversing the eye and the resultant image. For example, one means of evaluating the quality of a refracting system is the focal spot. This can take the form of an Airy disk (Figure 6.51) or focal spot shape (see also Chapter 3). Figure 6.52a shows the focal spot of an unexcised cornea. Figure 6.52b shows the focal spot after a cornea has undergone a relaxing incision procedure for astigmatism (Ruiz technique). Note the coma, evidenced by the tail emanating from the center. This patient experienced "ghosting of images" at 2 months post-operation.

This same cornea was further analyzed to produce various contour plots of the surface. Figure 6.53 is a profile of the cornea showing both major and minor meridians plotted against a reference sphere. The same data were used to draw the topographic map in Figure 6.54; this type of plot is more familiar to clinicians (or is getting to be). Figure 6.55 is an isometric surface map more familiar to optical engineers. However, the irregularities in the corneal surface can be readily seen. Note that these are not evident in the relatively low-resolution map in the previous figure. This is because the irregularities are of small magnitude and require data scaling to reveal. Thus, the contour map is a global view of the cornea showing gross deviations—like observing the Earth from space. The isometric map is a local view with enhanced data—like observing the Grand Canyon from a low-flying aircraft.

local
radius

reference
radius

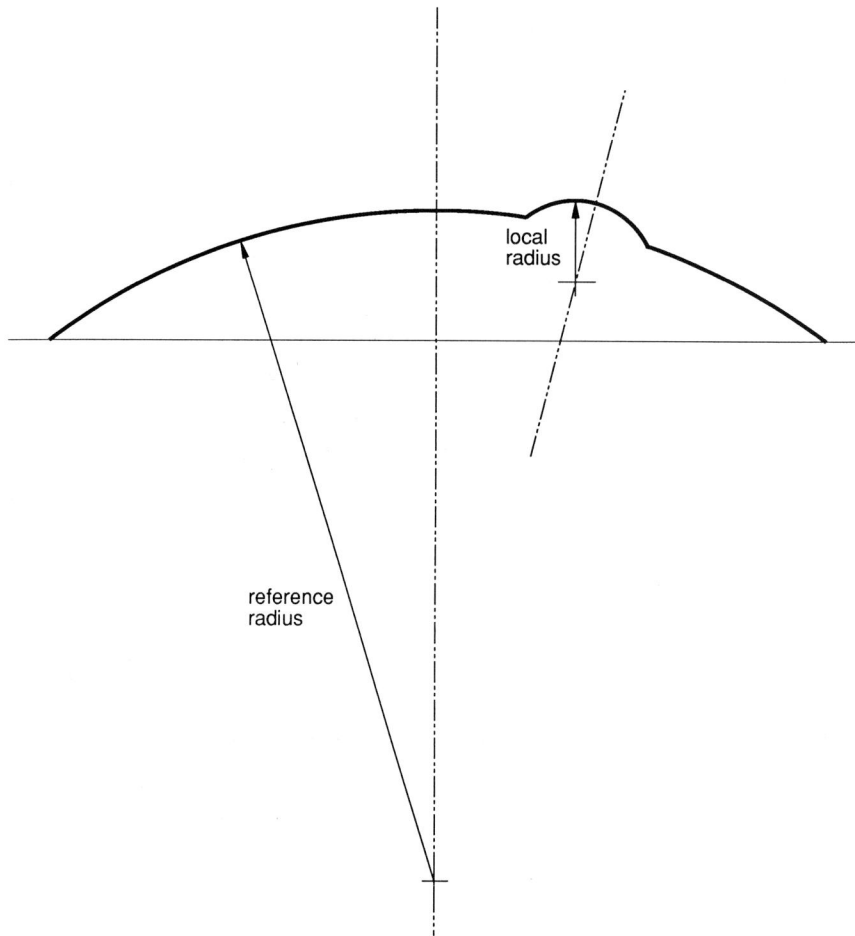

Fig. 6.50 The surface is drawn in
relation to a reference sphere.

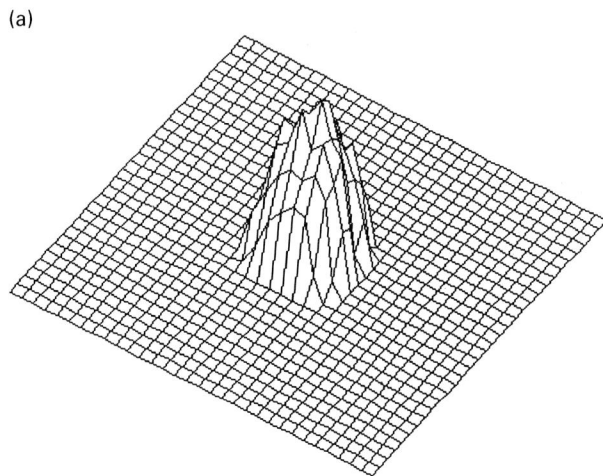

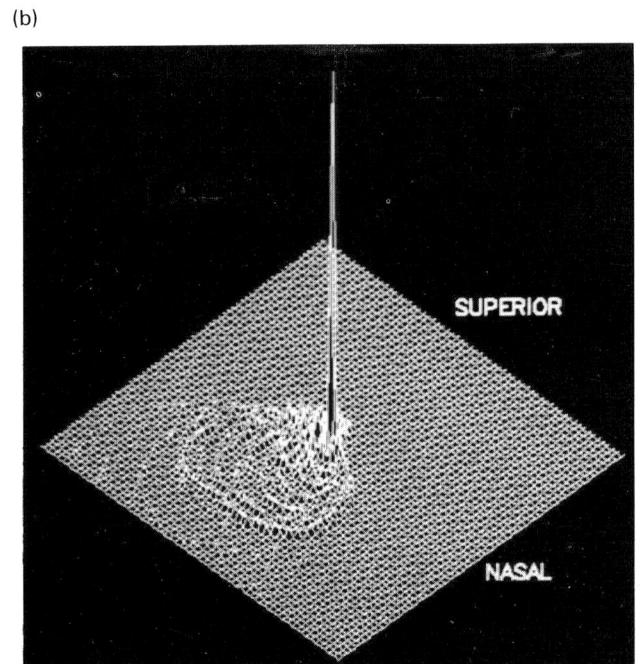

(a)

(b)

SUPERIOR

NASAL

Fig. 6.51 (a) Airy disk of an eye constructed from a surface hologram using a ray tracing program (BEAM4). Such an analysis can provide information as to the optical efficiency of the eye since basically it is the Strehl Ratio (S_r) that is being mapped. S_r is a measure of the size and relative brightness of the central Airy disk. (b) An Airy disk from a patient with keratoconus. Note the distortion of the pattern. (Courtesy of L. Maguire.)

(a)

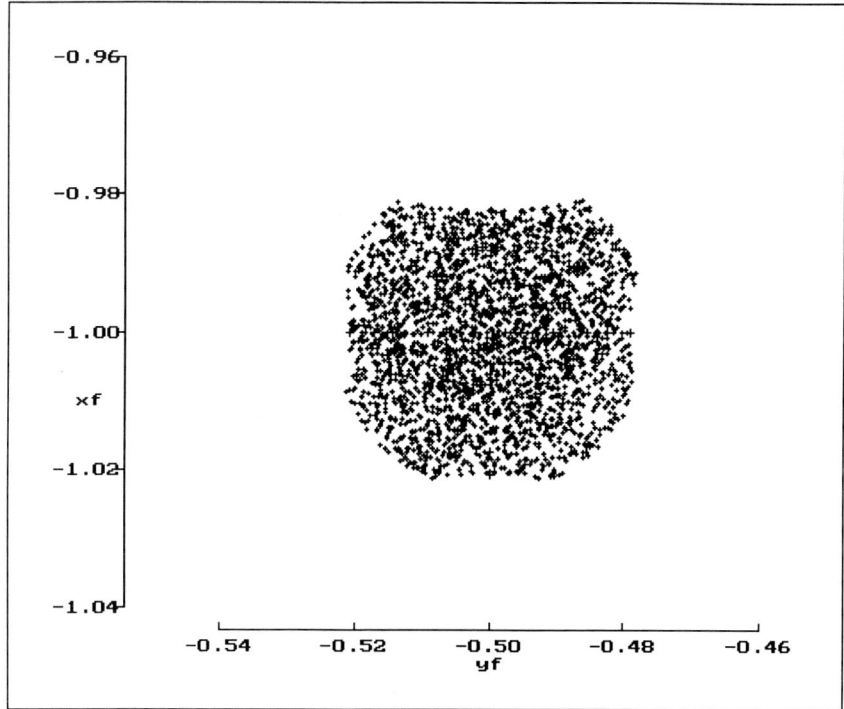

(b)

ruiz y frame 6 goes with frame 5 x
GEOMETRICAL ANALYSIS ZONAL SPOT DIAGRAM

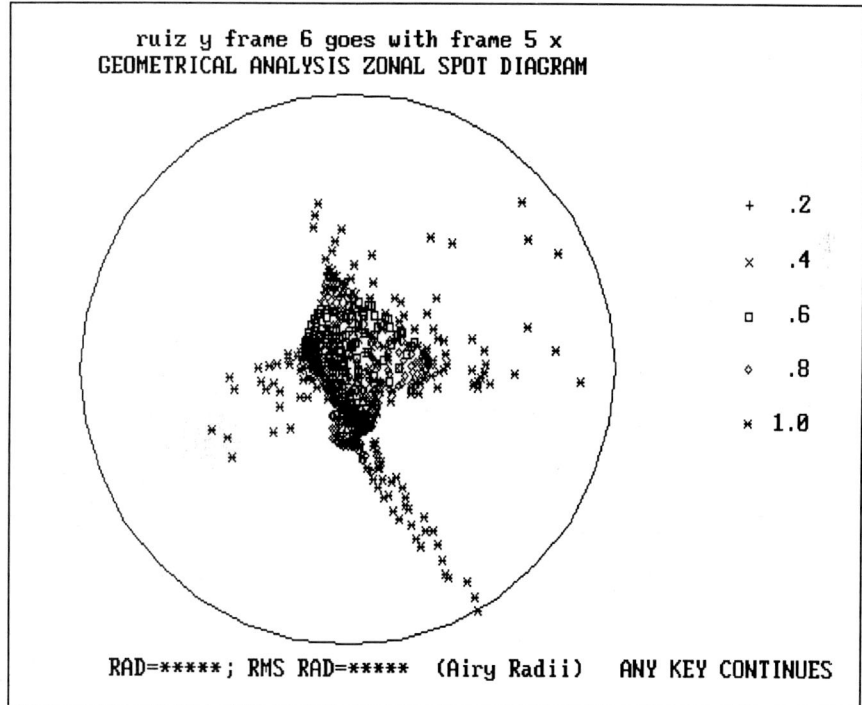

+ .2

× .4

□ .6

◇ .8

✳ 1.0

RAD=✳✳✳✳✳; RMS RAD=✳✳✳✳✳ (Airy Radii) ANY KEY CONTINUES

Fig. 6.52 (a) Pre-operative focal spot; (b) post-Ruiz focal spot. Note coma. By plotting the shape and size of the focal spot, tilt and coma can be detected and measured.

It is possible to produce a local contour map as well. Figure 6.56 shows such a map scaled to show the incisions in an eight-incision radial keratotomy case. To produce revealing surface plots such as these, the technician must have the data. Hence the emphasis on the accuracy of surface measurement, which is only possible with precision devices. Such precision is essential to obtain data to evaluate the modulation transfer function of an optical system. Figure 6.57 shows a modulation transfer function of a normal

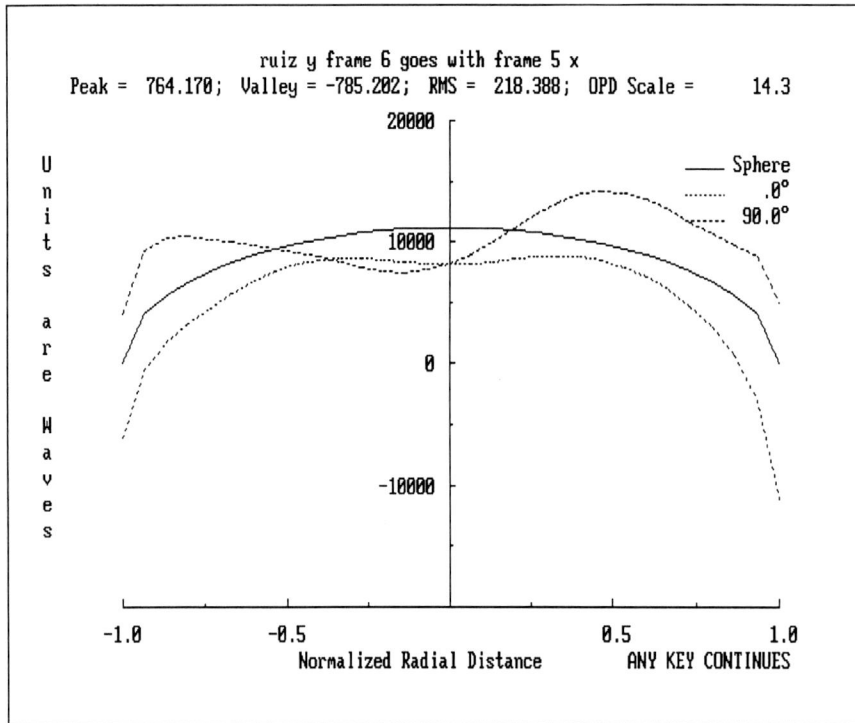

Fig. 6.53 Profile plot after a Ruiz procedure. Note how the surface major/minor meridian (dotted line) dips below (is flatter) and extends above (is steeper than) the reference sphere (solid line).

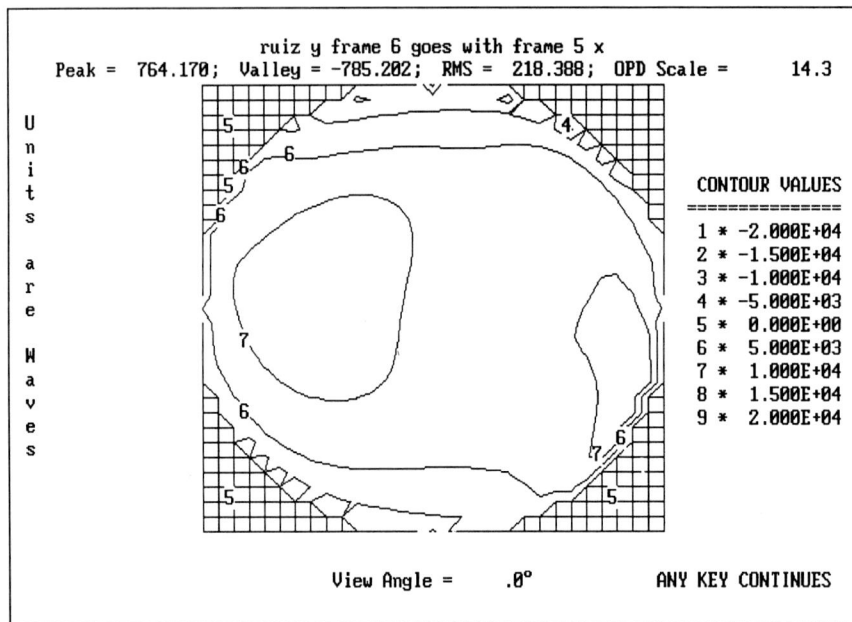

Fig. 6.54 Topographic map after a Ruiz procedure.

cornea using data obtained from the CLAS II device and the optical bench software BEAM4.

Corneal presentation schemes in general

As difficult as it might seem to achieve the three-dimensional reconstruction of the corneal surface from two-dimensional images, presentation of the resultant data in a meaningful fashion is more of a challenge. Itoi

and Maruyama [55] were the first (to our knowledge) to publish a wire mesh representation of corneas reconstructed from photokeratoscope analyses (Figure 6.58). This form allowed the observer to appreciate gross distortions of the cornea surface and was later refined by displaying deviations of corneal shape from a known sphere rather than presenting the corneal shape alone. Unfortunately, such presentation schemes failed to be easily interpretable. However,

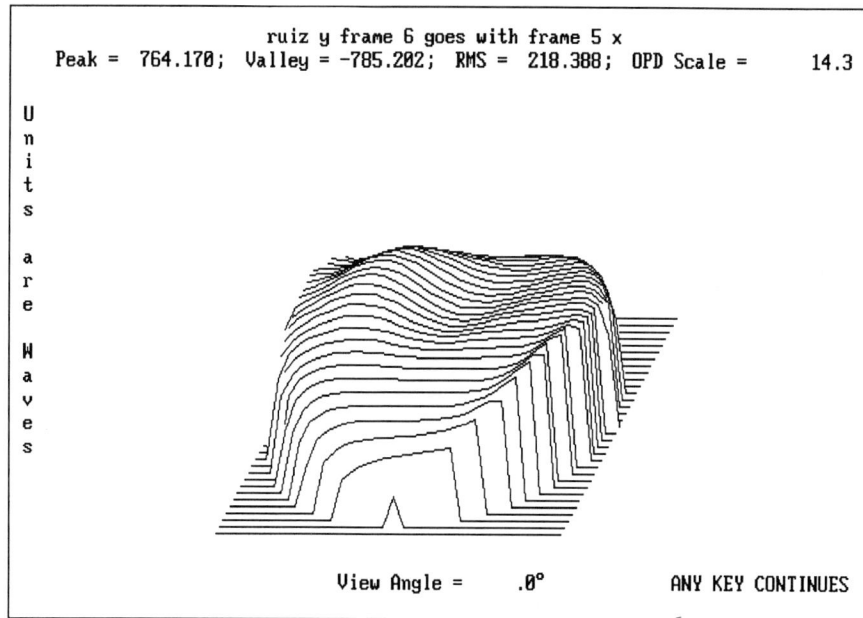

ruiz y frame 6 goes with frame 5 x
Peak = 764.170; Valley = -785.202; RMS = 218.388; OPD Scale = 14.3

View Angle = .0°   ANY KEY CONTINUES

Fig. 6.55 Isometric surface plot after a Ruiz procedure.

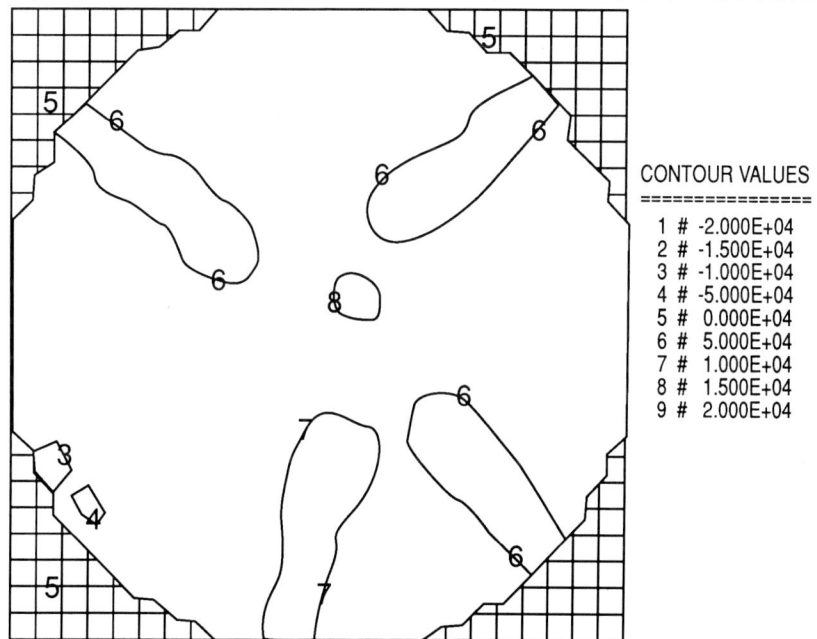

4.828; Valle = -4.712; RM = 1.653; OPD Scale= 2682.2

CONTOUR VALUES
================
1 # -2.000E+04
2 # -1.500E+04
3 # -1.000E+04
4 # -5.000E+04
5 # 0.000E+04
6 # 5.000E+04
7 # 1.000E+04
8 # 1.500E+04
9 # 2.000E+04

Fig. 6.56 Print-out of a local (scaled) contour map of an eight-incision radial keratotomy case (see also Figure 6.47).

View Angle = .0°

this beginning led to the development of the color-coded contour mapping scheme that is used in an increasing number of instruments. Color coding *per se* is not adequate in and of itself, however. The depiction of corneal topography using a color-coded mapping scheme must convey corneal shape information to be useful. To do so, it must be based on accurately obtained shape data, and interpretation of the presentation scheme must be straightforward and obvious

to the clinical audience. The color-coded contour map of corneal surface power is one step in the presentation of corneal topography.

What do some of these strange configurations mean, however? Do astigmatic corneas really look like bow-ties (Fig. 6.59)? How could anyone see through the center of that X? Is that really keratoconus? Of course the cornea does not look like a bow-tie (or a hot cross bun either). The bow-tie appearance is a mathematic

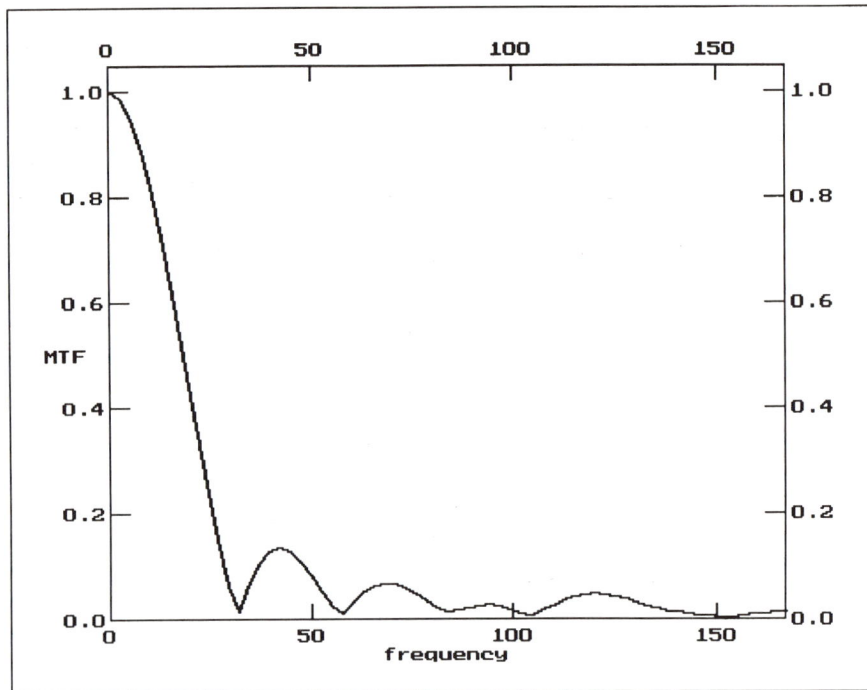

Fig. 6.57 Plot of modulation transfer function of an eye.

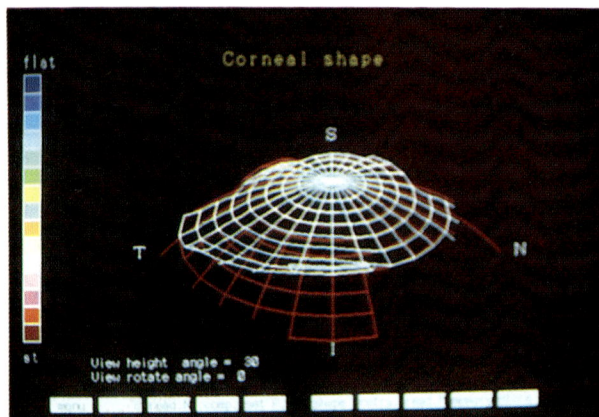

Fig. 6.58 Nidek system surface analysis based on Itoi and Maruyama's original work [52]. It overlays the plotted surface on top of a reference surface (red).

construct based both upon the resolution chosen for the map and the limitations of the mapping hardware (Figure 6.58). There are some practical considerations as well.

While it may be true that 16 million colors are potentially available for display on the monitors typically supplied with current systems, those colors are only available in systems equipped with 24-bit video cards. None of the current systems is so equipped. All current systems have 8-bit video display cards capable of displaying 256 colors, which is really enough. Too many colors, like too many chefs, can ruin the display by making it an incoherent gabble.

If one were to assign each and every color to each arbitrary change in the corneal curvature (and enough colors were available in the palette), that X-shaped or bow-tie central cornea would be shown as a gradual and smooth blend of colors from the steepest (red end) to the flattest (blue end) and no bow-tie figure would be seen. Beautiful to be sure but useless for our purposes—it would be almost impossible to choose one particular spot on the cornea which is of a specific curvature value. If we assign our colors to change at some larger and more practical value, the smooth blend changes to a series of steps and the X or bow-tie shape makes its appearance (Fig. 6.59).

Thus we must choose our scaling and mapping steps to match our requirements. If we are looking for irregularities to account for our patient's sub-normal visual results, we would use scaling and small steps. One the other hand, if we are merely looking at the general shape of the cornea pre- and post-surgery, scaling should be turned off and larger steps used for the map. In each case, additional types of analyses would be performed, such as modulation transfer function, focal spot mapping, etc. We must learn to use our new tools in a sensible and practical manner if they are to serve us in our quest to perfect our surgical art.

This new modality should provide a platform for launching even more useful presentation schemes in addition to the more quantitative analytical data needs, such as detailed above and by Dingeldein et al. [57]. The advent of modern analysis of corneal topography, coupled with the color-coded presentation schemes of

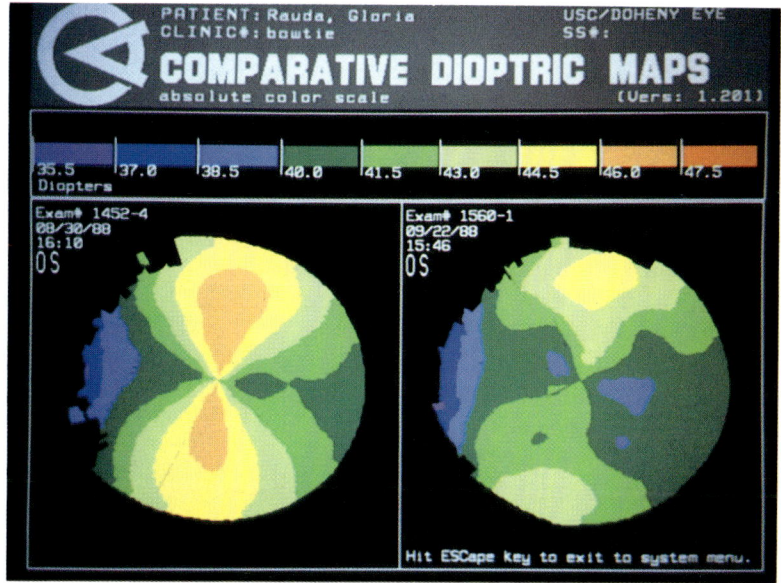

Fig. 6.59 Typical color-coded contour map of an astigmatism case showing "bow-tie" feature.

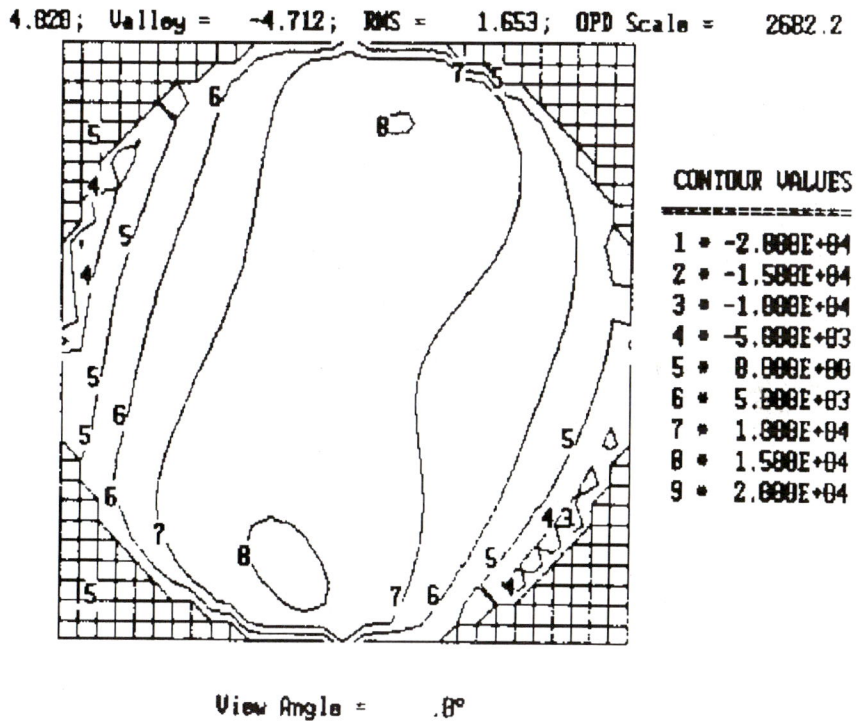

Fig. 6.60 A treasure map to new discoveries in refractive surgery.

corneal surface power distribution, have finally given corneal surgeons a tool that they can bring to practical clinical use [1,58,59] (Figure 6.60).

Validation of corneal topography devices

After all of the above discussion regarding the methods for the computerized reconstruction of the corneal surface from various automated approaches, it is essential to mention the importance for the validation of instruments. We cannot emphasize too strongly or too often the need for prospective purchasers of corneal topography equipment to insist upon certification data to verify the utility and accuracy of the equipment for the measurement of corneal shape. Validation of corneal topography analysis systems is slow in appearing, primarily because the best data are gathered by independent research laboratories and the publication process is lengthy by nature. Such a demonstration must include not only precision spherical surfaces, but aspherical surfaces such as done by Wang and co-workers [47]. The author has proposed a reflective peanut shell. This is not proposed entirely in jest. Take a look at an unhusked peanut. Not only has it an irregular shape but it is covered with multiple indentations. Such a surface would give a photokeratometer fits, yet some corneal surfaces can be quite as grotesque. A rasterstereographer might be able to handle it; surely a holographic unit could—at least most of it.

Assessing and describing the accuracy of corneal topographers presents a set of problems not previously encountered in keratometry. One of the major difficulties encountered is that current corneal topography analysis instruments have the potential to be more accurate than traditional methods used for the production of accurately defined aspherical surfaces, particularly holographic systems. This has the potential to confound certification studies. In the past, irregularities of these surfaces have not been a problem because the instruments that they were intended to calibrate lacked the sensitivity to detect many imperfections or alert one to inaccuracies. Where the concern was for an approximate average, as is the case in keratometry, relatively small irregularities of the calibrating balls were of little importance.

Clinicians tend to compare a new instrument to an old one with which they are familiar but in the case of corneal topographers such a comparison might be like checking the measurements of a micrometer with a common wooden yard stick. Perhaps the validation of corneal topography instruments for the purposes of Food and Drug Administration acceptance as with clinician acceptance should be judged on the basis of accuracy in permitting diagnosis of clinical shape anomalies.

References

1 McDonnell PJ, Garbus J, Lopez PF. Topographic analysis and visual acuity after radial keratotomy [see comments]. Am J Ophthalmol 1988;106:692–695.

2 McDonnell PJ, McClusky DJ, Garbus JJ. Corneal topography and fluctuating visual acuity after radial keratotomy. Ophthalmology 1989; 96:665–670.

3 Maguire LJ, Bourne WM. Corneal topography of early keratoconus. Am J Ophthalmol 1989;108:107–112.

4 Rowsey JJ, Balyeat HD, Monlux R, Holladay J, Waring GO, Lynn MJ. Prospective evaluation of radial keratotomy. Photokeratoscope corneal topography. Ophthalmology 1988; 95: 322–334.

5 Santos VR, Waring GOD, Lynn MJ, Holladay JT, Sperduto RD. Relationship between refractive error and visual acuity in the prospective evaluation of radial keratotomy (PERK) study. Arch Ophthalmol 1987; 105:86–92.

6 Maguire LJ, Lowry JC. Identifying progression of subclinical keratoconus by serial topography analysis. Am J Ophthalmol 1991;112:41–45.

7 Waring GO. Making sense of keratospeak II: conventional terminology for corneal topography. Refract Corneal Surg 1989; 5:362–367.

8 Helmholtz HLF. Ueber die Accomodation des Auges. Graefes Arch Ophthalmol 1954;1:1–74.

9 Dekking H. Fotografie der cornea opperwlakte Assen. Groninque th. med. 1930 No. 2, Van Gorcum, in Bcm, 91,360 (1930) no. 271,1930.

10 Gullstrand A. Photographisch-ophthalmometrische und klinishe untersuchungen uber die Hornhautrefraktion. Kongl Svenska Vet Akad Handl 1896; 28.

11 Klyce SD. Computer-assisted corneal topography. High-resolution graphic presentation and analysis of keratoscopy. Invest Ophthalmol Visual Sci 1984; 25:1426–1435.

12 Maguire LJ, Singer DE, Klyce SD. Graphic presentation of computer-analyzed keratoscope photographs. Arch Ophthalmol 1987; 105:223–230.

13 Bores L. Corneal Topography—the Dark Side of the Moon. In *Proceedings of the Soc Photo Inst Eng*, SA Benton (ed). The International Society for Optical Engineering, Los Angeles, 1991.

14 Miller D, Carter J. A proposed new division of corneal functions. The cornea. In: *Transactions of the World Congress on the Cornea III*, HD Cavanaugh (ed). Raven Press, New York, 1980.

15 Mandell RB. Corneal topography. *Contact Lens Practice*. Charles C Thomas, Springfield, 1981.

16 Scheiner C. *Occulus Hoc est: Fundamentum Opticum*. Daniel Agricolam, Innsbruck, 1619.

17 Kohlraush J. Uber die Messung des Radius der Vorderflache der Hornhaut am libenden menschlichen Auge. Okens Isis Jahrg 1840; 5:886.

18 Helmholtz H. *Treatise on Physiological Optics*, vol 1. J Southall (transl). Optical Society of America, New York, 1924.

19 Coccius A. *Ophthalmometrie und Spannungsmessung am kranksen Auge*. Leipzig, 1872.

20 Landolt E. *L'ophthalmomètre*. Congrès Periodique International des Sciences Médicales, Geneva, 1878.

21 Javal LE, Schiøtz HA. Un ophthalmomètre pratique. Ann Oculist 1881; 87:5.

22 Sutcliffe J. One position ophthalmometry. Optician Photogr Trades Rev 1907; 33(suppl):8.

23 Hartinger H. Optique physiologique. In: *Revue d'Optique*. Y LeGrand (ed). 1935.

24 Fincham EF. The changes in the form of the crystalline lens in accommodation. Trans Opt Soc Lond 1925; 26:239–269.

25 Berg F. Vergleichende Messungen der Form der vorderen Hornhautflache mit Ophthalmometer und mit photographischer Methode. Acta Ophthalmol 1929; 7:386–423.

26 Berg F. Bemerkungen zur Theorie der ophthalmmetrischen Messungen von Flachen-krummungen. Acta Ophthalmol 1929; 7:225–243.

27 Aubert H. Näher sich die Hornhautkrummung am meisten der Ellipse. Pfluegers Arch 1885; 35:597–621.

28 Tscherning M. *Physiological Optics*. C Weiland (transl). Keystone, Philadelphia, 1904.

29 Gullstrand A. Beitrag zur Theorie des Astigmatismus. Skand Arch Ophthalmol 1890; 2:269–359.

30 Reynolds A, Kratt H. The photoelectronic keratoscope. Contacto 1959; 3:53–59.

31 Feldman ST, Frucht-Pery J, Weinreb RN, Chayet A, Dreher AW, Brown SI. The effect of increased intraocular pressure on visual acuity and corneal curvature after radial keratotomy. Am J Ophthalmol 1989; 108:126–129.

32 MacRae S, Rich L, Phillips D, Bedrossian R. Diurnal variation in vision after radial keratotomy. Am J Ophthalmol 1989; 107:262–267.

33 Bores L. *Pseudo-accommodation Following Radial Keratotomy*. Quintum Forum, Bogota, Colombia, 1987.

34 Bonnett R. New method of topographical ophthalmometry, its theoretical and clinical applications. Am J Ophthalmol 1962; 39:227–251.

35 Duke-Elder S, Abrams D. The dioptric imagery of the eye. In: *System of Ophthalmology. V. Ophthalmic Optics and Refraction*, SS Duke-Elder (ed). CV Mosby, St Louis, 1970.

36 Duke-Elder S, Abrams D. Ophthalmic optics and refraction. In: *System of Ophthalmology*, SS Duke-Elder (ed). CV Mosby, St Louis, 1970.

37 Goode H. On a peculiar defect of vision. Trans Camb Phil Soc 1849; 8:493–496.

38 Placido A. Novo instrumento de esploracao da cornea. Periodico Oftalmol Pract 1880; 5:27–30.

39 Placido A. Novo instrumento par analyse immediate des irregularida des de curvatura de cornea. Periodico Oftalmol Pract 1880; 6:44–49.

40 Nordensen. Ann Oculist (Paris) 1883; 89:110.

41 Rowsey J. Ten caveats in keratorefractive surgery. Ophthalmology 1983; 90:148.

42 Rowsey JJ, Schanzlin DJ. Corneal topography. In: *Contact Lenses. The CLAO Guide to Basic Science and Clinical Practice*, OH Dabezies (ed). Grune & Stratton, Orlando, 1984.

43 Warnicki JW, Rehkopf PG, Curtin DY, Burns SA, Arffa RC. Corneal topography using computer analyzed rasterstereographic images. Appl Optics 1988; 27:1135–1140.

44 Gormley DJ, Gersten M, Koplin RS, Lubkin V. Corneal modeling. Cornea 1988; 7:30–35.

45 Doss JD, Hutson RL, Rowsey JJ, Brown DR. Method for calculation of corneal profile and power distribution. Arch Ophthalmol 1981; 99:1261–1265.

46 Wang J, Rice DA, Klyce SD. New reconstruction algorithm for improvement of corneal topographical analysis. Refract Corneal Surg 1989; 5:379–387.

47 El Hage SG. Computerized corneal topographer for use in refractive surgery. Refract Corneal Surg 1989; 5:418–422.

48 Arffa R, Warnicki JW, Rehkopf PG. Corneal topography using rasterstereography. Refract Corneal Surg 1989; 5:414–417.

49 Frobin W, Hierholzer E. Rasterstereography: a photogrammetric method for measurement of body surfaces. J Biol Photogr 1983; 51:11–18.

50 Koepfler AE. Moire topography in medicine. J Biol Photogr 1983; 51:3–10.

51 Foley JD, Van Dam A. *Fundamentals of Interactive Computer Graphics*. Addison Wesley, Reading MA, 1982.

52 Caceci MS, Cacheris WP. Fitting curves to data. Byte 1984; 9:340–362.

53 Adachi I. Real time analysis corneal keratometer. Thesis, United States Patent #4 692 003, Sept 8, 1987.

54 Gross GW, Baker P, Bores LD. Corneal topography via two wavelength holography. In *Proceedings of the Soc Photo Inst Eng*, SA Benton (ed). The International Society for Optical Engineering, Los Angeles, 1990.

55 Itoi M, Maruyama S. A new photokeratometry system. J Jpn Contact Lens Soc 1978; 20:119–124.

56 Dingeldein SA, Klyce SD, Wilson SE. Quantitative descriptors of corneal shape derived from computer-assisted analysis of photokeratographs. Refract Corneal Surg 1989; 5:372–378.

57 Lin DT, Webster RGJ, Abbott RL. Repair of corneal lacerations and perforations. Int Ophthalmol Clin 1988; 28:69–75.

58 Maguire LJ, Klyce SD, Singer DE, McDonald MB, Kaufman HE. Corneal topography in myopic patients undergoing epikeratophakia. Am J Ophthalmol 1987; 103:404–416.

7

The Beginning and the Evolution of Radial Keratotomy

There is nothing more difficult to take in hand, more perilous to conduct, or more uncertain in its success, than to take the lead in the introduction of a new order of things.
[Machiavelli]

We will begin our discussion of the surgical treatment of refractive disorders with radial keratotomy (RK)—which is only fitting—because the modern era of refractive surgery really began on 28 November 1978. It was on that date that the first RK in the western world was performed. Thus was inaugurated a period which, in only a few years, has seen more evolution in this field than has occurred in all the preceding centuries. Prior to that date, the flame was kept alive only by a select few stalwarts such as José Barraquer who worked in relative and unappreciated obscurity, and who carried the banner for all those who went before. The year 1978 saw refractive surgery thrust into the hands of the work-a-day ophthalmologist. More importantly, this surgery became available to the mainstream patient who now—and for the first time—had a viable, low-risk, alternative to ocular appliances.

This story is very much a personal one, inasmuch as I am the surgeon who performed that first case in 1978 (Table 7.1). Because I am also responsible for not a little of the early development of RK as well as the training of most of its practitioners, I hope that the reader will forgive the occasional use of the personal pronoun (Figures 7.1–7.3). It is, additionally, a story of deep-felt personal responsibility and anguish. Nevertheless, these pages are not the place for the darker side of this story: that part of the tale is best left for another time and another place.

RK is an elegant solution to a serious ocular deficit—myopia. By simply making partial-thickness, *ab externo*, corneal incisions, which radiate from a common center and whose length and depth are variable, the refractive surgeon can alter not only the shape of the cornea but the life of the patient as well. Having said that, what must be added is this: what looks simple—isn't. It is not enough just making the incisions: anyone can do that. Rather it is in the understanding of how, when, and where to make them that spells the difference between success and failure in this surgery. Thus, RK surgery can be likened to genius which has been described as "1% inspiration and 99% perspiration." In RK, as well as in refractive surgery generally, it is 10% *incision* and 90% *decision*, i.e. thinking before doing. To this end, it will be well to discuss how it is that this surgery works and how it was that the surgery evolved into what it is today.

Early history and development of radial relaxing incisions

To begin with, it must be understood that although there are some superficial resemblances, RK is not the Sato procedure. While a wagon and a truck resemble one another in that both have four wheels, one in each corner, that resemblance ends there—so it is with Sato's operation and RK.

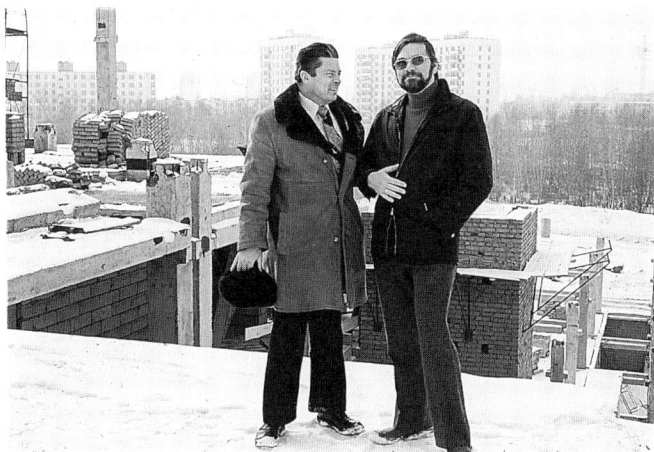

Fig. 7.1 Svatyslav N. Fyodorov and Leo D. Bores standing on the third floor of Fyodorov's unfinished institute in February 1976, the year RK was introduced to the western world (the first RK was performed in the west in November 1978). Only 135 cases had been performed up to that time.

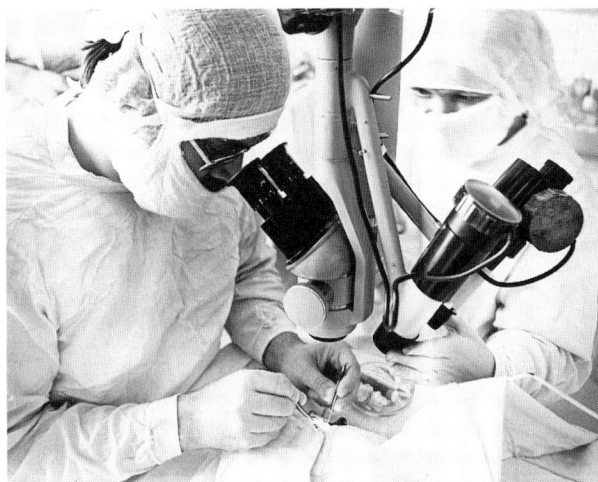

Fig. 7.2 The author performing his first RK in Moscow in 1976.

The Sato operation

Tutomu Sato, MD (Figure 7.4), late of Juntendo Medical College and a brilliant and gifted surgeon, himself called the operation posterior half-incision of cornea. It was originally conceived as a solution to the problem of keratoconus and was first reported by Sato in 1939 [1]; in this paper he described the results of such incisions in 10 eyes of eight patients. The technique was later applied to cases of regular astigmatism [2] and still later to spherical myopia itself. This method was not without precedent; Sato was familiar with the work of Lans [3] who stated that he had gotten the idea from something Snellen had proposed in 1869. However, whereas Lans confined his experiments to rabbits, Sato extended the method into humans.

While studying the subject of keratoconus under the guidance of Professor Shinobu Ishihara, inventor of the Ishihara Color Plates, in 1936, Sato noted the marked improvement in vision of a 20-year-old girl following spontaneous rupture of Descemet's membrane (Figure 7.5). Counting fingers vision, recorded 4 days after the rupture, improved to approximately 20/30 after 5 weeks of patching and medication. The corneal apex had not only flattened but had become more regular, as evidenced by its appearance with Placido's disk examination. Sato reasoned that he should be able to accomplish a better result through producing an artificial rupture of Descemet's by making an incision in the proper place. Thus he could control where the release of tension occurred and thereby retain and restore vision while forestalling an uncontrolled rupture [4–6].

Sato's operation for keratoconus was straightforward, effective, and considering the alternative, appropriate. The alternative, at least for most, was poor vision since corneal transplantation was proscribed by the religious beliefs of the Japanese. For others, it meant a long and expensive trip to either

Table 7.1 The results of the first radial keratotomies performed by Bores in the Soviet Union in 1976

| Patients | Pre-operative | | | | Post-operative | | | |
| | Refraction (D) | | Uncorrected vision | | Refraction (D) | | Uncorrected vision | |
	OD	OS	OD	OS	OD	OS	OD	OS
1	3.00	3.25	20/160	20/200	Plano	−0.25	20/20	20/25
2	4.50	4.50	20/200	20/200	Plano	Plano	20/25	20/25
3	3.75	3.25	20/200	20/160	Plano	−0.37	20/20	20/30
4	3.00	3.00	20/160	20/160	Plano	−0.25	20/20	20/25
5	7.00	7.25	20/400	20/400	−1.50	−1.25*	20/60	20/60
6	10.50	4.50	20/400	20/300	−4.00	Plano	20/200	20/20

*Reverted to −3.25 D OU (incisions too shallow). Remainder stable at 3 years.

(a)

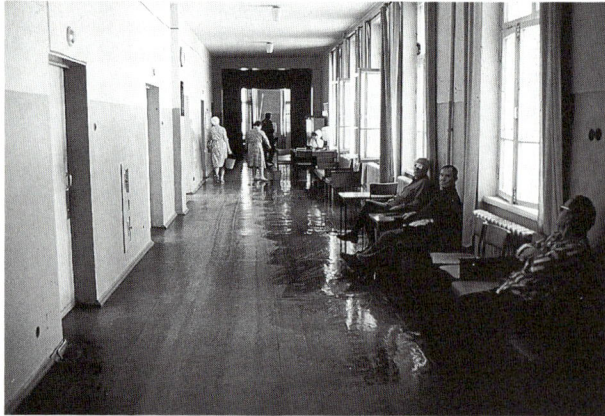

(b)

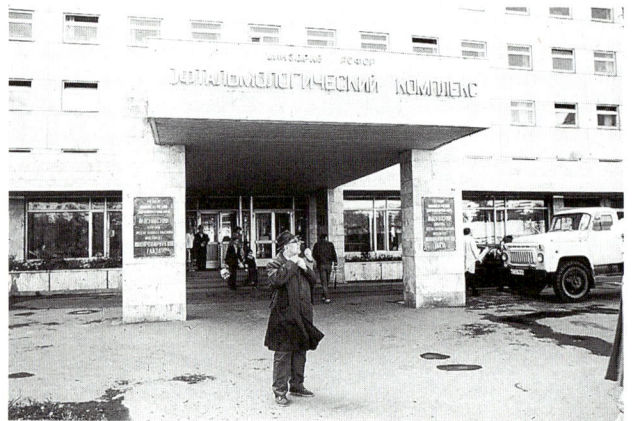

Fig. 7.3 (a) The main corridor of the original clinic—Hospital # 81, 10 Lobninskaya Street, Moscow. (b) The entrance to the Moscow Scientific Institute for Eye Microsurgery, 59a Beskudnikovsky Blvd.

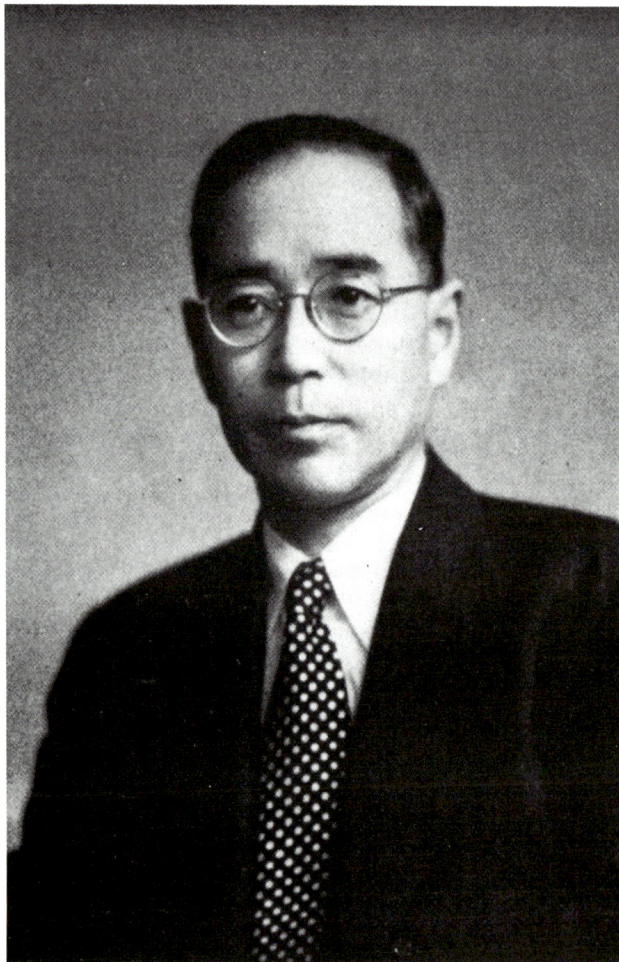

Fig. 7.4 Tutomu Sato, MD (Courtesy of A. Momose.)

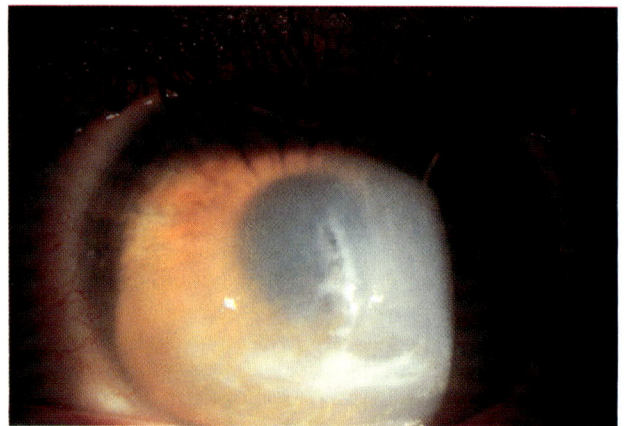

Fig. 7.5 A case of spontaneous rupture of Descemet's membrane in keratoconus.

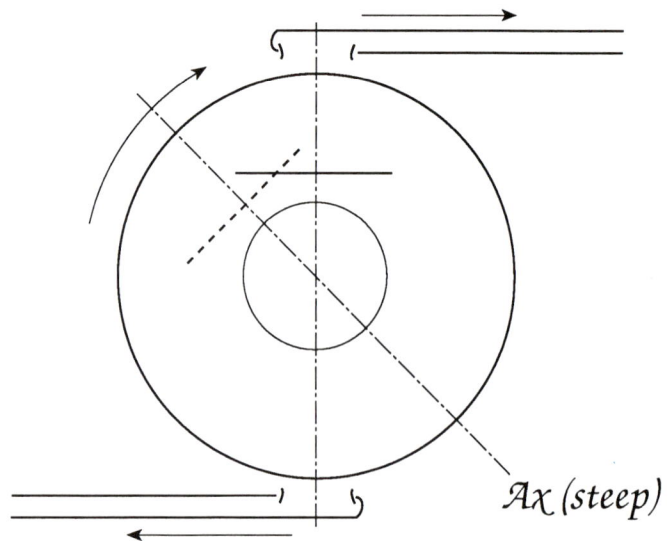

Fig. 7.6 Bridle sutures enabled the surgeon to rotate the eye as necessary.

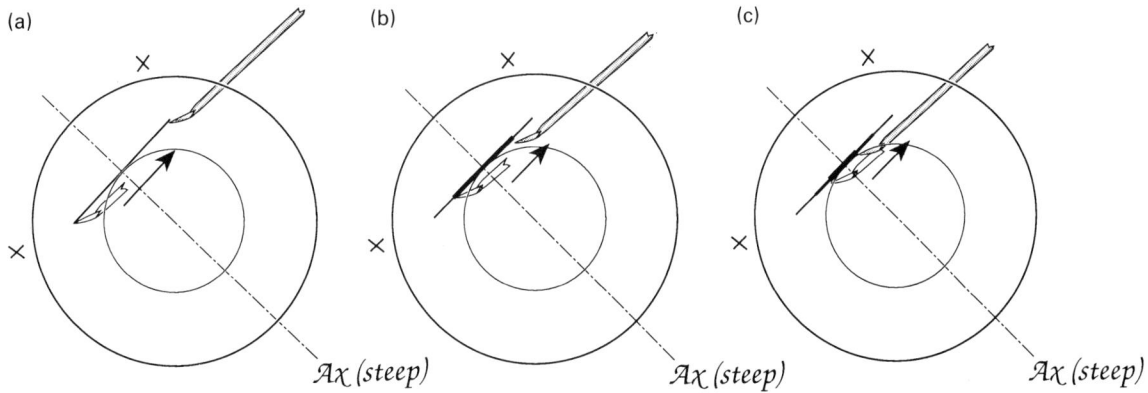

Fig. 7.7 (a) Internal transverse incisions were made tangential to the pupil. (b and c) Repeated passes were made as necessary.

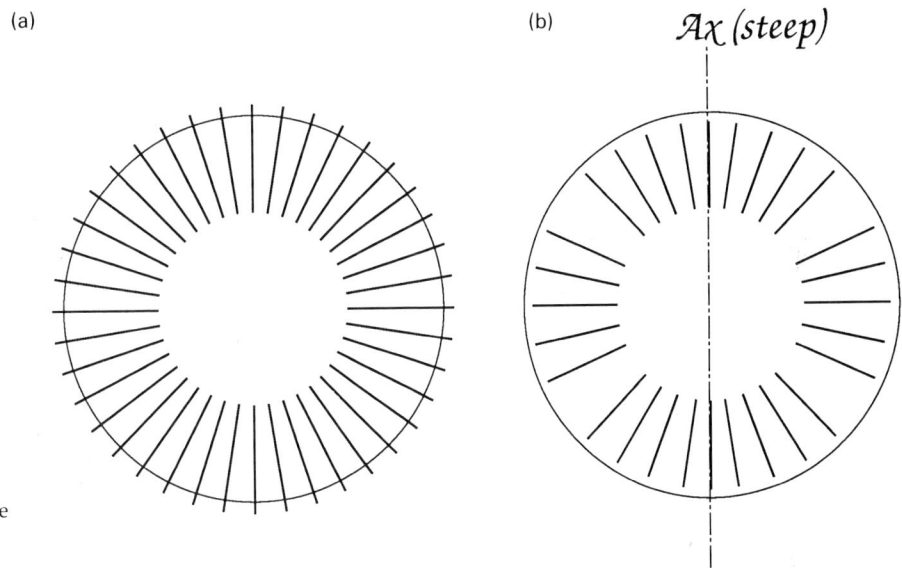

Fig. 7.8 (a) For spherical myopia, internal radiating incisions were followed by external radials. (b) In some cases of astigmatism, incisions were grouped.

Germany or the USA. Sato himself performed 200 of these cases between 1938 and 1943. It was widely used by Japanese ophthalmic surgeons and was taught to medical students after the war. Nevertheless, it was a technically difficult operation to perform. It required great skill on the part of the surgeon, necessitating incisions being made *ab interno*, through half the corneal thickness and in a straight line, close to the optic center. The method by which he performed these incisions for astigmatism is detailed in Chapter 9. For now we will confine our discussion to the extension of this technique to spherical myopia.

Sato found that anterior and posterior incisions made in the extrapupillary portion of the cornea resulted in a lengthening of the radius of the corneal curvature overlying the pupil. This of course reduced the corneal refractive power, making it relatively more hyperopic. In the rabbit eye, anterior incisions produced minimal central corneal flattening whereas posterior incisions produced a maximum flattening of

2 D [7]. Hence Sato was induced to employ incisions of this latter type when he extended this work into human eyes for mild myopia. For higher degrees of myopia, both anterior and posterior half-incisions were used.

Figures 7.6 through 7.8 show the method of performing this operation. Topical application as well as retrobulbar injection of anesthetic was used, the latter raising the specter of possible posterior bulbar perforation (see also Chapter 15). The latter anesthesia was to insure complete immobilization of the eye as well as to create slight proptosis of the globe, a method still advocated by some today (D. Shepard, 1988, personal communication). Bridle sutures were placed around the tendons of both vertical recti so as to be able to rotate the globe freely. The optic clear zone, approximately 6 mm in diameter, was delineated by making a loop of sterile gray human hair or fine white fishgut (this was later changed to a mark made with gentian violet) and placing it on to the cornea, centered

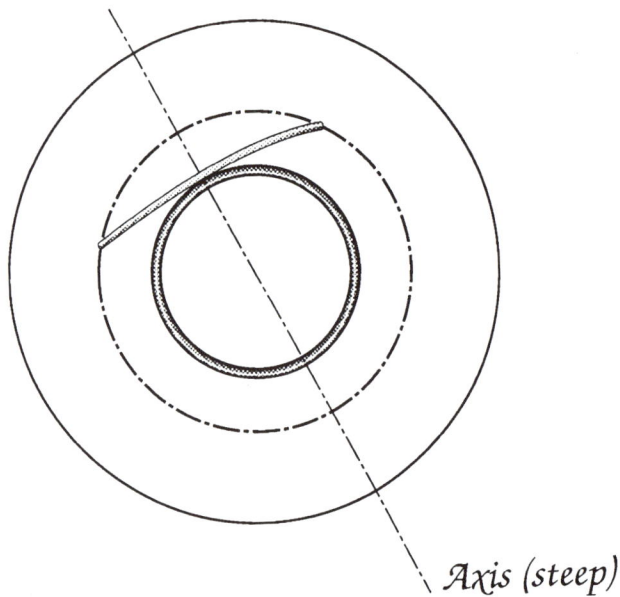

Axis (steep)

Fig. 7.9 A loop or length of human hair was used to delineate the optic clear zone and/or the extent of the T-cut.

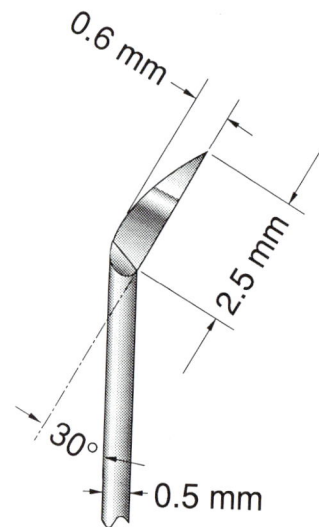

Fig. 7.10 Sketch of the blade of Sato's knife.

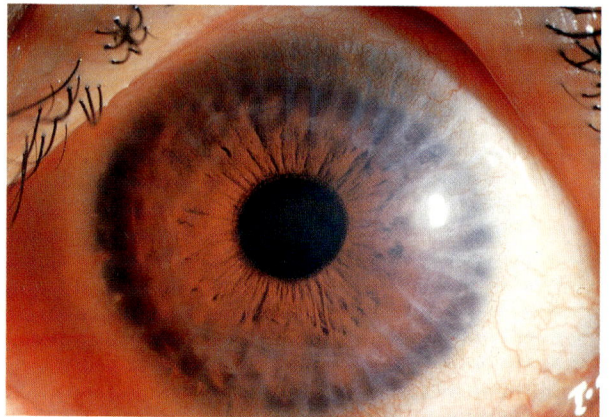

Fig. 7.11 The left eye of a 47-year-old female who had undergone the procedure of Sato 30 years previously. The other eye is similar. Distance visual acuity is 6/9, uncorrected. (Courtesy of A. Momose.)

on the miotic pupil (Figure 7.9). If astigmatism was also to be treated, four additional straight pieces of hair or gut (or dye marks) were laid in place on the major and minor meridians.

A specially designed knife (Figure 7.10) was then inserted into the anterior chamber at the superior limbus through a 2 mm scleral tunnel. This tunnel was important to minimize flattening of the anterior chamber—this type of incision is self-closing. Usually five to nine incisions were first made in the infero-posterior cornea, theoretically to 66% of its thickness (Figure 7.11). The operative word here is theoretically. The author has examined several of these patients and estimates the depth of the incisions as ranging from 20% to 95% of the corneal thickness. The center of the incision was used to make the estimate since there is a tendency in the Sato operation for both the beginning and end of the incisions to be shallower than the center. After each incision was made, from the limbus toward the center, the knife was disengaged by turning it to the side to prevent damage to the central clear zone. These incisions were followed by the same number made in the superior cornea by entering the anterior chamber at the inferior limbus. Finally nasal and then temporal incisions were added. Thus, some 20–36 incisions were made *ab interno*, with as many as six entries into the anterior chamber.

Posterior incisions alone were found to correct only an average of −1.2 D with a maximum of −4.5 D in the 35 cases reported in 1952 [8]. Therefore, in cases of myopia exceeding 2.0 D, an additional 40 incisions were made in a radial fashion through the anterior cornea from optic zone to limbal sclera. In this instance

a guarded knife similar to a Lancaster sclerotome (Okamura's knife) was utilized with the guard set to prevent perforation (Figure 7.12). How Sato determined the exact setting of this knife is not mentioned in any of his papers; however it was set to a uniform 0.6 mm in all cases. The average corneal thickness in the human at 6.0 mm is 640 μm; thus Sato was not far off, but was, in any case, too shallow. In this way, Sato and his associates obtained a mean correction of −3.0 D in a range from −1.12 to −7.0 D for the next 32 eyes. On the basis of this work, he drew two conclusions:

> We consider that this procedure, if properly performed, will safely cure myopia up to four diopters, and will produce marked improvement in myopia of from five to six diopters. This treatment, therefore, is efficacious for 95% of the

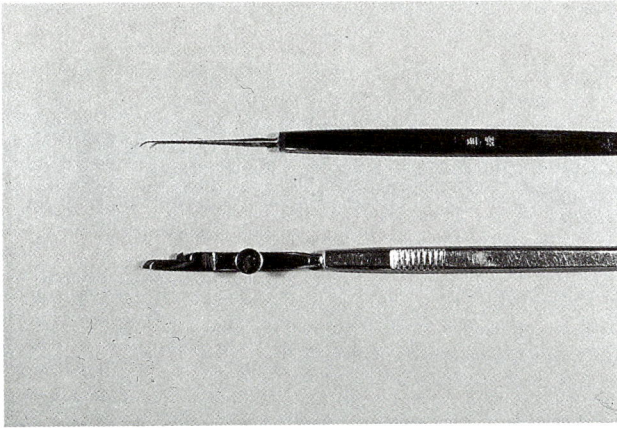

Fig. 7.12 Sato's knife (above); Okamura's knife (below). (Courtesy of A. Momose.)

myopic cases in Japan . . . no detrimental effects from this procedure have been observed, and none of the cases demonstrated any . . . loss of visual acuity.

His follow-up was only 5 months when he made this statement and both claims proved to be premature.

Akiyama [9,10] reported on the post-operative changes in two groups of eyes operated by the Sato method. The average change was 3.2 D in the first group of 172 eyes, with a range from -0.5 to -11.5 D, 70% of the eyes achieving an effect of -1.5 to -4.0 D. The average overall correction in the second group of 177 eyes was -2.8 D with a maximum of -10.5 D. In the eyes with over -4.0 D, the mean correction was -3.9 D. He concluded, as had Sato, that more than 35 posterior and more than 40 anterior incisions should be performed. He emphasized that posterior incisions should reach as deep as possible without perforation. From 1948 through 1959 (when contact lenses were introduced to Japan) Sato and his associates performed 681 similar cases, reporting similar results.

Unfortunately, the damage done to the corneal endothelium by posterior incisions frequently produced corneal opacification that only appeared 10–24 years later (Figures 7.13 and 7.14). In addition, certain technical deficiencies resulted in many low corrections in which the result did not warrant the risk of the surgery. Consequently, the surgery was abandoned. It was subsequently discovered that the reason for the corneal decompensation was the destruction of the

(a)

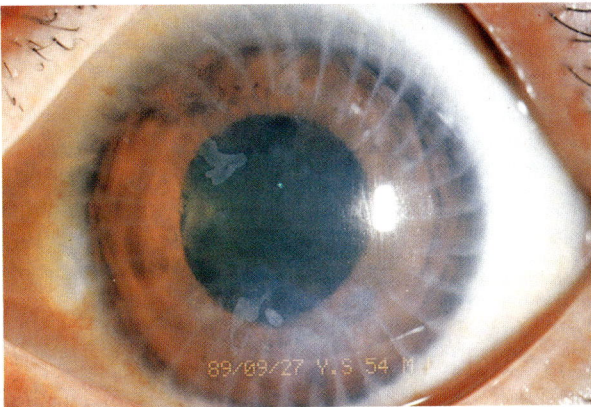

(b)

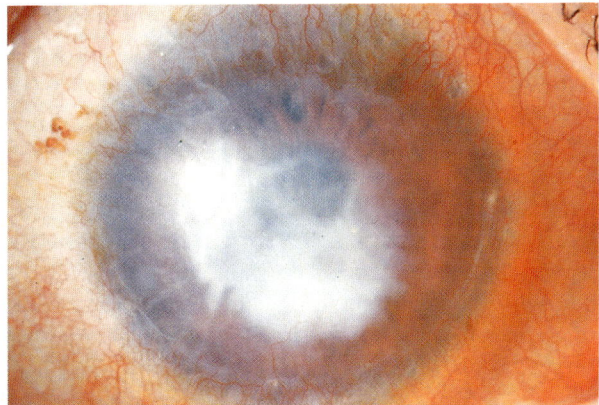

(c)

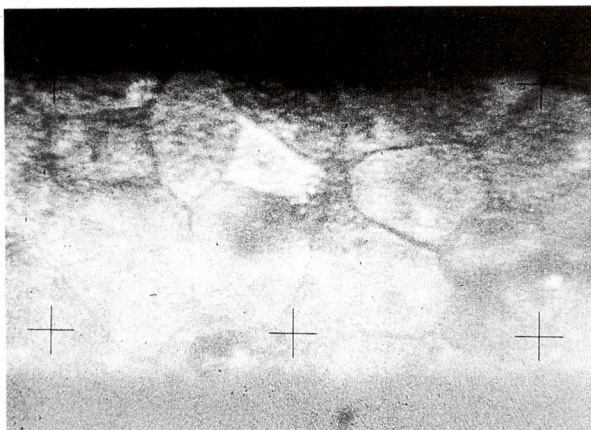

Fig. 7.13 (a) Moderate corneal decompensation following Sato's operation. (b) A more severe case with fibrous proliferation. (c) Peripheral endothelial cells in (b). (Courtesy of A. Momose.)

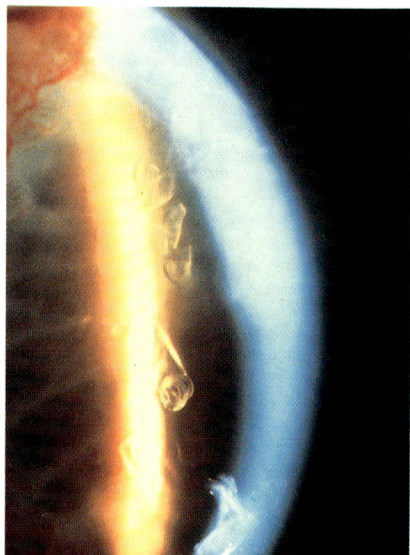

Fig. 7.14 The endothelial "tubes" and thickened cornea illustrate the cause of corneal decompensation in these cases.

corneal endothelial pump caused by the internal incisions—something never considered by the technique's author.

This should come as no surprise since the role of the corneal endothelium in maintaining corneal detumescence was almost completely unknown at the time. Neither were operating microscopes available. A film of Sato operating shows him wearing loupes. These provide only limited magnification and typically a small field of view. Operating in this fashion, it made sense to make the incisions from the posterior surface because presumably the knife tip could be seen more clearly as it approached the surface. Considering the fact that the corneal reaction must have been intense and with the availability of Okamura's guarded knife, to persist in this approach was brave—at the very least. It is obvious that the incisional depth must have

varied tremendously, as evidenced by the author's own examination of some of these patients. Additionally, Akiyama reported a range of corrections from 0 to −10.5 D. This effect and variability is respectively much less and much greater than that of present-day RK surgery, even with large clear zones.

Kanai, working at Juntendo University in Tokyo— the school where Sato was a professor—has followed 80 of the eyes of 50 patients (out of 281 myopic eyes upon which Dr Sato performed the operation after 1951) from 1971 through 1980. Sixty of the 80 eyes (75%) developed bullous keratopathy. It is assumed (without any evidence) that the remaining 581 eyes shared the same fate. Interestingly, in some patients in whom identical bilateral surgery was performed, only one eye developed bullous changes with resulting decrease in vision (see Chapter 15) [11].

When Kanai and his co-workers examined the ultrastructure of several corneal buttons removed from these patients at the time of keratoplasty, they found inter- and intra-cellular epithelial edema, disrupted epithelial basement membrane and Bowman's layer, increased inter-fibrillar spacing in the stroma, and abnormal collagenous material posterior to the normal portion of Descemet's membrane. The endothelium was absent in these cases.

That this problem occurred in a sizeable number of patients is not due to either the nature of Japanese corneas or the fact of incisions. That this was due solely to damaged endothelium can be seen in Japanese corneas operated with current RK techniques and with no endothelial involvement (Figure 7.15). In fact, despite the large number of cases of RK surgery which have been performed in the last 12 years, endothelial cell loss and consequent corneal decompensation have not been a factor (see also Chapter 15).

There has been considerable discussion of the Sato technique and its failure to produce good results coupled with its high complication rate in the form of

(b)

(a)

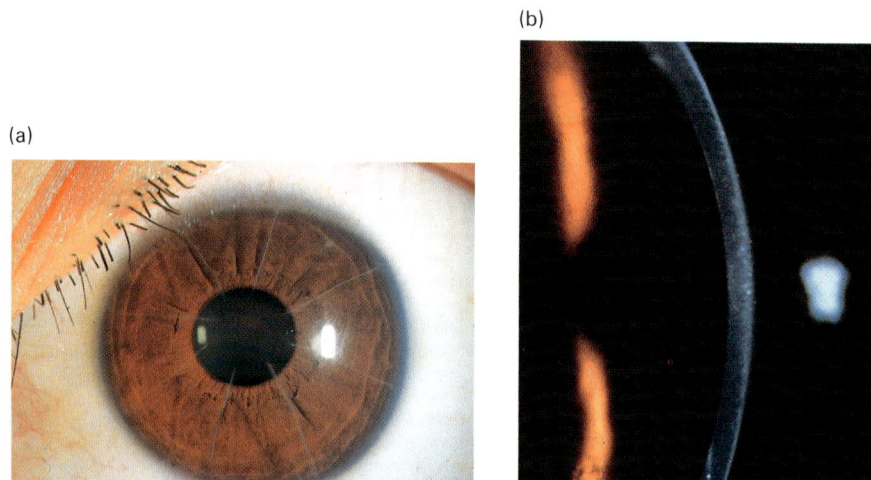

Fig. 7.15 RK in a Japanese patient. Note the total absence of endothelial involvement. (Courtesy of A. Momose.)

corneal decompensation [12]. It has been flatly stated that 80–85% of Professor Sato's cases resulted in some degree of corneal decompensation. But is this really true? It is not generally appreciated that not all of his cases were failures and that not all of the corneas became cloudy. I'm struck by the lack of completed follow-up in these cases. Only 281 (40% of 681) of the entire group of eyes—recall that Sato had performed 681 cases of this kind between 1951 and 1960—were studied and only 172 (61%) of that group were completely followed. In this group, 129 (75%) of the eyes developed bullous keratopathy. In short, 45% of the patients retained in follow-up developed this complication. The question has to be asked: what happened to the rest of the patients? We have been painted a picture of long lines of people requiring corneal transplantation as a result of this surgery. If there is truth in the observation that only problem patients can be counted on to return for follow-up, then the picture changes dramatically. For example, 129 eyes out of 681 is only 19%! High to be sure, but not the unmitigated disaster that has been described by so many, even if we were to double that number. Not withstanding, the procedure was stopped because the risks outweighed the benefits. Professor Momose, however, is of the opinion that the surgery fell into disuse for two reasons: the untimely death of professor Sato on 9 June 1960 at the age of 58, and the availability of contact lenses (A. Momose, 1990, personal communication).

Such a poor beginning has created considerable opposition to the adoption of a more modern and advanced technique—RK. This is particularly true among Japanese ophthalmologists who are loath to perform RK—only 10 are doing it at this writing. Many of these physicians are still confused between modern RK surgery and the procedure of Sato. They are not alone, as evidenced by the continued resistance to this surgery in the USA. Our better appreciation of the role of the endothelium in maintaining corneal clarity, coupled with advances such as the operating microscope, ultrasonic pachymeter, and more refined methods of corneal curvature measurement, has changed not only the performance of the surgery but its potential as well.

Early history and development of RK

RK had its beginning in 1973 after a chance observation of corneal flattening following ocular trauma in a child. Sasha was talking when he should have been listening, it seems—some school mate punched him in the eye, breaking the glasses he was wearing at the time. Svatyslav N. Fyodorov, MD, who at that time was director of the Hospital for Experimental Eye Surgery in Moscow, USSR, was stopped in the hallway by the

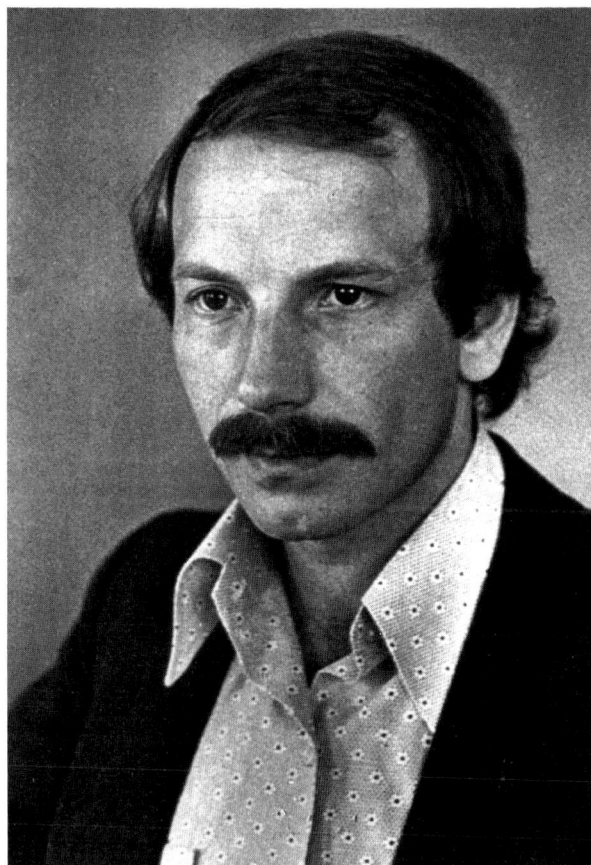

Fig. 7.16 V.V. Durnev, MD, Fyodorov's original co-worker in the development of RK.

patient who informed him that he could now see clearly without glasses in his injured eye. Professor Fyodorov examined the boy and found that he had a small curvilinear incision in the para-center of his left cornea, sparing the visual axis. The patient's myopia had been reduced 3D by this fortuitous accident. In characteristic Fyodorov fashion the professor mused: "*Chort vohz me*! If a fist can do this, so can I. After all, I'm an eye surgeon." Accordingly he began investigating the possibilities of such surgical intervention, assigning a young staffer named Valerie Durnev to the task (Figure 7.16).

A search of the literature turned up not only the work of Sato but of some Soviets as well, including Pureskin [13,14] who had duplicated Sato's work. Durnev and Fyodorov also repeated some of Sato's work in rabbits and at least once in a human subject, verifying most of Sato's findings, including a tremendous corneal reaction not reported by the Japanese surgeon (Figure 7.17). Consequently, posterior incisions were rejected out of hand. Continued study showed that combining deep anterior incisions with a smaller optical clear zone resulted in a more profound reduction in corneal curvature than had been reported by Sato [15,16].

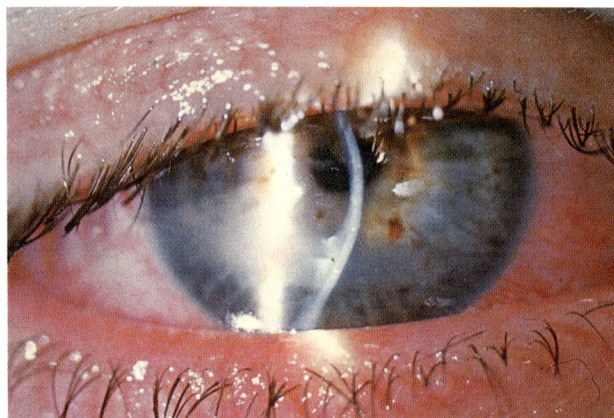

Fig. 7.17 One of Fyodorov's pre-RK patients with an internal T-cut. Note the extreme corneal reaction. Compare with Figure 6.2.

By October 1973, Fyodorov and Durnev had made several important changes in the surgery, to whit:

1 Varying the size of the optical zone from 2.0 (later enlarged to 3.0) mm to 6.0 mm, depending upon the degree of myopia (Figure 7.18).

2 Making all incisions from the external surface of the cornea—*ab externo*—thus minimizing the possibility of damaging the delicate endothelial cells (Figure 7.19). It was not certain at that time whether or not external incisions affected the endothelium. However, endothelial cell counts were made on all patients because of the concern that even incising the cornea from the outside might somehow act to produce cell damage. It was evident, however, from these examinations, that no significant cell loss was occurring and that the cell loss described in the cases of Sato was a consequence of direct trauma to the endothelium itself (Figure 7.20).

3 Basing incision depth on actual measurements of corneal thickness using optical pachymetry, and verifying the depth of the incisions with specially constructed gauges or "dipsticks" (Figure 7.21).

4 Using ultra-sharp disposable razor fragments to make the incisions. These incisions were made, at first, free-hand with an unguarded blade using special gauges called corneal dipsticks to check progress.

5 Limiting incisions to 32 made from the limbus, converging upon a pre-marked optical zone.

6 Using a microscope with all its advantages to do the surgery.

It was apparent from the beginning that the use of an unguarded blade would produce an incision of uneven depth and that this condition could be responsible for the variation in effect from patient to patient and the consequent difficulty in predicting the outcome. In addition, the smaller optical zones (2.0–2.5 mm) were difficult to center. Some of those patients complained of glare at night, and some of the incisions

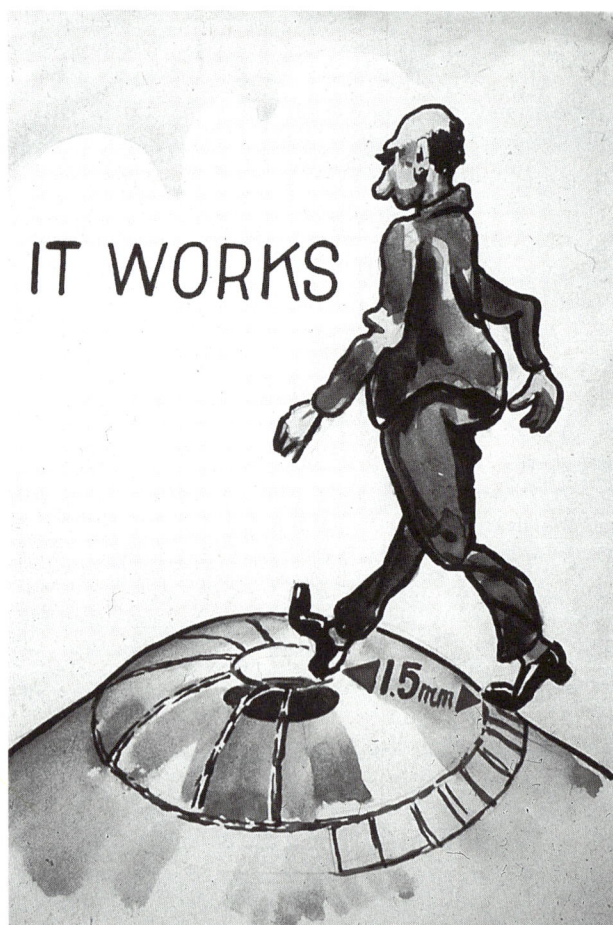

Fig. 7.18 Making the zone smaller than 6.0 mm works.

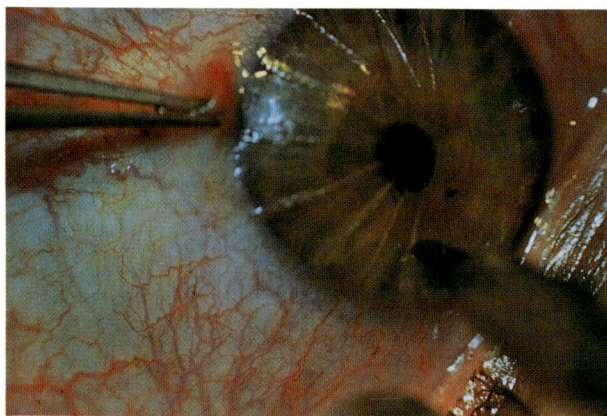

Fig. 7.19 Dosaged dissection of the circumferential ligament of Kokott scratched out in error, circa 1973.

tended to join up at the edge of the optical zone—especially those in whose corneas 32 incisions had been made. The first step in solving these problems was the fabrication of a micro-metrically adjustable knife handle which allowed precise control of incision depth (Figure 7.22). At the same time a marking device

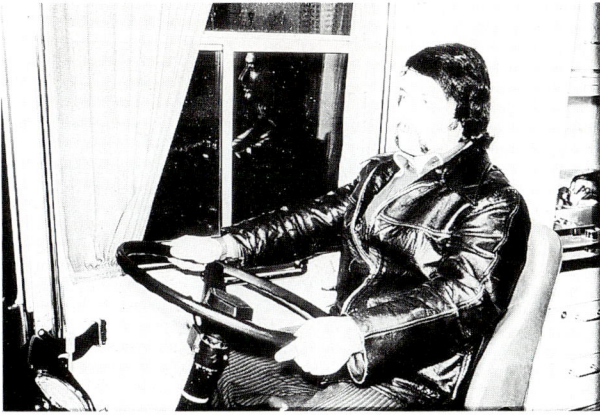

Fig. 7.20 The first RK patient—Mischa, the author's driver.

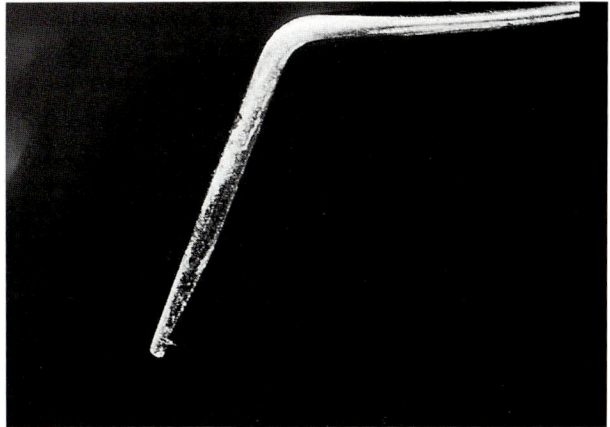

Fig. 7.21 Original Fyodorov dipstick.

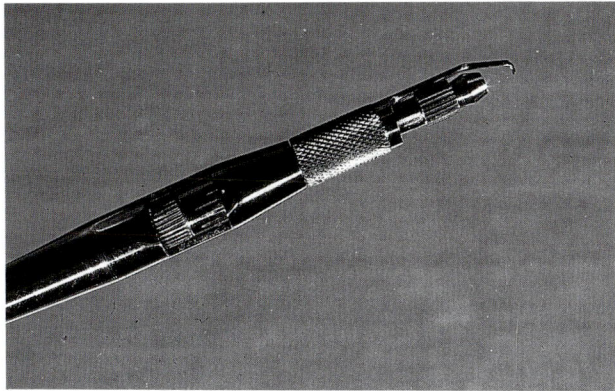

Fig. 7.22 Second-generation Fyodorov micrometer knife.

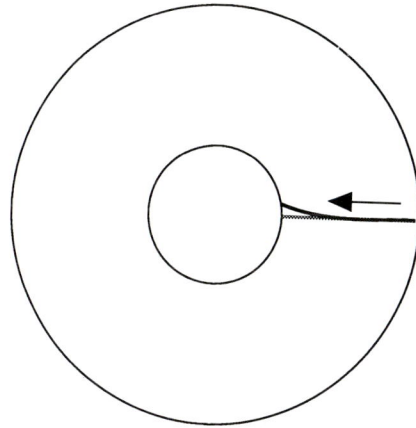

Fig. 7.24 Incisions made from the limbus tend to meet the central optical zone tangentially.

(a)   (b)

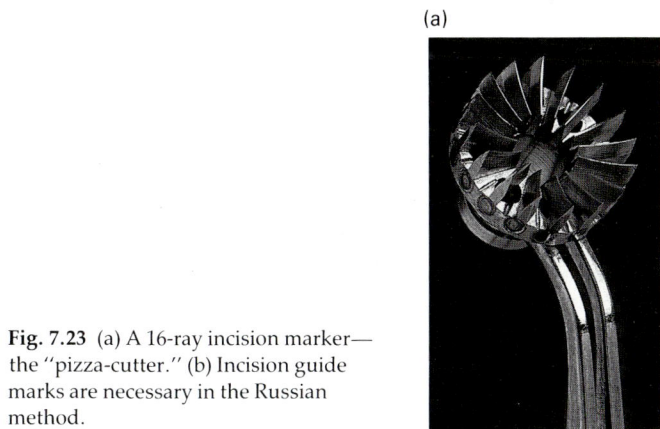

Fig. 7.23 (a) A 16-ray incision marker— the "pizza-cutter." (b) Incision guide marks are necessary in the Russian method.

(originally called a "pizza-cutter," an unfortunate choice of name because many people believed that this was the device that produced the incisions) was developed to make lines or marks upon the corneal surface, along which the surgeon could guide the knife (Figure 7.23). This was necessary in the Soviet method because incisions made from the limbus toward the center have a tendency to approach the optical zone tangentially like turbine blades instead of in a perpendicular manner (Figure 7.24).

Ongoing work with rabbit eyes suggested that a reduction in the number of incisions would not be

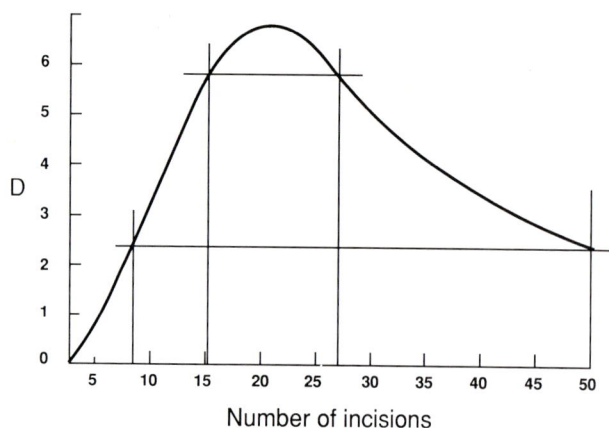

Fig. 7.25 Effect of incision number on outcome.

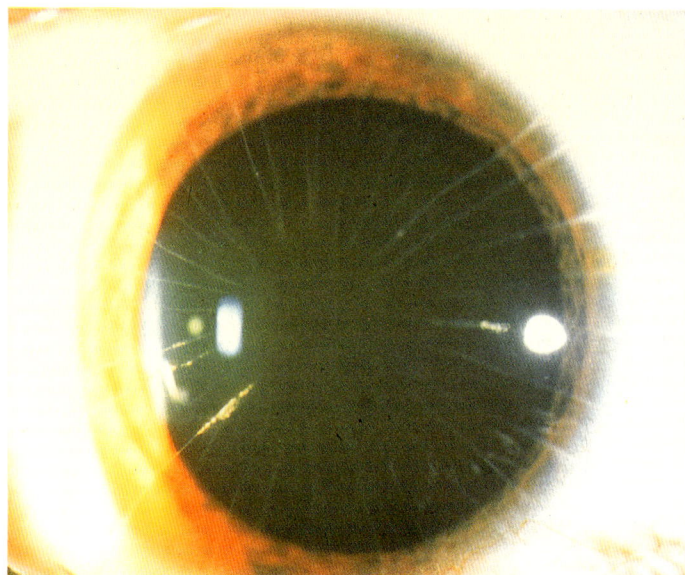

Fig. 7.26 Early 32-incision RK. Note that the central incisions join in some cases.

accompanied by any significant lessening of effect until the number of incisions fell below 16 (Figure 7.25). This was good news since one of the difficulties experienced in the early cases was that of keeping the ends of the incisions from joining up centrally (Figure 7.26). Cases with eight incisions not only showed a profound loss of effect (40–50%) but were also accompanied by a significant increase in surgically induced astigmatism. The reduction in number of incisions from 32 to 16, however, not only solved the problem of incisional merging but also, to a great extent, that of glare. In addition, comparing the results of 16 and 32 incisions of equal depth and length showed no significant difference in effect [17]. Additionally, it was found through application that increasing the number of incisions beyond 32 *decreased* the effect of the surgery. It is interesting to note that the effect of 40 incisions was almost identical to that of eight incisions. This phenomenon is undoubtedly one of the reasons for the poor overall results in the cases of Sato. The failure of more incisions (beyond a certain number) to produce a greater response has to do with the mechanism whereby the central corneal curvature is caused to flatten.

Mechanism of RK

The effects of the procedure depend upon the temporary structural weakening of the corneal periphery, thus allowing internal ocular pressure to move this area outward (Figure 7.27). This small movement of the periphery produces tension both upon the scleral ring and upon the unincised central clear zone. The scleral ring resists distortion and therefore most of the resultant force acts upon the central cornea. The effect of this force is to produce an increase in the chord length of the central arc with a concomitant reduction

in its sagittal height (Figure 7.28). In short, the corneal curvature becomes more flattened (Figure 7.29).

This flattening effect is dependent upon pressure acting on the tissue bands which lie between incisions and which connect the more flexible central clear zone with the relatively inflexible limbus. In materials science, it is sometimes seen that the modulus of elasticity of a material changes when its cross-sectional dimension also changes. As the section becomes thinner, the material will distort more before fracture occurs than will a thicker section—the material has become more stretchy or malleable. Thus, as the pressure acts upon the thinner corneal tissue bands seen in cases with high numbers of incisions, much of the tension is lost through stretching—the periphery bulges more—rather than acting upon the clear zone to induce flattening. Therefore, incisions in excess of 16 are superfluous and serve not only to reduce the ultimate effect of the surgery but may introduce additional problems such as glare or even irregular astigmatism (see also Chapter 15).

In the literature there are two models related to an estimation of curvature change due to RK surgery in which the cornea is considered as a uniform sphere. The model in the current discussion is based on the concept of effective thickness associated with cutting of fibrils by the incisions and is based on the analysis promulgated by Huang and co-workers [18]. These type of analyses are important in order to derive algorithms which can precisely predict the outcome of this surgery.

Figures 7.30 and 7.31 are tensor diagrams outlining the effect of incisions upon this theoretic thin corneal

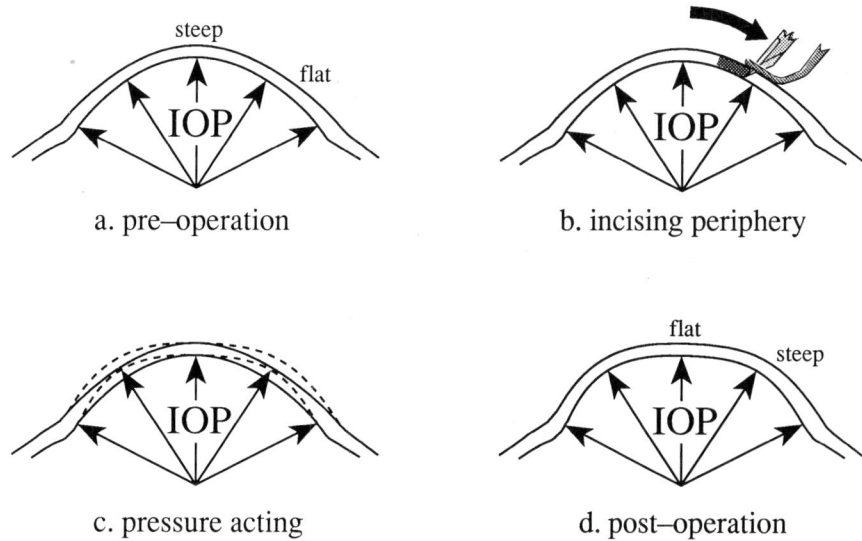

a. pre–operation

b. incising periphery

c. pressure acting

d. post–operation

Fig. 7.27 Mechanism of RK. (a) Pre-operation, the central cornea is steeper than the periphery. (b) The periphery is incised to weaken it. (c) The intra-ocular pressure pushes out on the weakened stroma, causing it to bulge (see Figure 7.28). (d) The result, post-operatively, is to steepen the periphery and flatten the center.

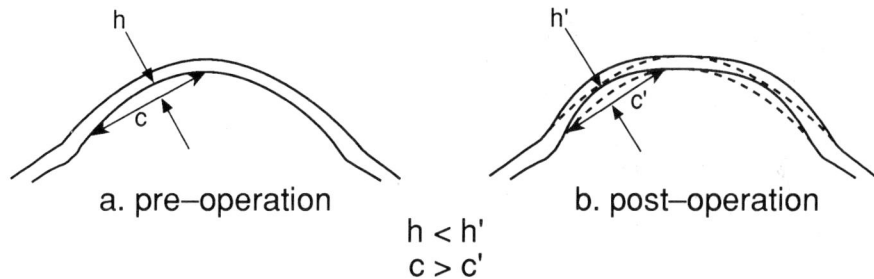

a. pre–operation

b. post–operation

h < h'
c > c'

Fig. 7.28 After surgery the bulging of the cornea shortens the chord length in the periphery and lengthens the chord in the center, flattening it.

shell. Figure 7.30 is a generalized tensor while Figure 7.31 is specific for a cornea undergoing RK. However, Kirchoff–Love assumptions, typically used to describe thin elastic plates, are inadequate for this purpose when dealing with impaired shells such as are found in the human cornea undergoing incisional weakening. Therefore, another method needs to be applied—transverse shear deformation analysis [19]. Moderate to severe transverse shear deformations appear in certain types of composite plates and shells in which the transverse shear modulus to in-plane elastic modulus ratios are very low. The cornea is an example of such a shell. These deformations become obvious in the vicinity of some locations such as partial-thickness incisions (Figure 7.32). Under certain circumstances, this local severe transverse shear deformation may rise sharply and influence the entire structural response. The mathematics of the analysis of such a shell are complex but are well-detailed by Reissner [20,21] and Whitney [22] for those so inclined.

There are many factors which, acting together, determine the extent to which the cornea will respond to this stromal weakening. Some of these are physical properties—such as modulus of elasticity—which are poorly understood or whose elucidation is lacking in

humans. However, there are some assumptions which can be made about these factors which appear to have a bearing on the mechanism of RK.

Early attempts at predicting the outcome

The problem of predictability was tackled by an extensive retrospective analysis of the patients in whom surgery had already been performed. From this analysis it was found that certain factors seemed to control the outcome of the surgery:

Optic zone—as the optic zone size decreased, the amount of correction increased (Figure 7.33).

Keratometry—as the corneal refractive power increased, the amount of correction also increased (Figure 7.34).

Corneal diameter—as the corneal diameter increased, there was a corresponding increase in the amount of the correction (Figure 7.35).

Corneal rigidity—as the cornea became stiffer, the amount of correction increased (Figure 7.36). This may seem illogical but it is, nevertheless, true and is the leading cause of over-corrections in patients over 40 years of age.

Practical coefficient of the surgeon—see below.

(a)

(b)

(c)

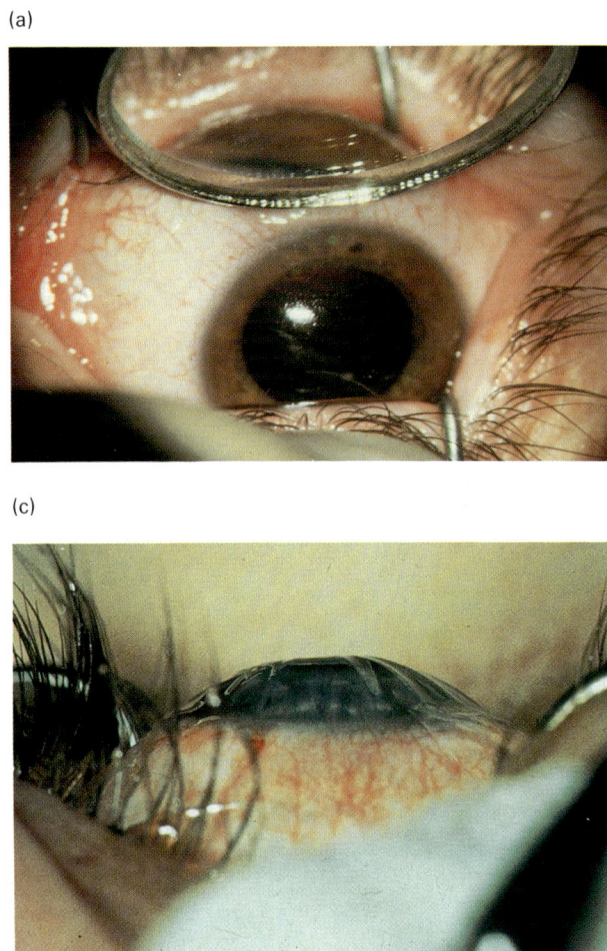

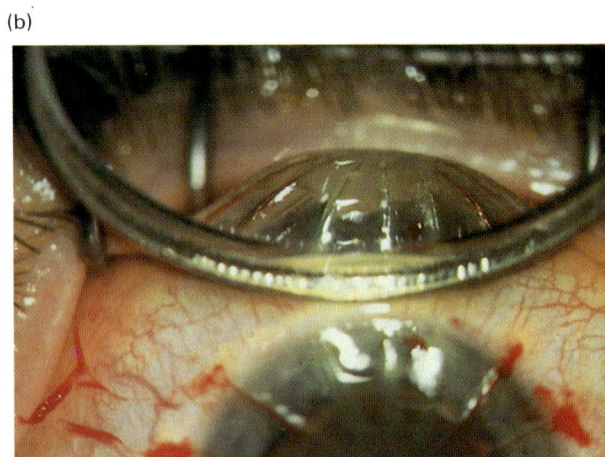

Fig. 7.29 (a) Pre-operative cornea—note the prolate shape. (b) Post-operative cornea—note the oblate shape. (c) Side view shows the flattening better.

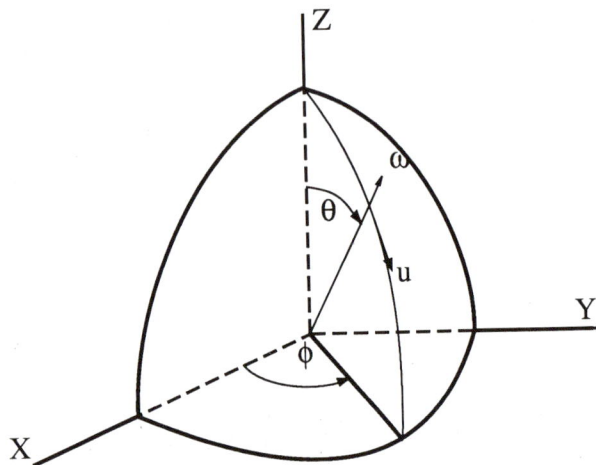

Fig. 7.30 General (simple) tensor diagram.

what was really being described was the effective depth of the incisions which increased as the surgeon became more skilled at making them and less timid in setting the blade (see the section on blades, below).

From these observations a formula was constructed:

$$P = \frac{\sqrt{D^2 + \frac{16}{3}\left(R - \sqrt{R^2 - \frac{D^2}{4}}\right)^2} - \sqrt{d^2 + \frac{16}{3}\left(R - \sqrt{R^2 - \frac{d^2}{4}}\right)^2}}{\sqrt{d^2 + \frac{16}{3}\left(R - \sqrt{R^2 - \frac{d^2}{4}}\right)^2}} \cdot K \cdot \alpha$$

This calculates the effect of surgery (P) given that: $D =$ the diameter of the cornea (in mm); $R =$ the radius of the cornea (in mm); $K =$ the coefficient of corneal rigidity, and $\alpha =$ the incisional depth coefficient. This allowed the surgeon to predict (within $\pm 1.00\,\text{D}$) the outcome of the surgery in most cases—at 1 year (Table 7.2). Other factors were eventually found to play a role and will be discussed later in this chapter.

Early changes in the technique

The author made some fundamental changes in the technique with that first case (described in the intro-duction) which had some far-reaching effects and

This latter factor, which eventually became known as the incisional depth coefficient, was an attempt to account for individual variations in the technique of the surgeon and was designed to be optimized as experience increased. It became quickly apparent that

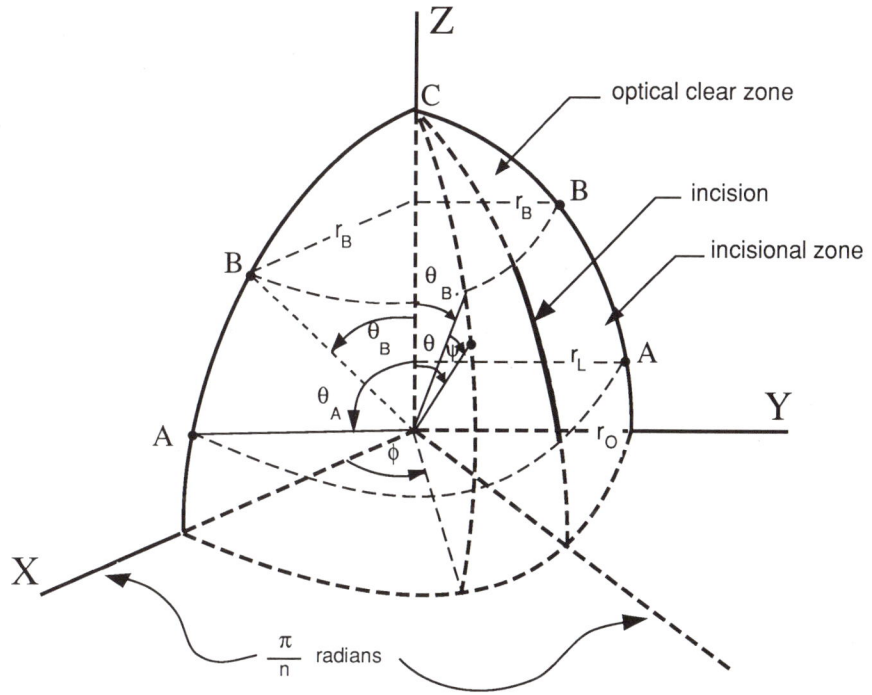

Fig. 7.31 Complex tensor diagram.

(a)

(b)

(c)

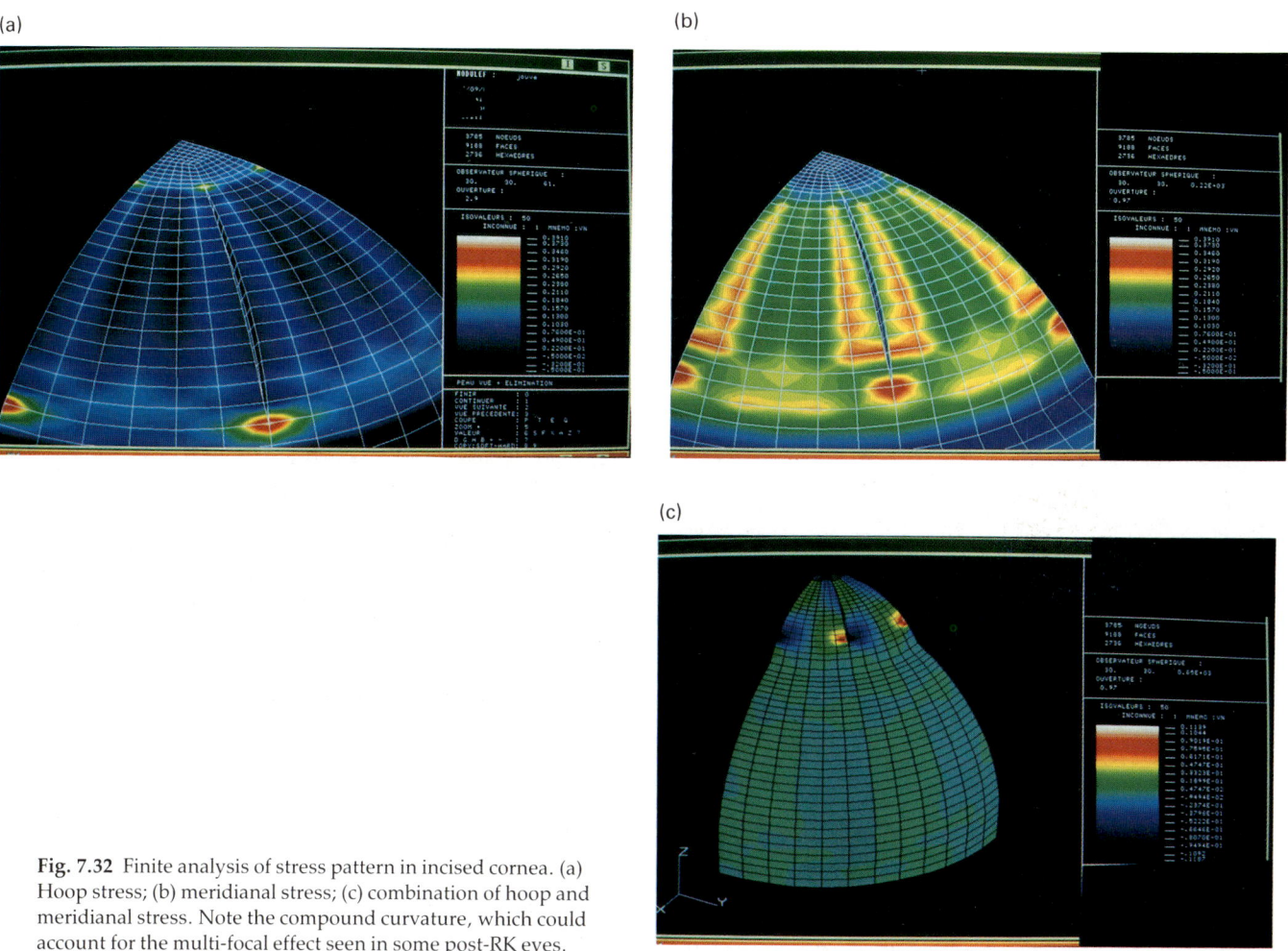

Fig. 7.32 Finite analysis of stress pattern in incised cornea. (a) Hoop stress; (b) meridianal stress; (c) combination of hoop and meridianal stress. Note the compound curvature, which could account for the multi-focal effect seen in some post-RK eyes.

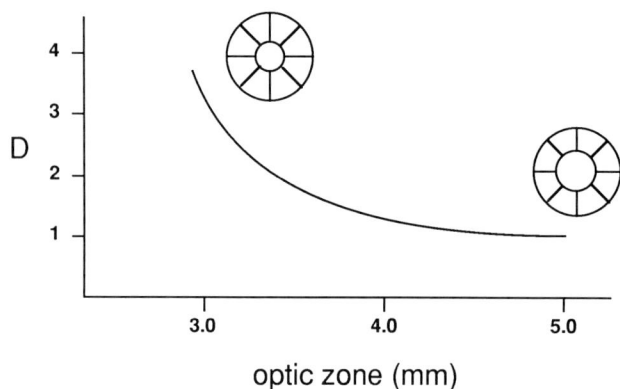

Fig. 7.33 Effect of changing optical zone size.

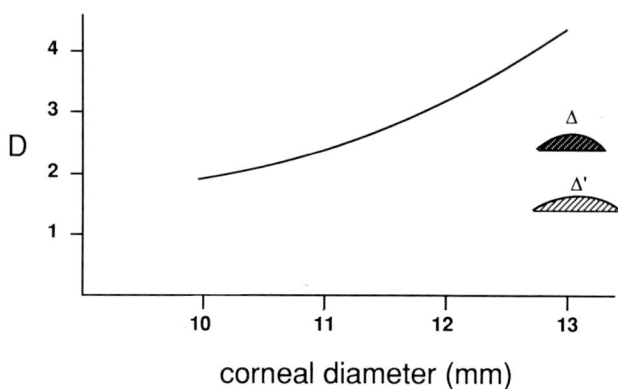

Fig. 7.35 Effect of corneal diameter.

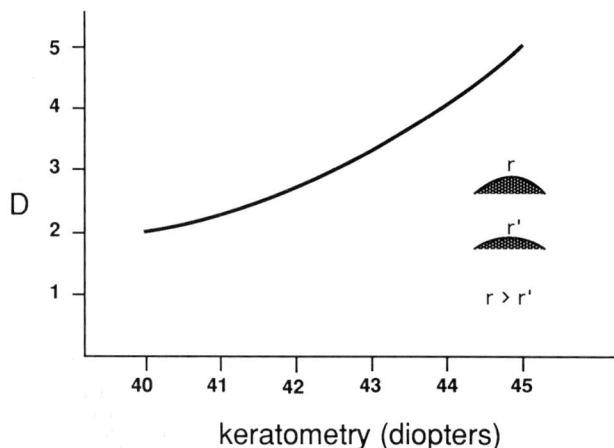

Fig. 7.34 Effect of corneal curvature.

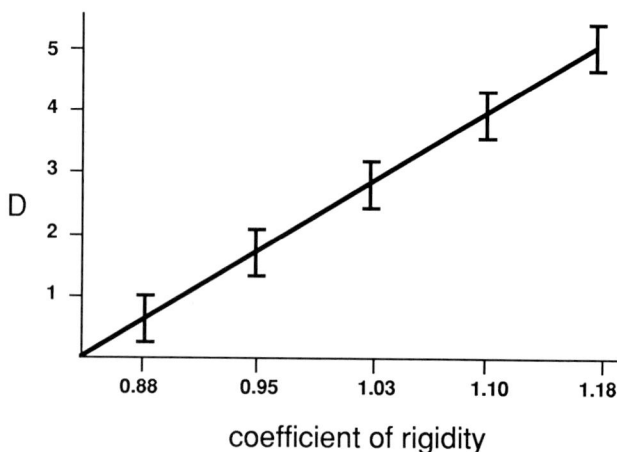

Fig. 7.36 Effect of corneal rigidity.

Table 7.2 The first nomogram used in radial keratotomy

Optical zone diameter (mm)	Effect (D)
4.5	0.75–1.25
4.0	1.50–2.00
3.5	2.25–2.50
3.0	>2.75

which forced a different perspective to be focused upon the subject of RK.

It was disturbing to me that the incisions were being made from the limbus toward the center. This methodology was then, as now, technically difficult and had the very real potential for causing a disaster should the patient move at the wrong instant, thus possibly causing an invasion of the optic zone or the optic axis. Even if the patient didn't move, making the incisions from limbus to center requires that pressure on the blade be released at the just the proper instant to prevent its stopping before the edge of the optical zone is reached. Attempts to re-start the blade in that event require that excessive pressure be placed on the knife to start it moving again. This is true even with

ultra-sharp crystalline blades, especially if the eye is soft. This excess pressure inevitably produces a sudden jumping forward of the blade as tissue resistance is overcome, almost always resulting in an invasion of the optical clear zone. Additionally, the incisions have a very real tendency to wander off-course and, unless each one is pre-marked, connect with the central zone mark in a tangential manner.

Therefore, beginning with my first solo case in 1978, all of the incisions were made from the central clear zone to the limbus, and all were made across from one another in pairs (i.e. 6 and 12, 3 and 9 o'clock, etc.), and not "around the clock." Doing it this centrifugal way eliminated the danger of invading the optical zone and the incisions were invariably very straight and perpendicular to the edge of the surgical clear zone. Another benefit of making the incisions in opposed pairs was that they spread around the effect of any incisional depth irregularity—a major concern given the quality of the blades used at that time. Because there is an ongoing change in corneal thickness during the surgery—something which begins to happen the moment Bowman's layer is incised—the order in which the incisions are made is of primary importance.

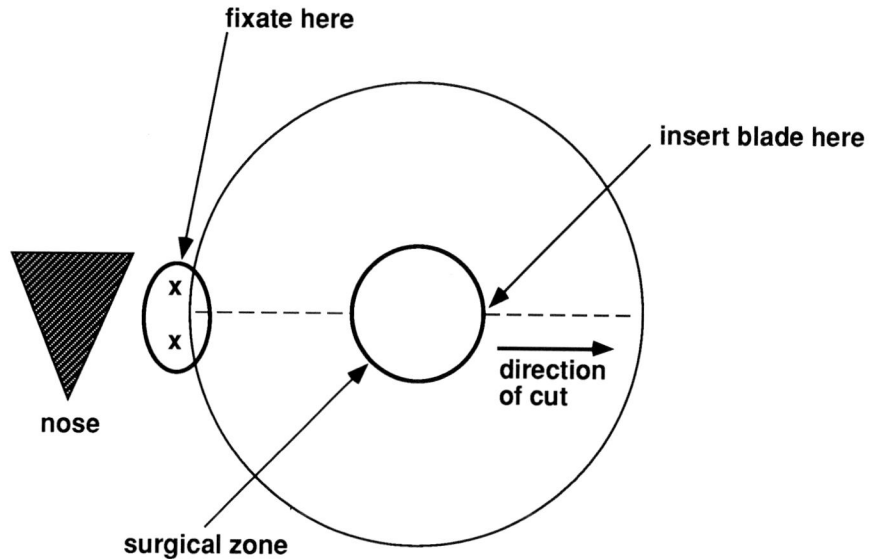

Fig. 7.37 Typical incision sequence: pairs of incisions with each member of the pair at 180° to its fellow.

In addition, the intra-ocular pressure of the eye decreases as each incision is made because the ciliary body is unable to keep pace with the increase in ocular volume which occurs as the incised tissue expands outward. It is reasonable, therefore, to expect that some variation in incision depth will occur with each additional incision as the resistance to cutting also decreases (see section on blades, below). While these incisional variations may be small by themselves, they have a cumulative effect and, being grouped or adjacent, will induce more or less flattening in a localized area, thereby producing irregular astigmatism. This is not just a theoretic concern.

Some of my early cases, which had been done in the Soviet manner, did indeed show just such astigmatism—especially the "wet" cases. It therefore made considerable sense to make incisions in horizontally opposed pairs, each incision in the pair being made 180° to the other (Figure 7.37). Making the incisions in this way also tends to reduce the chances of skipping an incision—something very likely to happen with pre-marking of the incision tracks as in the Fyodorov (out-to-in) or even in the Bores (in-to-out) technique. This is even more likely to occur with the neophyte keratotomist and one of the reasons the author recommends against such marking with his method. The marking material tends to obscure the incision track and may make it seem that an incision has been made when in fact it has not. Careful attention to this potential problem must be given when making incisions in the Russian manner where such pre-marking is essential.

Blades and pachymetry

At first, for a given blade setting—all else being as equal as possible—the initial surgical results obtained were different from what the Russians were reporting and so were the incisions. While I and my co-worker (William Myers, MD) were obtaining a good surgical effect initially, we were losing far more of it (56%) than Fyodorov had been reporting (20%). Our patients were also complaining of more glare at night. We also noted that our incisions were not as deep as the blade settings, and furthermore the shallower incisions were mainly to be found in the last eight incisions. It was obvious that the blade we were using at that time (Beaver #76a), whether because of its thickness, finish, or sharpness (or all three), was not cutting to its set depth. Also, the incisions were somewhat ragged and the resultant scars were slightly wider than seen with blades today. This, coupled with the fact that the eye became softer as more and more incisions were made (offering less resistance and therefore causing the tissue to "flow" away from the blade), resulted in shallow incisions from the outset, getting even shallower as the surgery went on.

It turned out that this incision shallowing was due in part to the direction in which the incisions were being made [23,24]. To logical types used to "dry-labbing" (resorting to theory without benefit of practical experience), that statement might not make sense—why would the direction of cut make any difference in the incision depth? The answer is, because the eye does not conform well to theory—the direction of the cut does make a difference and must be taken into account [25]. Binder has also suggested that centrifugal incision scars (in-to-out) tend to be thinner than centripetal (out-to-in) incision scars [26]. While the author has not noted this change in particular it could be that this is related to depth of the incision with a greater tendency of the incision to gape with deeper incisions. It should be added that greater incision depth and subsequent wider scarring may be operational in producing the progressive corneal flattening reported by some investigators (see also Chapter 15) [27,28], L.D. Bores, 1991, unpublished data).

The human cornea, as a rule, is thinner centrally than in the periphery, although there are exceptions to this rule. That fact introduces certain variables which affect the outcome of RK surgery; in fact, it affects *all* refractive surgical procedures. Whereas, while it may be true, as Barraquer teaches, that one cannot really change the shape of the cornea without involving Bowman's layer, it is equally true that the amount of ultimate curvature change is dependent upon distortion of the entire cornea, and that relates to tissue thickness.

The first factor to be considered is that the inner curvature of the cornea is less than that of the outer. Consequently, this surface is more myopic than the front and is arbitrarily given a value of -5.85 D. When this power is subtracted from the front surface curvature (in diopters), the effective power of the cornea is obtained (see the discussion in Chapter 5). The difficulty is that we have found that not all corneas behave the same way with respect to the gradient or delta of their thickness increase (or to put it another way, the decreasing radius of curvature toward the periphery). Naturally this leads to errors in obtaining the true refractive power of the cornea itself. However, until recently there has not existed nor has there really been a need for methods to measure that inner curvature (see also Chapter 6).

The second factor is that this variability in corneal thickness assures the surgeon that the incision is nowhere of uniform effect along its length—except in rare instances! It was this latter factor that led to the use of stepped incisions to overcome this handicap. This stepped incision technique, of course, led to the introduction of other variables into the equation and while solving some problems, created others in its wake.

It was evident—after examining the outcome of the early cases—that depth of incision was a major factor in the surgical result as well as in the variability of results seen in otherwise similar cases. Several attempts were made to solve that problem and ultimately it required an inversion in thinking to obtain the final solution. The first part of the solution was in recognizing that the practice of setting the blade based upon a percentage of the corneal thickness was not valid. While it is true that the relationship of incision depth to initial corneal thickness is constant with this method, the effectiveness of a given incision is not. I had been taking paracentral pachymetry measurements and setting the blade to 75% of that—the method used by the Soviets.

I at first reasoned that it would be a better idea to set the blade depth based upon the pachymetry *minus* a

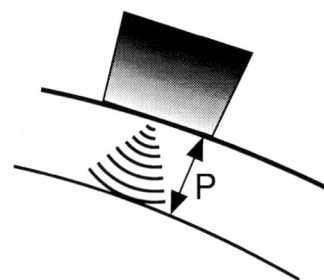

blade setting = P − .08 mm

Fig. 7.38 Early method of blade setting.

certain amount. When I reflected upon the fact that the amount of curvature change depended upon stromal weakening and that the degree of that weakening was, in turn, affected by incision depth, I quickly recognized that the ultimate factor in the amount of weakening was not the depth *per se* but the amount of tissue left uncut at the bottom of the incision. Hence it was logical to establish a given blade length by *subtracting* from the pachymetry a given amount and then using the result as the blade setting (Figure 7.38). In this manner, a specific amount of tissue would be left uncut at the bottom of each incision in each patient (i.e. the amount of tissue from the bottom of the incision to Descemet's membrane), at least at the beginning of the incision.

I had observed that while the paracentral readings varied markedly from patient to patient (within limits) and bore no predictable relationship to the central readings, the central readings were remarkably consistent among patients. Since the surgery works by exerting a pulling force upon the uncut central cornea, causing mostly flexion instead of stretch—thereby flattening the central curvature—it seemed logical that by making the uncut corneal lamella the same thickness for each patient, the variability from patient to patient would be reduced. To test this thesis, I operated on a series of patients in whom one eye was being done with the older method and the new technique used on the other. I found not only more consistent results in the latter group but, more importantly, greater corneal flattening occurred overall (Figure 7.39). This change did not, however, solve the need for maximizing the effect of the incision because the incision for the most part still became relatively more shallow toward the periphery.

To compensate for the additional shallowing still occurring in the last eight incisions, I began to extend the blade an additional 25 μm for the last eight incisions in the pattern (see also the section on wet versus dry, below). It was thus a natural extension of the previous thinking to take the further step of peripheral incision-deepening in all cases. No more

(a)

(b)

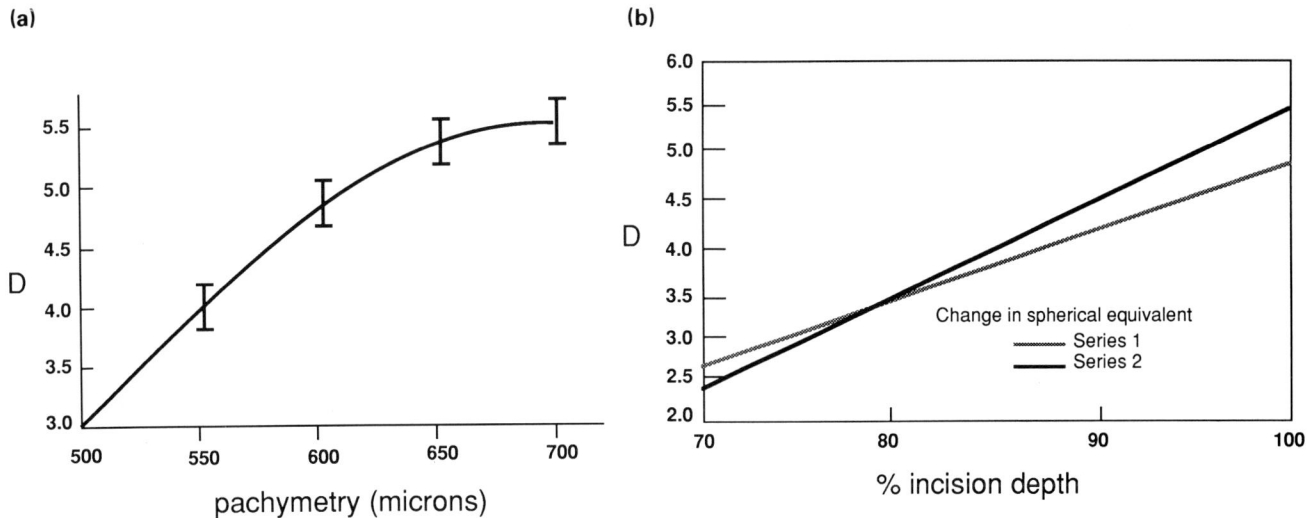

Fig. 7.39 Effect of deeper blade settings on outcome. ((b) Courtesy of M. Deitz.)

effective way has yet been devised to adjust the blade length dynamically or continuously while incising.

By examining a series of pachymetric measurements, it was determined that a significant change in corneal thickness occurred at approximately 6 mm from the optic center. This occurred again between 8 and 9 mm. Therefore, it was decided to make the incisions deeper in a step-wise manner. That is, each incision would be of one depth from the primary optical zone to 6.0 mm and another from thence to the limbus (Figure 7.40). In some cases, an intermediate step was made from 6 to 8 mm and from thence a deeper pass to the limbus. This technique resulted in considerably greater initial effect coupled with less surgical rebound [23]. This methodology was first applied in a series of patients in August 1979 and the results communicated to Fyodorov in November of that year. With certain modifications of this principle, permanent corrections of up to 14 D of myopia have been obtained with RK (see also Chapter 8).

At first this stepping was done by making the entire incision of one depth from the primary optical zone to the limbus. The blade would then be advanced the required length, re-inserted into the incision at 6.0 mm and the incision re-traced to the limbus, thereby deepening it. This method was, however, not without potential problems. If the re-deepening procedure was not carefully done, it was possible to produce an incision with a double bottom in the shape of an inverted Y (Figure 7.41). This could occur if too much pressure was applied to the knife handle both downward and tangentially, and also if fixation was not applied exactly at 180°. This did not occur either with free-hand deepening using a wound spreader or with a guarded blade if the blade was inserted carefully into the incision and the knife blade stroked gently to the

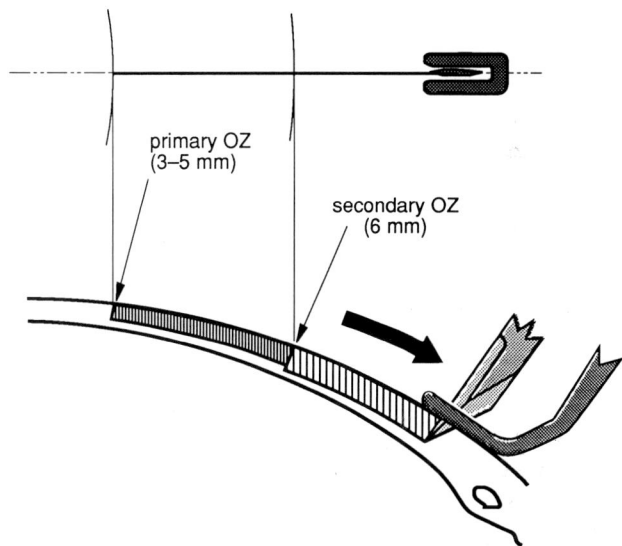

Fig. 7.40 Basic principle of the stepped incision.

limbus, allowing the sides of the incision to guide the blade. It is only when excess pressure is applied that the blade will wander; this is true even in making primary incisions. Sufficient pressure should be exerted so as to maintain firm but gentle contact between the knife jaw and the corneal surface, no more (see Chapter 8). In so doing, the incisions will be straight, perpendicular, and in the case of re-deepening, the knife will not fall into the incision. Myers labeled this the Bores "feather touch" technique. Incisional flaying was never shown to be a real occurrence except in one or two instances wherein the surgeon forced the effect to prove a point. The relatively dull edges of steel razor fragments used at that time made such a technique viable. With the

(a)

(b)

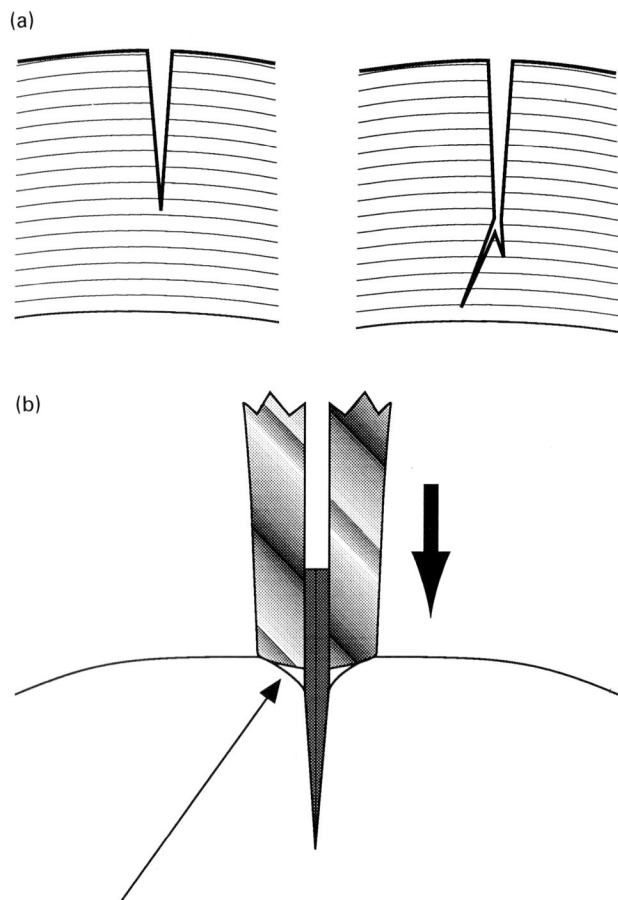

Fig. 7.41 (a) Y-shaped incision bottom. (b) The wound tends to open and spread.

advent of sharper blades, however—particularly those of crystalline materials such as sapphire or diamond—the danger of incision flaying became real. This reason, plus another, caused us to begin to make some of the incisions in a truly step-wise manner.

As our understanding of the dynamics of incision-making grew it became evident that the steel blades did not cut to the set depth except in the more peripheral parts of the incision. This was evidenced by the fact that incisions made from the limbus (the Fyodorov or Russian method) were deeper centrally than those made from the center (the Bores or American method) with the same setting. The reason for this phenomenon was soon apparent.

An examination shows the corneal stroma to be made up of an interlacing network of keratocytes arranged in layers (lamellae) akin to French pastry (Figure 7.42). Each of these keratocytes has a diameter of approximately 30 nm. The edge radius of a typical steel razor blade, however, is in the neighborhood of 1500 nm (Figures 7.43 and 7.44). Within and between

the cells there is fluid which is kept under very precise control by the endothelium to maintain corneal transparency. The presence of this fluid makes the tissue sponge-like. Not in the real sense that it is compressible because it is not, only in that it resembles a sponge in which fluid is interspersed between substance.

The cornea is also a very thin, dome-like structure that receives its support primarily from the limbus. When a blade is pressed against its surface, tissue resistance is finally overcome and the blade passes downward through the epithelium and Bowman's layer into the stroma. This resistance is not easily overcome because the tissue tends to bend over the relatively large blade edge radius (Figure 7.45). As the blade passes downward, it pushes tissue ahead of it until the tissue cannot move any more, whereupon the blade cuts through it. The resistance to tissue movement becomes less the deeper the blade penetrates until, rather than cut, the blade merely pushes the tissue ahead. With further movement downward, resistance to stretch occurs and the tissue will be cut (Figure 7.46a). If, however, the blade reaches its maximum depth before this point, the tissue will remain draped over the blade edge and will not be cut (Figure 7.46b).

Contrariwise, by introducing the blade into the thicker limbal tissue and moving it toward the center, the incision has reached its maximum effective depth well in advance of reaching the primary optical clear zone [25]. While this condition may have merit, cutting from the limbus carries with it some heavy penalties, both real and potential (see Chapter 15).

This also means that a blade of given length inserted into the cornea and drawn toward the periphery will penetrate less far initially than the same blade inserted at the limbus where there's more resistance. In the process of moving the blade it will eventually cut its way down almost to its set length. Therefore, when cutting from limbus to center (out-to-in) the maximum incision depth will be in the vicinity of the optical zone, whereas in the opposite direction (in-to-out), it will be somewhat shallower there (Figures 7.47 and 7.48). In order to get maximum depth with the American method the surgeon has to set the blade longer. We have found that while the length of the entire incision is important, that part of the incision closer to the optical zone is the most important. This area, which I have chosen to call the critical zone, extends from 3 to 6 mm (Figure 7.49). It is in this area that the maximum change in corneal curvature occurs [29]. In this transition zone, deep incisions permit a smoother curvature change without the formation of the so-called "knee" described in the earlier cases [30].

It seemed that a practical expedient to solve the problem of the blade's not cutting deep enough would be to add a blade factor or bias to the blade length. To

(a)

(b)

(d)

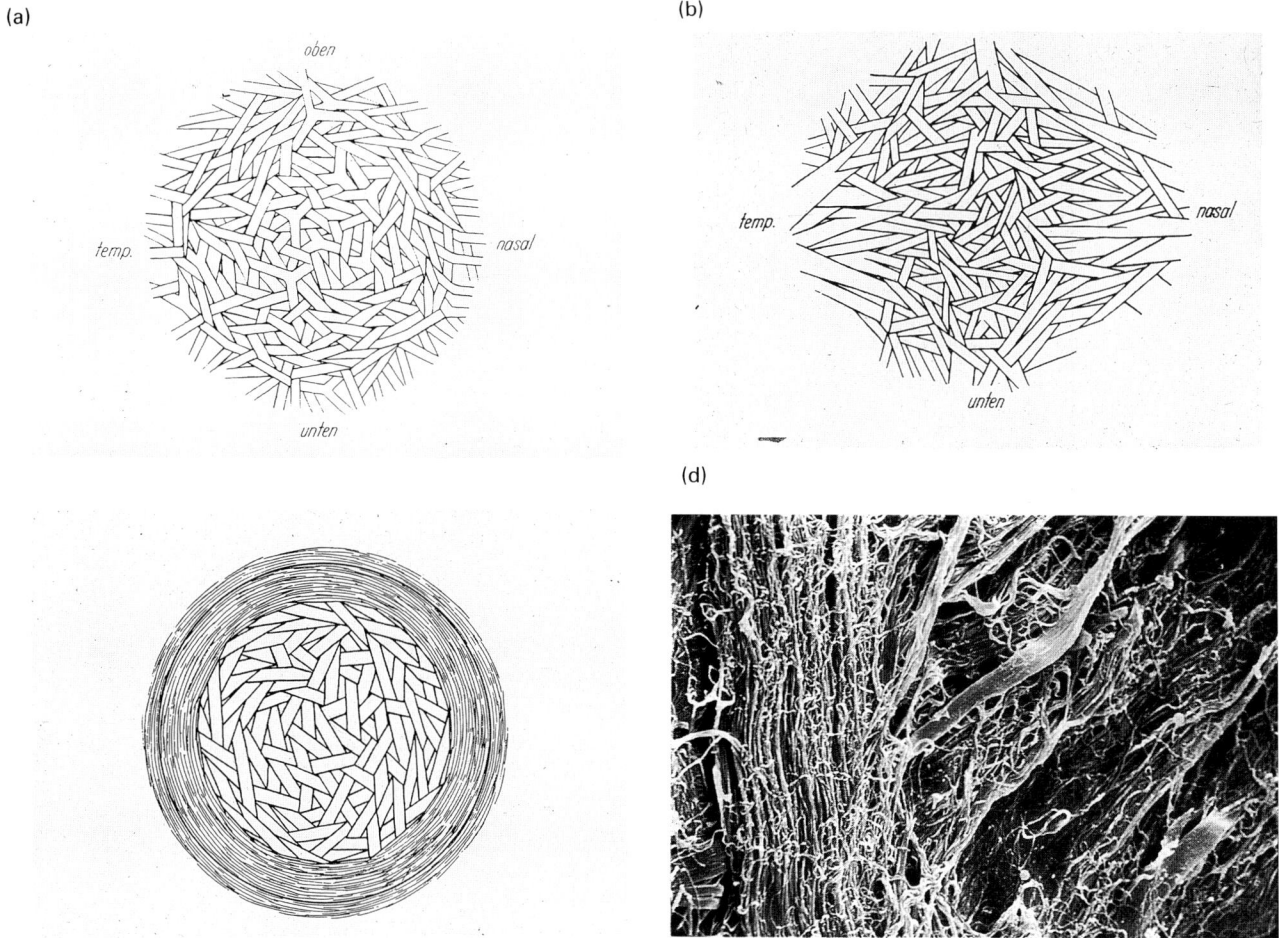

Fig. 7.42 (a and b) Kokott's dissection of the cornea revealing the interlaced arrangement of the keratocytes. (c) The deepest layers with the peripheral cells arranged in a circular manner—the so-called circumferential ligament of Kokott. (d) SEM of corneal stroma showing the same circular arrangement.

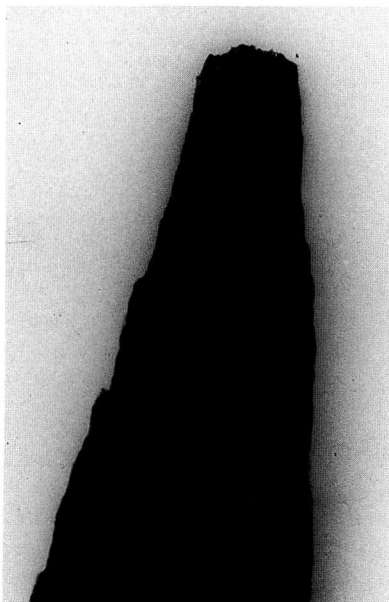

Fig. 7.43 SEM of typical razor blade.

test this theory we began adding small amounts to the blade setting for each case [23,24]. We continued to advance the blade length to attain maximum incision depth until we were setting steel blades up to 115% of the pachymetry. This additional blade length has been named blade bias and is blade-dependent, that is, each blade, regardless of material, requires that its own unique over-set factor be determined. Laboratory studies have shown that setting to 100% of the pachymetry yields an incision depth of 80–85% with most blades [31].

The advent of ultrasonic pachymetry

Initially, optical pachymetry was used to obtain the corneal thickness (Figure 7.50). This method of corneal thickness measurement is fraught with difficulties. It is not the least of its problems that it is not accurate, nor can it be used with unvarnished confidence off the visual axis, even with the Mishima–Hedbys pinlight

(a)

(b)

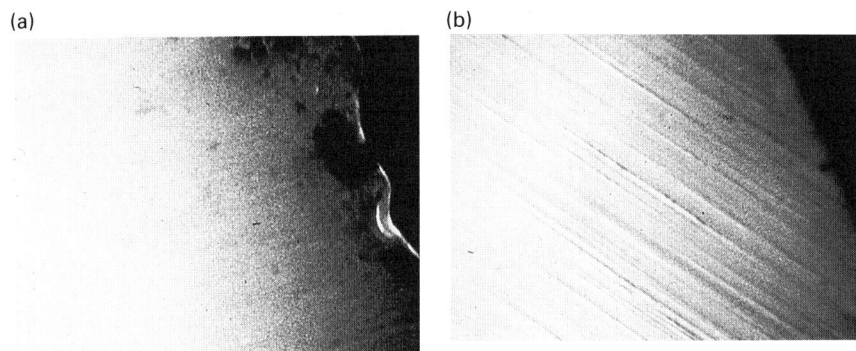

Fig. 7.44 (a) The edge of a typical razor blade fragment. (b) Honed steel blade designed for RK.

(a)

(b)

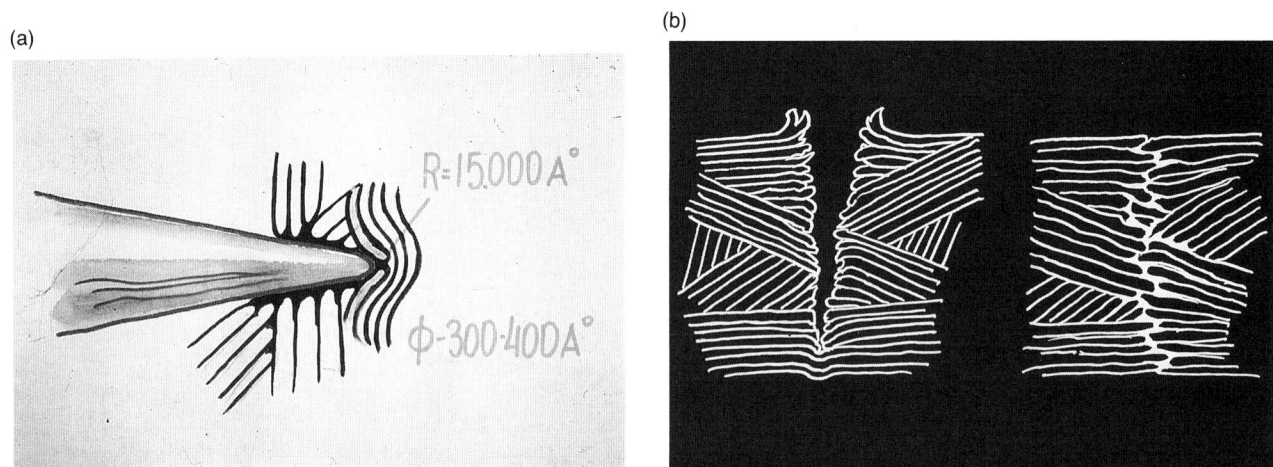

Fig. 7.45 (a) A dull steel blade pushes tissue ahead of it, tearing instead of cutting. (b) This results in wide, ragged scars.

(a)

(b)

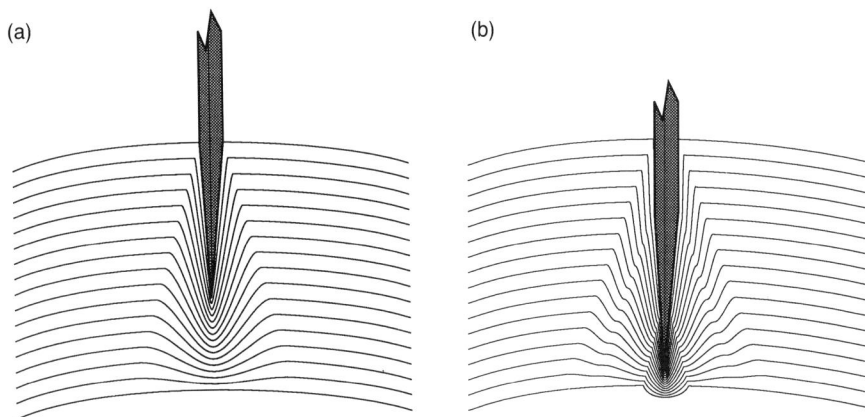

Fig. 7.46 (a) Stress lines as the blade pushes through tissue. (b) When the blade bottoms out, thinner layers remain uncut.

attachment [32]. This method can only measure in the horizontal meridian while incisions are made in all meridians. While we were able to get the optical pachymeter to function as an optical comparator, and with it did hundreds of cases with reasonable success, the method still wasn't exact enough for our purposes. Fortunately the problem was solved with the appearance of the ultrasonic corneal pachymeter, as

conceived by Kremer (Figure 7.51a,b). Originally a modification of an existing A-scan ocular biometer (Xenotech), it soon evolved into a stand-alone unit. The original Corneometer had a hollow, open-ended tip tapering to 1.5 mm, making it easy to place the probe accurately on the cornea (Figure 7.51c). For the first time, precise measurements of corneal thickness could be made with confidence anywhere on the

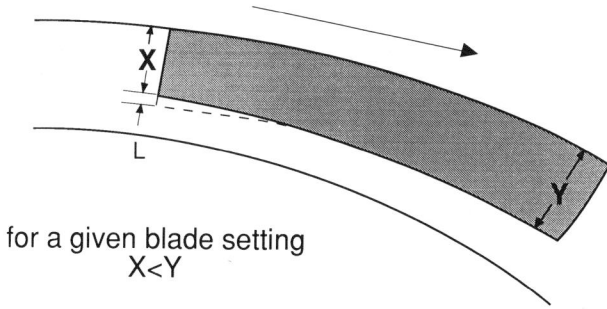

Fig. 7.47 Incision depth in American in-to-out technique.

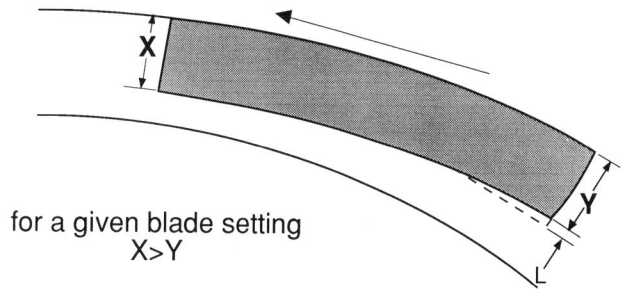

for a given blade setting
X<Y

Fig. 7.48 Incision depth in Russian out-to-in technique.

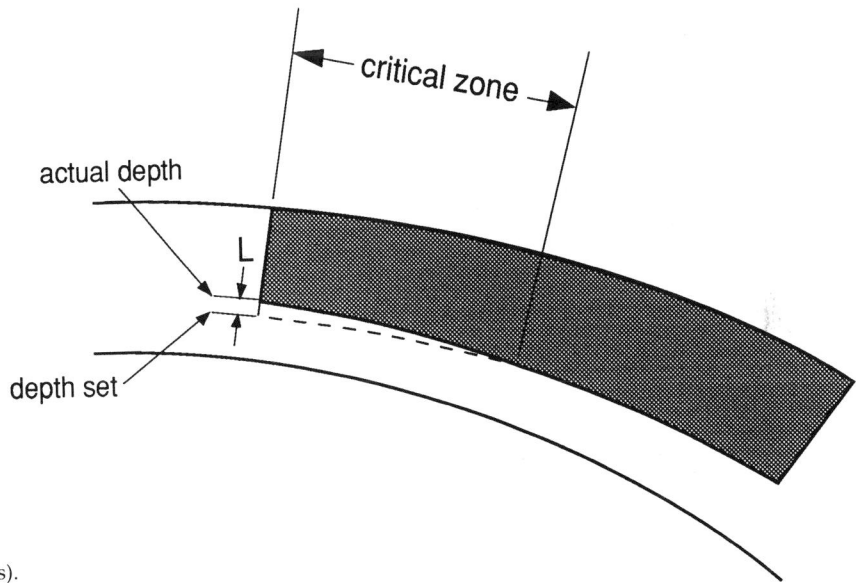

for a given blade setting
X>Y

Fig. 7.49 The critical zone (3–6 mm annulus).

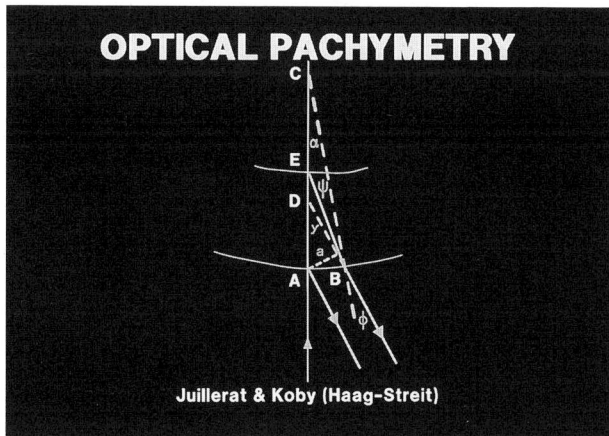

OPTICAL PACHYMETRY

Juillerat & Koby (Haag-Streit)

Fig. 7.50 The principle of optical pachymetry.

surface. A corneal thickness profile could also be generated by taking successive measurements (mapping) in any meridian (Figure 7.52).

It was by doing these mappings that a small piece of the puzzle fell into place. Because we now "understood" the cornea by virtue of our discovery of its sponge-like qualities we expected the micro-perforation rate to decrease. And so it did, for a time. However, as we kept increasing the blade length, we began to experience micro-perforations in unlikely places. For example, most were occurring in the corneal mid periphery and not always with the first deepening pass. Some occurred at around 9 mm and seemed to be mainly in the infero-temporal quadrant.

It was not enough to say that this was happening because continued corneal desiccation had caught up with us (see the section on wet versus dry, below). While this might explain such penetrations at the mid-periphery, it did not explain those in the far periphery. Some of these might also be explained through technical error such as too much blade pressure while making a stepped incision using the old method, but it was also occurring in cases where the newer technique was being used.

For years we had been taught that the cornea has a smooth thickness transition from center to limbus, in

(a)

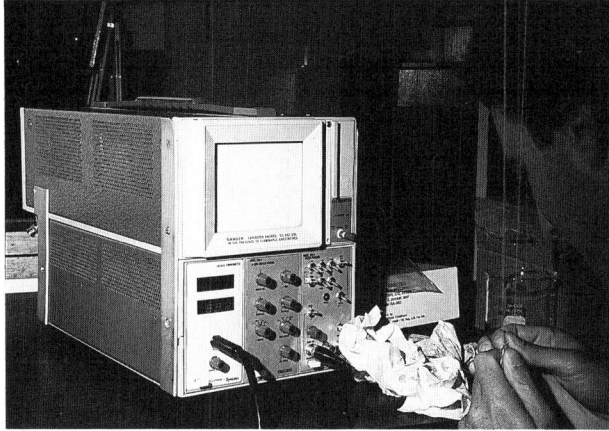

(b)

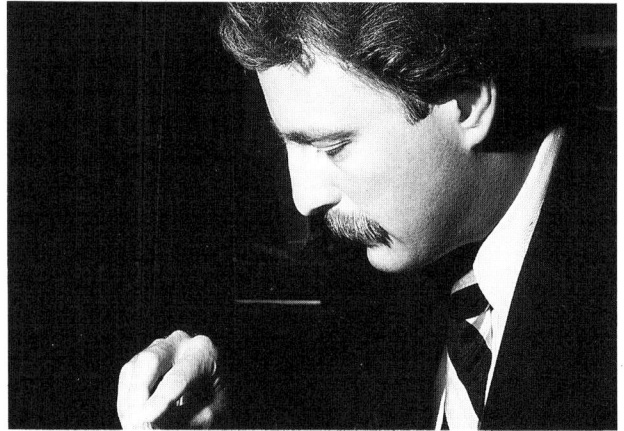

(c)

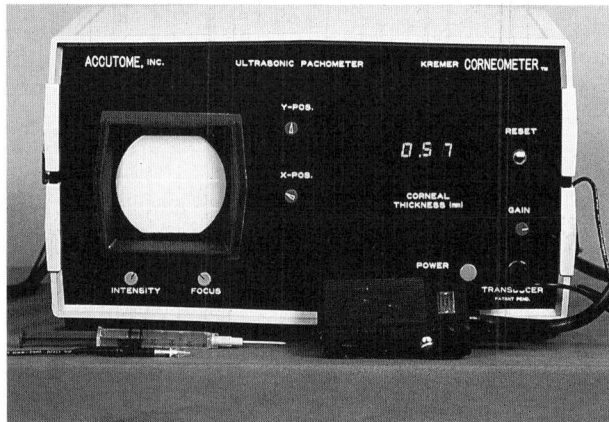

Fig. 7.51 (a) Modified Xenotech A-scan biometer used to make the first ultrasonic cornea thickness measurements. (b) Fred Kremer, MD, originator of ultrasonic pachymetry. (c) First commercial ultrasonic pachymeter.

the absence of corneal disease. However, ultrasonic corneal thickness mapping has shown that while this may be true in some eyes, for about 11% it is not. In older patients there is a tendency for the cornea to become thinner toward the periphery. In others, the thickness remains uniform until just before the limbus, where it thickens rapidly. Still others have been found to have small, abrupt areas of corneal thinning, which we have called corneal dimples. These dimples seem to occur at random and when first encountered were thought to be errors in measurement. An analysis of the distribution of these dimples showed a tendency to group in the mid-periphery in the infero-temporal quadrant (Figure 7.53). It was also in this quadrant that most of the instances of peripheral thinning could be found. In some cases, discovery of these areas before surgery—through mapping—allowed us to rotate our incisional pattern, thereby avoiding micro-perforations.

The search for the ideal blade

With the increased confidence that came with accurate pachymeter readings we again focused our attention

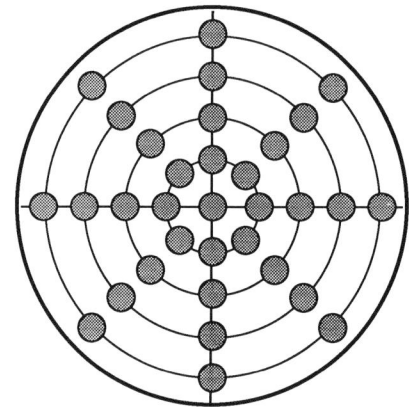

Fig. 7.52 Typical ultrasonic pachymeter mapping pattern.

upon the incisions. We soon abandoned the 76a Beaver blade in favor of razor fragments, particularly those of high carbon content, but the search for the ideal blade continued. A brief infatuation with the diamond promised much at first; however, until recently, the author has been uniformly disappointed with the

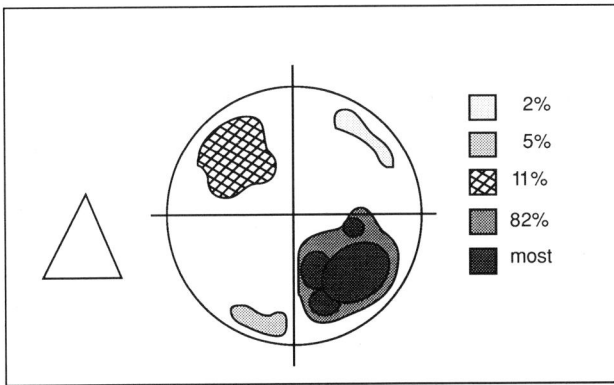

Fig. 7.53 Distribution of thin corneal areas (dimples).

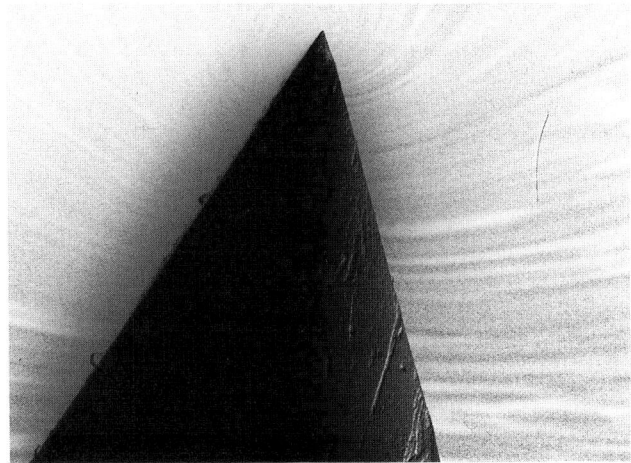

Fig. 7.54 SEM of sapphire RK blade.

performance of the guarded diamond knife. It does not seem to cut as well as steel razor fragments after it has been in use for many cases.

This need to over-set the blade was due, primarily, to the way the blades cut and partially to the pachymeter itself. The speed of sound through the cornea is not exactly known—estimates have ranged from 1540 m/s (the average speed through the human eye) to 1630 m/s [33,34]. The Corneometer had been pre-set to 1540 m/s at the beginning of our investigation. When we gradually advanced the speed setting to 1640 m/s (the current setting), we began to get more sensible readings—that is, the corneal thickness measurements began to relate more closely to the blade settings. This was so universal an experience that all instruments were re-called and re-adjusted to the faster speed.

This did not solve the entire problem, however. Blades still had to be over-set because of the characteristics of the corneal tissue and of the continued inadequacy of the blades being used. When I speak of inadequacy, I am speaking in relative terms, and I am talking about consistency. Certainly any blade will make an incision in the cornea. In RK surgery, however, we are talking about micro-meters—microsurgery in a very real sense—and any blade that does not cut exactly to where it is set is bound to be a disappointment.

As crystalline blades made their appearance the blade bias changed to 5–10% for diamonds and approximately 2% for sapphire blades. The sapphire bias is usually expressed in micro-meters rather than as a percentage, being typically 10 μm initially up to 70 μm as the blade becomes worn (this translates to a percentage bias of 1.5 to 15%). These crystalline blades cut deeper and smoother because their edge radius is typically 45 nm for diamond and ≤19 nm for sapphire (Figure 7.55). Except for some very fragile experimental sapphire blades, no blade has yet reached the ideal sharpness whereby it can be under-set to obtain

a 90–95% incisional depth. Recently, a new design diamond blade made especially for the author has come close—it has a blade bias of 0%.

It is the importance of small details such as this that sets refractive surgical techniques apart from others, and it is the attention to such details that sets the successful radial keratotomist apart from his or her fellows (Figure 7.56). To over-set a blade in order to maximize the incision depth while still not cutting through the cornea might seem illogical—nevertheless it works. Arriving at the settings to use was much easier than convincing colleagues to follow suit, however. It took demonstrations of the method during surgery to clinch the point. In the author's hands, such technique has reduced the mean perforation rate from 12% to 7%. Micro-perforation during this surgery is seen by some as undesirable to any degree. Hence the suggestion has been made to make the incisions shallow. Since the data from various authors have shown that deeper incisions produce a more profound and lasting effect, we will leave it to the reader to weigh the merit of this suggestion to prevent microperforations by under-setting the blade.

Progressive corneal flattening

There is one caveat that should be considered whenever the question arises: is deeper really better? While it has been stated, as well as shown, that deeper incisions produce an increase in ultimate effect, there may be a price to be paid for that depth increase—progressive hyperopia [27,28,35].

There is some evidence that deeper incisions may be associated with progression of effect. While progressive hyperopia will be covered in more detail in Chapter 16, it is appropriate to mention some aspects of the phenomenon at this juncture.

Fyodorov and the author had advocated, early in the history of RK, free-hand dissection of incisions to Descemet's membrane in cases of high myopia. As the quality of blades improved—particularly their tip geometry which allows the blade to penetrate more deeply at the beginning of an incision—and the accuracy of blade setting also increased, the number of cases in which free-hand deepening was mandated decreased. Added to this was the recognition that there was, as in all things, a ceiling or limit to the degree of myopia that could reasonably be expected to be eliminated by RK. The trend to cap-off the level of myopia amenable to RK incisions was also propelled by the advent of improvements in alternative refractive surgical techniques, such as keratomileusis-*in-situ*.

While the jury is still out on the question, it is reasonable to be alert to the possibility that incisions which approach closely or intersect with Descemet's membrane may actually induce progression in the effect of RK. It is my contention that incisions penetrating no greater than 95% of the corneal thickness will be shown to be safe with regard to progression of effect. However, the reader should carefully study the paragraphs on progressive hyperopia in Chapter 15 and consider that other factors are in play to produce this complication of the surgery (see also below).

Number of incisions

As stated earlier in this chapter, eight incisions were purposefully abandoned early on; they were revived as incisions got deeper. All accounts from individuals reporting "first experience" cases have stated that they have found little or at the most 10% difference between eight and 16 incisions. However, that hasn't been the author's experience. I have, for example, a group of 48 patients in whom eight incisions were done on one eye and 16 on the fellow eye, using the same technique. I found that the range of difference was 5–50%, with the mean 24.6%. This finding has been corroborated by Fyodorov and his group [36]. Eight or fewer incisions are used for all patients whose myopia is −4 D or less, for some whose myopia is −5 D, and very rarely for those whose myopia is greater (usually in astigmatic cases). Sixteen incisions are used for the remainder although four, six and 12 incisions are sometimes also used. Since it is more difficult to place the six- and 12-ray pattern symmetrically we use a specially designed marker to insure equal spacing of the incisions (see also Chapter 8). The six-incision cases have shown a mean difference in effect of 50% and the 12-incision cases 16% of that produced by 16 incisions.

Because of the physiologic changes that occur within the cornea after this surgery which seem to affect the outcome in second-stage surgery, we cannot recom-mend "sneaking up" on the myopia by staging the surgery. This method has been advocated by some as a preventive for over-correction [37]. That is, doing three or four incisions, waiting and then doing another three or four. For some reason, staging never seems to produce the same amount of ultimate correction as does using six, eight, or 16 primary incisions. While an occasional patient might be spared post-operative hyperopia by staging the incisions in this manner, still more will be subjected to additional surgery whose outcome will be even less predictable than the first go-around. Over-corrections are rare in the author's hands and Fyodorov has not reported this phenom-enon to any significant degree. Properly planned surgery assisted by computer prediction programs that take into account age, sex, keratometry, corneal diameter, depth of incision, and corneal rigidity are the best defense against over- and under-correction.

Incisional depth coefficients

Because of the greater changes in corneal curvature that were accompanying the newer methods of incision-making, the formulas began to fail in their ability to predict the outcome of the surgery. It was, therefore, necessary to generate three additional surgical coefficients. These factors were 1.6, 2.0, and 2.5. These coefficients related not only to the depth but also to the manner in which the incisions were made. In January 1980, we began (both here and in Fyodorov's clinic) to use these factors as follows:

1.3—used when 16 single-depth incisions were made to a depth approximately 70% of the corneal thick-ness at the primary optical zone. The operative word here is approximately—recall that with the advent of the subtraction/stepping technique I and my co-workers were not using percentages to set blade depth.

1.6—the same number and type of incisions were made with a blade set to produce an incision ap-proximately 90% of the corneal thickness at the primary optic zone.

2.0—used for 16 incisions with a deepening cut made in each incision from 6 mm to the periphery.

2.5—used for a case in which a stepped incision was made but also four or more incisions were deepened to Descemet's membrane, free-hand.

This latter free-hand deepening was performed at first with a tri-facet diamond knife. A diamond was initially used in these cases because it was felt that the sharpest blade available should be employed for this purpose—sapphire blade is currently being used. With a sharp blade very little pressure is needed to deepen a corneal wound, allowing the surgeon to maintain complete control of the incision. In addition the blade is transparent, allowing light into the bottom

(a)

(b)

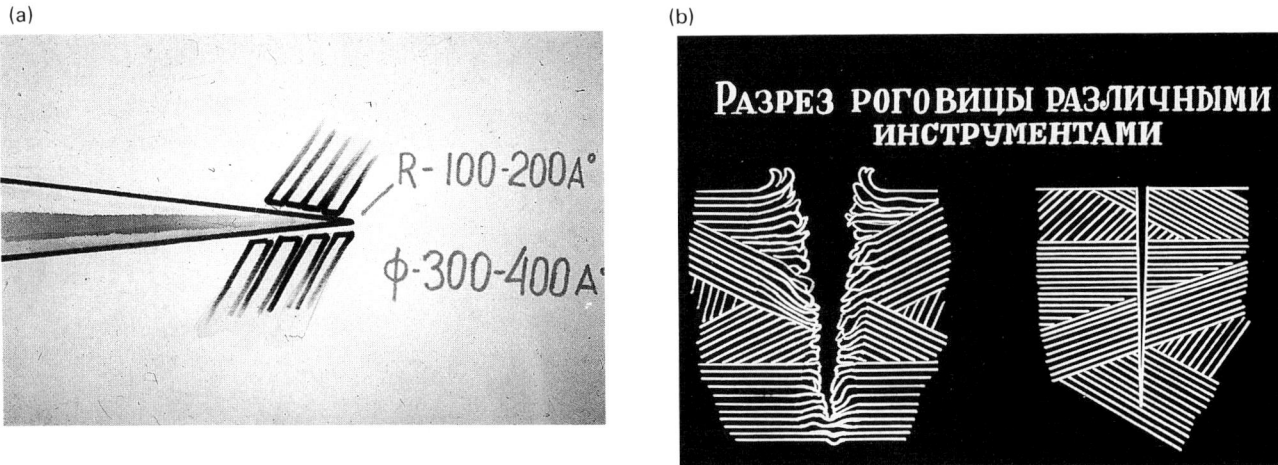

Fig. 7.55 (a) The cutting radius of the blade edge must be less than the diameter of tissue fiber to be cut. (b) A Russian slide showing the differences between incisions made with steel (left) and diamond (right).

of the wound and making it easier to see Descemet's membrane.

Wet versus dry

We found, almost serendipitously, that in patients in whom the cornea had not been kept wet during the surgery, the last eight incisions were much deeper than those in whom it had been kept wet. In some cases perforations occurred at the mid-periphery even when the blade was not extended.

We therefore performed surgery in a number of consecutive cases in which extended and non-extended blade settings with and without corneal wetting were done. Except to add anesthetic, which was blotted from the surface with micro-sponges almost immediately, no fluids were applied to the corneal surface in the non-wetted cases. In all cases of the dry technique without blade extension, the incisions were found to be deeper and more uniform throughout than incisions made in the old manner. In the wetted cases there was considerable variation in the individual incision depths—especially the last eight incisions. In those cases in which the blade was extended for the last eight incisions there was an improvement with respect to depth in the wetted cases, while in the non-wetted cases there was a tendency to perforate at incision number nine or 10. We therefore concluded that corneal wetting during the surgery would result in shallower incisions from swelling of the stroma due to tissue imbibition (Figure 7.57). Villasenor [38], in a series of experiments, showed that the incised corneas in monkey and human cadaver eyes thinned up to 25% of their original thickness within 25 min if not kept wet— almost 1%/min. One other advantage of the dry

technique was that the rate of operative epithelial stripping fell almost to zero.

There were, however, two other difficulties that required solution and which remain only partially solved today. The first is keratometry and the second is the so-called corneal rigidity.

The importance of central corneal curvature

There is still some discussion about the effect of the pre-operative corneal curvature on the outcome of RK surgery. Early work by Fyodorov and his colleagues [39,40] had indicated that it did affect the outcome. I have compensated for changes in corneal curvature from the beginning of my involvement with this surgical technique—I'm convinced that pre-operative K-readings affect the end result. When pre-operative keratometry was plotted against post-operative keratometry in a group of similar cases, an almost straight line resulted (Figure 7.58). If the pre-operative corneal curvature was *not* an influencing factor, there should have been less effect shown for the higher curvatures; however, there wasn't. There was instead, more effect shown, thus indicating that more compensation should have been made for steeper corneas. Therefore I am forced to conclude that pre-operative curvature is a factor in surgical outcome and I continue to compensate for it.

Corneal rigidity

The other factor, that of corneal rigidity, is still somewhat of a puzzler. All of us remember Freidenwald's constant when rigidity is mentioned. Freidenwald's constant seems to vary with the extent of the myopia and generally ranges between 0.018 and 0.025.

(a)

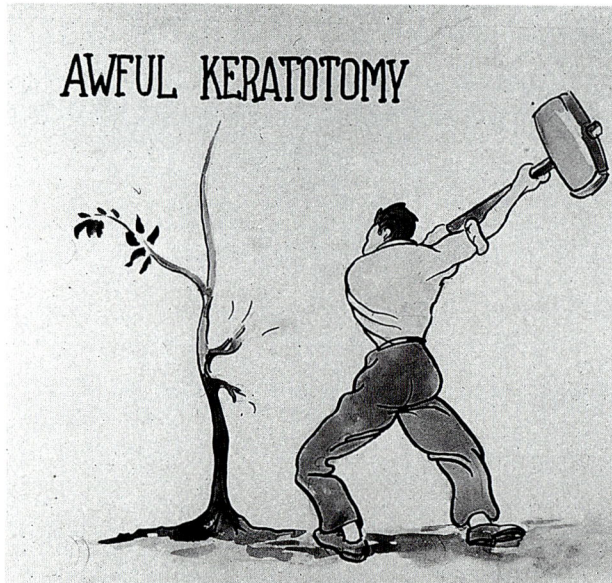

(b)

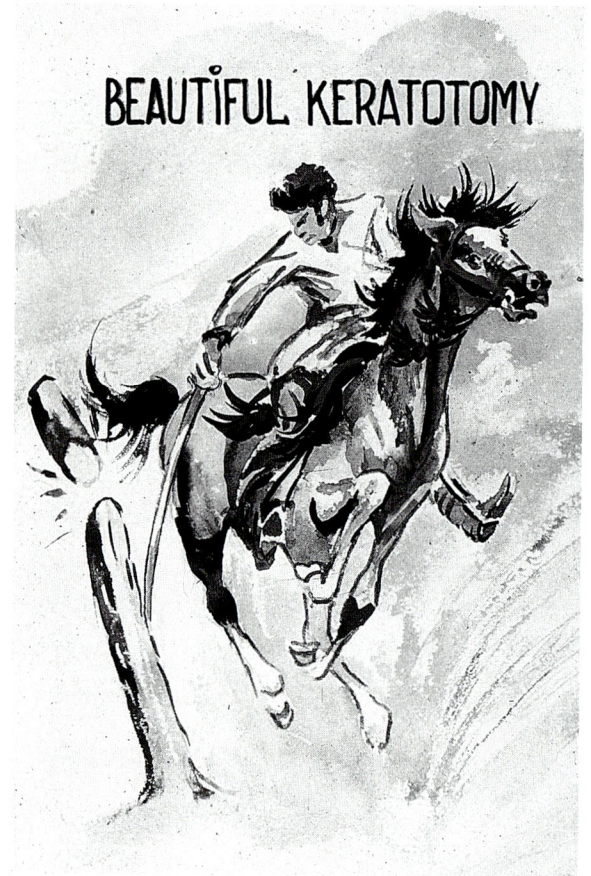

Fig. 7.56 (a) Awful keratotomy; (b) beautiful keratotomy. (Courtesy of S.N. Fyodorov.)

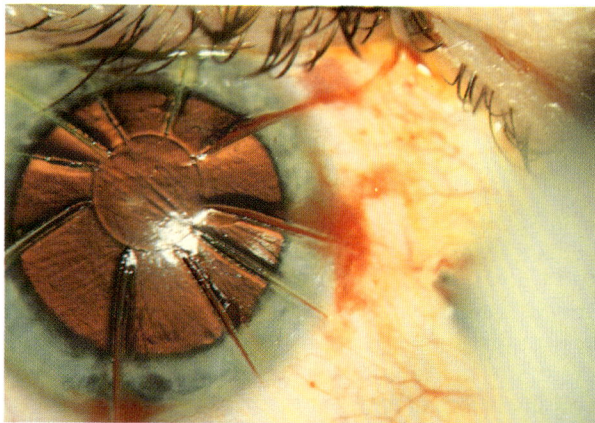

Fig. 7.57 Note the elevation of the incision edges in a wetted RK case.

Fyodorov used factors of 1.5, 0.96, 0.88, etc. What kind of constants was he talking about and where did he get them? He was really talking about the same thing that Freidenwald was, except that he measured it differently. Integration of this factor into the original formulas more accurately predicted the outcome of a

specific case. As the rigidity increased so did the effect of the surgery. In general, the rigidity increased with age, and was somewhat less at a given age for a woman than for a man. The difference is convergent, however, and beginning at age 45–46 the corneal rigidity is essentially the same for a man or a woman. That this variable is significant can be seen by examining the evidence described in Chapter 5.

Other factors

Other factors in the surgery were dealt with as they surfaced. The first cases were done with incisions that extended across the limbus. As the need for deeper incisions became apparent, concern grew for the angle structures. In addition such incisions tended to promote fibrous ingrowth at their most peripheral portions, producing conjunctival peaks at the limbus. Surprisingly these peaks were not accompanied by neo-vascularization except in some patients in whom soft contact lenses were fitted early (to stabilize the cornea) and only in those who wore extended wear lenses [41]. This problem vanished when the lenses were stopped or changed to daily wear, and thus

(a)

(b)

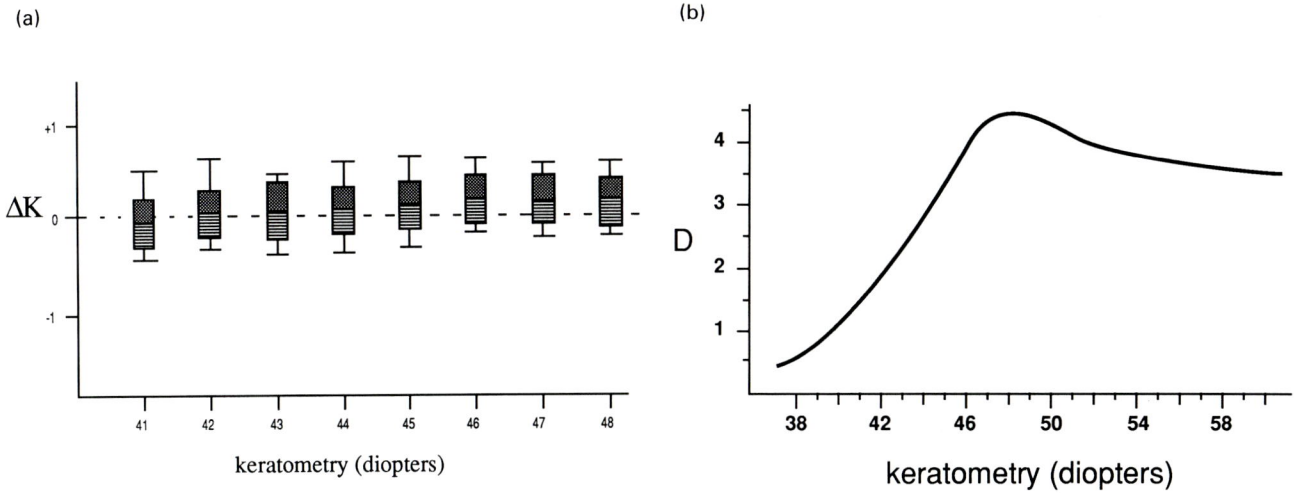

Fig. 7.58 (a) Effect of K-reading on outcome. (b) Steep corneal curvatures can decrease the effect.

Table 7.3 Results of a study on post-operative use of steroid drops (from J. Hayes)

	No steroids			Steroids		
	All	Males	Females	All	Males	Females
Number	25	13	12	33	21	12
Age (years)	33.6	34.6	32.5	36.5	36.3	36.7
Range of ages (years)	22–57	25–52	22–57	21–56	21–56	27–49
Pre-operative intra-ocular pressure	17.2	18.1	16.3	16.3	15.9	17.2
Pre-operative K(SE)	−5.66	−5.65	−5.68	−5.78	−5.11	−6.16
Range of corneal refraction	−3.62 to −8.00	−3.62 to −8.00	−3.75 to −7.62	−4.00 to −7.75	−4.00 to −7.75	−4.25 to −7.00
Delta corneal refraction	+3.99	+4.63	+3.29	+5.36	+5.44	+5.23
Range of the delta	+1.75 to +8.00	+1.75 to +8.00	+2.13 to +5.25	+3.12 to +10.12	+3.12 to +10.12	+3.25 to +8.00

seemed more related to oxygen deprivation in healing tissue than to the type of incision. The major factor in shortening these incisions was the theoretic, experimental, and clinical evidence which showed that perhaps this type of incision actually reduced the effectiveness of the surgery. We therefore began to make the incisions just to the capillary plexus and not beyond. We found that not only were the eyes quieter but the effect may well have been enhanced.

This experience prompted some workers to theorize that perhaps even shorter incisions would be just as effective, whereupon someone observed that if shorter incisions were the answer, why not just make punctures at the edge of the optical zone? Mendez has advocated the use of deliberate punctures through the cornea and has claimed 1 D of correction per puncture. Despite the reported success with such punctures, this methodology is *not* recommended. Some cases with short (3 mm) incisions have also been done and the results were reported to be satisfactory (Figure 7.59) [42]. However, no one, to the author's knowledge, is currently using this method.

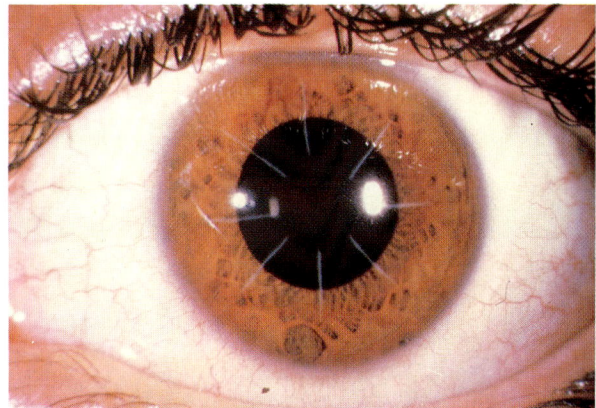

Fig. 7.59 Short (3 mm) incisions advocated by one surgeon to correct myopia on the grounds that computer simulations show that most of the effect of the incisions occurs in this area.

The author found, early on, that the use of steroid drops twice daily for 2 weeks following surgery enhanced the effect of the surgery and seemed to result in a smoother post-operative course withal. Consequently, the author recommends this course of action (see also Chapter 8). Table 7.3 submitted by John Hayes, MD summarizes his experience with two groups of patients: one not having received steroid therapy post-operation and another that did (J. Hayes, personal communication). It is evident from this study that steroids do indeed enhance the effect of the incisions. Paradoxically, if the steroid drops are used much beyond 2–3 weeks, it has been the author's experience that the overall effect is *diminished* in a significant number of cases. This led to such use in cases of over-correction (see Chapter 15). Prolonged use of steroids, while reported to enhance the effect do so by elevating the intraocular pressure (Shepard, personal communication). Other unpleasant side-effects of steroids have also been reported (see Chapter 15).

References

1 Sato T. Treatment of conical cornea (incision of Descemet's membrane). Acta Soc Ophthalmol (Jpn) 1939; 43:541.
2 Sato T. Experimental study on surgical correction of astigmatism. Juntendo Kenkyukai Zasshi 1943; 589:37.
3 Lans L. Experimentelle Untersuchungen uber die Entstehung von Astigmatismus durch nicht perforirende Corneawunden. (Experimental studies of the treatment of astigmatism with non-perforating corneal incisions.) Albrecht von Graefes Arch Klin Exp Ophthalmol 1898; 45:117–152.
4 Sato T. Experimental study of posterior half-corneal incisions for myopia. Acta Soc Ophthalmol Jpn 1951; 55:219.
5 Sato T. Experimental study of anterior and posterior half-corneal incisions for myopia. Rinsho Ganka 1952; 6:209.
6 Sato T, Akiyama K, Shibata H. A new surgical approach to myopia. Am J Ophthalmol 1953; 36:823–829.
7 Akiyama K. A new surgical approach to myopia. Acta Soc Ophthalmol Jpn 1952; 56:1142.
8 Akiyama K. Study of the surgical treatment for myopia. I. Posterior corneal incisions. Acta Soc Ophthalmol (Jpn) 1952; 56:1142–1150.
9 Akiyama K. Study of the surgical treatment for myopia. II. Animal experiments. Acta Soc Ophthalmol (Jpn) 1955; 59:294–312.
10 Akiyama K. Study of the surgical treatment for myopia. III. Anterior and posterior incisions. Acta Soc Ophthalmol (Jpn) 1955; 59:797–853.
11 Kanai A, Yamaguchi T, Yajima Y, Funahashi M, Nakajima A. The fine structure of bullous keratopathy after antero-posterior incisions of the cornea for myopia. Folia Ophthalmol (Jpn) 1979; 30:841–849.
12 Yamaguchi T, Kanai A, Tanaka M, Ishii R. Bullous keratopathy after anterior-posterior radial keratotomy for myopia. Am J Ophthalmol 1982; 93:600.
13 Pureskin NP, Boguslavskaia ES. Izmenenie krivizny rogovitsy putem ee perednikh i zadnikh neperforiruiushchikh nadrezov. (Changing corneal curvature through anterior and posterior nonpenetrating incisions.) Vestn Oftalmol 1967; 80:16–22.
14 Pureskin NP. Experimental investigation of possibilities of surgical treatment of myopia and astigmatism. Thesis, Moscow, 1968.
15 Durnev V. Decrease of corneal refraction by anterior keratotomy method with the purpose of surgical correction of myopia of mild and moderate degree. Tenth Meeting of Transcaucasian Ophthalmologists, Tbilisi, 1976.
16 Durnev V, Ermoshin A. Determination of dependence between the length of anterior radial non-perforating incisions of the cornea and their effectiveness. IV All Union Conference of Inventors and Rationalizers in the Field of Ophthalmology, Moscow, 1976.
17 Durnev V. Characteristic of the results of myopic surgical correction after performing 16 and 32 primary anterior radial non-perforating incisions. In: Surgery of Refractive Anomalies of the Eye, A Ivashina and S Kolmanovskii (eds). Moscow Scientific Research Institute for Eye Microsurgery, Moscow, 1981.
18 Huang T, Bisarnsin T, Schachar R, Black T. Corneal curvature change due to structural alternation by radial keratotomy. J Biomech Eng 1988; 110:249–253.
19 Chen Y. Transverse shear deformation in an impaired thin shell. Thesis, University of Texas, 1990.
20 Reissner E. Stress–strain relations in the theory of thin elastic shells. J Math Physics 1952; 31:109–119.
21 Reissner E. The effect of transverse-shear deformation on the bending of elastic plates. J Appl Mech 1945; 12:69–77.
22 Whitney J. The effect of transverse shear deformation on the bending of laminated plates. J Comp Materials 1969; 3:534–547.
23 Bores LD, Myers W, Cowden J. Radial keratotomy: an analysis of the American experience. Ann Ophthalmol 1981; 13:941–948.
24 Bores L. Historical review and clinical results of radial keratotomy. Int Ophthalmol Clin 1983; 23:93–118.
25 Melles G, Binder P. Effect of radial keratotomy incision direction on wound depth. Refract Corneal Surg 1990; 6:394–403.
26 Binder PS. What we have learned about corneal wound healing from refractive surgery (Barraquer lecture). Refract Corneal Surg 1989; 5:98–120.
27 Deitz M, Sanders D. Progressive hyperopia with long-term follow-up of radial keratotomy. Arch Ophthalmol 1985; 103:782–784.
28 Deitz M, Sanders D, Raanan M. Progressive hyperopia in radial keratotomy. Long-term follow-up of diamond-knife and metal-blade series. Ophthalmology 1986; 93:1284–1289.
29 Cowden JW, Bores LD. A clinical investigation of the surgical correction of myopia by the method of Fyodorov. Ophthalmology 1981; 88:737–741.
30 Rowsey JJ, Balyeat HD. Radial keratotomy: preliminary report of complications. Ophthalmic Surg 1982; 13:27.
31 Hernandez-Meijide R, Croxatto JO. Experimental radial keratotomy. J Refract Surg 1988; 3:224–226.
32 Mishima S, Hedbys B. Measurement of corneal thickness with the Haag–Streit pachymeter. Arch Ophthalmol 1968; 80:710–713.
33 Oksala A. Use of the echogram in the location and diagnosis of intraocular foreign bodies. Br J Ophthalmol 1959; 43:744–752.
34 Vanysek J, Preisova J, Obraz J. Ultrasonography in Ophthalmology. Butterworths, London, 1969.
35 Deitz M, Sanders D, Marks R. Radial keratotomy: an overview of the Kansas City study. Ophthalmology 1984; 91:467–478.
36 Fyodorov SN, Ivashina AI, Fedchenko OT, Moskvichev AL. Khirurgicheskaia korrektsiia miopicheskoi anizometropii metodom perednei keratomii. (Surgical correction of myopic anisometropia by anterior keratotomy.) Vestn Oftalmol 1984; 1:15–19.
37 Salz J, Villasenor A, Elander R, Reader A, Swinger C, Buchbinder M. Four-incision radial keratotomy for low to moderate myopia. Ophthalmology 1986; 93:727–738.

38 Villasenor RA, Salz J, Steel D, Krasnov M. Changes in corneal thickness during radial keratotomy. Ophthalmic Surg 1981; 12:341–342.

39 Fyodorov SN, Durnev VV. The use of anterior keratotomy method with the purpose of surgical correction of myopia. In *Practical Problems in Ophthalmic Surgery*, AI Ivashina (ed), Minister of Health, USSR, Moscow, 1977.

40 Fyodorov SN, Durnev VV. Operation of dosaged dissection of corneal circular ligament in cases of myopia of mild degree. Ann Ophthalmol 1979;11:1885–1890.

41 Binder P. The physiologic effects of extended wear soft contact lenses. Ophthalmology 1980; 87:745–749.

42 Schachar R, Black T, Huang T. Surgical implications of the theory of radial keratotomy. In *Radial Keratotomy*, R Schacher *et al.* (eds). LAL, Dennison, 1980.

Instrumentation and Technique of Radial Keratotomy

I hear and forget.
I see and hear and I remember.
However, when I see, hear and do,
I understand and succeed. [Anonymous]

Instrumentation

As we have repeatedly stated, this surgery is true micro-surgery. The outcome is not only dependent upon careful consideration of numerous, seemingly unimportant factors, but upon the instrumentation as well. Next to the pre-operative workup, the most important consideration in this surgery is the blade. In the beginning, razor fragments were used for this surgery. Because such blades were inconsistent in their quality, the search began immediately for an improved blade. While it is true that specially processed steel blades (such as the Katena K2-5550) are available today which surpass in quality any previously available razor fragment and in some cases even the early diamond blades, it is the consensus among most of the experienced practitioners of this surgery that some form of crystalline blade (not necessarily diamond) will produce the smoothest and deepest incision.

We have also repeatedly stressed that incision depth is a paramount factor in the outcome of radial keratotomy. As was pointed out first by Fyodorov and Durnev [1] and amply demonstrated since by the author and others, there are three factors which affect the depth of incision [2–6]. These are:

1 Blade length.
2 Blade sharpness.
3 Tissue resistance.

All of these factors are inter-related but only the first two can be controlled directly. The third factor can be compensated for to some degree by over-setting the blade.

Blades and blade handles

The ideal blade should have an extremely sharp point to penetrate to the maximum depth set instead of pushing the tissue ahead of it. In addition, the edge must be as sharp as possible to make an incision as smooth as possible. Depending upon the material, there seems to be a practical limit to the sharpness of the point and the edge. Steel does not readily take an edge much sharper than 100 nm (Figure 8.1). Material such as diamond can be taken to a theoretic limit of 2–5 nm in edge radius (Figure 8.2). Furthermore, in practical terms, diamond is extremely difficult to cut into slabs much thinner than 0.30 mm. Getting an edge radius less than 30 nm requires an expensive process which makes the price of such blades prohibitive. In addition, the bevel angle of the typical diamond blade is 43°, resulting in a snowplow effect while cutting (Figure 8.3). However, some newer blades have been able to reduce this to 35°. In fact the performance of the early diamond blades, in the author's hands, had been so disappointing that I, as well as many others, had gone back to the steel blade and was recommending

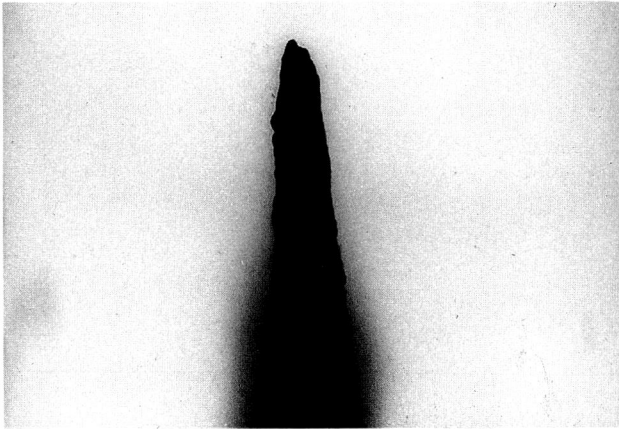

Fig. 8.1 SEM of a steel blade tip × 50.

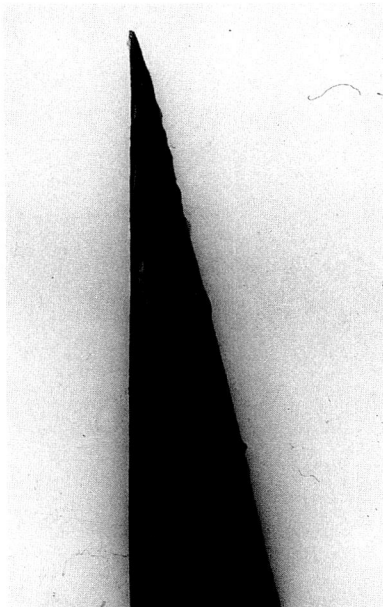

Fig. 8.2 SEM of a sapphire blade tip × 50.

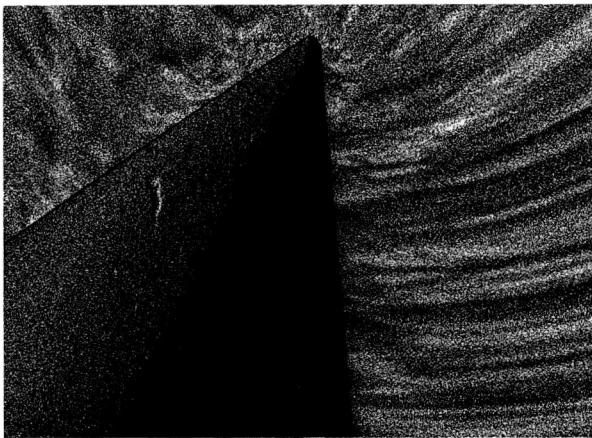

Fig. 8.3 SEM of the blade tip of a second-generation diamond blade × 400.

that beginning radial keratotomy surgeons not even consider the purchase of a crystal knife. This recommendation has since changed with the advent of the sapphire (see below) and newer diamond blades.

Ruby is second in hardness to diamond and is somewhat easier to work but it is difficult to get a uniform crystalline structure. I am very disappointed in its performance. Despite its hardness it does not seem to hold an edge well. In addition, it tends to drag when passed through tissue.

Sapphire has the same hardness characteristics of ruby but is easier to handle. Under the right circumstances it is possible to grow the crystal at a particular crystalline angle which, when sliced and chemically machined, produces a smooth, ultra-sharp edge, in many cases surpassing diamond and in all cases surpassing steel blades. Such a blade is commercially available under the trade name XTAL, and is marketed by the Katena Corporation.

Sapphire blades, while tougher than steel, still have a finite life and eventually must be replaced. Unless broken, the tip of such a blade wears evenly and smoothly, however. If the operator possesses an optical comparator (such as the DGH-800 Bores shadowgraphic blade gauge), it is possible to monitor the wear and compensate for it (see the section on optical or indirect gauges, below). Some sort of optical magnifier or comparator device is highly recommended as essential in the proper performance of incision-based refractive surgical procedures. This type of monitoring extends the life of the blade some three fold. In a busy practice this method will pay for itself very quickly in terms of blade life and successful surgery. Even at a worst case where 70–80 µm of bias must be used, such a blade will cut significantly more smoothly and evenly than any steel blade and many diamonds.

Diamond has an advantage over sapphire in that it is much harder. Properly cared for it can last considerably longer. Coupled with a shadowgraph-type gauge, one blade could last for many years. The problem with diamond has been that its very hardness has placed practical limits on the quality of the blade produced. Recently, manufacturers have been making great strides in improving quality. The Western Medical Products WMK-200 (LeCut) ultra-thin diamond blade, made to the author's specifications, is a quantum improvement over previous blades. It is only 0.15 mm in thickness with an included bevel angle of 33°, giving it an edge thickness of 22 nm—very similar to sapphire, up until recently the sharpest unicrystalline blades made. This double-edged blade is designed to fit into the Katena K2-6500 series handles and is completely interchangeable with the XTAL sapphire series blades.

It has ever been the practice, even with sapphire,

(a)

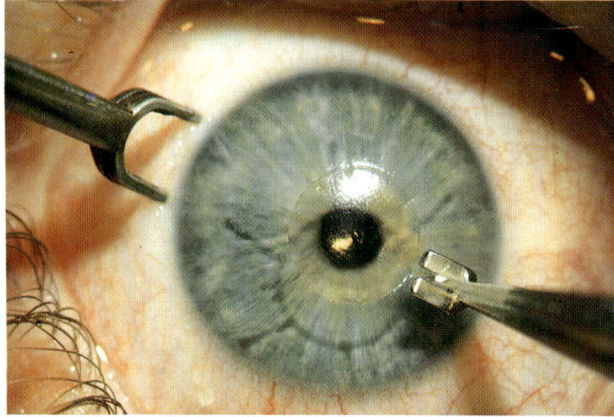

(b)

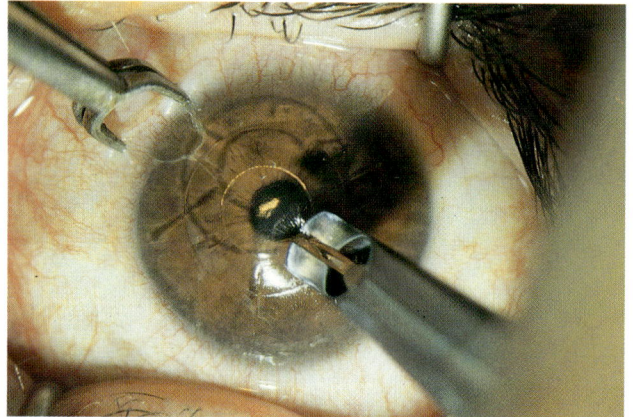

Fig. 8.4 (a) Katena footplate on cornea; (b) Micra (old style) footplate on cornea.

to set the blade longer than the measured corneal thickness. This overset (bias) has amounted to as much as 15% of the corneal thickness (typically 60–70 μm) with some diamond knives—best case. With the XTAL sapphire single-edged blade it is necessary to over-set the blade only 20–30 μm (0.02 mm) to insure adequate depth—best case. The new double-edged XTAL requires only a 10 μm best case over-set, while the WKM-200 diamond requires a bias of 0 μm. This latter bias requirement makes the WKM-200 the sharpest blade yet available for radial keratotomy with a price comparable to a similar double-edged sapphire blade. The ability to make consistently deep incisions is increasing the accuracy of our predictions considerably as well as increasing the surgical effect.

Another factor to be considered is blade inter-changeability, i.e. can the blade be removed from the handle to be replaced by another in case of breakage or dulling or if a different edge shape is needed? Most commercially available diamond knives presently lock the surgeon into a fixed handle/blade situation. This coupled with unreliability and high cost makes them, in my view, a second choice to an interchangeable sapphire blade or the new diamond from Western Medical.

The handle should have an open L-shaped (or sewing machine) foot with ample distance from the jaw or collet to the foot to allow an unobstructed view of the back of the blade for the Bores (American) technique or leading edge for the Fyodorov (Russian) technique (Figure 8.4). The footplate, in addition, should have the foot extend in front of the blade at least 1.0 mm (Figure 8.5) ahead of the leading blade edge and all footplate edges must be smooth and parallel, with all surfaces polished to a mirror finish. The slot for the blade should be wide enough to allow free movement of the blade during adjustment but not

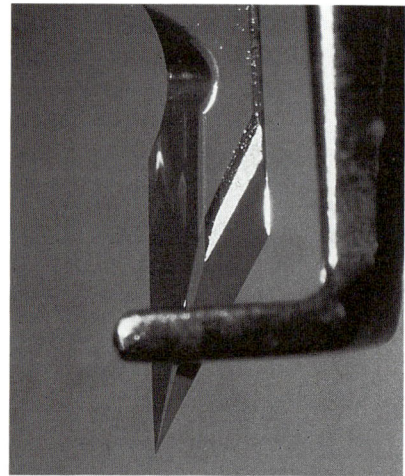

Fig. 8.5 The footplate on the Bores knife handle as supplied by Katena Instruments. Note the extension of the footplate ahead of the blade and that the curve of the footplate lies in front of the vertical cutting edge.

wide enough to trap debris or corneal tissue. Each half of the footplate should be between 0.75 and 1.00 mm in width; wide enough to provide adequate support and stability but not so wide as to obstruct the view of adjacent incisions. The spine of the blade should describe an angle of 90° to the footplate and should be set in sufficiently such that if the handle is tipped backward or forward a deeper cut does not occur. Some knives have the front curvature beginning at the center line of the blade, thus materially affecting the depth of the incision depending upon the direction of cut (Figure 8.6). The handle should allow smooth, continuous adjustment of blade length from a maximum of 1.0 to a minimum of −2.0 mm. Ideally, it should be equipped with a zeroing micrometer scale for fine adjustments of the blade once set (Figure 8.7).

(a)

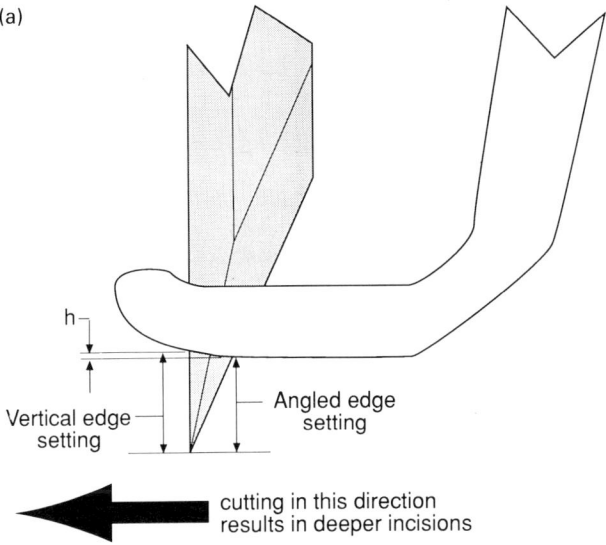

(b)

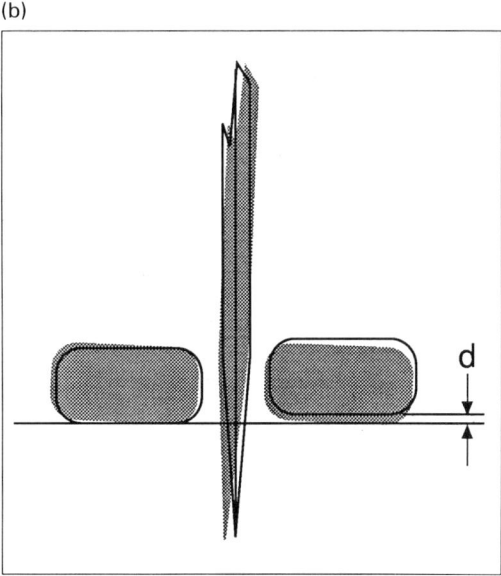

(c)

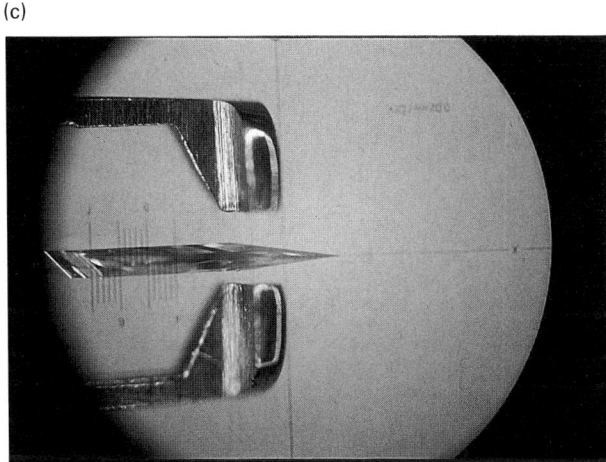

(d)

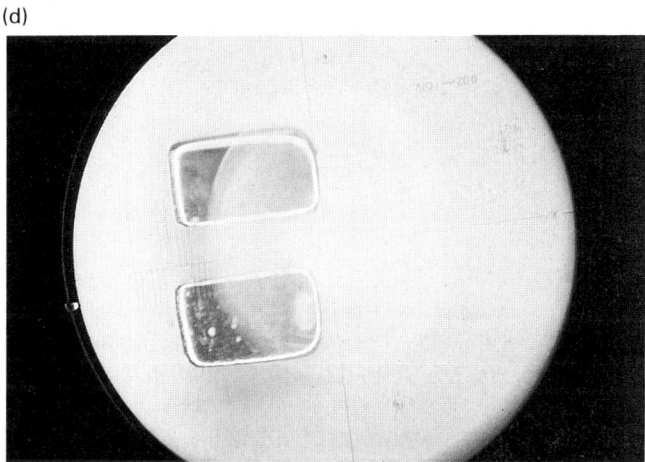

Fig. 8.6 (a) Difference between cutting with the vertical and angled blade edge. (b) Displaced footplates result in oblique incisions. (c and d) Using an optical comparator can readily detect displaced footplates.

(a)

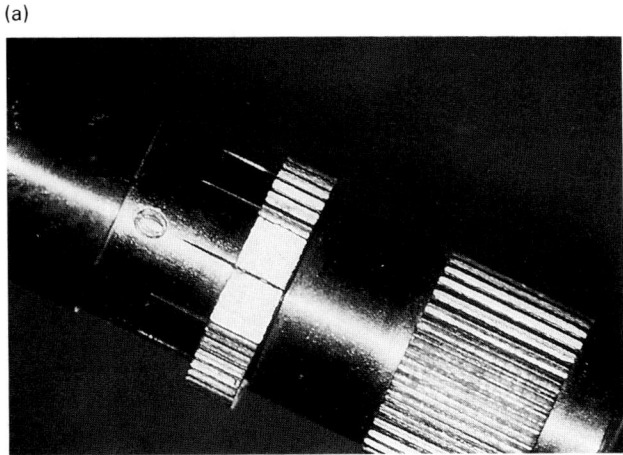

(b)

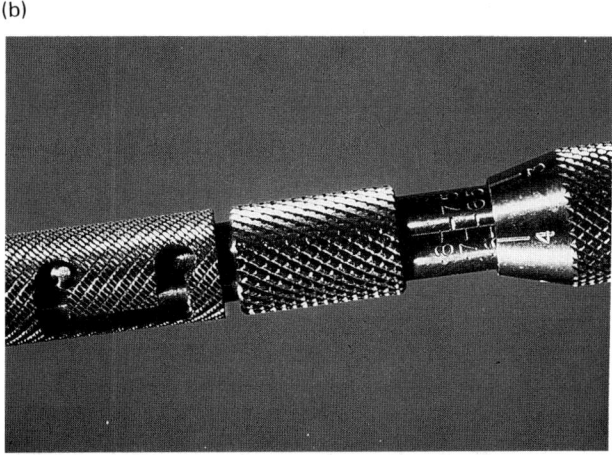

Fig. 8.7 (a) The micrometer adjustment dial on the Bores knife handle is used for fine adjustment once the blade is set with a gauge. (b) The micrometer adjustment on a typical fixed-blade diamond knife is used for all blade settings.

(a)

(b)

(c)

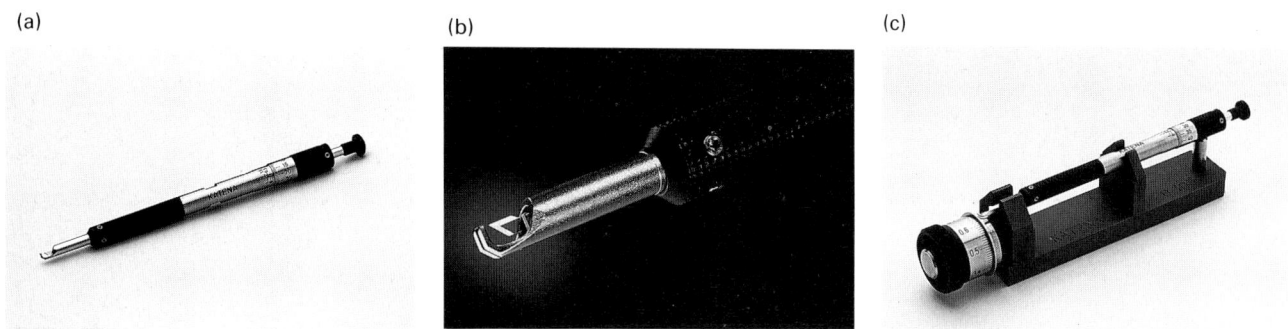

Fig. 8.8 (a) Typical micrometer diamond knife. (b) The footplate is short and does not extend sufficiently in front of the vertical blade edge. (c) Dial-type gauge and holder for this knife. This type of gauge is somewhat less prone to parallax errors when setting.

(a)

(b)

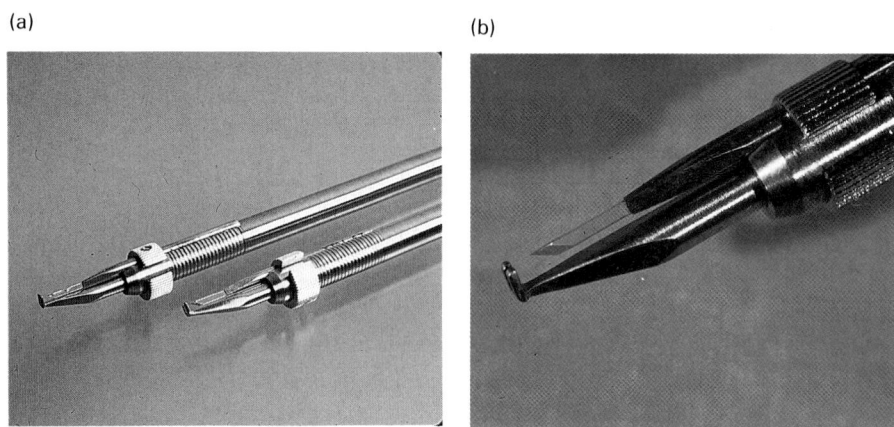

Fig. 8.9 (a) Author's knife handle design with vertical and angled blades—as manufacturered by Katena. (b) Note the open construction which allows excellent visibility of the blade, which is easily changed.

With this type of system the blade is advanced and checked against a gauge. After the proper length has been set the micrometer scale is zeroed. Each division on the micrometer barrel should correspond to some even multiple of a millimeter such as 0.01 or 0.0125 mm. However, no micrometer handle should be trusted to set the blade initially. The initial setting should *always* be checked against a proper gauge, preferably an optical one. There is too much play in any adjustment system to be completely accurate, particularly over a long range. However, with a zeroing micrometer barrel, small advances in the blade can be made with confidence. Because of this built-in play or looseness in the screw mechanism (backlash), always set the blade while advancing it. Never set the blade by backing up on the micrometer barrel and expecting the setting to be correct—it *never* will be. Always check the blade setting against a gauge (Figure 8.8).

The blade should be easily removed for cleaning and replacement. If it cannot be removed it should be able to be retracted sufficiently to clean it mechanically on all sides as well as allow access to the foot for cleaning without damaging the blade tip. Finally the handle should not be excessively heavy or bulky but should be able to be held easily in the fingers without fatigue.

The Bores XTAL micrometer knife handle, available from Katena (K2-6505 and -07), meets all the above requirements (Figure 8.9).

Handles with removable blades should be cleaned in an ultrasonic cleaner, from time to time, *with the blade removed*, rinsed with warm distilled water, and blown dry before storing in its carrier (K2-6555). *Do not ultrasonically clean any crystalline blade of whatever material.* Blades should be carefully rinsed in distilled water and wiped with a wet Weck-Cel or other microsponge. For stubborn residue, contact lens enzyme cleaner is useful. Avoid the use of potassium or sodium hydroxide, which tends to etch such blades. Blades can be stored in their original carriers or in the micrometer handle and can be steam or dry gas sterilized.

Blade gauges and gauging

As the quality of the blade edge has improved there is an ever-increasing emphasis upon the accurate measurement of the blade length. A precise, linearly stable gauge is a must. While many so-called coin gauges are sold with diamond and other knives, their only advantage is ease of use. Their disadvantages include measurement error due to parallax, error due

(a)

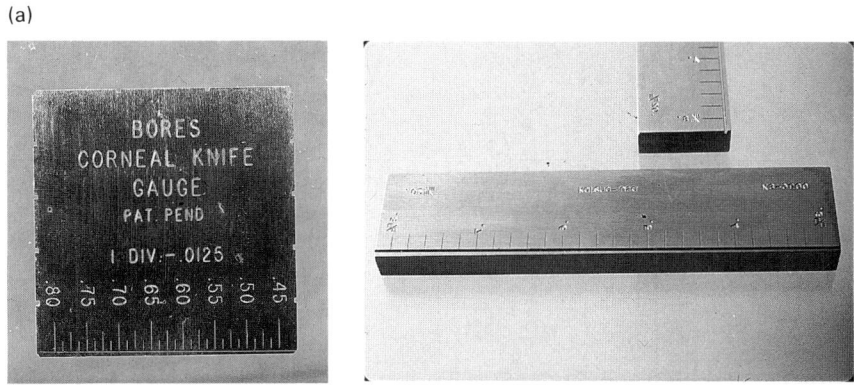

Fig. 8.10 (a) Bores corneal gauge block;
(b) Kremer corneal knife gauge.

to dimensional instability, and error in manufacturing. Unfortunately, many manufacturers have not gotten the message about the need for extreme accuracy in this surgery. Gauges do not lend themselves to mass production; that is why so many small gauge shops thrive in industry today.

Such instruments cannot be made of nylon, aluminum, glass, or combination materials. They cannot have the ticks photo-etched (at least with commonly available methods), as that leads to wide lines with imprecise edges. Gauges cannot be black-chromed to reduce glare—such a process will in time wear off, destroying the accuracy of the gauge. They must be made of stainless tool steel with the ticks scribed under a microscope by an expert in gauge-making.

Direct measuring gauges

Such a gauge block is the Bores Corneal Gauge Block (Figure 8.10), unfortunately no longer available. It was the first blade gauge made for this surgery and since 1979 this instrument has served as the standard for radial keratotomy blade gauges. This gauge is made of tool steel and is certified to an accuracy of $\pm 3\,\mu m$. If not used correctly, however, an erroneous measurement will result from this gauge, like any other. The measurement must be made from the edge of the block to the *front edge* of the scribed datum line (Figure 8.11). This is because the scribe marks were made with a flat-sided diamond scriber with the flat side held against the straight edge. This results in a half-V-shaped scribe mark whose straight edge is perpendicular to the gauge surface. Other gauges require the measurement to be made to the *bottom* of a V-shaped groove (Figure 8.12). Small changes in steel hardness can cause the scriber to rise and fall as it moves, changing the distance of the point from the straight-edge guide. In addition, the fact that the scriber is V-shaped prevents its being held perpendicular to the edge of the guide. Both of these problems result in wandering of the bottom of the V-groove with respect to the edge of the

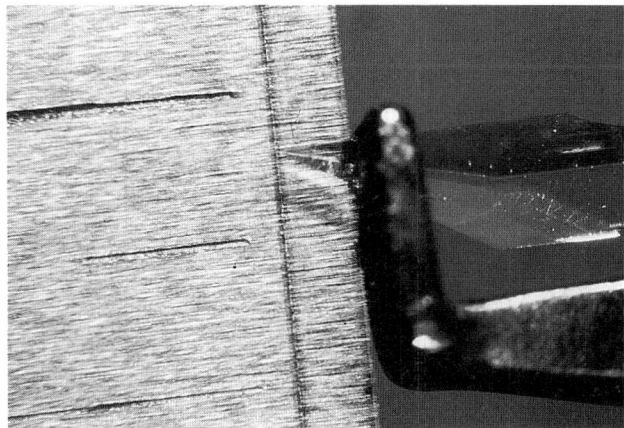

Fig. 8.11 Bores gauge in use with double-edged sapphire blade.

block and thus can produce errors in measurement. You should acquaint yourself with the characteristics of your gauge before using it in any event.

The Bores gauge has proved itself more than equal to the task of measuring blade settings but has disadvantages which make it difficult to use. Firstly, despite efforts to make it less so, this type of gauge is quite reflective. The resultant glare makes precise measurements difficult, but not impossible. This is a larger factor with the crystalline blades because of their transparency. Black chroming, while reducing the glare somewhat, will wear off in time, destroying the accuracy of the block. It is not generally appreciated that the finishing grind on the Bores block has produced the equivalent of a Ronchi ruling. This can be verified by tilting the block slightly under the microscope and observing the color changes. It will be noted that at a certain position the surface of the block takes on a rainbow hue. At this point the glare falls away to almost nil. That the surface is polarizing the light reflected from its surface can be appreciated by holding a diamond blade parallel to the measuring surface (Figure 8.13). The diamond becomes black (or very nearly so) because of cross-polarization. This phenomenon extends to the XTAL blade as well,

(a)

(b)

JGE

CK

JGE

CK

measurement is made
edge–to–edge

measurement is made
edge–to–bottom of V

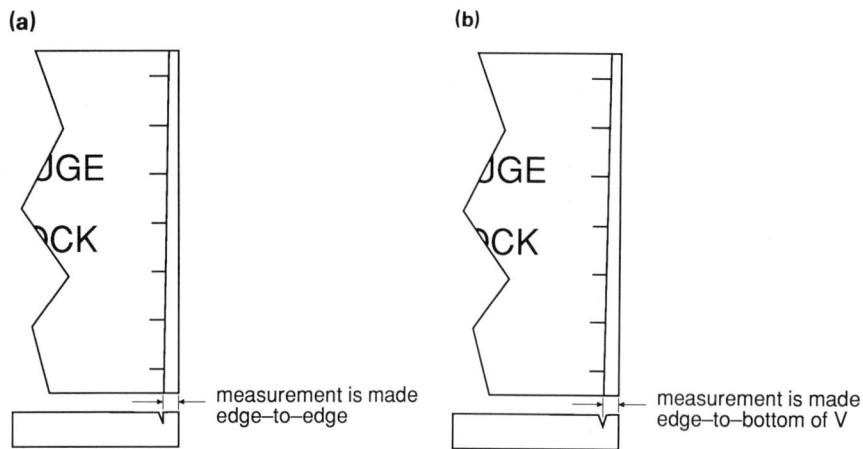

Fig. 8.12 (a) The scribe mark should be made with a flat-sided scriber. (b) A V-shaped scriber tends to wander.

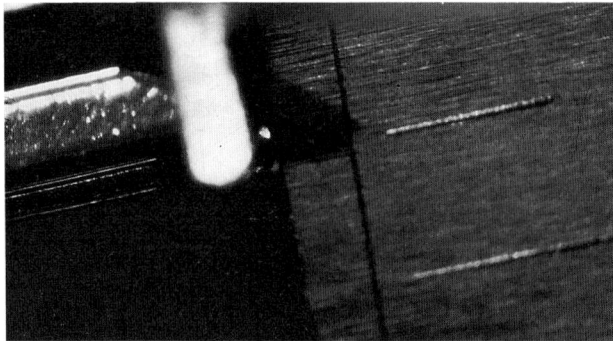

Fig. 8.13 Color change in blade caused by the cross-polarizing effect of the gauge finish and the crystal lattice of the blade.

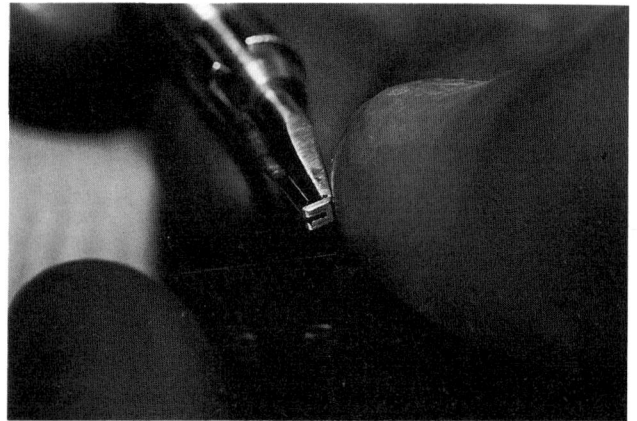

Fig. 8.14 In this single-edged sapphire the edge is rotated slightly to move the blade away from the gauge block. Measurement is taken along the back or spine of the blade.

making this block suitable for any blade the surgeon might be likely to use.

The block requires the user to steady the hands on some surface such as a Mayo stand, wrist rest, or even the patient's forehead to prevent "dinging" the blade edge against the steel block. As the blades have changed and their sharpness increased, the edges and tip have become thinner and more vulnerable. A mere touch of the blade against the gauge can render a crystalline blade useless for radial keratotomy, be it diamond or any other material. To prevent damage to the blade (a match can burn down a house) it must be carefully approximated to the gauge surface with the blade edge rotated upward slightly along its long axis (Figure 8.14). This brings the edge up and away from the block. Care must be taken not to press the blade against the block to avoid breaking the tip or the edge. If that happens the blade can still be used to make cataract sections, but little else.

This block (and others like it) is an expensive precision instrument and must be handled with care. Blocks should be stored in their original containers or in a specially padded plastic box and given a dip in instrument milk if the gauge is not going to be used for some time, to prevent rust. Remember that stainless steel is not rust-proof, just rust-resistant. The block

must not be allowed to come into contact with metallic objects.

There are limits to the resolution of the current operating microscope systems which further add to the problem in obtaining an accurate measurement. In addition, as the tips have become finer, difficulties in judging the tip end for measurement purposes have increased. The present life expectancy of a single-edged sapphire blade in experienced hands, in these circumstances, is about 80 cases. In inexperienced hands the average life of such a blade is about 10 cases. With the newer, sharper, thinner, double-edged blades this average falls to 30 and five cases respectively. It doesn't take long for this to add up; the author was changing one or more blades weekly using the steel gauge.

Optical or indirect gauges

For years devices called shadowgraphs or optical comparators have been used to examine and measure, under high magnification, objects made from transparent materials. These devices are usually quite large,

(a)

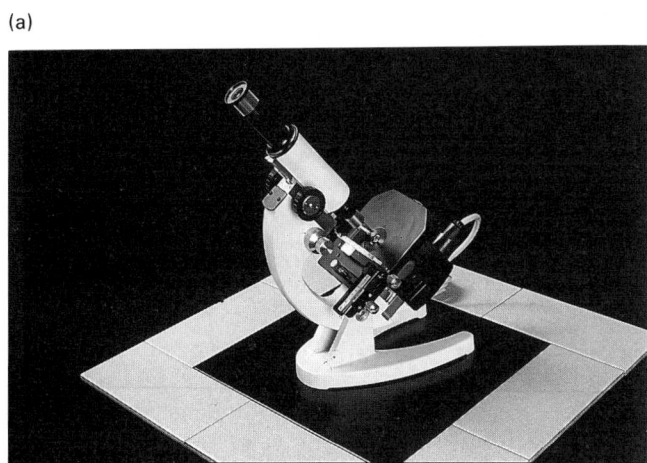

(b)

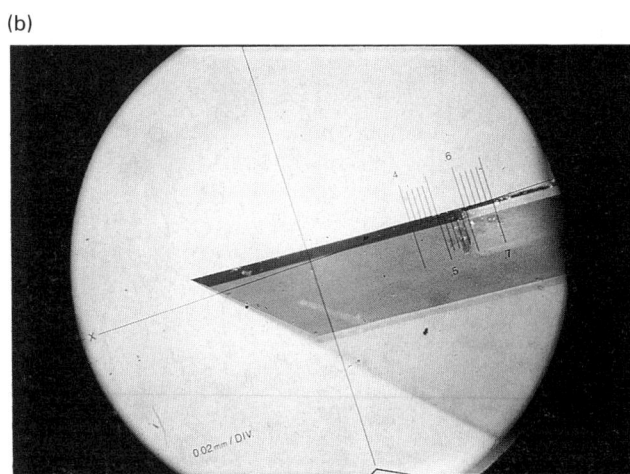

Fig. 8.15 (a,b) Magna diamond microscope and diamond blade.

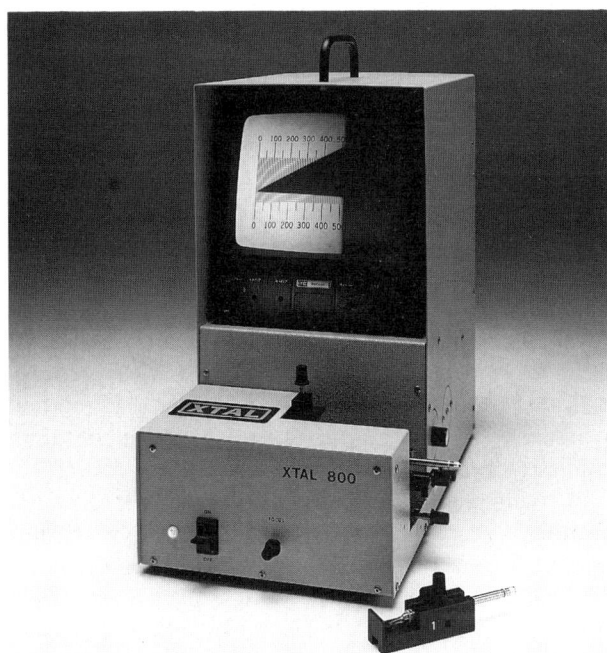

Fig. 8.16 Shadowgraph and knife carrier.

bulky, and very expensive. They do, however, provide a highly accurate means of measurement. An early attempt to emulate, inexpensively, the features of the shadowgraph was the Magna diamond microscopic blade gauge (Figure 8.15). While the device provides an excellent view of the blade and increases accuracy of measurement, it presents the very real hazards of blade damage and contamination of a sterile knife or blade. It is awkward in its use and vulnerable to dust. It is not recommended for use within the operating room but is adequate for pre-setting blades and examining their tips and edges for defects.

The DGH-800 Bores shadowgraphic blade gauge (Figure 8.16) was designed with three goals in mind:
1 Accuracy.

2 Ease of use.
3 Cost-effectiveness.
To this end the instrument is supplied with a special sterilizable carrier into which the knife handle and blade are placed and clamped. These carriers are available for almost all makes of knife handles and blades. The entire assembly can then be transferred on to the measuring stage for final setting of the blade. The DGH-800 provides a magnification of more than $190 \times$ which also allows inspection of the blade tip and edge. By using this device it is possible to triple the useful life of the XTAL sapphire blades. More importantly, the depth of the incisions will become more uniform, thereby increasing the confidence level of pre-operative calculations. Normal rounding of the blade tip can be readily seen and the compensating bias change made with ease (see below).

Fixation devices

Fixation of the eye is important to insure that all incisions are straight and perpendicular to the corneal surface. There are many devices on the market for this purpose. Any such device should be easily applied and removed and should not produce tissue damage. In addition, it must not interfere with the surgery.

The vacuum fixation devices based on the Barraquer fixation ring have not met these criteria—they always interfere with blade travel (Figure 8.17). For best results they must be used with peri-bulbar anesthesia because they produce considerable pain when the vacuum comes on. Also, the inner edge prevents the footplate of the knife from traveling its full length, requiring that the incisions be extended after the ring is removed. Expanding the inner opening to provide knife clearance requires enlarging the entire ring so as to provide an adequate suction surface. This results in a ring of such size that movement of the eye is greatly restricted, making some incisions awkward, if not

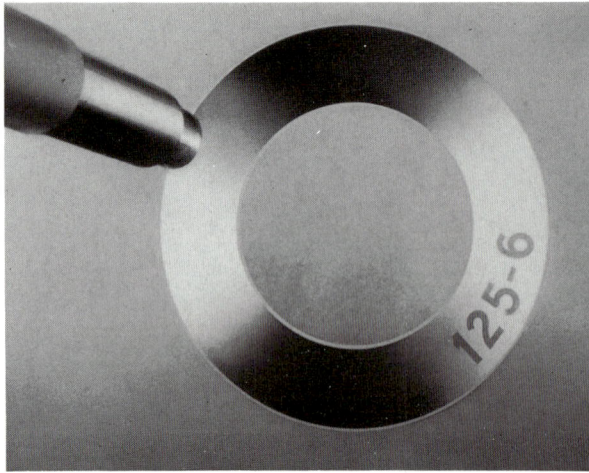

Fig. 8.17 Vacuum fixation ring.

impossible, to perform. It is not possible, for example, to rotate the eye downward without breaking suction and losing fixation. Considerable chemosis of the conjunctiva results from its use. These reasons, as well as the fact that it's expensive, and that the job can be done better and less expensively by other means, place this device on the not recommended list.

Another ring device, this one with a number of straight teeth arranged around its rim, is available from Katena—Thornton fixation ring K3-6165 (Figure 8.18). This is used by centering it over the front of the eye and pressing downward. This device has the advantage of pressurizing the eye, like the vacuum ring, but it does not cause the pain, hence peri-bulbar injection is unnecessary. It is easy to re-position as well. It shares with the vacuum ring the problem of being awkward to use, interferes with the surgery, and in the event of a micro-perforation makes matters worse.

Still another ring fixation device is based on the mechanism of the "twist-pick." This device is placed on to the eye with the handle rotated to one side. Pressing down against the eye and moving the handle to the 12 o'clock position screws it into the sclera, thereby allowing the eye to be pulled as well as pushed. In the event of a micro-perforation it acts like a Bonnocalto ring, supporting the eye instead of allowing it to collapse. Its rim is flared outward to minimize interference with the knife jaw. It shares the disadvantages of all ring devices, however, in that it is awkward to use if kept in one position and interferes with movement of the eye. It is available from Katena as the Bores twist fixation ring (K3-6160). It has proved to be more useful in performing penetrating keratoplasties than in refractive surgery.

Fixation of the eye is easily obtained by use of a forceps applied to the limbus. Forceps which grasp the cornea or incision edge (such as the Bracken) are not recommended because of the possibility of tearing the tissue. I designed, and had made for me, a double-pronged fixation forceps (Katena K5-3250). This forceps has a double set of 0.12 mm corneal–scleral teeth placed 3.0 mm apart. To use, the forceps is applied to the conjoint tendon at the limbus at 180° to the incision to be made (Figure 8.19a). The double fixation points prevent undue ocular rotation without the corneal distortion a wider jaw would produce, especially in a soft eye. Some ocular rotation will occur allowing the track of the incision to remain straight. Forceps that totally prevent some ocular rotation usually require the surgeon to make compensating moves with the knife to keep the incisions straight.

A wide-jawed forceps such as the Bores wide fixation forceps (K5-3280) provides the cross-limbus fixation essential to making straight transverse incisions, as in the Ruiz procedure (Figure 8.19c). Here

(a)

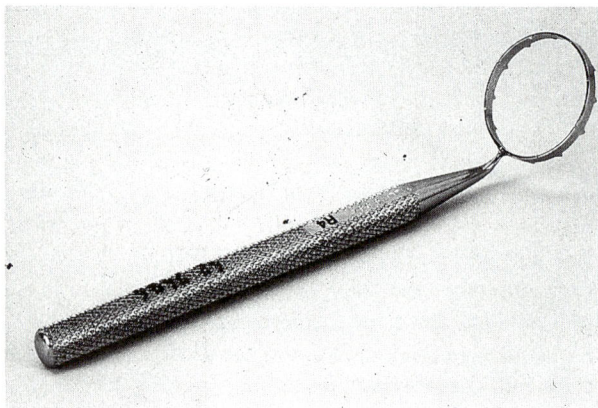

(b)

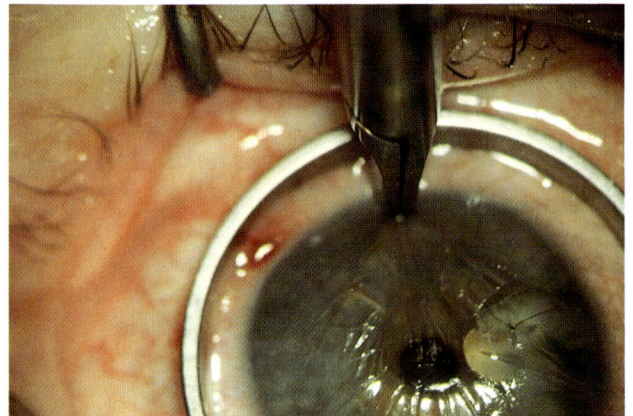

Fig. 8.18 (a) Thornton fixation ring; (b) ring in use. Note how close it is to the limbus, which interferes with knife travel. This photo shows another disadvantage of the ring, if a leak occurs.

(a)

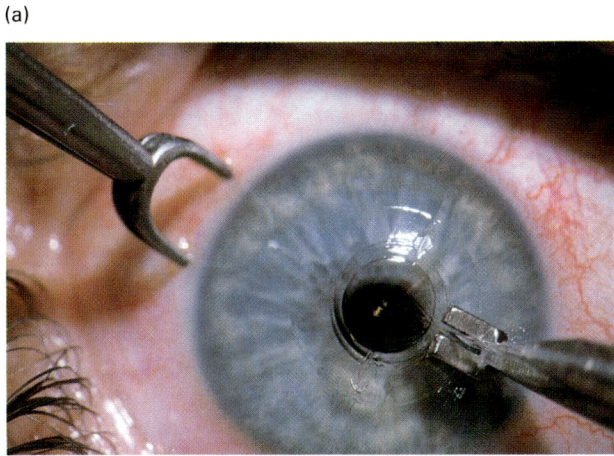

(b)

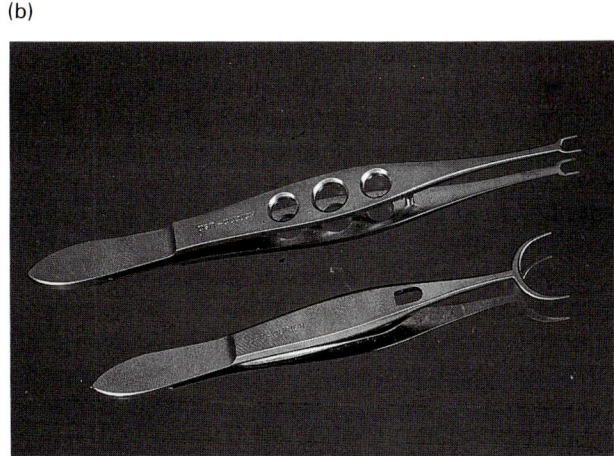

(c)

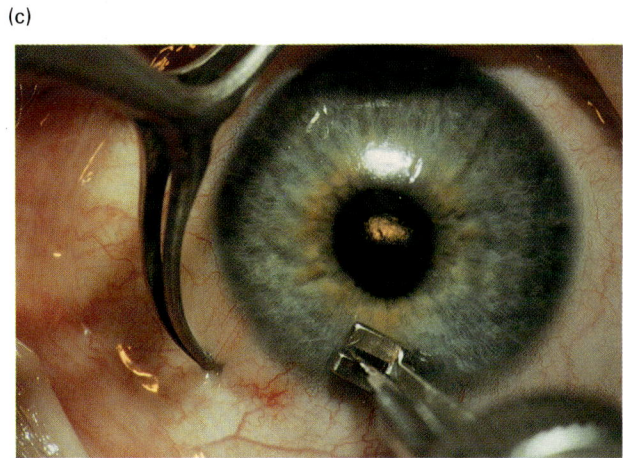

Fig. 8.19 (a) Bores fixation forceps (narrow) in use; (b) narrow and wide fixation forceps; (c) advantage of the wide forceps.

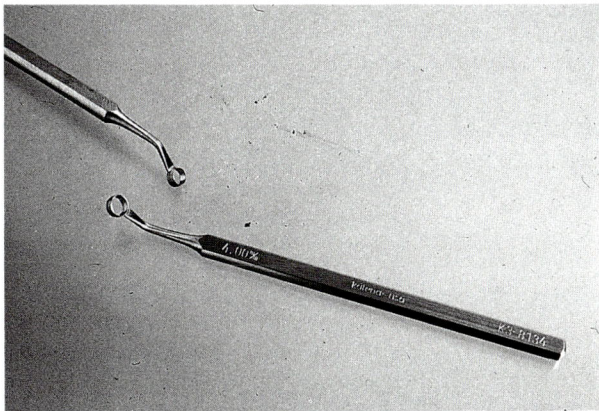

Fig. 8.20 Bores Lo-Profile optical zone marker.

the eye must be prevented from rotating to inhibit the natural tendency of the incision to curve. These instruments are also available with angled jaws for those who prefer it. Compressor devices, such as the Mendez ocular compressor, that squeeze the eye in order to increase intra-ocular pressure are to be avoided.

Optical zone and other markers

Corneal optical zone markers are available from various vendors. Some of these markers are not accurate (especially those for astigmatism), having been formed by stretching over a mandrel. The worst of these were the double-ended variety. Others are obviously made for people with size 2 hands. The best markers on the market today, in my opinion, are those supplied by the Katena Instrument Company (Figure 8.20).

The ideal spherical corneal marker is a perfect circle accurate to 0.05 mm and made in 0.25 mm increments from 3.0 mm to 5.0 mm, and in 0.50 mm increments from 5.50 to 8.0 mm. Of these, the most used will be the 3.0, 3.5, 4.0, 4.5, and 6.0 mm markers (Figure 8.21). However, eventually all of the sizes will find use in a busy refractive surgery practice. These should have an outside bevel to an edge sharp enough to mark the cornea with a fine narrow mark without cutting into the corneal surface. The markers can be shallow, but if deeper than 3.0 mm should be wider at the top (have a conical shape) so as to provide a clear view of the entire ''business end'' of the marker. Deeper markers should

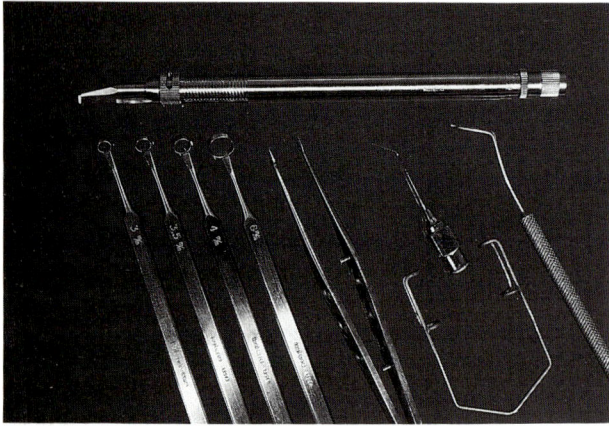

Fig. 8.21 Basic instrument set showing minimal number of markers required.

be provided with openings in their sides to allow light to enter so as better to visualize the corneal surface. A good example is the Fyodorov series of surgical zone markers (Figure 8.22).

Cross-hairs or other centering aids are useful but not essential, and frequently are inaccurately aligned. Sizes should be clearly marked on each marker, particularly astigmatism markers. All markers, especially those for astigmatism, must be handled with care to prevent damage that may distort their shapes. Double ring markers have been produced and can be especially useful for the starting surgeon (Figure 8.23). Those of 3.0 and 6.0, and 3.5 and 6.0 mm will prove to be the most useful. An occasional use will be found for a triple marker with rings at 3.0, 6.0, and 8.0 mm.

Special devices for marking the incision lines or spacing are available as well (Figure 8.24). However, all of these, with one exception, are optional. The one exception is the six-blade incision marker (Katena K3-8880; Figure 8.25). While it is possible to make four, eight, or 16 incisions evenly spaced by eye, it is not quite so easy to judge accurately the 30 or 60° between incisions in six- or 12-incision cases. Coating the bottom of this marker with brilliant green or gentian violet will enhance their usefulness, at least for the beginner or when demonstrating the surgery. The

(a)

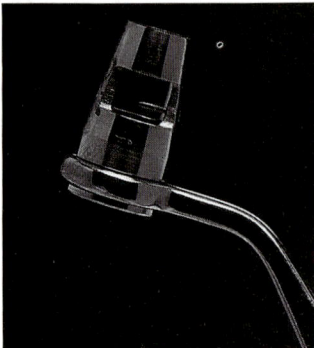

(b)

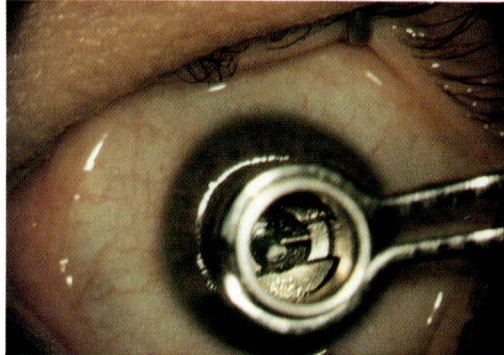

Fig. 8.22 (a) Fyodorov "bore-sight" marker; (b) the marker tapers and has an aiming stud.

(a)

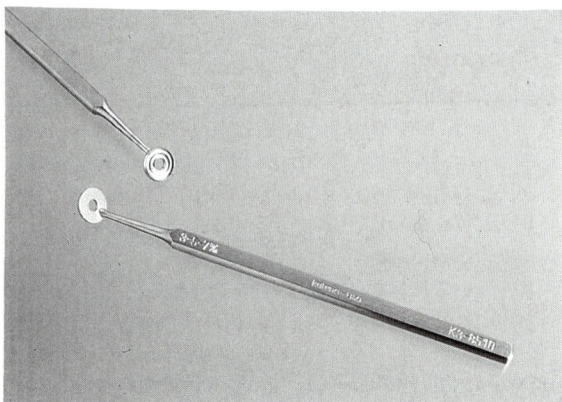

(b)

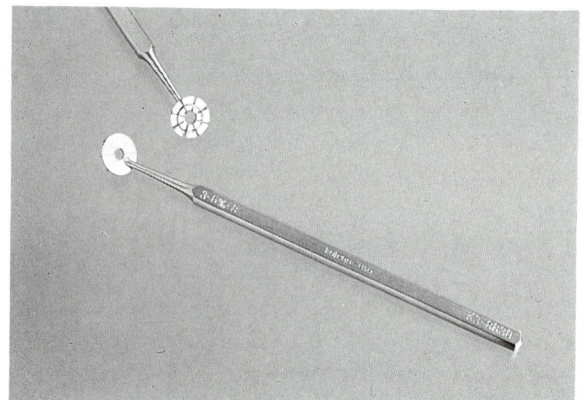

Fig. 8.23 (a) Double and triple ring markers; (b) double ring/incision markers.

(a)

(b)

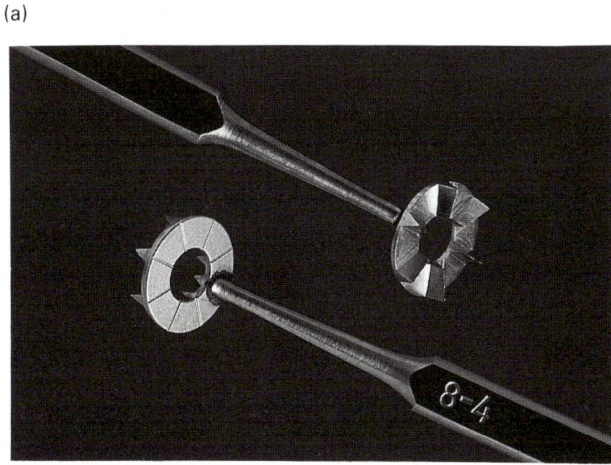

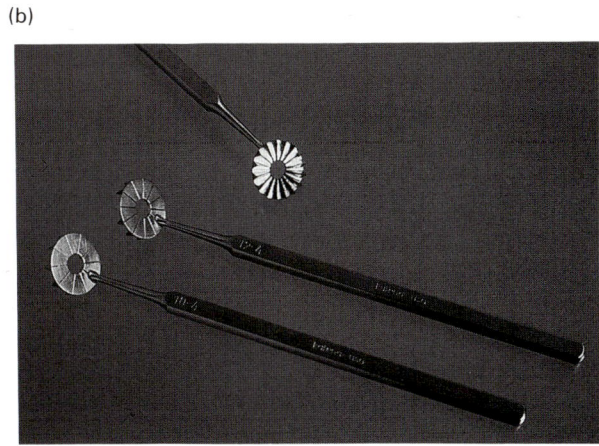

Fig. 8.24 Incision markers: (a) six and eight; (b) 10 and 12 incisions.

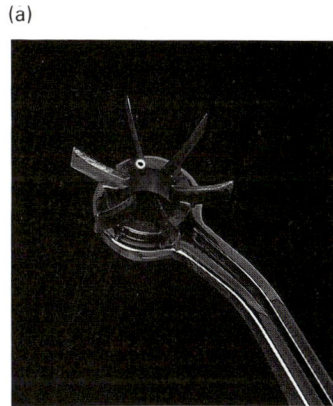

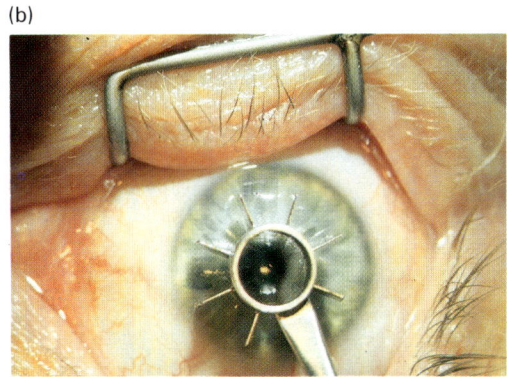

(a)

(b)

Fig. 8.25 (a) Fyodorov six-ray incision marker; (b) in use.

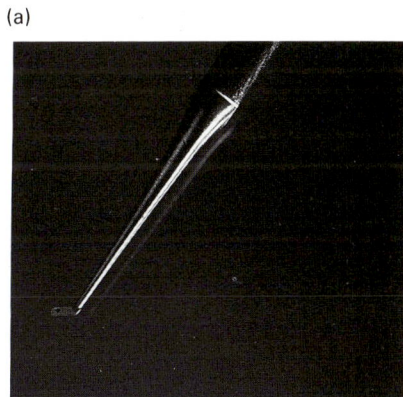

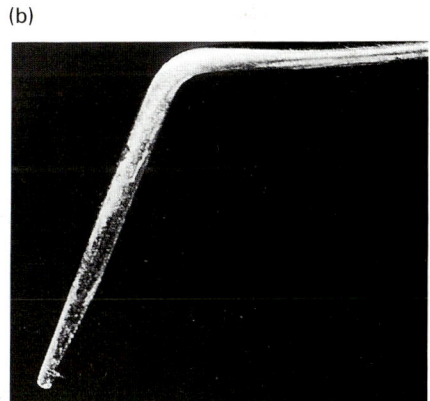

(a)

(b)

Fig. 8.26 (a) Deitz hockey stick; (b) Fyodorov dipstick.

more experienced surgeon will find the central ends of the marks sufficient to align the incisions.

Other useful instruments

There are some other instruments that the surgeon will find of use. A thin, flexible, flat-sided probe, such as the Deitz incision depth gauge (Katena K3-9600, -10, -20) is handy (Figure 8.26). This "hockey stick" is used to measure the relative depth of incisions and check the continuity of the incision bottom, especially for snags from improperly stepped incisions (Figure 8.27). Though available with three different blade widths, only one—K3-9620—is really needed. It is also useful for marking the optic center during optical zone marking and is recommended for this purpose over sharp needles.

Incision spreaders are used in rare cases of higher

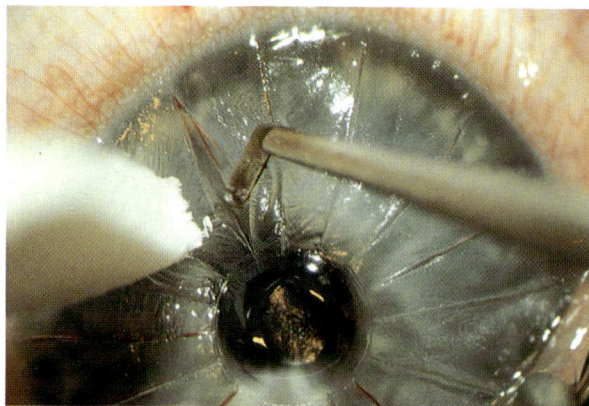

Fig. 8.27 Checking the wound with the dipstick.

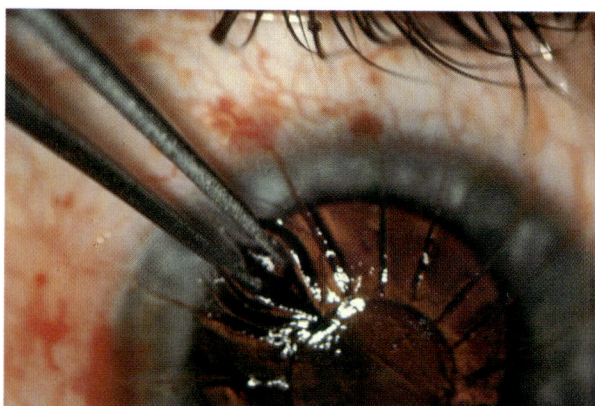

Fig. 8.28 Bores incision spreader in use.

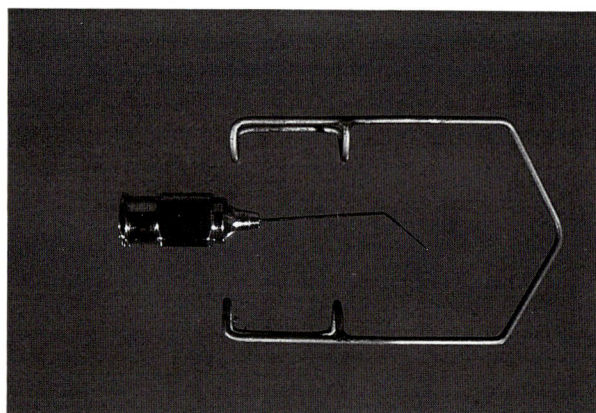

Fig. 8.29 Barraquer-type wire lid speculum; small-bore irrigating cannula.

myopia to deepen previously made incisions (Katena K5-6800). These instruments should be angled to provide an unobstructed view of the bottom of the incision (Figure 8.28). They should also be provided with an adjustable stop to prevent over-spreading the wound. Those made with large teeth (inverted Colibri forceps) should not be used because of the extensive tissue damage that can result if the eye moves. A newer type of spreader with diamond (or carborundum) chips on the outer surfaces of the spreader provides greater friction against slipping without the danger of tearing tissue.

A small-bore irrigating cannula with a rounded tip and flattened bore (Rainin 27 gauge cannula, Katena K7-3580) is used to cleanse the incisions of debris post-operatively. Such an irrigation stream should be gentle and directed along the incision to flush the wound toward the limbus.

A wire lid speculum of the Barraquer type (Katena K1-5010) is recommended for supporting the lids (Figure 8.29). It should not be one with solid blades as

this type will pop out with a blink. The Guyton-Park or rigid-type speculum is not recommended because it is too traumatizing to the lids and levator aponeurosis. Seven cases of upper lid ptosis caused by levator damage have been reported, clearly implicating this type of lid speculum [7].

A suitable tray-case should be obtained of a size adequate to hold a basic set of surgical instruments without their being bashed together and damaged. If the lid is removable for auto-claving, so much the better. Spare instruments can be put up in sterile bags, preferably those with one clear side. Alternately, they can be placed in steel parts cabinets with padded plastic drawers.

Predicting the outcome of radial keratotomy

The surgery of radial keratotomy is fairly straightforward. It is, however, not without its pitfalls. Careful attention to details and pre-operative planning can eliminate most of these. It is paramount for the new keratotomist to choose a single guru whose technique and philosophy will be followed to the letter. Do not alter or modify this technique unless or until your own results begin to match theirs. Only then is it safe for you to go off on your own.

The successful outcome of radial keratotomy surgery depends upon the careful integration of numerous factors [8], as amply demonstrated by the mediocre and unpredictable results of the PERK study, which didn't do this. These factors are:

1 Degree of myopia.
2 Curvature of the cornea—keratometry.
3 Degree of corneal asphericity (corneal shape—the difference between the peripheral and central corneal curvatures).
4 Corneal rigidity (elasto-tonometric coefficient).
5 Corneal diameter.

6 Age of the patient.
7 Sex of the patient.
8 Size of the optical zone.
9 Number of incisions.
10 Depth of the incisions.
11 Intra-ocular pressure.
12 Thickness of the cornea—pachymetry.
13 Degree of corneal toricity (astigmatism).

It does not take much perspicacity to realize that it requires more than a crystal ball to integrate this number of variables (Figure 8.30). It also does not take too much mental energy to realize that a "look-up" table such as used in the PERK study [9] cannot cope adequately with the problem either. Even nomograms are less than ideal because all cases will require multiple iterations and nomograms are done manually. While all surgeons may start out using nomograms with the best of intentions, the amount of paper work required with this method rapidly becomes onerous to the point where even a saint would look for short cuts. This is compounded by the necessity for the surgeon to perform the calculations him- or herself—this is one area of ophthalmology that cannot be delegated successfully.

Computers and refractive surgery

A word or two about establishing surgical parameters in refractive surgery. It is not possible to determine adequately how many incisions to make or what the optimum optical zone size should be without a computer. Look-up tables have been tried and found wanting. There is just too much data to be accounted for and correlated for two-dimensional tables, and multi-dimensional tables are too cumbersome and prone to look-up error. While it is true that good results have been reported by resorting to half-measures, it is well to heed an old Russian proverb: Better is the natural enemy of good enough.

Data accumulate rapidly and a paper grid lock can occur leading to a tendency to take short cuts with both data gathering and processing. An effective computer program and timely data analysis can prevent error and increase the efficacy of your surgery. The computer program that you choose to use, however, should be selected with the surgical technique in mind. Each program has been tailored for a specific surgeon's approach to making relaxing incisions. If you select a particular piece of software, you are also selecting that particular surgeon's technique.

It is just not possible to "mix and match" with this surgery. You cannot be eclectic in your surgical approach and expect any prediction software to be effective under those circumstances. You must adopt the calculation and surgical method of a particular, experienced surgeon and follow his or her method

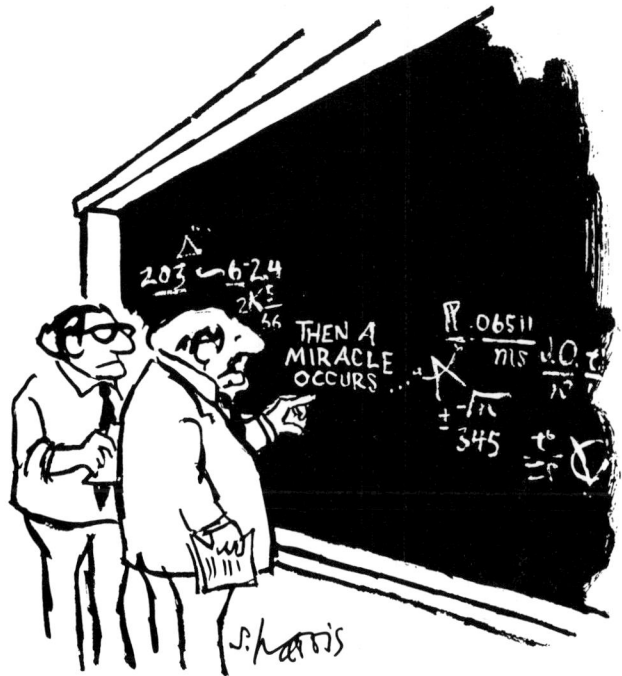

"I THINK YOU SHOULD BE MORE EXPLICIT HERE IN STEP TWO."

Fig. 8.30 More than a miracle is needed to calculate radial keratotomy parameters.

assiduously until such time that you have become absolutely confident in your understanding of all the nuances of this surgery. Then and only then will it be possible for you to "vary the theme" and strike off on your own.

The optical zone

Of all the factors that affect the amount of post-operative flattening of the cornea, the incisional length is one of the most important. All things being equal, the length of the incisions is controlled by the size of the surgical clear or optical zone. This is the central free zone left uncut, from which the incisions radiate toward the periphery of the cornea. These optical zones are either circular (in the case of spherical myopia) or elliptic (in cases of astigmatism, under certain circumstances). It is in the selection of these optical zones that the beginning keratotomist has the most difficulty.

There is a definite inverse relationship between the diameter of the optical zone and the degree of myopia in the patient's optical system. The selection of the size of the primary optical zone is based (for the most part) upon the patient's spectacle refraction, although the amount of astigmatism in the patient's optical system

Table 8.1 First radial keratotomy surgical guide

Optical zone diameter (mm)	Effect (D)
4.5	0.75–1.25
4.0	1.50–2.00
3.5	2.20–2.50
3.0	>2.75

may not bear any direct relationship to the astigmatism on the cornea (as measured by keratometry). Remember that we are correcting the refraction of the optical system by altering the corneal surface—much like fitting a contact lens for the same purpose.

To assist in the selection of these optical clear zones a series of tables was initially constructed (Table 8.1). These soon gave way to nomograms which take into consideration as many as six separate parameters (Figure 8.31) [10]. However, the accuracy of these nomograms has been shown to be inadequate for many cases of spherical myopia and well-nigh impossible in cases with astigmatism. Furthermore, one has to be drawn for more than one optical zone choice. Continuing work on this problem produced the first of

the Fyodorov formulas—Formula I. Shortly thereafter, the Durnev–Fyodorov–Bores formula (Formula II) made its appearance. Both of these formulas are used to predict the outcome of the surgery: the first by calculating the degree of myopia expected to be corrected, and the second, more useful Formula II, calculates the size of the optical zone to be used to affect a given amount of myopia.

The formulas

Formula I

$$P = \frac{\sqrt{D^2 + \frac{16}{3}\left(R - \sqrt{R^2 - \frac{D^2}{4}}\right)^2} - \sqrt{d^2 + \frac{16}{3}\left(R - \sqrt{R^2 - \frac{d^2}{4}}\right)^2}}{\sqrt{d^2 + \frac{16}{3}\left(R - \sqrt{R^2 - \frac{d^2}{4}}\right)^2}} \cdot K \cdot a$$

This calculates the effect of surgery (P) given that: D = the diameter of cornea (in mm); R = the radius of the cornea (in mm); K = the coefficient of corneal rigidity; and a = the incisional depth coefficient. This formula calculates the resultant reduction in myopia to be expected after 12 months for a given combination of factors. It is especially useful in cases where the

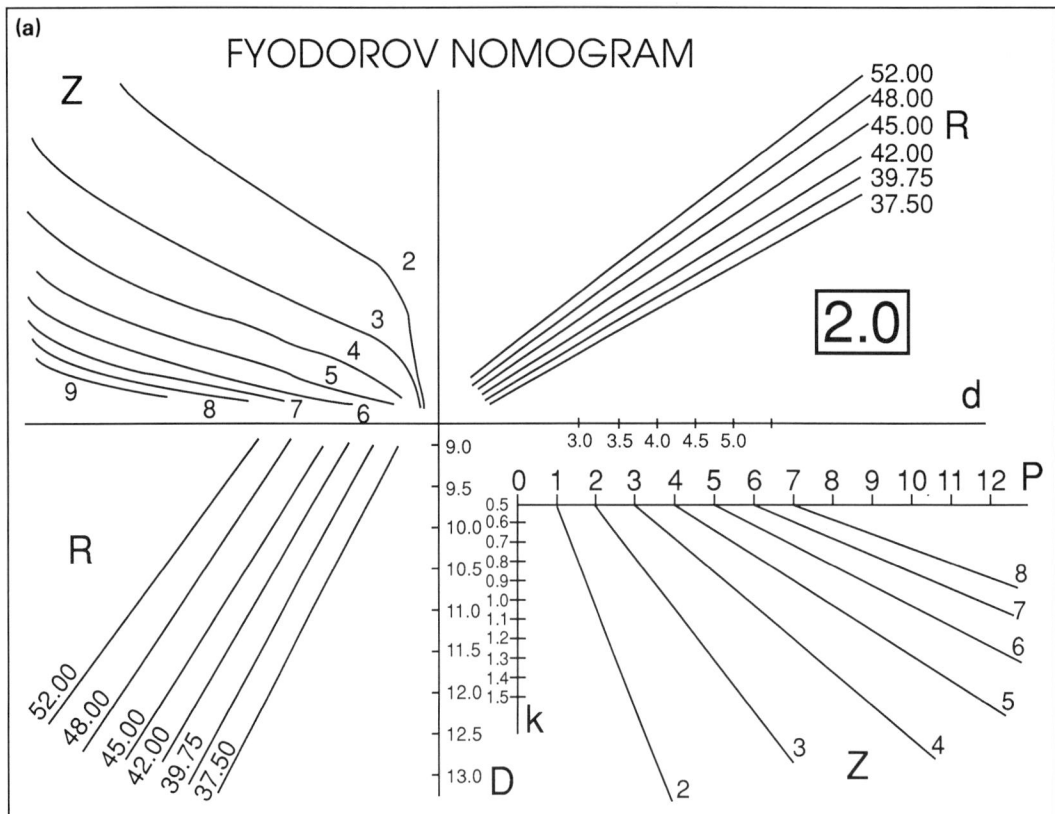

Fig. 8.31 (a) Fyodorov nomogram. (b–g) Using the Fyodorov nomogram to determine a surgical zone. (b) Select the myopia on the P line, and the rigidity on the K line. (c) Drop perpendiculars from both points. The intersection is the Z-point. (d) Draw a horizontal line to intersect the K-reading. (e) A vertical is drawn from that point to the upper Z-point. (f) A horizontal is drawn from the Z-point to intersect with the upper K-reading. (g) A vertical is dropped from that point to intersect the d line—the optical zone size.

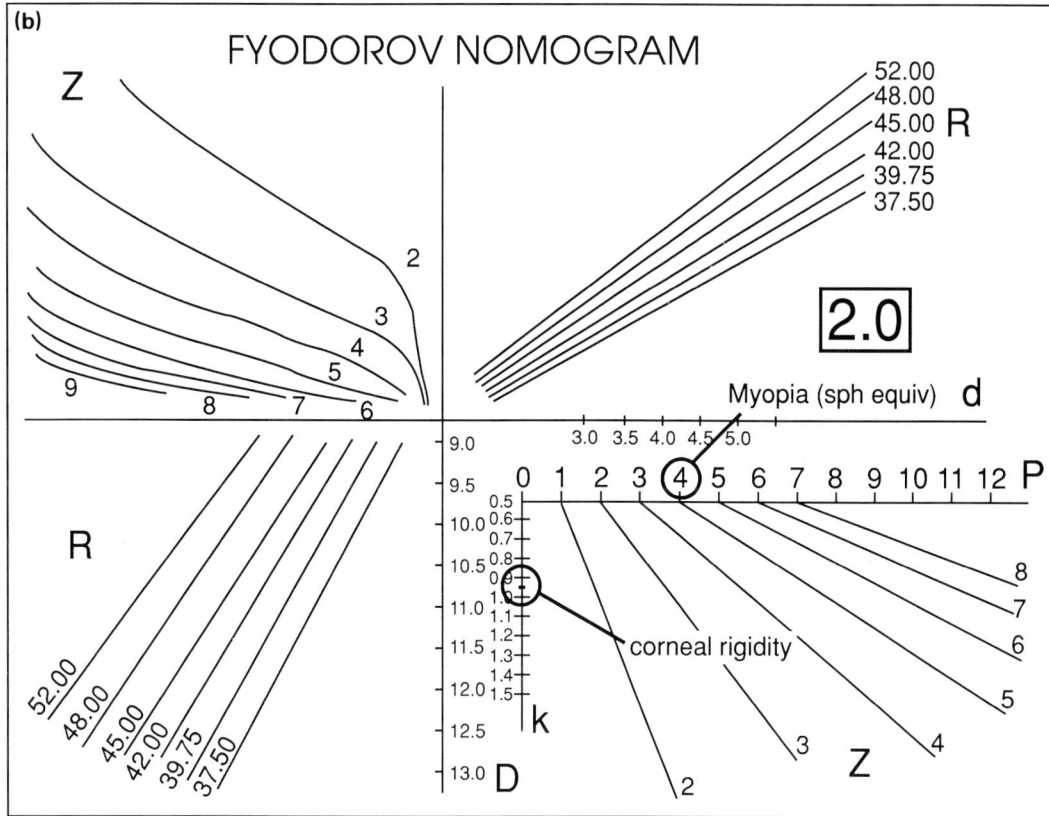

(b) FYODOROV NOMOGRAM

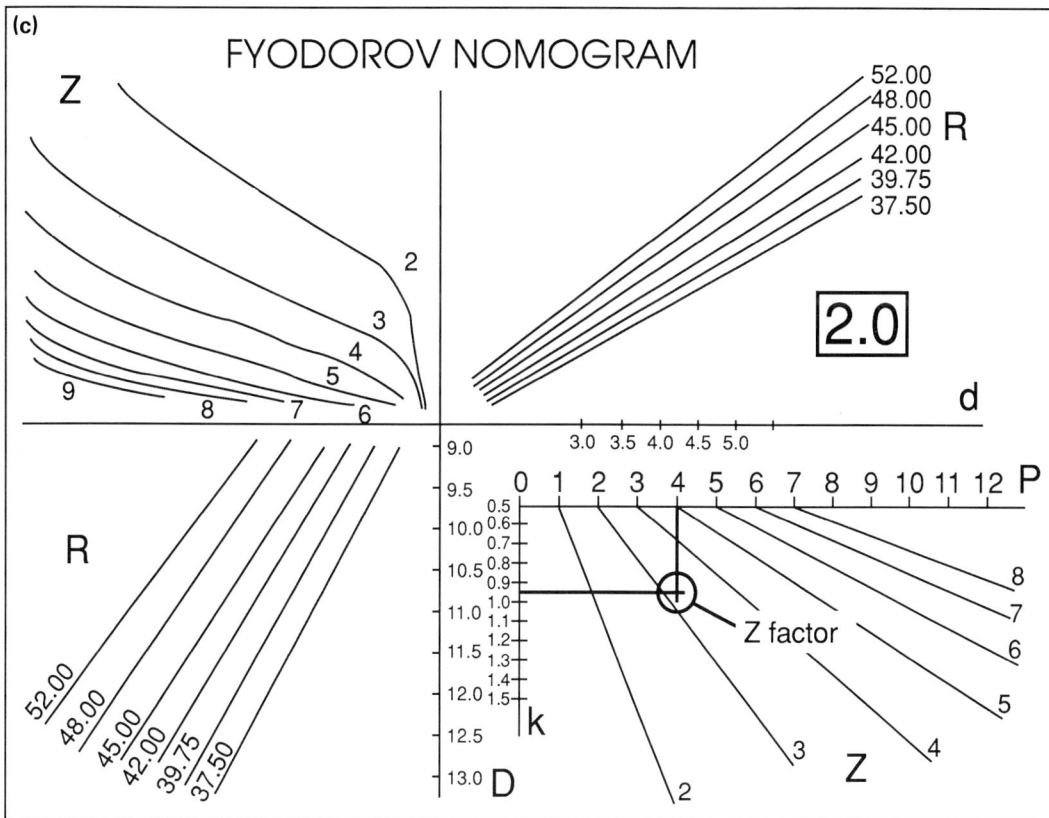

(c) FYODOROV NOMOGRAM

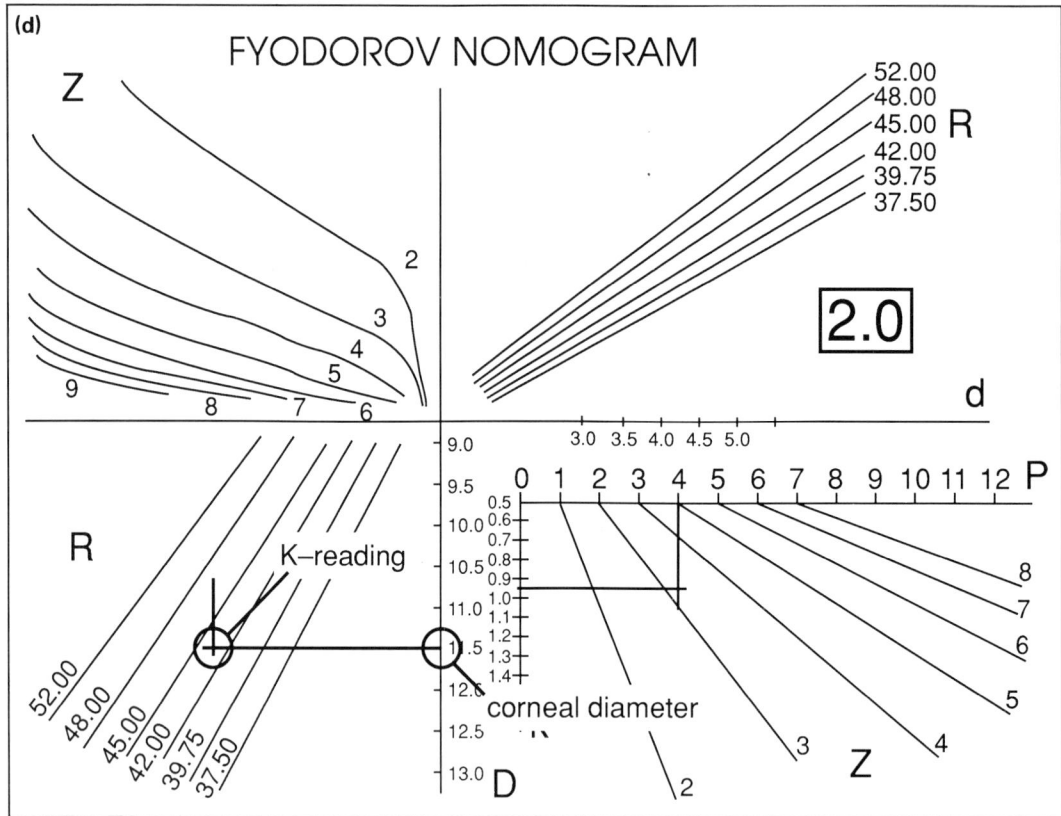

(d) FYODOROV NOMOGRAM

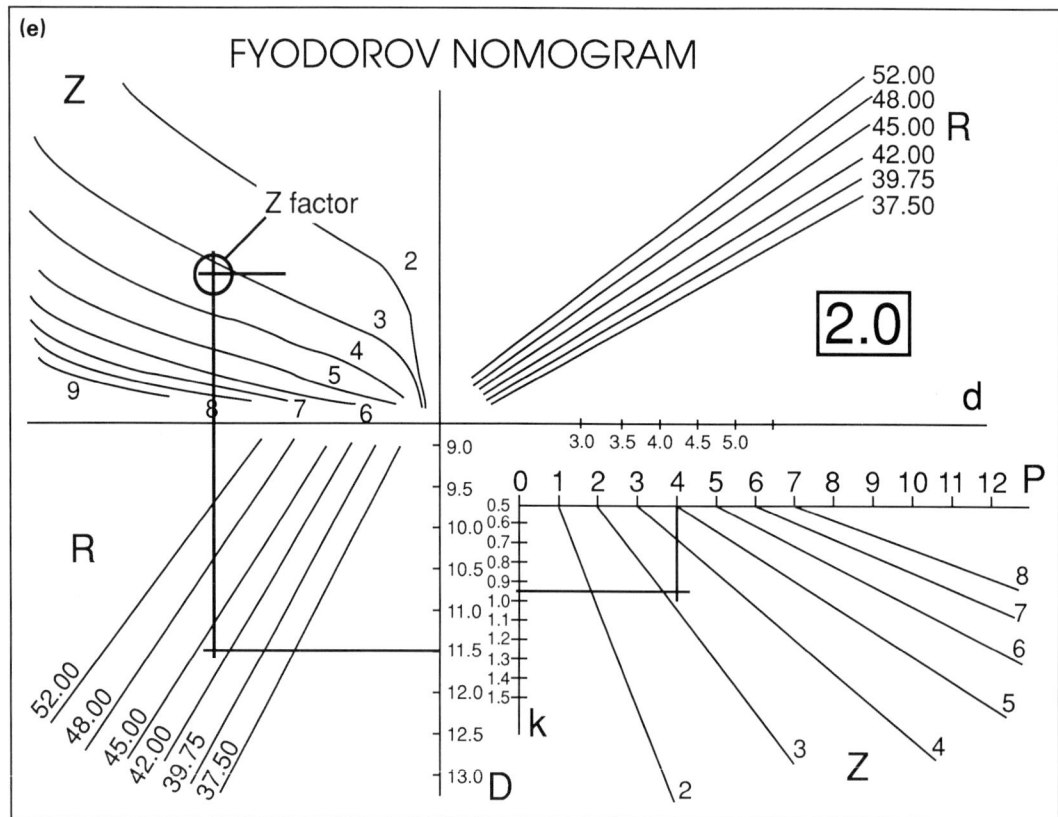

(e) FYODOROV NOMOGRAM

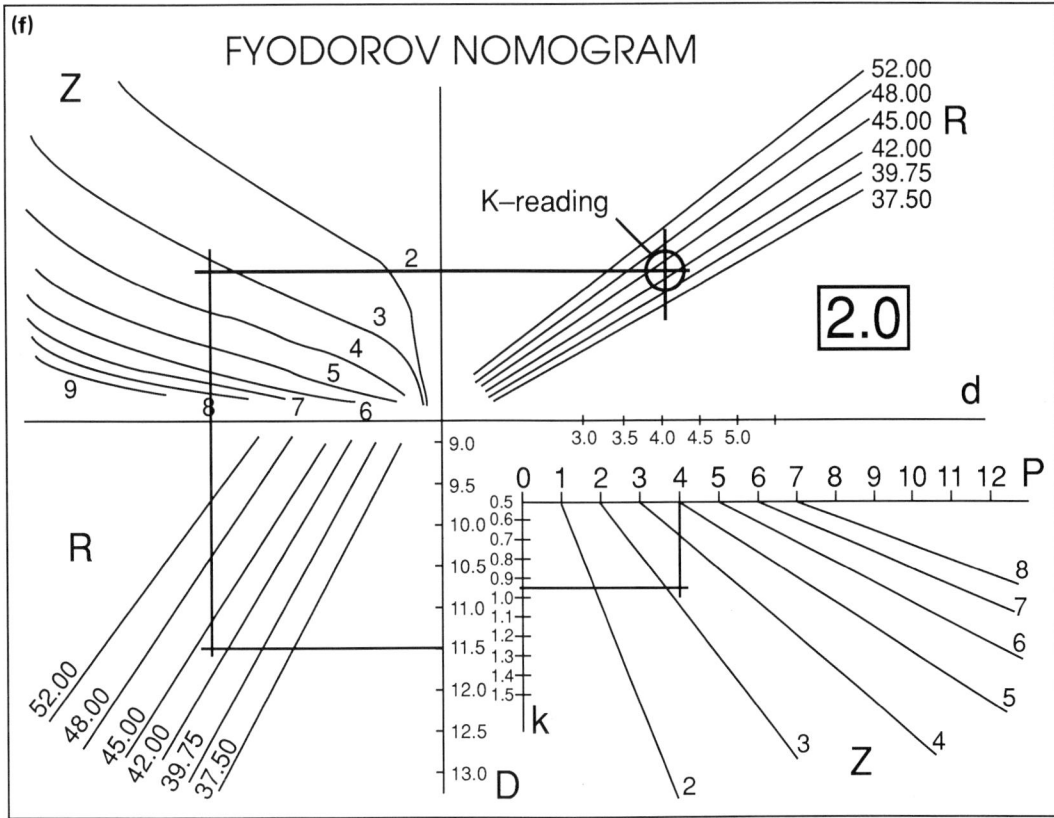

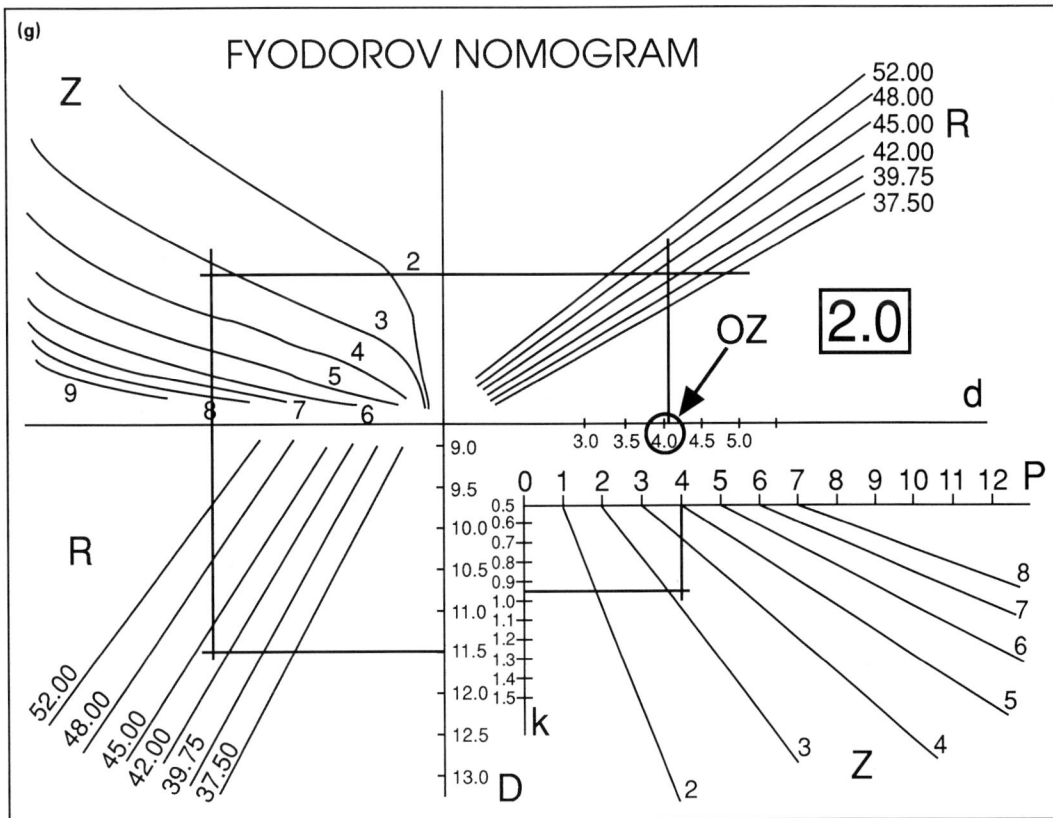

minimum size optical zone (2.75 mm) has to be used for a given correction. It will allow the surgeon to give the patient a reasonable expectation of the surgical outcome. It is incorporated into the RK DataMaster computer program (see below).

Formula II

$$d + \sqrt{-96R^2 - 3A + \sqrt{64R^2 \cdot (6(24R^2 + 2A))}}$$

where:

$$A = \left(D^2 + \frac{16}{3}\left(R - \sqrt{R^2 - \frac{D^2}{4}}\right)^2\right) \cdot \left(\frac{K\alpha}{P + K\alpha}\right)^2$$

This calculates the optical zone size (d) given that P = myopia (in D); R = the radius of the cornea (in mm); K = the coefficient of corneal rigidity; and α = the incisional depth coefficient. This formula will calculate the optical zone needed to correct fully a given amount of myopia. It will sometimes result in an optical zone much smaller than 2.75 mm. In that case, Formula I is used with the minimal size optical zone (2.75 mm) to predict how much correction can be reasonably expected. This formula is also incorporated into the RK DataMaster computer program and automatically switches to Formula I when the calculated primary optical zone is less than 2.75 mm with 16 incisions (maximum surgery).

Both formulas require the surgeon to input six factors:
1 The keratometry, both horizontal and vertical.
2 The corneal diameter.
3 The corneal rigidity.
4 The number of incisions to be used.
5 The incisional depth coefficient.
6 The size of the surgical optical zone (Formula I), or the amount of myopia (Formula II).

Using the formulas

It is necessary to make a number of measurements of each eye in order to use the formulas properly. Failure to take these factors into account leads to widely disparate results and causes confusion and disappointment, not only to the patient but to the surgeon as well. Furthermore, it promotes the notion that this surgery is not predictable.

Incisional depth coefficient

This factor, originally called "the surgeon's practical coefficient of correction," has created a great deal of confusion by virtue of being misunderstood. Simply stated, each coefficient represents the effect upon the surgical outcome by the depth of the incision. These factors are fixed in Formulas I and II. In each case the coefficient represents the depth of the incision as a factor of the thickness of the cornea, at the edge of the optical free zone. The confusion arises because of the way in which these coefficients were originally expressed:

Factor 1.3 (1.29)

The earliest coefficient, Factor 1.3 was originally described as representing an incision that was approximately 75% of the corneal thickness at the edge of the primary optical zone, which is usually 3.00 mm (minimum 2.75 mm). However, the factor was never used in that fashion. Instead, it was always used to describe any single-depth incision made by a blade set to the thickness of the cornea (measured at the edge of the optical zone) which resulted in an incision whose depth was approximately 70–80% of the corneal thickness. This was true regardless of the size of the optical zone. In short, it represented the shallowest practical incision that could be made with any hope of producing a significant—but not maximum—effect. Any incision shallower than this would produce less than 60% correction of the myopia and would be likely to regress in effect greatly over time. Typically this depth of cut is arrived at by setting the blade at 100% of the pachymetry. This early teaching of the author has been established by laboratory studies [11].

Subsequently, three other fixed coefficients were evolved (see also Chapter 7). It is vital that the surgeon understand these factors and their relationship to each other and to the actual incisions.

Factor 1.6 (1.62)

Factor 1.6 represents the deepest practical single-depth incision that can be made with a guarded blade. This factor describes any incision made by a blade set to the depth of the cornea at the edge of the optical zone which results in an incision whose depth is approximately 90–95% of the corneal thickness.

Factor 2.0

Factor 2.0 was used when making any two-stage (stepped) incision at maximum depth. That is, it describes two 1.6 factor incisions strung together with the second blade setting determined by the depth of the cornea at the edge of a secondary optical zone, which is usually 6.0 mm in diameter. Initially this deepening was accomplished by cutting over the previously made incision with an appropriately set blade starting at 6.0 mm. However, while this technique seemed to work satisfactorily with steel blades, it often resulted in incisions whose nether regions were "flayed" and whose depth was uneven. Crystalline blades, by virtue of their sharpness which occasioned instances of incisions wandering out of the track and by accompanying increases in micro-perforations and soft eyes, caused the technique to be changed (see the section on stepped incisions, below).

Factor 2.5

Factor 2.5 originally described incisions made using a 2.0 factor in which four, eight, or 16 incisions (or 20 in astigmatism cases) were deepened, free-hand, to Descemet's membrane. This factor has since changed to represent a three-step incision in which each step is made at maximum depth, that is, 90–95%. It is useful to consider this incision as three 1.6 coefficient incisions strung together to make one. Consequently, free-hand incision deepening is no longer a requirement and may actually be undesirable.

As the technique of radial keratotomy evolved, it was quickly found that the blades being used did not actually cut to the depth they were set. It became necessary to over-set the blades in relation to the ultrasonic pachymetry, that is, set them longer than the cornea was thick. Needless to say this promoted, in many surgeons, tachycardia and hyperventilation—at least at first. This over-setting is, however, an absolute necessity and is explained in Chapter 7.

Until recently this meant that a 1.3 factor represented an incision made by a sapphire (or similarly sharp) blade set to 100% of the corneal depth at the edge of the first optical zone. A 1.6 factor was the same blade set at the pachymetry +10 μm. As can be appreciated, the amount of myopic correction was increased because of the increased depth of the incisions which resulted from this over-setting. While holding the depth of the incisions constant, compensation is made by either decreasing the number of incisions or by increasing the size of the primary optical zone or both.

Currently the coefficients have the following meaning:

Coefficient 1.3—requires a blade setting which produces a corneal incision of approximately 75% at the edge of the primary optical zone. This is true of fresh steel and used sapphire blades. Slight under-setting of a fresh sapphire and/or diamond may be required, especially the LeCut diamond.

Coefficient 1.6—requires a blade set so as to produce an incision with a minimum depth of 90–95% at the edge of the primary optical zone. With the LeCut diamond this would be a setting of 100% of the pachymetry. The new sapphire blade requires an overset of 10 μm and steel and some diamond blades may need to be over-set 5–15%.

Coefficient 2.0—requires incisions of two steps, each step of coefficient 1.6 with the primary optical zone of variable size (up to 5.0 mm) and the secondary fixed at 6.0 mm (7.0 mm if the primary is 5.0 mm).

Coefficient 2.5—requires incisions having three steps. Each segment of the incision is to be at coefficient 1.6 and fixed zones at 6.0 and 8.0 mm (7.0 and 9.0) respectively.

Figures 8.32–8.35 graphically illustrate the relationship of these coefficients and should clarify the situation. Regardless of the method of blade setting,

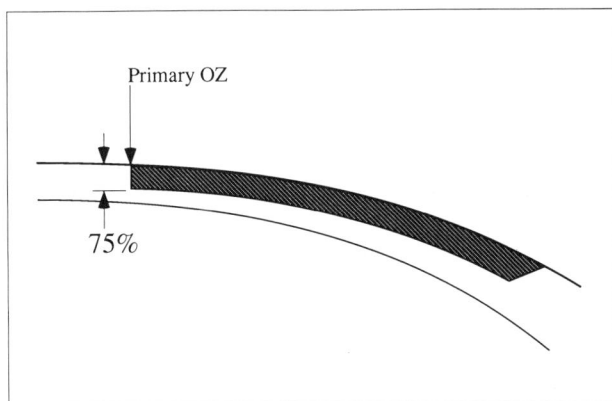

Fig. 8.33 Factor 1.6.

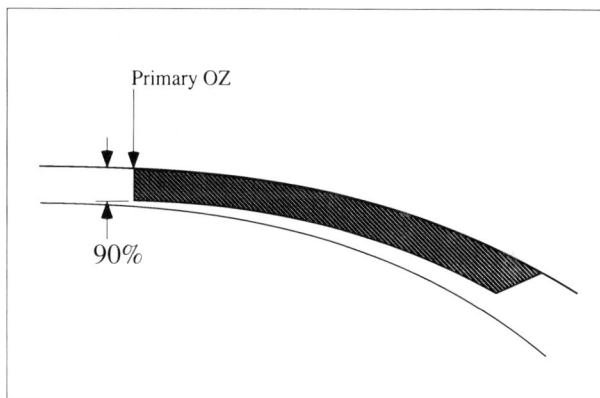

Fig. 8.32 Incisional depth (ID) factor 1.3.

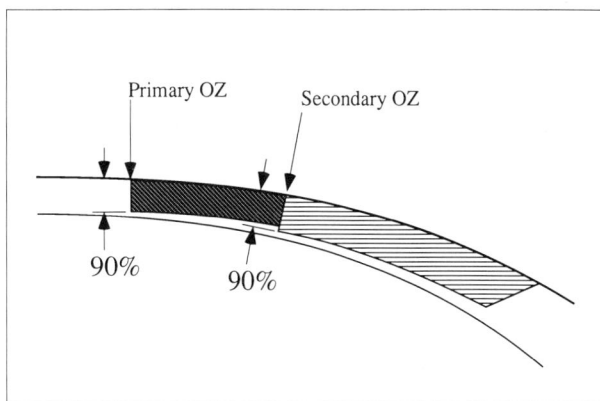

Fig. 8.34 Factor 2.0.

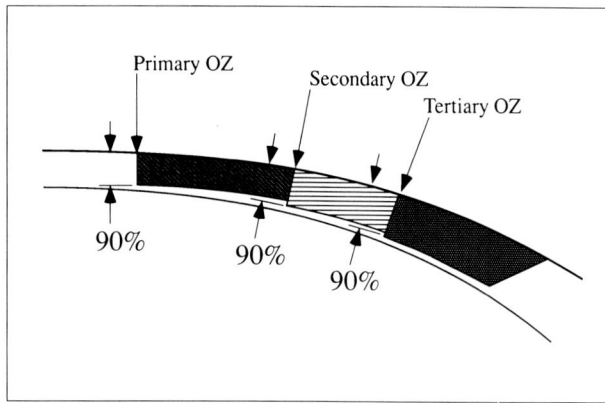

Fig. 8.35 Factor 2.5.

Table 8.2 Initial blade bias by type

Blade type	Typical bias (% of initial pachymetry)	Typical bias* (μm)	Blade setting* (pachymetry + bias)
Steel razor fragment	15	75	575
Honed steel	7–10	35–50	535–550
Diamond—old style	10–15	50–75	550–575
LeCut	0	None	500

* Example assumes a paracentral pachymetry of 500 μm.

these relationships are held constant both to the corneal thickness and to each other. It should be obvious that the method of blade setting used to accomplish these incision depths is dependent upon blade quality as well as design and necessitates evaluation of these factors individually for each type of blade, whether steel, diamond, or sapphire. Table 8.2 summarizes the settings with commonly used blade types.

Corneal diameter

This is a factor that, while significant, fortunately is not a large one—yet it must be considered. Most patients will be found to have corneas that fall within the 11.5–12.0 mm range, measured white-to-white. The actual measurements should be made at four points: in the vertical (6 to 12 o'clock), horizontal (3 to 9 o'clock), 45 and 135° meridians, and then averaged. A difference of 1.0 mm in corneal diameter represents about 1 D in actual refraction effect.

Corneal rigidity

This is another factor that many surgeons have ignored, either out of ignorance of its significance or because instruments to measure it have been generally hard to

Table 8.3 Pre-calculated mean corneal rigidity coefficient

Myopia (D)	Sex	Age (years) 25	35	45
1.5	Male	0.95	1.02	1.12
	Female	0.92	1.00	1.11
3.0	Male	0.90	0.95	1.04
	Female	0.88	0.90	1.03
5.0	Male	0.86	0.90	0.99
	Female	0.81	0.87	0.98
7.0	Male	0.80	0.82	0.96
	Female	0.70	0.78	0.95

obtain (Table 8.3). This factor is second only to the size of the optical zone in its influence on the outcome of the surgery. This parameter is related to aging—the rigidity seems to increase in older individuals and is reflected in the generally higher effect seen in these patients (the method of determining scleral or corneal rigidity is described in Chapter 5). The decrease in elasticity of corneal tissue, as evidenced by the cornea's resistance to deformation, causes most of the tension produced by the weakening of the peripheral cornea to be translated as a flattening of the central cornea instead of stretching—both in the center as well as peripherally. In addition, contraction of the healing scar meets more resistance to its tendency to produce flattening of the peripheral cornea (see also Chapter 7). This latter tendency could account for the progression of effect reported in some series [12].

Number of incisions

The number of incisions directly affects the outcome of the surgery—the fewer incisions, the less the effect. Using 16 incisions as 100%, 12 incisions will produce 15%, eight incisions 25%, and six incisions 50%—less effect. Making 32 incisions produces less than a 2% additional effect on the outcome of the surgery [13], while more than 32 incisions will produce a decrease in the effect; this helps to explain the failure of Sato's method (Figure 8.36). These ratios were arrived at by the retrospective evaluation of more than 15 000 cases over a period of several years and have been reinforced by an ongoing evaluation of patient data.

Additionally, as the number of incisions decreases, the incidence of operatively induced astigmatism increases. This was especially a problem in the earlier cases and caused Fyodorov and the author to abandon eight incisions—at least for a time.

Keratometry

Despite some suggestions to the contrary, corneal curvature remains one of the significant factors in

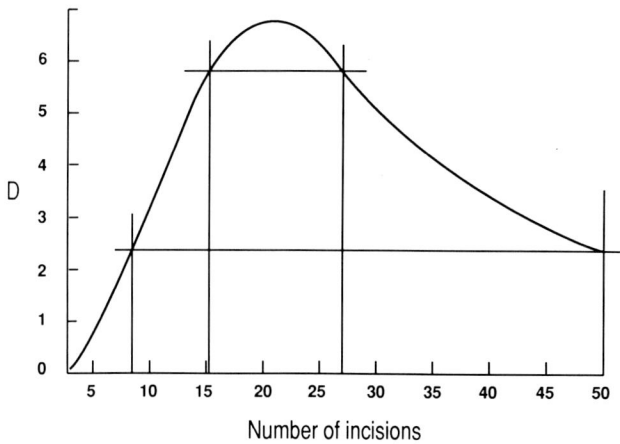

Fig. 8.36 The effect of the number of incisions on the surgical outcome.

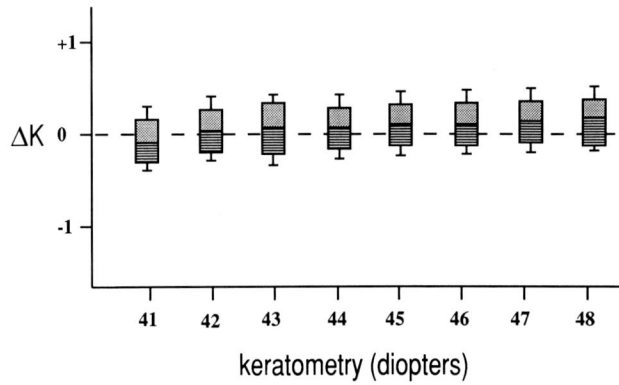

Fig. 8.37 Pre-operative K-readings make a difference.

determining the outcome of the surgery. Sufficient time has elapsed to bear this out (this factor is discussed in more detail in Chapter 5). Graphs plotted of cases in which compensation has been made for changes in curvature show a curve that is almost flat.

If it were true that corneal curvature has no effect, then those cases in whom the optical zone was opened (widened) in compensation should show less effect, all other things being equal. However, such cases show a slight rise to the curve in the higher keratometry ranges showing that there has probably been insufficient compensation for the keratometry (Figure 8.37). Since none of the other investigators commenting upon this relationship have considered age, corneal rigidity, etc. in their surgery, their cases are not truly representative and would naturally not show any significant effect due to corneal curvature. The work of Sanders and Marks [14] doing multiple regression analyses is beginning to corroborate our findings. It must be emphasized again that this surgery is microsurgery whose outcome depends upon an integration of a number of seemingly small, outwardly insignificant, and apparently unrelated factors which, when combined, result in significant changes in corneal curvature.

Summary of patient workup

Eligible patients must be at least 18 years of age with non-progressive myopia. They must be free of corneal or adnexal disease. They should have intra-ocular tensions greater than 12 mmHg and scleral rigidity greater than 0.75. They must have realistic expectations of the surgery and have signed an informed consent (see also Chapter 5).

All candidates for this procedure receive the following workup in the author's clinic prior to the surgery:

1 Refraction (manifest—cycloplegic where warranted).
2 Glare testing.
3 Ophthalmometry.
  (a) Conventional keratometry (central and peripheral).
  (b) Photokeratoscopy (Corneoscope).
  (c) Holographic topography (CLAS-II).
4 Intra-ocular pressure by applanation.
5 A-scan ocular biometry (axial length).
6 Corneal rigidity measurement—direct using the Maklokov tonometer.
7 Ultrasonic pachymetric corneal mapping.
8 Determination of handedness.
9 Corneal diameter measurement.
10 Routine ophthalmic evaluation.

We will examine a number of typical cases of spherical myopia and detail the parameter calculation, surgical decision-making process and the technique of surgery required in each case under examination. The optical zone size will be calculated using the RK DataMaster program on an IBM-PC/AT. From this program will be selected the optimal incision depth coefficient/optical zone(s)/incision number/configuration for the case. There are other computer programs available to aid you in calculating surgical parameters. These typically call for slightly larger optical zones than does the RK DataMaster (Figure 8.38).

The RK DataMaster program was written by the author for this surgery and uses modified versions of Formulas I, II, and the Ruiz algorithms (Figure 8.39). It will accept and process all of the data, calculates the theoretic scleral rigidity, allows editing of current and previously entered records, prints out the results per eye, and stores the data in standard disk files for later processing. This program is suitable for low to moderate myopia (cases recommended for the surgeon getting started in radial keratotomy) as well as complex cases of mixed astigmatism and allows the surgeon reasonably to predict the outcome of the surgery.

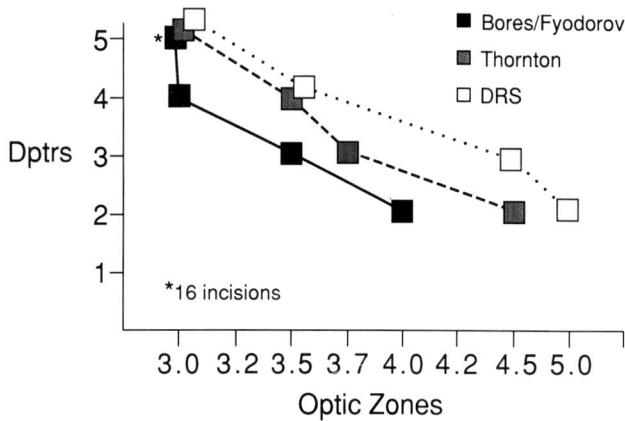

Fig. 8.38 Comparison of three popular radial keratotomy computer programs and recommended surgical zone sizes.

These algorithms are a result of extensive collaboration of the author and the Moscow Scientific Institute of Ophthalmic Microsurgery and the evaluation of over 15 000 cases of radial keratotomy. They are accurate to within ±1.00 D in better than 85% of cases in the author's hands and are especially useful for combined myopic astigmatism and higher degrees of myopia. Recently the Ruiz astigmatism calculations were integrated into the system so as to provide calculations for up to 8 D of associated myopic astigmatism.

The program takes into account the six factors previously mentioned, plus the following:

1 Age and sex of the patient.
2 Intra-ocular pressure.
3 Size of the intermediate (second and third) optical zones.
4 Depth of the incisions (for stepping).
  (a) primary.
  (b) secondary.
  (c) tertiary.
5 Pachymetry.
  (a) central.
  (b) paracentral.
  (c) mid peripheral.
  (d) para-peripheral.
  (e) limbal.
6 Axial length of the eye.
7 Astigmatism of the eye.

The program automatically calculates the scleral rigidity by extrapolating a mean statistical rigidity, taking into account age, sex, and amount of myopia. These calculations are based upon patient evaluations using measurements taken with the Maklakov tonometer in over 600 cases. The program also calculates the zones needed for astigmatism cases for most incisional configurations (see also Chapter 9) and suggests the particular type of incisions to use (i.e. stepped, etc.).

The program will not draw out the incisional configurations for the surgeon. It is highly recommended that the surgeon personally draws out for him- or herself these configurations on the surgical workup forms to avoid potential error.

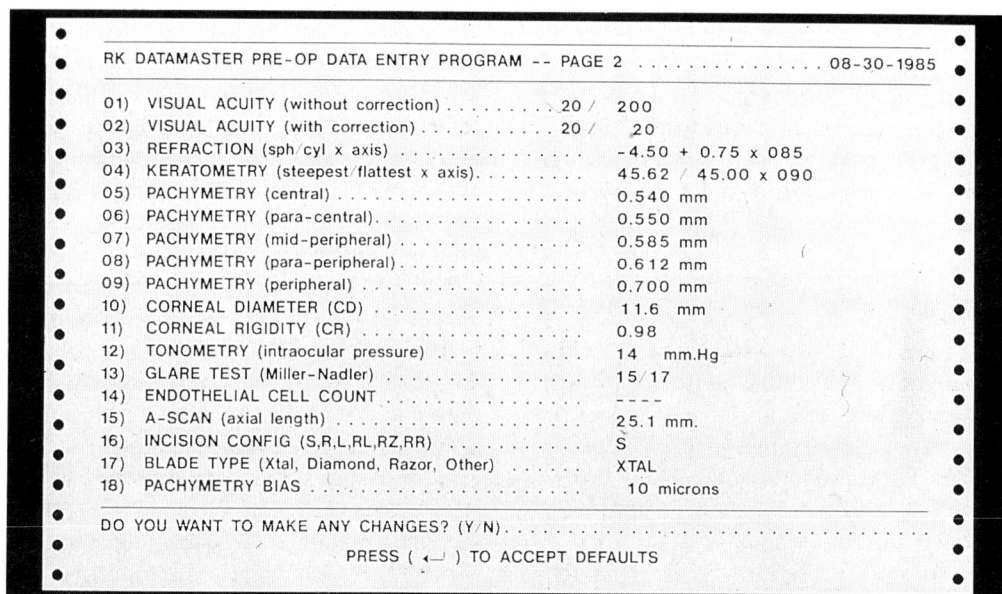

```
RK DATAMASTER PRE-OP DATA ENTRY PROGRAM -- PAGE 2 ............. 08-30-1985

01)  VISUAL ACUITY (without correction) ........ 20 /   200
02)  VISUAL ACUITY (with correction) .......... 20 /    20
03)  REFRACTION (sph/cyl x axis) ............     -4.50 + 0.75 x 085
04)  KERATOMETRY (steepest/flattest x axis). .......  45.62 / 45.00 x 090
05)  PACHYMETRY (central) ...................     0.540 mm
06)  PACHYMETRY (para-central). ..............     0.550 mm
07)  PACHYMETRY (mid-peripheral) .............     0.585 mm
08)  PACHYMETRY (para-peripheral). ...........     0.612 mm
09)  PACHYMETRY (peripheral) ................     0.700 mm
10)  CORNEAL DIAMETER (CD) ................      11.6  mm
11)  CORNEAL RIGIDITY (CR) ................     0.98
12)  TONOMETRY (intraocular pressure) ........     14   mm.Hg
13)  GLARE TEST (Miller-Nadler) ............      15/17
14)  ENDOTHELIAL CELL COUNT ...............      - - - -
15)  A-SCAN (axial length) ................      25.1 mm.
16)  INCISION CONFIG (S,R,L,RL,RZ,RR) ........      S
17)  BLADE TYPE (Xtal, Diamond, Razor, Other) ......  XTAL
18)  PACHYMETRY BIAS ....................        10 microns

DO YOU WANT TO MAKE ANY CHANGES? (Y/N) .....................

              PRESS ( ↵ ) TO ACCEPT DEFAULTS
```

Fig. 8.39 Example of a computer print-out from RK DataMaster.

```
┌──────────────────────────────────────────────────────────────┐
│                                                                │
│  RK DATAMASTER PRE-OP DATA ENTRY PROGRAM ............. Page 2  │
│                                                                │
│  01) VISUAL ACUITY (without correction) ............ 20/ 200   │
│  02) VISUAL ACUITY (with correction) ............... 20/ 20    │
│  03) REFRACTION (sph/cyl x axis) ................... -2.50 sphere │
│  04) KERATOMETRY (steepest/flattest x axis) ........ 44.25/43.75x90 │
│  05) PACHYMETRY (CP) ............................... 0.535     │
│  06) PACHYMETRY (PC) ............................... 0.560     │
│  07) PACHYMETRY (MP) ............................... 0.600     │
│  08) PACHYMETRY (PP) ............................... 0.723     │
│  09) PACHYMETRY (FP) ............................... 0.789     │
│  10) CORNEAL DIAMETER (CD) ......................... 11.8 mm   │
│  11) CORNEA RIGIDITY (CR) .......................... 0.95      │
│  12) TONOMETRY (intraocular pressure) .............. 17 mmHg.  │
│  13) GLARE TESTER (Miller-Nadler) .................. 16/17     │
│  14) ENDOTHELIAL CELL COUNT ........................ ------    │
│  15) A-SCAN (axial length) ......................... 24.5 mm.  │
│  16) INCISION CONFIG (S,R,T,L,RL,RZ,RR,RT) ......... S         │
│  17) BLADE TYPE (Xtal, Diamond, Razor, other) ...... LeCut     │
│  18) PACHYMETRY BIAS ............................... 100%      │
│                                                                │
│  ─────────────────────────────────────────────────────────    │
│          PRESS <  ◄─┘  > TO ACCEPT DEFAULTS                    │
│                                                                │
└──────────────────────────────────────────────────────────────┘
```

low degree myopia

typical corneal rigidity

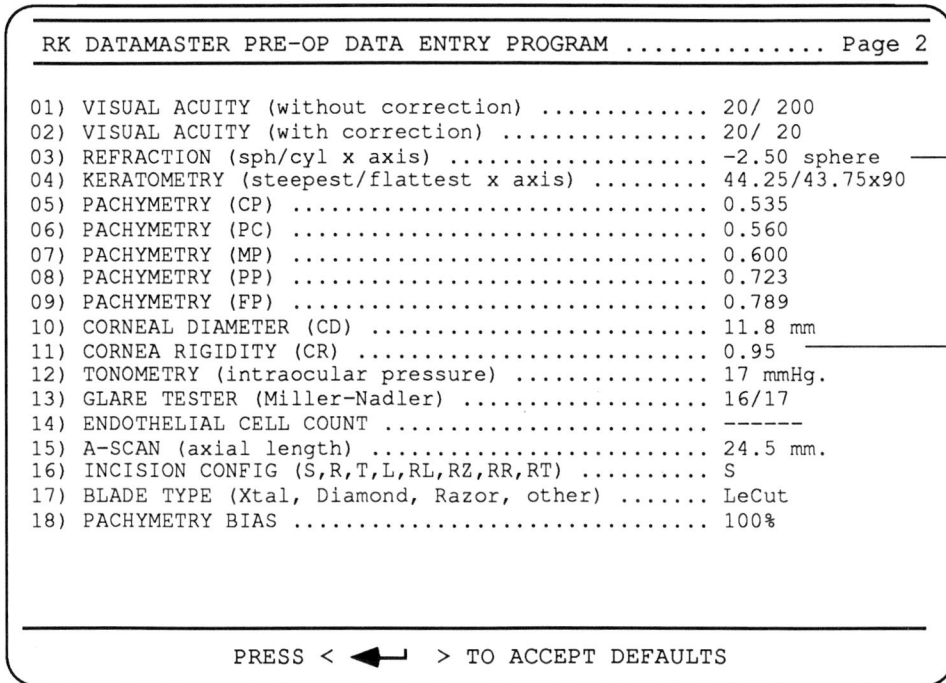

Fig. 8.40 RK DataMaster input screen #2—case 1.

Decision making in radial keratotomy

The examples considered within this section will be entirely confined to spherical cases. The specialized incisional patterns used for the treatment of astigmatism will be discussed in the chapter on that subject (Chapter 10). The beginning surgeon is admonished not to attempt the correction of astigmatism through any surgical means until he/she is completely familiar with the results of incisions in cases of simple myopia.

Case 1

The first case to be considered in our exercise is that of a 22-year-old male myopic patient whose pre-operative workup is entered into the computer as shown in Figures 8.40 through 8.42.

Once the operator has chosen the surgical parameters for the case, the computer will display a summary of the case and give the operator a chance to correct or review the data input (Figure 8.43). The surgical data and incisional configuration are drawn on the surgical workup sheet (Figure 8.44).

Case 2

In the next case, we will change only the amount of myopia (Figures 8.45 through 8.49). Note that the corneal rigidity has also changed. The operator will choose the incisional depth, number of incisions,

and primary optical zone as before. In addition, a secondary optical zone will probably be necessary.

Case 3

Again, only the amount of myopia and corneal rigidity have been changed (Figures 8.50 through 8.53). Take careful note, however, of the way in which the optical zones and incision numbers have changed.

Case 4

Here the myopia has been changed to a degree that exceeds that which can reasonably be expected to be fully corrected by radial keratotomy (Figures 8.54 through 8.57). This case will require maximum surgery even to get a partial correction. This type of case is explored below. Such cases are best avoided or corrected by other means.

Surgery—the technique of radial keratotomy

The following description of surgical techniques is of those used by the author and represents more than 15 years of experience with this surgery. These procedures have been considerably refined from the original method and should not prove too arduous for the average surgeon, providing that the proper instruments are used and the surgeon does not

```
┌─────────────────────────────────────────────────────────────────┐
│  RK DATAMASTER PRE-OP CALCULATION SUMMARY .......... 07-04-1990   │
│                                                                   │
│  George Sigafoos - Left eye -- S PROCEDURE -                      │
│  ─────────────────────────────────────────────────────────────   │
│     ID ------- 6         8         12        16  Incisions        │
│  ─────────────────────────────────────────────────────────────   │
│    1.3        3.25      3.75      4.00      4.50                   │
│  ─────────────────────────────────────────────────────────────   │
│    1.6        3.75      4.50      4.75      5.00                   │
│  ─────────────────────────────────────────────────────────────   │
│    2.0        4.50      5.00      5.25      5.75                   │
│  ─────────────────────────────────────────────────────────────   │
│    2.5        5.25      5.75      6.00      6.50                   │
│  ─────────────────────────────────────────────────────────────   │
│  NOTE:CHOOSE THE SURGICAL OZ FROM THE HIGHLIGHTED ZONES IN THE    │
│  TABLE ABOVE.                                                     │
│                                                                   │
│  These have already been rounded to the nearest 0.25 mm.          │
│  ─────────────────────────────────────────────────────────────   │
│  Do you wish to print this table? (Y/N) ....................  ▓   │
└─────────────────────────────────────────────────────────────────┘
```

Fig. 8.41 RK DataMaster input screen #3—case 1.

(a)

```
CHOOSE INCISION COEFFICIENT (ID)  .............1.3
```

(b)

```
CHOOSE # OF INCISIONS  (NI) .......................  6
```

(c)

```
CHOOSE 1ST SURGICAL OZ  ...................... 3.75 mm
```

Fig. 8.42 RK DataMaster input screen #3: (a) incisional depth coefficient input; (b) prompt for number for incisions; (c) choose primary optical zone.

attempt to "wing it" or improvise. The surgery is performed under topical anesthesia in a pre-medicated patient. Sedation is provided by the administration of diazepam (Valium) in a dose appropriate to the patient (Figure 8.58). Generally this will be 10 mg given orally approximately 30–40 min prior to surgery. Be advised that significant quantities of this chemical can still

be found in the blood 24 hours after ingestion. The patient should be cautioned accordingly.

The patient is placed supine upon the operating table and the eye is prepped with full-strength Betadine solution (Figure 8.59). Betadine preparation is not recommended because it contains soap which is extremely hard on the corneal epithelium. The microscope is then

```
RK DATAMASTER PRE-OP SURGICAL DATA SUMMARY ......... 07-04-90

SURGICAL PARAMETERS - FOR George Sigafoos LEFT EYE -- S PROCEDURE


1) INCISIONAL DEPTH COEFFICIENT .................... 1.3
2) SINGLE DEPTH INCISIONS ......................... 6
3) 1st RADIAL OPTIC ZONE .......................... 3.75 mm
4) 2nd RADIAL OPTIC ZONE .......................... NONE
5) 3rd RADIAL OPTIC ZONE .......................... NONE


Pachymetry -- CP:     PC:    4 mm:   5mm:    MP:     PP:     FP:

        .535    .560   .573    .587   .600    .723    .789

COMPUTED #1 BLADE SETTING ..... 0.560 mm
COMPUTED #2 BLADE SETTING ..... 0.000 mm
COMPUTED #3 BLADE SETTING ..... 0.000 mm


Do you wish to review the data? (Y/N) ....................... ▓
```

this coefficient means that the shallowest, single depth, incisions are to be made

these measurements are calculated by the computer

Fig. 8.43 RK DataMaster summary screen—case 1.

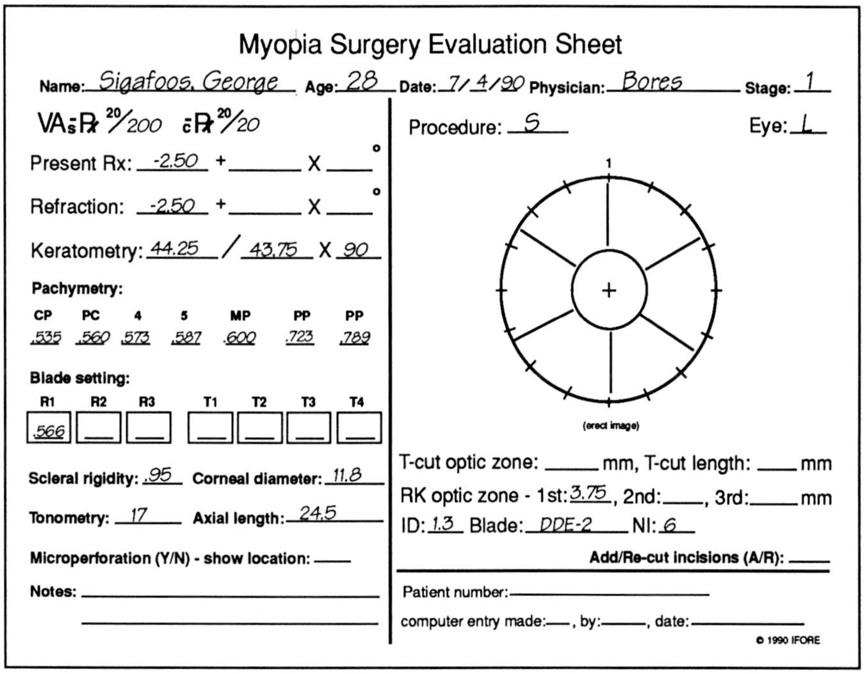

Myopia Surgery Evaluation Sheet

Name: _Sigafoos, George_ Age: _28_ Date: _7/4/90_ Physician: _Bores_ Stage: _1_

VA: s R̄x ^{20}/200 c̄ R̄x ^{20}/20

Present Rx: _-2.50_ + _____ X _____°

Refraction: _-2.50_ + _____ X _____°

Keratometry: _44.25_ / _43.75_ X _90_

Pachymetry:

CP	PC	4	5	MP	PP	PP
.535	.560	.573	.587	.600	.723	.789

Blade setting:

R1	R2	R3	T1	T2	T3	T4
.566						

Scleral rigidity: _.95_ Corneal diameter: _11.8_

Tonometry: _17_ Axial length: _24.5_

Microperforation (Y/N) - show location: _____

Notes: _____

Procedure: _S_ Eye: _L_

(erect image)

T-cut optic zone: _____ mm, T-cut length: _____ mm

RK optic zone - 1st: _3.75_, 2nd: ___, 3rd: _____ mm

ID: _1.3_ Blade: _DDE-2_ NI: _6_

Add/Re-cut incisions (A/R): _____

Patient number: _____

computer entry made: ___, by: ____, date: _____

© 1990 IFORE

Fig. 8.44 Typical pre-surgical workup sheet—case 1.

centered and adjusted and the surgeon scrubs up. At the author's clinic we have successfully used Septisol skin prep foam for this purpose for years. Draping is done using an aperture drape supplied by Alcon.

The anesthetic used is 0.5% tetracaine, followed by 1.0% non-buffered Pontocaine drops. Any additional anesthesia required during the case is provided by the application of additional 0.5% tetracaine. Occasionally for patients complaining of discomfort from fixation (particularly in second-stage cases), 10% cocaine solution is applied to the limbus on a cotton pledget or applicator.

```
RK DATAMASTER PRE-OP DATA ENTRY PROGRAM ............. Page 2

   01) VISUAL ACUITY (without correction) ............ 20/ 200
   02) VISUAL ACUITY (with correction) ............... 20/ 20
   03) REFRACTION (sph/cyl x axis) ................... -5.00 sphere
   04) KERATOMETRY (steepest/flattest x axis) ........ 44.25/43.75x90
   05) PACHYMETRY (CP) .............................. 0.535
   06) PACHYMETRY (PC) .............................. 0.560
   07) PACHYMETRY (MP) .............................. 0.600
   08) PACHYMETRY (PP) .............................. 0.723
   09) PACHYMETRY (FP) .............................. 0.789
   10) CORNEAL DIAMETER (CD) ........................ 11.8 mm
   11) CORNEA RIGIDITY (CR) ......................... 0.86
   12) TONOMETRY (intraocular pressure) ............. 17 mmHg.
   13) GLARE TESTER (Miller-Nadler) ................. 16/17
   14) ENDOTHELIAL CELL COUNT ....................... ------
   15) A-SCAN (axial length) ........................ 24.5 mm.
   16) INCISION CONFIG (S,R,T,L,RL,RZ,RR,RT) ......... S
   17) BLADE TYPE (Xtal, Diamond, Razor, other) ...... LeCut
   18) PACHYMETRY BIAS ............................... 100%


          PRESS <  ◄┘  > TO ACCEPT DEFAULTS
```

higher myopia — 03) REFRACTION

as the myopia increases, the rigidity decreases — 11) CORNEA RIGIDITY

Fig. 8.45 RK DataMaster input screen #2—case 2.

```
RK DATAMASTER PRE-OP CALCULATION SUMMARY ......... 07-04-1990

George Sigafoos - Left eye -- S PROCEDURE -

   ID ------- 6         8         12         16  Incisions

   1.3      1.75      2.00      2.25       2.50

   1.6      2.00      2.25      2.50       2.75

   2.0      2.50      2.75      3.00       3.25

   2.5      3.00      3.25      3.50       4.00

NOTE:CHOOSE THE SURGICAL OZ FROM THE HIGHLIGHTED ZONES IN THE
TABLE ABOVE.

These have already been rounded to the nearest 0.25 mm.


Do you wish to print this table? (Y/N) ....................█
```

note rightward shift in highlighted OZ's

Fig. 8.46 RK DataMaster input screen #3—case 2.

```
    CHOOSE 2ND SURGICAL OZ  ..................... 6.00 mm
```

Fig. 8.47 RK DataMaster input screen #3—case 2.

```
RK DATAMASTER PRE-OP SURGICAL DATA SUMMARY .......... 07-04-90

SURGICAL PARAMETERS - FOR George Sigafoos LEFT EYE -- S PROCEDURE

1) INCISIONAL DEPTH COEFFICIENT .................... 2.0
2) SINGLE DEPTH INCISIONS ........................... 8
3) 1st RADIAL OPTIC ZONE ............................ 2.75 mm
4) 2nd RADIAL OPTIC ZONE ............................ 6.00 mm
5) 3rd RADIAL OPTIC ZONE ............................ NONE

Pachymetry -- CP:    PC:    4 mm:   5mm:    MP:     PP:     FP:

              .535   .560   .573    .587    .600    .723    .789

COMPUTED #1 BLADE SETTING ..... 0.560 mm
COMPUTED #2 BLADE SETTING ..... 0.600 mm
COMPUTED #3 BLADE SETTING ..... 0.000 mm

Do you wish to review the data? (Y/N) .....................
```

this factor indicates that single stepped incisions will be made (note 2nd OZ)

note also that there are 2 blade settings

Fig. 8.48 Surgical parameter summary—case 2.

Myopia Surgery Evaluation Sheet

Name: Sigafoos, George Age: 28 Date: 7/4/90 Physician: Bores Stage: 1

VA s Rx 20/200 c Rx 20/20

Present Rx: -5.00 + ______ X ______°

Refraction: -5.00 + ______ X ______°

Keratometry: 44.25 / 43.75 X 90

Pachymetry:

CP	PC	4	5	MP	PP	PP
.535	.560	.573	.587	.600	.723	.789

Blade setting:

R1	R2	R3	T1	T2	T3	T4
.560	.600					

Scleral rigidity: .86 Corneal diameter: 11.8

Tonometry: 17 Axial length: 24.5

Microperforation (Y/N) - show location: ____

Notes: ____________

Procedure: S Eye: L

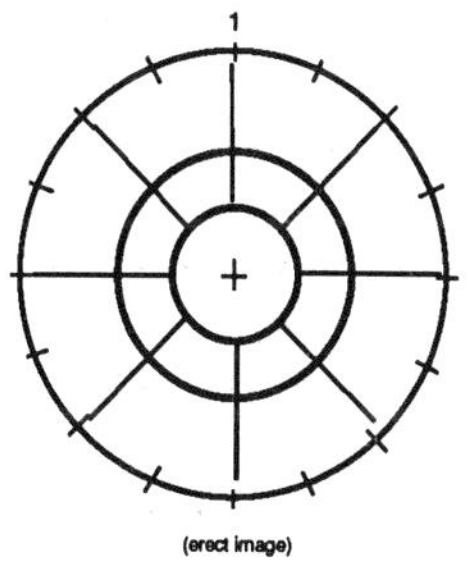

T-cut optic zone: ____ mm, T-cut length: ____ mm

RK optic zone - 1st: 2.75, 2nd: 6.00, 3rd: ____ mm

ID: 2.0 Blade: DDE-2 NI: 8

Add/Re-cut incisions (A/R): ____

Patient number: ____________

computer entry made: ___, by: ____, date: ________

© 1990 IFORE

Fig. 8.49 Surgical workup sheet—case 2.

The instrument tray is placed to the surgeon's right side. This tray is a standard auto-clave tray measuring 8 × 16 in (20 × 40 cm) supplied by the auto-clave manufacturer (Castle). The bottom of this tray is lined with suitable padding. The basic instruments (supplied for every case) are: 50 ml Pyrex glass beaker; Fyodorov dipstick (or Deitz hockey stick—Katena K3-9600); fixation forceps (Katena K2-3250); 27-gauge Rainin irrigating cannula (Katena K7-3580); Barraquer wire lid speculum (Katena K1-5010); an adjustable knife handle with blade in plastic sterilizer box; and Weck-Cel swabs. To this collection are added the

```
┌─────────────────────────────────────────────────────────────┐
│                                                               │
│   RK DATAMASTER PRE-OP DATA ENTRY PROGRAM ............. Page 2 │
│                                                               │
│   01) VISUAL ACUITY (without correction) ............ 20/ 200 │
│   02) VISUAL ACUITY (with correction) ............... 20/ 20  │
│   03) REFRACTION (sph/cyl x axis) ................... -6.50 sphere │
│   04) KERATOMETRY (steepest/flattest x axis) ........ 44.25/43.75x90 │
│   05) PACHYMETRY (CP) ............................... 0.535   │
│   06) PACHYMETRY (PC) ............................... 0.560   │
│   07) PACHYMETRY (MP) ............................... 0.600   │
│   08) PACHYMETRY (PP) ............................... 0.723   │
│   09) PACHYMETRY (FP) ............................... 0.789   │
│   10) CORNEAL DIAMETER (CD) ......................... 11.8 mm │
│   11) CORNEA RIGIDITY (CR) .......................... 0.83    │
│   12) TONOMETRY (intraocular pressure) .............. 17 mmHg.│
│   13) GLARE TESTER (Miller-Nadler) .................. 16/17   │
│   14) ENDOTHELIAL CELL COUNT ........................ ------  │
│   15) A-SCAN (axial length) ......................... 24.5 mm.│
│   16) INCISION CONFIG (S,R,T,L,RL,RZ,RR,RT) ......... S       │
│   17) BLADE TYPE (Xtal, Diamond, Razor, other) ...... LeCut   │
│   18) PACHYMETRY BIAS ............................... 100%    │
│                                                               │
│                                                               │
│           PRESS <  ◄─┘  > TO ACCEPT DEFAULTS                  │
│                                                               │
└─────────────────────────────────────────────────────────────┘
```

myopia is approaching the upper limit for this surgery

cornea is more elastic (lower rididity coefficient)

Fig. 8.50 RK DataMaster input screen #2—case 3.

```
┌─────────────────────────────────────────────────────────────┐
│                                                               │
│   RK DATAMASTER PRE-OP CALCULATION SUMMARY ......... 07-04-1990 │
│                                                               │
│   George Sigafoos - Left eye -- S PROCEDURE -                 │
│                                                               │
│     ID ------- 6       8       12       16   Incisions        │
│                                                               │
│    1.3      1.25    1.50    1.75    2.00                      │
│                                                               │
│    1.6      1.50    1.75    2.00    2.25                      │
│                                                               │
│    2.0      2.00    2.25    2.50    2.75                      │
│                                                               │
│    2.5      2.25    2.75    2.75    3.25                      │
│                                                               │
│   NOTE:CHOOSE THE SURGICAL OZ FROM THE HIGHLIGHTED ZONES IN THE│
│   TABLE ABOVE.                                                │
│                                                               │
│   These have already been rounded to the nearest 0.25 mm.     │
│                                                               │
│                                                               │
│   Do you wish to print this table? (Y/N) ..................▓  │
│                                                               │
└─────────────────────────────────────────────────────────────┘
```

extreme rightward shift means more and deeper incisions

Fig. 8.51 RK DataMaster results screen #3—case 3.

additional markers, forceps, etc. as required in a specific case (Figure 8.60).

The blade used is the LeCut, double-edged unicrystalline diamond blade (WMK-200) in the adjustable knife handle by Katena Instruments (K2-6505). The identical blade is also available in the micrometer diamond knife by KOI. The sapphire blade (Katena K2-6513) mounted in the same Katena micrometer handle is also recommended. There are two other blades available from Katena for this handle. One has a

```
RK DATAMASTER PRE-OP SURGICAL DATA SUMMARY .......... 07-04-90

SURGICAL PARAMETERS - FOR THE LEFT EYE -- S PROCEDURE

1) INCISIONAL DEPTH COEFFICIENT ..................... 2.5
2) SINGLE DEPTH INCISIONS ........................... 12
3) 1st RADIAL OPTIC ZONE ........................... 2.75 mm
4) 2nd RADIAL OPTIC ZONE ........................... 6.00 mm
5) 3rd RADIAL OPTIC ZONE ........................... 8.00 mm

Pachymetry -- CP:    PC:    4 mm:   5mm:    MP:     PP:     FP:

             .535   .560   .573    .587    .600    .723    .789

COMPUTED #1 BLADE SETTING ..... 0.560 mm
COMPUTED #2 BLADE SETTING ..... 0.600 mm
COMPUTED #3 BLADE SETTING ..... 0.720 mm

Do you wish to review the data? (Y/N) .....................
```

this factor indicates that each incision will be stepped twice (note that there are 3 OZ's)

there are 3 blade settings as well

Fig. 8.52 Surgical parameter summary—case 3.

Myopia Surgery Evaluation Sheet

Name: Sigafoos, George Age: 28 Date: 7/4/90 Physician: Bores Stage: 1

VA s̄ ℞ 20/200 c̄ ℞ 20/20 Procedure: S Eye: L

Present Rx: -6.50 + ____ X ____°

Refraction: -6.50 + ____ X ____°

Keratometry: 44.25 / 43.75 X 90

Pachymetry:

CP	PC	4	5	MP	PP	PP
.535	.560	.573	.587	.600	.723	.789

Blade setting:

R1	R2	R3	T1	T2	T3	T4
.560	.600	.720				

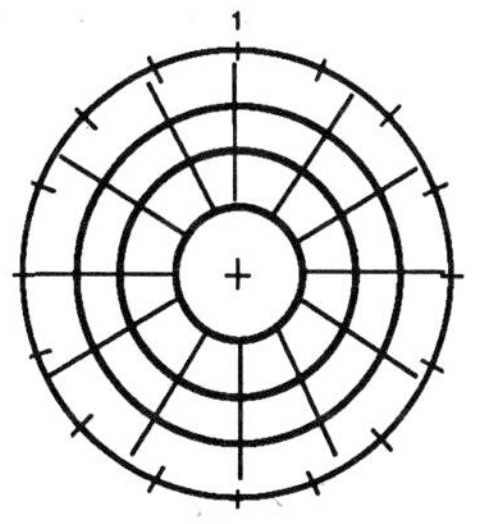

Scleral rigidity: .83 Corneal diameter: 11.8

Tonometry: 17 Axial length: 24.5

Microperforation (Y/N) - show location: ____

Notes: ____

T-cut optic zone: ____ mm, T-cut length: ____ mm

RK optic zone - 1st: 2.75, 2nd: 6.00, 3rd: 8.00 mm

ID: 2.5 Blade: DDE-2 NI: 12

Add/Re-cut incisions (A/R): ____

Patient number: ____

computer entry made: ____, by: ____, date: ____

© 1990 IFORE

Fig. 8.53 Pre-operative workup form—case 3.

single, 30° angled cutting edge designed for the Bores (American) method of incising (from the optical zone to the periphery), K2-6501. The other has a vertical cutting edge for use with the Fyodorov (Russian) technique (from the periphery toward the center), for re-incising old wounds and for making T or transverse incisions) K2-6511 (Figure 8.61). The single-edged blades are recommended for the beginning surgeon as they are more durable.

The blade is set utilizing the XTAL-800 shadowgraphic blade gauge which magnifies the tip approximately 200 times. While coin or other gauges can, with

```
┌─────────────────────────────────────────────────────────────┐
│  ─────────────────────────────────────────────────────────   │
│  RK DATAMASTER PRE-OP DATA ENTRY PROGRAM ............. Page 2  │
│                                                               │
│  01) VISUAL ACUITY (without correction) ............. 20/ 200 │
│  02) VISUAL ACUITY (with correction) ................ 20/ 20  │
│  03) REFRACTION (sph/cyl x axis) .................... -8.00 sphere ──
│  04) KERATOMETRY (steepest/flattest x axis) ......... 44.25/43.75x90 │
│  05) PACHYMETRY (CP) ................................ 0.535    │
│  06) PACHYMETRY (PC) ................................ 0.560    │
│  07) PACHYMETRY (MP) ................................ 0.600    │
│  08) PACHYMETRY (PP) ................................ 0.723    │
│  09) PACHYMETRY (FP) ................................ 0.789    │
│  10) CORNEAL DIAMETER (CD) .......................... 11.8 mm  │
│  11) CORNEA RIGIDITY (CR) ........................... 0.80 ──  │
│  12) TONOMETRY (intraocular pressure) ............... 17 mmHg. │
│  13) GLARE TESTER (Miller-Nadler) ................... 16/17    │
│  14) ENDOTHELIAL CELL COUNT ......................... ------   │
│  15) A-SCAN (axial length) .......................... 24.5 mm. │
│  16) INCISION CONFIG (S,R,T,L,RL,RZ,RR,RT) .......... S        │
│  17) BLADE TYPE (Xtal, Diamond, Razor, other) ....... LeCut    │
│  18) PACHYMETRY BIAS ................................ 100%     │
│                                                               │
│  ───────────────────────────────────────────────────────     │
│                                                               │
│          PRESS <  ◄─┘  > TO ACCEPT DEFAULTS                    │
└─────────────────────────────────────────────────────────────┘
```

not only is the myopia very high, but ...

... the corneal rigidity is very low

Fig. 8.54 RK DataMaster input screen #2—case 4.

```
┌─────────────────────────────────────────────────────────────┐
│  ─────────────────────────────────────────────────────────   │
│  RK DATAMASTER PRE-OP CALCULATION SUMMARY ......... 07-04-1990 │
│                                                               │
│  George Sigafoos - Left eye -- S PROCEDURE -                  │
│  ───────────────────────────────────────────────────────     │
│                                                               │
│                                                               │
│                                                               │
│  USING 16 INCISIONS AND AN INCISIONAL DEPTH COEFFICIENT OF 2.5│
│  NO OPTICAL ZONE EQUALS OR EXCEEDS 2.75 mm.                   │
│                                                               │
│  THE MAXIMUM MYOPIA THAT CAN BE REDUCED IN THIS CASE IS 7.51 D.│
│                                                               │
│                                                               │
│                                                               │
│  ───────────────────────────────────────────────────────     │
│                                                               │
│  Do you wish to print this table? (Y/N) ................... ▓ │
└─────────────────────────────────────────────────────────────┘
```

Fig. 8.55 RK DataMaster input screen #3—case 4.

care, be utilized, the fineness and the fragility of the blade tip make such usage hazardous from the standpoint of both setting accuracy and blade longevity. The blade is over-set according to the desired incisional depth coefficient as well as the blade type and style and the condition of the blade tip. This over-set (bias) is typically 10 µm in new sapphire blades and zero for the LeCut diamond. After about 10 cases, the tips on sapphire blades become rounded, requiring an increase in the blade bias to maintain adequate in-

```
RK DATAMASTER PRE-OP SURGICAL DATA SUMMARY .......... 07-04-90

SURGICAL PARAMETERS - FOR George Sigafoos LEFT EYE -- S PROCEDURE

1) INCISIONAL DEPTH COEFFICIENT .................... 2.5
2) SINGLE DEPTH INCISIONS ........................... 16
3) 1st RADIAL OPTIC ZONE ............................ 2.75 mm
4) 2nd RADIAL OPTIC ZONE ............................ 6.00 mm
5) 3rd RADIAL OPTIC ZONE ............................ 8.00 mm

Pachymetry -- CP:    PC:    4 mm:   5mm:    MP:     PP:     FP:

              .535   .560   .573    .587    .600    .723    .789

COMPUTED #1 BLADE SETTING ..... 0.560 mm
COMPUTED #2 BLADE SETTING ..... 0.600 mm
COMPUTED #3 BLADE SETTING ..... 0.720 mm

Do you wish to review the data? (Y/N) .....................
```

Fig. 8.56 RK DataMaster summary screen—case 4.

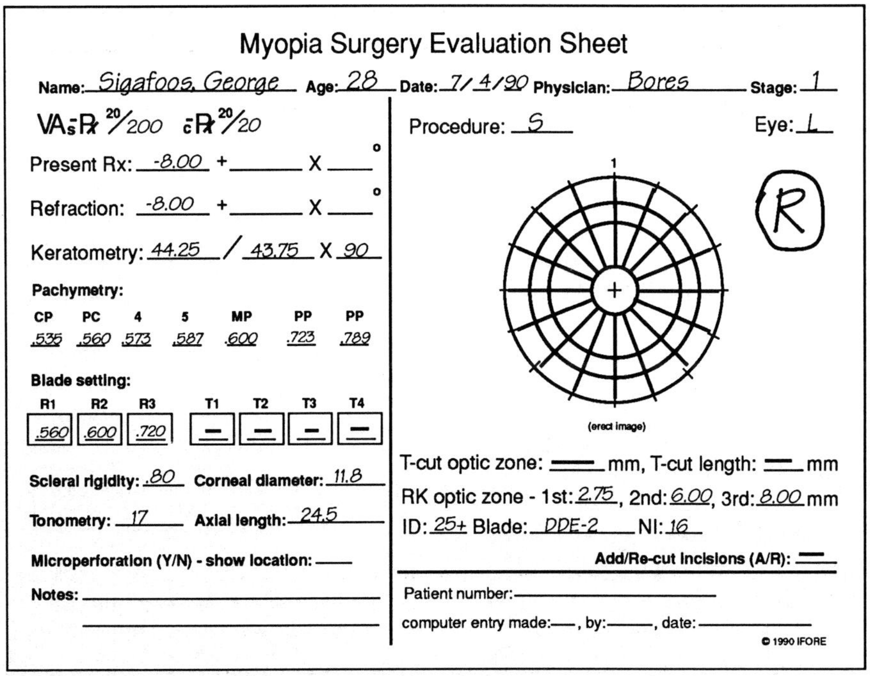

Myopia Surgery Evaluation Sheet

Name: Sigafoos, George Age: 28 Date: 7/4/90 Physician: Bores Stage: 1

VAsRx 20/200 cRx 20/20

Procedure: S Eye: L

Present Rx: -8.00 + ____ X ____°

Refraction: -8.00 + ____ X ____°

Keratometry: 44.25 / 43.75 X 90

Pachymetry:

CP	PC	4	5	MP	PP	PP
.535	.560	.573	.587	.600	.723	.789

Blade setting:

R1	R2	R3	T1	T2	T3	T4
.560	.600	.720	—	—	—	—

Scleral rigidity: .80 Corneal diameter: 11.8

Tonometry: 17 Axial length: 24.5

Microperforation (Y/N) - show location: ——

Notes:

T-cut optic zone: —— mm, T-cut length: —— mm

RK optic zone - 1st: 2.75, 2nd: 6.00, 3rd: 8.00 mm

ID: 25+ Blade: DDE-2 NI: 16

Add/Re-cut Incisions (A/R): ——

Patient number:

computer entry made: ——, by: ——, date: ——

Fig. 8.57 Pre-operative workup sheet—case 4.

cision depth—the diamond has not shown this same wearing pattern. This blunting is subtle and is impossible to detect under the operating microscope. Such blades, however, can continue to be used satisfactorily until the bias exceeds 70 μm or the tip breaks, in which case such a blade can still find use in cataract surgery.

Using the instrument is quite simple. First, it must be placed in an easily accessible location. This location will depend upon the volume of surgery the surgeon is

(a)

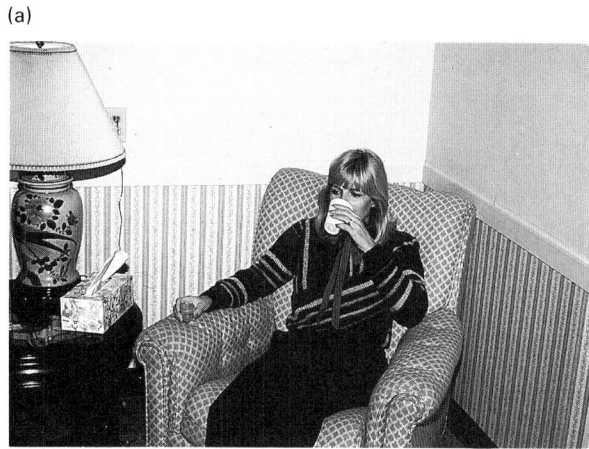

(b)

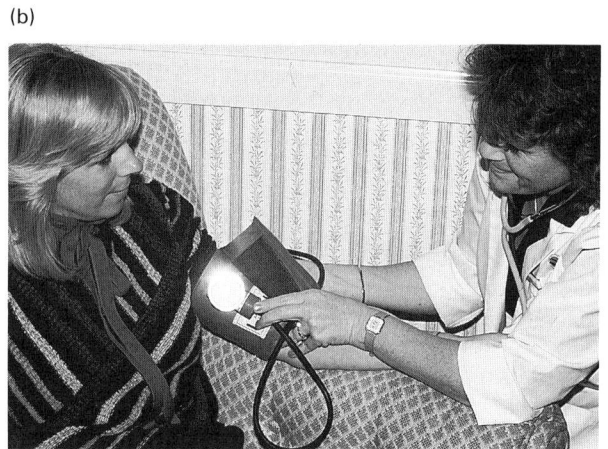

Fig. 8.58 (a) Patient taking oral sedation; (b) blood pressure is checked pre- and post-operation in all cases.

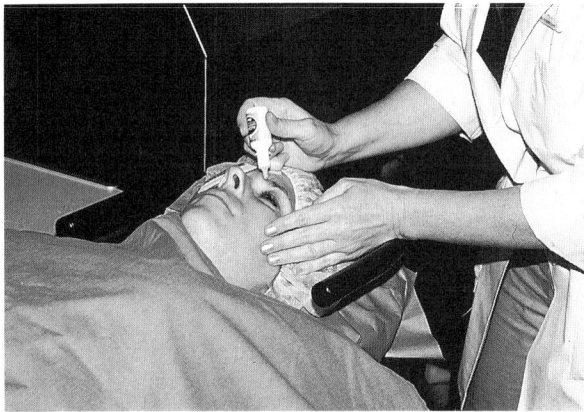

Fig. 8.59 Topical anesthetic is applied prior to prepping the eye.

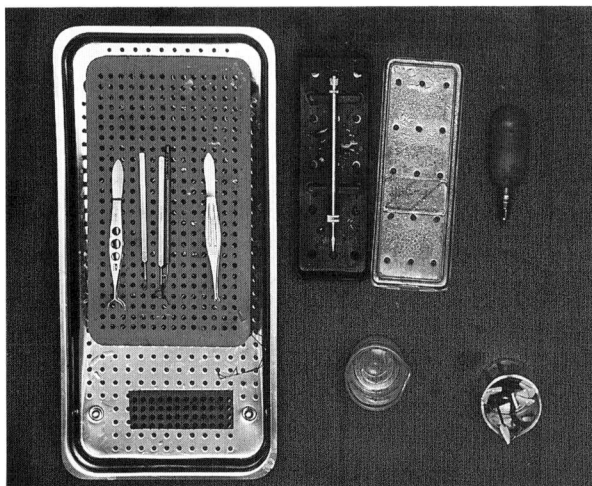

Fig. 8.60 Instrument tray set up for radial keratotomy.

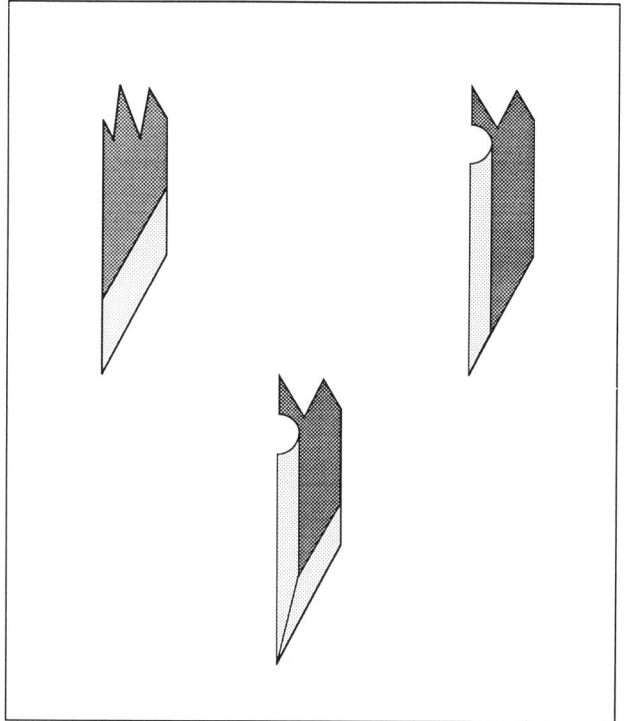

Fig. 8.61 Crystalline blade configurations.

currently doing on a daily basis and the number of knife handles and blades available. If fewer than six cases are performed daily, the device can be placed in the instrument room and the blade pre-set before

sterilization for each case. Experiments have shown that there is no measurable change in the settings after autoclaving with the XTAL/Katena handle combination. After setting, the handle is removed from the carrier and replaced into the sterilizing box, being careful not to disturb the micrometer screw. Each instrument tray is labeled with the patient's name. Care must be taken to prevent mismatching blade and patient, however. I prefer to have the instrument in the operating room where I use it to set the blade prior to and during the case. The device is placed on a small glove table to my right on top of a

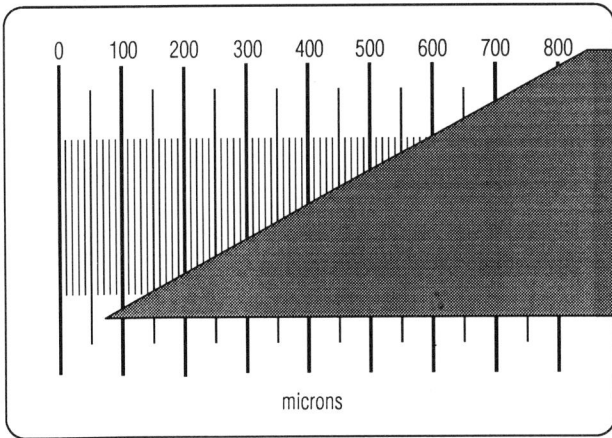

Fig. 8.62 Blade on screen in the shadowgraph.

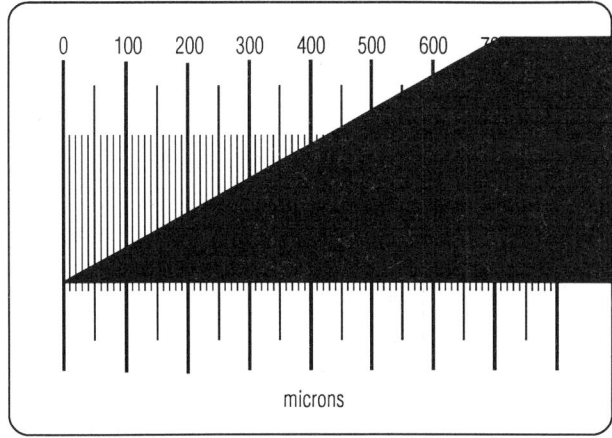

Fig. 8.63 Blade aligned with zero point on reticle.

(a)

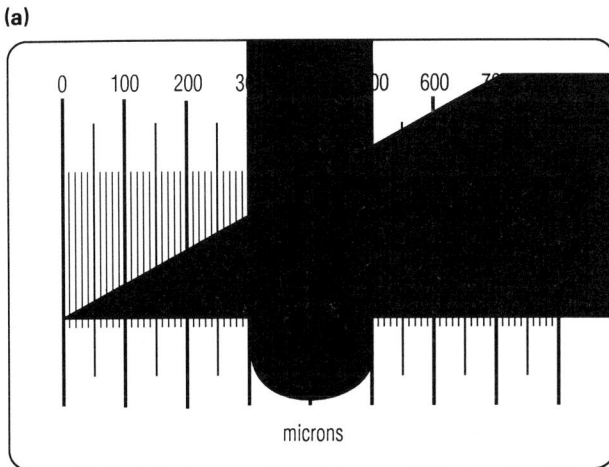

(b)

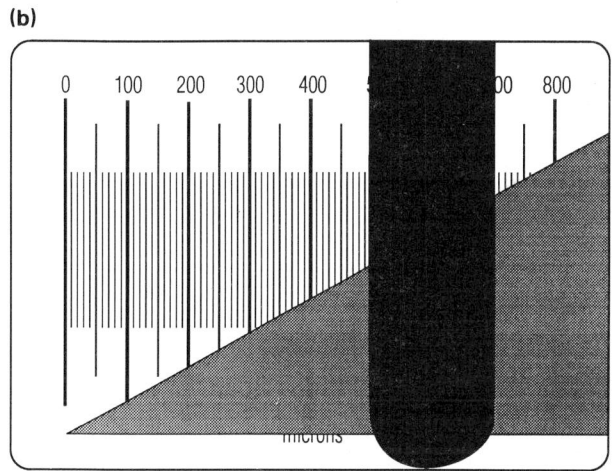

Fig. 8.64 (a) The footplate is moved into view; (b) the blade stage may have to be moved down to get the blade edge or footplate junction on screen.

sterile drape sheet such as a Barrier table cover. The eight auto-clavable silicone knob covers are placed over the adjustment and locking knobs.

Before initial use and from time to time, the calibration of the gauge should be checked using the special block provided with the instrument. Place the block on to the measurement stage and lock it in place with the locking knob. Adjust the focus, brightness and contrast controls until the reticle is crisp. The calibration bars should be super-imposed over the reticle ticks. If there is no correspondence, check to see that the block is properly seated on the stage. If you are unable to align the calibration and measuring reticles, notify the company. Do not try to adjust the calibration of the instrument yourself!

To set the blade using the Katena handle, the handle is placed into the shadowgraph carrier with the back of the footplate facing up. The blade shank then fits into the groove which has milled in the bottom of the

carrier, keeping the handle from rotating. The locking plate is then slid across the handle and the knob tightened, securing the handle in the holder. The block is then transferred to the measuring stage and locked in place. This stage can be rotated while the carrier and blade are locked to it. This allows the operator to check for defects in the blade and for any misalignment, either in the blade or in the footplates.

Adjust the stage up–down, in–out until the tip of the blade can be seen on the screen (Figures 8.62 and 8.63). Then retract the footplate until the blade protrudes through the footplate (Figure 8.64). Bring the blade shadow into sharp focus and adjust the stage until the tip of the blade just touches the zero point and the back edge of the blade is in full view and super-imposed upon the reticle. Next adjust the blade length by turning the adjustment screw on the blade handle. This moves the footplate and not the blade. Adjust the focus until the junction of the blade back and the footplate is well-seen and the bottom edge of the footplate is coincident with the measurement desired. Remove your hands from the controls and insure that the tip is still touching the zero point—you may have to re-focus. It will be found helpful, at this juncture, to reduce the brightness and contrast settings of the TV monitor so as to clarify the reticle lines as well as the blade edges and tip.

Please note in the case of double-edged blades: if you back up with your blade at this setting (i.e. cut with the vertical edge), your incision will be deeper than the setting because of the footplate curvature previously described (Figure 8.65). This is very important and must *never* be forgotten. Experienced surgeons can use this situation to increase the depth of the initial portion of their incisions by *gently* backing up to the edge of the optical zone.

If you are using the Russian (out-to-in) technique then this is your initial setting. If, however, you are using the Bores (in-to-out) method, the setting may need adjusting. Using the vertical adjustment knob, lower the blade until the slanted cutting edge/footplate junction comes into view. Adjust the focus and note the difference, if any, in the measured setting. With the current production Katena handles it may be that the measured length is from 10 to 30 μm *less* at this point. This is because the front curve of the footplate on this knife begins approximately in the middle of the blade and sweeps upward. Therefore, any measurement taken there (vertical edge) will be longer than one taken at the slanted blade edge where the footplate is more flat (and perpendicular to the midline of the blade). If you were to use the blade at this setting from in-to-out, the resultant incision would be shallower than that measured. Now elevate the blade until the straight edge comes into view and adjust the focus, checking to see that the blade is still zeroed. Now *lengthen* the blade the exact amount of the difference previously noted by turning the adjustment screw on the handle. This is your blade setting.

The adjustment knob of the handle is then turned until the footplate appears on the screen; in the Katena/WMK Bores-style adjustable knife handles the blade remains stationary while the footplate moves. Keep turning the knob until the bottom of the footplate aligns with the slanted edge of the knife blade. It may be necessary to lower the stage slightly to bring the edge down to the reticle. In that case the tip will no longer be touching the zero point. It will be necessary to move the stage up and down to check the zero point while making the final adjustment in blade setting.

You will find that while, at first, this method of setting may seem cumbersome, it will give the most accurate and reliable readings from setting to setting and is easily mastered. If you try to set the blade while looking at the slanted edge you will find that the tip

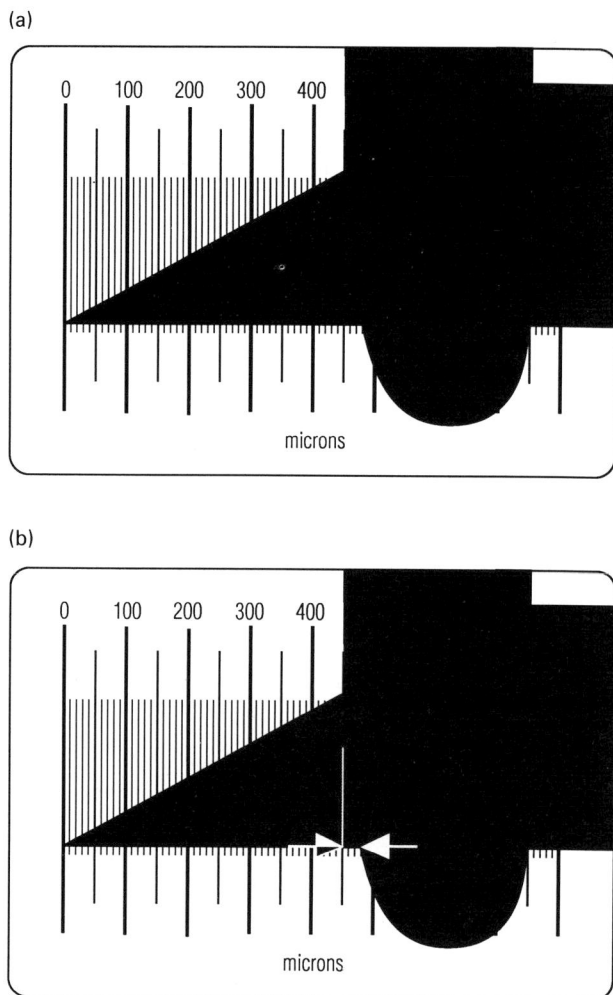

(a)

(b)

Fig. 8.65 (a) Measure along the vertical blade edge for incisions with the vertical edge and along the angled edge for incisions to be made with that edge; (b) note the difference in the two readings—this is typical for most knives.

will be off-screen. You will then not know if you have introduced any lateral movement into the system sufficient to move the blade tip off zero. Remember that the stage is sprung to dampen vibrations and can be shifted if pressure is applied. The author uses this methodology on all his cases, even for the settings of each of the Ts in the Ruiz procedure. The method is highly accurate and the comparator device is recommended to the refractive surgeon (Figure 8.66).

Now unlock the carrier and, grasping it by the handle-locking knob, remove it from the stage. If the handle is sterile, sliding the carrier out will be the safest maneuver. When free of the stage, grasp the *carrier* (not the knife handle) and lift it to a sterile surface. Since the bottom of the carrier is no longer sterile at this point, make sure always to set it down in the same place. I use a violet skin marking pencil to outline a safe "landing" area for the stage. You could

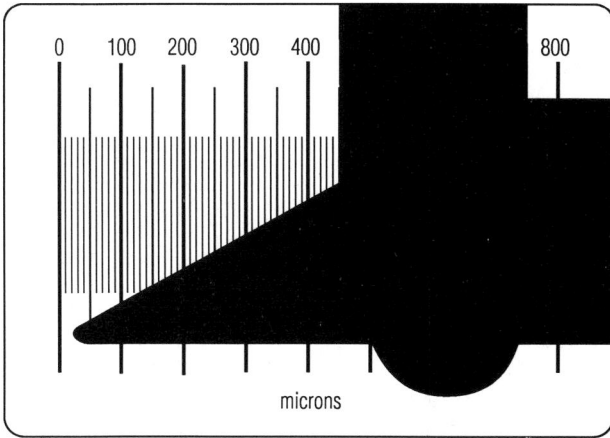

Fig. 8.66 It is very easy to see any blade defects—such as this rounded tip—with a shadowgraph. Such a defect would be missed under the microscope and would render any blade setting with a micrometer wrong.

simply place the carrier on to a 4 × 4 as well. Unlock the carrier and pick up the handle in such a way as to cause the head to rise first. Pushing down on the exposed end of the handle will accomplish this and prevent damage to the blade. Remove the knife and lay it in place it in the sterilizing box temporarily.

Practice these maneuvers with a discarded blade until you become proficient with them. Always check the calibration before each measuring session and be certain that the blade tip is coincident with zero when you are finished adjusting the blade. Keep the instrument covered when not in use and take care not to bump it or drop it while moving it. Try to keep it in one

place and not move it at all. This is a precision device and must be treated as such.

Establishing the optic center (fixation axis)

The patient is then asked to fixate upon the microscope light filament, whereupon the fixation point is marked with a blunt instrument, taking care to compensate for any parallax errors that may exist in the microscope system (Figure 8.67). This is the patient's visual axis or optic center. The light reflex seen through the Zeiss operating microscope is rectangular in shape. Because of two factors, the location of the light reflex will be displaced from the real locus of the optic axis. Figure 8.67 illustrates the appearance of the reflex from the right ocular of the microscope. Because of parallax within the microscope, the reflex will be displaced laterally (in this case, to the right). In addition, the position of the exit point of the light beam causes the patient to have to look down slightly in order to center the light's image. This causes the light reflex to be slightly higher than its true position. The rule of thumb for positioning the optic center mark is as follows:
1 Have the patient look at the light.
2 The surgeon fixates with one eye.
3 The mark is made in the upper corner opposite the fixating eye of the physician (Figure 8.67).

The Weck ophthalmic operating microscope typically produces two points of light on the corneal surface. In this case the procedure is similar, except that the surgeon alternately opens and closes the eyes each time, marking the spot between the light reflexes. When both eyes are fixating, two marks will be seen.

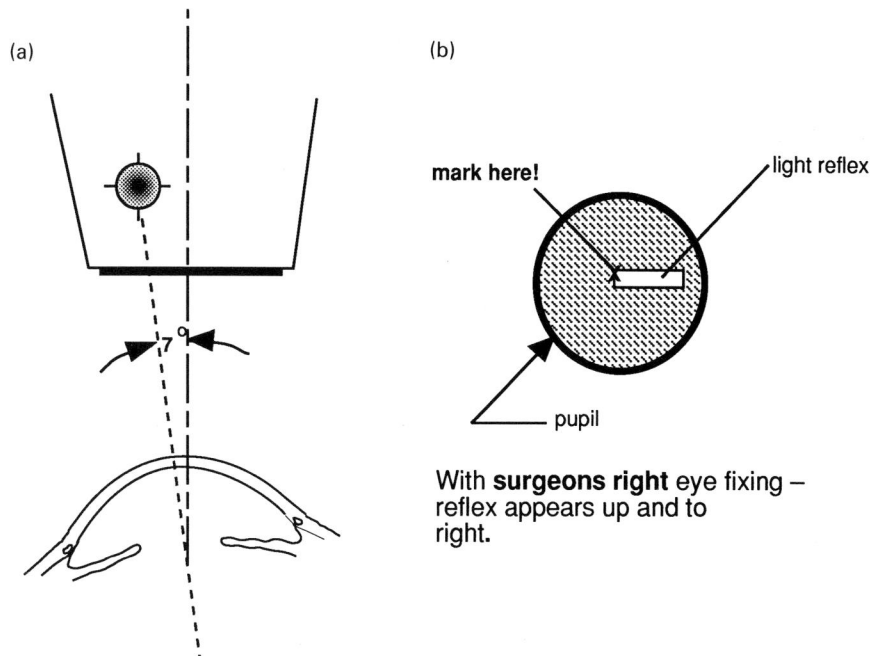

Fig. 8.67 (a) Microscope light reflex is typically higher than the visual axis; (b) the pupil is typically eccentric to the visual axis.

(a)

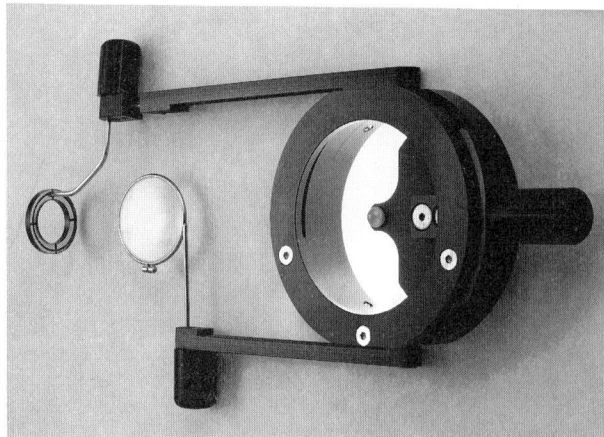

(b)

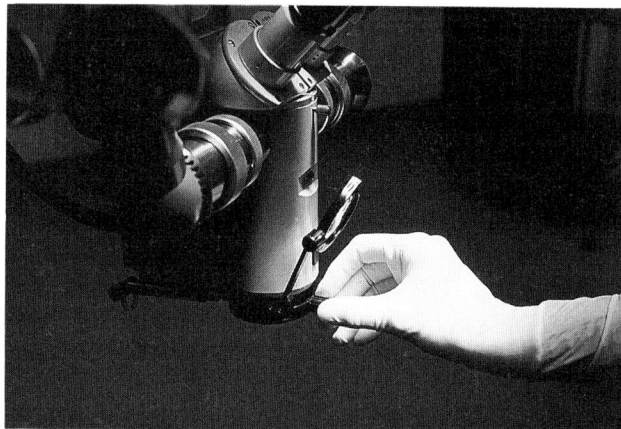

(c)

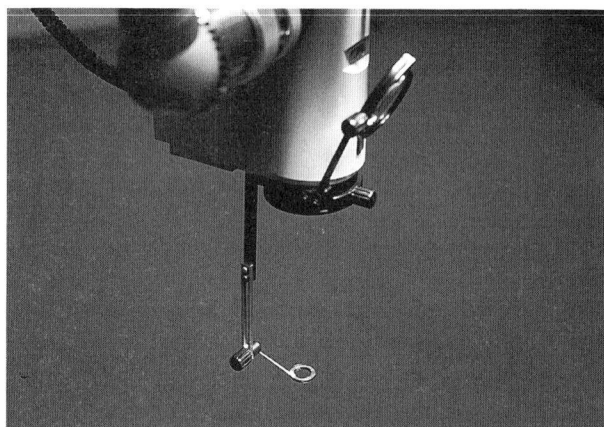

Fig. 8.68 (a) Martin aximeter from Mastel Precision Surgical Instruments. A magnifying lens and a surgical keratometer are also part of the instrument. (b and c) The apparatus attached to the microscope.

The optic center lies between the two. Mastel has made a rather nifty device which clamps on to the Zeiss operating microscope (Figure 8.68). This company also makes a complete line of radial keratotomy instrumentation including some of the most delicate and precise low-profile optical zone markers (Figure 8.69).

The main optical zone is then marked concentric to the optic axis, not to the pupil (Figure 8.70). This is extremely important because the pupil is not concentric with the optic axis of the eye (Figure 8.71). To verify the centration of the optic center and optical zone marks, the patient is asked to look away and then back at the light. Any discrepancy is corrected. The mid peripheral zone—if any—is then marked (Figure 8.72). Mark incisions if desired and the surgery begins (Figure 8.73).

A double-pronged corneal–scleral forceps designed for this purpose (Katena K5-3250) is applied to the limbus at the 3 o'clock position with the left hand for fixation (Figure 8.74). The blade tip is then inserted into the cornea exactly at the edge of the primary optical zone at the 9 o'clock position. The incision is carried to the mid-zone if there is one (see the section

on stepped incisions, below) or to the capillary plexus at the limbus. The back of the blade is your guide and should align with the mid-zone (if stepped) or capillary arcade (if single-depth).

The instruments are then switched to the other hand and the second incision made 180° to the first. The third incision is begun 90° to the first two. The surgeon continues in this manner until all incisions have been made (Figures 8.75 through 8.77).

One must also be sure that the knife footplate is perpendicular to the corneal surface and in contact with it at all times. This is especially important in the periphery where beginning surgeons have a tendency to keep the knife handle perpendicular to the floor of the operating room and not to the corneal surface— they forget that the corneal surface is curved. This tendency is clearly evident when the incisions are examined with the slit-lamp—almost all of them tend to curve up and become shallow in the extreme periphery. We have, therefore, suggested that novice surgeons should exert extra pressure against the cornea in the periphery to insure maximum depth of the incision there.

(a) (b)

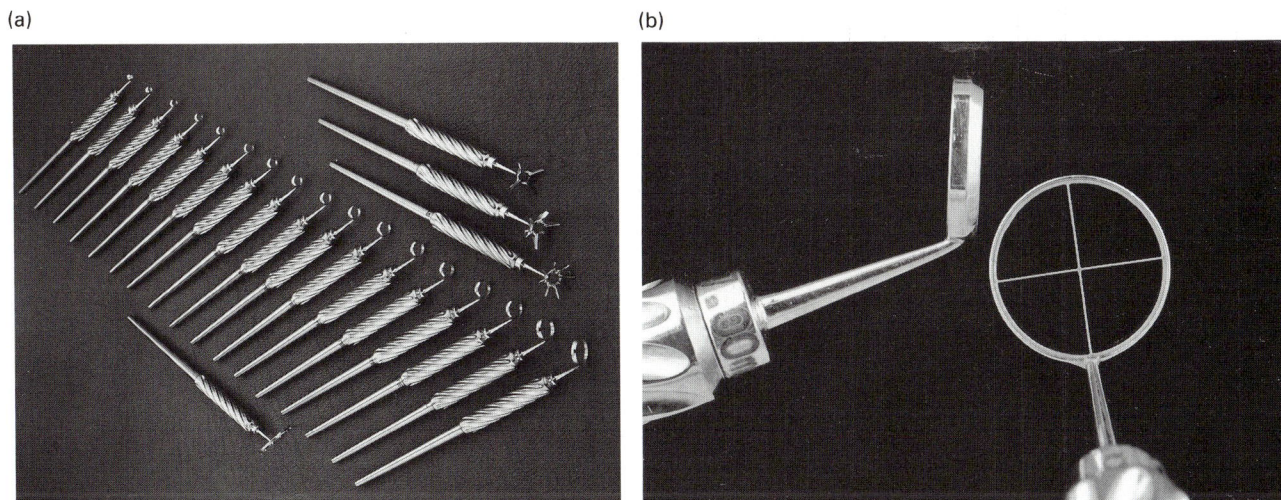

Fig. 8.69 (a) Light-weight, low-profile Mastel radial keratotomy markers. (b) Close-up of the optical zone markers.

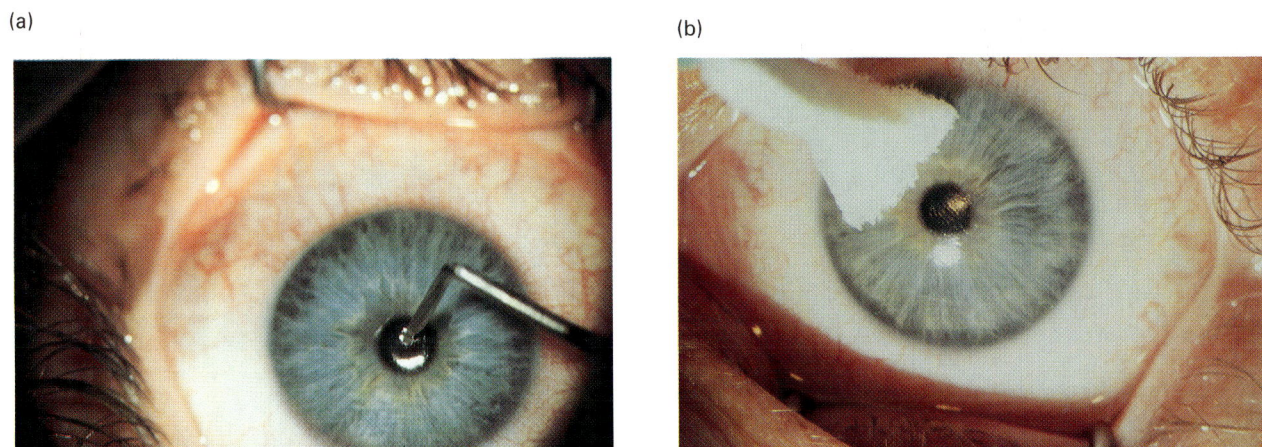

(a) (b)

Fig. 8.70 (a) Mark the optic center with a blunt instrument—a dipstick or Deitz hockey stick is ideal; (b) wipe off the cornea with a moistened WeckCel sponge to reveal the mark.

This has prompted some "experts" to assert that the extra pressure compresses the cornea, causing the incisions to be made deeper. They carry this notion a step further and recommend that extra pressure throughout will insure extra incision depth. While it is true that incisions will be deeper doing this, the cause is solid footplate–cornea contact, not tissue compression. I've not been able to demonstrate that normal corneal tissue is compressible to any degree, nor have I found any evidence in the literature to support the notion that it is.

Extra pressure, however, if carried to extreme may actually be harmful to the cornea by inducing bending of the endothelial cells. This is possibly the origin of the 22% endothelial cell loss reported by Hoffer and co-workers [15]. Video tapes of surgery being performed on the eyes included in that study show that

excess pressure was exerted in these cases, causing deep furrowing of the cornea along the wound track. A similar study, reported by Smith and Cutro [15] and using my technique, showed a net cell gain demonstrating that no cell loss had occurred. It is not necessary to exert much pressure at all against the cornea using the "feather touch" technique. Simply keeping the footplate in contact with the corneal surface and arcing the knife handle to follow the curvature is sufficient to produce incisions of even depth throughout (Figure 8.78).

Stepped incisions

If a stepped incision is required, the blade is re-set in the shadowgraph to the proper length, again oversetting as required. The blade is inserted into the end

(a)

4.0 mm circle

optic center

nose

pupil

(b)

(c)

(d)

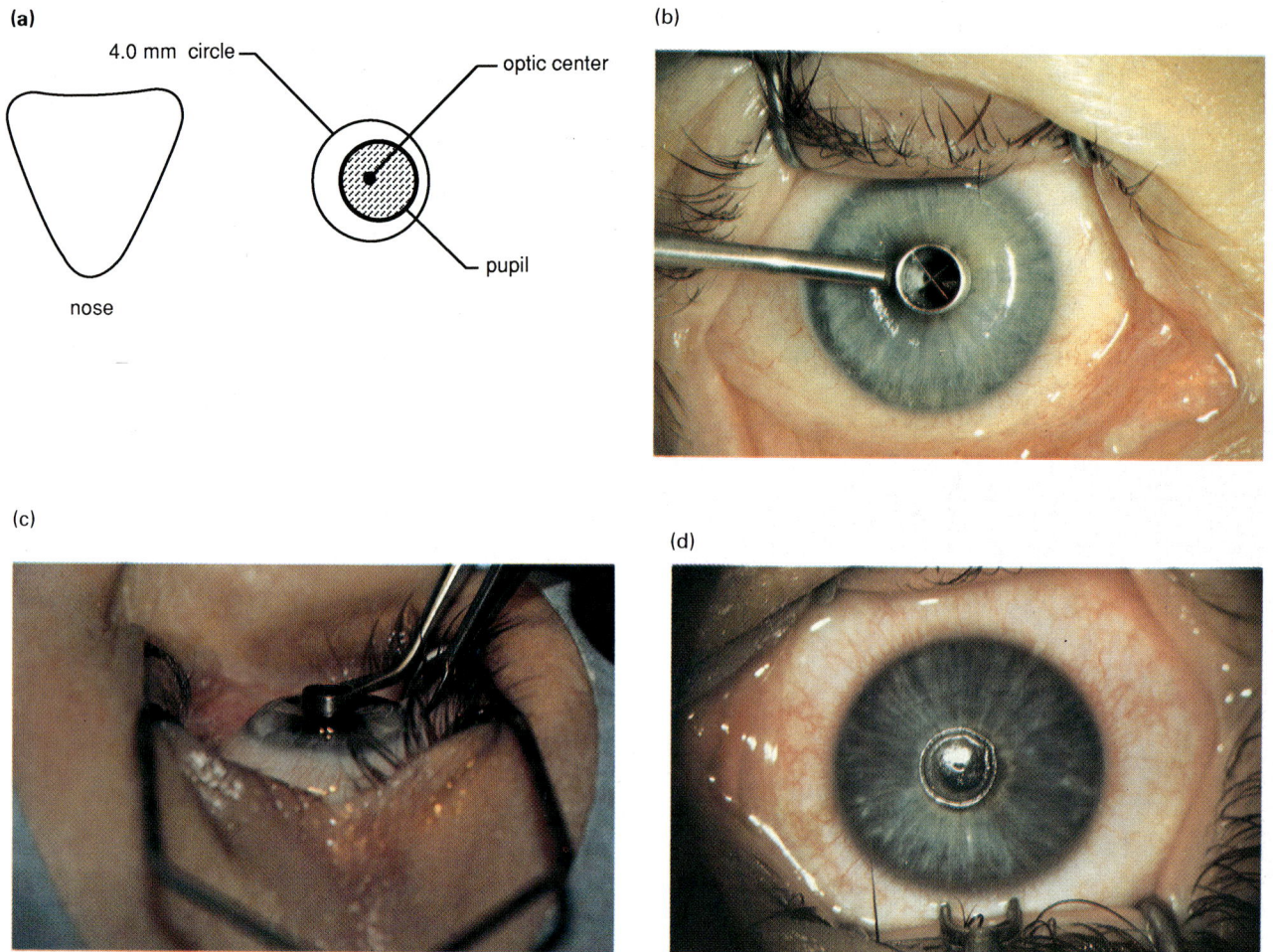

Fig. 8.71 (a) Mark the surgical zone concentric to the optic center. (b) A cross-hair is helpful. (c) Press the marker against the cornea with a slight rocking movement. Do *not* rotate the marker. (d) A dry cornea shows up the mark very clearly.

of the previously made incision just behind the edge of the mid-zone and the incision continued to the limbus. If the blade is drawn up gently to the end of the previous incision before extending it, the transition will be smooth and no tag or "stalagmite" will be left behind (Figures 8.79 through 8.83).

After all the incisions have been made, a Fyodorov dipstick (or similar instrument) is used to insure that no over-lapping tissue tags are left behind in stepped incisions (Figure 8.82c). If any are found, they must be incised so as not to leave a constricting band around the mid-zone, thereby reducing the effect of the surgery or even inducing astigmatism.

The Russian way

There are times when it may be necessary or desirable to do things the Russian way—that is, to make incisions from the limbus to the center. We will explain why this is necessary in our discussion about re-cutting over old incisions (see the section on second-

stage surgery, below). High myopia (greater than −7.0 D) is another (see Case 4 above). Since we have already stated that the practical upper limit of radial keratotomy is somewhere around −6.0 to −6.5 D, it might be asked why we discuss cases with more myopia than that. We are discussing them because there may be times when radial incisions are warranted in high myopia. The patient, for example, may decide that part of a result is better than staying myopic and may not wish to opt for MKM. Furthermore, despite what has been described as the practical upper limit of radial keratotomy, this statement does not mean that such cases are impossible to correct; it just means that they are less likely to be fully corrected. Less likely does not mean not likely, in any case. It should go without saying, though, that such a case should not be one of the first you try.

The Russian (Fyodorov) method requires a blade with a vertical cutting edge, a knife handle with an open foot (Katena/WMK), and a wide fixation forceps. It also requires that special markers be used to provide

(a)

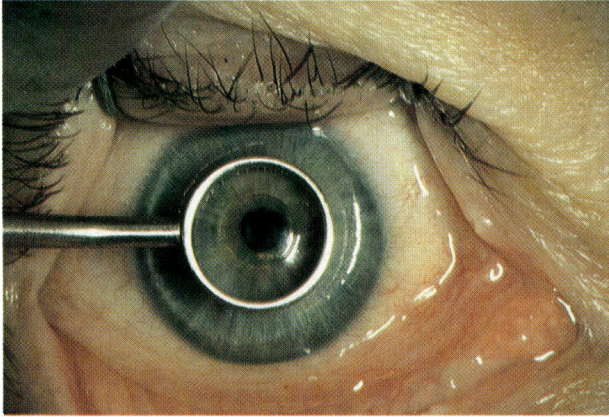

(b)

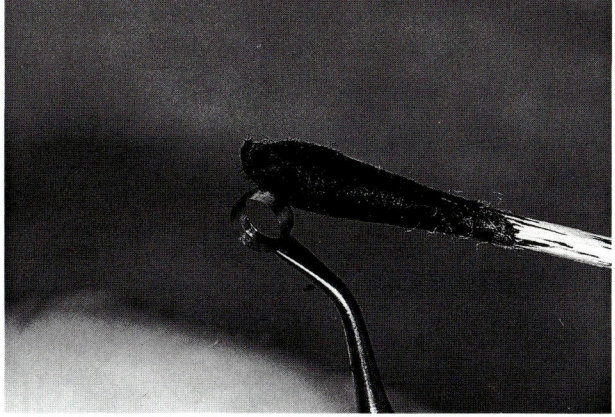

(c)

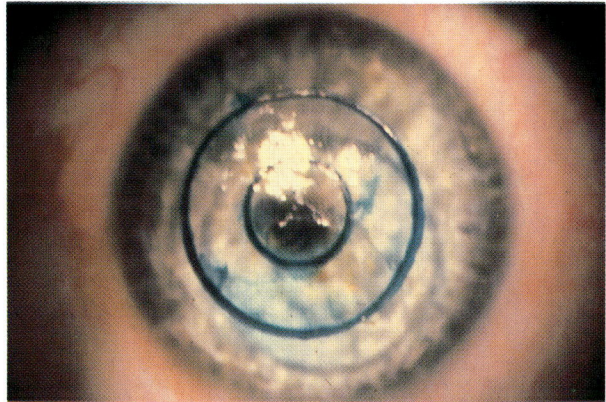

Fig. 8.72 (a) The mid peripheral zone (if any) is marked concentric to the first. (b and c) Coating the markers with brilliant green or a gentian violet skin marking pen can make the marks more vivid.

guidelines for making the incisions. There are any number of such markers on the market—I prefer those made by Katena (since most were made to my specifications). In addition, some sort of dye should be applied to the marker blades to stamp indelible marks on to the corneal surface (Figure 8.84). These are necessary because the Russian method is somewhat slower to perform and the impressions of the marker blades alone will fade before the case is completed. Fyodorov uses a 1% tincture of brilliant green but the author prefers a gentian violet skin marking pen (Katena K20-4500) because the marks are more readily seen on the cornea. This is applied to the optical zone and incision markers and allowed to dry thoroughly. Absolute alcohol is used to make the tincture of brilliant green and if any gets on the cornea it will destroy the epithelium, so make sure it's dry.

The optic center is marked in the usual way and the blade set to the corneal thickness of the largest optical zone to be used. Make sure, if using the shadowgraph, that the readings are taken at the juncture of the vertical blade edge and the footplate. Next the surgical (optical) zones are marked, starting with the smallest.

Since the smallest zone will almost always be 2.75 or 3.00 mm and the incisions will have steps at 6 and 8 mm respectively, a triple ring marker with these dimensions can be purchased for this purpose. Once the zones are marked, the incision guides are stamped on to the corneal surface. Fixation is made in the same manner as in the Bores technique—directly across from the incision at the limbus. If you are using a wide or limbal fixation forceps, fix the cornea at 12 and 6 o'clock. In any case make the first incision the horizontal one at 9 o'clock if the left eye and 10.30 if the right eye. It is important to do this because the central optical zone is shifted slightly nasally but the corneal thickness taper is not. Insert the blade at the limbus with the slot in the footplate straddling the incision mark (Figure 8.85).

Holding the eye steady and watching the corneal surface just in front of the blade, move the blade forward. It is futile to attempt to watch the leading edge of the diamond and sapphire blades—they are too fine to see under the microscope. However, it is easy to see the incision being made, especially as the tissue separates and flows away from the blade edge

(a)

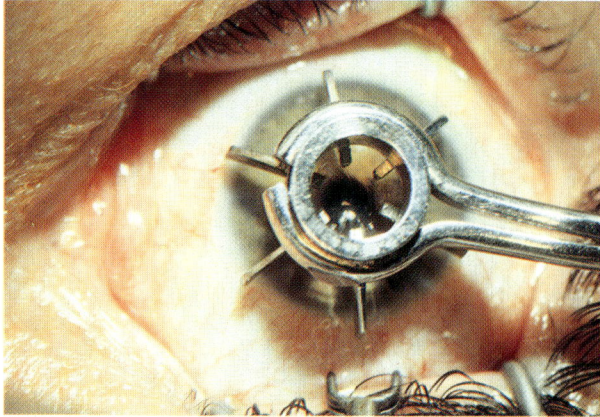

(b)

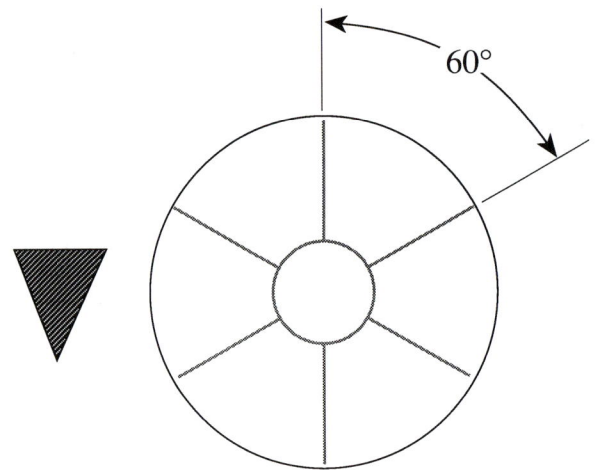

(c)

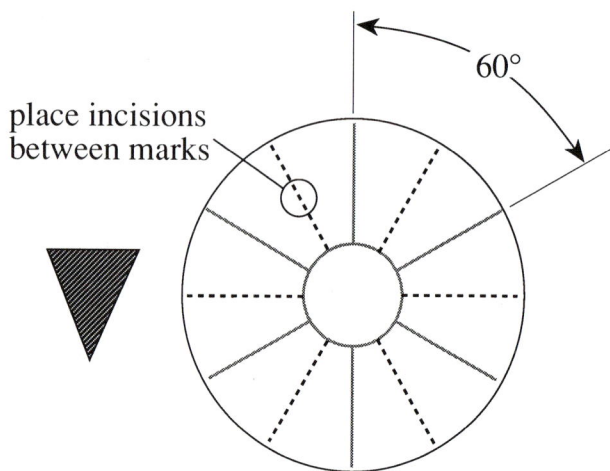

place incisions
between marks

Fig. 8.73 (a) Mark incisions as desired (see text). (b) A six-ray marker is useful because it is hard to line up incisions exactly at 60°. (c) For a 12-incision case, incisions are easily made between the six marks.

like water being cleaved by the prow of a boat. As the blade approaches the first zone mark pay very careful attention to the incision. Keep the blade moving until the first hint of aqueous appears, then stop immediately and remove the blade. Wait while the cornea in that area swells, sealing the wound—it should take no longer than a minute or two. You will be surprised just how far past that first mark it is possible to go. Note the point at which aqueous appeared and make all the rest of the incisions to that point, saving the infero-temporal one to the last. You will appreciate the "feather touch" technique here because using it is very unlikely to promote leakage from the micro-perforation. The perforation will be very much a micro one, in contra-distinction to what would be the case if the "ham-handed" ultra-heavy pressure technique were used (Figure 8.86). Herein it is vital that all incisions be made 180° apart.

When the first-step incisions are completed, re-set the blade to the corneal thickness at the secondary zone. Don't forget to add any blade bias that may be necessary. Re-insert the blade just behind the end of each previous incision—saving the one with the micro-perforation until last—and carry the incision toward the next zone, all the while watching for aqueous; stop and remove the blade in that event. Note that point and proceed. When all incisions have had the second step made, re-set the blade to the pachymetry at the primary optical clear zone (2.75 or 3.00 mm).

By now the eye will be much softer than it was at the beginning. Now you will likely find that fixation behind the blade, thereby pulling the cornea under the footplate, provides better control and a smoother cut (Figures 8.87 and 8.88). Carry each incision up to the central optical clear zone.

Caution! This end point is not that clear-cut (no pun intended). The tissue tends to roll under the footplate obscuring the edge of the zone. Watch the marked edge. As it passes under the tip of the footplate, begin easing the forward movement of the knife, stopping

(a)

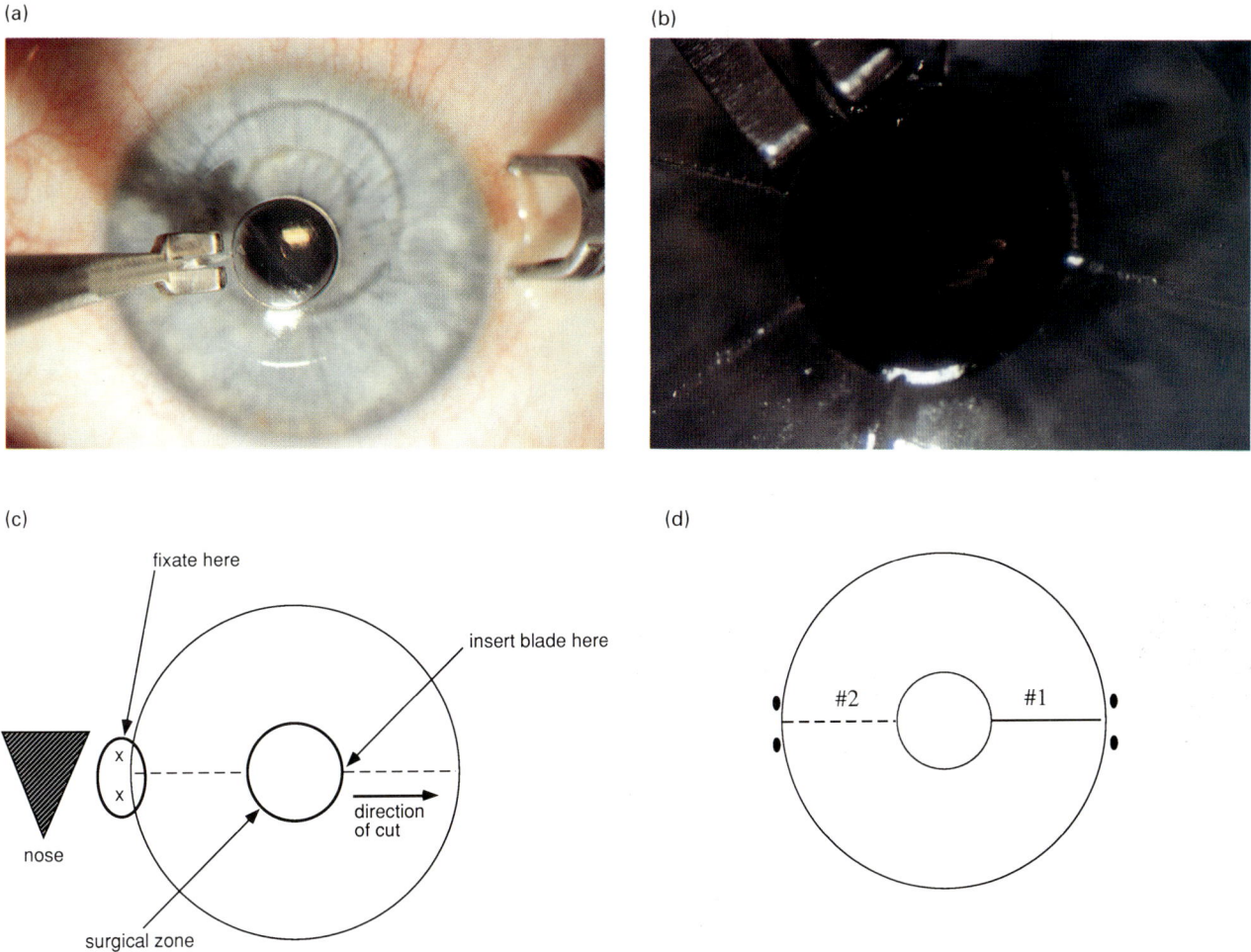

(b)

(c)

fixate here

insert blade here

x
x

direction
of cut

nose

surgical zone

(d)

#2   #1

Fig. 8.74 (a) Fixation is at the limbus, 180° to the incision. (b) The blade tip is inserted exactly at the edge of the surgical clear zone. (c,d) Make the first two incisions the horizontal ones.

when the mark completely disappears under the footplate. Remove the blade and you should find that the incision has stopped exactly on the mark.

If you find that you are consistently over-shooting the end point, use a central marker whose diameter is 0.25 mm greater than the smallest zone you are trying to achieve. Because the eye is soft more care will need to be taken to keep the incisions straight. Speed is a hindrance here—it only makes matters worse. Make your incisions with a slow, steady, and even pace. Do not be surprised if the terminal portion of the incisions tends to be curved or slightly irregular; although experience will minimize this effect, it is almost inevitable. Do not allow any incision to veer into and join another incision, however.

Second-stage surgery—dealing with under-corrections

The response of the eye to relaxing incisions, as in any biologic system, produces a typical Gaussian curve.

That is, while most corneas flatten to a narrow range of predicted values clustering around emmetropia, there are a fair number that do not—some fall on the plus side of emmetropia while some fall on the negative. Those that fall on the plus side—are over-corrected (or, more properly, have over-responded)—are more difficult to correct; there is no eraser on a scalpel, after all. The correction of such errors is dealt with in Chapter 15. Because there is no straightforward manner to correct hyperopia as yet, the RK DataMaster algorithms have been weighted so as to skew any calculation errors to the negative or myopic side. Therefore, if you use the author's technique you will find that, on balance, you will be contending with more cases requiring a second stage of the surgery but fewer over-corrections. This, however, is better than the alternative—an over-correction. It is a simple matter to lengthen, deepen, or add additional incisions in under-correction. Incisions cannot be erased in the event of an over-correction.

Some authors—with the best of intentions, no

(a)

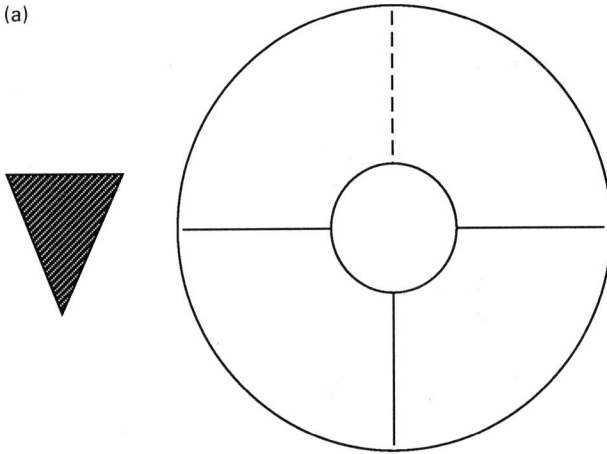

(b)

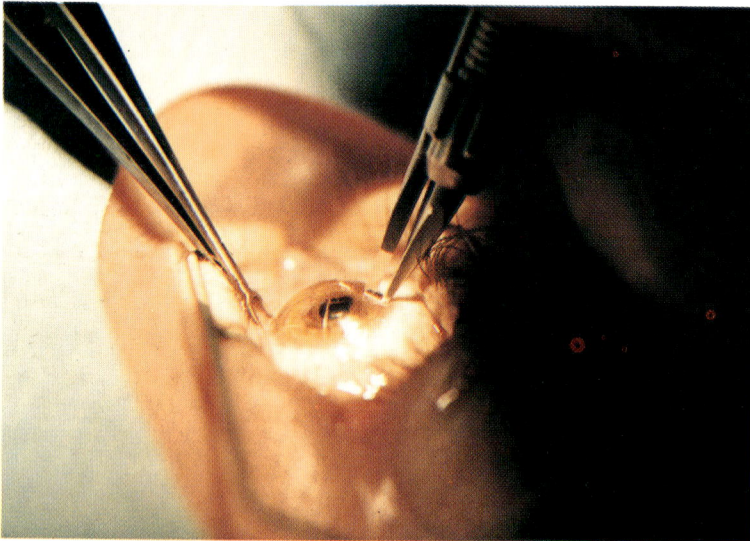

Fig. 8.75 (a,b) The 12 o'clock incision is the third to be made.

doubt—have advocated staging the surgery, at least in certain cases, to avoid the possibility of an over-correction. By this they mean that the patient receives half of the incisions (usually four) and then after a suitable period of time has elapsed, the remainder (also usually four) of the incisions are added, if needed. This sounds like a good idea, especially if one is concerned about over-corrections, but, ultimately, it is not a good idea. An impartial observer could be forgiven for concluding that the surgeon who took this approach was either unsure of the technique or was less than convinced of the validity of the surgery itself. If the former, then it would seem prudent to adopt another method of parameter selection and if the latter, perhaps it would be better if the surgeon stopped doing the surgery altogether.

There are enough variables in the equation to con-

tend with without introducing another—which is exactly what happens once Bowman's layer is incised. No one has yet devised a formula to take into account the profound changes which occur in the cornea once this has happened, especially when days or weeks have passed. All suggestions made to contend with the corneal shape after this event are purely empiric. One fact does seem irrefutable, however, and that is that the second group of incisions never results in the same effect as when all incisions are made at the same time. My advice, therefore, is to go for the whole of the myopia all at once and to do the non-dominant eye first. After a suitable period of time, do the second eye, making any necessary adjustments in the technique to secure an even better result. Do it this way even if mono-vision is the plan. Since, as Robert Burns put it, "The best laid schemes o' mice an' men, gang aft

(a)

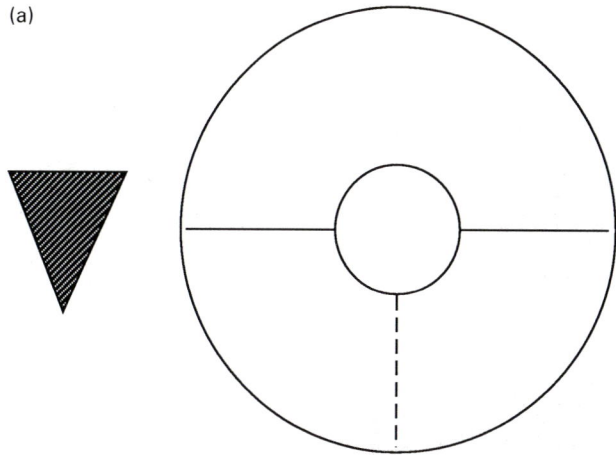

(b)

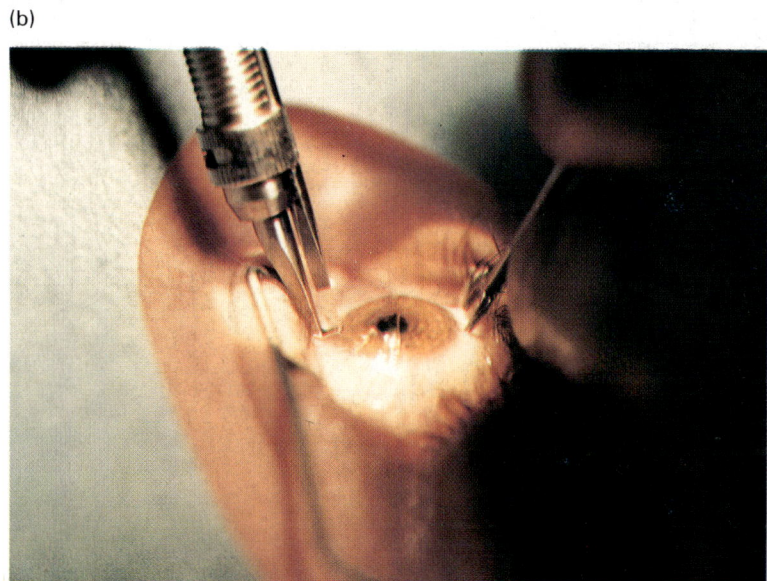

Fig. 8.76 (a,b) The fourth incision is made at 6 o'clock. Only the gentlest downward pressure is used.

a-gley," this mind-set will keep the surgeon out of hot water most of the time. For this and other reasons, do not perform simultaneous surgery (see below).

Having said all this, what's a person to do in the event of having "missed the mark"? The first piece of advice (and the second and third) is not to be in a hurry. The next is to learn how to evaluate the depth of the incisions, upon which all depends. Figure 8.89 illustrates the appearance of radial keratotomy incisions at the slit-lamp and their approximate depths. The observer should keep in mind several points. Firstly, early on, corneal edema can distort the appearance of incision depth, making incisions appear far deeper than they are. Since such edema can persist upward of a year, the task might seem impossible except that most of the edema subsides within the first 3–4 weeks. Consequently, it is essential that new

pachymetry readings be taken before additional surgery is performed. Usually a central reading is sufficient because the cornea swells up uniformly—add the difference to the old pachymetry measurements to get the new thicknesses. Secondly, the appearance of the incisions depends upon whether the slit-beam is coming from the nasal or temporal side of the eye. Incisions seen with the slit-beam on the nasal side will seem somewhat shallower than if viewed from the temporal.

To add incisions or to deepen them, that is the question. If the incisions are shallow, either from plan or from inadvertence, it will be well to deepen them as soon as possible, that is, within the first 30 days postoperation. To deepen incisions requires a steady hand and a sharp blade with a vertical cutting edge because the incisions have to be traced over from limbus to

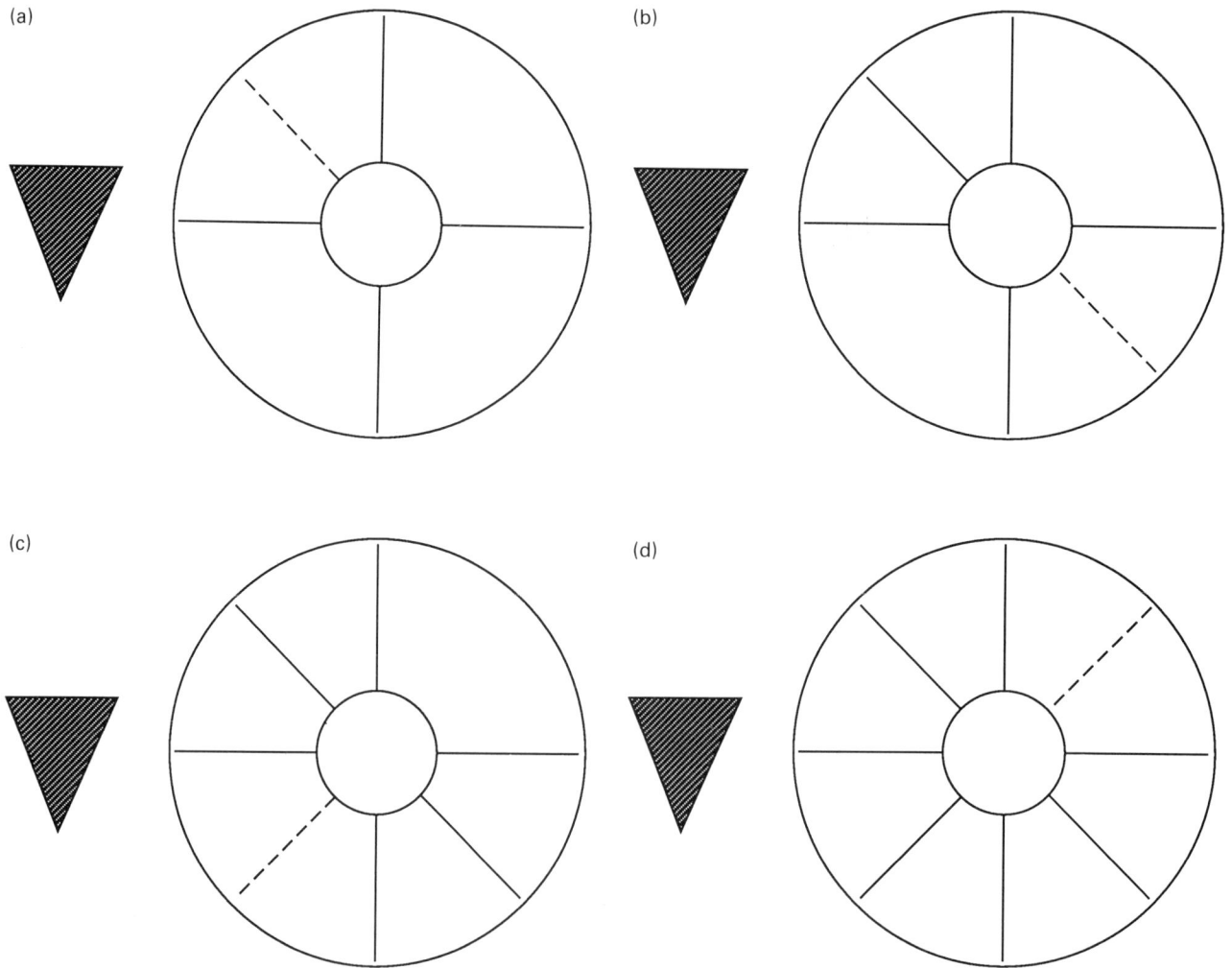

Fig. 8.77 (a) The fifth incision is made downward and nasally. (b) Incision 6 is made up and out (supero-temporal). (c) The seventh incision is made in the upper nasal quadrant. (d) The infero-temporal incision is *always* last.

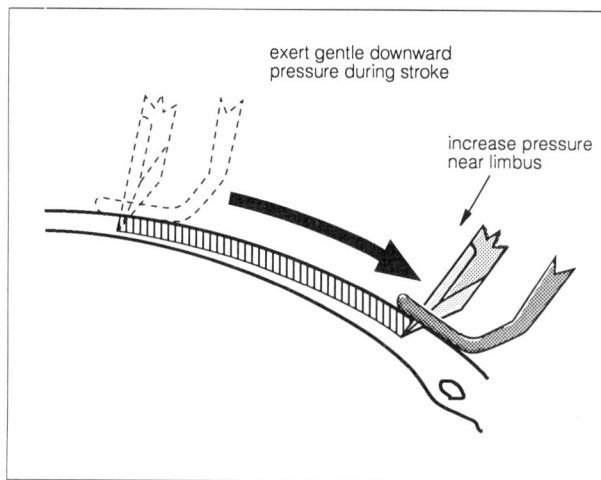

exert gentle downward
pressure during stroke

increase pressure
near limbus

Fig. 8.78 Keep the footplate against the corneal surface.

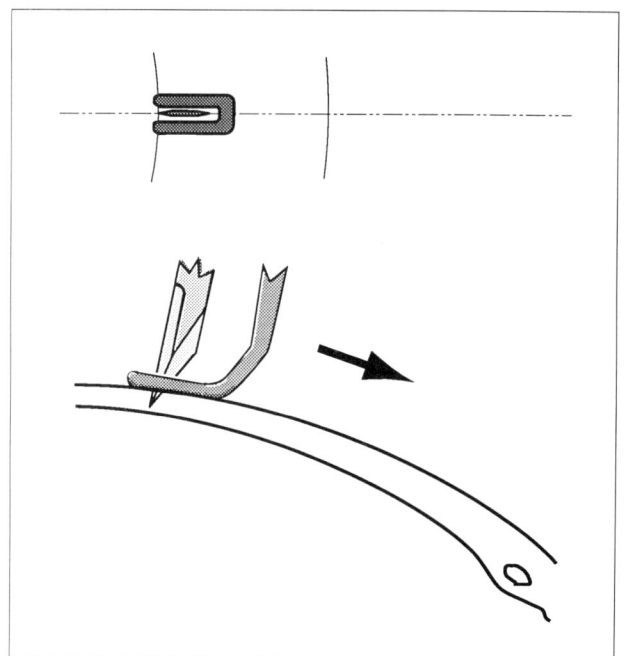

Fig. 8.79 (*Right*) Insert blade tip exactly at the edge of the primary optical zone as before.

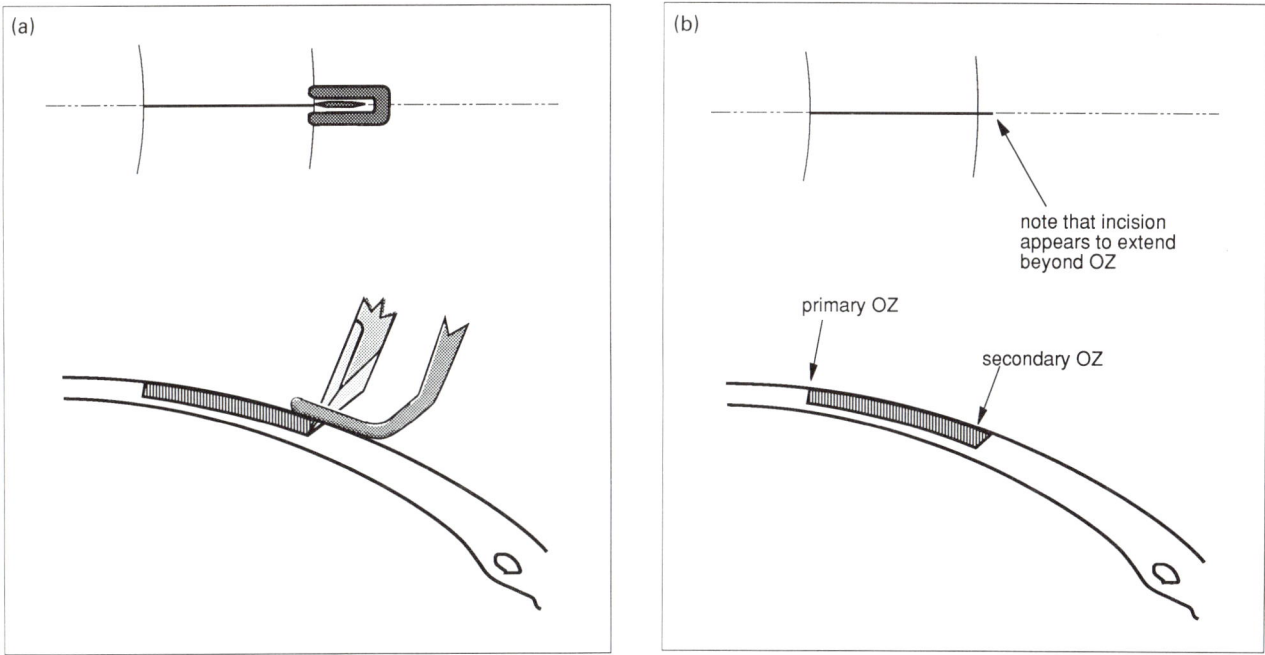

Fig. 8.80 (a) Stop at the secondary zone. (b) The incision will appear to extend beyond the secondary zone.

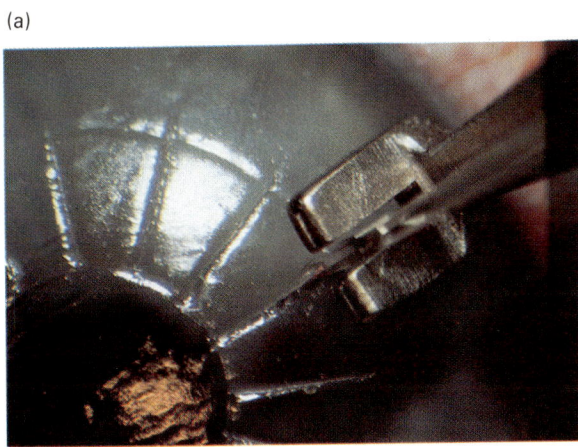

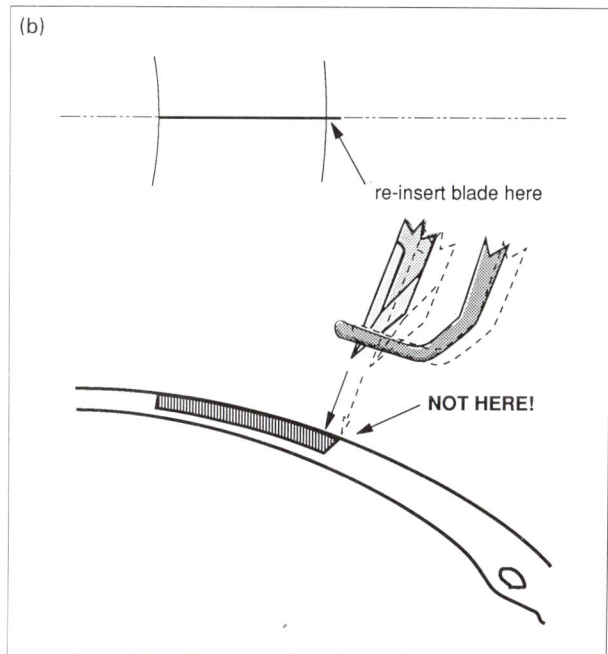

Fig. 8.81 The second step starts inside the first, not at the end.

center. Do not even think of doing this using a angled blade and moving from center to limbus—it will not work. It doesn't work because the surgeon will not be able to see the incision well enough to stay within it and it will not work because angled blades are almost impossible to keep from wandering out of the incision.

Figure 8.90 illustrates the technique of incision deepening. Note that fixation behind the blade is recommended. This is especially crucial for beginners in this technique. The surgeon will find that he/she will have much better control over both the direction and end point of the incision doing it this way—corneal rippling is completely avoided.

If the surgeon has an extremely sharp blade at his or her disposal and some experience, the same thing can be accomplished using a wide, limbal fixation forceps.

(a) re-inserting blade here …

… and making the incision

(b) re-inserting blade here …

… results in — a stalagmite!

(c)

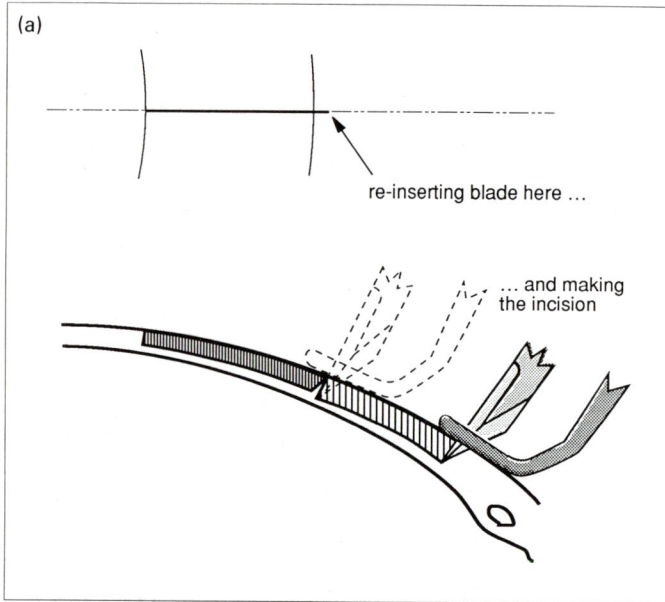

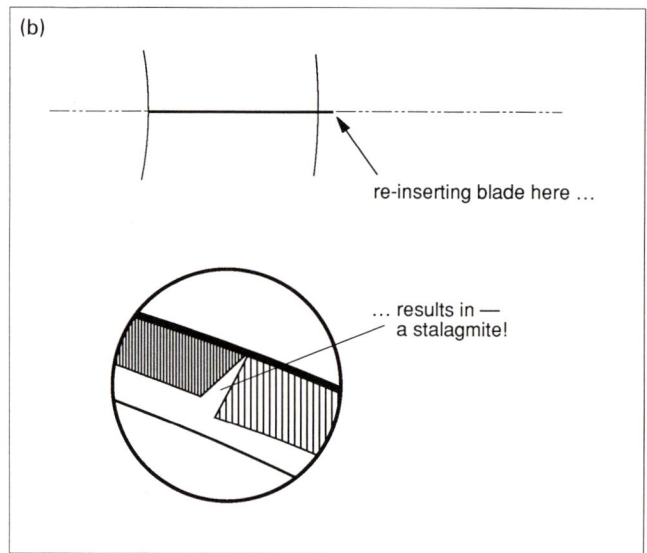

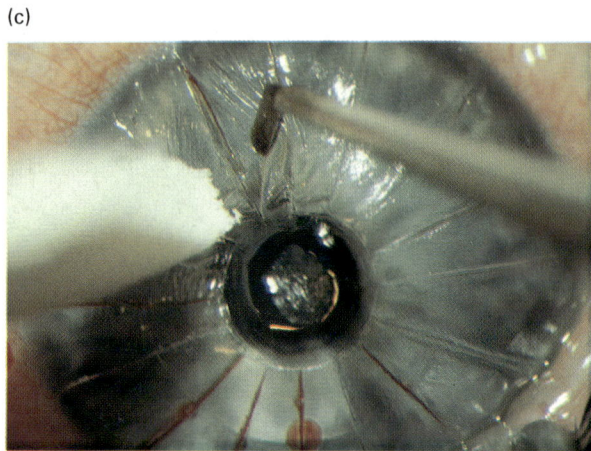

Fig. 8.82 (a) Inserting the blade at the end of the first incision results in (b and c) a stalagmite (between dipstick and swab).

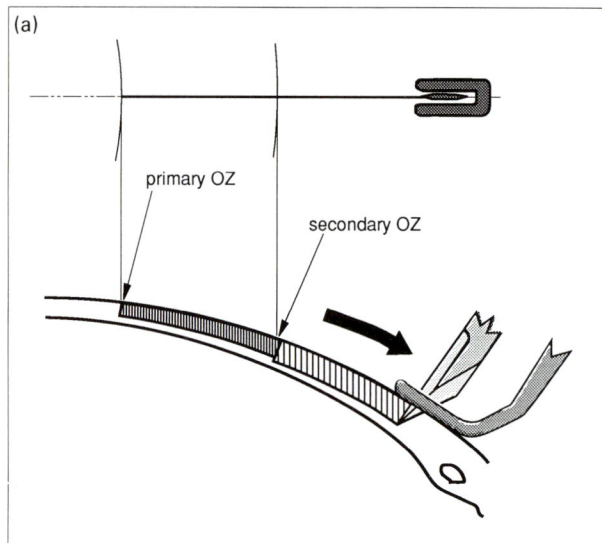

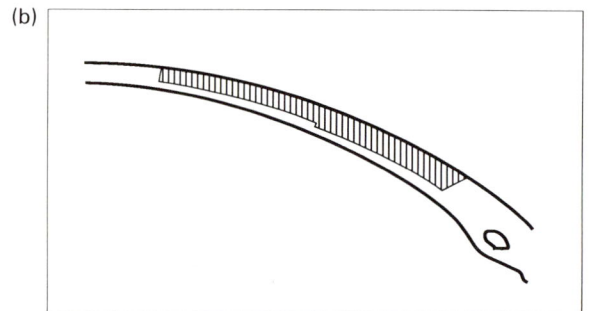

(a) primary OZ

secondary OZ

(b)

Fig. 8.83 Proper stepping technique. (a) Insert the blade just inside the previous incision. (b) Continue the incision to the limbus if the two-step procedure is being used.

(a)

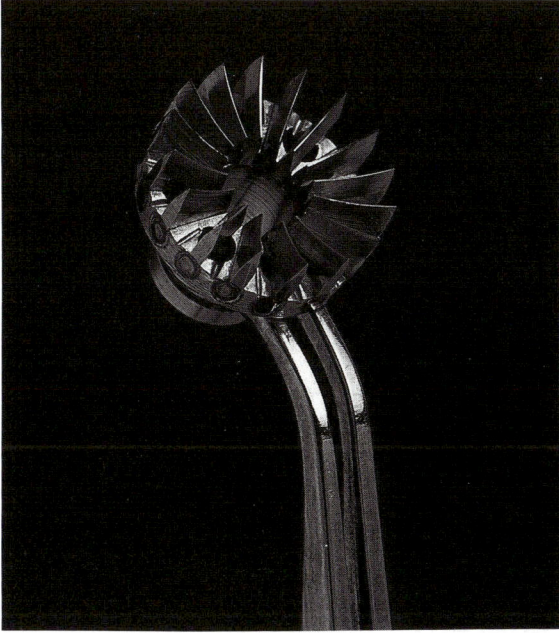

(b)

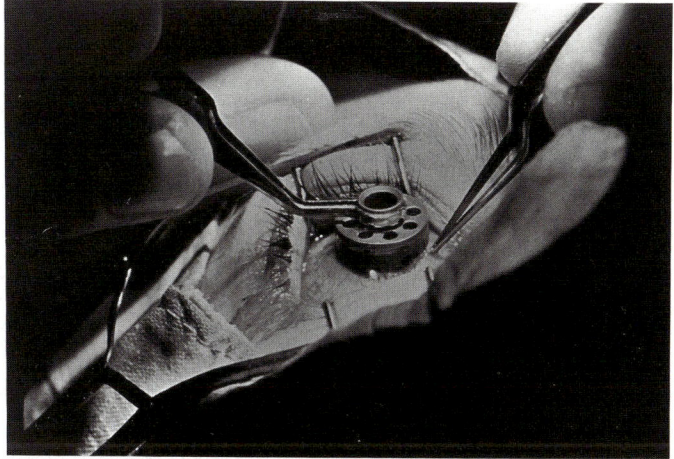

(c)

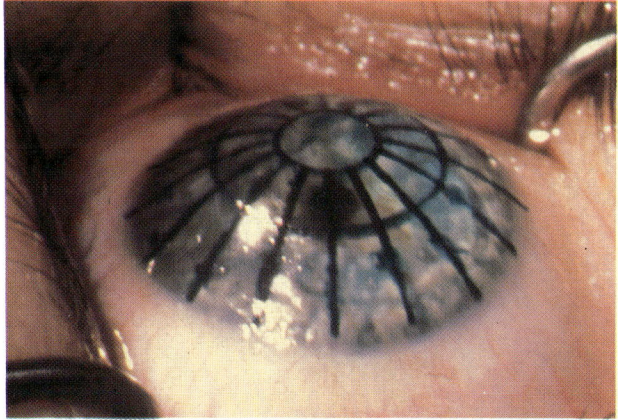

Fig. 8.84 (a) The ''pizza cutter'' (16-ray marker) is used to mark guidelines; (b) applied to the eye; (c) the marked cornea.

(a)

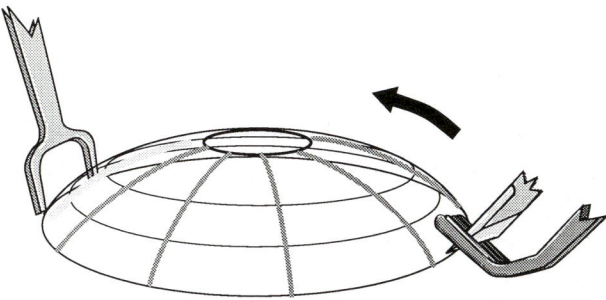

(b)

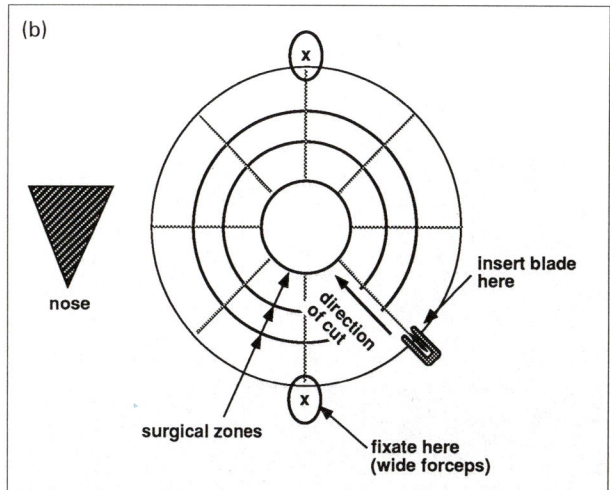

nose

insert blade here

direction of cut

surgical zones

fixate here (wide forceps)

Fig. 8.85 (a) Insert the blade at the limbus. (b) Incisions are made toward the center.

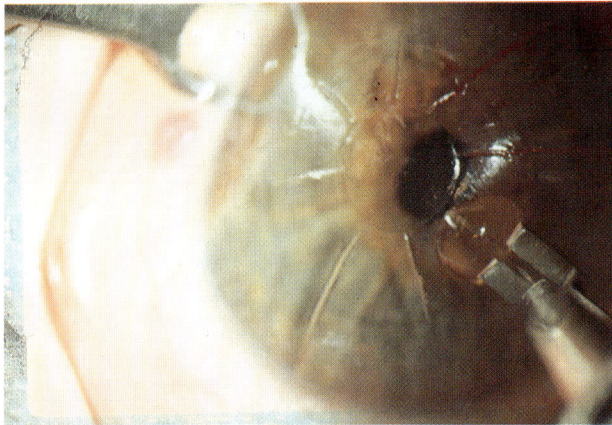

Fig. 8.86 The blade is carried forward until a micro-perforation occurs.

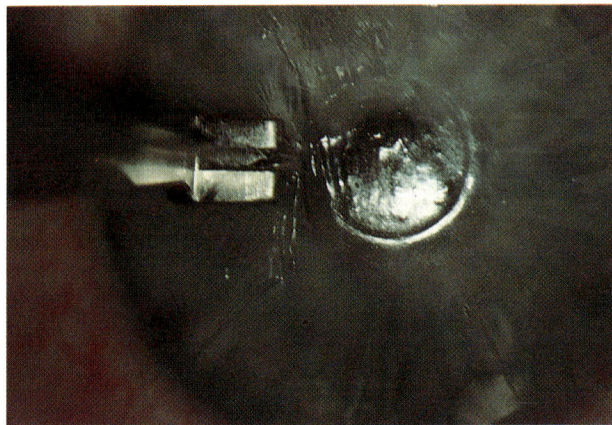

Fig. 8.88 Sharp blades, wide fixation and a steady hand result in straight and even incisions.

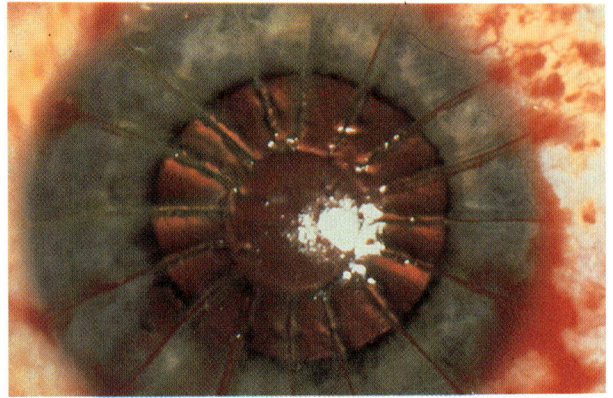

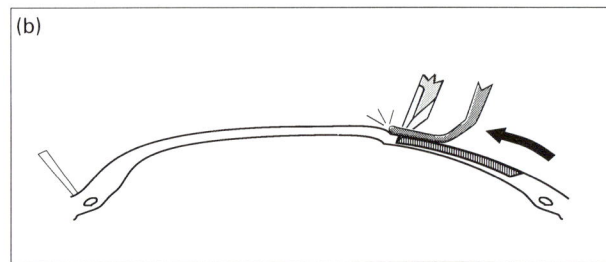

(b)

Fig. 8.87 (a and b) A "bow wake" or wrinkles will occur unless fixation is behind the blade or with limbus-to-limbus fixation.

Note, however, that the fixation points must be behind the end point. Such deepening can either be single-depth or in steps; just remember to set the blade according to the corneal thickness of the end point. One other tip (or pearl if you will): re-cut alternate incisions only—do not attempt to deepen them all. This is especially important where there have been 12 or more incisions made primarily. The eye will become

extremely soft very quickly and attempts to re-cut adjacent incisions will very likely end with one or more of them hook-shaped where the blade has inevitably wandered out of the track, or worse, join another incision.

Of course, all this could be avoided if the incisions were made deep enough in the first place. Practically every surgeon I know has had difficulty with the recommendation (nay necessity) that blades be set longer than the corneal thickness. The entire idea seems so illogical. However, if we were letting logic alone guide us, we would know that radial keratotomy can't work—but of course if does; so much for logic. At any rate, most surgeons will, therefore, not over-set the blade in their first few cases, thus obtaining less than ideal results. Some few of these will blame the procedure rather than their own timidity. Once they start over-setting, however, their results start getting up to speed. It is also true, though, that some eyes will not react to the surgery as predicted—a case requiring single-depth incisions will turn out to need increased depth in the periphery. The eye will always be right, however, so take some comfort from that.

If the incisions are of an adequate depth throughout, incisions can still be re-cut to lengthen them. In this case, fixation behind the blade is essential because absolute control of the end point is a must. In the previous example, the incisions are merely being deepened, not lengthened, and the blade will stop almost by itself when the inner extremity of the cut has been reached—especially if the surgeon is using what William Myers, MD, calls the Bores feather touch technique. In this technique, only sufficient pressure is exerted against the cornea to maintain contact between the knife handle footplate and the corneal surface. This method minimizes corneal distortion, rippling and blade wandering; our object is to incise the cornea, not bludgeon it.

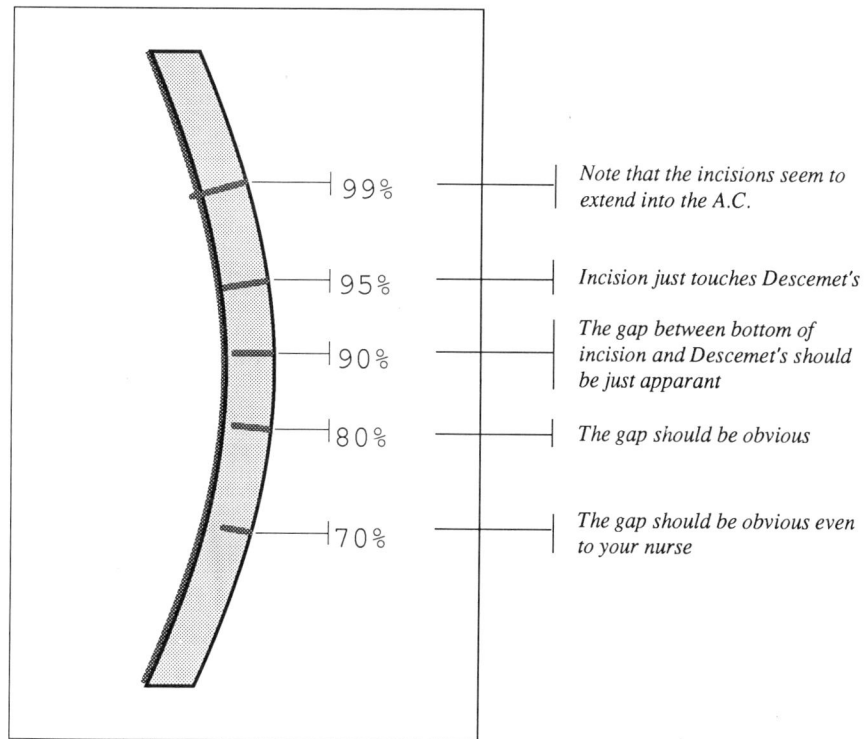

99%	*Note that the incisions seem to extend into the A.C.*
95%	*Incision just touches Descemet's*
90%	*The gap between bottom of incision and Descemet's should be just apparant*
80%	*The gap should be obvious*
70%	*The gap should be obvious even to your nurse*

Fig. 8.89 Estimating incision depth at the slit-lamp. Slit-beam should be finely focused.

All of the above suggestions should be carried out within the first 30 days after the initial surgery or after waiting for at least 6 months. Doing additional surgery in the intervening period can result in no further effect at the very least, and to complete loss of effect at the most. I am not quite sure why this should be so, but both Fyodorov and I have experienced just that in some of our earlier cases. If the surgery is not re-done within 30 days, the keratotomist is admonished not to do any additional surgery until at least 6 months have elapsed. There are three good reasons for this. The first is that whatever seems to be affecting the cornea after 30 days has lost that influence by 6 months. Secondly, and more importantly, some corneas will seem to lose ground between 5 and 6 months, only to gain back the effect lost. Some eyes have had additional surgery done prematurely in ignorance of this phenomenon— to the everlasting sorrow of both surgeon and patient. Thirdly, the cornea will be much more stable at this time and the incision scars firmer.

Assuming that the initial incisions were of adequate depth and length and their number does not exceed eight, the only alternative left is to add more incisions. There are no hard and fast rules that apply in such a case but there are some guidelines which can be of help. Typically, although the additional incisions will not gain the patient as much as if all the incisions had been done together, the difference will only be 20% if the new incisions are made in the same manner as the old. Depending upon the amount of under-correction,

it may be possible to make the new cuts longer or deeper than the old. Avoid doing both in a patient over 40 years of age if the residual is less than 25% of the original myopia, though. In this case it would be best to "sneak up" on the myopia and do it in stages.

Calculate the surgical parameters using the new myopia as well as the new K-readings. This technique will call for slightly more surgery than if the old Ks are used. However, this should not be sufficiently greater to increase the hazard of over-correction unduly. The pachymetry must be repeated as in re-cutting incisions except that the central reading may not reflect the additional corneal thickness that may exist near the old incisions. It is advisable to do a partial mapping of the corneal thickness at each of the main zones between the old incisions. The surgery can then be done as if the cornea had not been previously incised.

Post-operative management

Irrigation of the incisions with a gentle stream of BSS follows completion of the case (Figure 8.91). Look at each incision in turn: some will be filled with red blood cells while others will appear to be clean. These latter may be leaking and are clean-looking because the flow of aqueous has washed them out. In these incisions or in those in which a micro-perforation is known to exist, irrigation should be very gentle indeed. It is not a good idea either to extend the perforation or to cause fluid to be forced into the eye.

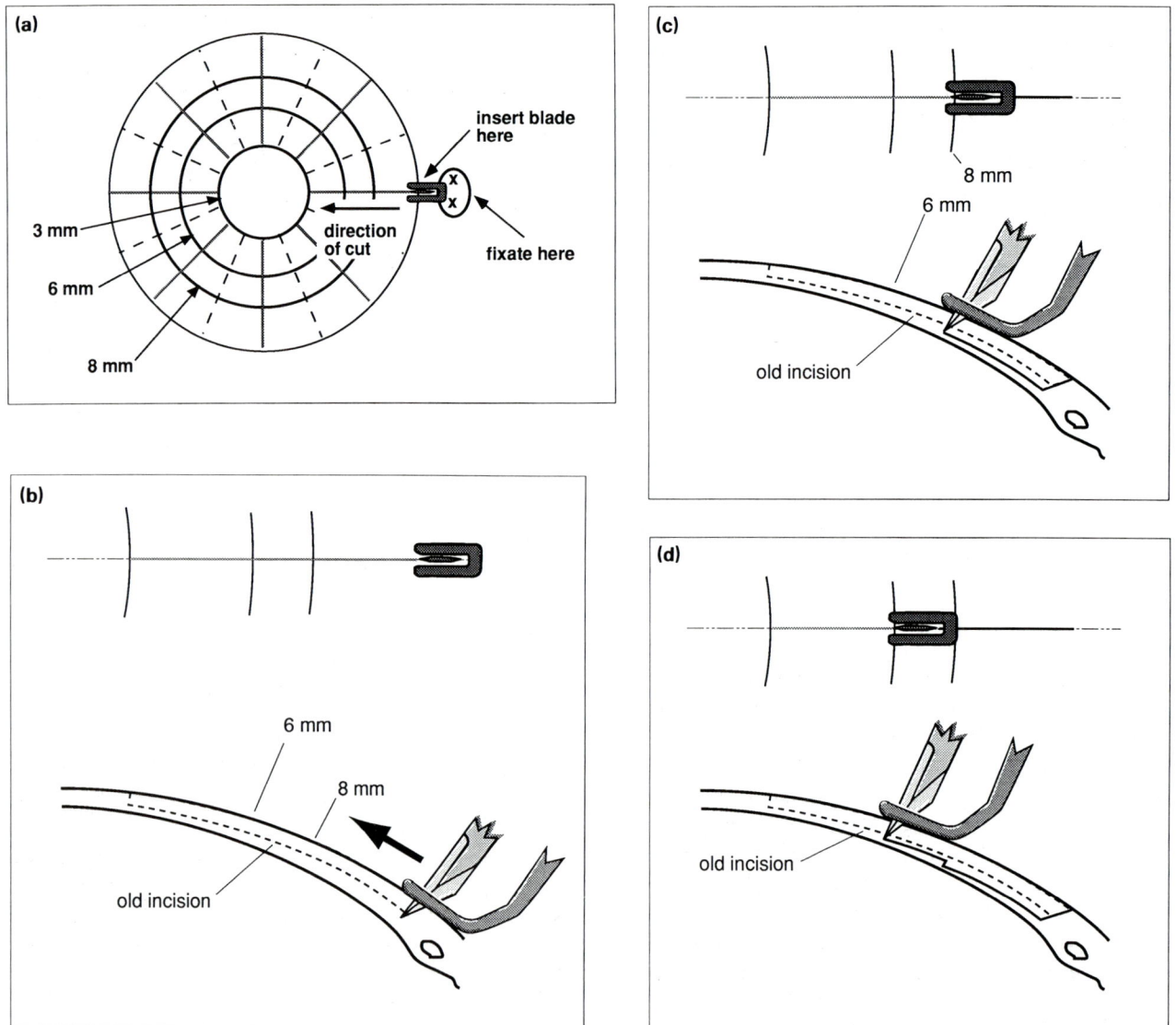

Fig. 8.90 Re-cutting over old incisions. (a) Straddle the old incision at the limbus. Re-cut alternate incisions. (b) Cut toward the tertiary optical zone. Re-set the blade and (c and d) continue the incision.

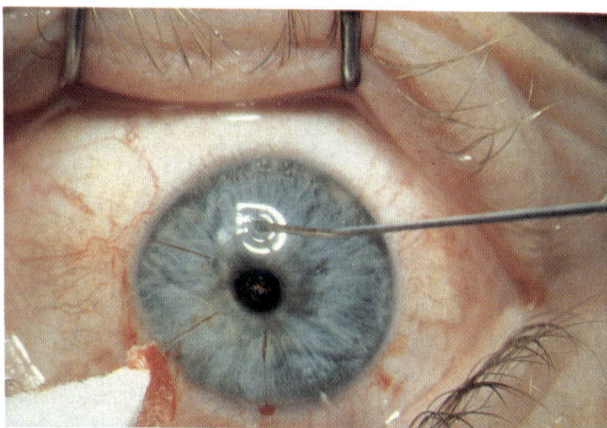

Fig. 8.91 Gently irrigate with balanced salt solution all but the incisions which have a micro-perforation.

In all cases, antibiotic drops are instilled into the cul-de-sac followed by a cycloplegic/mydriatic such as 1% cyclopentolate or 5% homatropine. If a perforation has occurred near the limbus and blood has entered the AC or if you have any doubts, a sub-conjunctival injection of 20 mg Garamycin is warranted. Usually a light patch is all that is necessary but in cases of a perforation or flat chamber, a pressure dressing may be warranted as well (Figure 8.92). In these cases, 1% atropine drops are advised instead of the milder cycloplegics. The patient, in that case, is told to leave the dressing in place until morning rather than removing it in 2 hours as is usual. If there has been a perforation or if one is suspected, begin the patient on a regimen of Keflex (cephalosporin, or some other broad-spectrum antibiotic) 500 mg b.i.d. for at least 5

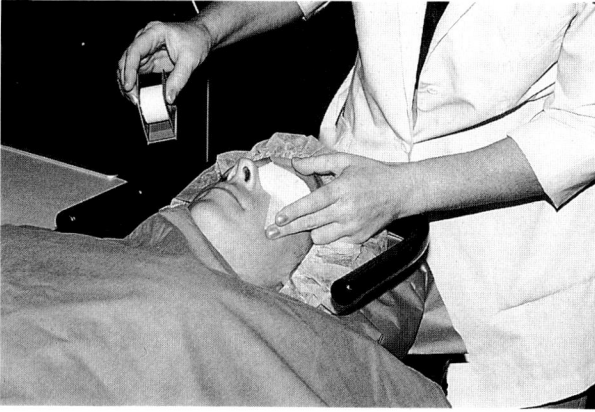

Fig. 8.92 Patch the eye for no more than 2 hours (see text).

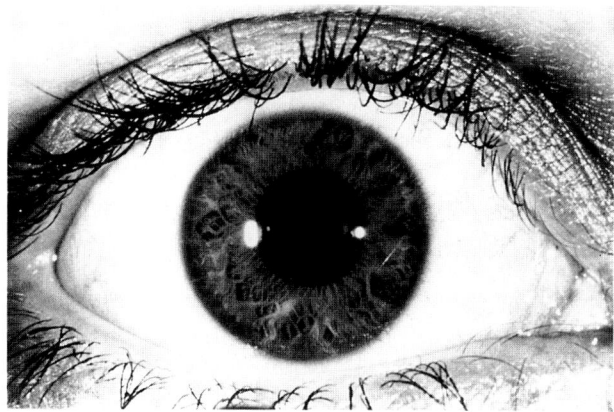

Fig. 8.93 A beautiful post-operative radial keratotomy eye.

days. Persons allergic to penicillin can be prescribed tetracycline or other antibiotic of choice.

Light analgesia, such as aspirin/codeine, should be enough to help the patients with any post-operative discomfort they may have. It has been my experience that at least 50% of those who complain of post-operative pain find that it subsides when the patch is removed. Cases with flat chambers or very soft eyes, on the other hand, will be found to be more comfortable with the patch. In these cases it may be well to send them to bed with some extra diazepam (Valium). Generally speaking, all cases will benefit from 3–4 hours of sleep immediately following the surgery.

All patients should be examined the next day (Figure 8.93). Putting a drop of proparacaine (Ophthaine, Alcaine, etc.) in the operated eye will facilitate this examination. The visual acuity can be taken at this visit but the result is not meaningful, except that I tend to be somewhat disappointed if they see better than 20/25. This usually, but not always, is an indication that a full correction has not been obtained. The rule of thumb is: morning vision blurry—good news; morning vision good—bad news. The refraction on the day following is usually spurious, ranging from highly myopic to highly hyperopic. The K-readings are a jumble as well. The patient should be encouraged, advised and begun on an antibiotic–steroid combination (the author's preference is tobramycin-dexamethasone—Tobradex) eye drop to be used b.i.d. for 2 weeks. This combination (or similar) has been used by myself in all cases (Maxitrol was used in the first cases) of radial keratotomy in my hands. I have found that the addition of the steroid not only promotes patient comfort but also enhances the effect, even in steroid non-responders. The only time that I have stopped this drop before time has been in those evidencing an allergic response and in one or two cases showing extreme over-correction at 1 week. In no case

is usage beyond 14 days warranted or desired. These is some circumstantial evidence that use at 6–8 weeks might cause a loss of effect.

In this vein, a word of caution. Some "experts," taking note that the effect of the surgery is enhanced with an increase in intra-ocular pressure, have advocated and used high-steroid drop dosages for upwards of a year in cases of under-correction. In so doing they have induced glaucoma and in some cases, cataract, to increase the effect of their inadequate surgical technique. I find no medical, moral or ethical reason to subject a patient to such increased risk of harm to gain a diopter or so of additional myopic correction. I have treated some of these unfortunates, first discontinuing the offending medication. Fortunately, in all but one case, the increased effect disappeared over time while in the remaining case the patient's best vision continues at a line less than preoperation, probably due to the residual cataract, despite the almost full myopic correction.

As I have said before, there are limitations to the correction that can be obtained by making relaxing incisions in the cornea. Some eyes respond in much lesser degree regardless of our skill and efforts—so be it. The difference between a good surgeon and a mediocre one is that the good surgeon not only knows when not to cut but also when to accept reality and quit. The practice of refractive surgery is not an Olympic struggle wherein points are awarded for the greatest amount of diopters corrected. It is, rather, a humanistic science wherein the welfare of the patient is still paramount and the patient's ultimate well-being guides our behavior.

The second eye can usually undergo surgery at 1 week. That time should be sufficient to ascertain where the patient's cornea is going to be at 1 year. At first, it may be better to let 30 days elapse until you are more comfortable with this surgery—that is for you to decide; many of us did just that. Except in experienced hands, it is not a good idea to do the surgery before 7 days. Likewise, I find no justification for performing the surgery on both eyes on the same day. Not only is the risk of infection not justified, but even in the best of hands mistakes in judgment and execution can occur. Furthermore, the patient can well tolerate the delay between eyes and the temporary anisometropia which results. In the event that the patient experiences intolerable glare he or she can still function with one eye until it subsides. Additionally, how could you explain bilateral over-corrections when it could have been avoided by delaying surgery on the fellow eye?

Further follow-up visits should be scheduled at 1, 6, and 12 months with complete evaluations—vision, Ks, topography, glare testing, refraction and symptoms—recorded. Spectacles, if needed, can usually be prescribed at 1 month but contacts, particularly soft, should wait 8 weeks or more.

Results

A surgical procedure is difficult to study in the classical sense—it is always on the move, like a positron. The uncertainty principle enters into this type of examination. If we stop the evolution of the surgery to examine it in a so-called controlled study, we end up by becoming paleo-ophthalmologists studying "ancient" eye surgery. If we try to study it on the fly we cannot apply the scientific method because each case is slightly different. Therefore, we can only get a feel of the efficacy of the surgery—some uncertainty remains. If a segment of the investigators insist on an attempt to study the surgery by adopting strict guidelines, while the remainder continue to alter and improve the technique, then the first investigative group are faced with a dilemma: can they morally deny the latest treatment to their patients on the grounds that the study must be kept pure? The second group have an equally important dilemma: are they exposing their patients to needless risk?

There is no absolute answer which is fitting because there are no absolutes in biologic processes—there are only approximations. The science of bio-statistics is really a stochastic art form full of assumptions and definite maybes. As the amount of data increases, an idea of the behavior of a biologic system can be obtained and from this idea certain guidelines can be constructed to assist individuals working with that system.

Therefore, I cannot give you any "truths." What I can do is present you with some data that have been gathered in what I believe to be an accurate and trustworthy way and let you decide for yourselves. In this manner I hope not to convince you that I am right because I have long since stopped worrying about my

Table 8.4 Myopia range in the first three RK groups

Pre-operative myopia (D)	Group 1	Group 2	Group 3
2.00–4.00	58	136	68
4.25–6.00	18	91	47
6.25–10.00	21	76	35
	97	303	150

Table 8.5 Resultant visual acuity (VA) in cases of low (−2 to −4 D) myopia in three groups (262 patients)

Uncorrected post-operative VA	Group 1	Group 2	Group 3
20/20–20/25	41 (70)	118 (87)	83 (93)
20/30–20/40	14 (25)	14 (10)	2 (3)
20/50–20/70	3 (3)	4 (3)	3 (4)
<20/70	1 (1)	—	—
Mean uncorrected VA	0.80	0.88	0.90

Percentages in parentheses throughout tables 8.5–8.22.

Table 8.6 Resultant visual acuity (VA) in cases of moderate (−4 to −6 D) myopia in three groups (156 patients)

Uncorrected post-operative VA	Group 1	Group 2	Group 3
20/20–20/25	7 (40)	58 (64)	33 (71)
20/30–20/40	2 (11)	15 (16)	7 (14)
20/50–20/70	4 (22)	2 (2)	5 (11)
<20/70	5 (27)	16 (18)	2 (4)
Mean uncorrected VA	0.40	0.50	0.55

data convincing anyone. Data are never convincing—only experience, or in its absence, prejudice, will result in a judgment being made. But I do hope to give you pause; to open your eyes just a little wider; to open your mind wider still; and to make your experience a little broader.

Results of surgery using "current" methodologies versus "older" techniques have been summarized in Tables 8.4–8.7. Instead of subjecting the reader to all the whys and wherefores (the reader is referred to the current literature for that) [2] I will just touch upon some salient points and utilize the rest of the space to discuss some areas of difference and conjecture on the future.

Group 1 consists of eyes which were among the first to have had the surgery performed outside of the Soviet Union. These and the patients in Group 2 had their surgeries done in the same way and with the same blades, except that those in Group 2 had the blades set using the Bores method of over-setting and some had peripheral incision-deepening. All patients in these groups had 16 incisions. The patients in Group 3 had surgery using Sputnik razor blades set at

Table 8.7 Resultant visual acuity (VA) in cases of high (−6 to −10 D) myopia in three groups (132 patients)

Uncorrected post-operative VA	Group 1	Group 2	Group 3
20/20–20/25	2 (10)	14 (18)	8 (25)
20/30–20/40	4 (18)	15 (20)	12 (33)
20/50–20/70	3 (13)	30 (39)	11 (32)
<20/70	12 (57)	17 (22)	4 (11)
Mean uncorrected VA	0.29	0.40	0.50

Table 8.8 Summary of surgical results and overall vision in all three early groups

	Group 1	Group 2	Group 3
Mean K change			
3 months	3.09 D	4.79 D	6.32 D
12 months	1.74 D	4.23 D	5.44 D
ΔK/ΔR	1.21 D	1.18 D	1.23 D
Residual refraction	3.12 D	1.18 D	0.88 D
Emmetropic eyes (± 0.50 D)	24 (25)	179 (59)	96 (64)
Hyperopic eyes	3 (3)	0	1 (<1)
Myopic eyes	70 (72)	124 (41)	47 (31)
Uncorrected post-operative VA			
20/20–20/25	50 (40)	137 (45)	80 (53)
20/30–20/40	20 (21)	61 (20)	35 (23)
20/50–20/70	10 (10)	64 (21)	23 (15)
<20/70	17 (18)	41 (14)	12 (8)
Mean uncorrected VA	0.29	0.50	0.58

VA, Visual acuity.

Table 8.9 Post-operative sequelae

	Group 1	Group 2	Group 3
Subconjunctival hemorrhage	39 (41.2)	22 (7)	2 (3)
Upper lid edema	16 (16.4)	48 (15.8)	24 (16)
Epithelial defect	11 (11.3)	18 (5.9)	5 (3)
Stromal edema			
14 days	90 (92.8)	91 (30)	35 (23)
14–30 days	29 (28.9)	26 (8.8)	8 (5)
Over 30 days	0	0	0
Cells/flare			
Trace	5 (5.4)	15 (4.9)	7 (5)
Significant	0	0	0
Photophobia			
14 days	14 (14.4)	297 (98)	138 (92)
14–21 days	4 (4.2)	15 (5.2)	6 (4)
Keratitis (mild)	1 (1)	6 (1.9)	3 (2)
Fibrous proliferation	1 (1)	0	0
Night glare			
<3 months	87 (89.7)	273 (90.3)	136 (91)
>3 months	3 (4)	12 (4)	3 (2)
Visual fluctuation			
<3 months	90 (92.8)	271 (89.4)	141 (94)
>3 months	6 (1.9)	30 (10)	18 (12)
Induced astigmatism >6 months	3 (3.2)	2 (0.6)	2 (1)
Neo-vascularization	<4%	<6.3%	<3.1%
Endothelial cell count	14 (14.4)	297 (98)	138 (92)

Table 8.10 Patient age distribution in the second RK series

Age range (years)	n
18–23	215
24–40	969
41–65	259
66 and older	5

Table 8.11 Range of myopia in the second RK series

Range of myopia (D)	n
2–4	676
4–6	438
6–8	235
8–10	99
Total cases reviewed	1448

Table 8.12 Resultant visual acuity (VA) in cases of low (−2 to −4 D) myopia in the second series

Uncorrected post-operative VA	n
20/20–20/25	636 (94)
20/30–20/40	20 (3)
20/50–20/70	20 (3)
<20/70	
Mean uncorrected VA	0.90

Table 8.13 Resultant visual acuity (VA) in cases of moderate (−4 to −6 D) myopia in the second series

Uncorrected post-operative VA	n
20/20–20/25	324 (74)
20/30–20/40	70 (16)
20/50–20/70	26 (6)
<20/70	18 (4)
Mean uncorrected VA	0.62

Table 8.14 Resultant visual acuity (VA) in cases of high (−6 to −8 D) myopia in the second series

Uncorrected post-operative VA	n
20/20–20/25	63 (27)
20/30–20/40	82 (35)
20/50–20/70	78 (33)
<20/70	12 (5)
Mean uncorrected VA	0.58

Table 8.15 Resultant visual acuity (VA) in cases of very high (−8 to −10 D) myopia in the second series

Uncorrected post-operative VA	n
20/20–20/25	21 (21)
20/30–20/40	28 (28)
20/50–20/70	37 (37)
<20/70	13 (14)
Mean uncorrected VA	0.40

Table 8.16 Summary of surgical results in the second series

Parameter	Result
Regression of K	−17%
Mean ΔK	−6.21 D
Residual refraction	−0.75 D
Emmetropic eyes (±0.50 D)	1043 (72)
Hyperopic eyes	43 (3)
Myopic eyes	362 (25)

Table 8.17 Post-operative sequelae in the second series

	n
Epithelial defect	27 (1.9)
Stromal edema	
14 days	326 (22.5)
14–30 days	66 (4.6)
>30 days	1 (0.07)
Cells/flare	
Trace	7 (0.49)
Significant	1 (0.07)
Photophobia	
14 days	1303 (90)
14–21 days	43 (3)
Keratitis	3 (0.02)
Night glare	
<3 months	1303 (90)
>3 months	43 (3)
Visual fluctuation	
>3 months	1390 (90)
>3 months	540 (37.2)
Induced astigmatism	10 (0.69)
Neo-vascularization	6 (0.41)
Endothelial cell loss	(4.2)

Table 8.18 Patient age distribution in the third RK series

Age range (years)	n
18–23	111
24–40	396
41–65	120
66 and older	5
Total	632

Table 8.19 Resultant visual acuity (VA) in cases of low (−2 to −4 D) myopia in the third series

Uncorrected post-operative VA	n
20/20–20/25	232 (88)
20/30–20/40	16 (6)
20/50–20/70	16 (6)
<20/70	
Total cases	264

Table 8.20 Resultant visual acuity (VA) in cases of moderate (−4 to −6 D) myopia in the third series

Uncorrected post-operative VA	n
20/20–20/25	160 (79)
20/30–20/40	16 (8)
20/50–20/70	12 (6)
<20/70	10 (1)
Total cases	203

Table 8.21 Resultant visual acuity (VA) in cases of high (−6 to −8 D) myopia in the third series

Uncorrected post-operative VA	n
20/20–20/25	49 (33)
20/30–20/40	51 (34)
20/50–20/70	42 (28)
<20/70	8 (5)
Total cases	150

Table 8.22 Resultant visual acuity (VA) in cases of very high (−8 to −10 D) myopia in the third series

Uncorrected post-operative VA	n
20/20–20/25	4 (25)
20/30–20/40	4 (25)
20/50–20/70	5 (36)
<20/70	1 (14)
Total cases	15

maximum using ultrasonic pachymetry and the "dry" technique. Approximately 20% of the patients in this group had eight incisions only. Patients that had re-operations are not included in this series. All patients with myopia greater than 8 D had stepped incisions. Your attention is called to Table 8.8 which shows the resultant visual acuities in these groups. Group 3 is remarkably similar to the long-term Russian results, and those of Nirankari and co-workers [17].

Table 8.23 Post-operative sequelae in the third series

	n
Epithelial defects	13
Stromal edema	
14 days	142
14–30 days	17
Over 30 days	0
Cells/flare	
Trace	4
Significant	0
Photophobia	
14 days	554
14–21 days	3
Keratitis	1
Night glare	
<3 months	620
>3 months	332
Visual fluctuation	628
Neo-vascularization	0

Endothelial cell counts show very little change. Cell "losses" are well within the error of counting (Table 8.9). Areas near micro-perforations are remarkably free of either cell loss or cellular distortion. We have not seen the cellular changes in humans that were reported by Yamaguchi *et al.* in animals [18].

Tables 8.10 through 8.17 show the results in a later and larger series of patients undergoing radial keratotomy. In all cases blades were Sputnik razor fragments over-set approximately 15%, based on ultrasonic pachymetry.

The last series shown are all cases performed using XTAL sapphire blades over-set up to 15% using a shadowgraph and ultrasonic pachymetry (Tables 8.18 through 8.23).

Complications of a serious or threatening nature have been rare with this surgery to date. Most can be traced to "pilot error" and/or inexperience and are not inherent in the procedure itself (see also Chapter 16). Considering that an estimated 600 000+ cases have been performed here and abroad (at this writing), the incidence of serious trouble is very low indeed.

The future of radial keratotomy

The future for radial keratotomy surgery looks very bright to me. We have advanced light years in the short time since this surgery was first introduced. Work is going forward with sophisticated instrumentation that will provide us with simultaneous surface corneal maps and thickness measurements (see Chapter 6). This will enable us, for the first time,

to obtain the inside corneal curvature. There are prototypes for knives that automatically adjust themselves to the corneal thickness, which is being monitored continuously by ultrasound. Newer materials are being studied for knife blades that have extreme edge sharpness; this will change not only this surgery but others as well.

References

1 Fyodorov SN, Durnev VV. Operation of dosaged dissection of corneal circular ligament in cases of myopia of mild degree. Ann Ophthalmol 1979; 11:1885–1890.

2 Bores LD, Myers W, Cowden J. Radial keratotomy: an analysis of the American experience. Ann Ophthalmol 1981; 13:941–948.

3 Cowden JW, Bores LD. A clinical investigation of the surgical correction of myopia by the method of Fyodorov. Ophthalmology 1981; 88:737–741.

4 Bores L. Radial keratotomy. I. A safe, effective way to correct a handicap. Surv Ophthalmol 1983; 28:101–105.

5 Bores L. Historical review and clinical results of radial keratotomy. Int Ophthalmol Clin 1983; 23:93–118.

6 Deitz M, Sanders D, Marks R. Radial keratotomy: an overview of the Kansas City study. Ophthalmol 1984; 91:467–478.

7 Linberg JV, McDonald MB, Safir A, Googe JM. Ptosis following radial keratotomy. Ophthalmology 1986; 93:1509–1512.

8 Lynn M, Arentson J, Asbell P. Factors affecting outcome and predictability of radial keratotomy in the PERK study. Arch Ophthalmol 1987;105:42–51.

9 Fyodorov SN, Agronovsky A. Long term results of anterior radial keratotomy. J Ocul Ther Surg 1982; 1:217.

10 Durnev V, Ermoshin A. Determination of dependence between the length of anterior radial non-perforating incisions of the cornea and their effectiveness. IV All Union Conference of Inventors and Rationalizers in the Field of Ophthalmology, Moscow, 1976.

11 Hernandez-Meijide R, Croxatto JO. Experimental radial keratotomy. J Refract Surg 1988; 3:224–226.

12 Deitz M, Sanders D. Progressive hyperopia with long-term follow-up of radial keratotomy. Arch Ophthalmol 1985; 103:782–784.

13 Durnev V. Characteristic of the results of myopic surgical correction after performing 16 and 32 primary anterior radial non-perforating incisions. In: *Surgery of Refractive Anomalies of the Eye*, A Ivashina and S Kolmanovskii (eds). Moscow Scientific Research Institute for Eye Microsurgery, Moscow, 1981.

14 Sanders D, Marks R. Prospective clinical study of radial keratotomy. Ophthalmology 1982; 89:1292–1293.

15 Hoffer KJ, Darin JJ, Pettit TH, Hofbauer JD, Elander R, Levenson JE. UCLA clinical trial of radial keratotomy. Preliminary report. Ophthalmology 1981; 88:729–736.

16 Smith RS, Cutro J. Computer analysis of radial keratotomy. CLAO J 1984; 10:241–248.

17 Nirankari VS, Katzen LE, Richards RD, Karesh JW, Lakhanpal V, Billings E. Prospective clinical study of radial keratotomy. Ophthalmology 1982; 89:677–683.

18 Yamaguchi T, Asbell P, Ostrick M, Safir A, Kissling G, Kaufman H. Endothelial damage in monkeys after radial keratotomy performed with a diamond blade. Arch Ophthalmol 1984; 102:765–769.

9
Surgical Management of Astigmatism

The scientific reasons for preferring one testimonial to another are, no doubt, sometimes very strong. They are not, however, strong enough to prevail upon our passions, our prejudices or our interests, or to overcome that lightness which is common to all grave men. So that we always present facts in a manner that is either prejudiced or frivolous.
[Anatole France, *Penguin Island*]

The correction of astigmatism has been the subject of much interest down through the years. Thomas Young was probably the first to describe the defect itself (in his own eyes) in 1801 while the first astigmatic spectacles were made to order for the astronomer George Airy in 1825—about the same time an enterprising and observant clergyman named Goodrich had some made for himself in New York (see Chapter 2). Prior to these attempts, astigmatism was compensated for by fitting spherical spectacles alone—a compromise at best [1]. The idea of performing surgery to correct this disorder came late.

We will examine the historical record primarily to glean whatever pearls we may from the information collected and secondarily to admire from afar the audacity of some of our early colleagues. In this chapter we will have occasion to mark, from time to time, the lessons to be learned from this early work. For all of the techniques we currently use are really not new at all but stem from our predecessors' careful observations of specific corneal reactions to injury.

In this chapter the author has used the term congenital to describe astigmatism unassociated with disease and/or trauma—iatrogenic or no. The author is not especially enamored of the term and has no objection if readers choose to discard it for their own pet expression but it seems to fit the situation reasonably well.

The first surgical attempts (paleo-ophthalmology)

Most discussions on this topic start out with reference to Snellen, Lans, and Bates, giving the reader the pardonable impression that these three gentlemen were in the forefront of the surgical correction of astigmatism. And so they were, but they were not the first to attempt such surgery. Donders described astigmatism following cataract extraction in 1864, thus it seems natural to ascribe the astigmatism to the corneal incision [1]. The wonder is that no one thought about trying to surgically correct astigmatism of any stripe before 1869.

Snellen's "suggestions"

The author is unable to substantiate that the Dutch ophthalmologist, Herman Snellen of Utrecht, ever performed surgery for astigmatism—although he defined both with-the-rule (W-T-R) and against-the-rule (A-T-R) astigmatism in 1869 [2] (see also Chapter 2). He did, however, suggest that a corneal section running perpendicular to the steepest meridian would induce an opposite astigmatism which would then neutralize the first, though he made no mention of the effect such an incision might have on the opposite

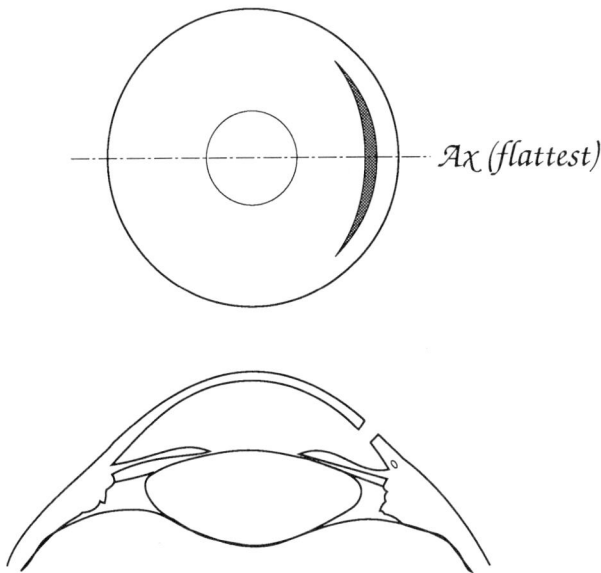

Fig. 9.1 The crescentic corneal resection of von Galezowski.

meridian—a process called coupling [2]. Thus Snellen has the distinction of describing the principle of what we now call T-cuts, besides being the inventor of the Snellen optotypes [3,4].

Xavier Galezowski and "half-moon" corneal wedge resections

Around the time Fukala performed his first clear lens extraction for myopia in 1890, Galezowski attempted to flatten the cornea by resecting half-moon-shaped wedges out of the stroma—unsuccessfully, according to Fukala [5] (Figure 9.1). Since this was segmental surgery (with no sutures), the supposition is that this was an attempt at flattening myopic astigmatism through relaxation. If so, then Galezowski performed the first wedge resection for astigmatism; if not, it still pre-dates any other recorded attempts at the surgical correction of myopia.

Schiøtz and limbal transverse perforating incisions

The next case report pre-dated that of Lans by some 13 years. In 1885, Hjalmar August Schiøtz, a Norwegian ophthalmologist, reported the case of a 33-year-old man with 19.5 D of post-operative aphakic astigmatism. Four months after the original surgery, Schiøtz made a 3.5 mm, limbal, penetrating, Graefe knife section in the steepest corneal meridian, which gradually reduced the astigmatism to 7 D 1 month later [6]. Schiøtz is, of course, better known for other contributions. The wonder is that he did not pursue this idea. Perhaps it was a response to a single need.

Whatever the reason, Schiøtz has the distinction of being the first to carry out the previous ideas of Snellen but went no further with it.

Bates and his transverse non-perforating incisions

William Horatio Bates was a physician who practiced at the New York Eye Infirmary in the late 19th century, specializing in diseases of the head. For five years, 1886–1891, he taught ophthalmology at the New York Post-graduate Medical School and Hospital, leaving after a "personality conflict" with the director, Roosa [7]. Actually the dispute centered around Bates' claim that myopia could be surgically cured and Roosa's insistence that it could not. Roosa resolved the debate by banishing Bates.

In 1894 Bates published a suggestion for a surgical procedure to correct astigmatism [8]. In this paper he evaluates, succinctly, five cases of iatrogenic and one case of traumatic astigmatism. He goes on to set down some basic principles or propositions of astigmatic surgery, which this author has dubbed Bates' axioms:

1 A corneal incision lengthens the radius of curvature of that meridian which is at right angles to the line of the incision, and does not flatten any other meridian. The astigmatism produced is a regular astigmatism, and is corrected by a convex cylinder at an axis parallel to the line of the incision.

2 The immediate result is greater than the ultimate result.

3 The astigmatism produced is permanent after a length of time—at least a month after the cornea has healed.

4 The amount of astigmatism produced is greater near the center of the cornea.

5 The amount of correction can be regulated by the number, depth, and length of the incisions [8].

In this Bates obviously recognized the ability of relaxing incisions to produce flattening of steep curvatures—independently and before Lans. It is not likely that Bates had access to the work of Schiøtz (although it is possible).

He then describes two cases in which such incisions were made. In the first case, a 14-year-old girl with simple astigmatism of 2.5 D and the steep axis at 75°, he marked the 165° axis with adhesive tape and made a Graefe knife incision parallel to the tape. He notes that no aqueous escaped, hence the incision was partial-thickness. Within 5 days the vision had improved but was not wholly satisfactory because he repeated the surgery, this time making the non-perforating incision more central on the cornea. He repeated the surgery thrice more—once 20 days after the second incision; once 6 weeks later; and the last time 2½ weeks after that. He does not stipulate whether these incisions were re-cuts or in addition to those previously made.

He apparently ceased when he did because no further change by ophthalmometry was noted and the patient saw well enough. Eighteen months after the initial surgery the vision was said still to be improved and scars were not discernible to cursory examination.

The next case was that of a 23-year-old physician with a refraction of $-1.25 - 0.75 \times 100°$ in both eyes. The astigmatism could not be measured with the ophthalmometer. Thus Bates operated for system or total astigmatism, not for corneal astigmatism—a concept still valid today. Bates made a shallow, transverse incision at 100° on the tempo al side of the cornea in the right eye. One day later, the procedure was repeated on the left eye. Six months after that, the patient retained good, unaided visual acuity with minimal scarring. Thus Bates was the first to describe and use non-perforating T-cuts—as we know them today—as well as perform repeat surgery for undercorrections.

Faber and idiopathic astigmatism

In 1895, another Dutch ophthalmologist named Faber used an anterior, penetrating, transverse, semi-arcuate limbal incision, 6 mm in length (and perpendicular to the plus cylinder axis), in a 19-year-old to treat his congenital astigmatism. Faber succeeded in reducing the patient's astigmatism from 1.5 D to 0.75 D and improving his uncorrected vision sufficiently—from 20/60 to 20/25—to permit the patient to attend the military academy from which he had been rejected [9]. Today (at least for now) such surgery would result in quite a different outcome—in the USA refractive surgery makes one ineligible for military service. Faber concluded that such techniques work but that the predictability would be uncertain. An interesting note is that Faber declared this procedure to be new and that he'd never heard of anyone performing such an operation before this.

Lucciola and L-incisions

The first European surgeon to utilize non-perforating incisions was Lucciola of Turin, Italy [10]. He reported 10 cases of non-perforating corneal incisions made *parallel* to the steeper meridian in order to correct astigmatism. He detailed the influence of the type and location of the incisions as well, thus establishing himself as the first to use L-cuts.

Thus, by 1896 two concepts have been established: the first is that incisions *perpendicular* to the steep meridian flatten that meridian and second is that the same thing can be accomplished with incisions *parallel* to the steep meridian. Additionally, these incisions need not be full-thickness.

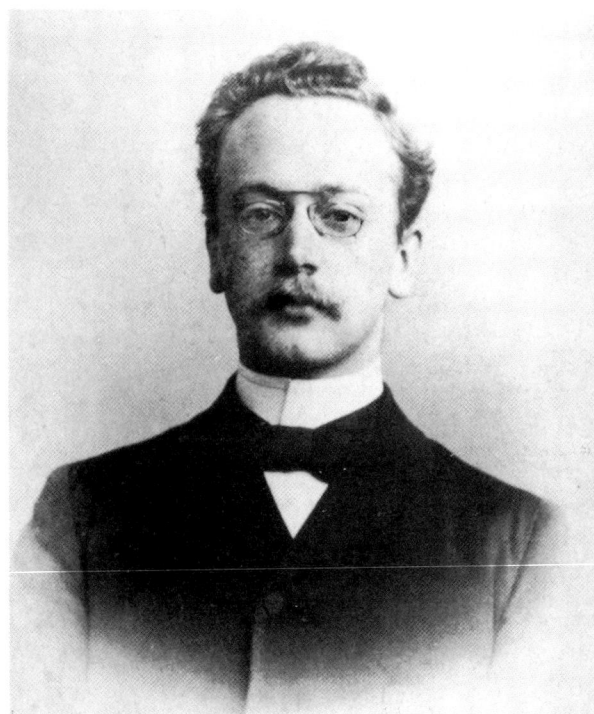

Fig. 9.2 Leendert Jan Lans, the first ophthalmologist to perform systematic studies of refractive surgery in 1896.

Lans and the coupling effect

Although not the first to perform surgery for astigmatism, still another Dutch ophthalmologist, Leendert Jan Lans, was the first to perform systematic studies of refractive surgery at the University of Utrecht in 1896 (Figure 9.2). In 1888 he enrolled as a student at the University of Leiden. He received his doctor's degree cum laude from the university in 1897 by defending a thesis entitled *Experimentelle Untersuchungen uber die Entstehung von Astigmatismus durch nicht perforirende Corneawunden* (Experimental Studies of the Treatment of Astigmatism with non-perforating Corneal Wounds). This work was done at the Snellen's clinic in Utrecht where he had made a training arrangement, though his thesis advisor was Willem Koster, eye department chairman at Leiden. Utilizing carefully planned experimentation in rabbits, he evaluated patterns of keratotomy, keratectomy, and thermokeratoplasty, thereby establishing (along with Bates) the basic principles which would serve as the root of modern astigmatic surgery. He also showed that flattening in the meridian perpendicular to a transverse incision would be associated with steepening in the opposite meridian—the first description of coupling (see the section on Sato, below). He, independently of Bates, found that deeper and longer incisions would have a greater effect. In his paper he also admitted that he got the idea from Snellen and cited the work of Pfluger and Doganof using parallel incisions *à la* Lucciola [11]. However, he was unable to obtain satisfactory results with incisions so he turned instead to cautery. He utilized a fine tip to make two cauterized bands 2 mm by 4–8 mm across the selected meridian on rabbit cornea. After 4 months' follow-up he concluded that such application could produce refractive changes up to 6 D but that these changes were highly labile and reversible within the first 4–8 weeks post-application. Beyond these few experiments and this paper there is nothing further on the matter. He eventually settled in Arnhem where he never again returned to the subject of refractive surgery.

Loose gears sink careers

Why is it that this idea of Bates (and later that of Lans) was apparently ignored? Lans was certainly respected. After receiving his doctorate he completed his training with Snellen; no black cloud followed him around. Bates himself appears to have been an above-average physician as well as a competent surgeon. In 1886 he published a reasonable paper on the treatment of deafness [12]. Later, he conducted a study in which he demonstrated the value of sutures to close the cataract wound—an important innovation for that time [13]. Bates was a peculiar fellow, nevertheless, and was probably his own worst enemy. By 1891 he had begun his unyielding infatuation with his own ideas, and he wasn't quiet about it. He thus joined that select group of brilliant, and meritorious scientists and physicians who have sometimes forsaken the orthodox and familiar scientific method for more esoteric, unorthodox, and often bizarre thinking. In short they take counsel of their own beliefs to the exclusion of other views. In that, however, they follow in the footsteps of the great Claudius Galenus and are thereby in good, if misguided, company. Bates may have eventually become in the vernacular, "looney tunes," but that looniness was singular, involving mostly the topic of myopia. He did good work in other areas and published creditable papers on other topics, hence he does not deserve to be shunted into the back alley of ophthalmology—his astigmatism axioms are still valid today.

But surgery for astigmatism was not just ignored in the USA; it seems it was ignored everywhere else as well. With the exception of a few isolated instances, it took 42 more years—more than a generation—before reports of similar cases made their appearance in the medical literature.

Wray's reprisal of Lans' technique

In 1914, Wray used cautery *à la* Lans to correct a case of 6 D of hyperopic astigmatism [14]. The patient was a 19-year-old whose refraction was plano +6.00 × 180°

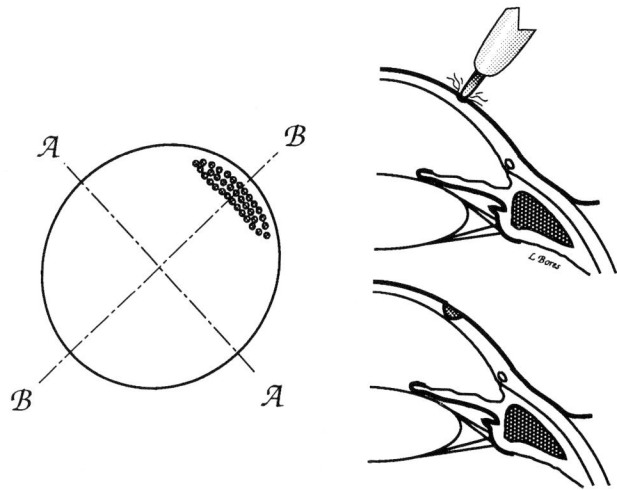

Fig. 9.3 Wray's cautery for hyperopic astigmatism.

OU. A linear-type cautery was performed twice in the right eye on the hyperopic meridian inferior to the corneal apex. This was not successful, succeeding only in causing the astigmatism to rotate 30°. Somewhat better results were obtained in the left eye with four applications of what Wray called superficial burns (probably non-linear) and sufficiently peripheral so as "not to interfere with reading" (Figure 9.3). The refraction improved to +0.50 + 1.00 × 180° at 1 year with vision of 6/6. Wray blamed the poor result on the right to involvement of Bowman's but it's more likely that the result was due to the scars being too superficial.

Meier and the case of the peeled cornea

In 1917, Weiner reported a method of corneal peeling for keratoconus which he attributed to Meier. It consisted of resecting a two-thirds-thickness elliptical strip approximately 4 × 12 mm from the cornea [15]. Burr took this idea somewhat further by removing a full-thickness section of cornea [16]. Weiner later modified this to making a 6–7 mm incision about 1 mm from the limbus. A section of cornea, 1.5 mm wide at center and tapering toward each end, was removed. The wound was then sutured closed [17].

O'Connor, Bock, and corneal cautery

O'Connor was not as sanguine as *Herr Doktor* Lans in the use of cautery for cases of high astigmatism—only half his patients showed any improvement and those were unstable. Cases of keratoconus fared somewhat better [18,19]. One year later (1939), Bock published his work with high-frequency cautery on the rabbit cornea (see also Chapter 14). Within a few weeks, however, the corneas had regained their pre-operative curvatures [20].

(a)

(b)

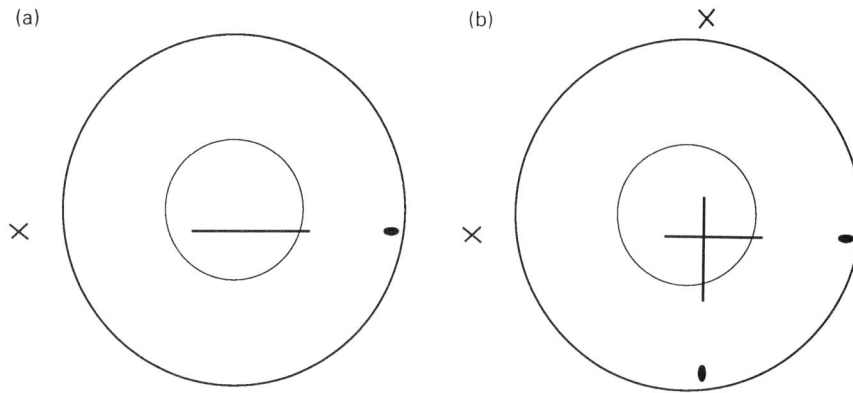

Fig. 9.4 Sato's operations for keratoconus—original pattern.

Sato and his posterior half-incisions for astigmatism

Tutomu Sato began his work with keratoconus using posterior incisions (see Chapter 7 for more details). While studying the subject of keratoconus under the guidance of Ishihara in 1936, Sato noted a marked improvement in the vision of a 20-year-old woman following spontaneous rupture of Descemet's membrane. He felt that he could do better with a knife and proceeded to demonstrate it. He reported his first 10 cases in 1939 in the Japanese literature [21]. His technique consisted in making one, sometimes two or three horizontal incisions across the corneal paracenter from the posterior side using a modification of de Lapersonne's knife—now called Sato's knife—introduced through the lateral limbus (Figure 9.4). While making internal incisions was original, he was probably aware of Lans' work. At that time, much of the Japanese case-work was being published in the German literature—Japanese surgeons studied in Germany as well. Fukala's first case reports give an address for him in Pilsen-Karlsbad. Hence, Sato was probably also aware of Kokott's 1938 work on elucidating the anatomic structure of the cornea [22]. This last point is important as it may have influenced Sato's decision to use posterior incisions in the first place.

Sato's operation for keratoconus was straightforward, effective, and, considering the alternative, appropriate. It became widely used in Japan (A. Momose, 1990, personal communication). Gilbert introduced it in France under the name *débridement de la Descemet's* [23]. Linder [24] and Hruby [25] also reported good results. Gilbert used a Graefe knife to make the incisions while Linder modified Sato's knife and also sharpened the tip of Bowman's canaliculotome, which he claimed was a safer instrument. Nevertheless, it was a technically difficult operation to perform. It required great skill on the part of the surgeon, necessitating incisions being made *ab interno*, through half the corneal thickness and in a straight line, close to the optic center. However, between

1939 and 1943, he performed 200 such operations successfully [26,27].

The specially designed knife was then inserted into the anterior chamber at the limbus through a 2 mm scleral tunnel [28]. These internal incisions were almost always followed by external incisions made between the internals with a guarded blade.

Sato devised a cross-wise technique for very advanced keratoconus which he reported in 1942 [29]. This technique was later modified and applied to the correction of congenital astigmatism using a standard incision length of 4.00 mm. Sato reported that in the rabbit eye, anterior incisions produced minimal central corneal flattening whereas posterior incisions produced maximum flattening. Hence he was encouraged to use posterior incisions preferentially [30]. In this same paper he first described radial incisions made from the posterior side—a modification or extension of Lans' original idea (see above)—thus this was not the début of radial incisions, as has been proposed.

Of his early 19 cases of surgery for congenital astigmatism in the human eye, Sato achieved 0.5–0.75 D of flattening in three eyes; 1.0 D in seven eyes; 3.0 D in one eye; 4.0 D in four eyes; 6.0 D in one eye; and no correction in three eyes [27]. Respectable numbers to be sure, but if he counted total change (including coupling) those numbers are not quite so impressive and are, in fact, troubling (see below). The phenomenon of coupling cannot be ignored, as we shall see when we discuss tangential incisions further on, and can be disastrous (see the section on the technique of the Ruiz Procedure, below).

In 1950, he reported his technique in the American literature, describing at the time T- and V-incisions for astigmatism [31]. These T-cuts were exactly that—Ts (Figure 9.5). He declared the T- and V-shaped incisions to be unsatisfactory due to wide edge separation, thick scars and irregular astigmatism. This finding has been corroborated by later surgeons (see also the section on current methods for the control of astigmatism, below).

With a radial incision in the rabbit, Sato was able to

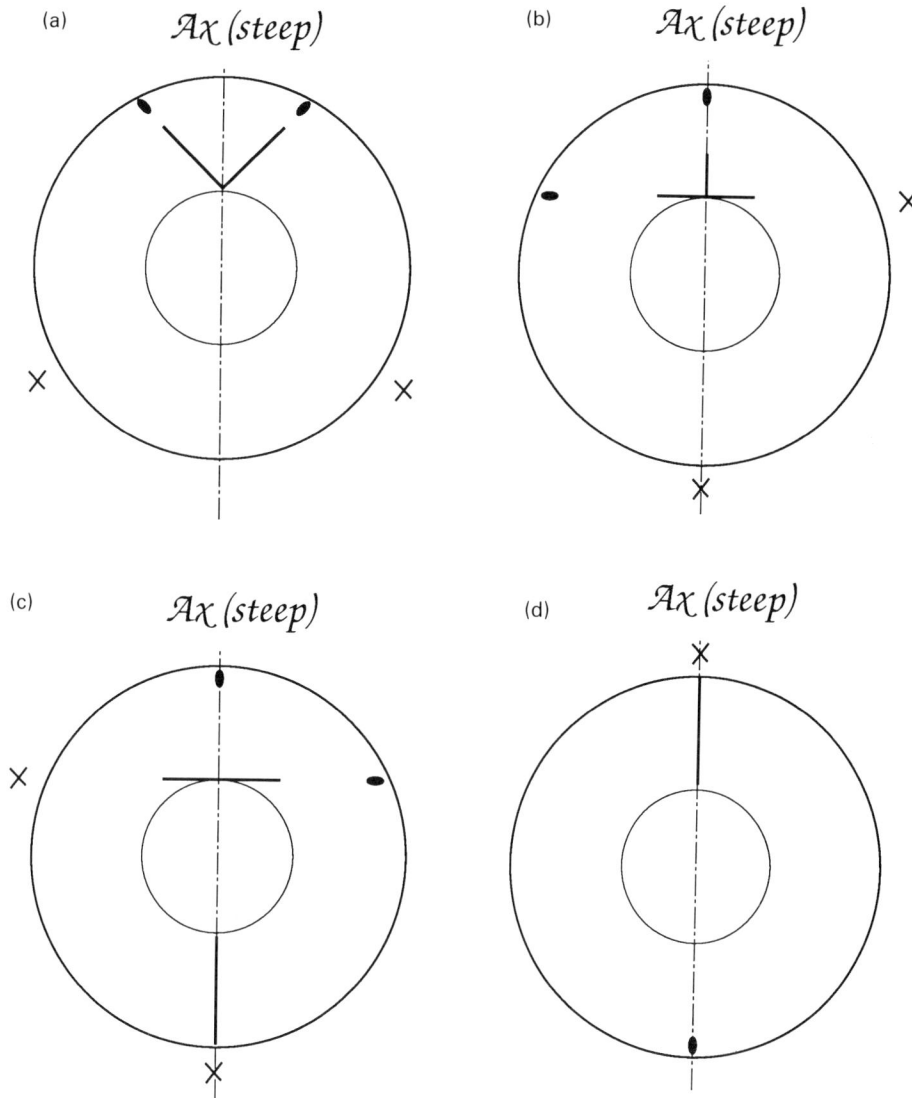

Fig. 9.5 Sato's operations for keratoconus—1950 pattern.

correct as much as 4 D of astigmatism but succeeded in only eliminating half that much in the human. With a transverse incision (T-cut), he demonstrated in the rabbit that while in one case, he obtained a flattening of 4 D in the meridian crossed by the T-cut, 3.5 D of steepening was induced in the opposite meridian— 7.5 D of corneal change had occurred in all. Thus the fact of incisional coupling was noted and described again. He found (as did Lans before him) that deeper incisions produced more flattening in the steep meridian and longer incisions more steepening in the flat meridian. He suggested that this phenomenon would be useful in compound astigmatism. The author believes that this was an error in translation and that he really meant *mixed* astigmatism, which makes more sense. He also made this telling statement: "There is no difference in the effect of surgical treatment between corneal and lenticular astigmatism" [27].

In another paper the same year, this time in the Japanese literature, he reported cases in which a lamellar dissection of the cornea was combined with a posterior incision tangential to the steep axis (Figure 9.6) [31].

His second paper in the American literature described the improved technique of tangential half-incisions (Figure 9.7). In these cases he dilated the pupils with atropine and made the incisions just inside the pupillary margin [32].

Sato was enthusiastic about his "new" technique and said as much [33]. However, he reckoned without the endothelial destruction his surgery had produced (see Chapter 7 for details). Considering the fact that the corneal reaction must have been intense (see the description of Fyodorov's early efforts in Chapter 7), to persist in this approach was brave, at the very least. Sato should be given much credit, however, for

(a)

Ax (steep)

(b) Ax (flatter)

Ax (steeper)

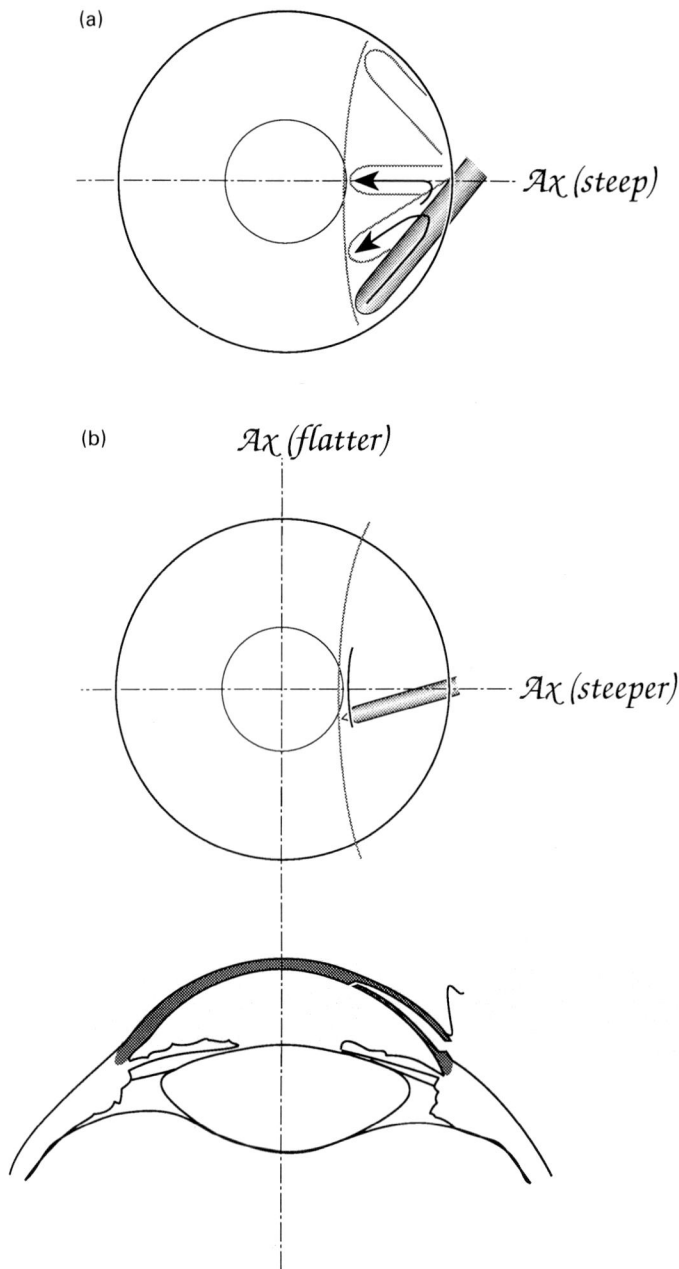

Fig. 9.6 Sato's lamellar dissection procedure.

many of his ideas were successful and his work did not escape notice, even if some of the notice was unfavorable.

The evolution of surgery for astigmatism

There were, of course, others who involved themselves in this subject, for better or for worse, using various techniques and modalities.

Troutman's wedge resection for post-keratoplasty astigmatism

Troutman pioneered the technique of corneal wedge resection post-keratoplasty in 1970, utilizing a razor blade knife to excise a crescent of tissue centered on the flattest meridian adjacent to the graft–host junction [34,35]. The technique is detailed below (see the section on wedge resections for hyperopic astigmatism—revisited).

Jensen introduced a double-bladed knife for more precise control of wedge resections and proposed a more quantifiable determination for the correction of large and small degrees of astigmatism [36].

Radial relaxing incisions

In 1973 Fyodorov and co-workers began utilizing external radial relaxing incisions to correct myopia. At the same time various arrangements of incisions were studied in an effort to correct astigmatism [37]. It was found that, as Sato had pointed out, transverse incisions whose separation and length varied were effective in reducing small amounts of myopic astigmatism. From this work a number of other configurations were suggested for this purpose as well. Many of these are in use today.

Basic principles and patient workup

Astigmatism surgery is still evolving in technique and further study is needed. None the less, many patients who cannot be rehabilitated with conventional optical measures benefit significantly from surgical treatment of their astigmatism. The author considers a surgical alternative for any amount of astigmatism which exceeds 20% of the associated spherical component or, in cases of simple myopic astigmatism, when the astigmatism exceeds 0.50 D. The lower degrees are only approached if they are oblique, A-T-R, and/or are symptomatic. An astigmatic refractive error in the range of 1.00–2.00 D might be expected to reduce uncorrected visual acuity to the 20/30–20/50 range and greater than 2.00–3.00 D should reduce uncorrected visual acuity to the 20/70–20/100 range [38]. However, the author has seen cases of mixed astigmatism reaching as high as 2.5 D whose unaided visual acuity has been 20/30. The refractive surgeon must be careful in these cases, particularly if this is the result of previous refractive surgery—beware not to violate Bores' First Rule. Less than careful selection of surgical parameters might well reduce the astigmatic component in, for example, a case whose refraction is $-2.50 + 2.50 \times 45$ such that the result is -2.50 D of spherical myopia. Thus you will have reduced the cylinder along with the unaided vision. Such a patient

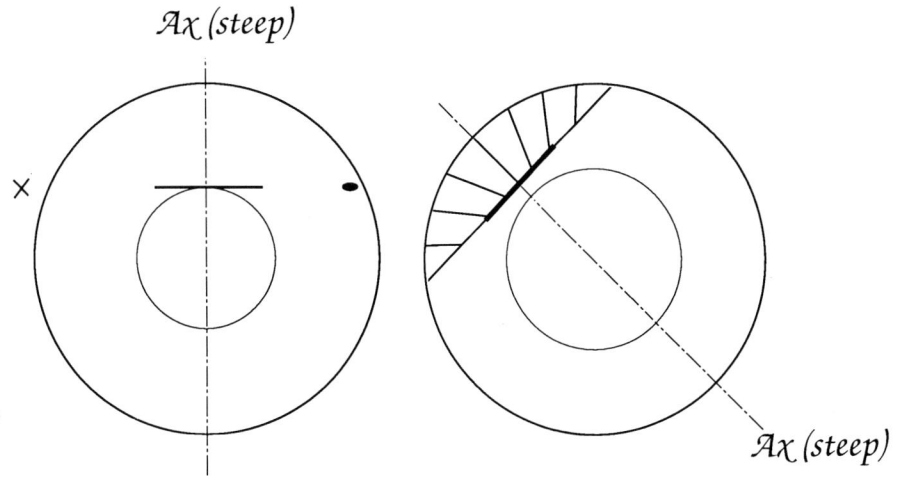

Fig. 9.7 Sato's single external T-incision alone and combined with internal radials for astigmatism.

will be difficult to convince that surgery has been successful.

Astigmatism following cataract surgery is less common today with the smaller incisions being used. Still, small-incision surgery is not universal, thus post-cataract astigmatism will continue to be encountered. Cases of astigmatism greater than 3 D were reported to be 10% in a series reported by Jaffe and Clayman [39]. High astigmatism after keratoplasty is even more common, with astigmatism greater than 1.00 D being the norm [34].

Despite the attention that astigmatism has received, its treatment remains less than straightforward. To produce a lasting effect through surgery, the aspiring refractive surgeon must have a complete grasp of the fundamentals of surgical correction of spherical errors. He or she must also be experienced with this modality and obtaining good, predictable results with spherical errors before attempting astigmatic corrections. While the cornea is somewhat forgiving in nature, there is less margin for error in astigmatism than for spherical cases, by several orders of magnitude. You are advised *not* to tackle even the simplest case as your initiation into refractive surgery. You are also advised to read the basic rules and dicta of refractive surgery which, if adhered to, will keep you out of "hot water".

Caveats

Astigmatism chasing

One of the biggest mistakes that can be made by refractive surgeons is the tendency to keep adding incisions in an effort to control the astigmatism. They begin by chasing the astigmatism and end by themselves being controlled by it.

The usual scenario is this: the patient is operated on for astigmatism—especially with T-cuts—and post-

operatively the astigmatism reappears in a different location (see Chapter 15). Sometimes it's greater, sometimes it's the same degree. Without waiting for things to simmer down, forgetting the lessons learned (if they ever were learned), the surgeon blithely adds another T-cut or two. The astigmatism now turns up in another meridian. By now the prudent surgeon would realize that things are not under control and stop, heeding Bores' Ninth Rule. But not our neophyte and certainly not our stalwart "expert" surgeon, for whom it's full speed ahead. He or she adds another T-cut or two, and so on. They are often puzzled to find after the surgery a patient with unstable, sometimes irregular, often hyperopic, astigmatism. This could all have been avoided in the first place. The author is unable to discover the need for haste here. The patient has had the original problem for years and now is likely to have an added one for some years to come. Please heed the moral of this tale: wait until things have stabilized before using your knife and thereby obey Halstead's maxim.

There is one other error the author sees quite frequently—unpaired T-cuts. Such incisions make no sense theoretically or practically. The corneal surface is toroidal and regular in its toricity. Symmetric surfaces demand symmetric surgery. One unpaired T-cut, especially at 6–7 mm, produces an asymmetric surface change. If the corneal thickness were even across its entire extent, such incisions might possibly produce an even curvature change. The normal cornea is not of even thickness, thus curvature changes from an unpaired T-cut will not be regular. The fact that the K-readings have changed in the presence of such an incision or that a patient's vision may be improved is not proof of the correctness of such application. Examination of such surfaces with sensitive ultra-sonographic topography shows asymmetry of the corneal center. It is known that relaxing incisions can

(a)

𝒜–𝒜 **long** axis, **least** curvature, **least** myopic.
𝓑–𝓑 **short** axis, **most** curvature, **most** myopic.

(b)

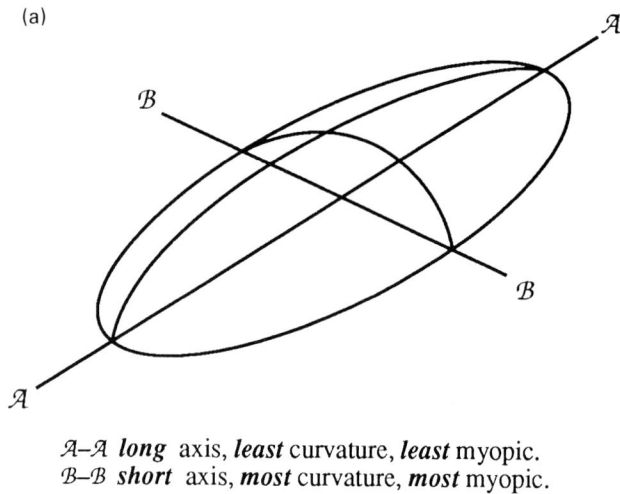

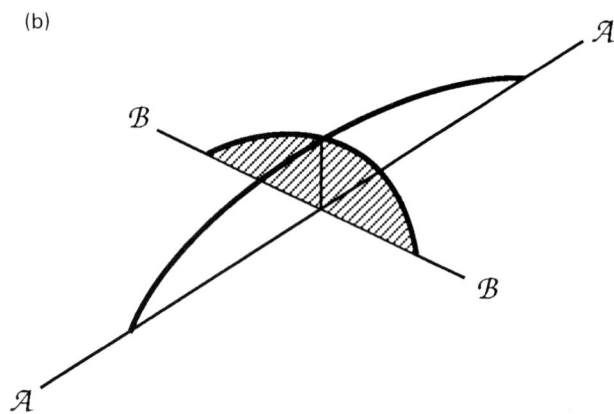

Fig. 9.8 Astigmatic meridians.

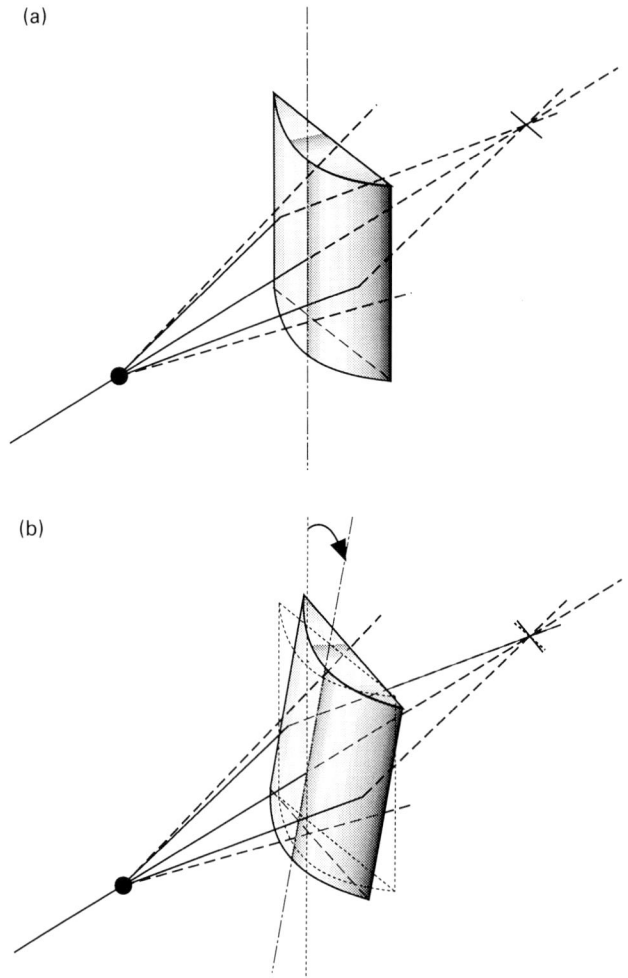

(a)

(b)

Fig. 9.9 The principle of cylinder lens.

produce multi-focal surfaces—good vision may be a happenstance related to that event [40]. K-readings are not a good criterion for the presence or absence of small areas of irregularity either; their resolution is too coarse and they are not reliable for non-spherical surfaces; even photokeratography can miss small irregularities.

Astigmatism—by way of review

To undertake the treatment of astigmatism by the method of using relaxing incisions (or, for that matter, by any technique), the surgeon must understand that he or she is dealing with a regular toroidal surface. In a regular toroidal surface two extremes of curvature can be identified.

1 The curvature of least radius.
2 The curvature of greatest radius.

For the sake of discussion we will call these curvatures major (flatter) and minor (steeper). Since these curves can be represented by lines in a plan view of the

surface (that is, a head-on view) we can call these lines (curves) major and minor axes (Figure 9.8). These terms will be most helpful later on in the discussion. However, do not confuse these axes with the axes of astigmatism, since, in fact, they correspond to the astigmatic meridians (because they represent the long and short axes of an ellipse; see below).

In the case of a cylindrical refractive surface, the refractive power of the cylinder is manifest at a right angle (90°) to its axis (Figure 9.9). This power axis is referred to as the meridian of the cylinder. Thus in a case whose refractive error is −6.00 + 3.00 × 90°, the cylindrical axis is at 90° whereas the meridian is at 180° (Figure 9.10). That meridian is relatively flat in its curvature (since that is the plus meridian). The minus axis is at 180° but its meridian is at 90°. The 90° meridian therefore has the steepest curvature (it's more myopic). That's where all the action is. All the fancy configurations for myopia, incision placement, etc. are oriented on the plus cylinder axis—hence Bores' Fifth Rule of refractive surgery: *Plus cylinder notation must*

(a)

M' -3.00 D

(b)

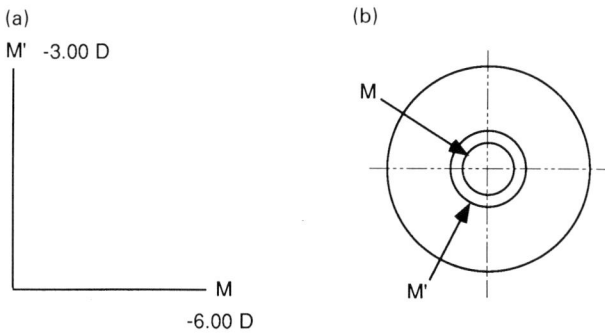

Fig. 9.10 (a) Power diagram; (b) two zones for astigmatism.

always be used in planning myopic astigmatism surgery and the reverse for hyperopic astigmatism.

Assuming a toroidal surface with a major and minor axis, imagine a planar section being made through this surface. In a plan view this slice would be parallel with the floor. If we were then to turn the piece over and look at it (or trace its edge on to a piece of paper), we would find that the resulting shape would be that of an oval or, more properly, an ellipse (Figure 9.11). The short side of the ellipse would represent the minor axis and correspond to the greater (steepest, least radius) surface curvature on the surface, whereas the long side would represent the major axis and correspond to the lesser (flattest, most radius) surface curvature. Sections perpendicular to the surface along the major and minor axis illustrate this point.

Patient workup

The basic workup for astigmatism is that for spherical myopia (see Chapter 5) with some additions and special precautions. Unless you or your refractionist are particularly good at manifest refractions, cycloplegic examinations are recommended in these cases. As you become more familiar with the process of dealing with astigmatism, a return can be made to manifest refractions. This is especially important in mixed or compound astigmatism. The Jackson cross cylinder must be used to refine the cylinder axis for the same reasons of accuracy. The keratometry readings should all be done by the same person and the axis clearly defined. This is easier to do with small mire instruments such as the Haag-Streit ophthalmometer. In fact, its purchase should be a priority for any keratotomist.

There is a definite relationship between the diameter of the surgical optical zone and the degree of myopia of the patient's optical system. The selection of the size of the primary optical zone is based, for the most part, upon the patient's spectacle refraction. The amount of astigmatism in the patient's optical system may not bear any direct relationship to the astigmatism on the

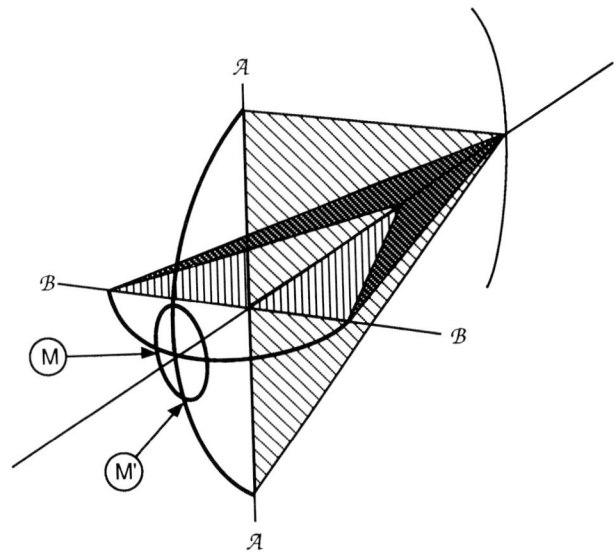

Fig. 9.11 The resultant optical zone required is elliptic in shape.

cornea (as measured by keratometry). Remember, we are correcting the refraction of the total optical system by altering the corneal surface—much like fitting a toroidal contact lens for the same purpose.

The problem often arises as to what should be done when the K-readings do not match the refraction. In practice this seldom becomes a problem. Generally speaking, in higher degrees of astigmatism where the curvature and axis are more critical, the refraction will correspond quite closely to the Ks. The Ks should always be used when the astigmatism is high and a clear-cut refractive result is not possible. In smaller amounts of astigmatism where the problem is less critical, the refraction should *always* be taken over the Ks. In mixed astigmatism the solution may be less clear-cut because the unaided vision is usually quite good in these cases. An incorrect assessment of the parameters could result in a loss of uncorrected vision post-operatively. The best rule-of-thumb is always to operate for total astigmatism. Trust the cross-cylinder to refine the cylinder axis.

In some cases the photokeratometer may be of help because the axis of astigmatism is the critical factor here (L.A. Ruiz, 1989, personal communication). However, it takes skill to interpret the photos— although it is a skill that can be acquired in time. Be especially watchful for any indications that the limbus is less than circular. While rare, an elliptic limbus requires special techniques to deal with adequately and each case has to be assessed individually. There are no hard and fast rules here (see the section on the technique of the Ruiz procedure, below). A photokeratometer and/or other surface mapping device should be in the armamentarium of all keratotomists, despite its shortcomings (see Chapter 6). There are cases in which nothing but experience will be of help. When in doubt, do not hesitate to seek advice regardless how trivial the problem may seem.

In some instances, particularly those in which the patient has been wearing contact lenses, your refraction may not match that of the patient's spectacles. Here common sense should prevail. Generally speaking, if patients see well and comfortably with their glasses it is safe to assume that they will also be comfortable after surgery using their old spectacle refraction in lieu of yours. Unless there is some compelling reason to alter the situation, go with the present prescription.

It is very important that the cornea be as stable as possible prior to the surgery. Therefore, contact lenses should be out as long as practical but in no case less than 1 week (Table 9.1). This goes for soft lenses as well; these are known to cause corneal warpage in as little as 20 hours [41]. If patients have no back-up spectacles, have them remove the lens from one eye for the required period. Warn them that they may experience some difficulty with depth perception and to be especially careful while driving.

Keratometry after corneal surgery

Typically, when the full thickness of the cornea has been involved—as in penetrating keratoplasty—ordinary K-readings will be as reliable as ever they were. However, after lamellar surgery, such as keratomileusis, where only the anterior curvature has been altered, K-readings are inaccurate and may underestimate the true refractive power and astigmatism by 11% or more (see Chapter 6 for a more detailed explanation) [42]. This again emphasizes the author's admonition that refractive surgery demands an accurate means of evaluating the true corneal curvature.

Instrumentation

This discussion concerns itself mostly with those instruments used for astigmatism surgery and which are adjunctive to the basic tools of refractive surgery. The reader is referred to Chapters 7 and 8 for a more in-depth description of basic instrumentation.

Incision depth is a paramount factor in the outcome

Table 9.1 Contact lens removal schedule

Lens type	Minimum time*
Hard	1 week
Soft	48 hours
Ortho-K	6 months

*See text.

of radial keratotomy for spherical myopia—it is no less important in the control of astigmatism. As was pointed out first by Fyodorov and co-workers and has been amply demonstrated since by many others, there are three factors which affect the depth of incision. We reiterate:
1 Blade length.
2 Blade sharpness.
3 Tissue resistance.

All of these factors are inter-related but only the first two can be controlled directly. The third factor can be compensated for in some degree by over-setting the blade and by pressurizing the eye.

Blades and blade handles

As has been stated repeatedly, this surgery is true micro-surgery. The outcome is dependent not only upon careful consideration of numerous, seemingly unimportant factors, but also upon the instrumentation. Next to the pre-operative workup, the most important consideration in this surgery is the blade. In the beginning, razor fragments were used (see also Chapter 7). Because such blades were inconsistent in their quality, most surgeons today use some form of crystalline blade.

While it is true that specially processed steel blades (such as the Katena K2-5550) are available today which surpass in quality any razor fragment and in some cases even some older diamond blades, it is the consensus among most of the experienced practitioners of this surgery that some form of crystalline blade (not necessarily diamond) will produce the smoothest and deepest incision. Being able to make consistently deep incisions is increasing the accuracy of our predictions considerably.

Angled blades are not an appropriate choice for making transverse incisions, nor are the less sharp steel blades. A vertical-edged crystalline blade provides the exquisite sharpness required for precise control of the length and depth of transverse incisions. An extra-sharp, double-edged blade such as the XTAL sapphire blade (Katena K2-6512) or the Western Medical Products WMK-200 ultra-thin LeCut diamond blade is a real asset and is highly recommended. On the other hand, the author has not had a good experience with the square diamond blades advocated by Thornton [43].

A knife handle with a slightly longer than normal footplate is useful as well. Most of the current diamond blade holders do not provide a sufficiently clear and unobstructed view of the blade edge and operative area. Even if you have a favorite diamond knife, consider purchasing the Katena K2-6500 for astigmatism surgery. Keep this blade and handle sequestered and use it for astigmatism only.

Fixation devices

Fixation of the eye is especially important in astigmatism cases to insure that all incisions are straight and perpendicular to the corneal surface. There are many devices on the market for this purpose. Any such device should be easily applied and removed and should not produce tissue damage. In addition, it must not interfere with the surgery.

Fixation forceps

The narrow double fixation forceps prevents ocular rotation without the corneal distortion a wider jaw would produce, especially in a soft eye. However, it does not provide sufficient stability for transverse incisions. For these cases, a wide-jawed forceps such as the Bores wide fixation forceps (K5-3280) provides the cross-limbus fixation essential to making straight (or arcuate) transverse incisions, as in the Ruiz procedure (see Chapter 8). These instruments are also available with angled jaws for those who prefer that configuration (Figure 9.12).

Optical zone and incision markers

Cross-hairs or other centering aids are useful but not essential, and frequently are inaccurately aligned. Sizes should be clearly marked on each marker, particularly astigmatism markers. All markers, especially those for astigmatism, must be handled with care to prevent damage that may distort their shapes.

Astigmatic optical zone markers

Despite the fact that the effective optical zone in astigmatism is an ellipse, there are few occasions where an actual elliptical zone need be marked (Figure

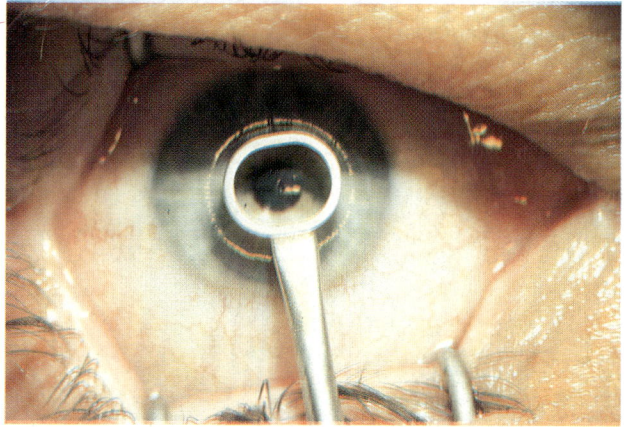

Fig. 9.13 Oval optical zone marker (Katena).

9.13). In these cases, the following markers may prove the most useful:

1 3.00×3.50 mm (Katena K3-8060).
2 3.00×4.00 mm (Katena K3-8062).
3 3.00×4.50 mm (Katena K3-8064).
4 3.00×5.00 mm (Katena K3-8066).
5 3.50×4.00 mm (Katena K3-8068).
6 3.50×5.00 mm (Katena K3-8070).

Incision markers

Special devices for marking the incision lines or spacing are available as well. However, all of these, with two exceptions, are optional. One exception is the six-blade incision marker (Katena K3-8880). While it is possible to make four, eight, or 16 incisions evenly spaced by eye, it is not quite so easy accurately to judge the 30° or 60° separation between incisions in six- or 12-incision cases. Coating the bottom of these

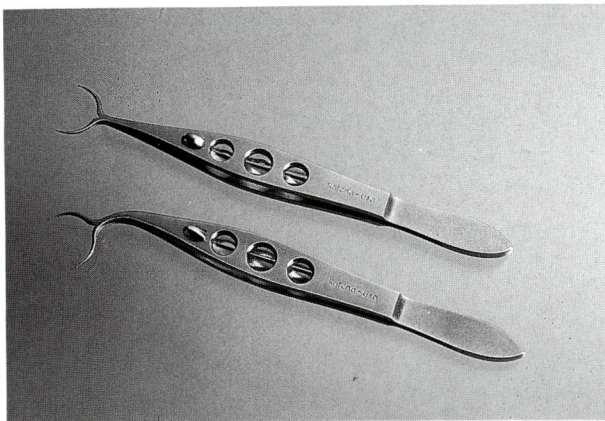

Fig. 9.12 Straight and angled wide fixation forceps.

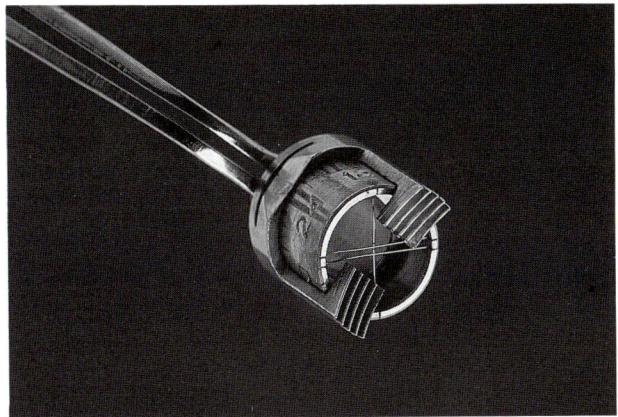

Fig. 9.14 Fyodorov L-marker.

(a)

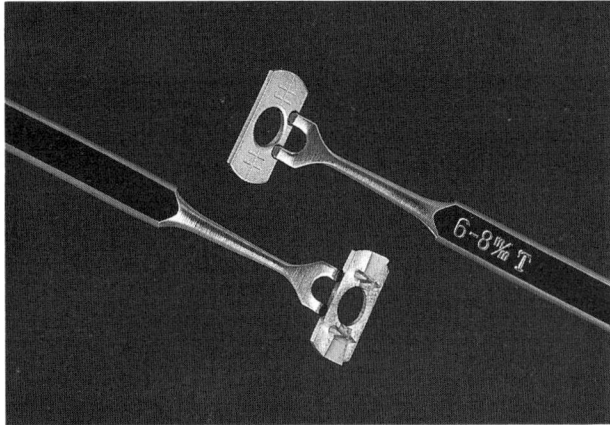

(b)

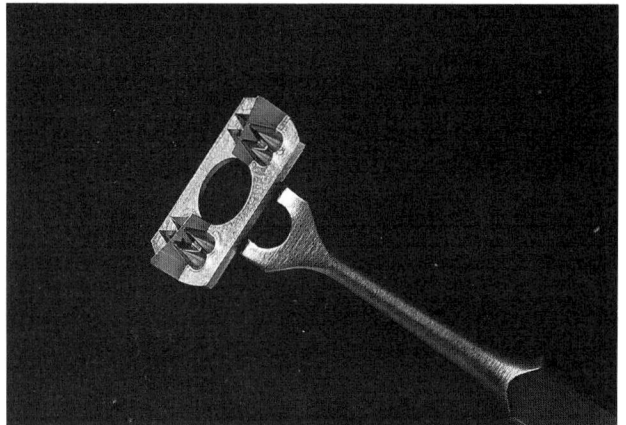

(c)

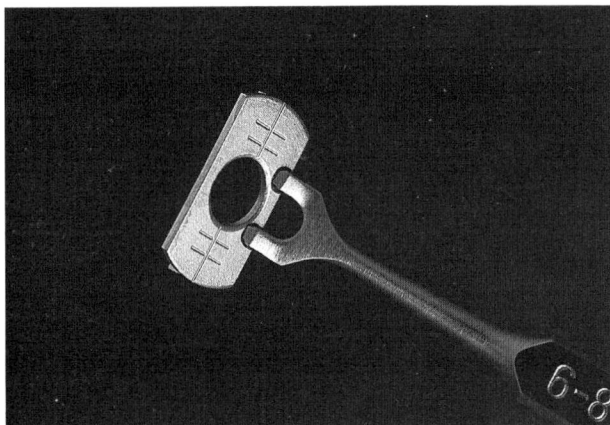

(d)

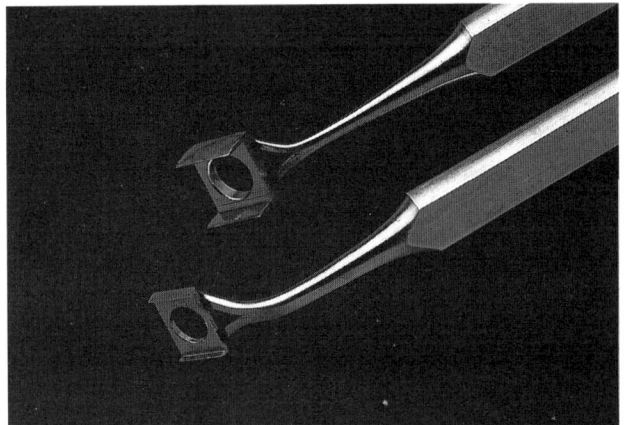

Fig. 9.15 (a–d) Single and double T-markers (Katena).

markers with brilliant green or gentian violet will enhance their usefulness—at least for the beginner. The more experienced surgeon will find the beginning of the marks sufficient to align the incisions. The other exception is the L-incision marker (see method RL below) (Figure 9.14).

Because a vertical cutting blade is used to make the transverse T-incisions, the cutting is done in reverse (toward the open end of the footplate). It is necessary to use a guideline to insure that the incision is straight and of the proper length. There are numerous guide markers available for marking individual and clustered T-incisions, with and without radials. I recommend the Katena series of markers as being durable and accurate for this purpose (Figure 9.15). In lieu of such markers, a new Castroviejo-type caliper (Katena K3-9010) and Dietz "hockey stick" (Katena K3-9620) marker can be used to scribe lines on to the corneal surface.

Special markers

Special markers such as the Bores/Ruiz, Bores L-markers, etc. will be discussed under individual configurations.

Axis marker

The Bores axis marker (Katena K3-7910) is a must for astigmatism surgery (Figure 9.16). This can be used in conjunction with a Mendez protractor (Katena K3-7900) or Zeiss eyepiece reticle to mark the axis of cylinder.

The Zeiss astigmatism reticle

The Zeiss astigmatism reticle (Figure 9.17) is supplied in a matched set of 10-power high-point oculars by Zeiss (reticle No. 30-55-83). Originally designed for use in fitting toric contact lenses, it serves admirably in the eyepiece tube of any Zeiss operating microscope. These can also be adapted to fit into a Weck scope.

(a)

(b)

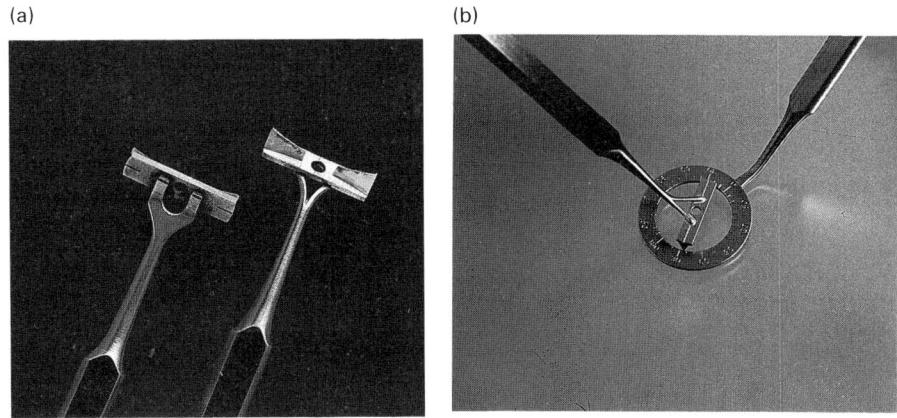

Fig. 9.16 (a) Bores axis marker; (b) used with Mendez protractor.

For those of you with Zeiss operating scopes who cannot get or don't want the expense of the first reticle, there are some other reticles available which can be purchased for your eyepieces. Zeiss reticle 30-55-98 is designed for a 12.5× eyepiece. It has a ruler in the center and is marked off into 12 segments corresponding to 15° increments. If the eyepiece is aligned so that 12 and 6 o'clock marks are coincident with the 12 and 6 o'clock positions of the patient's cornea, the patient's cylinder axis can be closely approximated. This reticle must be factory-installed, however.

Using the Zeiss reticle

This reticle consists of a precisely engraved optical flat with a cross-hair in the center. The long arm of the cross-hair is marked off in equal increments from 0 to 15. At the bottom edge of the reticle is engraved a 90° protractor, off-set 10°. Further, the protractor is marked in major divisions of 10° and minor divisions at 2° in increments from 0 to 90° on one side, and from 0 to 110° on the other. Riding in a groove under this protractor is a steel ball whose diameter is exactly 20°. When placed into the usual angled eyepiece of the Zeiss operating microscope, this ball will self-center. The reading is made off the right-hand side of the steel ball.

With the patient supine and looking at the co-axial light reflex, the eyepiece is rotated until the right edge of the ball is aligned at 90° (or 0) on the reticle. The operating microscope is then aligned sagittally with the patient's head such that the zero mark corresponds to 12 o'clock on the patient's cornea—it helps to have marked this position at the slit-lamp, prior to surgery. The eyepiece is then rotated to correspond to the axis of astigmatism (Figure 9.18).

The microscope is adjusted to place the cross-hair of the reticle on to the previously marked visual axis. This is done by aligning and locking the microscope head in place and then grasping the barrel of the eyepiece

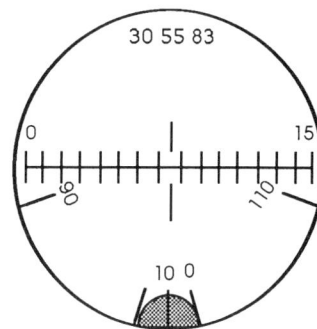

Fig. 9.17 Zeiss reticle.

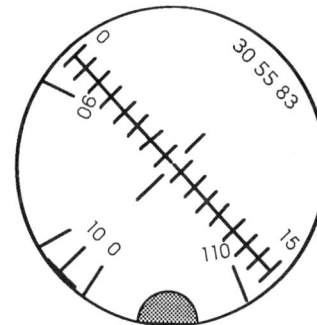

Fig. 9.18 Zeiss reticle rotated.

(below the adjustment collar) and rotating it until the cross-hair is properly aligned. It is helpful to set this eyepiece in such a way that the long arm of the cross-hair is parallel to the cylinder axis (this is not always possible). This is important—study the drawing of this reticle to understand why this is so. By aligning the reticle in this way you have provided yourself with an additional reminder of the orientation of the steep or flat meridian—the axis you're going to be working in. Sometimes it is not possible to use the reticle in this manner: that's where the axis marker comes in.

Remember: in myopic astigmatism, the *short* side of the *ellipsoid* corresponds to the *plus cylinder axis*. (If you have forgotten why this is so, please refer back to the beginning of the review section on astigmatism). Some astigmatism markers have a cross-hair or aiming stud to assist in this alignment. The elliptic optical zone marker is then aligned using the cross-hair as a guide to proper orientation and the primary zone is marked.

The Fenzl reticle

Another product is the Fenzl reticle (Figure 9.19). This is an engraved glass reticle which can be placed into any microscope eyepiece (instructions are provided). While not as elegant as the previously described Zeiss, it is serviceable and infinitely better than nothing. You will need two of these—one for the microscope and one for your slit-lamp. This reticle is basically used in the same manner as the Zeiss product.

Mendez protractor

The Mendez degree gauge (Katena K3-7900) can be used to assist the surgeon in marking the axis of the cylinder (see above). In this case the 12 o'clock position of the patient's cornea should be determined either at the slit-lamp or under the operating microscope. The device is then placed on to the anesthetized cornea and the 0 or 90° mark aligned with the 12 o'clock point on the cornea. The axis marker is then rotated within the protractor ring and aligned with the proper tick mark.

Other useful things

See also Chapter 8 for other essential instruments. The Thornton ruled marker is useful as a generic T-marker for transverse incisions of various lengths (Figure 9.20).

Current methods for the control of astigmatism

Wedge resections for hyperopic astigmatism— revisited

This method is not this author's favorite way to control astigmatism—there are better, more predictable methods (namely relaxing incisions) to do this. Still, there are times when nothing else will do. Thus, it is important that every refractive surgeon knows how to perform this surgery. Troutman introduced this technique in 1970 to treat post-keratoplasty astigmatism [35]. Despite all the best efforts, post-keratoplasty astigmatism still plagues us. This is not the place to discuss the merits of double-running versus interrupted sutures, etc., however. We can leave that for

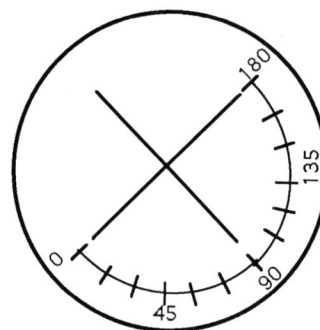

Fig. 9.19 Fenzl reticle.

textbooks on keratoplasty techniques. Suffice it to say that we do not yet have a handle on the problem, and considering what we have learned thus far from refractive surgery, we may never solve it. Nevertheless, if the problem is ever solved the author will predict, for the record, that the answer will come from the ongoing work with refractive surgical procedures.

Before beginning a more detailed description of this technique, the student should be reminded that astigmatism surgery is a giant can of worms which can be dealt with successfully only by approaching it in a rational way while being prepared for occasional irrational results. It is true that some methods are more predictable than others, but wedge resections are not in that category.

This procedure steepens flat axes (even though the incision in transverse to the meridian) because this a *resection* of tissue with subsequent suturing—hence the chord of the arc is shortened, and when the chord of an arc is shortened, the arc is steepened. The rule of thumb for this surgery is that for every 0.1 mm of resection, 0.67 D of cornea will be steepened– theoretically. We say theoretically because 1.0 mm of resection should gain you 10 D of correction except that it doesn't, it gets you somewhat less. How much less is anyone's guess—sometimes a lot, sometimes a little. Usually, for astigmatism equal to or less than 10 D, a little more surgery is needed, while for more than 10 D, a little less is required. In any event, no resection width should exceed 1.5 mm; thus the procedure tops out at about 15 D, although as much as 27 D of correction has been reported [44], which is a lot of astigmatism in anyone's book. Better you should not be too exuberant with this surgery in any event; if you've under-corrected go back and do a little more by shaving down one side of the resection, on the limbal side. The object is to reduce the astigmatism to manageable proportions. Manageable could mean glasses, contact lenses,

(a)

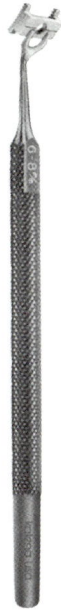

(b)

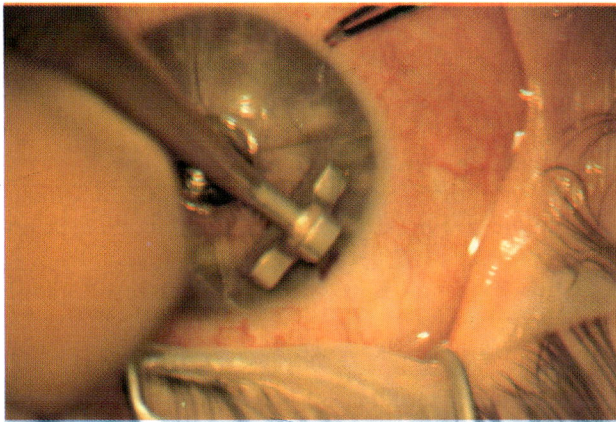

(c)

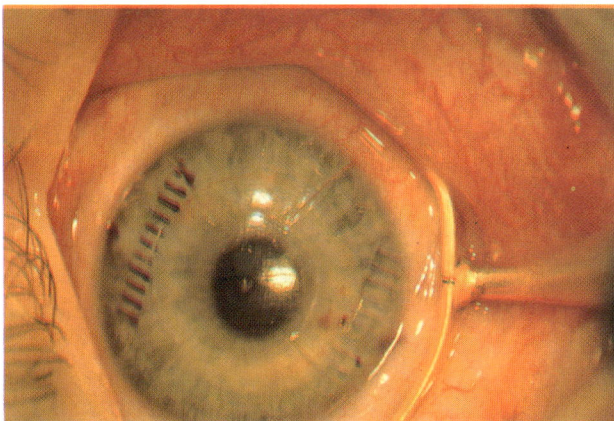

Fig. 9.20 (a–c) Thornton ruled T-marker.

or more predictable relaxing incisions (see the section on relaxing incisions; and also wedge versus Ruiz, below).

Be also cognizant of Bores' axiom: "Beware pushing down the curvature too much over *here*; it might pop up over *there* under an assumed name." That means that anything you do to one meridian will be reflected (in its true sense) in the opposite meridian at a ratio of about 2:1. That is, 1 D of *steepening* at 90° will be accompanied by 0.50 D of *flattening* at 180°. Thus for every 0.67 D of steepening there will be a corresponding 0.33 D of flattening, or 1 D of total cylinder will be induced. Better you should keep the 2:1 relationship in mind and not add up the vectors since typically we're concentrating on one meridian and are trying to get rid of lots of cylinder. It does you no good to reduce 10 D in one meridian just to induce 5 D in the other—balance is the key here. Maybe you should only try for 7.50 D of correction. That would leave you with, for example, a residual of +2.50 D in the original meridian and you would have induced +3.75 D in the other, opposite meridian (which is only 1.25 D difference), ultimately. Thus the final refraction would be +2.50 + 1.25 × whatever axis. In suppose you could try to figure out the exact relationship so as to end up with a plano result (or even slightly minus) but you'd go crazy trying to cut the exact incision width to accomplish it. For a patient who was plano +10.00 before surgery, that's an improvement anyone can live with. Be aware that some patients with mixed astigmatism, even up to 2.5 D, can record uncorrected vision as good as 20/30. An over-correction of the astigmatism is always induced in any case with this surgery because of the compression induced by the suturing.

The corneal astigmatism should be stable for about 6–8 weeks after complete keratoplasty suture removal. Pachymetry is performed over the graft scar. Take several readings so a thin spot won't surprise you. In performing this surgery, a surgical keratometer is almost essential to success. Retrobulbar or general anesthesia should also be employed.

To proceed, first establish the meridian of the hyperopic cylinder by photokeratoscopy and/or ophthalmometry (see Figure 9.21 for a method of modifying the faceplate of the photokeratometer). Prior to surgery, seat the patient at the slit-lamp and lightly mark the 12 o'clock position on the cornea, near the limbus, bedore administering the retrobulbar. If the patient is already anesthetized, you will have to rely on remembered landmarks. With the patient on the operating table and anesthetized, align the microscope eyepiece reticle with the 12 o'clock mark on the cornea (see the section on using the Zeiss reticle, above). In lieu of the reticle, use the Mendez protractor for the next step.

Prepare and drape the patient and insert the wire lid speculum. Coat a Bores astigmatism axis marker with brilliant green (make sure that it dries) or gentian violet. Align the axis marker with the hyperopic (flat) meridian using the reticle or Mendez protractor and mark the meridian (Figure 9.22). Next coat the blades of an eight- or four-ray radial keratotomy incision marker with dye. Align the marker with the flat meridian and mark the cornea. Now you have both the axis of cylinder and incision extent demarcated (the extent should be 90°—3 clock hours): you are ready to take the next step.

Good fixation is a must in wedge resection. A very good method of fixation for this surgery is the vacuum suction ring of Barraquer (used for MKM) with or without keratome guides. If using the ring, the author suggests that you reverse the handle from the method described by Troutman and have it positioned at 6 o'clock. Apply the vacuum and hold the handle with your non-dominant hand.

The incisions can be made with a single-blade, guarded, radial keratotomy diamond knife or the special double-blade device described by Troutman— the author uses the former for the first incision. Both methods will be described.

Single-blade method

Set the guarded blade so as not to produce a perforation. If the diamond blade is a new LeCut, under-set it about 5–10 μm. Here's where the Bores shadow-graph shines (see Chapter 8); the Baribeau microscope can also be used. Insert the blade tip at one end of the incision and, using the vertical knife edge, incise a curvilinear incision just inside the graft–host junction, using the scar as a guide.

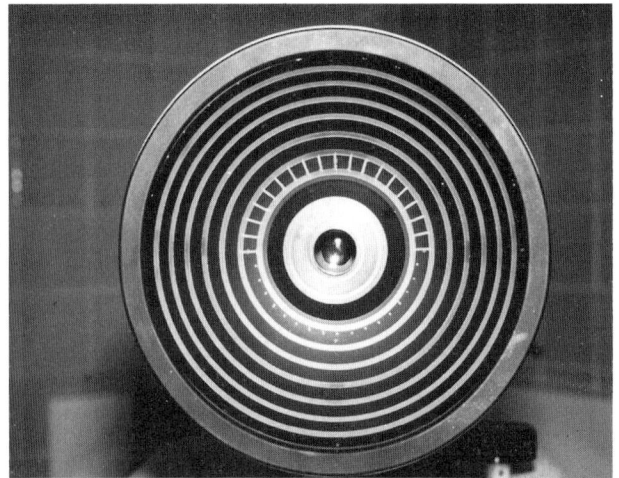

Fig. 9.21 Modified keratoscope faceplate *à la* Ruiz.

The next part of the incision is make free-hand with a naked blade. If you have the Katena handle (K2-6700), you can remove the blade from the guarded handle and use it. Otherwise the author suggests the Katena K2-6705 in the same handle. Using a caliper, mark the widest extent of the wedge along the astigmatic meridian toward the limbus so that the incisions parallel the scar. It may help to use a fresh skin-marking pencil to trace out the incision. Trace the mark with the blade partially through the stroma. Then deepen the cut, angling toward the first incision. Avoid perforation at this juncture to insure an even section. The suction ring can now be released. Finish the resection of the wedge with Vannus or other scissors.

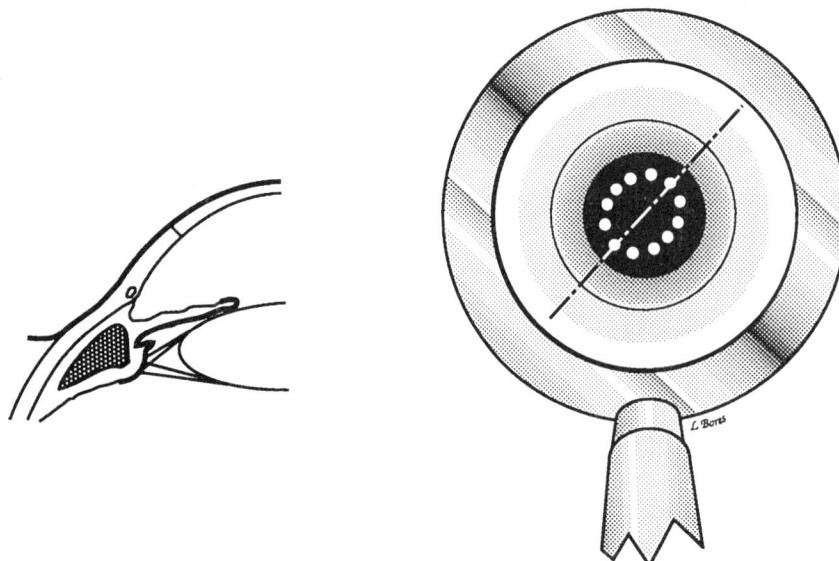

Fig. 9.22 Establishing the hyperopic meridian.

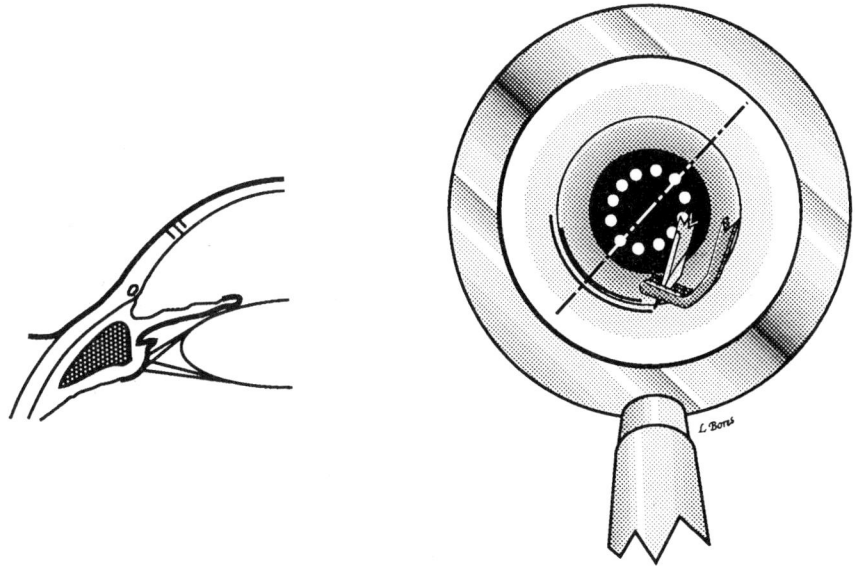

Fig. 9.23 Making the incisions.

Double blade technique

Using the double-blade diamond knife, trace out the incision as shown (Figure 9.23). You will probably have to do this in stages to avoid entering the AC. Using the free-hand blade, extend the inner incision to join the outer. Complete the resection as described above. You will probably find that the first method yields a more even wedge than the second.

Completing the resection

A knife needle or 15° razor knife is used to make a paracentesis to reduce the intra-ocular pressure. This will facilitate suture closure of the wedge without tension—something which should be avoided at all costs. Care should be taken in aphakic eyes if vitreous is present in the AC. In this case inject a *small* amount of air or Healon to push the vitreous away from the cornea. The wedge is closed with 8–10 10-0 nylon sutures placed through-and-through (Figure 9.24). Start peripherally and work toward the center. Troutman suggests tying each loop with a double slip knot, tightening them in pairs beginning in the periphery and working centrally [45]. If you have a surgical keratometer, the knots are tied so as to convert the pre-operative ellipse into one with the opposite shape and extent. The extent of this over-correction should be about 50% of the original. The sutures are then locked and the knots pulled below the limbal corneal surface.

Unfortunately, in the past, this considerable over-correction compromised vision during the "sutures-in" period, sometimes lasting up to a year. Troutman has advocated the use of compensatory compression sutures to reduce the inevitable (and necessary) astigmatic over-correction resulting from this surgery. Two or more interrupted sutures are placed across the graft scar, 60° from each end of the closed wedge. These are tightened until the reversed ellipse becomes circular (Figure 9.25). These will remain until the resection sutures are removed—generally at 6 months—although if the patient is comfortable they can remain for longer periods. Expect some reversal of effect when the sutures are completely removed. Mean residual astigmatism in the author's few cases was approximately 3 D.

Relaxing incisions for myopic astigmatism: basic principles

Relaxing incisions have a venerable position in the hierarchy of astigmatism surgery, being among the first to be seriously applied to the problem. First used in controlling iatrogenic astigmatism, they were eventually used in congenital astigmatism as well. They have the distinct advantage of being eminently controllable through their length and depth, are easier to perform and result in a much more rapid diminution of the astigmatic error. Typically, these procedures can be done under topical anesthesia and since suturing is avoided, the results can be more readily anticipated.

The object of myopic astigmatism surgery is to produce corneal flattening proportional to the degree of myopia. Since the degree of the myopia is proportional to the degree of curvature of the corneal surface (all else being equal), then more flattening force must be exerted in the axis of greatest corneal curvature to reduce the myopic astigmatism. Figure 9.26 is representational of a myopic astigmatic optical surface.

Note that the flattening force has to be applied to the short side of the ellipse, with less force being applied to the long (flatter) side of the ellipse in order to

(a)

(b)

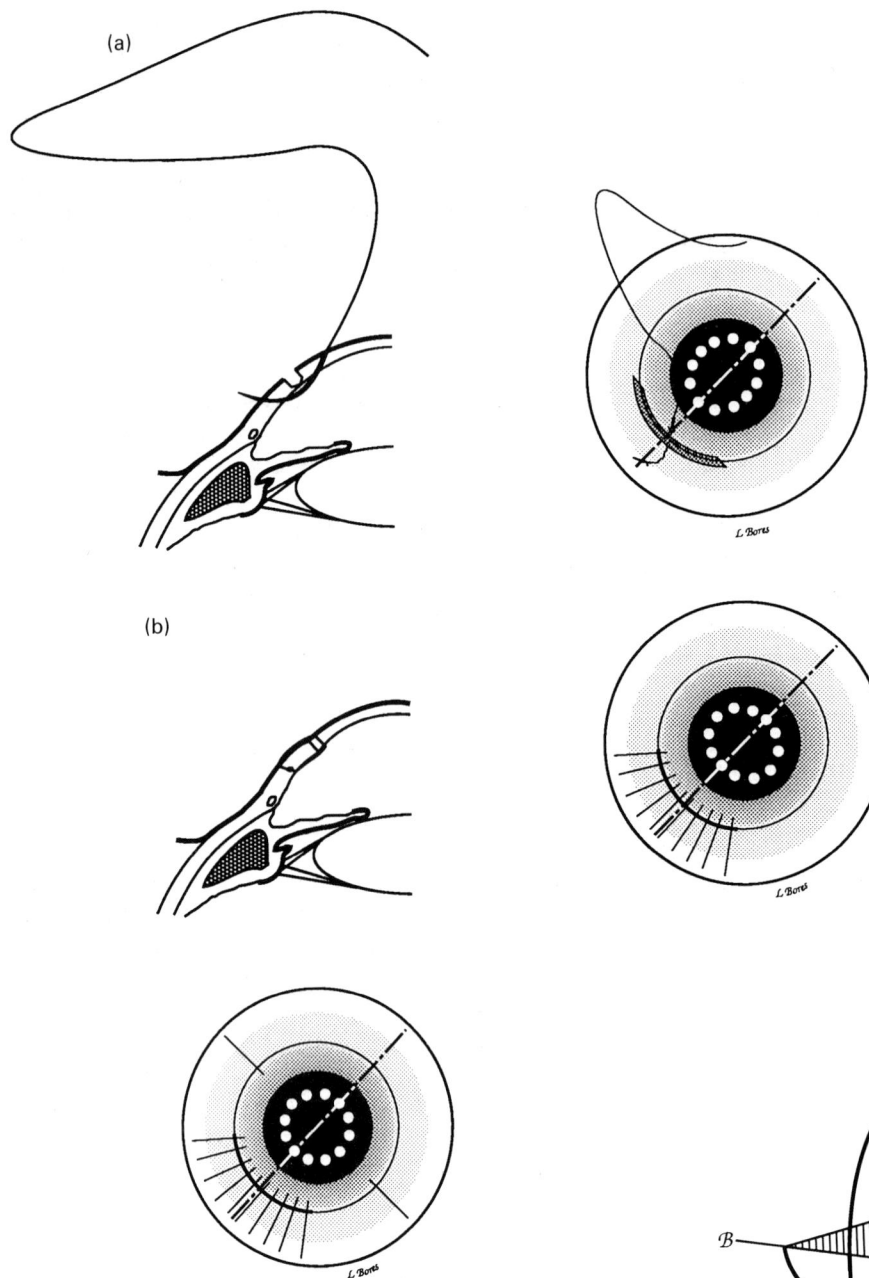

Fig. 9.24 (a) Sutures are through-and-through; (b) they are tied sufficiently tight to close the wound. Note the reversal of the astigmatism.

Fig. 9.25 Compression sutures are placed at 90° to the hyperopic axis to relieve the inevitable but temporary over-correction.

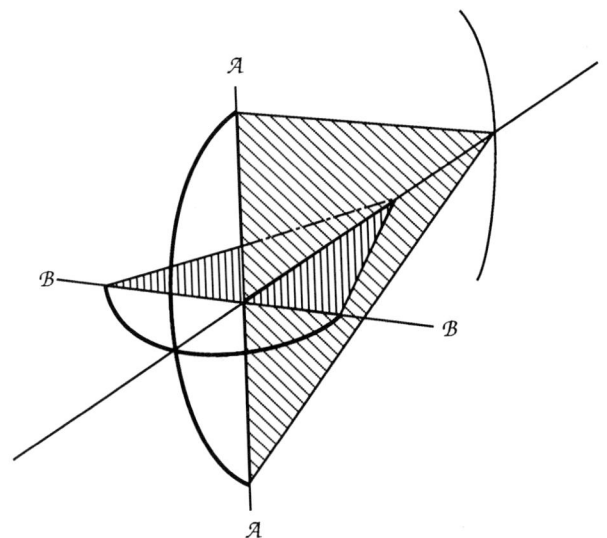

Fig. 9.26 Simple myopic astigmatism.

bring all points to a focus upon the retina. In radial keratotomy surgery this flattening force is created by peripheral bulging (i.e. increasing peripheral corneal curvature) in an amount proportional to the central curvature, caused by the structural weakening of the cornea by the incisions. This is the same principle applied in quadrantic (arcuate) intra-cicatricial relaxing incisions used in post-keratoplasty astigmatism (see below).

The degree of peripherall bulging is directly related to the length (and depth) of the incisions. Therefore, a long incision placed parallel to the short axis will cause greater peripheral bulging and correspondingly greater central flattening along that axis. Since we are dealing with a toroidal surface, the degree of curvature diminishes as we approach the flatter axis from the steeper, and therefore the required incision length becomes shorter.

For all practical purposes the limbus can be considered circular (although there are exceptions). Therefore, graduating the length of the incisions produces an optical zone that has the shape of an ellipse. In classic, early radial keratotomy, such elliptic optical zones were advocated in the control of corneal astigmatism [46]. However, transverse incisions and circular optical clear zones—with or without accompanying radial incisions—have since been found to be more efficient and predictable. Thus the circle is complete and we're back to where we began in 1894.

The size of the optical zone is, of course, related to the amount of correction desired. That is, a $-6.00 + 3.00 \times 90°$ refractive error will need the clear zone diameter along the steeper axis to be of a size required to correct 6 D of myopia, while the diameter along the flatter axis (90° to the steeper) must be of a size to correct 3 D.

Thus, in classic radial keratotomy, to correct astigmatism associated with myopia, we would need merely to make an elliptic optical zone of appropriate dimensions to obtain the correction desired. In principle this is how it works. In practice, however, it has been found necessary to make certain modifications in the arrangement of the incisions depending upon the amount of total astigmatism present.

Peripheral deepening is done in the same manner as in spherical myopia (see also Chapter 8). However, for the most part circular mid-zones seem to produce a better result than elliptic ones.

Decision making

The author uses his own computer program to calculate the surgical parameters for astigmatism surgery.

In a previous chapter (Chapter 8) we have pointed out the importance of not being eclectic (Bores' Fourth Rule). It is *not* possible to "mix and match" with this surgery and expect any prediction software to be effective under those circumstances. Thus while we have reviewed some of the other software available for this purpose (see Chapter 8), our current discussion will confine itself wholly to how the author carries out the decision-making process. Therefore, the examples we will be using concern the output of the RK Data-Master program and no other. The RK DataMaster programs are capable of evaluating cases of simple, compound and mixed myopic astigmatism. A number of cases will be shown to demonstrate this capability. Figure 9.27 illustrates the incisional configurations covered by the program.

From the calculation display is selected the optimal incision depth coefficient/optical zone(s)/incision number/surgical configuration for the case. However, the program will not draw out the astigmatic incisional patterns for you. This is a deliberate omission designed so as to prevent mistakes made resulting from erroneous input. Too many people assume that if the computer says a thing, it must be so. Remember GIGO (garbage in—garbage out).

The prudent keratotomist will draw out the incisional configuration for every astigmatic case *prior* to the day of surgery. This should be done after calculating the surgical parameters. It is too easy to place the incisions off-axis otherwise. *Do not rely upon a drawing made by a computer from the data that you have input.* This is so vital as to be worth repeating. It might be more convenient to have a computer do this but there have been instances where invalid data have been used to construct a drawing, resulting in surgery being placed in the wrong axis. There have also been instances in which the input data were changed but not the

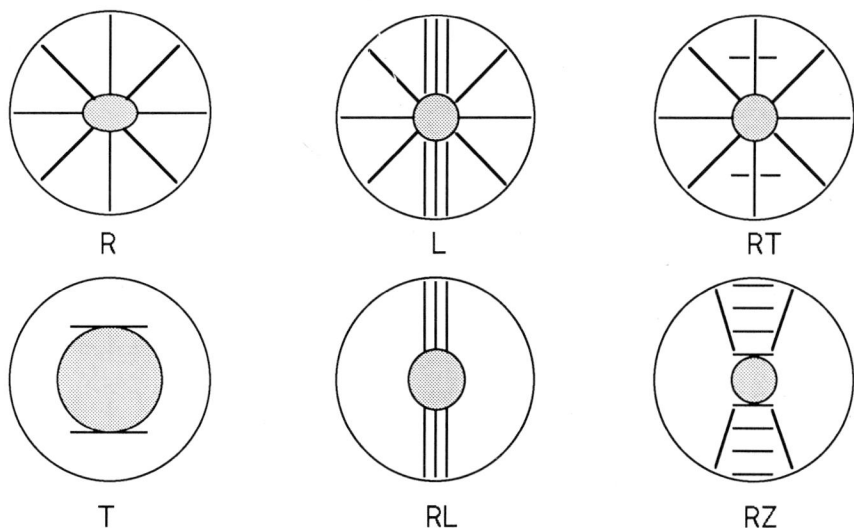

Fig. 9.27 Current incisional configurations for astigmatism.

drawing. It takes little imagination to follow that scenario to its end. Furthermore, by drawing out the configuration yourself, you are forced to consider the data in the light of your experience. Never, never, delegate this chore—*never*! Comes a denouement, reliance upon your technician is no defense. The author has caught errors in the data in too many instances for there to be any call to ease up on this advice, and the technicians at the Bores Eye Institute are very experienced. We are all human and subject to making errors—keep that in mind.

There should be a separate surgical sheet made up for each eye, on to which all pre-operative parameters are entered (see the Appendix for an example of such a workup sheet). Your technician can fill out the pre-operative parameters, which you should check against the original workup. *Do not hesitate to question any data that seem to be at variance with experience.* Use these data to input into the computer.

The author does these calculations himself and has written RK DataMaster in a way that it is not convenient for a technician to do. It is not safe to let your assistant do it anyway. There are some decisions to be made while running the program that only the surgeon can make. It is possible to do as many as 20 such calculations within 30 min, including the data print-out, so it is not an onerous task. Once you have made your decisions as to what surgical parameters you will use, enter them on to the sheet using a black or dark blue felt-tip pen—something that will show up well. This sheet will be posted later next to your operating microscope and must be clearly legible.

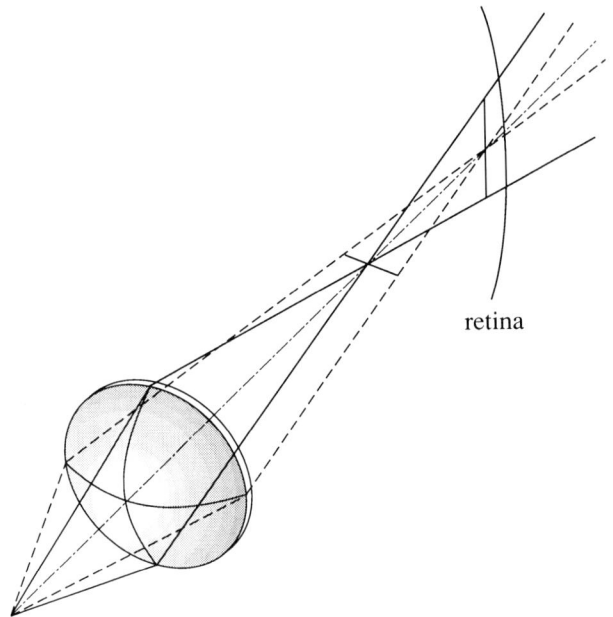

retina

Fig. 9.28 Compound myopic astigmatism.

Case workup examples

Case 1—RT procedure

This is a case of low-grade, compound, myopic astigmatism (Figure 9.28). The computer has suggested an RT (radial transverse) procedure but it is possible to perform the surgery another way.

```
RK DATAMASTER PRE-OP DATA ENTRY PROGRAM ............. Page 2

01) VISUAL ACUITY (without correction) ............ 20/ 200
02) VISUAL ACUITY (with correction) ............... 20/ 20
03) REFRACTION (sph/cyl x axis) ................... -3.50+1.50x45
04) KERATOMETRY (steepest/flattest x axis) ........ 45.25/43.75x45
05) PACHYMETRY (CP) ............................... 0.535
06) PACHYMETRY (PC) ............................... 0.560
07) PACHYMETRY (MP) ............................... 0.600
08) PACHYMETRY (PP) ............................... 0.723
09) PACHYMETRY (FP) ............................... 0.789
10) CORNEAL DIAMETER (CD) ......................... 11.8 mm
11) CORNEA RIGIDITY (CR) .......................... 0.95
12) TONOMETRY (intraocular pressure) ............. 17 mmHg.
13) GLARE TESTER (Miller-Nadler) ................. 16/17
14) ENDOTHELIAL CELL COUNT ........................ ------
15) A-SCAN (axial length) ........................ 24.5 mm.
16) INCISION CONFIG (S,R,T,L,RL,RZ,RR,RT) ........ RT
17) BLADE TYPE (Xtal, Diamond, Razor, other) ..... LeCut
18) PACHYMETRY BIAS .............................. 100%


               PRESS <  ←  > TO ACCEPT DEFAULTS
```

astigmatism is less than the sphere

Fig. 9.29 RT procedure—page 2.

```
╭─────────────────────────────────────────────────────────────────╮
│                                                                   │
│  RK DATAMASTER PRE-OP CALCULATION SUMMARY .......... 07-04-1990   │
│                                                                   │
│  George Sigafoos - Left eye -- RT PROCEDURE                       │
│  ─────────────────────────────────────────────────               │
│                                                                   │
│      Sphere portion of procedure --                               │
│                                                                   │
│          RADIAL incisions ....................... 8               │
│          1st optic zone ......................... 4.25 mm         │
│          2nd optic zone ......................... 6.00 mm         │
│                                                                   │
│                                                                   │
│      Cylinder portion of procedure --                             │
│                                                                   │
│          TRANSVERSE incisions (T-cuts) per side .. 1              │
│          Length of T-cut ...................... 2.50 mm           │
│          1st T-cut optic zone ................. 6.00 mm           │
│          CONFIGURATION AXIS ................... 45 degrees        │
│                                                                   │
│  ─────────────────────────────────────────────                   │
│                                                                   │
│  Do you wish to print this table? (Y/N) ....................▓     │
│                                                                   │
╰─────────────────────────────────────────────────────────────────╯
```

this procedure has at least two radial OZs

Fig. 9.30 RT procedure—page 3.

Myopia Surgery Evaluation Sheet

Name: *Sigafoos, George*   Age: *28*   Date: *7/4/90*   Physician: *Bores*   Stage: *1*

VAs℞ ²⁰/200 c̄℞ ²⁰/20   Procedure: *RT*   Eye: *L*

Present Rx: _-3.50_ + _1.50_ X _45_ °

Refraction: _-3.50_ + _1.50_ X _45_ °

Keratometry: _45.25_ / _43.75_ X _45_

Pachymetry:

CP	PC	4	5	MP	PP	PP
.535	.560	.573	.587	.600	.723	.789

Blade setting:

R1	R2	R3	T1	T2	T3	T4
.570	.600	—	.590	—	—	—

Scleral rigidity: _.90_ Corneal diameter: _11.8_

Tonometry: _17_ Axial length: _24.5_

Microperforation (Y/N) - show location: ____

Notes: _____

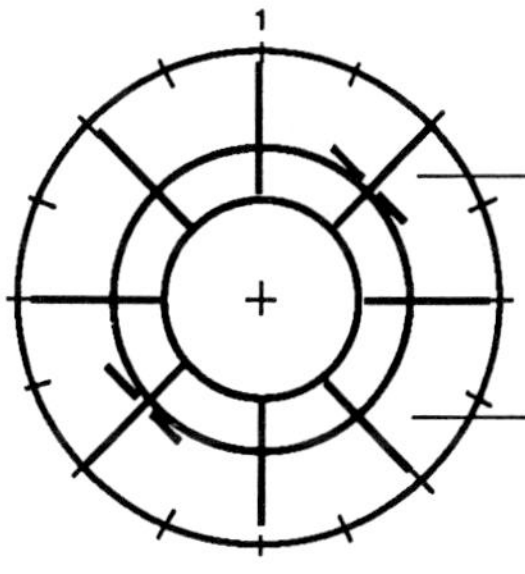

_____

T-cut optic zone: _6.00_ mm, T-cut length: _2.50_ mm

RK optic zone - 1st: _4.25_, 2nd: _6.00_, 3rd: ___ mm

ID: _2.0_ Blade: _DDE-2_ NI: _10_

Add/Re-cut incisions (A/R): __

Patient number: _____

computer entry made: __, by: ___, date: _____

© 1990 IFORE

T–cuts break at the radials

radials are **always** stepped, hence the 2 OZs

Fig. 9.31 RT procedure—surgical workup sheet.

Generally, the computer suggests what Dr Bores would normally do, but we'll look at the alternative when we finish with the RT case.

Page 2 displays the data input while page 3 presents the results of the calculation (Figures 9.29 and 9.30).

It is recommended that you fill out a form similar to the one shown in Figure 9.31 after determining the surgical parameters for the case. An example suitable for copying can be found in the Appendix.

The prudent keratotomist will draw out the in-

```
RK DATAMASTER PRE-OP CALCULATION SUMMARY .......... 07-04-1990

George Sigafoos - Left eye -- RL PROCEDURE -

   ID ------- 10          12          14          Incisions

   1.3        4.25        4.50        3.5x4.25

   1.6        4.75        5.00        4.00x5.25

   2.0        5.50        5.75        4.50x6.00

   2.5        6.25        6.50        5.00x6.75

NOTE:CHOOSE THE SURGICAL OZ FROM THE HIGHLIGHTED ZONES IN THE
TABLE ABOVE.

These have already been rounded to the nearest 0.25 mm.


Do you wish to print this table? (Y/N) ....................
```

note that OZ becomes elliptical when parallel incisions exceed 3 per side

Fig. 9.32 RL procedure—page 3, low-grade astigmatism.

Myopia Surgery Evaluation Sheet

Name: _Sigafoos, George_ Age: _28_ Date: _7/ 4/90_ Physician: _Bores_   Stage: _1_

VA s Rx ^{20}/200 c Rx ^{20}/20

Present Rx: _-3.50_ + _1.50_ X _45_ °

Refraction: _-3.50_ + _1.50_ X _45_ °

Keratometry: _45.25_ / _43.75_ X _45_

Pachymetry:

CP	PC	4	5	MP	PP	PP
.535	.560	.573	.587	.600	.723	.789

Blade setting:

R1	R2	R3	T1	T2	T3	T4
.590	—	—	—	—	—	—

Scleral rigidity: _.90_ Corneal diameter: _11.8_

Tonometry: _17_ Axial length: _24.5_

Microperforation (Y/N) - show location: ——

Notes: _____

Procedure: _RL_   Eye: _L_

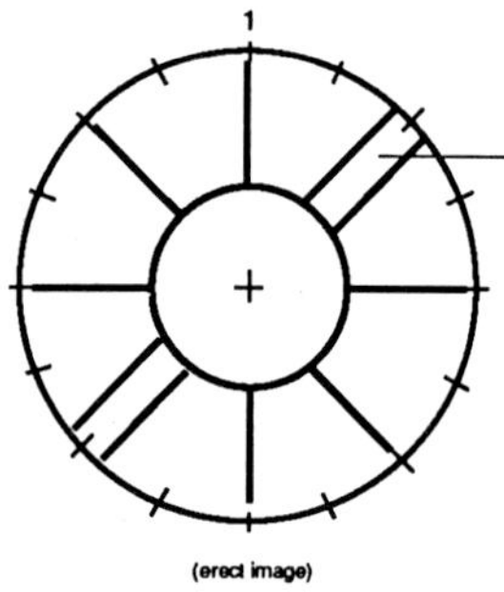

incisions parallel the **plus** astigmatic axis

(erect image)

T-cut optic zone: ——mm, T-cut length: ——mm
RK optic zone - 1st: _4.75_, 2nd: ——, 3rd: ——mm
ID: _1.6_ Blade: _DDE-2_   NI: _10_

Add/Re-cut incisions (A/R): ——

note number of incisions

Patient number: _____

computer entry made:——, by:——, date:————

© 1990 IFORE

Fig. 9.33 RL procedure—surgical workup sheet—case 1.

```
RK DATAMASTER PRE-OP CALCULATION SUMMARY ......... 07-04-1990

George Sigafoos - Left eye -- R PROCEDURE -

   ID ------- 6          8          12          16  Incisions

  1.3      2.50x3.75   2.75x4.25  3.00x4.50  3.50x5.00

  1.6      3.00x4.25   3.25x4.75  3.50x5.00  4.00x5.50

  2.0      3.50x5.00   4.00x5.50  4.25x5.75  4.50x6.25

  2.5      4.00x5.50   4.50x6.25  4.75x6.50  5.25x6.75


NOTE:CHOOSE THE SURGICAL OZ FROM THE HIGHLIGHTED ZONES IN THE
TABLE ABOVE.

These have already been rounded to the nearest 0.25 mm.


Do you wish to print this table? (Y/N) ....................
```

note that OZs are not round

Fig. 9.34 R procedure—page 3—case 1.

Myopia Surgery Evaluation Sheet

Name: _Sigafoos, George_ Age: _28_ Date: _7/4/90_ Physician: _Bores_ Stage: _1_

VA: s Rx ^{20}/200 c Rx ^{20}/20

Present Rx: _-3.50_ + _1.50_ X _45_ °

Refraction: _-3.50_ + _1.50_ X _45_ °

Keratometry: _45.25_ / _43.75_ X _45_

Pachymetry:

CP	PC	4	5	MP	PP	PP
.535	.560	.573	.587	.600	.723	.789

Blade setting:

R1	R2	R3	T1	T2	T3	T4
560	590	600	—	—	—	—

Scleral rigidity: _.90_ Corneal diameter: _11.8_

Tonometry: _17_ Axial length: _24.5_

Microperforation (Y/N) - show location: ___

Notes: _____

Procedure: _R_   Eye: _L_

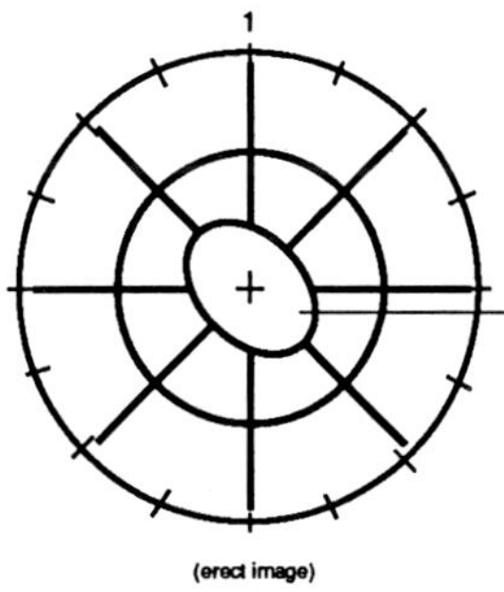

elliptical (oval) OZ

(erect image)

T-cut optic zone: ___ mm, T-cut length: ___ mm
RK optic zone - 1st: _3.25x4.75_, 2nd: _6.00_, 3rd: ___ mm
ID: _2.0_ Blade: _DDE-2_ NI: _8_

Add/Re-cut Incisions (A/R): ___

Patient number: _____

computer entry made: ___, by: ___, date: _____

© 1990 IFORE

Fig. 9.35 R procedure—surgical workup sheet—case 1.

```
┌─────────────────────────────────────────────────────────────────┐
│                                                                   │
│  RK DATAMASTER PRE-OP DATA ENTRY PROGRAM ............. Page 2      │
│                                                                   │
│  01) VISUAL ACUITY (without correction) ............. 20/ 200     │
│  02) VISUAL ACUITY (with correction) ................ 20/ 20      │
│  03) REFRACTION (sph/cyl x axis) .................... -1.50+1.50x45│
│  04) KERATOMETRY (steepest/flattest x axis) ........ 45.25/43.75x45│
│  05) PACHYMETRY (CP) ................................ 0.535        │
│  06) PACHYMETRY (PC) ................................ 0.560        │
│  07) PACHYMETRY (MP) ................................ 0.600        │
│  08) PACHYMETRY (PP) ................................ 0.723        │
│  09) PACHYMETRY (FP) ................................ 0.789        │
│  10) CORNEAL DIAMETER (CD) .......................... 11.8 mm      │
│  11) CORNEA RIGIDITY (CR) ........................... 0.95         │
│  12) TONOMETRY (intraocular pressure) ............... 17 mmHg.     │
│  13) GLARE TESTER (Miller-Nadler) ................... 16/17        │
│  14) ENDOTHELIAL CELL COUNT ......................... ------       │
│  15) A-SCAN (axial length) .......................... 24.5 mm.     │
│  16) INCISION CONFIG (S,R,T,L,RL,RZ,RR,RT) .......... T            │
│  17) BLADE TYPE (Xtal, Diamond, Razor, other) ....... LeCut        │
│  18) PACHYMETRY BIAS ................................ 100%         │
│                                                                   │
│  ───────────────────────────────────────────────────────────     │
│           PRESS < ◄── > TO ACCEPT DEFAULTS                         │
│                                                                   │
└─────────────────────────────────────────────────────────────────┘
```

astigmatism equals sphere

Fig. 9.36 T procedure—page 2—case 2.

```
┌─────────────────────────────────────────────────────────────────┐
│                                                                   │
│  RK DATAMASTER PRE-OP CALCULATION SUMMARY ......... 07-04-1990     │
│  ───────────────────────────────────────────────────────────     │
│  George Sigafoos - Left eye -- T PROCEDURE                        │
│  ───────────────────────────────────────────────────────────     │
│                                                                   │
│                                                                   │
│     Cylinder portion of procedure --                              │
│                                                                   │
│         TRANSVERSE incisions (T-cuts) per side .. 1               │
│         Length of T-cut ........................ 2.50 mm          │
│         1st T-cut optic zone ................... 6.00 mm          │
│         CONFIGURATION AXIS ..................... 45 degrees       │
│                                                                   │
│                                                                   │
│  ───────────────────────────────────────────────────────────     │
│  Do you wish to print this table? (Y/N) ....................█     │
│                                                                   │
└─────────────────────────────────────────────────────────────────┘
```

typical T–cut OZ

Fig. 9.37 T procedure—page 3—case 2.

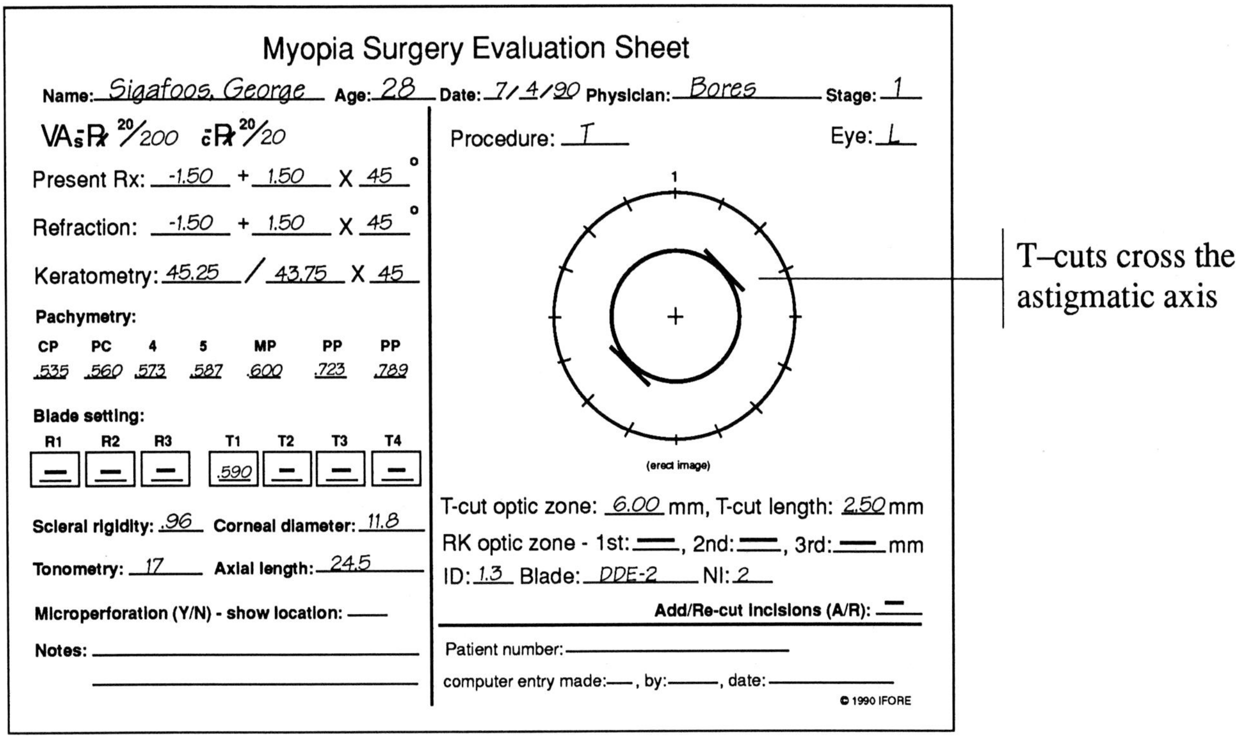

Myopia Surgery Evaluation Sheet

Name: *Sigafoos, George* Age: *28* Date: *7/4/90* Physician: *Bores* Stage: *1*

VA: R $\frac{20}{200}$ c̄R $\frac{20}{20}$

Present Rx: *-1.50* + *1.50* X *45* °

Refraction: *-1.50* + *1.50* X *45* °

Keratometry: *45.25* / *43.75* X *45*

Procedure: *T* Eye: *L*

(erect image)

T—cuts cross the astigmatic axis

Pachymetry:

CP	PC	4	5	MP	PP	PP
.535	.560	.573	.587	.600	.723	.789

Blade setting:

R1	R2	R3	T1	T2	T3	T4
—	—	—	.590	—	—	—

Scleral rigidity: *.96* Corneal diameter: *11.8*

Tonometry: *17* Axial length: *24.5*

Microperforation (Y/N) - show location: ——

Notes: _____

T-cut optic zone: *6.00* mm, T-cut length: *2.50* mm

RK optic zone - 1st: ——, 2nd: ——, 3rd: —— mm

ID: *1.3* Blade: *DDE-2* NI: *2*

Add/Re-cut incisions (A/R): —

Patient number: ——————————

computer entry made: ——, by: ——, date: ——————

© 1990 IFORE

Fig. 9.38 T procedure—surgical workup sheet—case 2.

cisional configuration for every astigmatic case prior to the day of surgery. It is too easy to place the incisions off-axis otherwise. This should be done after calculating the surgical parameters. Do not rely upon a drawing made by a computer from the data that you have input. This is so vital as to be worth repeating. There have been instances where invalid data have been used to construct a drawing in which the input data were changed later but not the drawing. It takes little imagination to follow that scenario to its end. By drawing out the configuration by hand you are forced to consider the data in the light of your experience. Never delegate this chore!

Case 1—RL procedure

Figures 9.32 and 9.33 illustrate the computer output if the RL (radial longitudinal) procedure is chosen for the procedure type instead of RT.

Case 1—R procedure

It is also possible to choose to do the procedure as an R incision type (Figures 9.34 and 9.35). Method R (for radial, formerly called A) was the first astigmatic incision configuration to be used. Its use is limited to up to 1.00 D of astigmatism. Generally speaking, that amount of astigmatism, especially if W-T-R, is often eliminated by performing straightforward spherical surgery. It has been found that as much as 1.50 D of

astigmatism can be lost in spherical surgery if the incisions are deep enough and there are 16 of them because of the tendency of the cornea to become spherical when incised. In this tendency the eye is obeying Pascal's law for fluid-filled spaces. It is probably this tendency of the cornea that accounts for the low incidence of induced post-operative astigmatism seen in this surgery. It has been the author's experience that patients tend to be a little more comfortable with a small amount of residual W-T-R astigmatism, however. Therefore, the need for this amount of W-T-R correction is not great. It is useful in oblique or A-T-R astigmatism and can be employed by the neophyte to lower greater amounts of astigmatism safely (up to 2.00 D, in which case 0.5 or 1.00 D will be corrected).

Case 2—T procedure

The next case is one of simple astigmatism. There are two possible configurations that may be used; however, the computer will suggest that a T configuration be employed (Figures 9.36 through 9.38). T-incisions affect both the major and minor axes so their lengths must be carefully controlled—so be advised. It is easier to get into trouble with T-incisions than with any other.

The depths of the incisions are expected to be no greater than 85% of the corneal thickness. Note that this is somewhat shallower than usually called for in radial keratotomy surgery. This depth is especially critical for T-cuts. It has been shown convincingly that deeper transverse incisions are prone to cause progressive flattening of the meridian and some increase in curvature in the opposite axis (see the discussion under the Ruiz procedure for further details). Usually only one transverse T-incision is made on each side but in some rare cases there may be two incisions per side.

Case 2—L procedure

By grouping the incisions into parallel bundles as in Method L (longitudinal), as much as 2.00 D can be corrected (Figures 9.39 and 9.40). This was the second configuration to be tried. While technically easier to perform, it seems less predictable and titratable than some other configurations. Methods L (longitudinal) and T (transverse) produce about the same amount of astigmatic correction—1.75 D—but the T method has a somewhat greater range of variance and is more incision depth-sensitive.

Case 3—RZ procedure

Method RZ (Ruiz or trapezoidal) of astigmatic correction combines semi-radial and tangential incisions to flatten the steepest meridian of the cornea. The technique controls different degrees of astigmatism by varying the size of the optical zone and the length of the transverse corneal incisions. The optical zones

used vary from 2.75 to 5.00 mm and the length of the transverse incisions varies from 1.5 to 5.00 mm.

It is very useful for myopic astigmatism in amounts from -2.50 D and above, and can be combined with six radial incisions (Method RR), to correct spherical myopia and is quite predictable and stable (Figures 9.41 through 9.43). Difficulties reported with this surgery are often due to the fact that the incisions are made either in excess of 85% depth or are too long.

There is an aspect to this technique that must be carefully borne in mind: the length of the incision not only affects the flattening in the steep axis, it also affects the opposite axis by steepening its curvature! This surgery can induce myopic astigmatism in the opposite axis very handily. This can be very dangerous. If the length of the transverse component is not carefully chosen and controlled, it is possible to reverse the astigmatism. This property makes the procedure very useful in mixed myopic astigmatism. For example: $-2.00 + 4.00 \times 90$ ($+2.00 - 4.00 \times 180$) can be converted to a plano sphere by judicious lengthening of the T-cuts (see below). In fact, the Ruiz procedure is the only technique currently available that can do so in a predictable manner. The Ruiz incision flattens the steeper meridian in an approximate ratio of 6:1 (see section on wedge versus Ruiz, below).

Case 3—T procedure

This possibility is shown out of interest (Figures 9.44 and 9.45). While paired T-cuts can be used in this

```
RK  DATAMASTER  PRE-OP  CALCULATION  SUMMARY ..........  07-04-1990

George Sigafoos - Left eye -- L PROCEDURE -

   ID ------- 4         6          8         10   Incisions

   1.3       4.25      4.50       5.00       5.25

   1.6       4.75      5.00       5.50       5.75

   2.0       5.50      5.75       6.25       6.50

   2.5       6.00      7.00       7.00       7.25

NOTE:CHOOSE THE SURGICAL OZ FROM THE HIGHLIGHTED ZONES IN THE
TABLE ABOVE.

These have already been rounded to the nearest 0.25 mm.

Do you wish to print this table? (Y/N) ................... ▨
```

OZ s are usually large

Fig. 9.39 L procedure—page 3—case 2.

Myopia Surgery Evaluation Sheet

Name: _Sigafoos, George_ Age: _28_ Date: _7/4/90_ Physician: _Bores_ Stage: _1_

VA: s℞ 20/200 c̄℞ 20/20

Present Rx: _-1.50_ + _1.50_ X _45_ °

Refraction: _-1.50_ + _1.50_ X _45_ °

Keratometry: _45.25_ / _43.75_ X _45_

Pachymetry:

CP	PC	4	5	MP	PP	PP
.535	.560	.573	.587	.600	.723	.789

Blade setting:

R1	R2	R3	T1	T2	T3	T4
.590	—	—	—	—	—	—

Scleral rigidity: _.99_ Corneal diameter: _11.8_

Tonometry: _17_ Axial length: _24.5_

Microperforation (Y/N) - show location: ——

Notes: _____

Procedure: _L_ Eye: _L_

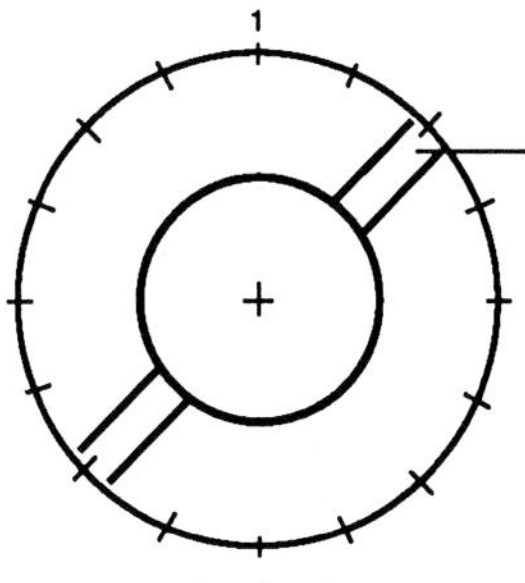

(erect image)

incisions are parallel

T-cut optic zone: ___ mm, T-cut length: ___ mm
RK optic zone - 1st: _4.75_, 2nd: ___, 3rd: ___ mm
ID: _1.6_ Blade: _DDE-2_ NI: _4_
Add/Re-cut incisions (A/R): ___

Patient number: _____

computer entry made: ——, by: ——, date: _____

© 1990 IFORE

Fig. 9.40 L procedure—surgical workup sheet—case 2.

```
RK DATAMASTER PRE-OP DATA ENTRY PROGRAM .............. Page 2


01) VISUAL ACUITY (without correction) ............ 20/ 200
02) VISUAL ACUITY (with correction) ................ 20/ 20
03) REFRACTION (sph/cyl x axis) .................... -2.50+2.50x45
04) KERATOMETRY (steepest/flattest x axis) ......... 45.25/42.75x45
05) PACHYMETRY (CP) ................................ 0.535
06) PACHYMETRY (PC) ................................ 0.560
07) PACHYMETRY (MP) ................................ 0.600
08) PACHYMETRY (PP) ................................ 0.723
09) PACHYMETRY (FP) ................................ 0.789
10) CORNEAL DIAMETER (CD) .......................... 11.8 mm
11) CORNEA RIGIDITY (CR) ........................... 0.95
12) TONOMETRY (intraocular pressure) .............. 17 mmHg.
13) GLARE TESTER (Miller-Nadler) .................. 16/17
14) ENDOTHELIAL CELL COUNT ........................ ------
15) A-SCAN (axial length) ......................... 24.5 mm.
16) INCISION CONFIG (S,R,T,L,RL,RZ,RR,RT) ......... RZ
17) BLADE TYPE (Xtal, Diamond, Razor, other) ...... LeCut
18) PACHYMETRY BIAS ............................... 100%




       PRESS <  ◄┘  > TO ACCEPT DEFAULTS
```

astigmatism equals sphere

Fig. 9.41 RZ procedure—page 2—case 3.

```
RK DATAMASTER PRE-OP CALCULATION SUMMARY .......... 07-04-1990

George Sigafoos - Left eye -- RUIZ PROCEDURE


RUIZ optical zone ...................... 4.0 mm
TRANSVERSE incision (ladders) LENGTH .... 1.5 mm
CONFIGURATION AXIS ..................... 45 deg
Estimated residual refraction .......... 0.2 dptrs




Do you wish to print this table? (Y/N) ....................
```

note ladder length

Fig. 9.42 RZ procedure—page 3—case 3.

Myopia Surgery Evaluation Sheet

Name: _Sigafoos, George_ Age: _28_ Date: _7/4/90_ Physician: _Bores_ Stage: _1_

VA: sR ^{20}/200 cR ^{20}/20   Procedure: _RZ_   Eye: _L_

Present Rx: _-2.50_ + _2.50_ X _45_ °

Refraction: _-2.50_ + _2.50_ X _45_ °

Keratometry: _45.25_ / _42.75_ X _45_

Pachymetry:

CP	PC	4	5	MP	PP	PP
.535	.560	.573	.587	.600	.723	.789

Blade setting:

R1	R2	R3	T1	T2	T3	T4
—	—	—	.570	.590	.710	.780

Scleral rigidity: _.90_ Corneal diameter: _11.8_

Tonometry: _17_ Axial length: _24.5_

Microperforation (Y/N) - show location: ___

Notes: _____

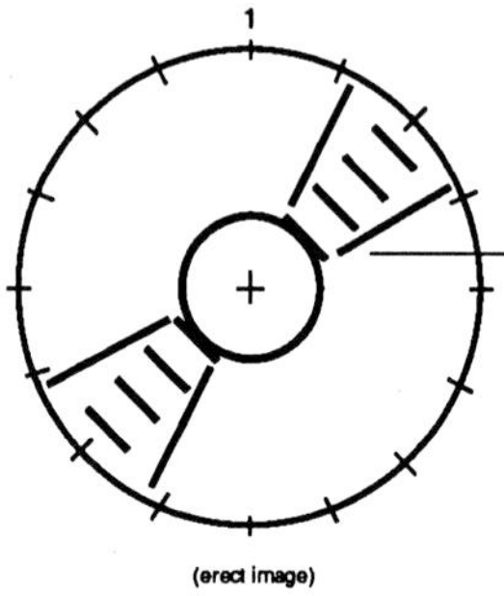

radials **do not** join the ladders

(erect image)

T-cut optic zone: _4.00_ mm, T-cut length: _1.5_ mm
RK optic zone - 1st:__, 2nd:__, 3rd:__ mm
ID: _1.3_ Blade: _DDE-2_ NI: _12_

Add/Re-cut incisions (A/R): __

Patient number: _____
computer entry made:__ , by:___, date: ____
© 1990 IFORE

Fig. 9.43 RZ procedure—surgical workup sheet—case 3.

```
RK DATAMASTER PRE-OP CALCULATION SUMMARY ......... 07-04-1990

George Sigafoos - Left eye -- T PROCEDURE
_____



     Cylinder portion of procedure --

        TRANSVERSE incisions (T-cuts) per side .. 2
        Length of T-cut ....................... 2.50 mm
        1st T-cut optic zone .................. 5.00 mm
        2nd T-cut optic zone .................. 7.00 mm
        CONFIGURATION AXIS ....................   45 degrees




     _____

Do you wish to print this table? (Y/N) ...................▓
```

note there are 2 T–cut OZs

Fig. 9.44 T procedure—page 3—case 3.

Myopia Surgery Evaluation Sheet

Name: *Sigafoos, George* Age: *28* Date: *7/4/90* Physician: *Bores* Stage: *1*

VA: s̄Rx 20/200 c̄Rx 20/20

Present Rx: *-2.50* + *2.50* X *45* °

Refraction: *-2.50* + *2.50* X *45* °

Keratometry: *45.25* / *42.75* X *45*

Procedure: *T*   Eye: *L*

Pachymetry:

CP	PC	4	5	MP	PP	PP
.535	.560	.573	.587	.600	.723	.789

Blade setting:

R1	R2	R3	T1	T2	T3	T4
—	—	—	.580	.650	—	—

Scleral rigidity: *.95* Corneal diameter: *11.8*

Tonometry: *17* Axial length: *24.5*

Microperforation (Y/N) - show location: —

Notes: ____

T-cut optic zone: *5/7* mm, T-cut length: *2.50* mm
RK optic zone - 1st: —, 2nd: —, 3rd: — mm
ID: *1.3* Blade: *DDE-2* NI: *4*
Add/Re-cut incisions (A/R): ____

Patient number: ____
computer entry made: —, by: —, date: ____
© 1990 IFORE

(erect image)

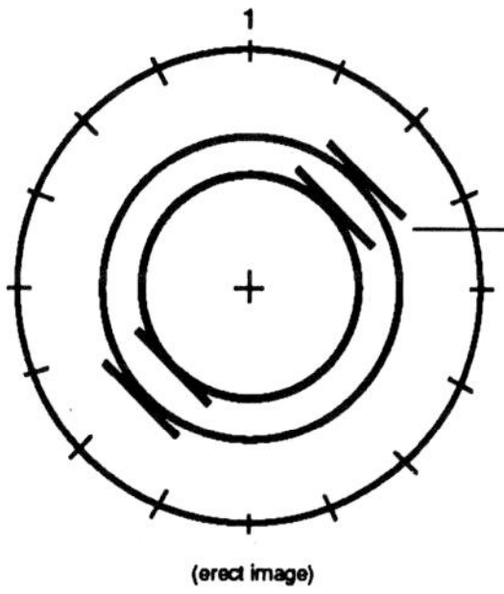

paired T–cuts, 2.5 mm length on each side

Fig. 9.45 T procedure—surgical workup sheet—case 3.

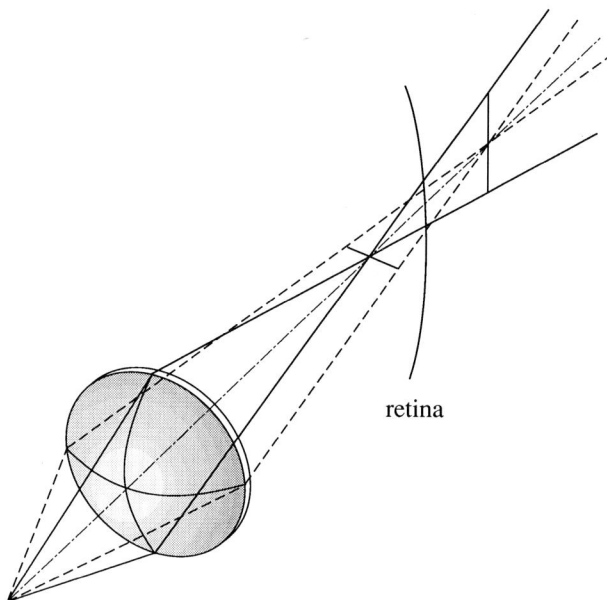

Fig. 9.46 Mixed astigmatism.

manner, there are better methods available. There are, however, instances where such a technique may be the best of choices.

Case 4—RZ procedure

The next two cases illustrate the use of the RZ method in mixed astigmatism (Figure 9.46). This procedure is the only form of relaxing incision technique effective

for this type of astigmatism. The degree of associated hyperopia has been varied to illustrate the changes made in the incisions (Figures 9.47 through 9.49).

Case 5—RZ procedure

Here the hyperopic component is much higher requiring longer transverse (ladder) incisions to be made (Figures 9.50 through 9.52). Further discussion of this will be found in the section on technique, below.

Case 6—RR procedure

If there is spherical myopia associated with the astigmatism (compound myopic astigmatism; Figure 9.53), it can be attenuated with six radial incisions added on either side of the trapezoidal incisions and arranged around an appropriate optical zone or zones. This procedure is called the RR (radial Ruiz) procedure. The optical zone size for this part of the surgery is automatically calculated in the RK DataMaster program. A six-ray radial marker is invaluable to mark the position of the six incisions. Cases 6 and 7 are examples of such calculations (Figures 9.54 through 9.59).

Case 7—RR procedure

Finally, it has been said before but it will be repeated: the use of these programs pre-supposes a working knowledge of the surgical technique of radial keratotomy as practiced and taught by L.D. Bores, MD and

```
RK DATAMASTER PRE-OP DATA ENTRY PROGRAM .............. Page 2

01) VISUAL ACUITY (without correction) ............ 20/ 200
02) VISUAL ACUITY (with correction) ............... 20/ 20
03) REFRACTION (sph/cyl x axis) ................... -3.00+4.00x45
04) KERATOMETRY (steepest/flattest x axis) ........ 45.00/41.50x45
05) PACHYMETRY (CP) ............................... 0.535
06) PACHYMETRY (PC) ............................... 0.560
07) PACHYMETRY (MP) ............................... 0.600
08) PACHYMETRY (PP) ............................... 0.723
09) PACHYMETRY (FP) ............................... 0.789
10) CORNEAL DIAMETER (CD) ......................... 11.8 mm
11) CORNEA RIGIDITY (CR) .......................... 0.90
12) TONOMETRY (intraocular pressure) .............. 17 mmHg.
13) GLARE TESTER (Miller-Nadler) .................. 16/17
14) ENDOTHELIAL CELL COUNT ........................ ------
15) A-SCAN (axial length) ......................... 24.5 mm.
16) INCISION CONFIG (S,R,T,L,RL,RZ,RR,RT) ......... RZ
17) BLADE TYPE (Xtal, Diamond, Razor, other) ...... LeCut
18) PACHYMETRY BIAS ............................... 100%


            PRESS <  ◄┘  > TO ACCEPT DEFAULTS
```

astigmatism greater than sphere

Fig. 9.47 RZ procedure—page 2—case 4.

```
RK DATAMASTER PRE-OP CALCULATION SUMMARY .......... 07-04-1990

George Sigafoos - Left eye -- RUIZ PROCEDURE


RUIZ optical zone ...................... 4.0 mm
TRANSVERSE incision (ladders) LENGTH .... 3.5 mm
CONFIGURATION AXIS ..................... 45 deg
Estimated residual refraction ........... .04 dptrs




Do you wish to print this table? (Y/N) ....................
```

ladder length is increased

Fig. 9.48 RZ procedure—page 3—case 4.

Myopia Surgery Evaluation Sheet

Name: _Sigafoos, George_ Age: _28_ Date: _7/4/90_ Physician: _Bores_ Stage: _1_

VAsRx 20/200 cRx 20/20   Procedure: _RZ_   Eye: _L_

Present Rx: _-3.00_ + _4.00_ X _45_ °

Refraction: _-3.00_ + _4.00_ X _45_ °

Keratometry: _45.00_ / _4150_ X _45_

Pachymetry:

CP	PC	4	5	MP	PP	PP
.535	.560	.573	.587	.600	.723	.789

Blade setting:

R1	R2	R3	T1	T2	T3	T4
—	—	—	.570	.590	.710	.780

Scleral rigidity: _.90_ Corneal diameter: _11.8_

Tonometry: _17_ Axial length: _24.5_

Microperforation (Y/N) - show location: —

Notes: _____

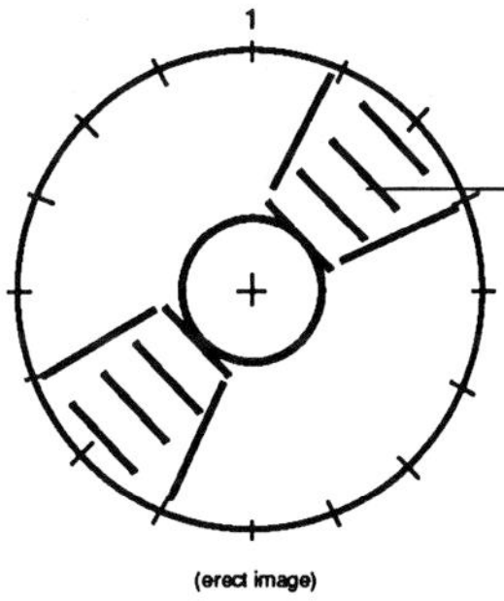

longer ladders

T-cut optic zone: _4.00_ mm, T-cut length: _3.50_ mm
RK optic zone - 1st:—, 2nd:—, 3rd:— mm
ID: _1.3_ Blade: _DDE-2_ NI: _12_
Add/Re-cut incisions (A/R): —
Patient number: _____
computer entry made:—, by:—, date:——
© 1990 IFORE

Fig. 9.49 RZ procedure—surgical workup sheet—case 4.

```
┌─────────────────────────────────────────────────────────────┐
│                                                               │
│  RK DATAMASTER PRE-OP DATA ENTRY PROGRAM ............. Page 2 │
│ ─────────────────────────────────────────────────────────────│
│                                                               │
│  01) VISUAL ACUITY (without correction) ............ 20/ 200  │
│  02) VISUAL ACUITY (with correction) ................ 20/ 20  │
│  03) REFRACTION (sph/cyl x axis) .................... -3.00+5.00x45 │
│  04) KERATOMETRY (steepest/flattest x axis) ........ 46.00/41.50x45 │
│  05) PACHYMETRY (CP) ................................ 0.535    │
│  06) PACHYMETRY (PC) ................................ 0.560    │
│  07) PACHYMETRY (MP) ................................ 0.600    │
│  08) PACHYMETRY (PP) ................................ 0.723    │
│  09) PACHYMETRY (FP) ................................ 0.789    │
│  10) CORNEAL DIAMETER (CD) .......................... 11.8 mm  │
│  11) CORNEA RIGIDITY (CR) ........................... 0.90     │
│  12) TONOMETRY (intraocular pressure) .............. 17 mmHg.  │
│  13) GLARE TESTER (Miller-Nadler) .................. 16/17     │
│  14) ENDOTHELIAL CELL COUNT ........................ ------    │
│  15) A-SCAN (axial length) ......................... 24.5 mm.  │
│  16) INCISION CONFIG (S,R,T,L,RL,RZ,RR,RT) ......... RZ        │
│  17) BLADE TYPE (Xtal, Diamond, Razor, other) ...... LeCut     │
│  18) PACHYMETRY BIAS ............................... 100%      │
│                                                               │
│ ─────────────────────────────────────────────────────────────│
│          PRESS <  ←┘  > TO ACCEPT DEFAULTS                    │
└─────────────────────────────────────────────────────────────┘
```
astigmatism greater than sphere

Fig. 9.50 RZ procedure—page 2—case 5.

```
┌─────────────────────────────────────────────────────────────┐
│                                                               │
│  RK DATAMASTER PRE-OP CALCULATION SUMMARY .......... 07-04-1990│
│ ─────────────────────────────────────────────────────────────│
│  George Sigafoos - Left eye -- RUIZ PROCEDURE                 │
│ ─────────────────────────────────────────────────────────────│
│  RUIZ optical zone ..................... 4.0 mm               │
│  TRANSVERSE incision (ladders) LENGTH .... 5.0 mm             │
│  CONFIGURATION AXIS ..................... 45 deg              │
│  Estimated residual refraction .......... .16 dptrs           │
│ ─────────────────────────────────────────────────────────────│
│                                                               │
│  Do you wish to print this table? (Y/N) ................▓     │
└─────────────────────────────────────────────────────────────┘
```
ladder length is increased

Fig. 9.51 RZ procedure—page 3—case 5.

Myopia Surgery Evaluation Sheet

Name: _Sigafoos, George_ Age: _28_ Date: _7/4/90_ Physician: _Bores_ Stage: _1_

VAsPx 20/200 cPx 20/20

Procedure: _RZ_   Eye: _L_

Present Rx: _-3.00_ + _5.00_ X _45_ °

Refraction: _-3.00_ + _5.00_ X _45_ °

Keratometry: _46.00_ / _41.50_ X _45_

Pachymetry:

CP	PC	4	5	MP	PP	PP
.535	.560	.573	.587	.600	.723	.789

Blade setting:

R1	R2	R3	T1	T2	T3	T4
—	—	—	.570	.590	.710	.780

Scleral rigidity: _.90_ Corneal diameter: _11.8_

Tonometry: _17_ Axial length: _24.5_

Microperforation (Y/N) - show location: ——

Notes: ——————

(erect image)

T–cuts (ladders) should not exceed 5 mm length

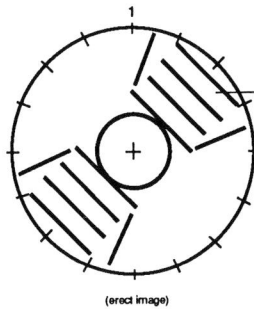

T-cut optic zone: _4.00_ mm, T-cut length: _5.00_ mm

RK optic zone - 1st: ——, 2nd: ——, 3rd: —— mm

ID: _1.3_ Blade: _DDE-2_ NI: _12_

Add/Re-cut Incisions (A/R): ——

Patient number: ——————

computer entry made: ——, by: ——, date: ——————

© 1990 IFORE

Fig. 9.52 RZ procedure—surgical workup sheet—case 5.

retina

Fig. 9.53 Compound myopic astigmatism.

S.N. Fyodorov, MD. The results of these calculations are to be used as guidelines to the proper performance of the surgery but are no substitute for the experience and surgical judgment of the surgeon.

Basic preparation, caveats, and methods

The surgery is performed under topical anesthesia in a pre-medicated patient—beware retro-bulbar injections. The anesthetic used is 0.5% tetracaine, followed by 1.0% non-buffered tetracaine (Pontocaine) drops. Any additional anesthesia required during the case is provided by the application of additional 0.5% tetracaine. Occasionally for patients complaining of discomfort from fixation (particularly in second-stage cases), 10% cocaine solution is applied to the limbus on a cotton pledget or applicator. Sedation is provided by the administration of oral diazepam (Valium) in a dose appropriate to the patient. Generally this will be 10 mg given approximately 30–40 min prior to surgery.

As in spherical cases, the workup is taped or otherwise placed next to the operating microscope in plain view of the surgeon. The patient is placed supine upon the operating table and the eye is prepped with full strength Betadine solution (Betadine preparation is not recommended because it contains soap which is extremely hard on the corneal epithelium). The microscope is then centered and adjusted and the surgeon scrubs up. At the Bores Eye Institute we have successfully used Septisol skin preparation foam for this purpose for years. Draping is done using the aperture drape supplied by the Alcon Company (102320).

The blade used is a Bores, double-edged uni-crystalline sapphire or diamond blade (Katena K2-6513, or the Western Instruments WMK-200, LeCut) mounted in the Katena (Bores) micrometer handle (K2-6505).

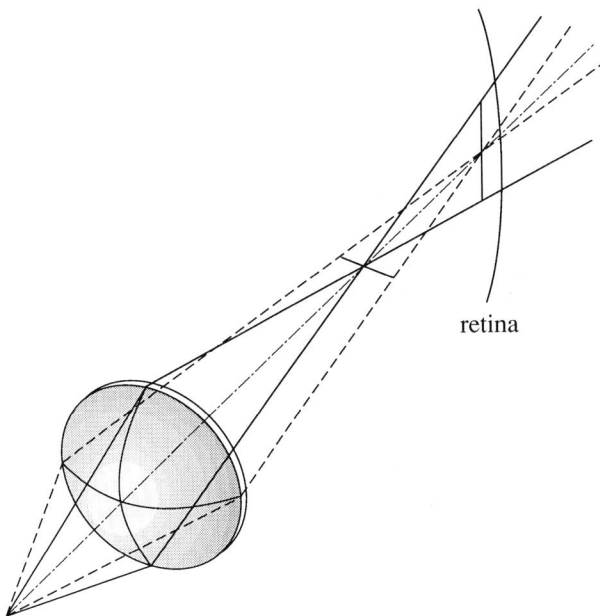

```
┌─────────────────────────────────────────────────────────────┐
│                                                               │
│  RK DATAMASTER PRE-OP DATA ENTRY PROGRAM ............. Page 2 │
│                                                               │
│  01) VISUAL ACUITY (without correction) ............. 20/ 200 │
│  02) VISUAL ACUITY (with correction) ................ 20/ 20  │
│  03) REFRACTION (sph/cyl x axis) .................... -4.50+2.50x45 │
│  04) KERATOMETRY (steepest/flattest x axis) ......... 45.25/42.75x45 │
│  05) PACHYMETRY (CP) ................................ 0.535    │
│  06) PACHYMETRY (PC) ................................ 0.560    │
│  07) PACHYMETRY (MP) ................................ 0.600    │
│  08) PACHYMETRY (PP) ................................ 0.723    │
│  09) PACHYMETRY (FP) ................................ 0.789    │
│  10) CORNEAL DIAMETER (CD) .......................... 11.8 mm  │
│  11) CORNEA RIGIDITY (CR) ........................... 0.95     │
│  12) TONOMETRY (intraocular pressure) ............... 17 mmHg. │
│  13) GLARE TESTER (Miller-Nadler) ................... 16/17    │
│  14) ENDOTHELIAL CELL COUNT ......................... ------   │
│  15) A-SCAN (axial length) .......................... 24.5 mm. │
│  16) INCISION CONFIG (S,R,T,L,RL,RZ,RR,RT) .......... RR       │
│  17) BLADE TYPE (Xtal, Diamond, Razor, other) ....... LeCut    │
│  18) PACHYMETRY BIAS ................................ 100%     │
│                                                               │
│                                                               │
│                                                               │
│         PRESS <  ◄─┘  > TO ACCEPT DEFAULTS                     │
│                                                               │
└─────────────────────────────────────────────────────────────┘
```

moderate myopia and astigmatism

Fig. 9.54 RR procedure—page 2—case 6.

```
┌─────────────────────────────────────────────────────────────┐
│                                                               │
│  RK DATAMASTER PRE-OP CALCULATION SUMMARY ......... 07-04-1990 │
│                                                               │
│  George Sigafoos - Left eye -- COMBINED RK/RUIZ PROCEDURE     │
│                                                               │
│  RUIZ optical zone ...................... 4.0 mm              │
│  TRANSVERSE incision (ladders) LENGTH .... 1.5 mm             │
│  CONFIGURATION AXIS ..................... 45 deg              │
│                                                               │
│  CHOOZE OZ FOR 6 RADIAL INCISIONS --   ID:    OPTICAL ZONE:   │
│                                                               │
│                                       1.3       4.75          │
│                                       1.6       5.50          │
│                                       2.0       6.00          │
│                                       2.5       6.75          │
│                                                               │
│  NOTE:CHOOSE THE RADIAL INCISION OZ FROM THE HIGHLIGHTED ZONES │
│  IN THE TABLE ABOVE.                                          │
│                                                               │
│  These have already been rounded to the nearest 0.25 mm.     │
│                                                               │
│  Do you wish to print this table? (Y/N) ..................▓   │
│                                                               │
└─────────────────────────────────────────────────────────────┘
```

note length of ladders

only one OZ available

Fig. 9.55 RR procedure—page 3—case 6.

There are two other blades available for this handle. One has a single, 30°, angled cutting edge designed for the American (Bores) method of incising from the optical zone to the periphery—K2-6501. The other has a vertical cutting edge for use with the Russian (Fyodorov) technique from the periphery toward the center, for re-incising old wounds and for making T-incisions—K2-6511. The single-edged blades are recommended for the beginning surgeon as they are more durable. The blade is set utilizing the XTAL-800,

Myopia Surgery Evaluation Sheet

Name: _Sigafoos, George_   Age: _28_   Date: _7/4/90_   Physician: _Bores_   Stage: _1_

VA̱s R̶x ²⁰/₂₀₀ c̄ R̶x ²⁰/₂₀   Procedure: _RR_   Eye: _L_

Present Rx: _-4.50_ + _2.50_ X _45_ °

Refraction: _-4.50_ + _2.50_ X _45_ °

Keratometry: _45.25_ / _42.75_ X _45_

Pachymetry:

CP	PC	4	5	MP	PP	PP
.535	.560	.573	.587	.600	.723	.789

Blade setting:

R1	R2	R3	T1	T2	T3	T4
.580	—	—	.570	.590	.710	.780

Scleral rigidity: _.90_   Corneal diameter: _11.8_

Tonometry: _17_   Axial length: _24.5_

Microperforation (Y/N) - show location: ——

Notes: _____

_____

note that there are 2 OZ s — one for the astigmatism, one for the sphere

(erect image)

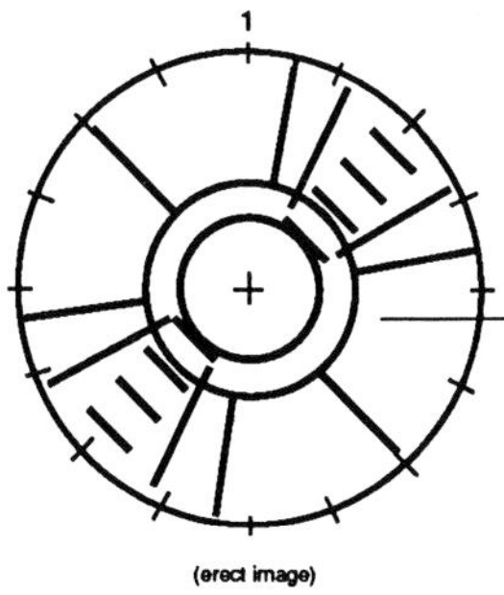

T-cut optic zone: _4.00_ mm, T-cut length: _1.5_ mm

RK optic zone - 1st: _4.75_, 2nd: ——, 3rd: —— mm

ID: _1.3_ Blade: _DDE-2_   NI: _18_

Add/Re-cut incisions (A/R): __—__

Patient number: _____

computer entry made: ——, by: ——, date: ——

© 1990 IFORE

Fig. 9.56 RR procedure—surgical workup sheet—case 6.

```
RK DATAMASTER PRE-OP DATA ENTRY PROGRAM .............. Page 2


01) VISUAL ACUITY (without correction) ............ 20/ 200
02) VISUAL ACUITY (with correction) ................ 20/ 20
03) REFRACTION (sph/cyl x axis) ................... -10.00+5.50x45
04) KERATOMETRY (steepest/flattest x axis) ........ 47.00/42.00x45
05) PACHYMETRY (CP) ............................... 0.535
06) PACHYMETRY (PC) ............................... 0.560
07) PACHYMETRY (MP) ............................... 0.600
08) PACHYMETRY (PP) ............................... 0.723
09) PACHYMETRY (FP) ............................... 0.789
10) CORNEAL DIAMETER (CD) ......................... 11.8 mm
11) CORNEA RIGIDITY (CR) .......................... 0.80
12) TONOMETRY (intraocular pressure) ............. 17 mmHg.
13) GLARE TESTER (Miller-Nadler) ................. 16/17
14) ENDOTHELIAL CELL COUNT ........................ ------
15) A-SCAN (axial length) ........................ 24.5 mm.
16) INCISION CONFIG (S,R,T,L,RL,RZ,RR,RT) ......... RR
17) BLADE TYPE (Xtal, Diamond, Razor, other) ...... LeCut
18) PACHYMETRY BIAS .............................. 100%



           PRESS <  ◄┘  > TO ACCEPT DEFAULTS
```

myopia and astigmatism both high

be sure that proper configuration has been entered

Fig. 9.57 RR procedure—page 2—case 7.

Bores shadowgraphic blade gauge (see the section on instrumentation, above). The blade is over-set according to the desired incisional depth coefficient and the blade type and style (see Chapter 8).

Establishing the optic center and marking the surgical zones are accomplished as usual. Keep in mind that it is frequently the case that the optic center is displaced somewhat nasally. This is normal. Do not

```
RK DATAMASTER PRE-OP CALCULATION SUMMARY ......... 07-04-1990

George Sigafoos - Left eye -- COMBINED RK/RUIZ PROCEDURE


RUIZ optical zone ..................... 3.0 mm
TRANSVERSE incision (ladders) LENGTH .... 1.5 mm
CONFIGURATION AXIS ..................... 45 deg

CHOOZE OZ FOR 6 RADIAL INCISIONS --    ID:      OPTICAL ZONE:

                                       1.3        1.75
                                       1.6        2.25
                                       2.0        2.50
                                       2.5        3.00

NOTE:CHOOSE THE RADIAL INCISION OZ FROM THE HIGHLIGHTED ZONES
IN THE TABLE ABOVE.

These have already been rounded to the nearest 0.25 mm.


Do you wish to print this table? (Y/N) ....................
```

only one OZ available for the radial portion

Fig. 9.58 RR procedure—page 3—case 7.

Myopia Surgery Evaluation Sheet

Name: Sigafoos, George   Age: 28   Date: 7/4/90   Physician: Bores   Stage: 1

VA: sRx 20/200 cRx 20/20

Present Rx: -10.00 + 5.50 X 45°

Refraction: -10.00 + 5.50 X 45°

Keratometry: 47.00 / 42.00 X 45

Pachymetry:

CP	PC	4	5	MP	PP	PP
.535	.560	.573	.587	.600	.723	.789

Blade setting:

R1	R2	R3	T1	T2	T3	T4
.560	.600	.720	.570	.590	.710	.780

Scleral rigidity: .80   Corneal diameter: 11.8

Tonometry: 17   Axial length: 24.5

Microperforation (Y/N) - show location: —

Notes: _____

Procedure: RR   Eye: L

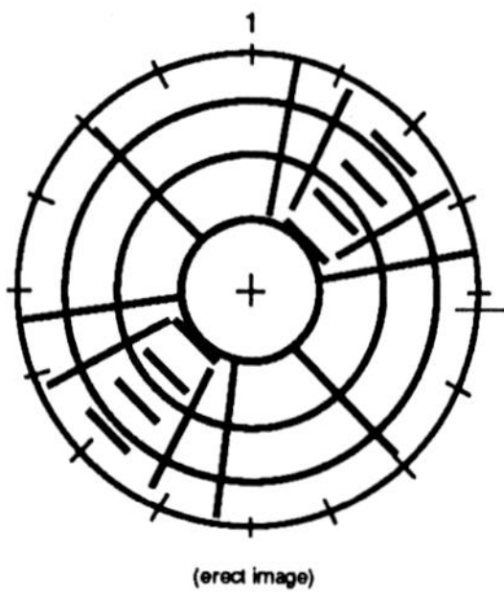

(erect image)

T-cut optic zone: 3.00 mm, T-cut length: 1.5 mm
RK optic zone - 1st: 3.00, 2nd: 6.00, 3rd: 8.00 mm
ID: (2.5) Blade: DDE-2   NI: 18
Add/Re-cut incisions (A/R): —

Patient number: _____
computer entry made:—, by:—, date:—
© 1990 IFORE

there are 3 OZ s in this case (see incisional depth coefficient — circled)

Fig. 9.59 RR procedure—surgical workup sheet—case 7.

(a)

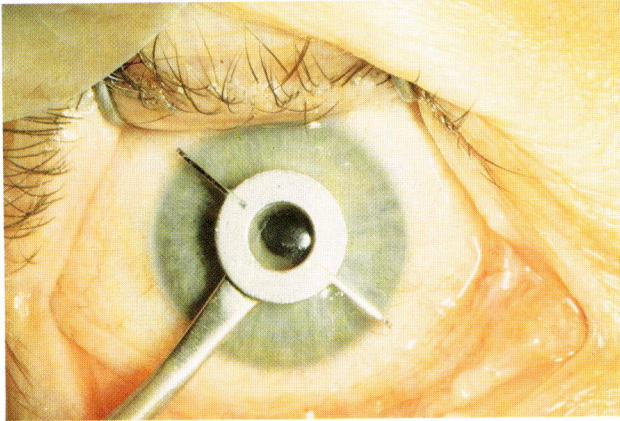

(b)

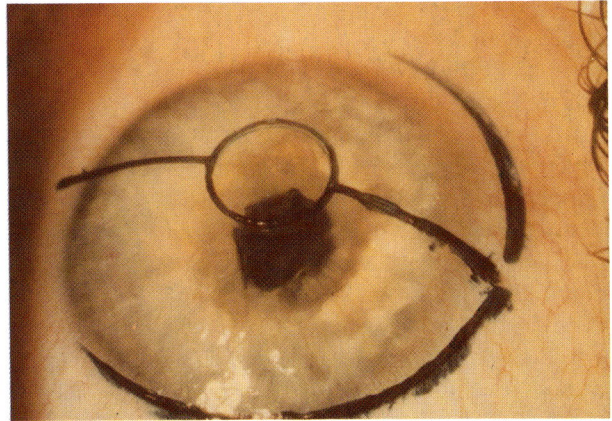

Fig. 9.60 (a) The axis is marked on the cornea after the visual axis is spotted. (b) It helps to use some dye on the marker.

position the incisions in the anatomic center of the cornea or induced oblique astigmatism will result.

Marking the steep meridian

The correct plus cylinder axis is checked by referring to the workup sheet and repeating the axis to the circulating nurse or assistant. The axis is verified by the assistant by reference to the patient's original record. To avoid mistakes, only the particular patient's record is brought into the operating theater. Following this the patient is again requested to fixate on the microscope light and without holding the patient's eye, the axis of the cylinder is marked with the axis marker. To do this properly, some sort of reticle is necessary in the microscope eye piece. There are several products available for this purpose (see the section on instrumentation, above).

Regardless of the device used, some method must be employed to orient the surgeon properly with respect to the 12 and 6 o'clock positions of the patient's cornea. This is readily done by seating the patient at the slit-lamp with the eye anesthetized and the head held vertical. With the patient looking straight ahead, the 12 and 6 o'clock positions are marked off on the cornea near the limbus. The patient is then taken into the operating theater.

The Bores axis marker is aligned with the chosen orientation device and pressed on to the corneal surface marking the plus axis (Figure 9.60). It is helpful to coat the blade of the marker with gentian violet or brilliant green first to make a more noticeable mark. This is most important in cases of re-operations where sometimes an old incision can be mistaken for the axis mark.

The primary optical zone is then marked concentric

to the fixation point, not to the pupil. This is extremely important because the pupil is not concentric with the optic axis of the eye. To verify the centration of the optic center with the optical zone mark, the patient is asked to look away and then back at the light. Any discrepancy is corrected and the mid peripheral zone(s), if any, are then marked and the surgery begins.

The basic surgical technique is similar to that utilized in marking for spherical myopia; however, one additional factor has been introduced—axis of plus cylinder. Because the optical zone in astigmatism can be an ellipsoid (with a long and a short dimension), any elliptic marker must be applied to the cornea with the narrow side aligned with the plus cylinder axis (Figure 9.61).

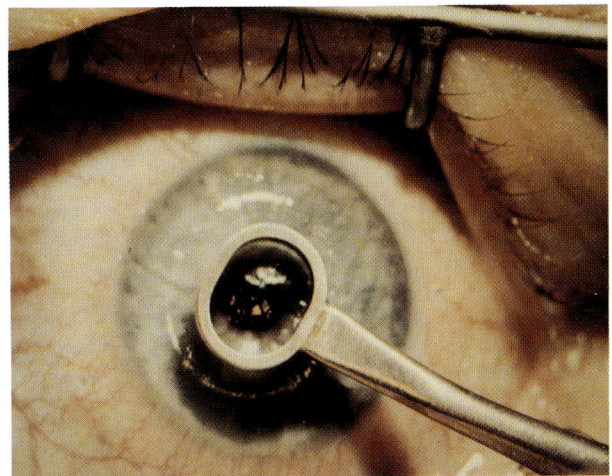

Fig. 9.61 The primary optical clear zone is then marked. Note, in the case of an elliptic zone, that the narrow portion is perpendicular to the axis.

If a third zone is to be used (i.e. the incision is to have three steps as in a case needing a 2.5 incisional depth coefficient), this zone is usually marked *after* the first part of the incision is made. Experience has shown that marking this zone before-hand often finds the mark faded-out before it's time to reference it. This is especially the case with beginning surgeons. If that happens to you and you don't choose to wait to make that last mark, use dye to make the mark last longer.

If a perforation is encountered, the surgery can be continued if extensive leakage does not occur and the eye does not get too soft; otherwise the case must be abandoned. Further surgery should be postponed for at least 2 weeks. Most patients, even in the face of a severe leak (very rare), will have a deep AC the following morning. No attempt at free-hand deepening should be made in any case with a leak and a shallow or flat chamber. Suturing should rarely be necessary.

Patients receive a course of steroid-antibiotic (Tobradex) drops b.i.d. for 2 weeks. Patients with perforations receive oral broad-spectrum antibiotics (Keflex) and mydriatics for an appropriate period of time. Patients are followed at 2, 4, 8, 12, 26, and 52 weeks when possible. Any necessary second-stage surgery is deferred for at least 6 months (see also Chapter 8).

Radial keratotomy—surgical techniques and methods

Method R

Method R (for radial, formerly called method A; Figure 9.62) was the first configuration to be employed by Fyodorov. Its use is limited to up to 1.00 D of astigmatism. Generally speaking, however, that amount of astigmatism, especially if it's W-T-R, is often eliminated by performing straightforward spherical sur-

gery. It has been found that as much as 1.50 D of astigmatism can be lost in spherical surgery if the incisions are deep enough and there are 16 of them, because of the tendency of the cornea to become spherical when incised. In this tendency the eye is obeying Pascal's law for fluid-filled spaces. It is probably this tendency of the eye that accounts for the low incidence of induced post-operative astigmatism seen in spherical surgery.

It has been the author's experience that patients tend to be a little more comfortable with a small amount of residual W-T-R astigmatism. Therefore, the need for this amount of W-T-R correction is not great and thus the R-procedure finds little application. It is useful in oblique or A-T-R astigmatism and can be employed by the neophyte to lower greater amounts of astigmatism safely (up to 2.00 D, in which case 0.5, or 1.00 D will be corrected).

This surgery is the simplest of all the configuration types to perform and is a good way for the new physician to get his/her "feet wet." The axis of plus cylinder is marked on the cornea in the manner previously described. An elliptic optical zone marker is used for the first or primary optical clear zone. If the computer calls for a secondary incision deepening or step, the optical zone for that step is a standard zone marker—usually a 6 mm (sometimes a 7 mm). Rarely will an 8 mm marker be required. The necessary surgical zones are marked and the incisions are made with a standard blade as if performing a simple case for spherical myopia.

Method RL

By grouping the incisions into parallel bundles as in Method RL (for radial longitudinal, formerly B; Figure 9.63) as much as 2.00 D can be corrected. This was the second astigmatic configuration Fyodorov tried. While technically more difficult to perform, it is more pre-

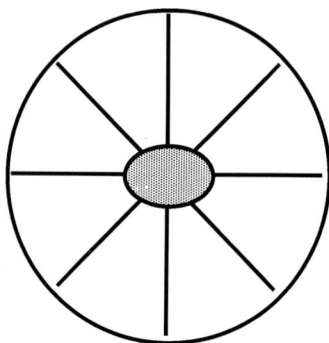

Fig. 9.62 R configuration.

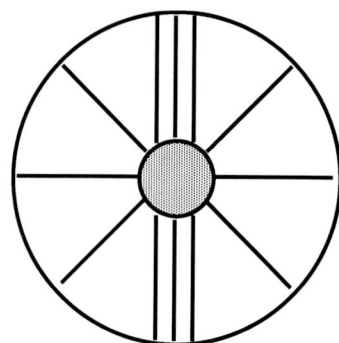

Fig. 9.63 RL configuration.

(a)

(b)

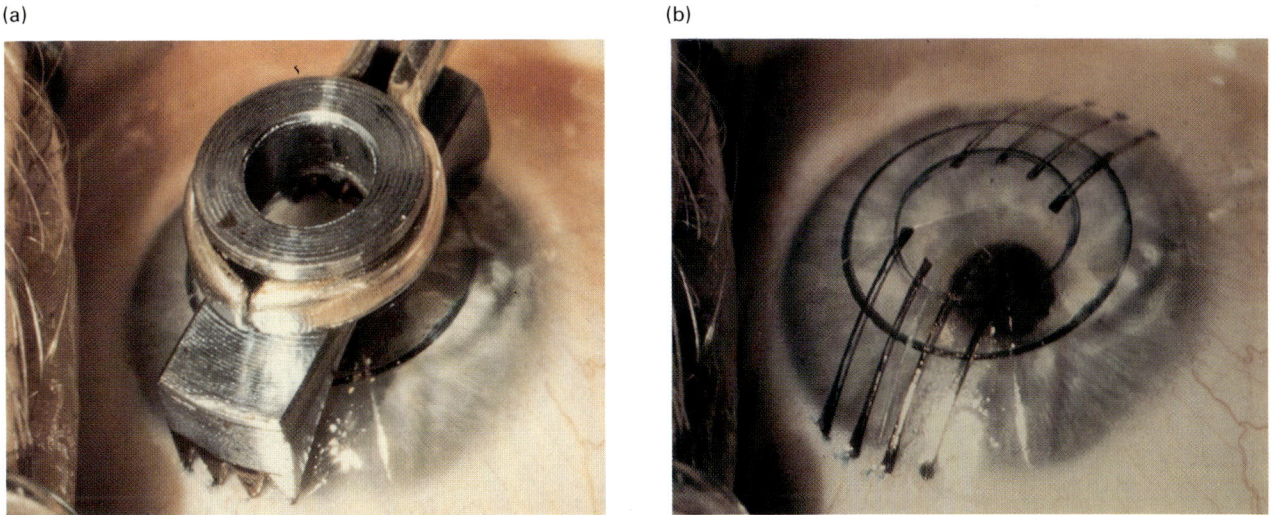

Fig. 9.64 (a) The parallel incision positions are marked with a special marker after the optical zones; (b) dye applied to the markers will help.

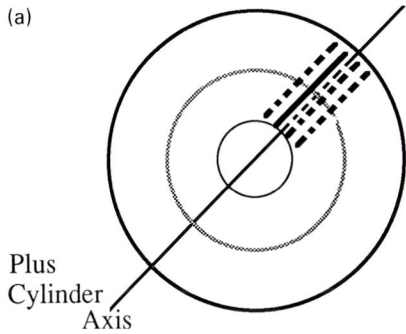

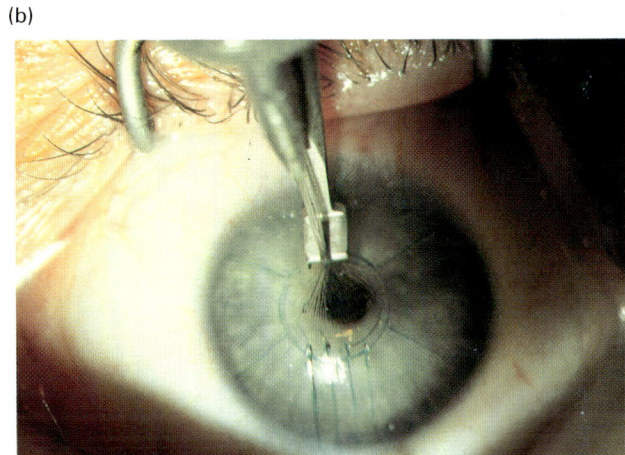

(b)

(a)

Plus
Cylinder
Axis

Fig. 9.65 (a,b) RL procedure—first incision.

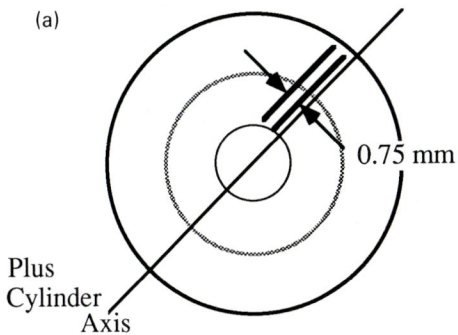

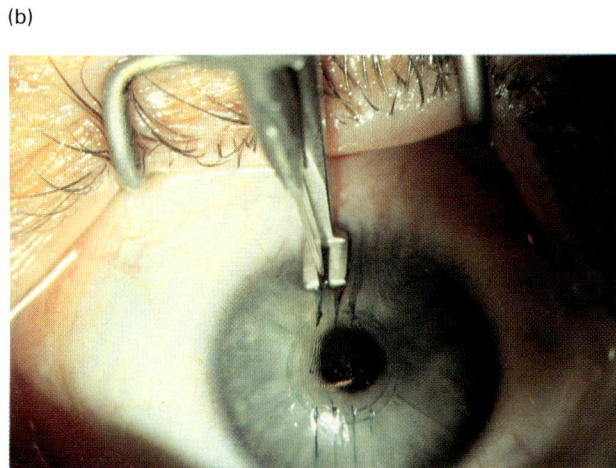

(b)

(a)

0.75 mm

Plus
Cylinder
Axis

Fig. 9.66 (a,b) RL procedure—second incision.

dictable and titratable than some other configurations. It also has the advantage that coupling is minimal. When concerned about over-correction, this is the procedure of choice. The amount of astigmatic correction is controlled, not only by the length of the incisions, but also by the number of incisions made.

Optical zone marking resembles that of the R-procedure (although it is possible to use a plain spherical marker for the primary optical zone in simple myopic astigmatism). Secondary zones are also marked in the same manner. It is helpful to use some sort of parallel marker to help with the incision spacing. The special parallel markers from Katena Instrument Company (K3-8050, K3-8052), fit the bill. The use of a limbus-to-limbus fixation forceps (Katena K5-3280) can make performing this procedure much easier. Figures 9.64 through 9.70 illustrate the manner in which this surgery is performed—in this instance, a case of compound myopic astigmatism. Note that the parallel incisions are all made first and all the incisions are made on one side at a time. Note also that the incisions are made from the inside of the pattern out. This is important. Do not make two incisions and then try to put one in between. The tissue is too unstable and your incision will inevitably run into one or the

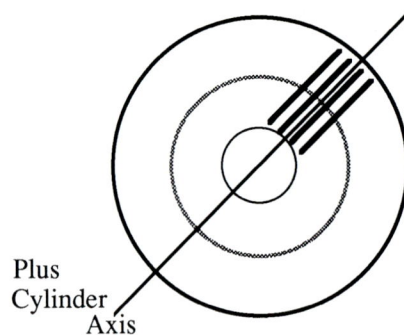

Plus
Cylinder
Axis

Fig. 9.68 RL procedure—fourth incision.

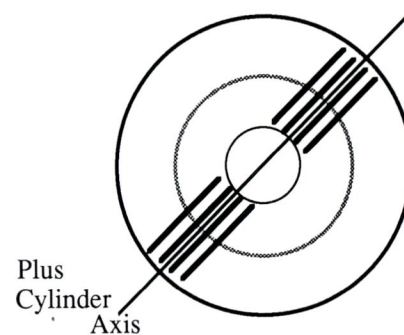

Plus
Cylinder
Axis

Fig. 9.69 RL procedure—parallel incisions complete.

(a)

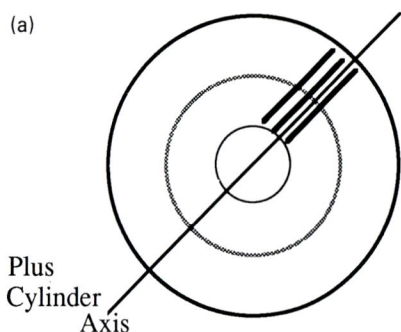

Plus
Cylinder
Axis

(b)

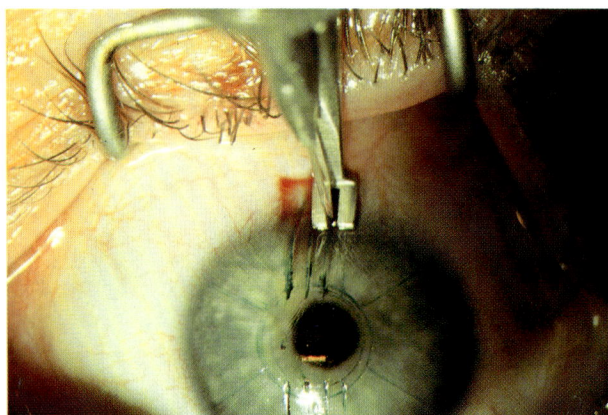

Fig. 9.67 RL procedure—third incision.

(a)

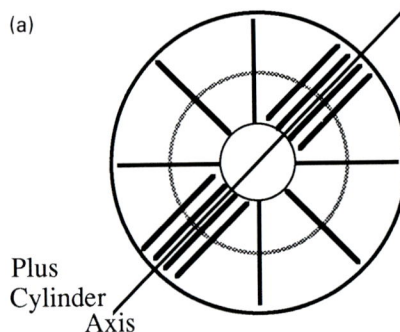

Plus
Cylinder
Axis

(b)

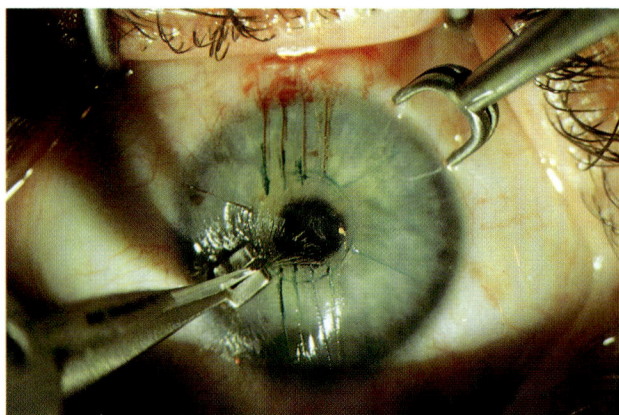

Fig. 9.70 RL procedure—radial incisions added.

other of the previous ones. Needless to say, a very sharp blade is mandatory for this technique to succeed.

Neither the L- or RL-configurations are recommended for post-MKM astigmatism for the reason that delamination of the lenticule could easily occur between incisions.

Methods L and T

Methods L (longitudinal) and T (transverse; Figure 9.71) produce about the same amount of astigmatic correction—1.75 D—but the T-method has a greater range of variance. Furthermore, T-incisions affect *both* the major and minor meridians so their lengths must be carefully controlled (Figures 9.72 through 9.74). The parallel cuts are made in the manner described above. The T-incisions will be discussed below (the RT procedure). The mathematics for the T-incisions are as follows:

$$S_T = \sqrt{\frac{0.8497 - P_0 - L_T^4}{(20800 + 373 \cdot T)(H_1 + H_2) \cdot B}}$$

$$B = \frac{664}{D_1 + D_2 - 0.53} - \sqrt{\left(\frac{664}{D_1 + D_2 - 0.53}\right)^2 - \frac{L_T^4}{4}}$$

$$- \frac{332}{D_2} + \sqrt{\left(\frac{332}{D_2}\right)^2 - \frac{L_T^4}{4}}$$

where S_T = distance between T-incisions; L_T = length of incisions (in mm); P_0 = true intra-ocular pressure (in

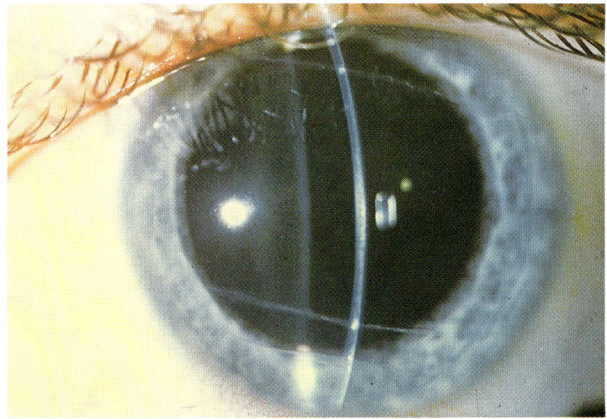

Fig. 9.72 T-incisions.

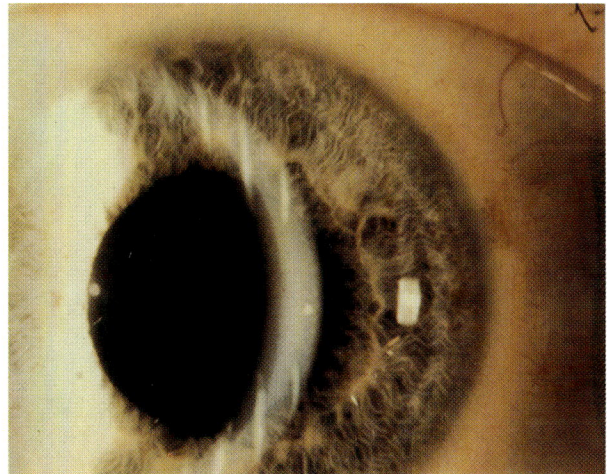

Fig. 9.73 L-incisions.

mmHg); D_1 = K-reading (steep); D_2 = K-reading (flat); H_1 = central corneal thickness (in mm); H_2 = peripheral corneal thickness (in mm); and T = age of patient (in years).

Method TR

Method TR (transverse radial; Figure 9.75) was the third method employed by Fyodorov for myopic astigmatism and was found to correct as much as 6.00 D. However, it is extremely difficult to perform, tends to produce isolated columns of corneal tissue which are very unstable and thus is not recommended but is shown for historical reasons. The areas of incisional intersection are a source of difficulty producing wide scars and longer-lasting corneal instability (Figure 9.77; see also Chapter 15). If the T portion is made secondarily (after 6 months), the intersection

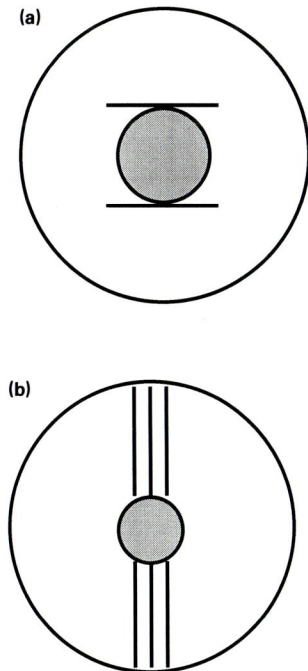

Fig. 9.71 (a) T configuration; (b) L configuration.

(a)

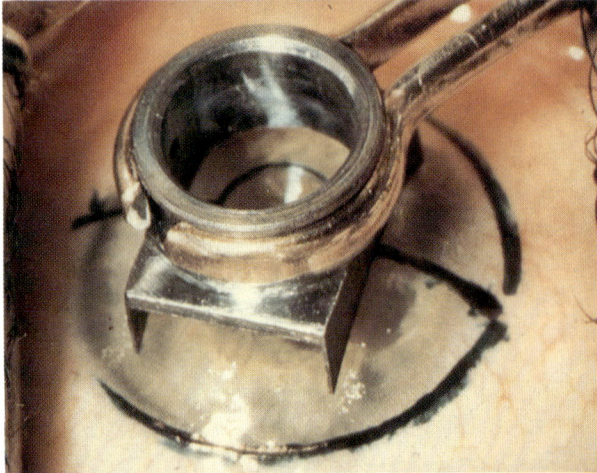

(b)

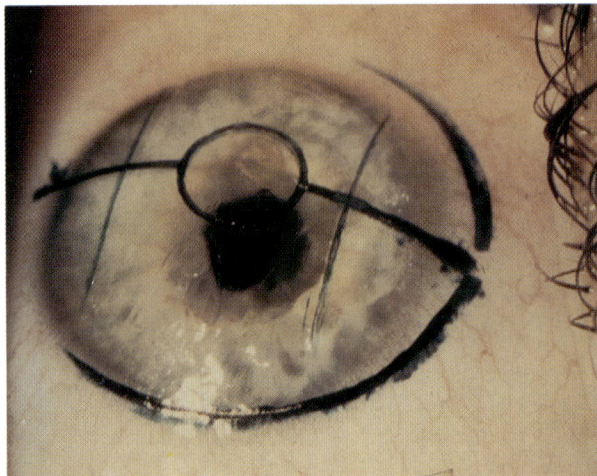

(c)

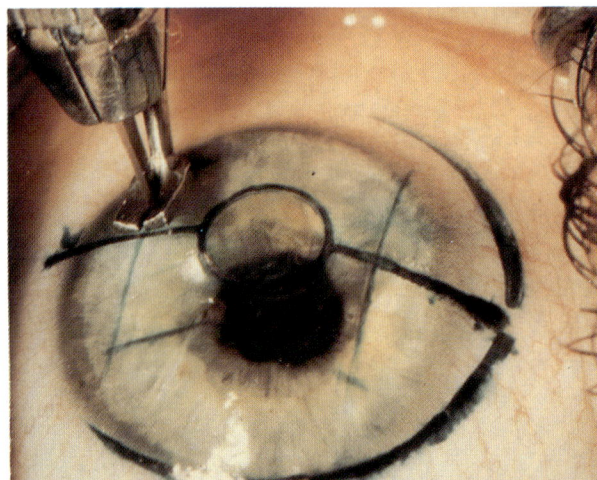

Fig. 9.74 Making T-incisions: (a) marking; (b) marks; (c) incision making.

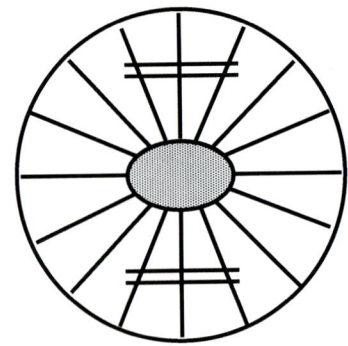

Fig. 9.75 TR configuration.

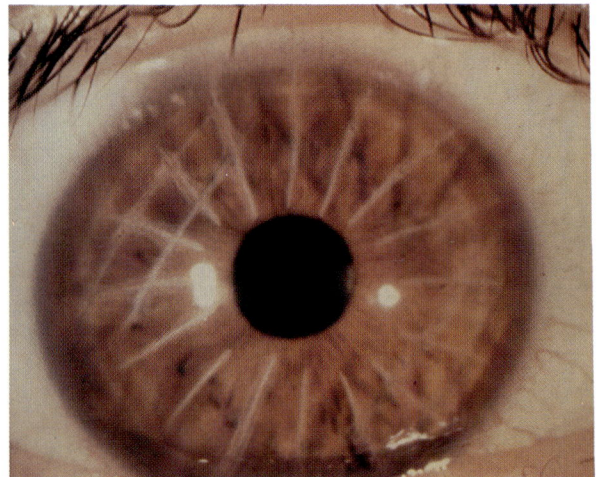

Fig. 9.76 Note wide scars at the incisional intersections.

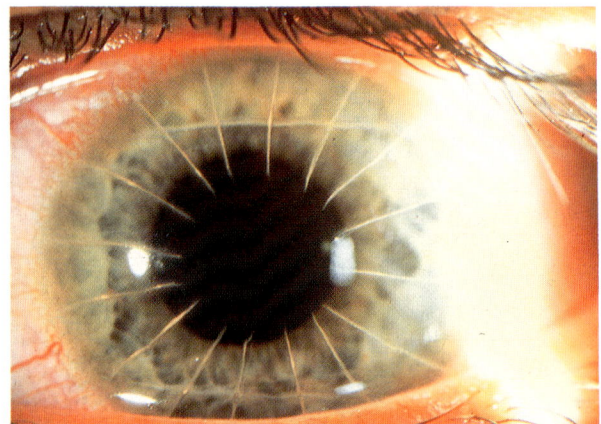

Fig. 9.77 If the T-incisions are made when the radials are partially healed, the intersection scarring is minimal.

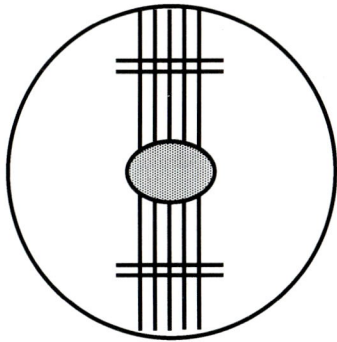

Fig. 9.78 TL configuration.

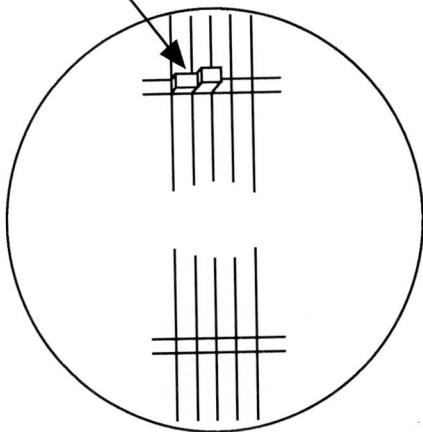

isolated corneal "dice" swell and are easily damaged or lost

Fig. 9.79 Corneal "dice"—loose and isolated elements of stroma.

melting is less (Figure 9.77). This technique and the Method TL have been supplanted by the RT procedure (see below).

Method TL

The same objection can be raised for Method TL (transverse longitudinal) (Figure 9.78) as for the TR method. Crossing of incisions is to be avoided as much as possible. If incisions must be crossed, the surgery should be planned in two stages and at least 3 months allowed to elapse between stages (Figures 9.79 and 9.80). There are currently much better methods to obtain the same results so these configurations are not recommended.

Method RT

Method RT (radial transverse; Figure 9.81), with radial incisions combined with non-joining or interrupted T-cuts, is widely used in compound myopic astigmatism and is recommended for astigmatism up to and including $-2.25\,\mathrm{D}$. There are numerous variations on this basic theme; however, the author uses the configuration shown and this is the one computed for in RK DataMaster. It is not possible to use standard look-up tables with this surgery. The computer program has to take into account the induced steepening of the flatter meridian and adjusts the spherical optical zone component accordingly.

This technique is derived from the TR procedure but differs in certain important details. To avoid confusion with the earlier method it has been designated the RT procedure (radial transverse). This procedure is useful in astigmatism associated with spherical myopia in

(a)

(b)

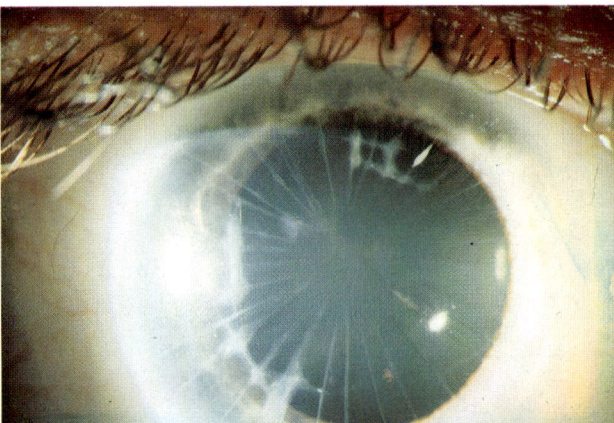
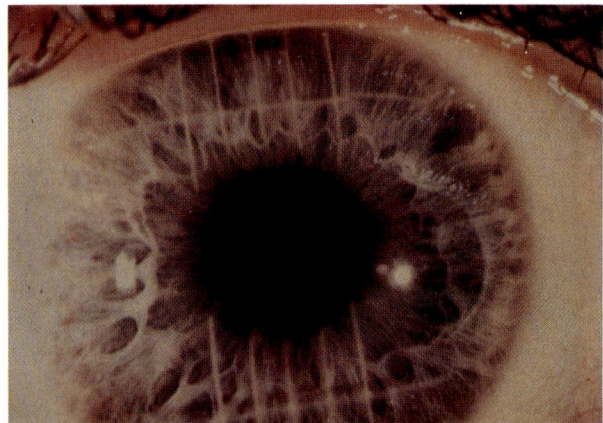

Fig. 9.80 (a) Wide intersection scars are the hallmark of T-incisions made too early. (b) Less scarring is encountered if the Ts are made later.

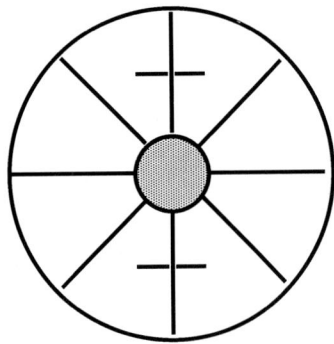

Fig. 9.81 RT configuration.

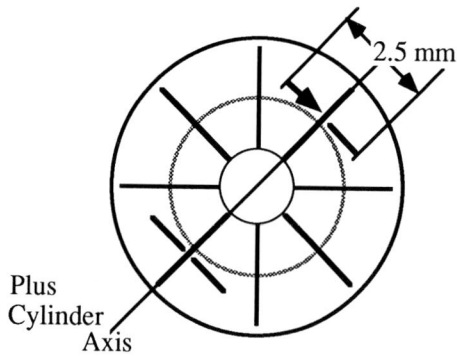

Plus
Cylinder
Axis

Fig. 9.82 RT procedure.

amounts up to 2.25 D. The amount of associated sphere can be any amount up to the limit correctable by eight incisions.

There are certain caveats that you should be aware of with this technique. First, the depths of the T-incisions are expected to be no greater than *85%* of the corneal thickness. Note that this is somewhat shallower than usually called for in radial keratotomy surgery. It has been shown convincingly that deeper transverse incisions are prone to cause progressive flattening of the meridian and some increase in curvature in the opposite axis—see the discussion under the Ruiz procedure for further details. In addition, the radial incisions are *always* stepped (or deepened) at 6 or 7 mm. The T-incisions are exactly 2.5 mm in length overall and do *not* join or cross the radials—at least in theory (Figure 9.82). Usually only one set of paired transverse (T) incisions is made but in some cases there may be two. Figure 9.83 shows a typical computer display for this procedure. This procedure is definitely *not* for the beginner.

The procedure is basically an eight-incision spherical case with the addition of the T-incisions. The radial incisions should all be made *before* the T-cuts, beginning with the pair on-axis followed by the pair at 90° to those, and then the remainder follow. The T-cut marks follow, *tangential* to the T-cut optical zone and centered on the axial incision. Make sure that these marks are perpendicular to the astigmatism axis. The use of

```
RK DATAMASTER PRE-OP CALCULATION SUMMARY ......... 07-04-1990

George Sigafoos - Left eye -- RT PROCEDURE


   Sphere portion of procedure --

      RADIAL incisions ....................... 8
      1st optic zone ......................... 4.25 mm
      2nd optic zone ......................... 6.00 mm


   Cylinder portion of procedure --

      TRANSVERSE incisions (T-cuts) per side .. 1
      Length of T-cut ........................ 2.50 mm
      1st T-cut optic zone ................... 6.00 mm
      CONFIGURATION AXIS ..................... 45 degrees


   Do you wish to print this table? (Y/N) ....................
```

this procedure has at least two radial OZs

Fig. 9.83 Computer summary of an RT procedure.

(a)

(b)

(c)

(d)

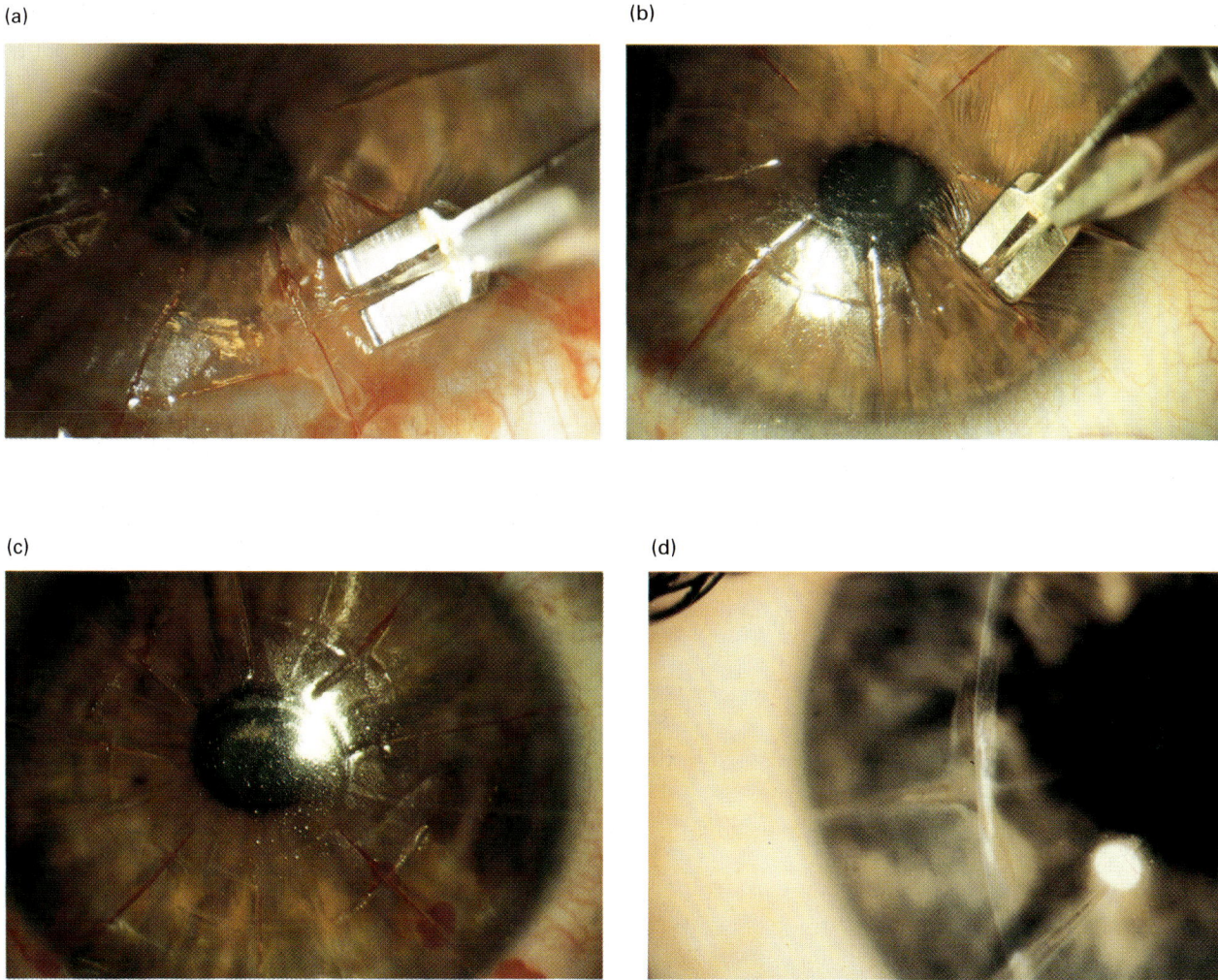

Fig. 9.84 (a–c) Note that the T-cuts are made *toward* the radial, stopping just short of intersection. (d) Entering the T-cut can produce wide gaping with associated wide scars and possible irregular astigmatism due to uneven healing.

brilliant green dye applied to the markers can be helpful here.

The eye is fixated employing wide forceps applied across the limbus perpendicular to the Ts. A vertical blade is then inserted into the cornea at the end of the T-mark and the incision made *toward the radial* (Figure 9.84). Making the incision away from the radial, while seemingly easier, does not work and causes the tissue to separate at the bottom of the radial. Use high magnification and stop just short of entering the radial. A small bridge of tissue should remain. It is not always possible to stop in time, even for the most skilled hands. However, experience will lower the incidence of radial incision entry. The edge of the radial tends to roll under the footplate of the knife. When you see this occurring—stop. A very sharp blade does not require as much pressure to be applied and this rolling moment is therefore minimized, making it easier to see and control the end point. It is for this reason that the

author suggests that the surgeon put aside a double-edged blade to be used *only* for T-cuts.

The radial incisions always have a step, therefore a "dipstick" of appropriate size is inserted into each wound and the uniformity of each incision gauged. Any unsatisfactory incisions are re-cut at this time. Occasionally, the beginning and end of stepped incisions will over-ride one another. That over-riding connection must be separated for best effect (see Chapter 8). Each wound is then gently irrigated with balanced salt solution.

Method RZ (Ruiz procedure)

Method RZ (Ruiz or trapezoidal) is very useful for simple myopic or mixed astigmatism in amounts from −2.50 D and above (Figure 9.85). It can be combined with six radial incisions (Method RR), to correct mixed myopic or compound astigmatism and is quite pre-

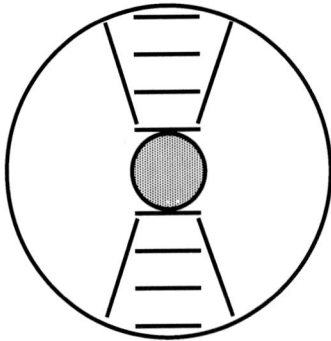

Fig. 9.85 RZ configuration.

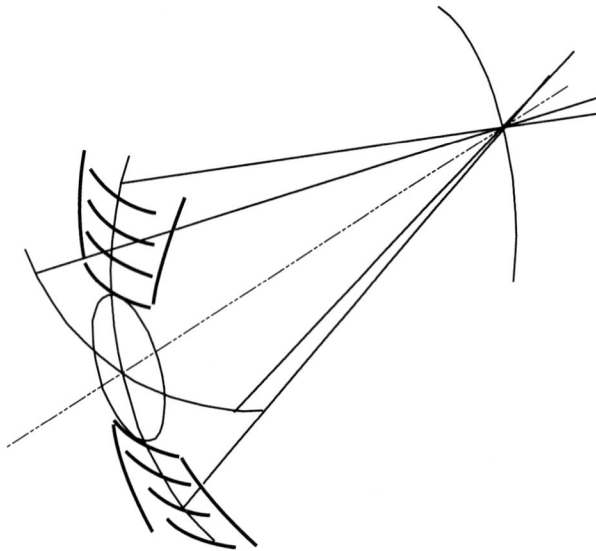

Fig. 9.86 Ruiz pattern incisions on the cornea.

dictable and stable. Difficulties reported with this surgery are often due to the fact that the incisions are either made deeper than 85% or are too long (or both). The Ruiz method of astigmatic correction combines semi-radial and tangential incisions to flatten the steepest meridian of the cornea (Figure 9.86). The technique was introduced by Luis Antonio Ruiz, MD, of the Clinica Barraquer, Bogota, Colombia and controls different degrees of astigmatism by varying the size of the optical zone and the length of the transverse corneal incisions. The optical zones used vary from 2.75 to 5.00 mm and the length of the transverse incisions varies from 1.5 to 5.00 mm. Up to 8 D of cylinder has been corrected by this method.

This surgery can induce myopic astigmatism in the opposite axis very handily. This fact makes it very useful in mixed myopic astigmatism. For example, $-2.00 + 4.00 \times 90°$ ($+2.00 - 4.00 \times 180°$), can be converted to plano by judicious lengthening of the T-cuts (see the section on decision making, above).

There is, however, an aspect to this technique that must be carefully borne in mind: the length of the incision not only affects the flattening in the steep axis, it also affects the opposite axis by steepening its curvature. This can be very dangerous—it can also be very useful. If the length of the transverse component is not carefully chosen and controlled, it is possible actually to reverse the astigmatism. Therefore, this operation is definitely not for the faint of heart, nor the imprudent. By taking care and utilizing computer analysis of the pre-operative data, it is possible to eliminate completely mixed astigmatism. In fact the Ruiz procedure is the only technique currently available that can do so in a predictable manner.

The Ruiz incision flattens the steeper meridian in an approximate ratio of 6:1. Troutman found that his wedge resection steepened the flatter meridian in a 2:1 ratio. That is, for every 2 D of flattening that occurred in the steeper meridian, 1 D of steepening was induced in the flatter meridian. An excellent discussion of this relationship has been detailed by Lee Nordan and, with permission, is abstracted below:

Wedge versus Ruiz

Consider a theoretical patient model with A-T-R astigmatism—that is, astigmatism at 180°. The vertical meridian (90°) will be flatter than the horizontal meridian (180°). If pre-operative keratometric readings are represented by H and V, where H is the reading in the horizontal meridian and V the reading in the vertical meridian, the total amount of astigmatism (A) is represented by $H - V$. X represents the dioptric change in the steepest meridian of a cornea undergoing either a Ruiz procedure or a wedge resection. If the astigmatism is fully corrected by the surgery then $A = 0$. According to Troutman, a wedge resection which *increases* the K-reading of the *flatter* meridian V by X will *decrease* the K-reading for the *steeper* meridian H by $X/2$ [35]. Therefore, in a wedge resection:

$$\left(H - \frac{X}{2}\right) - (V + X) = 0$$

$$\left(\text{steep} - \frac{X}{2}\right) - (\text{flat} + X) = 0$$

$$2H - X - 2V - 2X = 0$$

$$2(H - V) = 3X$$

$$X = \frac{2}{3}(H - V)$$

$$X = \left(\frac{2A}{3}\right) \{\text{because } A = H - V\}$$

In this model of A-T-R astigmatism, the vertical meridian, V, is steepened by two-thirds of the amount of the original astigmatism A. The horizontal meridian, H, is therefore flattened by one-third of the original astigmatism. It should be noted that, if properly performed, the wedge resection will steepen the meridian in which it is made—but only up to a certain point. Beyond that point, a wedge resection will actually flatten the meridian because of the effect of excessive tissue removal.

In the Ruiz procedure, $A = 0$ if the astigmatism is totally corrected as well. According to data obtained from patients in whom the surgery has been performed, the Ruiz procedure decreases the K-reading of the steeper meridian H by X, and increases the ·K-reading of the flatter meridian V by $X/5$. Therefore in the Ruiz procedure:

$$(H - X) - \left(V + \frac{X}{5}\right) = 0$$

$$5(H - V) = 6X$$

$$X = \frac{5}{6}(H - V)$$

$$X = \frac{5A}{6}$$

Thus, the steep meridian, H, is flattened by five-sixths of the total astigmatism $A(H - V)$, while the flatter meridian, V, is steepened by one-sixth A.

Both the wedge resection and the Ruiz procedure will correct astigmatism. However, there are other optical considerations that must be noted. Because it steepens the flatter meridian so dramatically, a wedge resection creates a significant myopic shift, increasing the myopic component of the refractive error by two-thirds of the pre-operative astigmatism.

Conversely, the Ruiz procedure primarily flattens the steeper meridian. The myopic shift in this case will only be one-sixth of the pre-operative astigmatic component. There is, therefore, a fourfold difference in the amount of myopic change induced in the spherical component between the two procedures (two-thirds divided by one-sixth).

If one considers the comparative effect of the two procedures on the spherical equivalent (SE), then the wedge resection shifts the SE toward the *myopic* side equal to one-sixth of the pre-wedge astigmatism. Recall that the SE of any optical system is equal to the spherical component minus one-half the astigmatic component. The pre-wedge SE would therefore equal the sphere $-(-A/2)$. The post-operative SE would then equal sphere $-(2A/3)$ since the wedge resection will shift the spherical component toward myopia by two-thirds the pre-operative astigmatism—assuming a perfect correction of the astigmatism. Therefore, since

$SE = S - A/2$, where S = sphere and A = astigmatism in diopters, then if $-5.00 + 1.00 \times 9$ (or $-4.00\ -1.00 \times 180$) then:

$$SE = -5 - \frac{1}{2}\left\{-4 - \left(-\frac{1}{2}\right)\right\}$$

$$SE = -5 - 0.5$$

$$SE = -4.50\,D$$

Thus the shift in SE can be expressed as the difference between the pre- and post-operative SEs in this manner:

$$\Delta SE = \left(\text{sphere} - \left(\frac{2}{3}A\right)\right) - \left(\text{sphere} - \frac{A}{2}\right)$$

$$= -\frac{2A}{3} + \frac{A}{2}$$

$$= -\frac{(-4A + 3A)}{6}$$

$$= -\frac{A}{6}D$$

The Ruiz procedure will create a *hyperopic* shift in the SE equal to one-third that of the pre-operative astigmatism. In this case the post-operative SE equals sphere $-(A/6)$ since the Ruiz procedure shifts the spherical component toward myopia by one-sixth of the preoperative astigmatism. Thus:

$$\Delta SE = \left(\text{sphere} - \frac{1}{6A}\right) - \left(\text{sphere} - \frac{A}{2}\right)$$

$$= -\frac{A}{6} + \frac{A}{2}$$

$$= \frac{(-2A + 6A)}{12}$$

$$= \frac{4A}{12}$$

$$= \frac{A}{3}D$$

Hence, the Ruiz procedure creates a hyperopic shift in the SE equivalent to one-third the pre-operative astigmatism.

Troutman states that the corneal wedge resection produces a shift toward hyperopia due to a shortening effect on the axial length of the globe [35]. It is unclear, however, whether Troutman was referring to the spherical component or the SE of the refraction. In either event, we can derive the amount of shortening required to produce the effect described. In Troutman's study, the amount of pre-wedge astigmatism

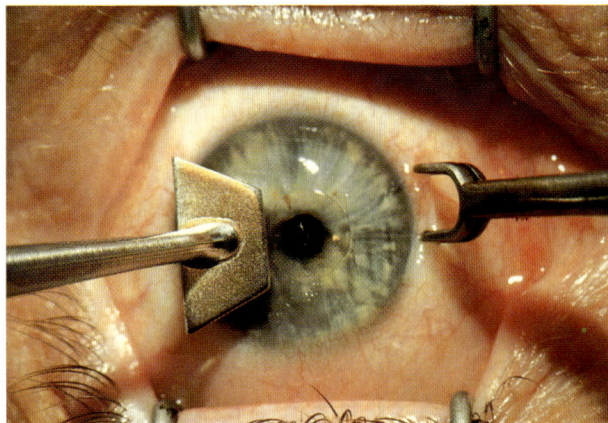

Fig. 9.87 A special marker is used for the Ruiz procedure.

averaged 11.4 D. Following the wedge resection, we have shown that the shift in SE will equal one-sixth that of the pre-operative astigmatism. Therefore, the mean shift will be almost 2 D:

$$-\frac{11.4}{6} = 1.9\,\text{D}$$

If we consider the spherical component alone, then the myopic shift will be 7.6 D:

$$-11.4 \cdot \frac{2}{3} = 7.6\,\text{D}$$

If we accept Rubin's approximation of axial myopia in a model eye, wherein 0.4 mm of axial elongation is equivalent to a dioptric change of 1.0 D, then the axial length in the first instance would be shortened 0.76 mm (0.4 × 1.9) and in the second, 3.04 mm (0.4 × 7.6) [47]. This clearly does not happen.

The Ruiz procedure is technically easier than a wedge resection and may be performed in combination with other refractive procedures, especially radial keratotomy. Furthermore, post-operative results for a Ruiz procedure are more predictable than for a wedge resection because sutures are not used. However, it is more variable in cases where the corneal architecture has been altered, as by previous surgery. Post-wedge resection, there is incisional relaxation as some sutures are cut and others biodegrade. Consequently the cornea regresses toward its pre-wedge astigmatism in an unpredictable manner.

The technique of the Ruiz procedure

Establishing the optic center is accomplished as usual; however, this procedure is particularly sensitive to decentration. Mark the optic axis carefully. Next a specially designed marker (Figure 9.87) is used to mark the positions and length of the transverse incisions.

Figure 9.88 shows a computer display for this procedure. This illustrates the surgical parameters for a simple case of myopic astigmatism without any spherical component. The 4.5 mm optical zone is the zone at which the first transverse incision will be made. Each succeeding incision is made at equally spaced intervals to the limbus.

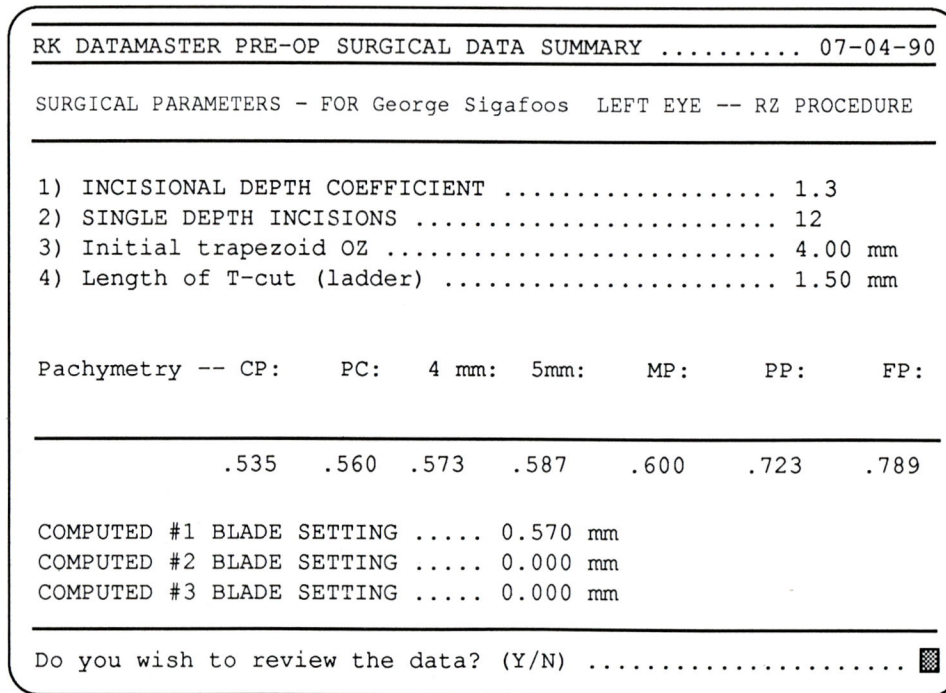

```
┌──────────────────────────────────────────────────────────────────────┐
│  RK DATAMASTER PRE-OP SURGICAL DATA SUMMARY .......... 07-04-90        │
│                                                                        │
│  SURGICAL PARAMETERS - FOR George Sigafoos  LEFT EYE -- RZ PROCEDURE   │
│                                                                        │
│                                                                        │
│  1) INCISIONAL DEPTH COEFFICIENT ................... 1.3               │
│  2) SINGLE DEPTH INCISIONS ........................ 12                  │
│  3) Initial trapezoid OZ .......................... 4.00  mm           │
│  4) Length of T-cut (ladder) ...................... 1.50  mm           │
│                                                                        │
│                                                                        │
│  Pachymetry -- CP:    PC:   4 mm:  5mm:    MP:     PP:      FP:         │
│                                                                        │
│                                                                        │
│              .535    .560  .573   .587   .600    .723     .789         │
│                                                                        │
│  COMPUTED #1 BLADE SETTING ..... 0.570 mm                              │
│  COMPUTED #2 BLADE SETTING ..... 0.000 mm                              │
│  COMPUTED #3 BLADE SETTING ..... 0.000 mm                              │
│                                                                        │
│  Do you wish to review the data? (Y/N) ...................... ▩        │
└──────────────────────────────────────────────────────────────────────┘
```

Fig. 9.88 Computer display for Ruiz (RZ) procedure.

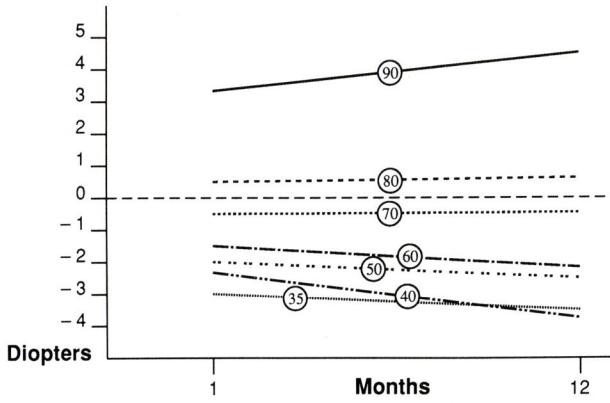

Fig. 9.89 Effect of incision depth of Ruiz "ladders" on outcome.

The transverse incisions are made first, using a crystalline blade with a vertical cutting edge. The blade is set to obtain an effective depth of cut of between 80 and 90%, as determined by ultrasonic pachymetry. Deeper incisions have been shown to result in progressive flattening with this procedure, while shallower incisions have the opposite effect (Figure 9.89). The computer predictions assume an 85% incision depth. The eye must not be allowed to rotate, so trans-limbal fixation using a Katena K5-3280 fixation forceps is

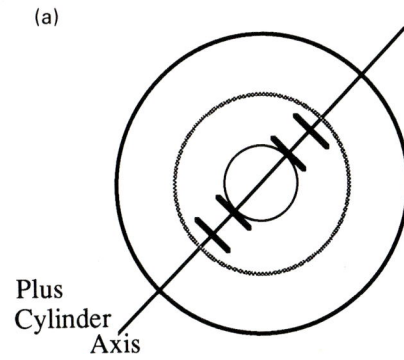

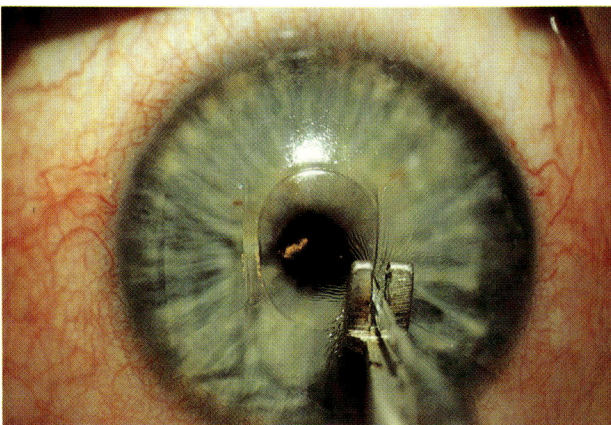

Fig. 9.90 (a,b) RZ procedure—first incision pair.

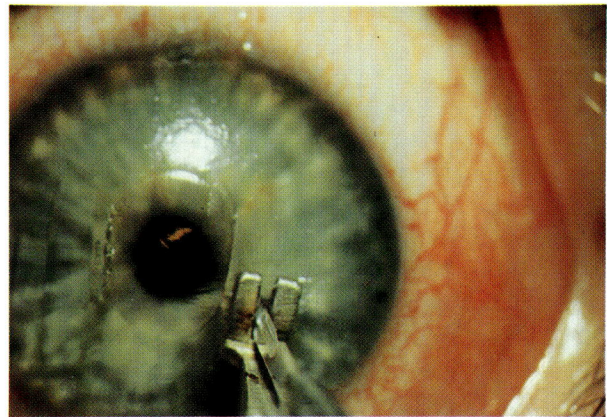

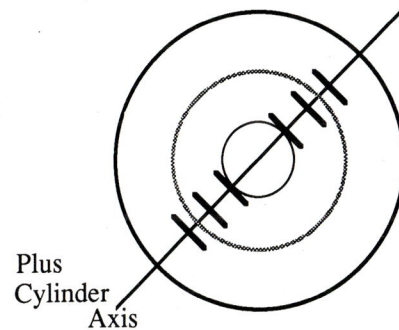

Fig. 9.91 (a,b) RZ procedure—second incision pair.

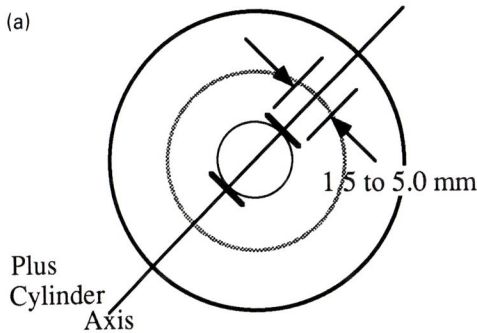

Fig. 9.92 RZ procedure—third incision pair.

recommended. The two central incisions are made first, the blade is advanced approximately 25 μm and the next two incisions are made. It is here that the XTAL shadowgraphic blade gauge is most useful. The blade is advanced for each succeeding transverse incision, proportionally to the corneal thickness at that point, until all eight (four on each side) "rungs" have been completed. It is important that the transverse incisions be evenly spaced and that the last one be as close to the limbus as possible. Figures 9.90 through 9.94 illustrate the various steps involved in this technique.

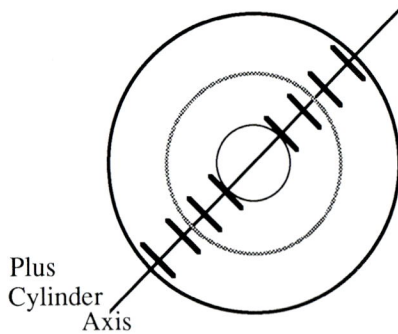

Fig. 9.93 RZ procedure—fourth incision pair.

The blade is switched for one with an angled cutting edge and set (or re-set if a double-edged blade) according to the corneal thickness at the primary astigmatic optical zone (in the example, 4.5 mm). The semi-radial incisions are then made at an angle of 20–22° normal to the inner tangential incision (Figure 9.95). These incisions must start *under* the outer ends of the inner ladder rung and they must not connect with them. Making the incisions at the ends of the ladder rungs effectively increases their length. Connecting the incisions can produce wide scars and irregular healing which can lead to increased glare and irregular astigmatism (Figure 9.95). Long T-cuts also gape considerably and take longer to heal (Figure 9.96). In higher degrees of astigmatism the radial portion of the Ruiz pattern can be made in a stepped manner.

In certain instances, wherein the hyperopic component is effectively greater by far than the spherical component, a reversal of the pattern can be made (Figures 9.97 and 9.98). Thus in a case whose refraction is: $-0.05 + 5.00 \times 146$, a reversed Ruiz resulted in the following; $+1.50 + 0.50 \times 180$. The computer calculated the case as shown in Figure 9.99.

RR procedure

If there is spherical myopia associated with astigmatism in excess of 2.25 D, it can be attenuated with a six-incision radial pattern added between the trapezoidal incisions and arranged around an appropriate optical zone or zones (Figures 9.100 and 9.101). This procedure is called Method RR (radial Ruiz). The optical zone size for this part of the surgery is automatically calculated in the RK DataMaster program. A six-ray radial marker is invaluable to mark the position of the six incisions. These additional incisions have to be oriented correctly, as shown.

Do not mark the optical zone for the radials or the radials themselves until *after* the astigmatic portion of the procedure is completed. There is too much danger of mistaking the (usually smaller) radial optical zone for the (usually larger) astigmatic optical zone if all zones are marked at the same time.

In MKM cases, the radial incisions extend across the lenticular edge and can be stepped as in routine RR procedures. The T-incisions are arranged such that two fall within the lenticule and two fall outside (Figure 9.102). It is well to consider doing the RZ procedure in these cases only for astigmatism above 3 D. For astigmatism below this amount, use the RT procedure.

In skilled hands the Ruiz or trapezoidal incisions are an effective and predictable method of correcting simple myopic or mixed astigmatism over 2.25 D (to 6.00 D) with or without associated spherical error. The use of a computer to assist in determining the surgical parameters has all but eliminated the problem of induced astigmatism. This procedure is highly recommended to skilled and experienced refractive surgeons for the purpose for which it was designed. However, take care not to find yourself in the predicament shown in Figure 9.103. Beginning surgeons should avoid performing this or other forms of astig-

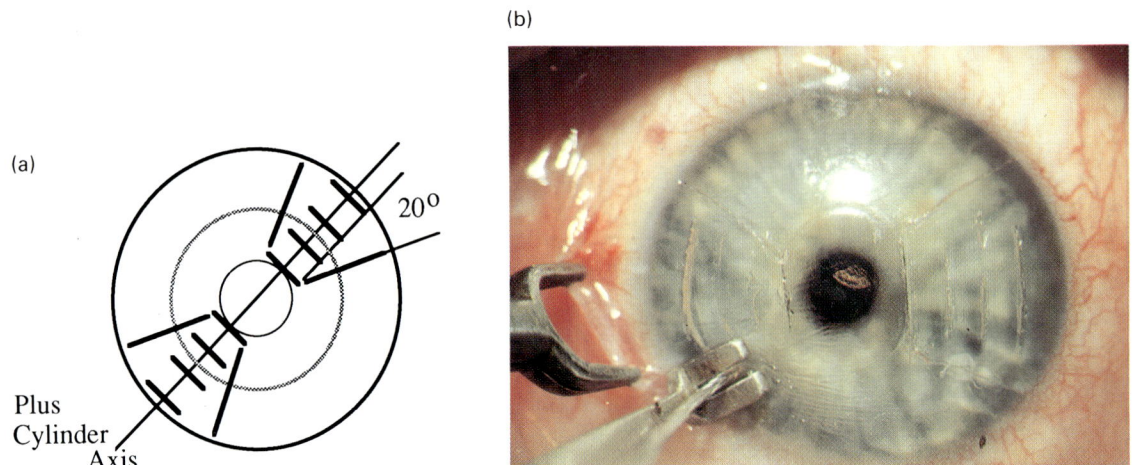

Fig. 9.94 (a,b) RZ procedure—semi-radial incisions added. Note that the semi-radials do not join the T-cuts.

(a)

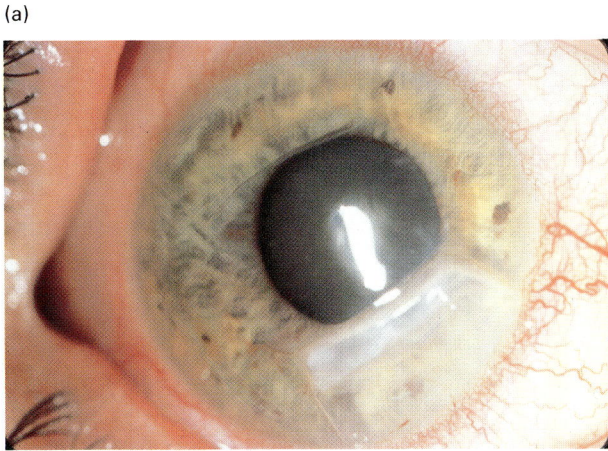

(b)

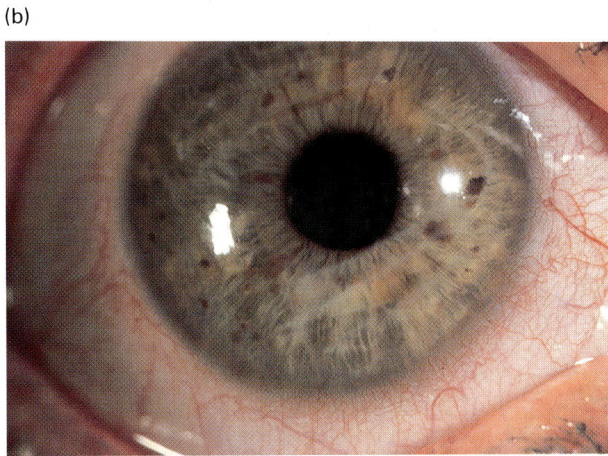

(c)

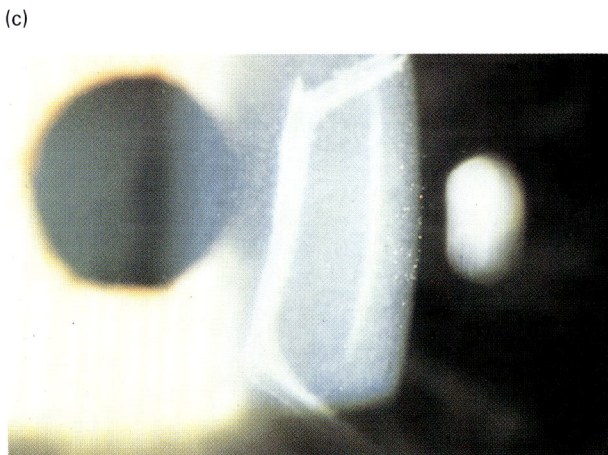

Fig. 9.95 (a) If the T-cuts join the radials, considerable edema can occur. (b) While this will subside in time, (c) wide scars usually result.

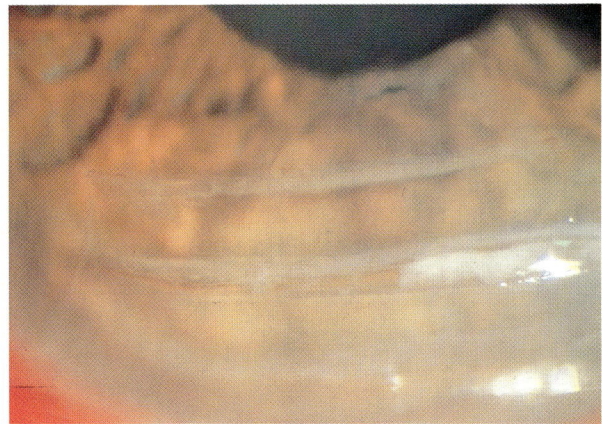

Fig. 9.96 Long T-cuts tend to gape.

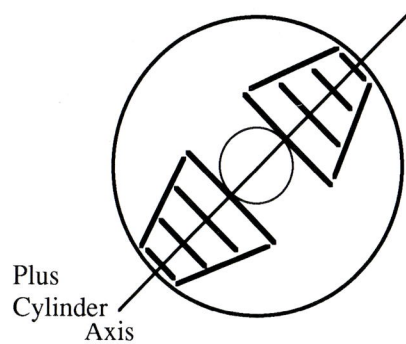

Plus
Cylinder
Axis

Fig. 9.97 Inverted Ruiz pattern.

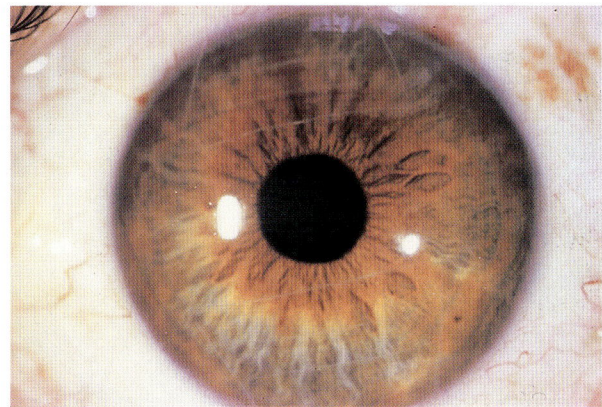

Fig. 9.98 Post-operative inverted Ruiz pattern.

matic refractive surgery until their skills and experience match their ambition.

Results with RK methods

Tables 9.2–9.8 summarize the author's results with the various configurations described above.

Variations of the trapezoidal procedure

Some variations of the basic incision pattern have been attempted. Figure 9.104 shows a configuration that has not proved to be sufficiently reliable. Lindstrom has described a technique he calls a delimited T procedure [48]. Essentially, it is a Ruiz (RZ) procedure with the

```
RK DATAMASTER PRE-OP CALCULATION SUMMARY ......... 07-04-1990

George Sigafoos - Left eye -- RUIZ PROCEDURE


RUIZ optical zone ....................... 4.0 mm
TRANSVERSE incision (ladders) LENGTH .... 5.0 mm
CONFIGURATION AXIS ...................... 45 deg
Estimated residual refraction .......... 2.50 dptrs




Do you wish to print this table? (Y/N) ....................
```

computer predicts a residual hyperopia

Fig. 9.99 Computer display showing Ruiz procedure and predicted results for mixed astigmatism.

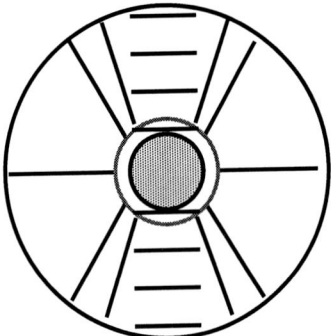

Fig. 9.100 Radial Ruiz (RR) configuration.

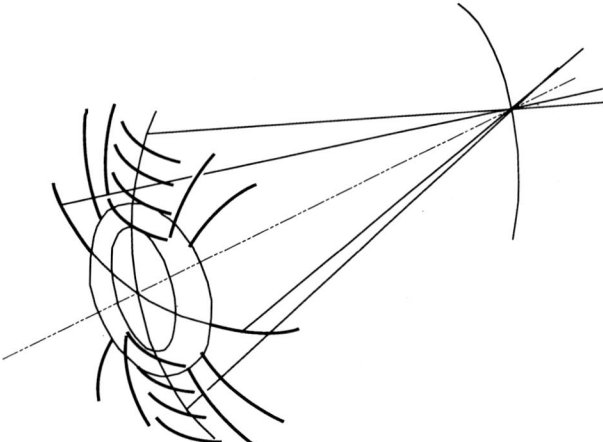

Fig. 9.101 Isometric of RR incision pattern on cornea.

elimination of the two outer T-cuts. Lindstrom has claimed that these outer incisions are not needed, based on work with cadaver eyes that seemed to show decrease of effect when these incisions were added. The author submits for your consideration the fact that a dead eye is not a dynamic, living structure—living eyes react somewhat differently to this surgery. Furthermore, Ruiz ([49], L.A. Ruiz, 1991, personal communication) and Bores ([50], L.D. Bores, 1991, unpublished data) have pointed out that stability of effect is increased in the presence of these outer incisions. Rowsey has corroborated the findings of Ruiz and Bores that varying the optical zone as well as adding the outer two incisions is effective in flattening the steep meridian [51].

Lindstrom uses a simplified method consisting of two paired incisions, either alone at 5 mm or with another pair at 7 to 8 mm (Figure 9.105). Note that Lindstrom varies the optical zone for the limiting radials, but keeps both the length and separation of the T-cuts constant [48]. In cases of post-keratoplasty astigmatism, he begins with a single pair of T-cuts at 5 mm. If an adequate effect is not obtained, he adds a second pair of T-cuts at 8 mm. While he states that post-operative steroids q.i.d. for 1 month can be used to enhance the effect, the trend of this technique is to progressive flattening—thus steroids should be used with caution. The author advises that the surgeon shoot for a slight under-correction and use steroids b.i.d. for 2 weeks only (see also Chapter 8).

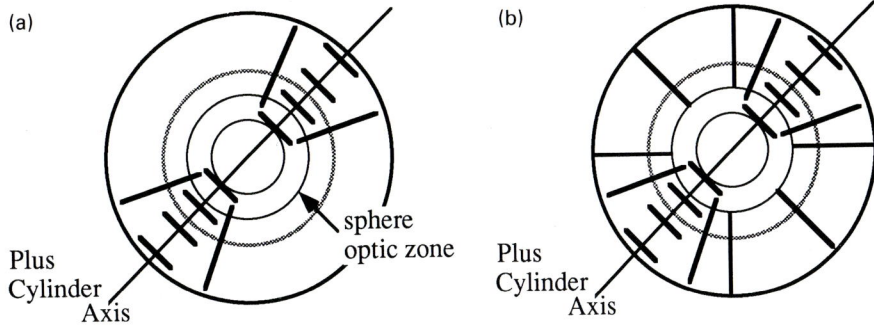

Fig. 9.102 RR procedure—showing the optical zone mark for radials to be added.

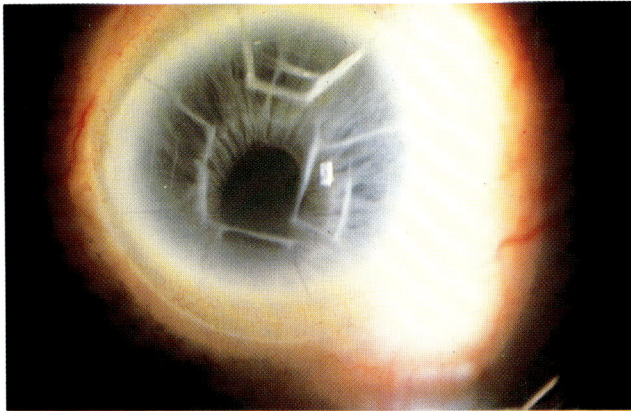

Fig. 9.103 Do not make a mistake in the axis or length of the T-cuts in the Ruiz procedure.

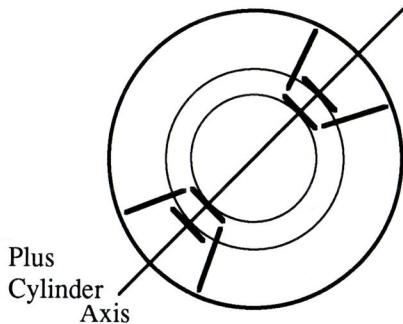

Fig. 9.104 Lindstrom's variation of the Ruiz procedure.

Table 9.3 Visual results of the application of T-cuts

Visual acuity	Pre-operative	Post-operative
20/200–20/50	47 (82%)	21 (36.8%)
20/40–20/33	10 (17.5%)	22 (38.4%)
20/25–20/20		14 (24.6%)
Total	57 (100%)	57 (100%)

Table 9.4 Refractive results of early application of L-cuts

Astigmatism	Pre-operative	Post-operative
0.0–0.75 D		22 (44%)
1.0–1.75 D	7 (14%)	21 (42%)
2.0–3.0 D	28 (56%)	6 (12%)
3.25–5.5 D	15 (30%)	1 (2%)
Total	50 (100%)	50 (100%)

Table 9.5 Visual results of early application of L-cuts

Visual acuity	Pre-operative	Post-operative
20/200–20/50	32 (64%)	13 (26%)
20/40–20/33	15 (30%)	24 (48%)
20/25–20/20	3 (6%)	13 (26%)
Total	50 (100%)	50 (100%)

Table 9.6 Pre-operative breakdown of patients by age and astigmatism

Parameter	n
Total cases	632
Age range	18–57 (31)
Dioptric range	75–8.25 D
Pre-operative astigmatism breakdown	
<1.5 D	158
1.5–2.5 D	387
2.5–4.0 D	67
4.0–8.0 D	22

Table 9.2 Early results of the application of T-cuts

Astigmatism	Pre-operative	Post-operative
0.0–0.75 D		12 (21%)
1.0–1.75 D	4 (7%)	27 (47.4%)
2.0–3.0 D	26 (45.6%)	14 (24.6%)
3.25–6.75 D	27 (47.4%)	4 (7%)
Total	57 (100%)	57 (100%)

Table 9.7 Pre-operative breakdown of astigmatism by procedure

Type	<1.5 D	1.5–2.5 D	2.5–4.0 D	4.0–8.0 D
R	126	1	—	—
L	28	73	—	—
T	4	3	—	—
RL	—	306	4	
TR	—	—	32	19
TL	—	—	11	
RZ	—	4	20	3
Total	158	387	67	22

Table 9.8 Post-operative breakdown of astigmatism by procedure

Type	<1.5 D	1.5–2.5 D	2.5–4.0 D	4.0–8.0 D
R	127	—	—	—
L	78	23	—	—
T	4	3	3	—
RL	271	36	7	—
TR	22	21	32	—
TL	8	3	—	—
RZ	21	3	3	—
Total	531	89	13	

Intra-cicatricial relaxing incisions

Relaxing incisions can be placed in the host–graft interface (scar) to correct post-keratoplasty astigmatism (Figure 9.106). In some instances—such as very high astigmatism—this is a better choice than trapezoidal incisions. The author particularly favors this approach in grafts whose edges are vascularized. This procedure was first described by Troutman and Swinger for correction of high astigmatism following keratoplasty, correcting up to 15.92 D of cylinder [34].

This technique can also be used for post-cataract astigmatism. The length of the incisions can vary from 70 to 90° (3 clock hours)—the author prefers the latter—with flattening:steepening ratios of 1:1 to 2:1. Stability usually occurs within 8 weeks and although others have reported lessening of effect if one waits too long after removing sutures [52], the author has not found this to be the case. On the contrary, the author has found increased stability and predictability when he had waited a minimum of 4 months post-suture removal to make these incisions. In any case, no surgery should be attempted after suture removal until the K-readings stabilize.

Compression sutures can be added to increase the gaping of the relaxing incisions in cases where insufficient flattening has occurred. This technique has the advantage of being titratable to some degree. The author has combined in-the-wound relaxing incisions with wedge resections in two cases of very high, second graft, post-PKP astigmastism, with good results.

Arcuate keratotomy

Merlin was the first surgeon to popularize the use of arcuate keratotomy as an alternative to straight transverse keratotomy [53]. The author is using the term arcuate keratotomy to describe arcuate incisions made perpendicular to the steep axis in clear cornea. We wish to distinguish this procedure from the method of Troutman. He based this preference on theoretic considerations, feeling that an arcuate incision would remain the same distance from the center of the cornea and would be less likely to have a distorting effect. He repeated a series of 205 eyes with arcuate keratotomies varying in length from 100 to 160° placed at optical zones between 5 and 7 mm. He found increasing efficacy with increasing length of incision up to 120°. In addition, the major effect occurred at a

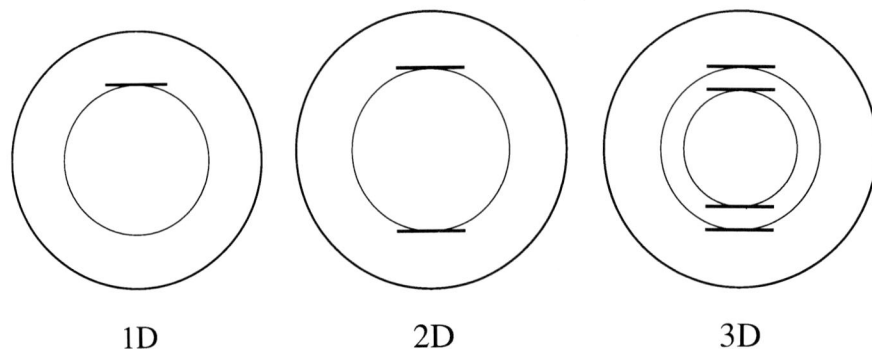

1D   2D   3D

Fig. 9.105 Lindstrom's variation of the T procedure.

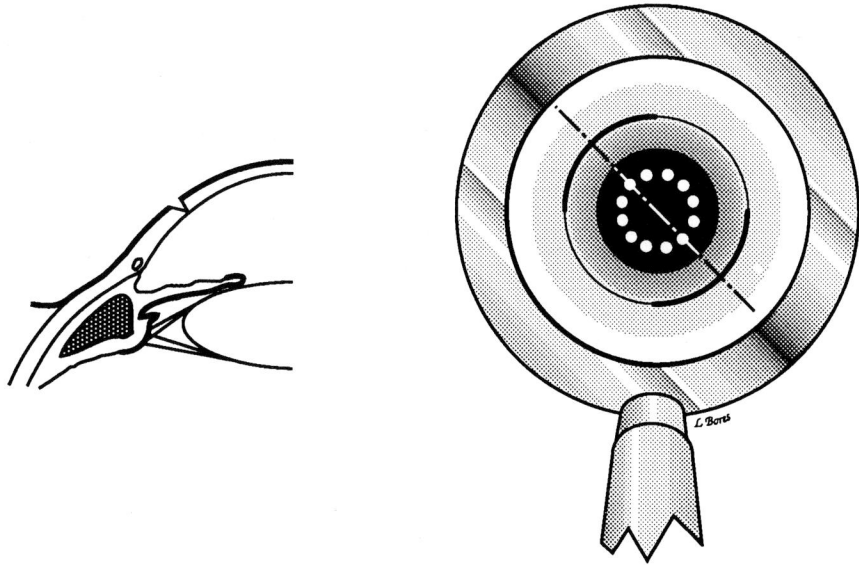

Fig. 9.106 Intra-cicatricial relaxing incisions.

zone of 5 mm. He found this to be a simple repro-ducible procedure and noted that there were some cases of over-correction. His results utilizing a pair of 100° length arcuate incisions at a 7 mm optical zone yielded a 2.10 D mean reduction in astigmatism. He, however, had only two eyes in this group.

Lindstrom has advocated this approach to the treatment of post-operative and congenital astig-matism and uses a simplified nomogram as a planning aid for this and straight-line T-cuts. He cautions the individual trying to use this nomogram that it will have to be tailored to the individual surgeon—good advice [54]. He admits to a predictive error of ±2 D. Such a margin of error in predicting the outcome of astig-matism surgery is somewhat high in the author's experience. Lindstrom has also designed a special marker for this procedure (Figure 9.107), available from Katena Instruments as K3-7996, 7 mm.

Topical anesthesia, as outlined above, is used in all cases. The procedure is logical and straightforward. The optic center is marked in the usual manner, as is the axis. The required optical zone is marked next. A six-ray marker is used to delineate the extent of a 60° arcuate incision—Lindstrom and the author do not make 120° incisions. An eight-ray radial keratotomy marker can be used to mark 90° and a 16-ray can be used for a 45° extent (Figure 9.108). The Lindstrom marker can also be used for this purpose. The begin-ning surgeon is warned about the use of such a marker. It is very easy to make the incision too long when confronted with all the tick marks this marker displays. The surgeon is advised to extend the ap-propriate tick marks with the skin-marking pen to avoid confusion. A caliper is used to strike off the

3 mm length of the straight T-incisions or the method of Lindstrom can be used (Figure 9.109).

The author sets the blade, as in all transverse in-cision cases, to 100% of the mean pachymetry at 5 or 7 mm as outlined in Chapter 8. If only astigmatism incisions are planned, mapping of the area around the planned incision site is sufficient. Arcuate incisions are always made at 7 mm. As with all astigmatism cases involving transverse incisions, only the very sharpest blade should be used. The eye is fixated with a limbus-to-limbus forceps. Beginning at one end of the transverse incision, insert the blade into the cornea, straddling the incision mark (Figure 9.110). Make each incision with a single smooth even motion of the blade—stopping exactly at the end of the mark. It is not a good idea to make the incisions in halves by starting in the middle and working out to the ends. You are likely to end up with an overlapping incision this way. Furthermore, it is possible for the bottom of the incision to invaginate up into the previous wound sufficiently that a penetration into the AC can occur. Transverse incisions are extremely difficult with a soft eye. The short slanted end of the beginning of each incision is of no moment; however, the square blade of Thornton may be used to make these incisions, obviating the possible problem of a slanted end point (Figure 9.111). Post-operative treatment is the usual (Chapter 8). Lindstrom's nomogram is shown in Figure 9.112.

The maximum correction the author has obtained with the arcuate method is 4.5 D and 5 D for the paired T-cuts. No over-corrections were obtained in the 18 cases in which this procedure was used. The author has not combined arcuate incisions with radials, so far

(a)

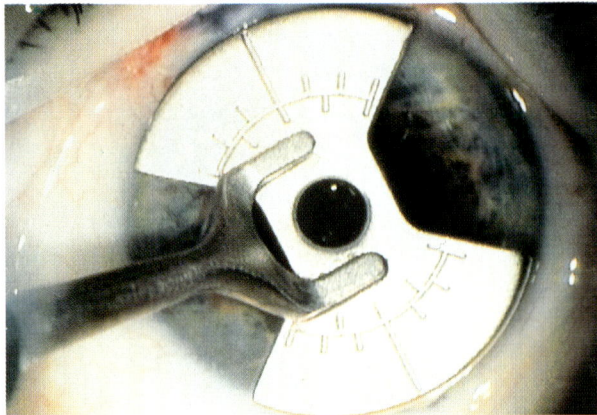

(b)

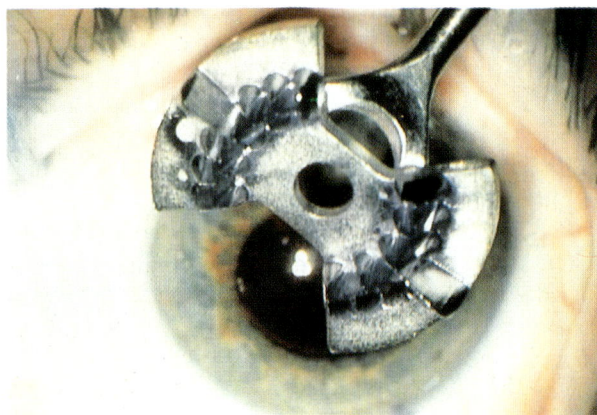

(c)

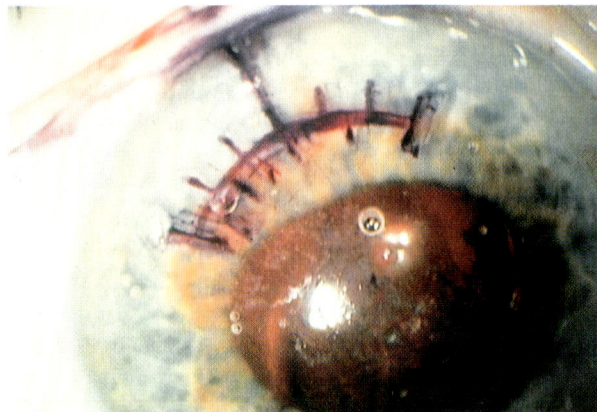

Fig. 9.107 (a–c) Lindstrom's arcuate incision marker.

being content with the results obtained with radial keratotomy methods (see above).

Over-view of relaxing incisions for astigmatism

The results obtained with these procedures confirm that straight transverse and arcuate non-perforating relaxing keratotomy incisions can be an effective tool for the reduction of naturally occurring and post-cataract astigmatism with or without associated spherical error. More classic approaches to post-keratoplasty astigmatism correction through the use of intra-incisional relaxing incisions with or without compression sutures may be a better alternative [34,55–60].

There is a significant range of effect with astigmatism surgery, with over-correction and under-correction being the rule. In addition, many patients continue to experience changes in their corneal topography and refraction beyond the expected time. This finding is especially true with cases involving T-incisions.

Thornton, using his own nomogram, analyzed 60 eyes with between 1.00 and 2.25 D of pre-operative astigmatism where an eight-incision radial keratotomy was combined with one to four straight transverse relaxing incisions. The transverse incision was placed between the radials. The mean pre-operative astigmatism was reduced from 1.50 to 0.40 D with a short follow-up period. The astigmatism was reduced in all but two of his patients. The highest pre-operative astigmatism attempted was 2.25 D in this series [58,61].

Park and Lee reported a series of 16 eyes where a transverse incision technique intersected the radial incision. The minimum astigmatism was 5.00 D. The mean pre-operative cylinder was 2.41 D and the mean correction was 1.92 D. All but one eye achieved a decrease in pre-operative astigmatism. The authors did not describe problems with intersection of the transverse incision with the radial incision. The effect decreased slightly with time, with a 23% reduction in effect at 10 months as compared to the first postoperative day [62].

Neumann also reported a series of eyes with transverse incisions placed at a 6 mm optical zone. His pattern was similar to the RT procedure in that the radial incision was interrupted at the transverse—in the RT procedure the transverse is interrupted at the radial. In 47 eyes with a mean age of 32.6 years, and a mean follow-up of 3 months, he found a mean reduction in astigmatism of 1.33 D with one or two T-incisions. Four eyes had no improvement and nine of the 47 eyes showed an increase in astigmatism. The maximum astigmatism treated was less than 2.75 D [63].

In a series of Lindstrom-pattern cases, 10 eyes with straight transverse relaxing keratotomy alone and 20 eyes with straight transverse relaxing keratotomy combined with radial keratotomy were evaluated. The mean follow-up in the transverse keratotomy alone group was 3.4 months and in the transverse and radial keratotomy group it was 7.7 months. A mean pre-operative cylinder of 5.30 D was reduced an average of

(a)   (b)   (c)

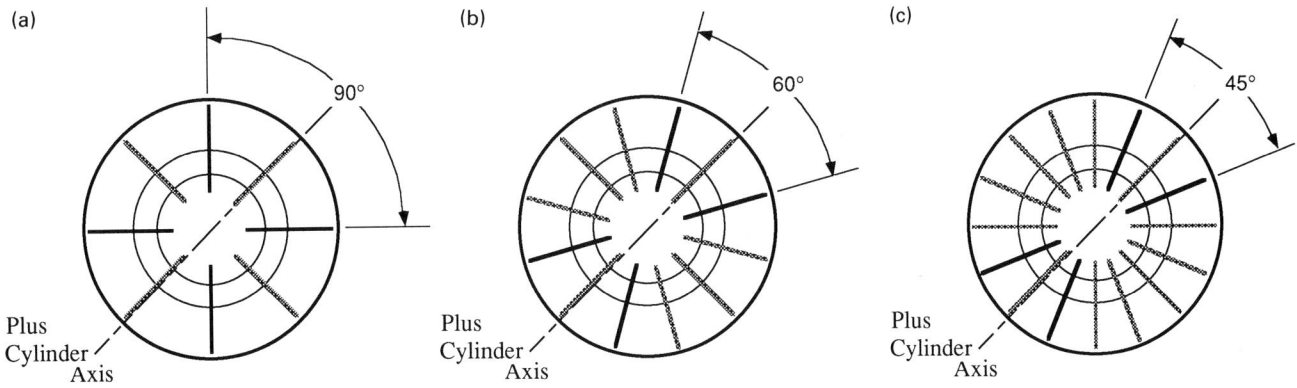

Fig. 9.108 (a–c) Various radial keratotomy incision markers can be used to delineate the extent of the required arcuate incision.

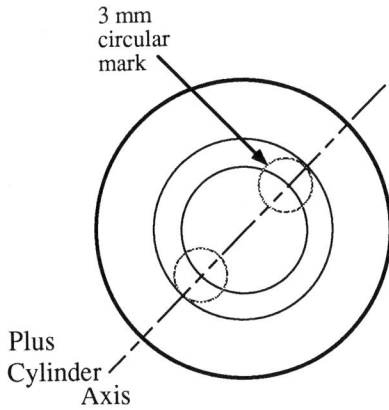

Fig. 9.109 Lindstrom's method using a 3 mm optical zone marker.

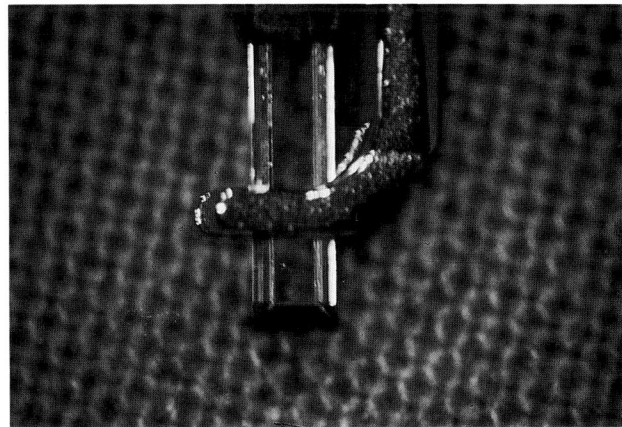

Fig. 9.111 The square diamond blade as recommended by Thornton.

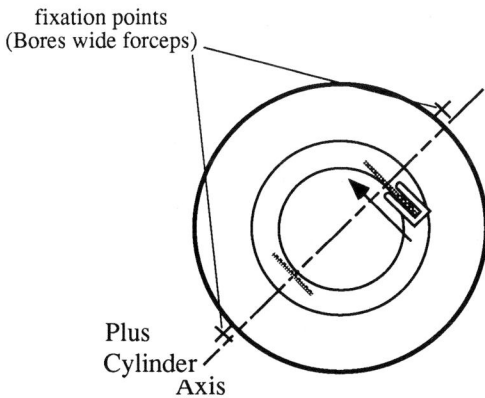

Fig. 9.110 A wide (limbus-to-limbus) fixation is necessary for precise incision control.

6.30 D in the astigmatism only group. In the combined compound myopia series, a pre-operative cylinder of 2.50 D was reduced an average of 2.90 D. The number of eyes which showed increased astigmatism was not presented. In this study, there was also a high degree of variability, which has persisted in more recent series ([64], R.L. Lindstrom, 1991, personal communication).

Currently published information, including the author's, is inadequate to determine whether straight or arcuate transverse relaxing keratotomy is superior. My results appear better with straight T keratotomy since I find that method easier to predict with pre-operative keratometry. Lindstrom has the opposite experience, preferring the arcuate Ts since he finds it easier to titrate with intra-operative keratometry (R.L. Lindstrom, 1991, personal communication). He found that 10 out of 24 patients operated with straight transverse incisions experienced over-corrections. This can be explained by his optical zone size which he tends to keep at 5.0 mm, occasionally adding an extra pair at 7.0 mm, and also by the length, which he keeps at 3 mm. The author rarely makes T-cuts at 5.00 mm except in cases utilizing the RZ method and then the Ts are only 1.5 mm in length.

The author was surprised to find such a low incidence of over-correction in Lindstrom's arcuate incision cases. Astigmatism reversal could not be evaluated because the post-operative residual cylinder axis was not reported. The author found that astigmatism tended to reverse itself in the majority of

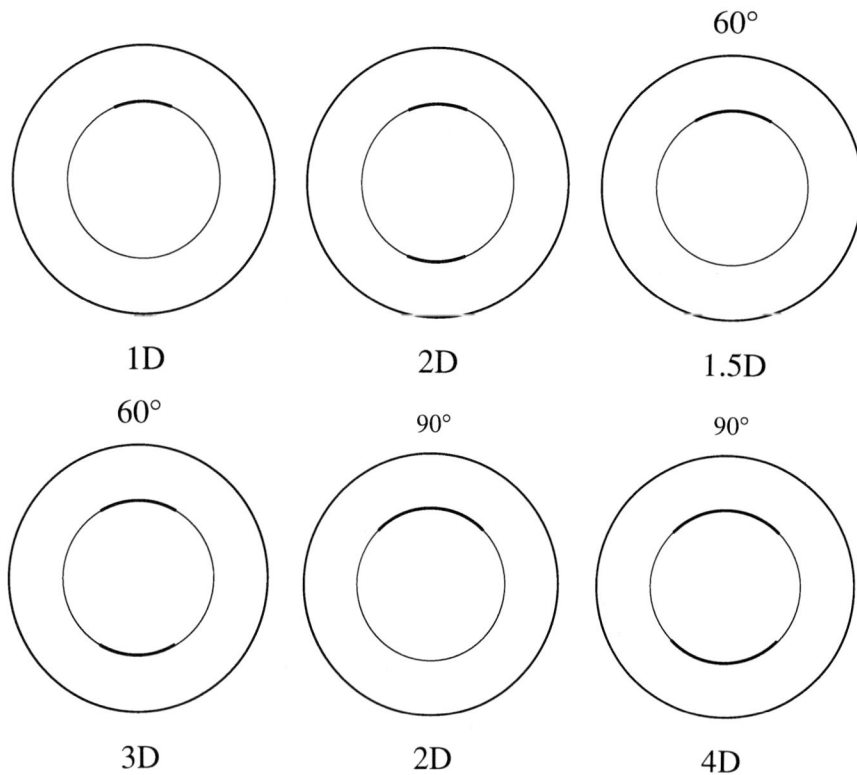

Fig. 9.112 Lindstrom nomogram for astigmatism to 4 D.

cases in which the arcuate method was applied *à la* Lindstrom. There is an explanation for this.

Arcuate incisions are advocated instead of straight T-incisions for the stated reason that the incision will thus be everywhere equidistant from the optic center. In this author's view, this may not be a good thing. Consider that the astigmatic surface has the shape of a regular toroid. As has been pointed out in our discussion of the nature of astigmatism (see the section on astigmatism—by way of review, above), there is a gradual lessening of corneal curvature as one progresses from the steeper meridian to the flatter. There is a direct relationship between incision length, or in the case of T-cuts, incision spacing, and the degree of the corneal curvature. That is, the steeper the curvature to be flattened, the longer the radial incision or the closer the spacing of the T-cut. Therefore the primary optical clear zone is smaller. Figures 9.113 and 9.114 illustrate this principle. Note that if one were to draw the extent of the variation of this clear zone on such a surface, it would take the shape of an ellipse. It should also be obvious that the meridians that are immediately off-axis require slightly larger optical zones.

This requirement is automatically met by a straight T-cut (Figure 9.113). Note that the ends of the T-cut, regardless of length, are farther away from the center than is the central portion. This is as it should be. Note also that such an incision most closely approaches a

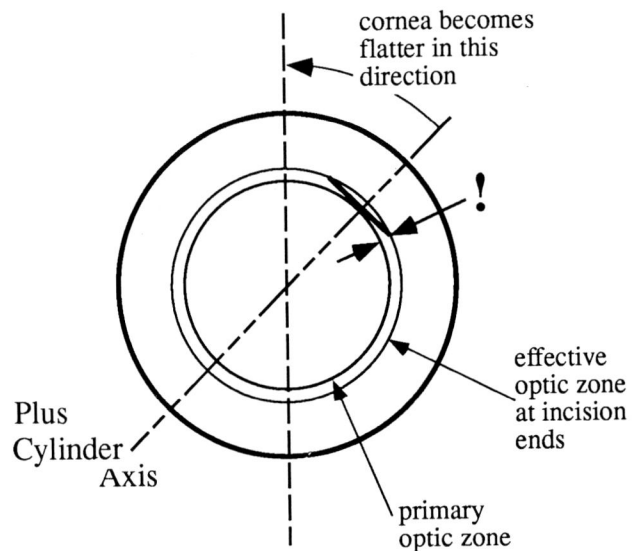

Fig. 9.113 The ends of the standard straight T-cut act at a greater distance than does the center.

tangent to the theoretic elliptic optical zone. As the T-cut gets longer and gets closer to the flatter meridian, other factors begin to manifest themselves and coupling occurs (see astigmatism discussion, above).

In an arcuate incision, regardless of length, all parts of the incision are equidistant from the center (Figure 9.114). This means that the ends of the incision, which

cornea becomes
flatter in this
direction

!

effective
optic zone
at incision
ends

Plus
Cylinder
Axis

primary
optic zone

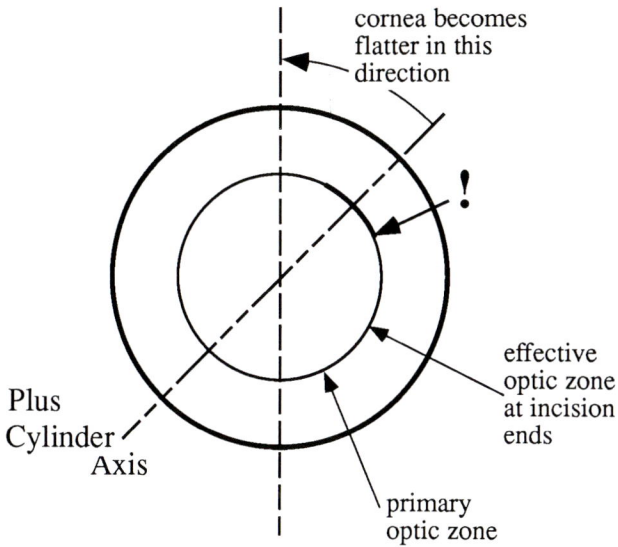

Fig. 9.114 An arcuate incision acts at the same distance throughout its length.

(a)

(b)

Fig. 9.115 (a,b) Hanna suction arcuate keratotomy trephine (K. Hanna, personal communication, 1992).

are off-axis, are closer to the optic center when they really should be farther away. Thus they are exerting much more influence per increment of length than a comparable straight T-cut—they are producing excess flattening precisely where less is needed. Theoretically, for a given optical zone and incision length, an arcuate cut should tend to produce more coupling effect. This is exactly what happens in the cadaver eye. This exact effect is not seen in the living eye for the reason that the optical zones typically called for are larger than used in T-cuts and also because living eyes display a different response to incisions than do cadaver eyes. Still, this aspect of arcuate cuts could help to explain the tendency the author has seen toward progression of effect (which can be explained by coupling and gradual reversal of the astigmatism). The length of these incisions undoubtedly plays a role as well. Bates

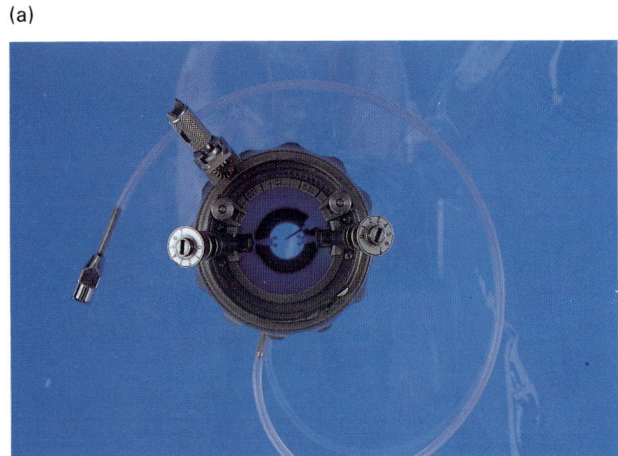

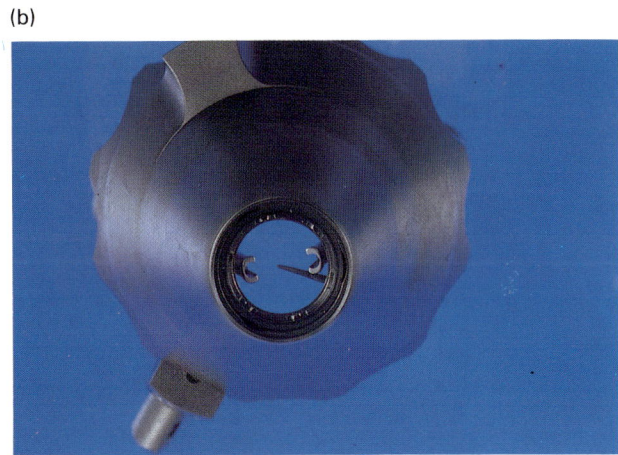

and Lans established the relationship of length to effect in both meridians almost 100 years ago.

Since arcuate incisions are somewhat harder to make accurately than straight Ts and for the reasons outlined above, the author urges caution in applying them.

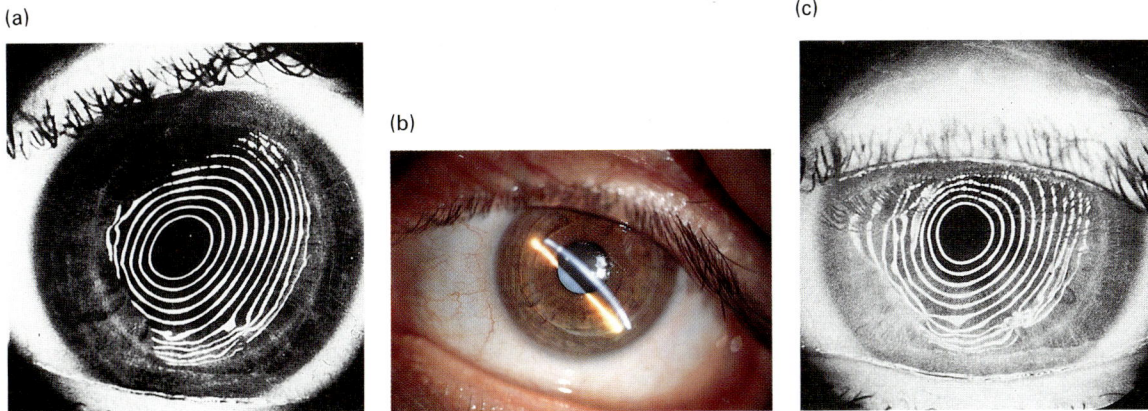

(a)

(b)

(c)

Fig. 9.116 (a) Pre-operative photokeratograph of astigmatism patient. (b) Eye post-surgery with the suction arcuate keratotomy trephine. (c) Post-operative photokeratograph of the eye in (b).

(a)

(b)

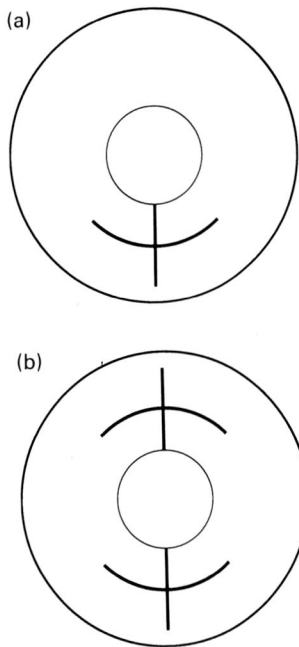

Fig. 9.117 Arciniegas and Amaya's method of radial arcuate incisions for low-order astigmatism.

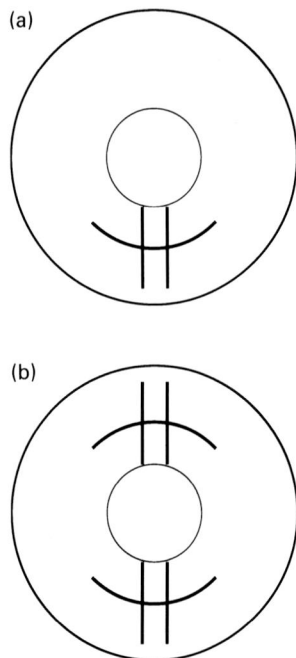

(a)

(b)

Fig. 9.118 Arciniegas and Amaya's method of radial arcuate incisions for higher-order astigmatism.

Fortunately, in those eyes where over-correction occurs, removal of the epithelial facet with compression suture placement can produce a good result in most cases (see Chapter 15). In under-correction, extension or deepening of an arcuate or T-type keratotomy incision or addition of further T-cuts is possible.

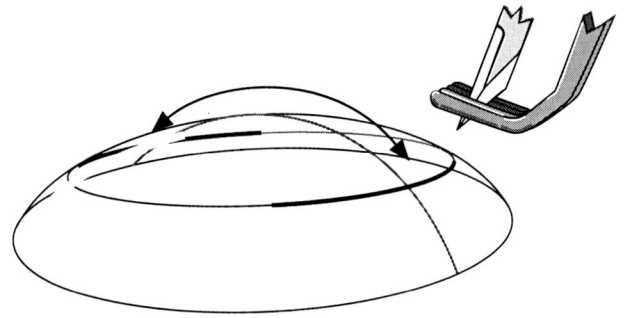

Fig. 9.119 The radial incision is made from the T-incision toward center and then from the T toward the limbus.

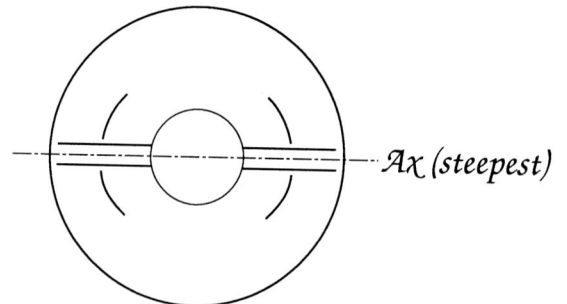

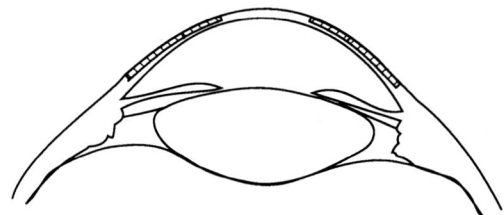

Fig. 9.120 A variation of the radial arcuate procedure using non-crossing incisions.

Hanna has devised a instrument which makes both limbs of the arcuate astigmatic pattern automatically. Similar to his suction trephine for penetrating keratoplasty, it is motor-driven (Figures 9.115 and 9.116) [65].

Combined arcuate–linear incisions

Arciniegas and Amaya [66] have devised a method for treating both spherical and astigmatic myopia by using arcuate incisions in conjunction with radials. The author has the same concerns for crossing incisions in this technique as expressed above in the discussion of the TR and TL procedures. The potential problems of arcuate incisions must always be kept in mind— especially in the lengths employed (Figures 9.117 through 9.120).

(a)

(b)

(c)

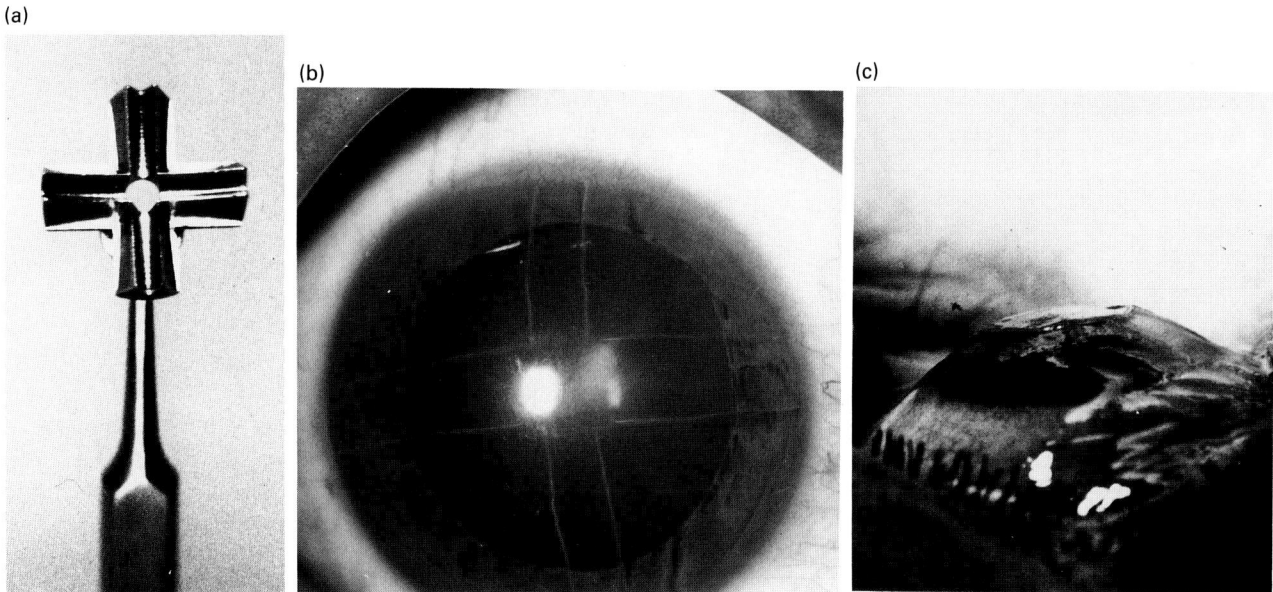

Fig. 9.121 (a) Marker for paired parallel incisions; (b) appearence of incisions on the cornea; (c) side view of eye showing profound flattening of the central cornea with this technique. (Courtesy of A. Arciniegas.)

Paired parallel incisions

In this technique, Arciniegas and Amaya [66] vary both the optical zone size and incision depth to effect changes in the curvature of both spherical and astigmatic corneas. Figure 9.121 illustrates the technique and results in human subjects. This technique is intriguing because it uses a minimum number of incisions to accomplish the task. Sufficient time has yet to elapse to prove the efficacy of this idea but it has merit and deserves trial.

Hyperopic astigmatism procedures

See also Chapter 15 for discussion of this subject.

Cauterization techniques (Figures 9.122 and 9.123)

These methods will be discussed in detail in Chapter 14.

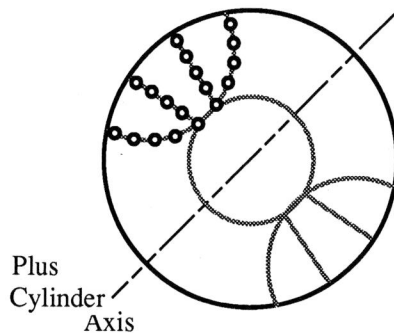

Fig. 9.122 Typical thermokeratoplasty (of Fyodorov) pattern for hyperopic astigmatism.

Ruiz quadrantic limbal incisions

Figure 9.124 illustrates a technique attempted by Ruiz in a few cases in an effort to control hyperopic astigmatism with relaxing incisions. The results were not satisfactory in the few cases attempted by the author and have since been abandoned.

Hexagonal keratotomy

The reader is referred to Chapter 14 for a discussion on attempts to control hyperopic astigmatism with this method.

References

1 Donders FC. *On the Anomalies of Accommodation and Refraction of the Eye*. WD Moore (transl). The Hatton Press, London, 1864.
2 Snellen H. Die Richtunge des Hauptmeridiane des Astigmatishen Auges. (The axis of the major meridians of the astigmatic eye.) Albrecht von Graefes Arch Klin Ophthalmol 1869; 15:199–207.
3 Brajkovich HL. Dr. Snellen's 20/20: the development and use of the eye chart. J Sch Health 1980; 50:472–474.
4 den Tonkelaar I, Henkes HE, van Leersum GK. The Utrecht Ophthalmic Hospital and the development of tonometry in the 19th century. Doc Ophthalmol 1988; 68:57–63.
5 Fukala V. Operative Behandlung der hochstgradigen Myopie durch Aphakie (Surgical treatment of high degrees of myopia through aphakia.) Graefes Arch Ophthalmol 1890; 36:230–244.
6 Schiøtz HA. Ein Fall von hochgradigem Hornhautastigmatismus nach Staarextraction. Besserung auf Operativem Wege. (A case of severe corneal astigmatism after cataract extraction. Improved by surgical means.) Arch Augenheilk 1885; 15:178–181.

(a)

(b)

(c)

(d)

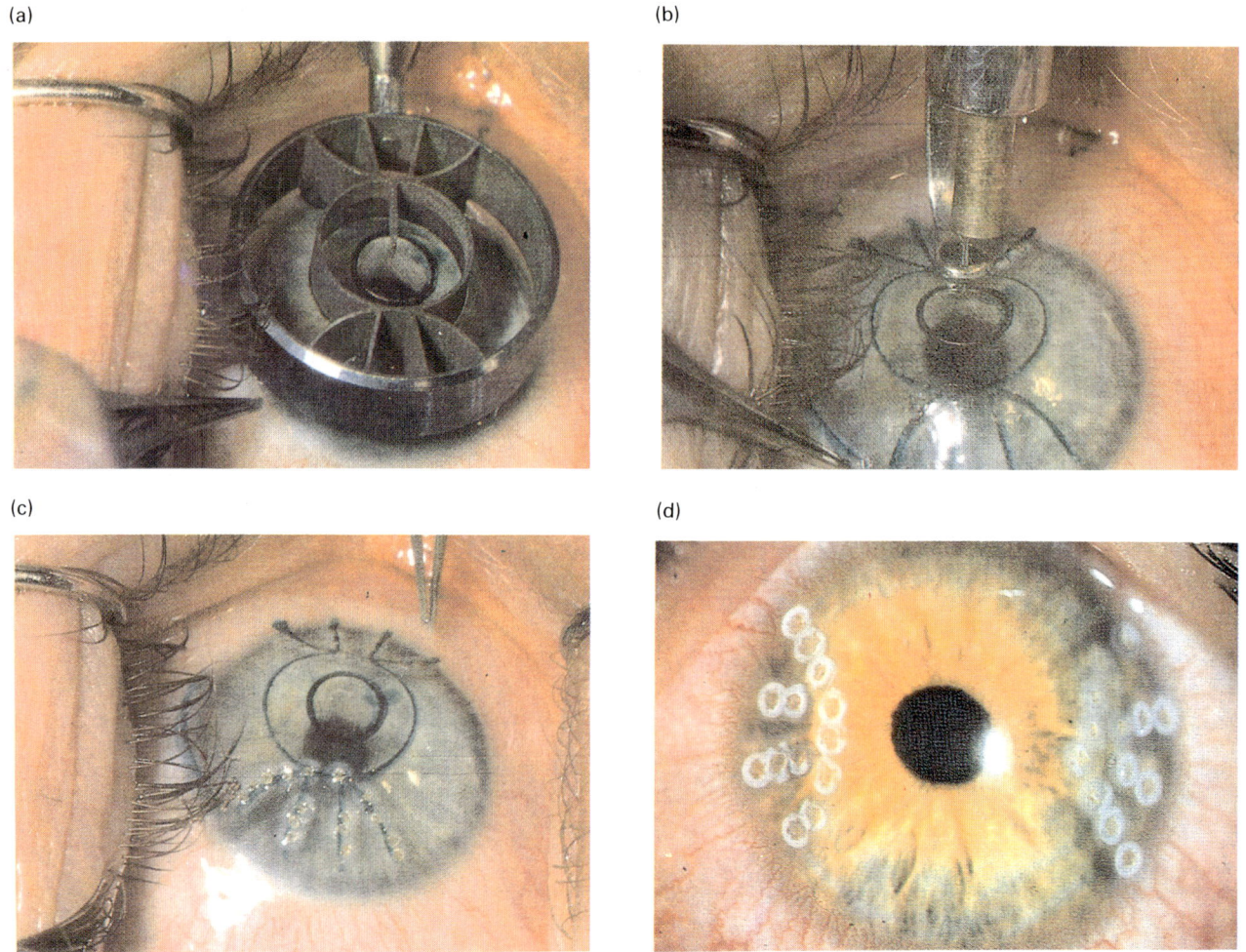

Fig. 9.123 The use of the Fyodorov method for astigmatism (a) A special pattern marker is used, aligning the marks with the plus (hyperopic) axis. (b) The prescribed number of thermal punctures is then made using the pattern as a guide. (c) Thermokeratoplasty for hyperopic astigmatism, immediately post-application. (d) The same eye at 24 hours post-surgery. (Courtesy of S.N. Fyodorov.)

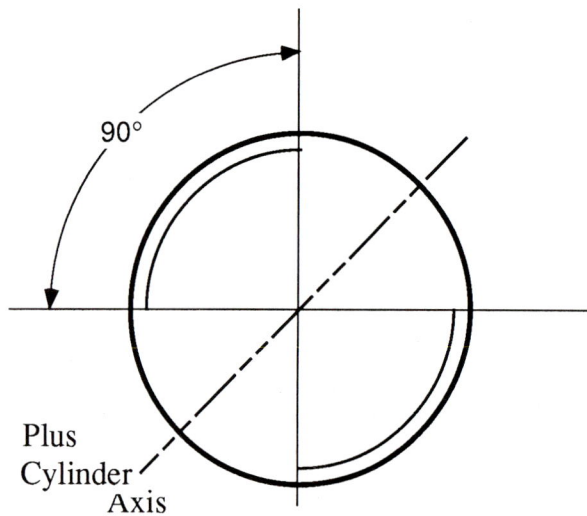

Fig. 9.124 Ruiz quadrantic arcuate incisions for hyperopic astigmatism.

7 Karatz MA. William Horatio Bates, MD, and the Bates method of eye exercises. NY State J Med 1975; 75:1105–1110.

8 Bates WH. A suggestion of an operation to correct astigmatism. Arch Ophthalmol 1894; 23:9–13.

9 Faber E. Operative Behandeling van Astigmatism. (Operative treatment of astigmatism.) Nederl Tijdschr v Geneesk 1895; 2:495–496.

10 Lucciola J. Traitement chirugical de l'astigmie. Arch Ophthalmol 1896; 16:630–638.

11 Lans L. Experimentelle Untersuchungen uber die Entstehung von Astigmatismus durch nicht perforirende Corneawunden. (Experimental studies of the treatment of astigmatism with non-perforating corneal incisions.) Albrecht von Graefes Arch Klin Exp Ophthalmol 1898; 45:117–152.

12 Bates WH. Operation for relief of persistent deafness. M Record 1886; 29:88.

13 Bates WH. Suture of the cornea after removal of the lens. Arch Ophthalmol 1898; 27:181.

14 Wray C. Case of 6 D of hypermetropic astigmatism cured by cautery. Trans Ophthalmol Soc (Lond) 1914; 34:109.

15 Weiner M. Meier's method of peeling of the cornea. Ophthalmol Year Book 1917.

16 Burr WS. Keratoconus; results of different types of operations. Trans Ophthalmol Soc (Lond) 1939; 59:480.

17 Weiner M. *Ophthalmology in the War Years*. Year Book Publishers, Chicago, 1946.

18 O'Connor R. Corneal cautery for high myopic astigmatism. Am J Ophthalmol 1933; 16:337.

19 O'Connor R. Corneal cautery for conic cornea and corneal astigmatism. Trans Pacific Coast Oto-Ophthalmol Soc 1938; 23:25–31.

20 Bock J. Uber Versuche, den Hornhautastigmatismus durch Stichelungen mit der Elecktrokoagulationsnadel zu beeinflussen. Wien Klin Wochenschr 1939; 2:971–974.

21 Sato T. Treatment of conical cornea (incision of Descemet's membrane). Acta Soc Ophthalmol (Jpn) 1939; 43:541.

22 Kokott W. Uber mechanisch-kunktionelle Strukturen des Auges. Graefes Arch Ophthalmol 1938.

23 Gilbert W. Zur Behandlung des Keratokonus nach Sato. Klin Monatsbl Augenheilkd 1943; 109:702–704.

24 Linder K. Nach Sato erfolgreich operieter Keratokonus. Wien Klin Wochenschr 1949; 61:653–654.

25 Hruby K. Zur Sato operation. Wien Klin Wochenschr 1949; 61:653–654.

26 Sato T. Ueber eine Operationsmethode zur Behandlung des Keratoconus (Descemetspaltung). Klin Monatsbl Augenheilk 1941; 107:234–238.

27 Sato T. Posterior incision of cornea; surgical treatment for conical cornea and astigmatism. Am J Ophthalmol 1950; 33:943–948.

28 Akiyama K. Study of surgical treatment for myopia. I. Posterior corneal incisions. Acta Soc Ophthalmol (Jpn) 1952; 56:1142–1150.

29 Sato T. Crosswise incisions of Descemet's membrane for the treatment of advanced keratoconus. Acta Soc Ophthalmol (Jpn) 1942; 46:469–470.

30 Sato T. Experimental study on surgical correction of astigmatism. Juntendo Kenkyukai Zasshi 1943; 589:37.

31 Sato T. Posterior half incision combined with the method of separating middle layers of cornea. Juntendo Med Assoc 1950.

32 Sato T, Akiyama K, Shibata H. Posterior half-incision of the cornea for astigmatism; operative procedures and results of the improved tangent method. Am J Ophthalmol 1953; 36:462–466.

33 Sato T, Akiyama K, Shibata H. A new surgical approach to myopia. Am J Ophthalmol 1953; 36:823–829.

34 Troutman RC, Swinger C. Relaxing incision for control of postoperative astigmatism following keratoplasty. Ophthalm Surg 1980; 11:117–120.

35 Troutman RC. Microsurgical control of corneal astigmatism in cataract and keratoplasty. Trans Am Acad Ophthalmol Otolaryngol 1973; 77:563–572.

36 Jensen RP, Jensen AC. Surgical correction of astigmatism by microwedge resection of the limbus. Ophthalmology 1978; 85:1288–1298.

37 Fyodorov SN. Surgical correction of myopia and astigmatism. Proceedings of the Keratorefractive Society Meeting 1980.

38 Duke-Elder S, Abrams D. Ophthalmic optics and refraction. In: *System of Ophthalmology*, SS Duke-Elder (ed). CV Mosby, St Louis, 1970.

39 Jaffe NS, Clayman HM. The pathophysiology of corneal astigmatism after cataract surgery. Ophthalmology 1975; 79: 615–630.

40 Maguire LJ, Bourne WM. Multifocal lens effect as a complication of radial keratotomy. Refract Corneal Surg 1989; 5:394–399.

41 Mobilia EF, Kenyon KR. Contact lens-induced corneal warpage. Int Ophthalmol Clin 1986; 26:43–53.

42 Swinger CA, Barker BA. Prospective evaluation of myopic keratomileusis. Ophthalmology 1984; 91:785–792.

43 Thornton SP. New diamond blade configuration for transverse incisions (instruments). Refract Corneal Surg 1989; 5:49.

44 Troutman RC. Primary astigmatism control using the Troutman surgical keratometer. In: *Current Concepts in Cataract Surgery. Selected Proceedings of Sixth Biennial Cataract Surgical Congress*, JM Emery and AC Jaconson (eds). CV Mosby, St Louis, 1980.

45 Troutman RC. Corneal ˙wedge resections and relaxing incisions for postkeratoplasty astigmatism. Int Ophthalmol Clin 1983; 23:161–168.

46 Fyodorov SN, Durnev VV. Surgical correction of complicated myopic astigmatism by means of dissection of circular ligament of cornea. Ann Ophthalmol 1981; 13:1.

47 Rubin ML. The induction of refractive errors by retinal detachment surgery. Trans Am Ophthalmol Soc 1976; 73:452–490.

48 Lindstrom R. Surgical correction of postoperative astigmatism. Indian J Ophthalmol 1990; 38:114–123.

49 Ruiz LA. *Surgical Treatment of Astigmatism*. American Academy of Ophthalmology, Atlanta, 1986.

50 Bores LD. *Surgical Management of Astigmatism*. Keratorefractive Society, Atlanta, 1986.

51 Rowsey JJ. Current concepts in astigmatism surgery. J Refract Surg 1986; 2:85–94.

52 Krachmer JH, Ching SS. Relaxing corneal incisions for postkeratoplasty astigmatism. Int Ophthalmol Clin 1983; 23:153–159.

53 Merlin D. Curved keratotomy procedure for congenital astigmatism. J Refract Surg 1987; 3:92–97.

54 Lindstrom RL. The surgical correction of astigmatism: a clinician's perspective. J Refract Surg 1990; 6:441–454.

55 Barner SS. Surgical treatment of corneal astigmatism. Ophthalm Surg 1976; 7:43–48.

56 Krachmer JH, Fenzl RE. Surgical correction of high postkeratoplasty astigmatism. Relaxing incisions vs wedge resection. Arch Ophthalmol 1980; 98:1400–1402.

57 Lavery GW, Lindstrom RL, Hofer LA, Doughman DJ. The surgical management of corneal astigmatism after penetrating keratoplasty. Ophthalm Surg 1985; 16:165–169.

58 Thornton S. Thornton guide for radial keratotomy incisions and optical zone size. J Refract Surg 1985; 1:29–33.

59 Mandel MR, Shapiro MB, Krachmer JH. Relaxing incisions with augmentation sutures for the correction of postkeratoplasty astigmatism. Am J Ophthalmol 1987; 103:441–447.

60 Sugar J, Kirk AK. Relaxing keratotomy for post-keratoplasty high astigmatism. Ophthalm Surg 1983; 14:156–158.

61 Thornton SP, Sanders DR. Graded non-intersecting transverse incisions for correction of idiopathic astigmatism. J Cataract Refract Surg 1985; 13:27–31.

62 Park K, Lee JJ. Surgical correction of astigmatism using paired T-incisions. Korean J Ophthalmol 1989; 3:61–65.

63 Neumann AC, McCarty GR, Sanders DR, Raanan MG. Refractive evaluation of astigmatic keratotomy procedures. J Cataract Refract Surg 1989; 15:25–31.

64 Agapitos PJ, Lindstrom RL, Williams PA, Sanders DR. Analysis of astigmatic keratotomy. J Cataract Refract Surg 1989; 15:13–18.

65 Saragoussi K, Hanna K, Goichot-Bonnat L, Hoang T, Besson J, Pouliquen Y. Astigmatisme post-keratoplastie et trepan DE Hanna: premiers resultats. Bull Soc Ophthalmol France 1987; 3:255–257.

66 Arciniegas A, Amaya LE. Combined semi-radial and arcuate keratotomy for correction of ametropia: a theoretical bioengineering approach. J Refract Surg 1988: 4:51–59.

10

Lamellar Refractive Surgery

Discovery consists of seeing what everybody has seen and thinking what nobody has thought. [Albert Szent-Gyorgi, *The Scientist Speculates*]

Briefly, lamellar refractive surgery seeks to modify the corneal shape through mechanic means. This process can take several forms:

1 Removing and re-shaping the resected tissue—*keratomileusis*.
2 Removing tissue and re-shaping the underlying stroma—*keratomileusis-in-situ*.
3 Attaching an appliqué to the corneal surface—*epikeratophakia*.
4 Removing tissue and sandwiching another material between—*keratophakia*.
5 Internal tissue ablation—*intra-stromal ablation*.

The latter method seeks to re-shape the surface via intra-stromal tissue ablation through use of photo-disruptive laser light. Hence it will be discussed in Chapter 11.

Of the remaining four methodologies, though keratophakia is the harbinger of the preceding three, it shall be discussed last.

The history of lamellar refractive surgery

The term refractive keratoplasty was coined in 1949 by Barraquer when he demonstrated that plastic surgery of the cornea could alter its refractive power in a pre-determined way [1]. Basically the initial procedure (Figure 10.1) called for double, non-penetrating, concentric, trephinations at 10 and 11 mm. The resulting annulus was resected and discarded. The central portion was then dissected to form a planar disk which was re-sutured to the eye, flattening the corneal curvature. The procedure was modified, in one case, to treat keratoconus except in this instance by substituting a thicker, homoplastic disk of donor cornea.

Keratomileusis and keratophakia are freeze-lathing procedures that had their beginnings in 1961 when Barraquer reported his first eight cases of allopathic keratophakia in human eyes followed in 1963 by keratomileusis [2]. The technique was introduced into the USA in 1977 by Richard Troutman, MD, professor and former chairman of the Ophthalmology Department of the Manhattan Eye and Ear Infirmary. In the ensuing years, relatively few cases have been performed in the States by relatively few surgeons.

Basic principles of lamellar refractive surgery

The premise is simple: remove or add sufficient material within the corneal stroma to alter the external curvature of that cornea without materially affecting Bowman's layer. This precept is violated by the technique of "Bowman's blasting" with the excimer laser, which totally obliterates that structure in the visual axis (Figure 10.2). Epithelium and Bowman's seem to have a special affinity—though "normal"

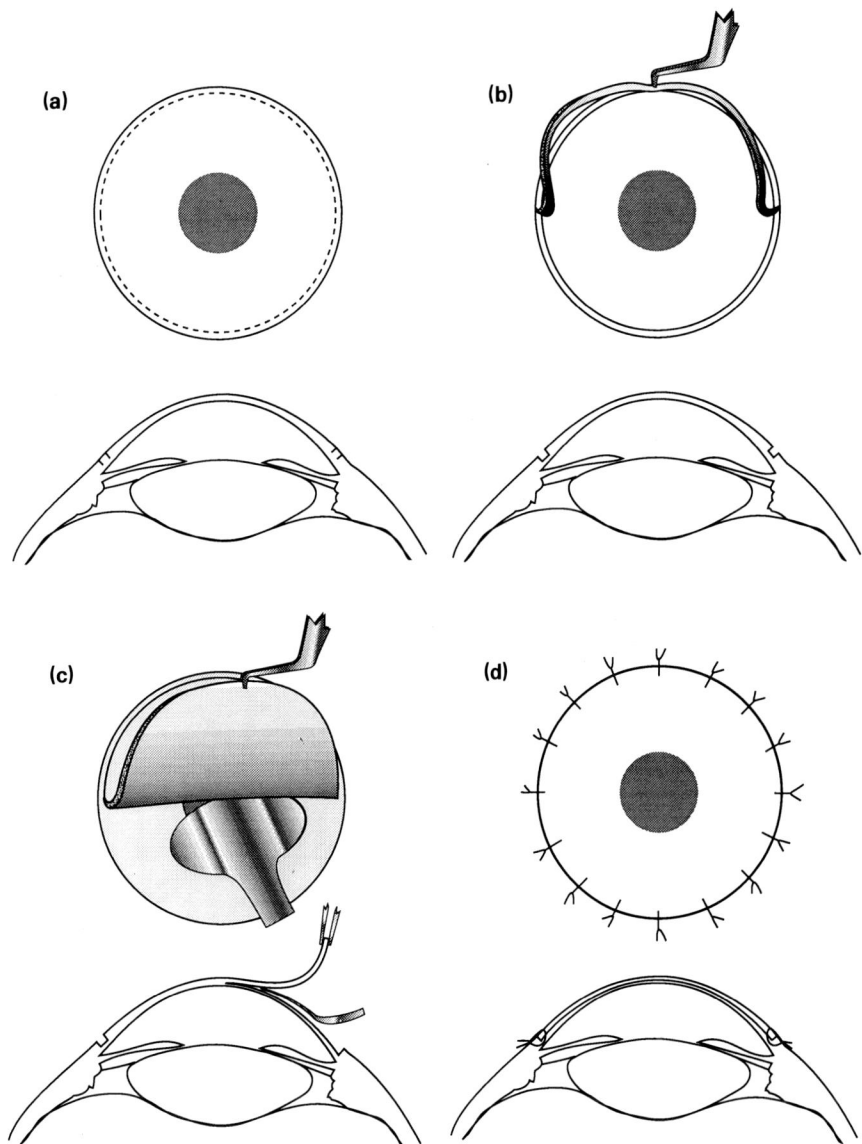

Fig. 10.1 Barraquer's lamellar stromectomy for myopia. (a) Two non-penetrating trephinations are made—10 and 11 mm in diameter. (b) The annular ring of stroma between is dissected and removed. (c) Next the central corneal stromal disk is dissected free. (d) This freed disk is then sutured to the periphery thereby flattening the central curvature. A similar method was used to treat keratoconus. In these cases a homoplastic disk was substituted for the patient's central stroma.

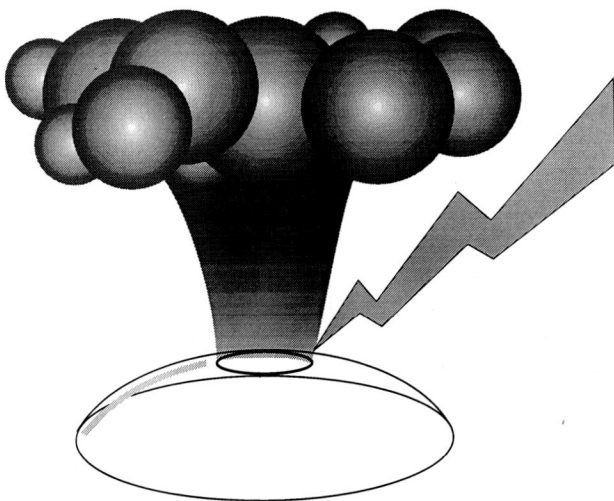

Fig. 10.2 Bowman's blasting—laser stromectomy.

appearing hemidesmosomes are reported following laser surface ablation (see Chapter 4). Considerable variability in result has been reported (see Chapter 11).

Merely stuffing material into a pocket made intra-stromally does not usually result in good effect either. Typically the resistance of Bowman's to distortion and/or stretch results in a change in the back surface curvature of the cornea, which may (or may not) alter the total refractive power. Consequently, all successful lamellar procedures involve a complete separation of Bowman's from its limbal connection. This allows the front corneal layer to adjust smoothly to the induced distortion and enhances the curvature change. Various techniques have been devised to accomplish the main goal. Some have been successful, some not. Our discussion will deal with most, if not all, such attempts.

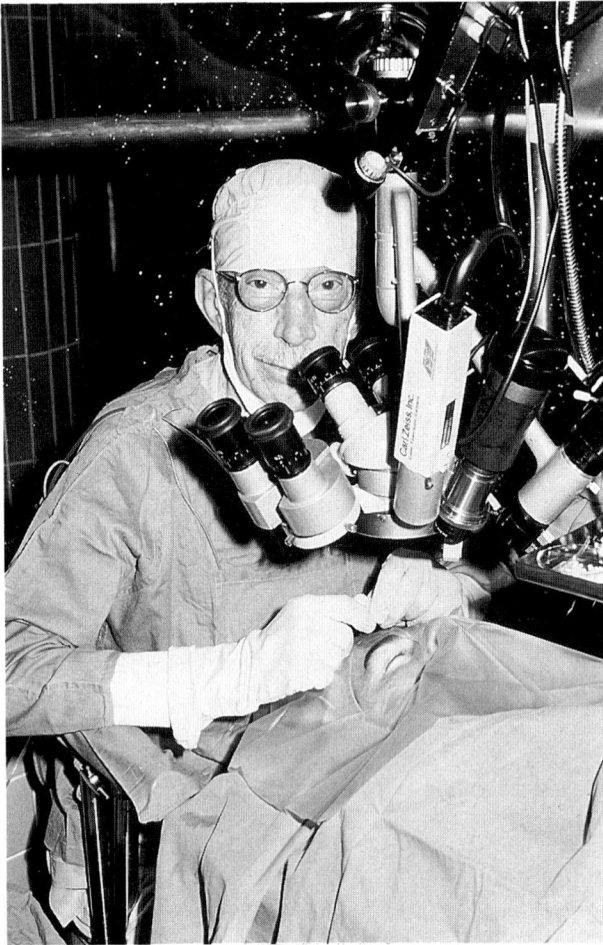

Fig. 10.3 Professor José Ignatio Barraquer—refractive surgery pioneer.

Keratomileusis

Approximately two score years ago, a young physician began a series of experiments that culminated in a surgical technique largely unappreciated and un-heralded even today. The procedure—keratomileusis; the physician—José Ignatio Barraquer (Figure 10.3). The term keratomileusis itself comes from the Greek words *keras* (horn-like—cornea) and *smileusis* (carving)—corneal carving. Over the years very few ophthalmologists have taken the trouble to learn anything about this operative technique; fewer have attempted to perform it; even fewer have mastered it. Attitudes toward practitioners of this "black art" are mixed. All are looked on as élitists or as ophthalmic buccaneers or even worse. This notion is intensified by the tendency of these "cultists" to gather together in tight little groups, to speak in tongues—angle α, base plate, non-torque suture, etc.—and are characterized by the thousand-yard stare of one who's *been there*.

Keratomileusis is an exhilarating, challenging, and elegant procedure whose performance is akin to flying:

long moments of joy punctuated by short periods of stark terror. Having said that, we hasten to add that it is also a rewarding and satisfying procedure whose anxiety-provoking potential is in direct proportion to experience. Still, the allusion to flying pretty much sums up how many feel about this operation—terrified. It is perceived to be a technically demanding and meticulous procedure whose path to completion is studded with minefields. It *is* that and more. There is no question that the operation of keratomileusis demands levels of skill exceeding that of any other in ophthalmology. There is no question that this technique is fraught with difficulties and carries with it a high potential for disaster. There is no question that this operation is not for the sunshine ophthalmologist (like the sunshine patriot: invincible in peace, invisible in war), the occasional surgeon or the multi-thumbed instant expert. There is also no question that, properly performed, this operation provides the dedicated refractive surgeon power over high degrees of myopia. With its encompassing ability to overcome hyperopia as well, it is a valuable tool withal.

This section is designed to increase the reader's knowledge about this technique as well as provide the student of refractive surgery with insight into its mechanism and performance. It is hoped that the knowledge gained will alleviate some of the understandable anxiety surrounding the procedure. Perhaps some of you will even be tempted to test the waters. This is all well but the author suggests that in that case readers should prepare themselves for possible failure. This technique is learnable and diligence and care will pay off.

If the reader carries away no more from reading this text than an enlightened view of this technique, then it will be time well spent, both for the reader as well as the author. Regardless, a study of this approach to corneal modulation is an essential precursor to understanding and performing other techniques such as epikeratophakia, keratophakia and laser corneal surface shaping.

Patient selection and workup

The basic requirements that a patient must meet to be eligible for refractive surgery have been outlined in Chapter 5. However, lamellar refractive surgical candidates have' additional requisites depending on the modality. For example, in autoplastic MKM (wherein the patient's own cornea will be lathed) the lower limit of refraction is −6 D and the upper limit should be −15 D if a complete correction is expected. Furthermore, there is a limit to the degree of flattening with MKM which has a floor of 33 D. Thus a −15 D patient should have a pre-surgical spherical equivalent K-reading of 48 D. If the patient has a higher myopic refraction, homoplastic MKM can be done. In such a case corrections of up to −30 D have been obtained. However, even with homoplastic MKM the effective optical zone becomes quite small and centration critical. In these cases the incidence of induced astigmatism is increased.

Corneal curvature can also affect the initial corneal disk resection. Excessively steep corneas—7.81 mm (47.54 D)—or excessively flat corneas—8.6 mm (39.24 D)—can make the resection more difficult.

The actual amount of ametropia *at the cornea* to be corrected (D_V in the calculations) must be the contact lens power or the spectacle power corrected for the vertex distance thus:

$$D_V = \frac{D_C}{1 - (VD)(D_C)}$$

Where VD = vertex distance in meters, and D_C = spectacle spherical equivalent. Hence, if the patient wears a −13 D spectacle whose vertex distance is 12 mm, then:

$$D_V = \frac{-13}{1 - (0.012)(-13)}$$

$$= \frac{-13}{1 - (-0.156)}$$

$$= \frac{-13}{1.156}$$

$$= -11.25 \text{ D at the cornea}$$

For a hyperopic patient wearing a +13 D spectacle at the same vertex distance, the power at the cornea would be +10.49 D.

Corneal thickness is also a factor. Generally speaking the higher the myopia, the greater the central corneal thickness should be, as measured ultrasonically. In any case, a cornea with a central thickness less than 0.45 mm (450 μm) should not have autoplastic keratomileusis, though a homoplastic keratomileusis might be done. Such thin corneas are rare and might be cases of sub-clinical keratoconus, in which event the surgery should be avoided altogether.

Instrumentation for keratomileusis

In classic keratomileusis, the key instrument of the surgery is the microkeratome. In keratomileusis-*in-situ* (see below), the key instrument is still the microkeratome. While it is true, in classic keratomileusis, that the power changes in the corneal tissue are produced by the operation of lathing, still, without a proper keratectomy, the operation fails. In keratomileusis-*in-situ* the correct use of the microkeratome is paramount to the success of the operation. Short cuts and "make-do" are not appropriate approaches to the use of this instrument. Despite the difficulty of its application, however, correct usage can be learned with a modicum of diligence and practice. You are encouraged to continue such practice until you are comfortable with the instrument. Figure 10.4 shows two typical microkeratome instrument sets.

Microkeratome

This instrument is based upon the principle of the carpenter's plane (Figure 10.5). The microkeratome head is divided into an anterior and posterior section in relation to the cutting blade. This blade is caused to oscillate at approximately 10 000 excursions/min by a precision, foot-switch-controlled, electric or gas turbine motor. The blade itself protrudes a fixed distance from the base of the keratome plane or head. The Steinway unit uses a fixed plate to control resection depth. In the SCMD unit, a threaded knob attached to a movable plate in the anterior portion of the head varies the relative protrusion of the blade;

(a)

(b)

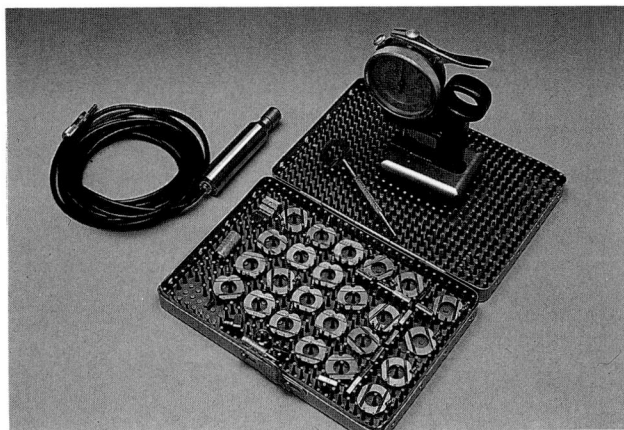
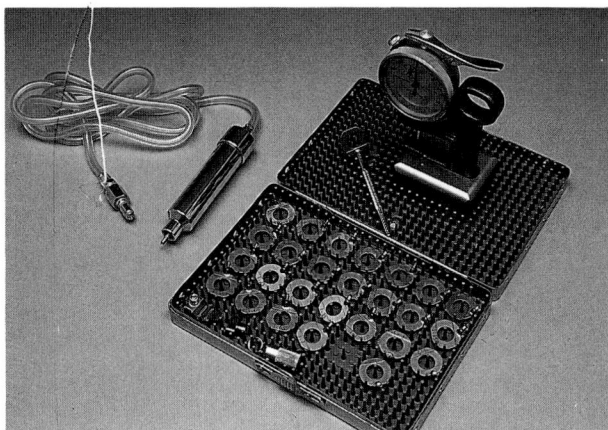

Fig. 10.4 Standard keratectomy sets. (a) Steinway *in-situ* set with electric motor handle; (b) SCMD *in-situ* set—gas turbine handle. Both instruments can be used with the cryo-lathe.

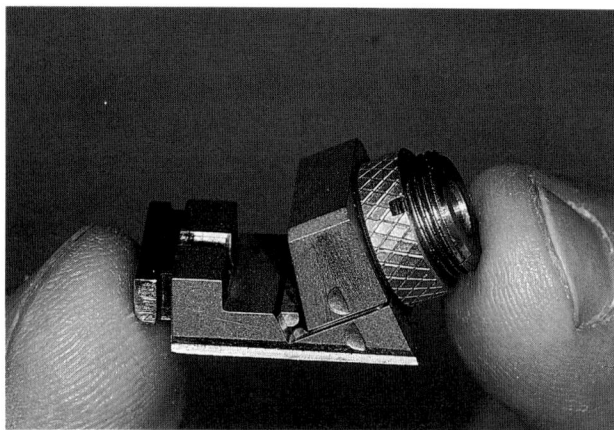

Fig. 10.5 The standard Barraquer microkeratome head.

this in turn alters the thickness of the tissue section removed. This head will be described further below. The Draeger microkeratome operates on a slightly different principle and will be discussed, along with the new Ruiz–Steinway keratome, in a separate section.

The sides of the microkeratome head have dovetail guides on either side along the bottom edge of the plane. These guides fit into corresponding guides in the pneumatic rings, and position the edge of the cutting blade at a constant 0.13 mm to the plane of the pneumatic fixation ring. The position of the posterior platform of the plane is held constant to prevent any modification of the intra-ocular pressure during the resection. The prototype of the current keratome used

(a)   (b)   (c)

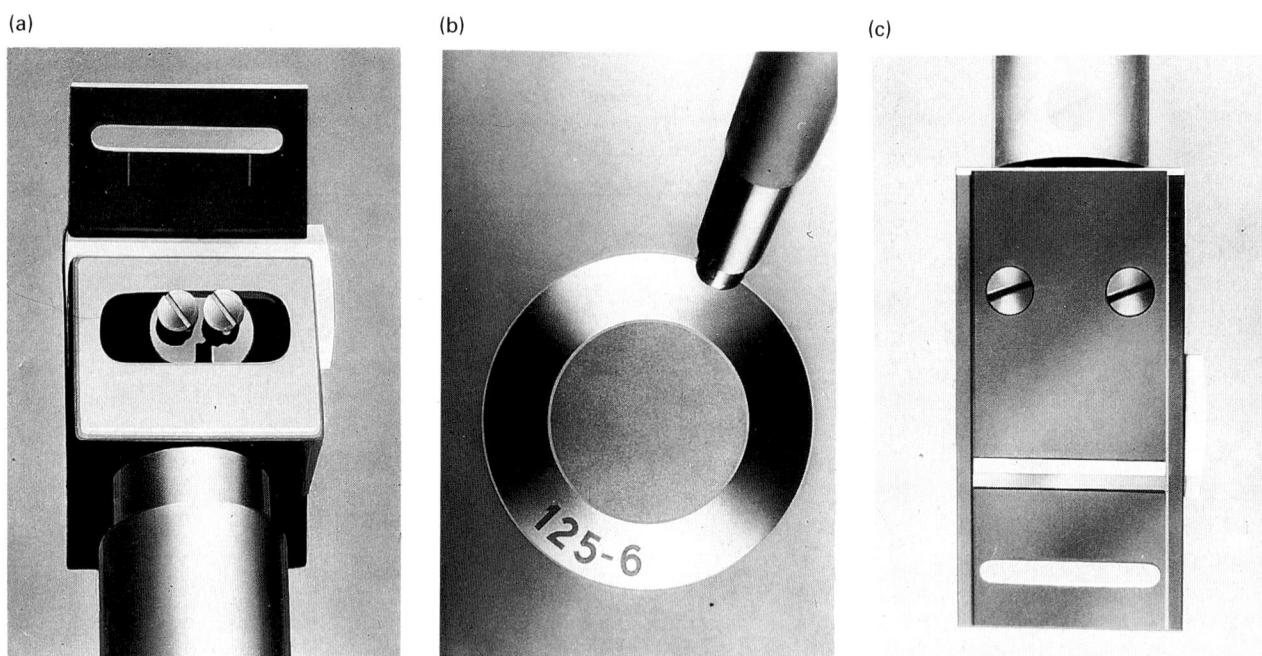

Fig. 10.6 (a,b) Top and bottom views of the prototype microkeratome. The blade is adjustable. (c) Prototype vacuum fixation ring. Note the absence of guides for the keratome (from Barraquer JI. Historia de la cirugia refractiva de la cornea. In: *Cirugia Refractiva de la Cornea*, Instituto Barraquer de America, Bogota, Colombia, 1989).

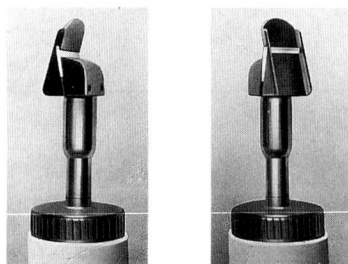

Fig. 10.7 Second-generation keratome head with dovetails, fixed blade, and provision for replaceable applanation plate (from Barraquer JI. Historia de la cirugia refractiva de la cornea. In: *Cirugia Refractiva de la Cornea*, Instituto Barraquer de America, Bogota, Columbia, 1989).

an adjustable blade, had no guiding dovetails and was passed across the surface of a flat-topped pneumatic fixation ring (Figure 10.6). The problems produced by this configuration were manifold. It was, for example, not possible to gauge precisely the thickness of the resection from case to case. The keratome was subsequently re-designed to provide both guides and a fixed-position blade (Figure 10.7). The resection thickness was (and still is) controlled by a variable-thickness applanator plate (Figure 10.8).

The dimensions of the microkeratome have been carefully selected in relation to the size of the human globe and the average corneal curvature. It is a sensitive and high-precision instrument manufactured from surgical stainless steel. It is easily disassembled

(a)

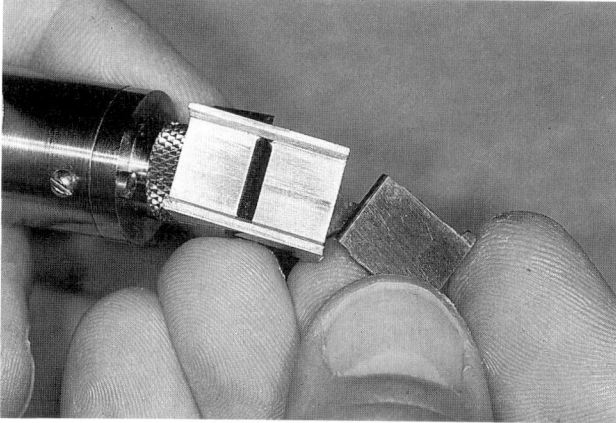

(b)

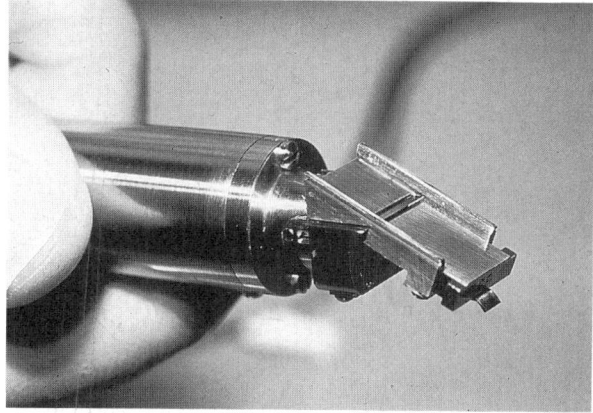

Fig. 10.8 (a) Resection depth (disk thickness) is controlled by interchangeable plates. (b) These plates snap into the anterior part of the keratome base.

(a)

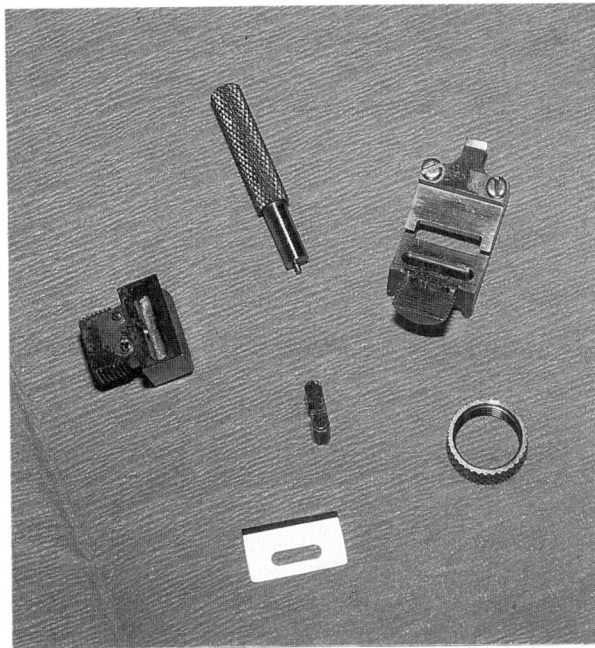

(b)

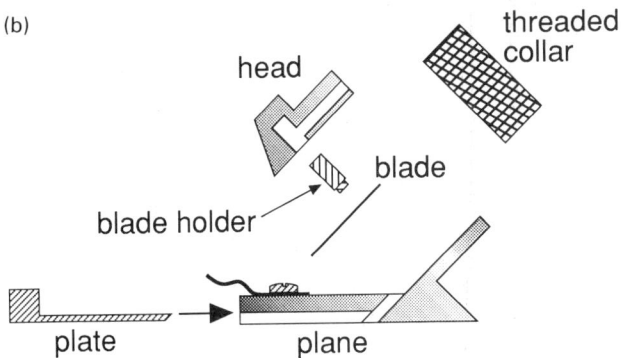

Fig. 10.9 (a) The five individual components of a standard microkeratome head. The short-shaft used to test the assembled head for binding is at the 12 o'clock position. (b) Exploded drawing of a standard keratome.

for cleaning and blade-changing. It should always be carefully cleaned and dried after each session and should never be stored assembled or wet. The microkeratome is disassembled by unscrewing the knurled ring at the rear using the pronged tool provided to start—finishing with the fingers.

The standard microkeratome head consists of six parts (Figure 10.9):

1 Head (posterior part) with shaft hole and blade holder slot.
2 Plane (anterior part) slotted for interchangeable plate.
3 Blade holder, slotted with blade boss.
4 Plate.
5 Blade, slotted.
6 Threaded fixation collar.

The head has a slot into which is fitted the blade holder (Figure 10.10). The blade holder is also slotted to engage the motor shaft which inserts through a hole drilled in the head. There are two pins protruding from the head which engage holes in the plane to insure complete alignment.

Head assembly

To assemble the head, fit the blade on to the holder. This can best be done by placing the head, slot upwards and shaft hole toward you, on to a soft surface such as a moistened microsponge instrument wipe (Murocel—do not use cotton 4 × 4s or a WeckCel as these tend to be very linty). Place the blade holder into the slot of the head with the holder slot facing the shaft hole and the small bosses facing up (Figure 10.11). Holding a fresh blade carefully by the side edges, place the blade on to the holder with the cutting edge facing forward. If the blade is single-edged, make sure that the bevel is facing up. Align the blade slot with the

(a)

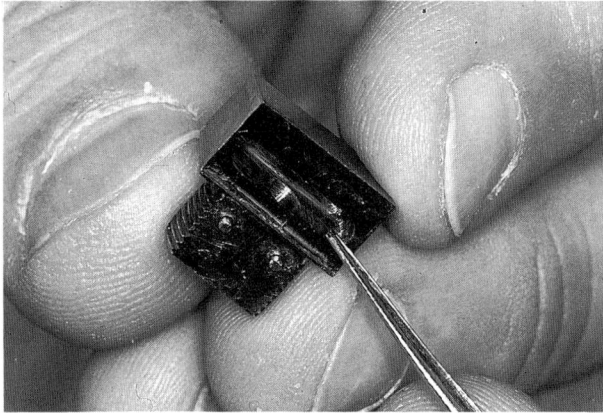

(b)

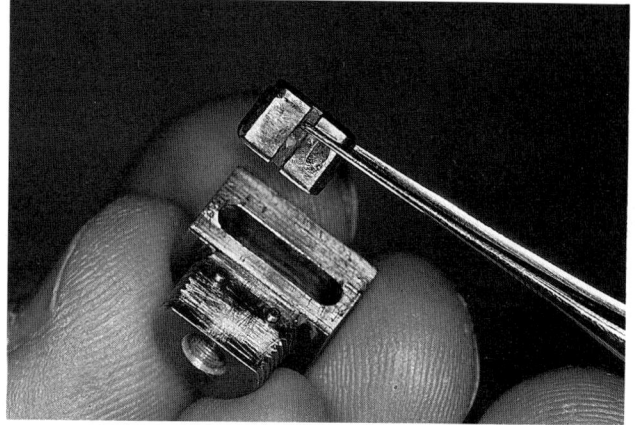

(c)

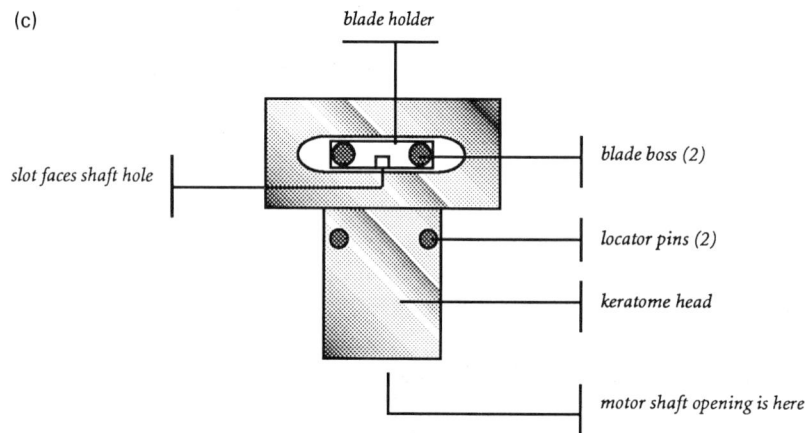

(d)

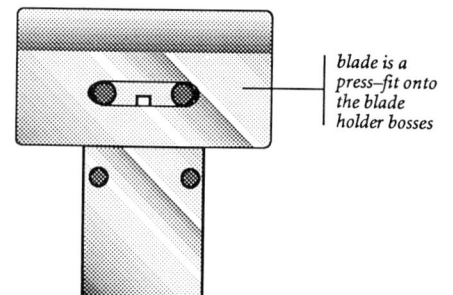

Fig. 10.10 (a) Upper portion of the head. Note the position of the drive shaft hole and the locator pins. (b) The blade holder. The slot accommodates the drive shaft. (c) Drawing of the head with the blade holder in place. (d) Drawing showing blade snapped on to the holder blade bosses.

holder bosses and press down—gently—until the blade is engaged. Next place the plane carefully on to the head, avoiding touching the blade edges to the head, and align the pins into the holes. Holding the assembly together between thumb and forefinger, screw the knurled ring on to the threaded end of the assembly. Make sure that the keyed portion of the ring faces outward. Use the tool provided to tighten the ring gently against the head assembly. Next the short-shaft section is inserted into the shaft hole, engaging the blade holder. Rotate the short-shaft between thumb and forefinger to insure that the blade oscillates freely. Any binding should be remedied by disassembling the unit and carefully re-assembling it. Inspect the blade edge at the microscope under high power. It will be necessary to replace the blade if it is nicked. The head for all standard design units is assembled in the same manner as the SCMD unit described above.

The microkeratome head is attached to the handle by screwing it into the handpiece. A small amount of special grease is applied to the eccentric pin at the very end of the motor shaft. The shaft is inserted into the keratome head which is then screwed into place until seated finger-tight. Apply power to the assembly by depressing the foot-switch. If the head rotates, tighten it more firmly. The microkeratome should operate freely. With practice, any problems with free movement of the shaft and blade can be detected by the sound. Pay strict attention to the sound of a properly functioning keratome while in your instruction lab.

The original microkeratome motor handle is smaller and must be gas-sterilized. The newer Steinway motor handle is slightly larger, operates at 12 V (instead of the 30 V of the original), is sealed and is therefore auto-clavable. It is also quieter and develops more torque by virtue of its non-cogging motor. Motor speed is not adjustable on either of these model motors.

The SCMD handle assembly consists of a stainless steel handpiece with integral gas supply hose and quick-release tubulature fitting. The unit is completely sealed and autoclavable and is designed to run on compressed nitrogen. Take care not to kink the supply

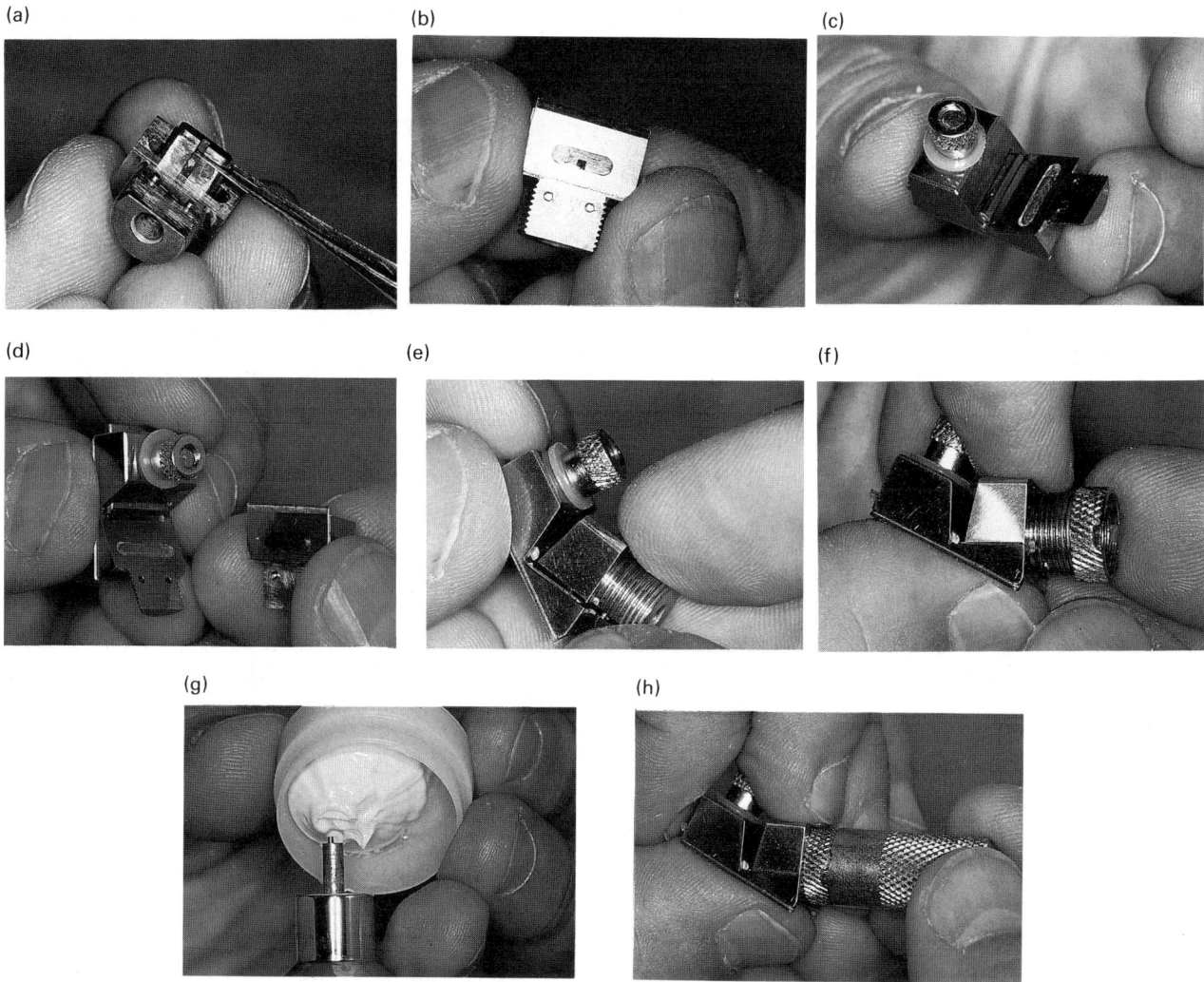

Fig. 10.11 Assembly of the SCMD microkeratome head. (a) The blade holder is inserted into the head with the drive slot facing the shaft hole. (b) The blade is then press-fit on to the blade holder bosses. It should fit snugly without undue pressure. (c) The plane portion of the keratome head. Note relieving slot to accommodate the blade bosses. (d,e) Line up the locator pins and assemble the top and bottom of the head taking care not to nick the blade edge. (f,g) Hold the head together while attaching the knurled collar. Tighten the collar with the assembly tool—finger-tight only. (h,i) Only the tiniest amount of lubricating grease should be applied to the drive shaft eccentric pin.

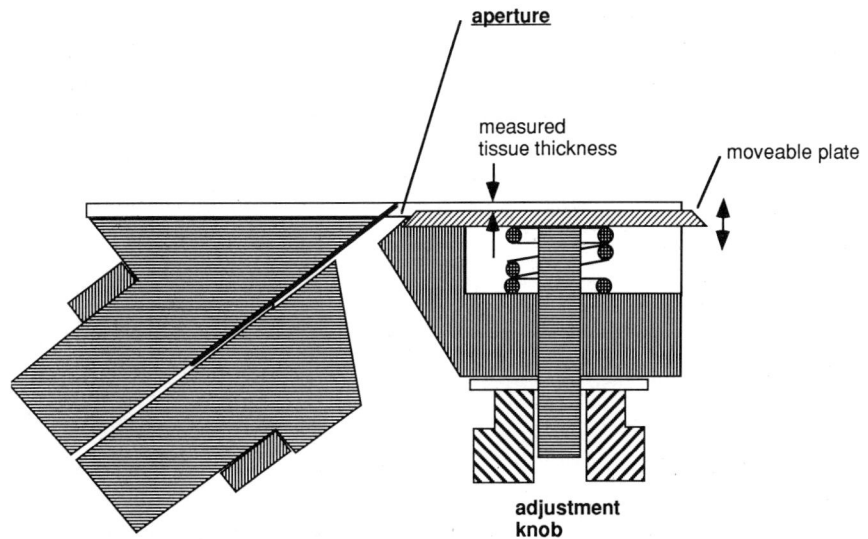

Fig. 10.12 The applanator plate ultimately determines the thickness of the tissue resected. The aperture between the blade edge and the end of the plate can also affect resection depth.

hose. The speed of this motor is adjustable but is set at the factory to run at approximately 16 000 rpm. Its only drawbacks are its weight, size and the fact that it is extremely noisy—sounding like a jet turbine (which in fact it is, in miniature). It also tends to vibrate at a high frequency which actually tends to help float the head through the guides on the fixation ring.

Plate

The thickness of the disk resected by the microkeratome is regulated by the plate. In the standard microkeratome head (for lathing) these plates are supplied in fixed sizes: 15, 20, 25, 30, 35, 40, and 45, corresponding to expected resections of 150–450 μm. Keratome sets designed for non-lathing procedures are supplied with slightly different plate sizes. There are other differences as well which will be discussed in the section on non-freeze lamellar techniques.

In practice the thickness of the resection will depend upon two factors: speed of movement of the head across the cornea and the diameter of the disk. Typically, the instrument will invariably produce a section 20–30 μm thicker than the plate size. Additionally, disks cut from human eye bank eyes can be expected to measure 20–40 μm *more* in thickness than those cut from living eyes. If the speed of the motor is less than 7000 rpm or the translation speed (speed of movement across the cornea) is too fast, the resultant sections will be thinner than expected.

If disks of different diameter are cut with the same plate, it will be found that the larger disk will be somewhat thicker than the smaller one. For example, using a #15 plate, the operator cuts a disk of 7.25 mm diameter. Typically, such a section will measure 170–180 μm in thickness. A disk cut with the same setting but with a 4.25 mm diameter will usually measure 140–150 μm in thickness.

It should be noted that the numbers engraved upon each of these plates refer to the nominal thickness of the disk expected to be resected *using that specific keratome head*—plus some additional amount. Despite the number engraved on the plate, a section of greater or lesser (usually greater) thickness will result. These plates are not transferable and cannot be used with other keratome heads, even those made by the same manufacturer. Each plate is custom-fitted to a specific head. This is only a potential problem unless, like the author, the surgeon has more than one microkeratome.

Some surgeons have become concerned by apparent inconsistencies in plate thicknesses after having measured various plates with a micrometer. Some plates have different numbers but are of the same thickness! This is easily explained by reference to Figure 10.12. Disk thickness is, of course, related to just how much blade edge is exposed below the plate.

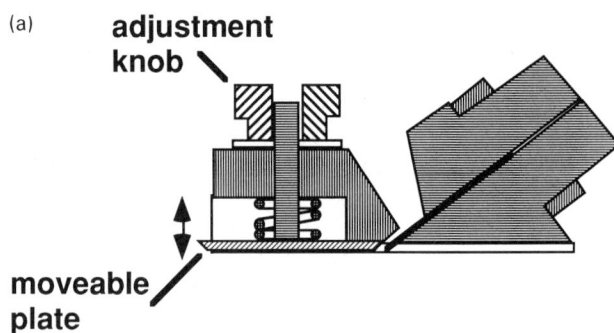

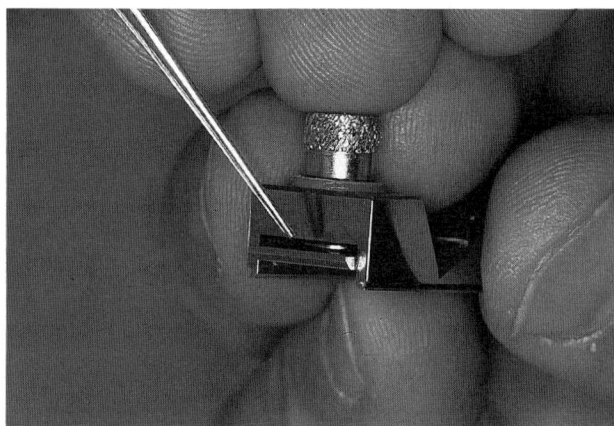

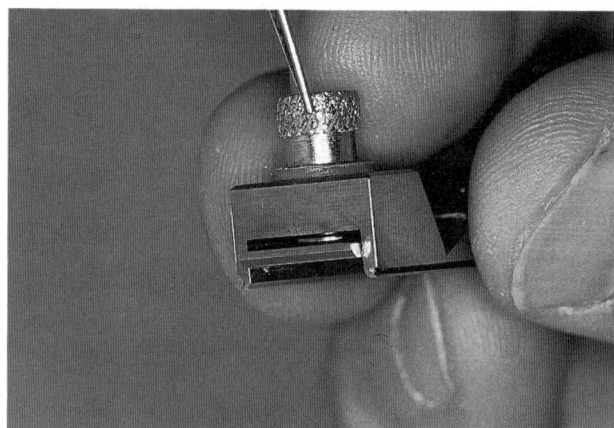

Fig. 10.13 (a) The SCMD adjustable plate microkeratome head. The plate (b) is adjusted by the knurled knob (c).

However, remember that this unit resembles a carpenter's plane. Thickness of the section is thus also related to the aperture or space between the blade edge and back edge of the plate. Thus if a plate is slightly shorter than another of the same thickness, the shorter plate will produce a slightly thicker section, all else being equal.

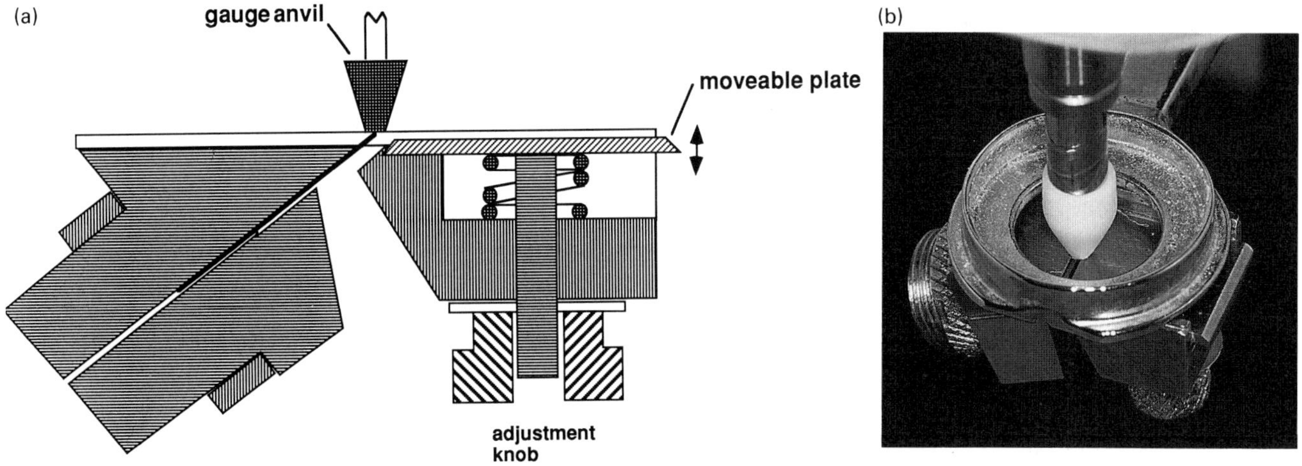

Fig. 10.14 (a,b) Lower the anvil on to the head behind the blade edge. Then gently slide the head toward the anvil, allowing it to climb up the back of the blade. It will stop when it gets to the top edge of the blade. This is the zero point.

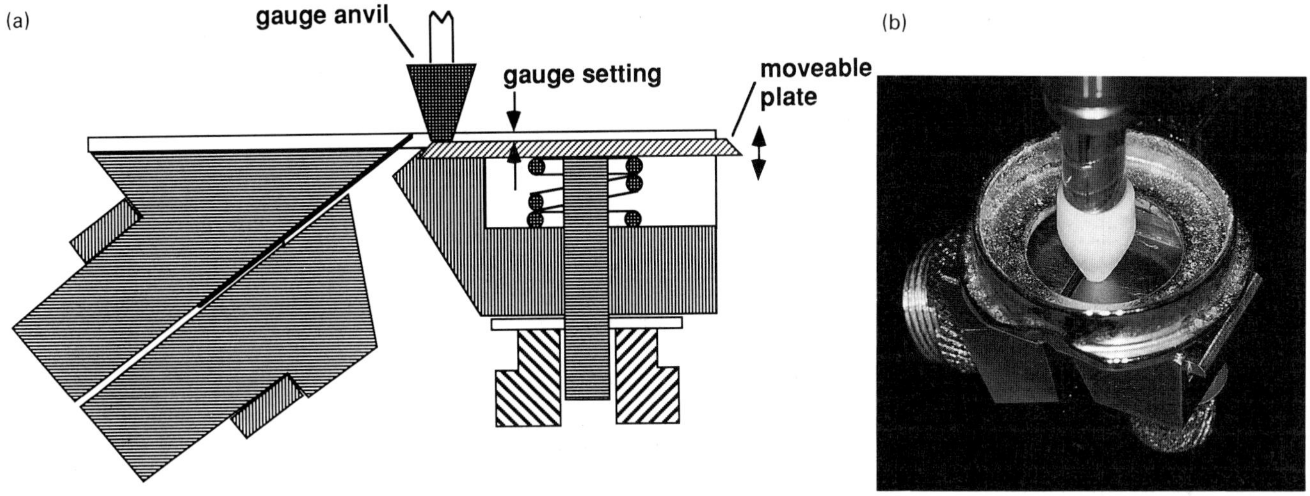

Fig. 10.15 (a and b) The head is moved and the anvil lowered on to the plate adjacent to the blade aperture. Don't let the side of the anvil touch the blade.

SCMD microkeratome head

In the case of the SCMD instrument, this disk thickness is determined by moving the plate up or down with the threaded adjustment knob (Figure 10.13). In practice this is accomplished by placing the detached head, upside down, into a special gauge ring mounted on a heavy support base. The system is zeroed by slowly lowering the Teflon anvil until it rests on the blade edge (Figure 10.14). The zero point is set and the gauge locked. The anvil is raised slightly above the blade and the head moved back slightly so that when the anvil is again lowered it will now rest on the surface of the moveable plate, adjacent to the blade (Figure 10.15). The head is grasped firmly and the knob turned to move the plate the desired distance (Figure 10.16). Once the correct thickness has been reached, the anvil is raised and the zero point re-

checked. Next the setting is re-gauged. It is very important that the plate–blade edge spacing be measured with the anvil as close to the blade as possible. Take care to insure that the anvil does not touch the blade. It is possible for it to be caught by the edge and held. In that case an erroneous setting will result.

Rule 1: The *plate* determines disk *thickness*.

To use the microkeratome in refractive surgery, a few complementary instruments—such as pneumatic fixation rings, applanation lenses, and a pre-surgical tonometer—are necessary.

Pneumatic fixation rings

Regardless of the precision of the microkeratome head, accurate sections cannot be obtained in the absence of

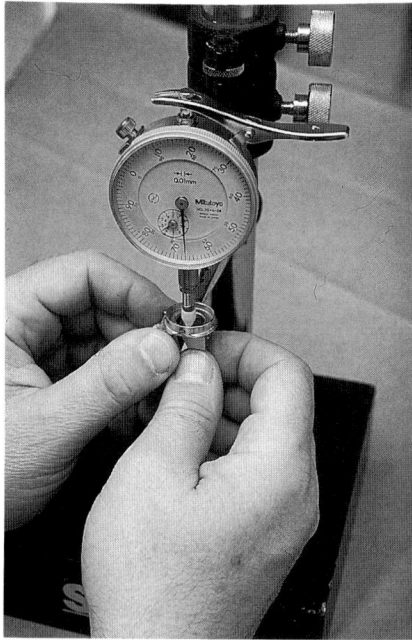

Fig. 10.16 The head is held firmly in the gauging ring while the plate is adjusted.

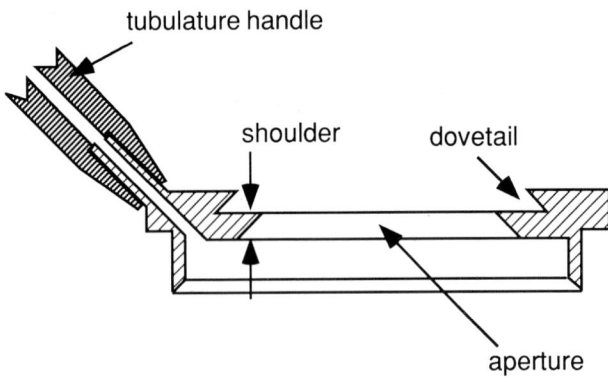

Fig. 10.17 Typical vacuum ring design. The internal shoulder varies in thickness to provide different resection diameters.

the vacuum guide, or fixation rings. These rings are designed not only to fixate the eye but to pressurize it as well. In addition, they provide a precise base against which the keratome acts to produce the proper thickness of tissue section as well as its diameter.

The primary function of the rings is to insure that the proper diameter tissue disk is cut.

Rule 2: *Rings* determine disk *diameter*.

The fixation ring is a short cylinder approximately 21 mm in diameter machined internally to fit snugly onto the eye (Figure 10.17). Those of you with lathing experience will note that the keratomileusis-*in-situ* rings are slightly larger than those provided with the lathe. The central opening of the rings is 11.5 mm, through which the cornea will protrude. The upper surface is highly polished to reduce friction and is provided with a ridge and double-dovetail keratome guide. The author prefers the easy off–on nature of the original Barraquer rings with a single dovetail—they're easier to disengage at the end of the keratectomy (Figure 10.18). Theoretically, this feature also makes it easier to lose contact with the ring surface. If this happens the section will be irregular in thickness. The argument in favor of the double guides is that they prevent the keratome from lifting off the ring surface. This makes it a cinch for the surgeon (especially the beginner) to maintain contact with the plate. While this is true, the double-guide rings also tend to bind, resulting in a jerky movement across the corneal surface. This also results in irregular resection thickness. That the concern surrounding the single dovetail is spurious is demonstrated by Figure 10.18. Rings can be supplied with either single or double guides.

The lower surface of the fixation ring is concave with a wide 360° groove (Figure 10.19). When applied to the globe and when a vacuum is applied via the ring tubulature handle, the ring adjusts to the globe and holds it with suction. The diameter of the ring–eye interface (12.5 mm) and the degree of vacuum supplied

(a) (b) (c)

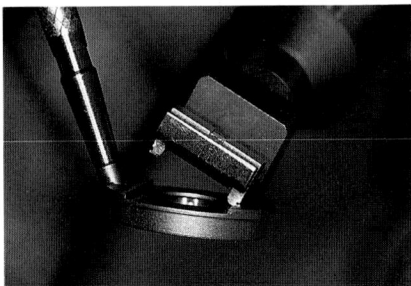 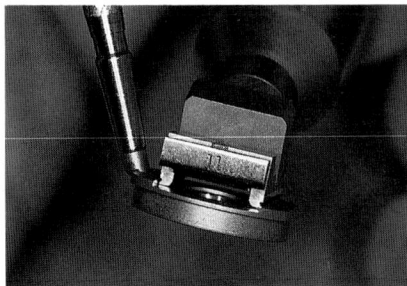 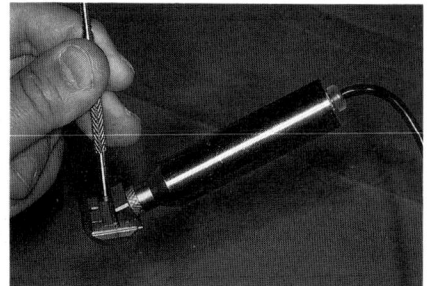

Fig. 10.18 (a,b) A single-dovetail guide allows easy engagement and disengagement of the keratome. (c) The only thing holding this assembled microkeratome securely in the fixation ring is a single-dovetail guide.

set, ranging from 0.4 (#4) to 1.80 (#18). In some cases, rings as low as #2 or #3 may be needed and are available as optional equipment depending upon the design and purpose of the set. It is advised that these be obtained when you take delivery of your equipment—*all rings have to be matched to a specific microkeratome*. The diameter of these rings is constant but their *internal* and *external height* vary. Inside each ring there is a small ledge or shoulder in which is cut the aperture of the ring. The thickness of this shoulder varies and increases as the ring number increases. Each ring is engraved with an identifying number which corresponds to the height of the upper ring surface as measured from the corneo-scleral contact point in 0.10 mm. The thickness (height) of this shoulder determines just how far the cornea protrudes through the central aperture and consequently the amount of cornea flattened by the plastic applanator lens. The lower the number, the more cornea that will protrude and the larger the diameter disk that will be cut. The *ring size*, then, determines the *diameter* of the resected corneal disk when used with the applanator lenses (see below).

The accompanying diagrams illustrate this point. In Figure 10.20 the shoulder height is low (thinner), therefore *L* is high. In this case, the area applanated will be large. In Figure 10.21, the shoulder height is high (thicker), therefore *L* is low. In this case, the area applanated will be small. If the applanated area is too large, less cornea must be drawn up into the ring to

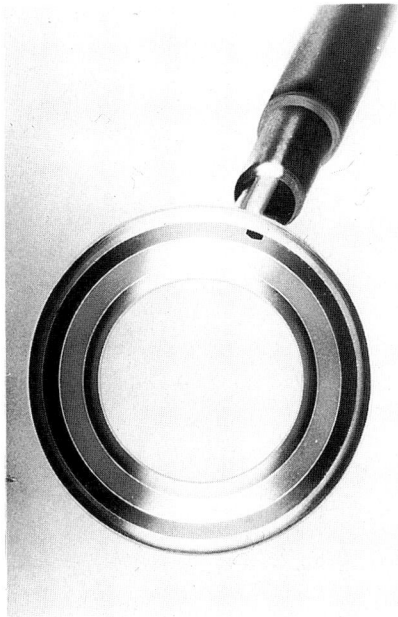

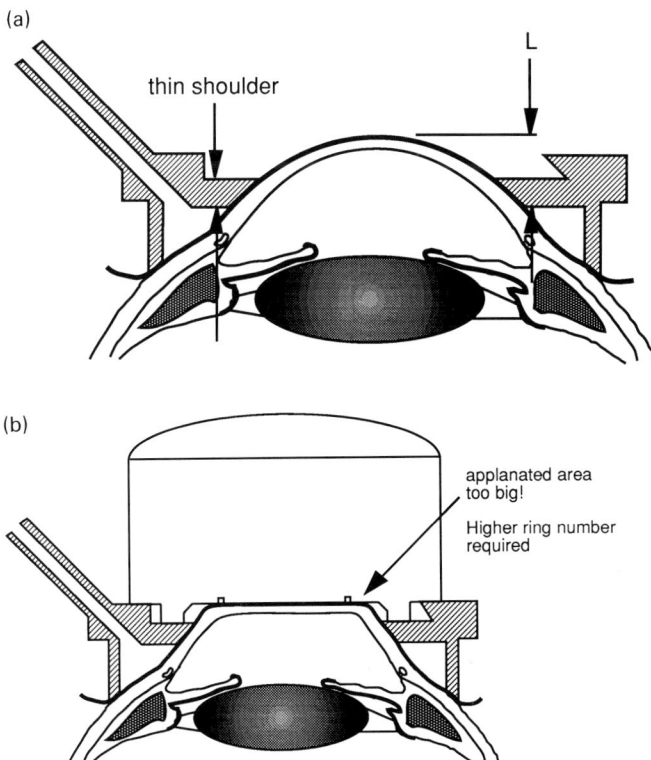

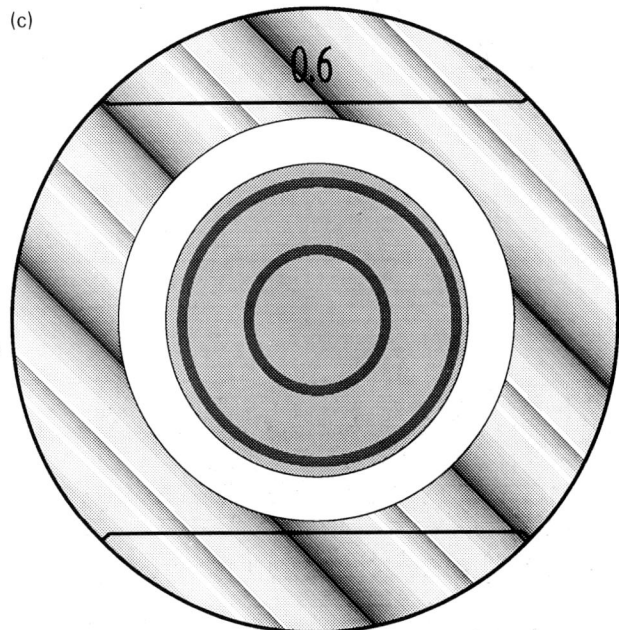

Fig. 10.19 The under-side of a vacuum fixation ring (prototype) (from Barraquer JI. Historia de la cirugia refractiva de la cornea. In: *Cirugia Refractiva de la Cornea*, Instituto Barraquer de America, Bogota, Colombia, 1989).

by the pump (22 inches of water) have been carefully selected to induce an intra-ocular pressure rise of 65 mmHg. Smaller (11.0 mm diameter) rings are used in pediatric cases and are available on special order.

There are some 10–25 rings, depending upon the

Fig. 10.20 In a low-numbered ring (thin shoulder), more cornea protrudes through the ring. (a–c) Now the applanated area is too large. Choose a slightly thicker (higher number) ring and try again.

(a)

(b)

(c)

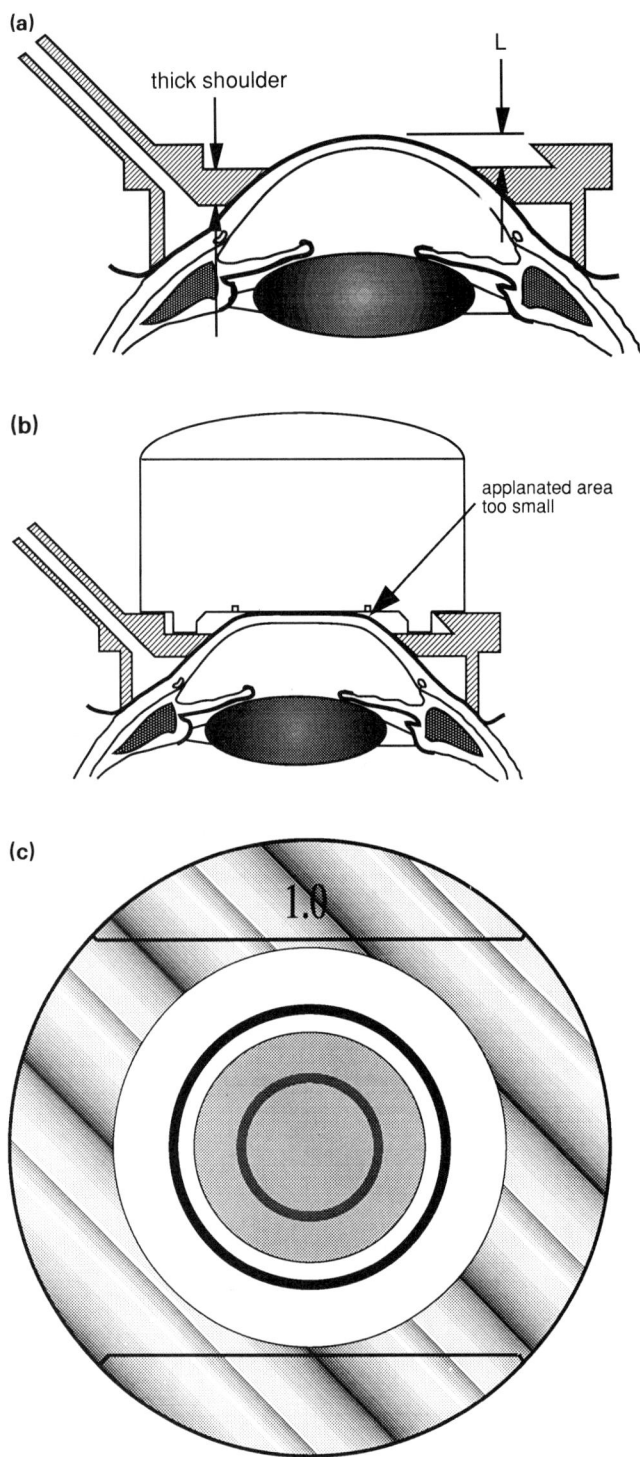

Fig. 10.21 In a high-numbered ring (thick shoulder), less cornea protrudes through the ring. (a,b) The applanated area is too small. Choose a lower number (thinner) ring and try again.

get a smaller diameter disk. In that case it will be necessary to select a ring having a *higher* number (thicker shoulder). Conversely, if the applanated area is too small, a *smaller* number ring (thinner shoulder) must be selected (Figure 10.21).

For example, when a disk diameter of 7.25 mm is desired, that applanator is selected. In applanators having two reticle rings (Bores-type), the outer, larger ring always measures 7.25 mm in diameter, therefore the applanator will be marked with the diameter of the *small* reticle. Next a fixation ring is selected that through experience will cause an area of cornea to be applanated (flattened) which measures 7.25 mm in diameter. Typically, a #8 (0.8 mm) ring will expose sufficient cornea to achieve this. Start the #8 and apply suction to the eye. Dry the cornea and apply the applanator (Figure 10.22).

The area flattened should just fit within or be slightly smaller than the inscribed circle. If the area is *too small*, more cornea needs to be exposed or the disk will be too small. Therefore a ring of *lower* height (thinner) needs to be used to attain the diameter desired. Try a #5 (0.5 mm). If the area is *too large*, less cornea needs to be exposed, therefore select a ring of *greater* height (thicker). Try a #10 (1.0 mm) ring.

Corollary to Rule 2: If the disk is too small, choose a lower-numbered ring and vice versa.

Applanator lenses

These lenses are measuring instruments designed to determine that the proper fixation ring is used so as to obtain a tissue disk of the correct diameter upon sectioning. Treat them accordingly.

Some of these lenses are made from PMMA and are to be cold-sterilized by soaking in CIDEX or a similar chemical disinfectant. Gas sterilization is not recommended because the carrier gas, freon, can craze the plastic surfaces, destroying their accuracy. Recently, autoclavable, clear plastic applanators have become available. Check with your supplier to make sure which type you have—don't assume.

Typically, the applanators will have an upper face made convex to serve as a magnifying loupe (Figure 10.23). The bottom surface has a matt finish and is inscribed with one or two circles (reticles). The larger of the circles in double-ring applanators is *always* 7.25 mm in diameter. These lenses are marked with the size of the smaller ring. Thus a 3.5 double-ring applanator has a 7.25 and 3.5 mm ring scribed on its under-surface. The smaller circles range in diameter from 3.5 to 5.0 mm in the keratomileusis-*in-situ* set. The applanator set for hyperopic lamellar keratotomy has single rings measuring from 4.8 to 6.8 mm in diameter. Standard applanators supplied for lathing typically have only one reticle, although double rings can be specified.

When these lenses are placed on to the fixation ring, the reticle is at the same height as that of the micro-keratome back plane—0.13 mm. Two indentations

(a)

(b)

applanated area
correct size

0.8

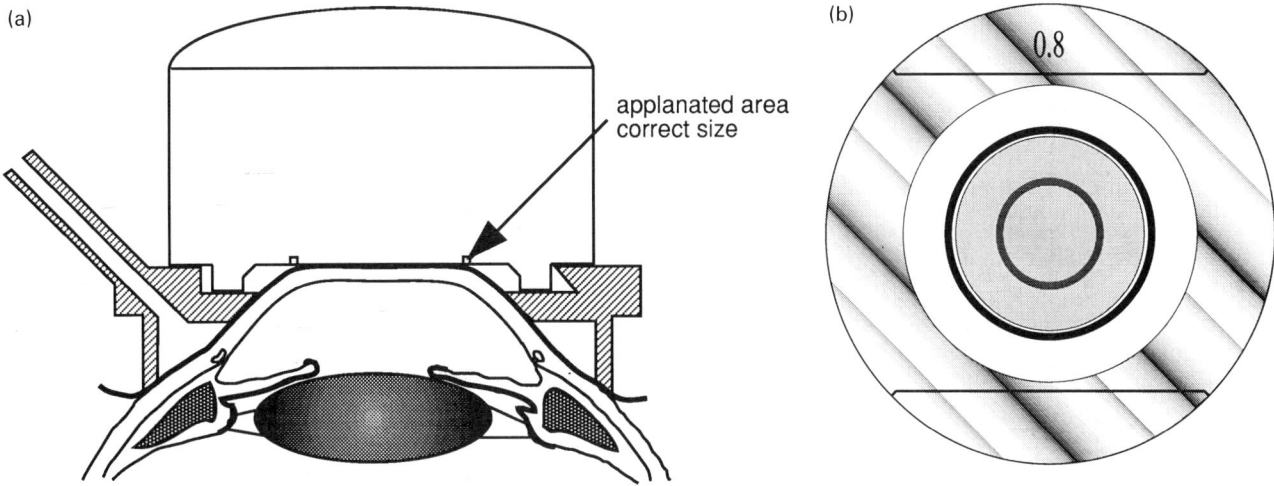

Fig. 10.22 (a,b) The #8 ring is the correct choice in this case. Note that the edge of the applanated area is slightly smaller than desired. This is necessary (but not critical in keratomileusis-*in-situ*) because the disk will have a diameter 0.2 mm in excess of that applanated.

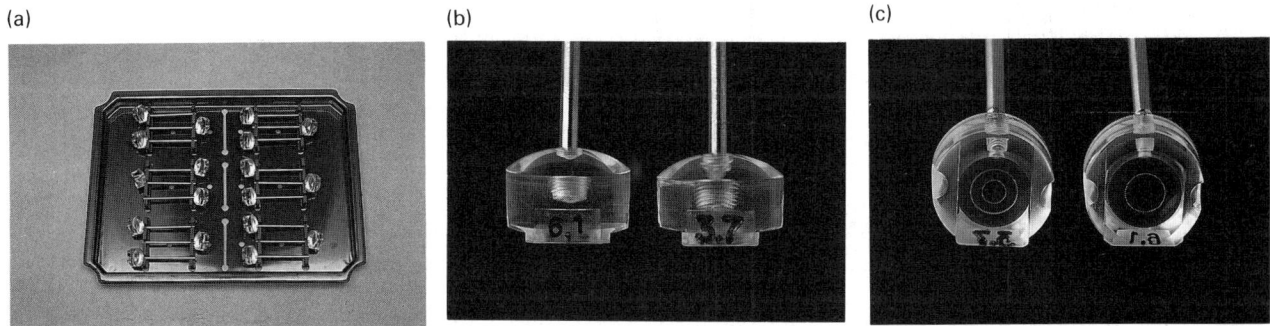

(a)

(b)

(c)

Fig. 10.23 (a) A set of plastic applanator lenses for MKM. (b,c) Double reticle applanators are marked with the size of the *smaller* reticle, the larger is always 7.25 mm.

have been made into the sides of the lenses to fit around the vacuum tubulature handle of the fixation ring (Figure 10.24). The applanator must contact the surface of the ring completely in order to insure that the measurements are correct (Figure 10.25). If contact is not made, an incorrect disk diameter will result—typically larger.

The disk diameter will need to be varied somewhat, depending upon the amount of ametropia to be corrected—the computer will determine the disk diameter. In keratomileusis-*in-situ*, for example, the diameter of the first section has been determined, optimally, to be 7.25 mm. While the ideal diameter of the first section should be 7.25 mm, there is no appreciable difference in outcome with sections varying from 6.0 to 8.0 mm in diameter. There appears to be a greater incidence of post-operative astigmatism with disks that are either larger or smaller than 7.25 mm, however. Disk diameters in classic keratomileusis should never be smaller than 7.0 mm.

To obtain a disk of the proper size, always begin

with a #8 ring and place it on to the eye insuring that there is sufficient clearance between it and the lid retractor so as not to interfere with passage of the keratome through the ring. Engage the suction foot

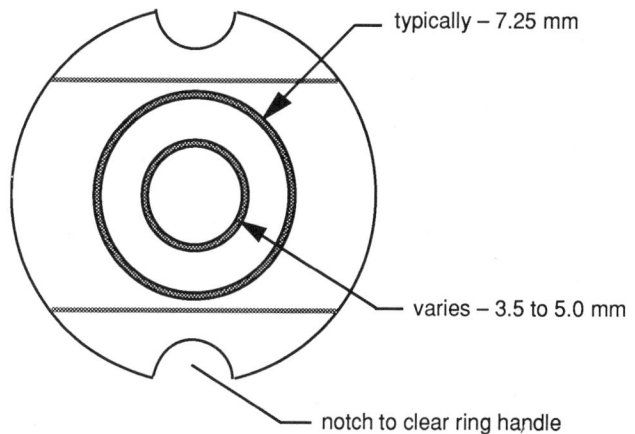

typically – 7.25 mm

varies – 3.5 to 5.0 mm

notch to clear ring handle

Fig. 10.24 The applanator is usually notched to clear the tubulature handle.

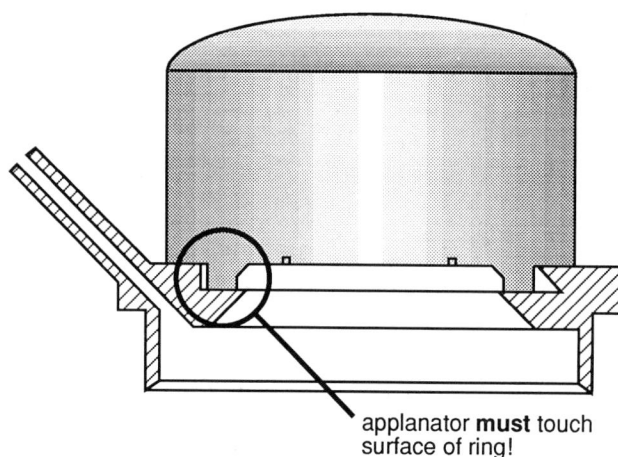

Fig. 10.25 The applanator lens has to be in contact with the ring surface to read correctly.

pedal and check the intra-ocular pressure with the surgical tonometer (see below). Then place the applanator lens on to the fixation ring. *Make sure the cornea is dry!* The applanated portion of the central cornea should just touch the inside edge of the inscribed ring. Ideally the applanated area should be approximately 0.2 mm less than the scribed ring because the actual diameter of the resected disk is always about 0.2 mm larger than measured. If the area is too small, then a smaller (lower-number) ring must be used. Try to select the ring size by observing the size of the applanated area. If it is just slightly undersize, then the next size down will probably do it. If it is markedly smaller, then select a ring several sizes smaller. Details on making the keratectomy will be discussed in the following section.

Try to make the choice of ring with as few reapplications of suction as possible so as to minimize intra-operative conjunctival edema and possible subconjunctival hemorrhage. Occasionally, repeated applications of suction during surgery will result in sufficient edema of the conjunctiva so as to prevent adequate fixation. In these cases a peritomy may be necessary or the case may have to be abandoned (see also Chapter 15). The same steps are taken for the second resection in keratomileusis-*in-situ*. Remember—keep the cornea dry when measuring with the applanator lenses to avoid errors.

Remember, also, that there is a subtle relationship between disk diameter and thickness. For a given plate, a large-diameter applanation (lower-numbered ring) will always result in a thicker disk. The flatter the corneal curvature, the smaller diameter will be the resultant corneal section. The reverse is also true. Don't forget that sections that are larger are slightly thicker as well.

Pre-surgical tonometer

To obtain a good resection with the microkeratome, the intra-ocular pressure must be raised momentarily and uniformly. Experience has shown that an intraocular pressure of approximately 65 mmHg is required at the moment of resection to obtain an optimum disk. The pressure will not be applied longer than 10 seconds and thus far there have been no secondary complications due to this. The pre-surgical tonometer has been designed to ascertain that the correct pressure has been obtained when the suction ring has been engaged.

The device is a cone-shaped lens made of methylmethacrylate, weighing approximately 10 g (Figure 10.26). The upper face is convex to act as a magnifier to facilitate reading the reticle. The narrow or bottom face has been given a matt finish and is inscribed with a reticle 0.38 mm in diameter.

Wipe the lower face with a damp micro-sponge to remove any trace of sterilizing solution. The instrument is then held vertically over the center of a *dry* cornea being careful not to touch the ring or lid retractor. This maneuver is aided by the loose plastic ring supplied with the device. Apply the instrument to the cornea. The applanated area should just fill the inscribed circle. A wet cornea will give a false reading so make sure that the cornea is dry.

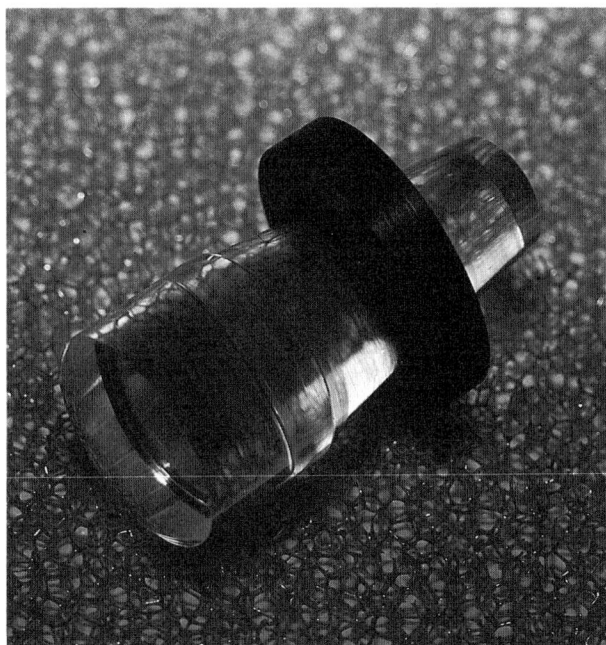

Fig. 10.26 The pre-surgical tonometer is in two parts: the applanator and the support ring.

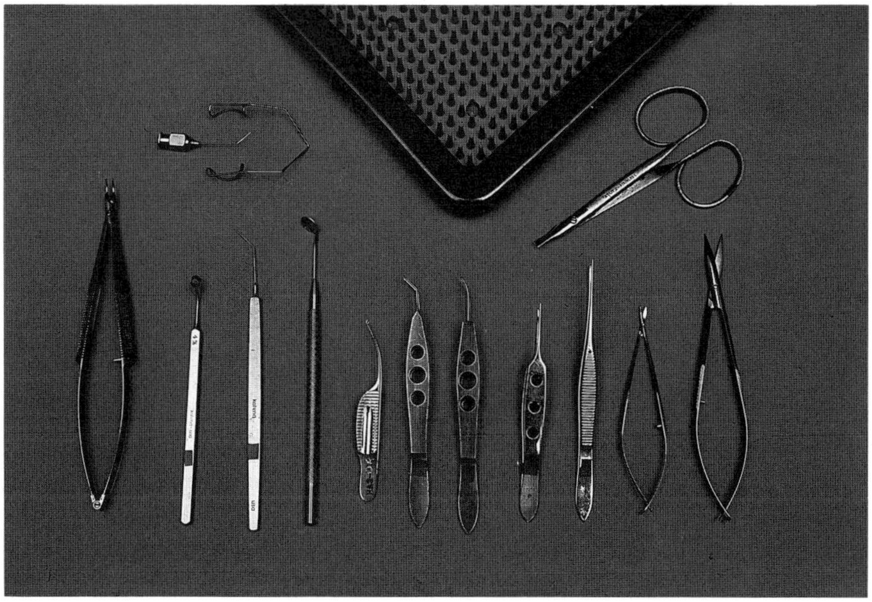

Fig. 10.27 Hand instruments for MKM. The only unfamiliar instrument should be the Barraquer lenticule spoon (fourth from the left, bottom). The radial keratotomy optical zone marker (4.0 mm) is used to circumscribe the pupil prior to making the tangential reference mark. The large rat-toothed forceps (third from right, bottom) is used to handle donor tissue. The needle holder (extreme left) is a Greishaber Barraquer needle driver.

Hand and special instrumentation

There are, in addition to the equipment described in the previous sections, certain other hand instruments and miscellaneous equipment used with this surgery (Figure 10.27). The first of these is the Barraquer lenticule spoon (Katena K3-4250). This instrument is also available from Western Instruments in titanium. While especially designed for retrieving disks from the kitton green preservative solution used during cryo-lathing, it is also extremely useful for handling the thin first disk in keratomileusis-*in-situ*. Since this tissue is only 130–150 µm in thickness, it is easily damaged by handling with the usual corneal tissue forceps such as a Colibri with 0.12 mm teeth. If you must handle the disk with forceps, a Pierse–Hoskins type is recommended and the pressure on the tissue should be very light—sufficient to hold but not crush the disk edge.

Another instrument that may be of considerable help, especially for the beginning surgeon, is the Bores–Ruiz bullseye marker from Western Instruments (see Figure 10.28). This maker is made of titanium and consists of an outer 10.5 mm ring joined and aligned with a smaller 4.0 mm ring fitted with a cross-hair and off-axis reference-marker blade. This marker is used by coating it with 1% tincture of brilliant green applied with a cotton bud and allowed to dry. This will produce a bright green, semi-indelible mark upon the corneal surface. If this is done, make sure that the alcohol has completely dried upon the marker before applying it to the cornea to avoid damaging the epithelium. A fresh skin-marking pen can also be used to coat the surfaces of the marker. This marker is aligned with the constricted pupil and

produces two concentric marks on the cornea which serve to assist in aligning the suction ring on the eye. In addition, the off-axis blade makes the parallel reference mark simultaneously.

A 4.0 mm marker such as the Bores optical zone marker for radial keratotomy (see Chapter 8) should also be included in the instrument set. This instrument is used to mark the cornea for hyperopic lamellar keratotomy and also to circumscribe the pupil prior to making the tangential reference mark.

The Hofman-Polack forceps is an optional instrument that some find useful in this surgery to prevent the tissue disk from rotating when placing the cardinal sutures. The author uses this forceps extensively in transplant surgery but does not find it essential in MKM.

A plastic moist chamber is essential for storing the disk/lenticule while cleaning the resection bed and making the second cut in keratomileusis-*in-situ* (Figure 10.29). A plastic corneal cap is needed to cover the resection while cleaning and/or lathing the tissue disk. A white porcelain crucible with lid is used to hold the cryo-preservative—kitton green. The white color makes it easier to see the disk in the solution. A stainless steel crucible with lid holds a balanced salt solution in a special heater block to thaw the lenticule after lathing.

An artificial anterior chamber completes the list of necessary equipment (Figure 10.29). This device is necessary for sectioning disks from preserved donor tissue when whole globes are not avaliable for back-up, for homoplastic keratomileusis, or when making epi-lenticules.

(a)

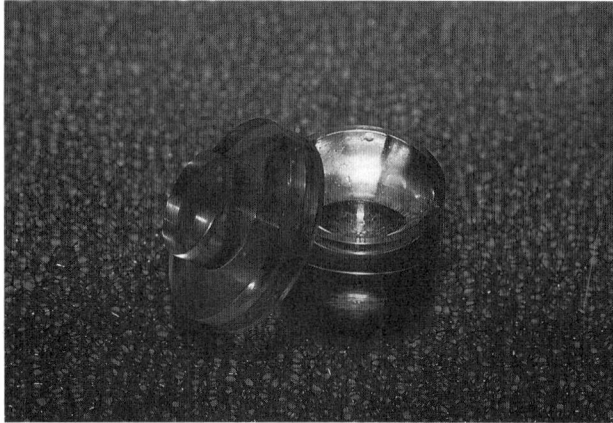

(b)

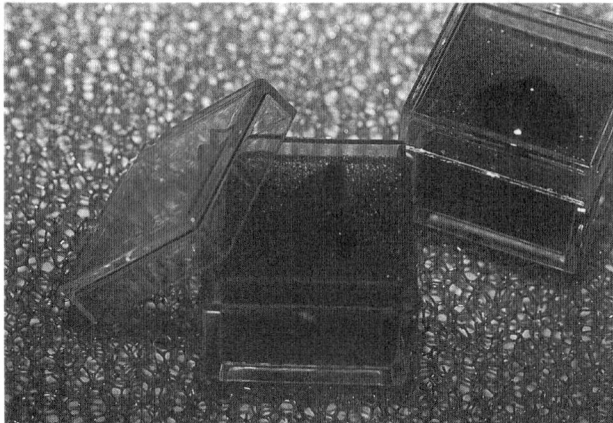

(c)

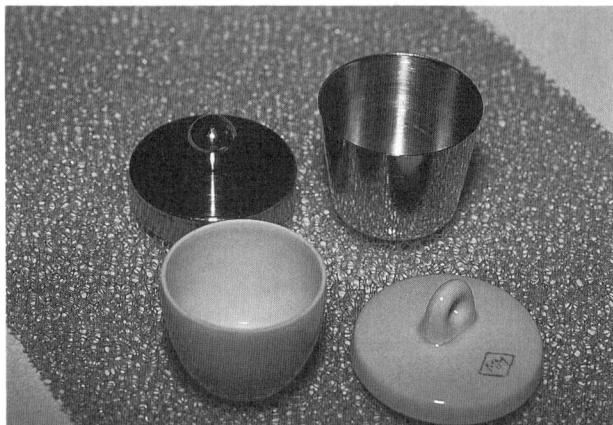

Fig. 10.28 Ancillary equipment. (a) Plastic moist storage chamber; (b) corneal dust cover; (c) the white crucible is for the cryo-preservative, the other is the tissue-thawing chamber.

Advances in microkeratome design

The keratectomy has always been the stumbling point in lamellar procedures. It is difficult to make consistently regular sections. Consequently, manufacturers have cast about in an effort to make that part of the procedure more precise and repeatable.

Draeger microkeratome

The Draeger microkeratome unit has a rotating blade powered by a geared motor (Figure 10.30). The head is driven across the cornea by a helical gear train which provides a smooth and even translation each time. The advantage of such a motor-driven translation system is, of course, the possibility of producing an even-thickness resection case after case. Disk diameter is regulated by an adjustable, transparent applanator plate. Disk thickness is selectable in several discrete increments by inserting a special shim analogous to the applanator plate of the standard keratome (Figure 10.31). The unit is very quiet. Prototypes tended to produce uneven-thickness sections due to instability of the rotating blade. Disks also tended to be slightly elliptic. The author has not found the new unit to possess these deficiencies. A special artificial anterior chamber/motor table allows the device to be used to cut disks from donor corneal buttons and produce non-lathed epi-lenticules (Figure 10.32).

Steinway–Ruiz automatic microkeratome

This unit differs from the other products of this company by being completely motor-driven (Figure 10.33). An external cogwheel system moves the microkeratome through the guide ring and across the cornea automatically (Figures 10.34 and 10.35). The unit depends upon the pressure of the eye to force the head against the dovetail guides and keep the gear in its track. When it moves it does so with a slightly tottering or drunken pitching movement. Theoretically, the unit should produce sections whose cut surface would be ridged. However, clinical experience has not shown this to be the case.

The new unit also incorporates a continuously adjustable suction ring (Figure 10.36). This theoretically allows the operator to retain the ring on the eye for the second section in keratomileusis-*in-situ*, thereby insuring proper centration. However, since the keratome plate has to be changed it is neither practical nor a good idea to leave the suction on the eye while this is done. It does cut down on the number of parts to keep track of, none the less.

The motor design incorporates a safety mechanism such that if the unit stalls in its movement, blade motion stops as well. This is an important safeguard

(a)

(b)

(c)

(d)

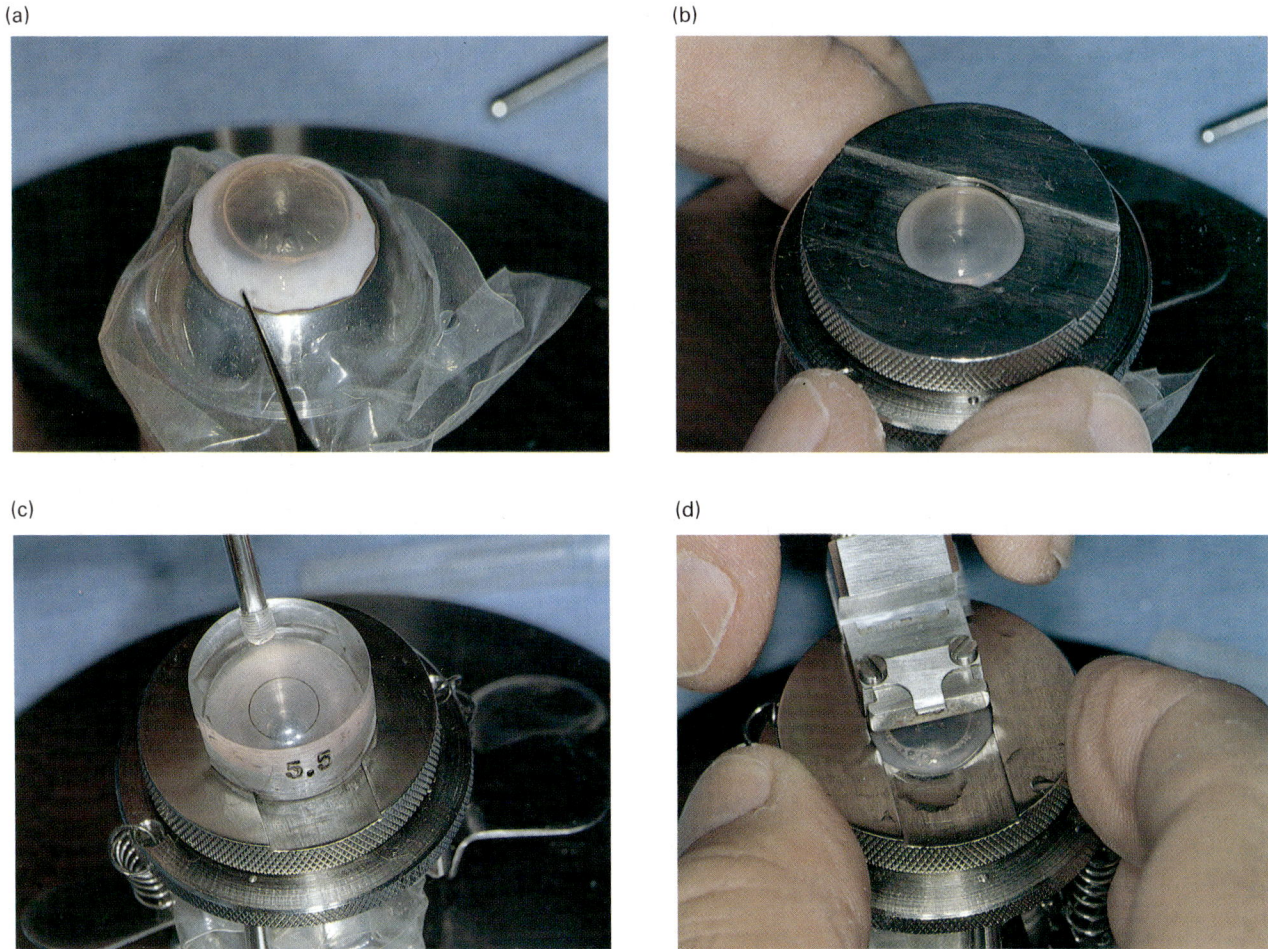

Fig. 10.29 Artificial anterior chamber. Thin rubber dam material is placed over the pressure chamber aperture and the chamber is filled with saline, expelling all air. (a) The donor cornea is centered over the chamber aperture. (b) The retainer ring is snapped over the tissue button completely covering the edges. The guide ring is then screwed on to the retainer. (c) The disk diameter is checked with the applanator. The diameter is controlled by screwing or unscrewing the guide ring. (d) Holding the guide ring firmly, the keratectomy is performed.

and prevents both cutting into the anterior chamber and the mangling of the resected disk. However, disengaging the unit from the tissue when this happens is not easy to accomplish without endangering the disk.

Most important is that the speed across the cornea is pre-set and constant from section to section. This completely eliminates the variability in sections made with the classic versions of this keratome which depended entirely upon operator skill. Since the most critical part of keratomileusis is the keratectomy, this device should open the door to a more widespread application of lamellar refractive surgery.

Surgical technique of classic keratomileusis

The surgery should be performed at a site in which dust has been strictly controlled. This is critical to avoid interface debris which has the potential to degrade vision. The floor model laminar flow filters manufactured by Stora Filterprodukter of Grycksbo, Sweden, have been recommended in the past for dust control. These units are currently not available in the USA or Canada. However, Oto-Med, of Lake Havasu, Arizona, is making a low-profile, high-efficiency, wall-hung unit which will serve even better. There are two units available—large and small. The larger unit can move 1600 cubic feet of air/min. In a recent test, the device reduced a room from 16 000 0.5 µm particles/cubic foot to 500 particles/cubic foot within 5 min. These units should be switched on a minimum of 1–2 hours before surgery is to take place—running full speed, although they can run at low speed over-night. At the author's clinic the units are run for a few hours each day. If you are using your own facility, floor mopping and dusting should be done while the filter

(a)

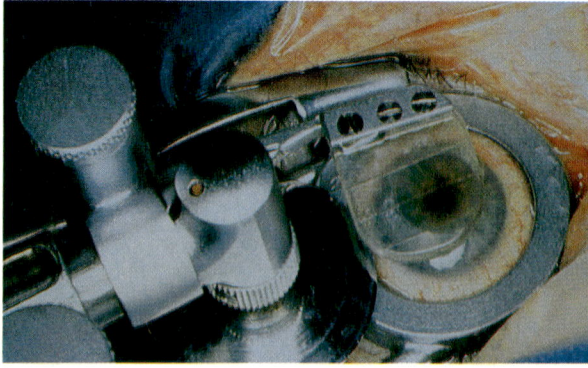

(b)

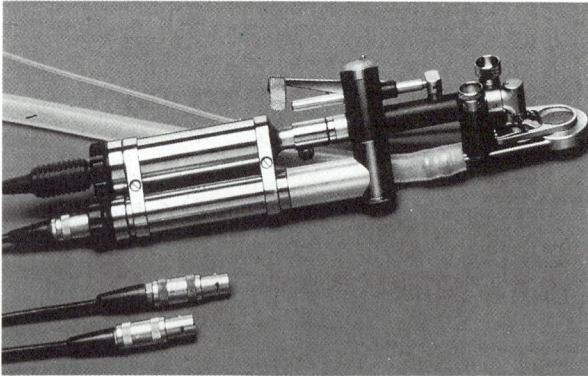

(c)

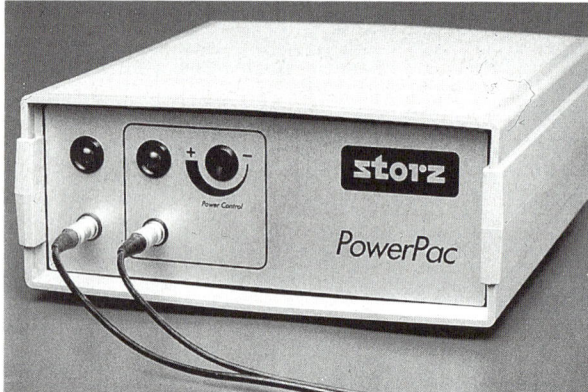

Fig. 10.30 (a,b) The Draeger microkeratome unit. It is powered by a compact power supply (c).

(a)

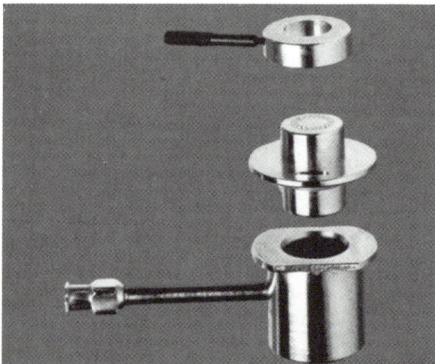

(b)

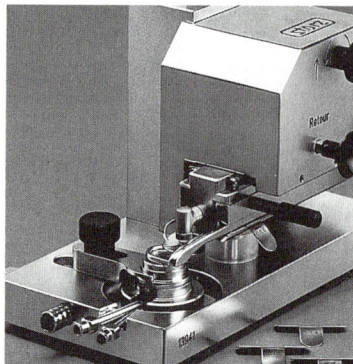

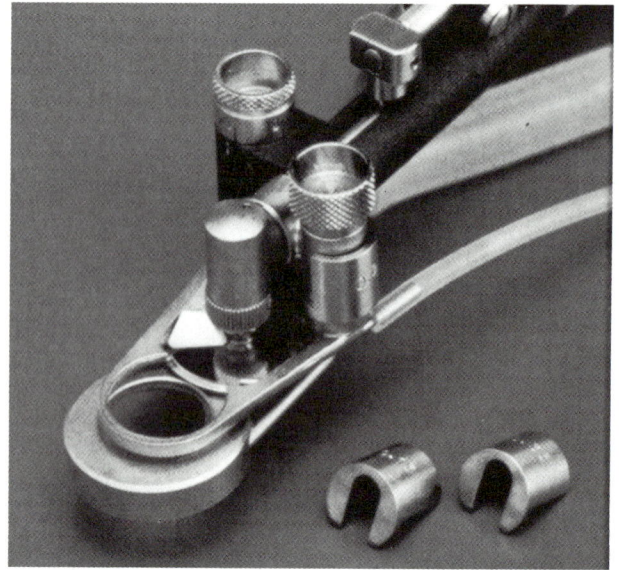

Fig. 10.31 Disk thickness is selectable by inserting special shims.

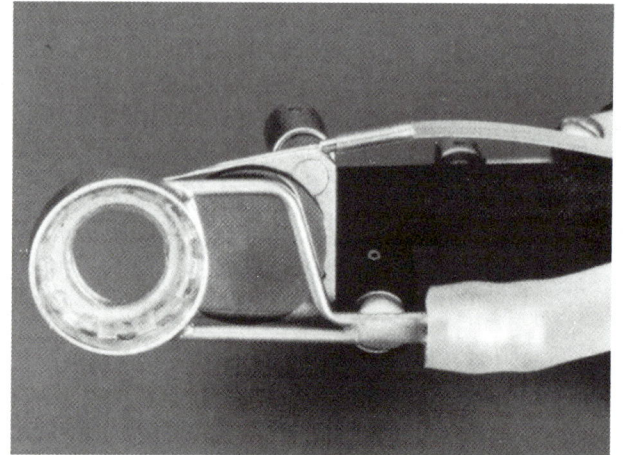

Fig. 10.32 The vacuum fixation ring is integral with the handpiece.

Fig. 10.33 The artificial anterior chamber (a) is inserted into the base of the motor table (b). Disk thickness is controlled by interchangeable plates. Disk cutting is automatic once the system is set up.

(a)

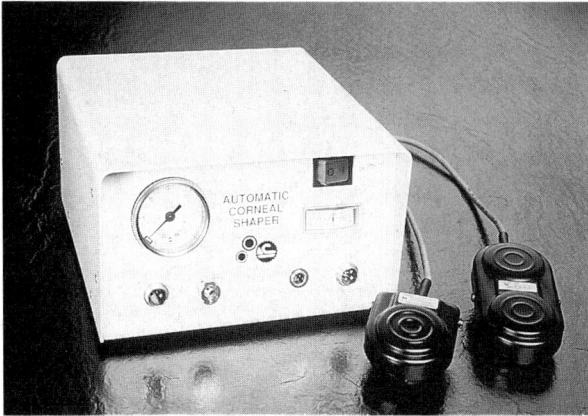

(b)

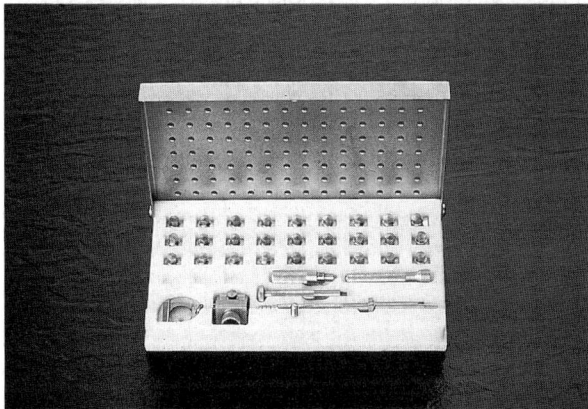

(c)

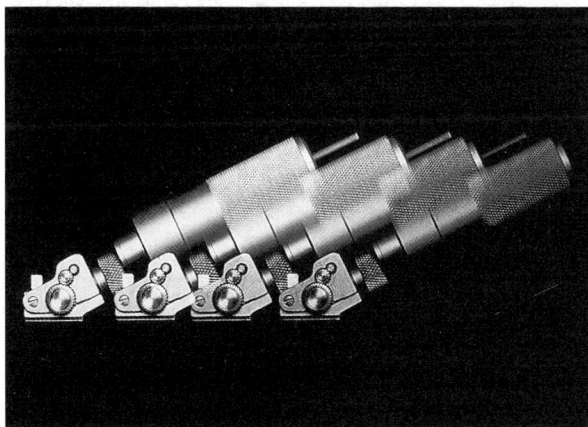

Fig. 10.34 (a–c) The Steinway–Ruiz automatic corneal shaper.

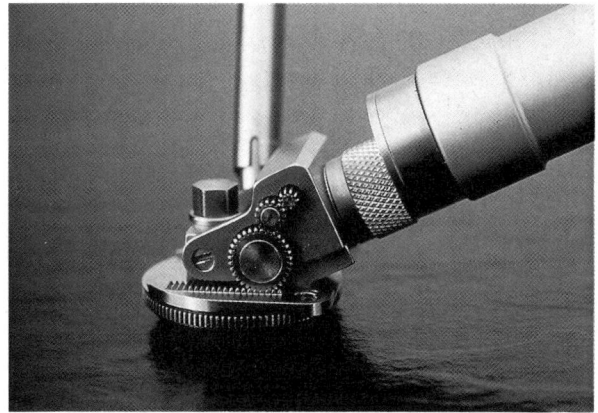

Fig. 10.35 This device is a gear-driven microkeratome.

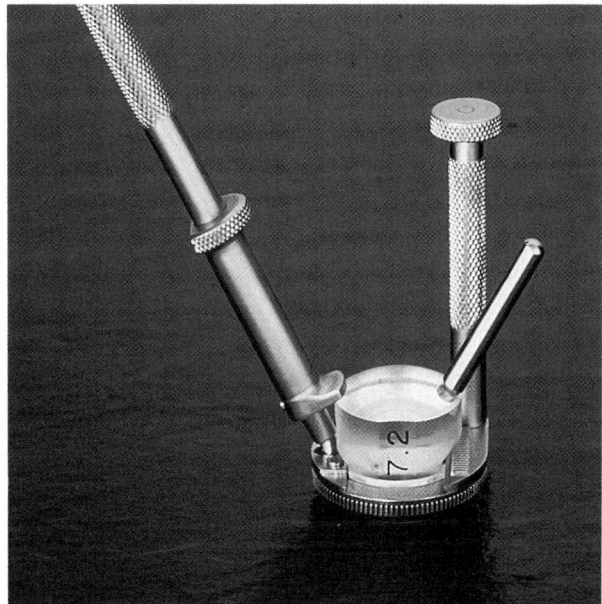

Fig. 10.36 The vacuum fixation ring is adjustable to produce the desired disk diameter.

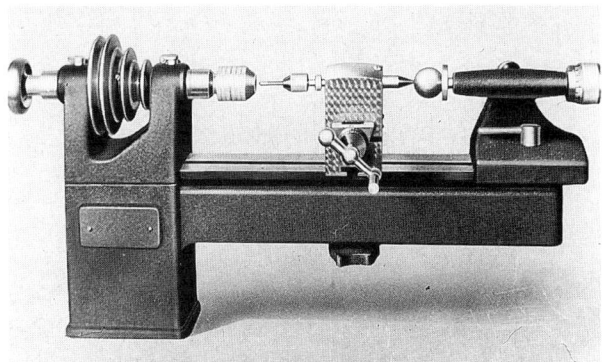

Fig. 10.37 Professor Barraquer's first lathe (from Barraquer JI. Historia de la cirugia refractiva de la cornea. In: *Cirugia Refractiva de la Cornea*, Instituto Barraquer de America, Bogota, Colombia, 1989).

is running at full speed. Sterile lintless drapes are required in the surgery and no gloves are to be worn when performing any of these procedures.

While the keratectomy may be a critical factor in the outcome of the case, the disk needs to be converted to

(a)

(b)

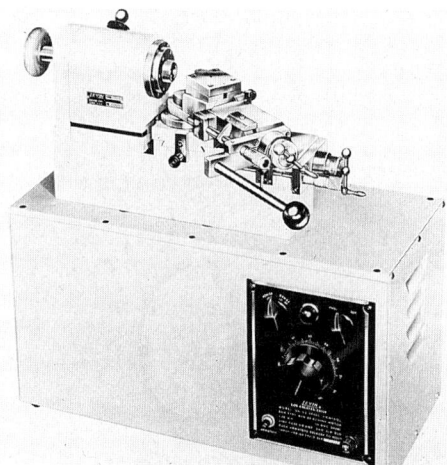

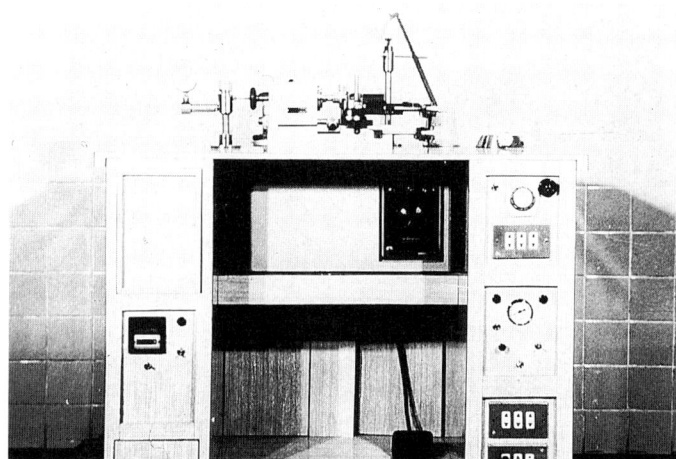

Fig. 10.38 (a) The Levin contact lens lathe. (b) The first cryo-lathe—a modified version of (a) with which the first human cases were performed (from Barraquer JI. Historia de la cirugia refractiva de la cornea. In: *Cirugia Refractiva de la Cornea*, Instituto Barraquer de America, Bogota, Colombia, 1989).

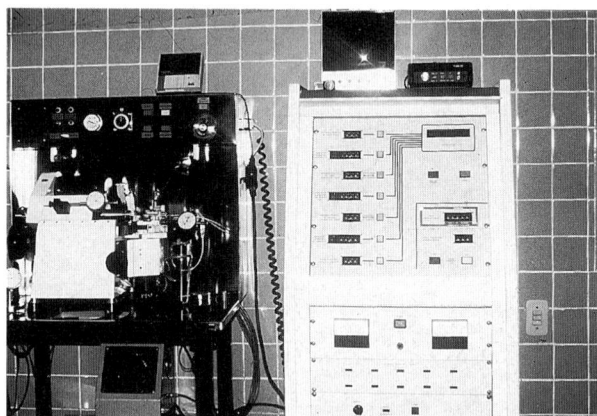

Fig. 10.39 The prototype of a completely computer-driven, automatic, cryo-lathe designed by Professor Barraquer (from Barraquer JI. Historia de la cirugia refractiva de la cornea. In: *Cirugia Refractiva de la Cornea*, Instituto Barraquer de America, Bogota, Colombia, 1989).

a lenticule—that's where the lathe comes in. In classic keratomileusis, therefore, the lathe is the instrument that produces the alteration of corneal curvature to achieve the desired effect. Barraquer's experimental work was performed on a modified jeweler's lathe (Figure 10.37). The actual lathe used for the first surgical cases was a modified Levin contact lens lathe (Figure 10.38). Today's lathe is much more sophisticated and tomorrow's promises to be more so (Figure 10.39). When the first of these cases were done, the cryo-lathe was not located in the surgical suite—it was in a laboratory some 3 km distant. Thus, after the resection was done the tissue was transported to the lab where, under sterile conditions, the calculations

were completed and the lathing performed. The tissue was then placed into a sterile vial to thaw and taken back to the surgical suite where it was returned to the eye (Figure 10.40). The first lenticules were not sutured in place but were kept in place by an inverted conjunctival flap. Ultra-fine suture material did not become available until almost 15 years later.

A number of calculations must be undertaken to complete the lathing. Various data are transferred into the computer where the calculations are performed. Table 10.1 lists the most common data points and their meaning. This list is not complete, nor is the discussion below a comprehensive guide to keratomileusis—only a formal course can cover all the details and provide the hands-on experience necessary to perform this surgery.

Lathe preparation

The lathe should be placed in an easily accessible location (Figure 10.41). Check the gas supply the night before, replacing tanks if the pressure falls below the recommended levels set by the manufacturer (Figure 10.42). Make sure that the tanks are secured within their holders and that the heating collars are properly attached to the lower part of each tank. Close and latch the tank access doors—tape them closed. It is not unusual for these doors to come open either through jarring or vibration. The electrical supply of the lathe is connected via safety interlocks to the doors. When the door is open, even slightly, power is disconnected from the lathe. If this happens during the case— trouble. If it happens during the UV cycle, the lathe sterilization will be incomplete and contamination of the patient's tissue is possible.

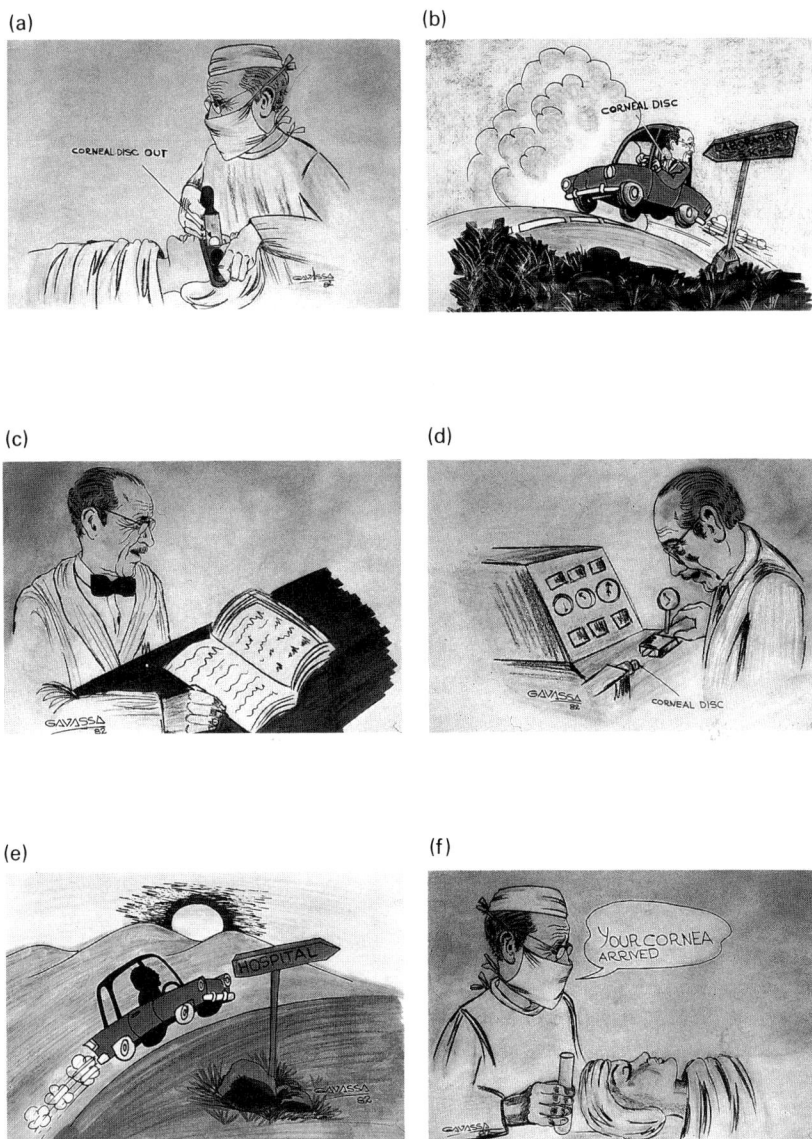

Fig. 10.40 (a–f) The first keratomileusis (from Barraquer JI. Historia de la cirugia refractiva de la cornea. In: *Cirugia Refractiva de la Cornea*, Instituto Barraquer de America, Bogota, Colombia, 1989).

Remove the front cover and turn on the main power switch—replace the cover. If the lathe is located in an area that can be accessed by others (hospital, outpatient surgical clinic, etc.) it is a good idea to chain the cover to the lathe via the handles. Set the timer for the UV sterilizer (on the back) to the recommended time (minimum 12 hours) and turn on the UV power switch. Make sure that the UV power is off before removing the cover at the end of cycle. On the day of surgery untape the doors and turn on both carbon dioxide tanks. Close and re-tape the doors. Remove the cover from the lathe and place it outside the operating room in a safe place. Make sure no one touches the lathe or front panel until the case(s) are completed. The author has a special shelf holding a monitor hooked up to the lathing computer. The monitor is situated directly in front of the surgeon. It is turned on at this time.

Delrin base plate preparation

Under sterile conditions (scrubbed and gowned) turn on all console power switches and zero all digital readouts (you can't zero the cutting radius digital readout). Make sure that the tissue freezing timer is off and re-set. Turn on the light. Put an 8.0 mm pre-sterilized delrin base plate into the headstock and secure it with the threaded ring. Pull out the headstock locking knob to disengage the head and spin it up to make sure it works. If you forget to pull out the lock, the drive belt

Table 10.1 Abbreviations used in lamellar keratoplasty discussions and calculations

Abbreviation	Definition
Alpha	The angulation of the lathe tool in relation to the axis of rotation (determines the limit of the optic zone (Zo))
D	Diopters
Db	Diameter of the delrin base (typically = 8.0 mm)
Dc	Diopters of spectacle correction
Dd	Disk diameter
Di	Initial anterior corneal curvature—in diopters
Dp	Displacement of the tool
Dv	Dioptric power at the corneal vertex (see text)
Ea	Thickness of the wing (in EPI and hyperopic lamellar keratotomy)
Ec	Central corneal thickness remaining after lathing
Ed	Thickness of the resected disk *before* preservation
Edp	Thickness of the resected disk *after* preservation
El	Thickness of the lenticule in hyperopia
Ezi	Thickness of the intersection zone (EPI and hyperopic lamellar keratotomy)
Rb	Radius of the base
Re	Radius of the resection base (inter-face)
Ri	Initial anterior corneal curvature—in millimeters (see Di)
Rt	Cutting radius
Zi	Intersection zone (EPI and hyperopic lamellar keratotomy)
Zo	Optical zone (diameter of the resection in keratomileusis and of the lenticule in keratophakia)

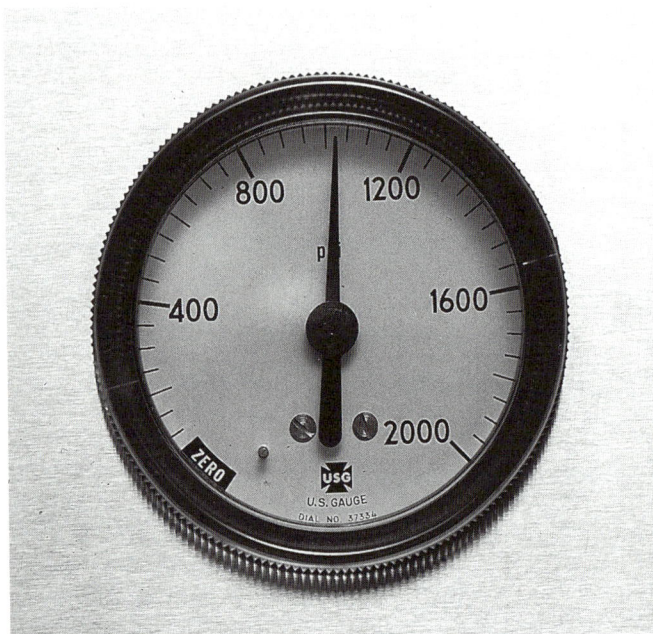

Fig. 10.41 The current model cryo-lathe as manufactured by Steinway Instruments, San Diego, CA. The monitor relays information from the central computer used to calculate the lathing parameters in each case.

is sure to come off the pulley. It's inside the lathe and not easy to get at.

The stop pin should be unlocked, as should the radius stop (Figure 10.43). Run the tailstock up toward the head until the tool just touches the delrin base. Make sure that the cutting radius is set to 8.02. Turn on the lathe and zero the displacement read-out. Set the displacement micrometer read-out to 20.00. Advance the tool and cut the base until the displacement read-out displays −2.50. A new base has to be cut at least this much to insure even and rapid freezing. Some surgeons forget this step and risk incomplete and/or prolonged freezing times.

(a)

(b)

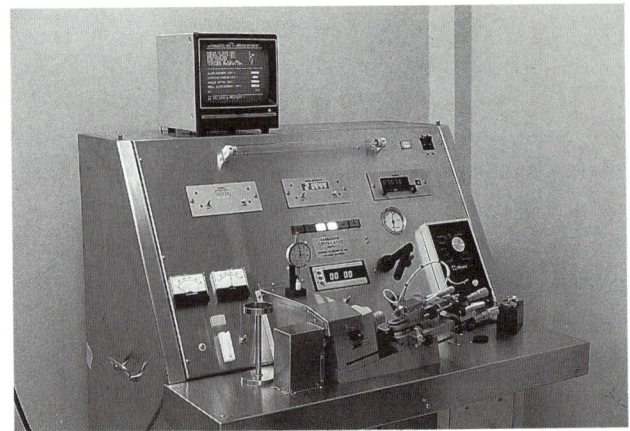

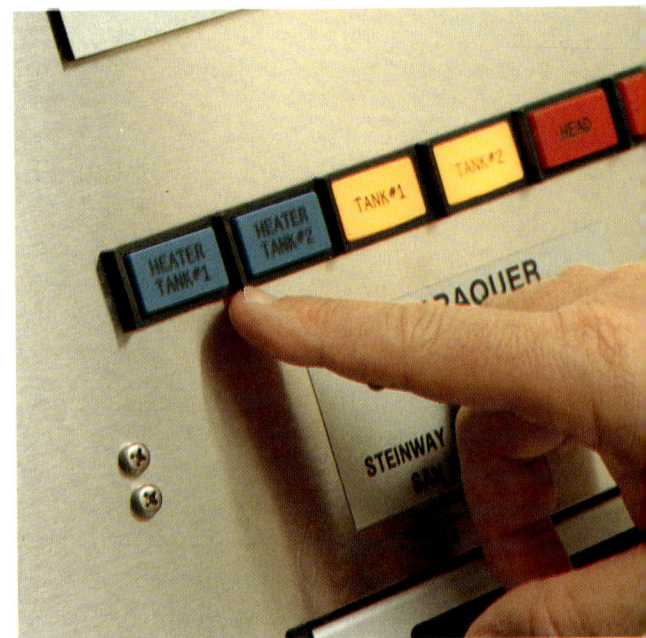

Fig. 10.42 (a) A fresh carbon dioxide tank should show a pressure of 1000 psi. (b) If the pressure falls to 800 psi, the tank heaters should be switched on.

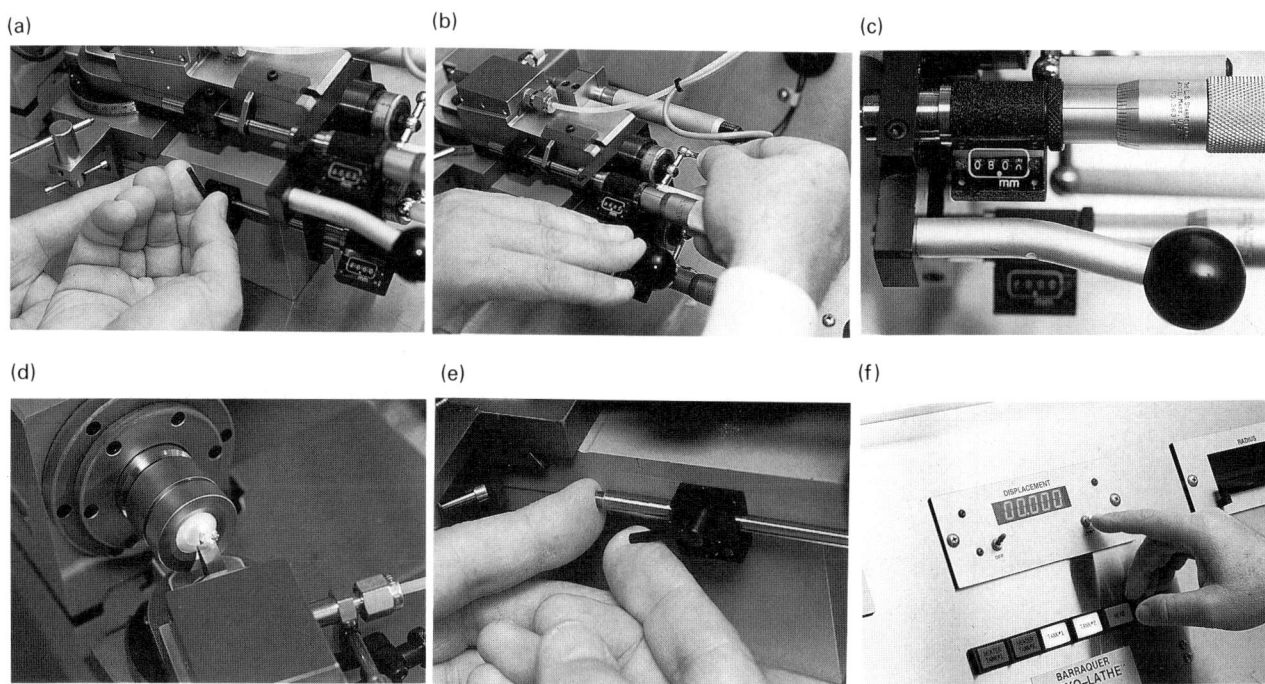

Fig. 10.43 Lathe set-up. (a) Unlock the displacement stop pin. (b,c) Set the initial cutting radius. (d) After cutting the base, make sure the displacement is still set and locked at 20.00. (e) Zero the displacement read-out. (f) Lock the stop pin.

Lock the stop pin. Advance the tool against the stop—the knob will be very difficult to turn but it will move a few thousandths. Re-set the displacement digital read-out and withdraw the tailstock. Bevel the edge of the delrin base by holding a blade lightly against its edge—this removes any "flash" that may remain after the base is cut. Turn on tanks 1 and 2 from the front panel: the system is now ready for the first case.

Pre-operative patient preparation

Approximately 1 hour prior to surgery, the patient should have two drops of 1% pilocarpine instilled in the operative eye. Repeat with one drop no less than 30 minutes before surgery if the pupil is not yet constricted. Using a miotic too soon before surgery presents the surgeon with congested conjunctiva which is more likely to bleed or interfere with using the vacuum fixation ring. Position the patient beneath the microscope and align the optics perpendicular to the patient's optic axis. If possible, prior to the administration of anesthesia, mark the optic center, outlined as follows. The patient is asked to fixate upon the microscope light filament whereupon the fixation point is marked with a blunt instrument, taking care to compensate for any parallax errors that may exist in the microscope system (Figure 10.44). To verify the centration of the optic center the patient is asked to look away from and then back to the light. Any discrepancy is noted and corrected.

Anesthesia is then administered. In hyperopic eyes, retro-bulbar anesthesia is safer than in myopic eyes. However, since some of these eyes will be hyper-corrected myopes, it is safer to use peri-bulbar anesthesia coupled with a modified Van Lint (or O'Brien or Nadbath) lid block or even general anesthesia. If using local anesthesia, perform the blocks yourself unless the anesthesiologist has demonstrated the ability to perform such blocks without excess lid or sub-conjunctival infiltration. To avoid possible injury, have the patient look down and out before inserting the needle into the orbital space. This maneuver swings the vulnerable posterior pole away from the needle tip but still allows infiltration of the cone (see Chapter 15). At the author's clinic, we use a mixture of 10.0 ml 4% plain Xylocaine, 4.0 ml bicarbonate and 5.0 ml 0.75% Marcain as our anesthetic medium.

The patient can now be prepped and draped for the procedure. For the prep, we recommend Betadine solution—full- or half-strength. Do *not* use Betadine preparation! Betadine preparation contains soap which is highly irritative to the conjunctiva and cornea—it can remove the corneal epithelium in a flash. If that happens, the case should be aborted. For a drape, we recommend the large 3M plastic incise adhesive drape, #1060. This is large enough to cover the field and to drape the Mayo stand placed over the patient's chest. More importantly, it is lintless. The surgeon should have prepped his or her hands in the usual manner for a full 10 min and be wearing *no gloves*! Hands should be

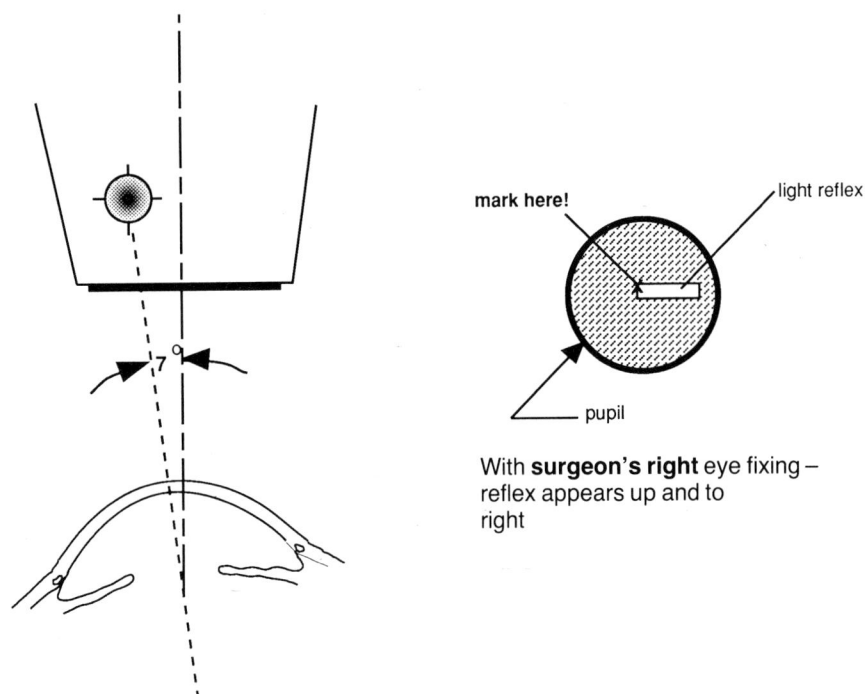

mark here!

light reflex

pupil

With **surgeon's right** eye fixing – reflex appears up and to right

Fig. 10.44 Marking the visual axis. The light reflex is displaced downward because of the microscope design. To verify the centration of the optic center the patient is asked to look away from and then back to the light. Any discrepancy is noted and corrected. The visual axis is located as shown. The optic axis is not concentric with the pupil. Note that the visual axis is eccentric to the pupillary margin. It will be helpful to mark a 4.0 mm optical zone with an appropriate radial keratotomy marker—it helps when lining up the fixation ring.

thoroughly rinsed in sterile water and dried on low lint or lintless towels.

The drape is opened with blunt scissors (taking care not to injure the lids or cut off any eye lashes), and a wire lid speculum is inserted between the lids. Insure that the vacuum fixation ring fits within the space provided by the speculum with some clearance at 12 and 6 o'clock. Neither the lids nor the speculum should encroach upon the ring so as to interfere with passage of the keratome. Be sure that the conjunctiva is flat and that there has been no anterior infiltration of the peri-bulbar anesthetic. If insufficient clearance is present, utilize an alternative form of lid retraction such as sutures. Take care with the placement of such sutures so as to prevent hemorrhaging.

A small canthotomy may be needed in some cases but this will be unusual. To perform a canthotomy, first insure that the area has been properly anesthetized. If it is found necessary to inject anesthetic, perform the injection at the posterior edge of the lateral orbit using the method of Van Lint. Next use a straight, medium Halstead hemostat and clamp the lateral canthal area. After a brief wait, remove the clamp and perform a small canthotomy—do not involve the bulbar conjunctiva. If done properly, very little, if any, bleeding will occur. Remember to suture the canthotomy at the close of the procedure.

Assemble the microkeratome under a good light making sure that all parts fit without forcing and that the blade moves freely. Be very careful of the blade both to protect its edge and to protect your fingers. Place the microkeratome (and handle) to the side in a

secure place. With the SCMD unit, do not attach the head to the handle until the plate has been set. Some surgeons recommend that these be placed within a special pocket of the operating gown. *Do not do this!* It is too easy for the blade to be damaged or lint and other particles to make their way into the microkeratome head. This goes for the rings as well. Do not put any of the rings into any gown pockets or pouches. Arrange these in a convenient place, in ascending order. Examine each one carefully for any signs of corrosion or accumulations of detritus. Clean any suspect areas and test the fit and movement of the microkeratome in each one that you are likely to use. The microkeratome must move freely through the rings without any binding or catching.

Test the vacuum by occluding the tube and depressing the vacuum foot pedal. The gauge should read 22 in. Then attach the ring handle and test the vacuum again. Attach one of the rings and re-test the vacuum by pressing the ring against your thumb with the vacuum pump on. It should hold on to your thumb as long as the vacuum pedal is depressed. Do not test the vacuum by putting the tubing into water. The system is not designed for this. Although there is a moisture trap in the system, it is a small one.

Centration of the resection

To begin the surgery, it will be necessary to mark the cornea to:
1 center and position the resection;
2 insure that the tissue is replaced epithelial side up.

To accomplish the first goal, a 4.0 mm radial keratotomy optical zone marker is applied to the cornea, concentric to a pre-made optic center mark. If the patient has already been anesthetized before marking the optic center, make the mark concentric and slightly nasal to the constricted pupil. This is extremely important because the pupil is not concentric with the optic axis of the eye.

Using a disposable needle (25-gauge), scribe a *tangential* reference mark on the corneal surface as shown in Figures 10.45 and 10.46a. Do *not* make more than one mark! This mark satisfies requirement number 2. Note that this mark is not made radially, as some of you may have been taught or read. This is because it is easier than you might think to replace the corneal disk upon the cornea *upside down!* If the reference mark is made in the manner illustrated, and the tissue is replaced incorrectly, the mark will appear as in Figure 10.46b. This is especially important in radial keratotomy hyper-corrections because of the

radial scars already present. It is easy to get confused, so be careful.

Plate selection

The typical section thickness for lathing should be around 300 μm—though 350 μm is not too thick. Avoid resections that leave less than 150 μm of tissue in the resection bed. Thin posterior sections are likely to result in progressive corneal ectasia which can reduce or eliminate the myopic correction and can even increase the myopia over time. This phenomenon is used to advantage in the hyperopic lamellar keratotomy procedure described below. Conversely, do not remove such a thin disk that when lathed, the center thickness is less than 120 μm. Such thin centers are often associated with irregular astigmatism due to wrinkling or actual freeze-cracking of Bowman's layer. The exact plate selection will depend upon the in-

(a)

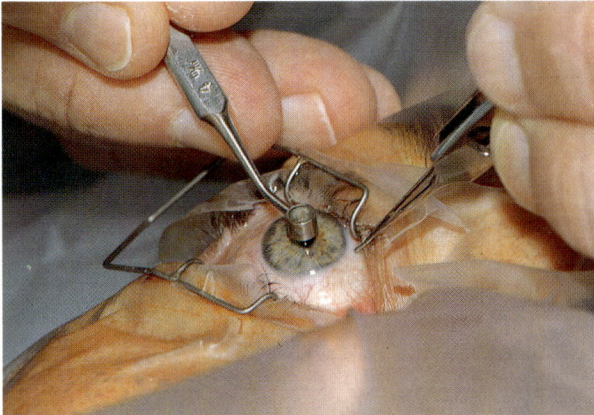

(b)

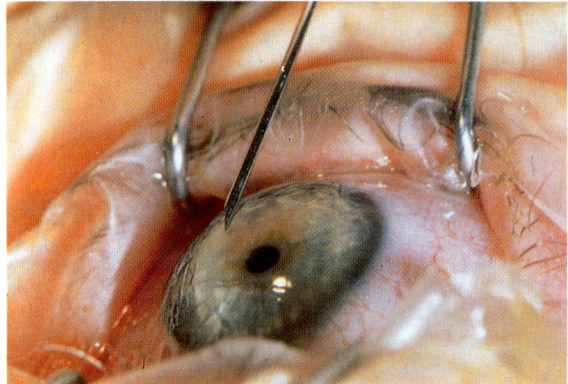

(c)

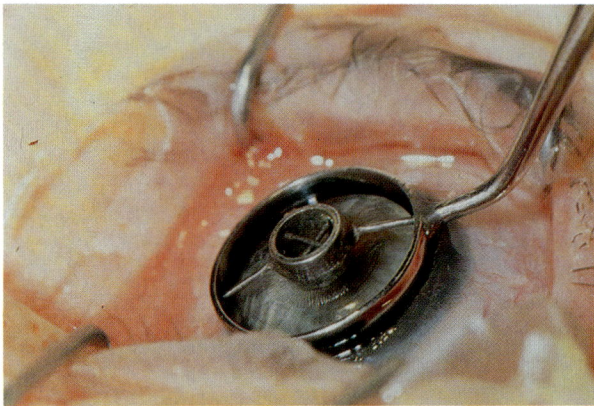

(d)

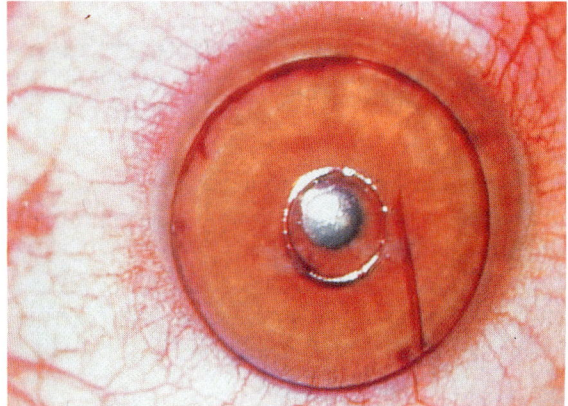

Fig. 10.45 Making the reference mark. (a) Make a 4.0 mm optical zone mark concentric to the optic center. (b) Use a fine-gauge needle held almost parallel to the corneal surface, taking care not to cut through Bowman's layer. This mark must be made tangential to the central zone—a gentian violet skin-marking pen can be used to enhance the mark. (c,d) An alternative is to use the Bores–Ruiz bullseye marker.

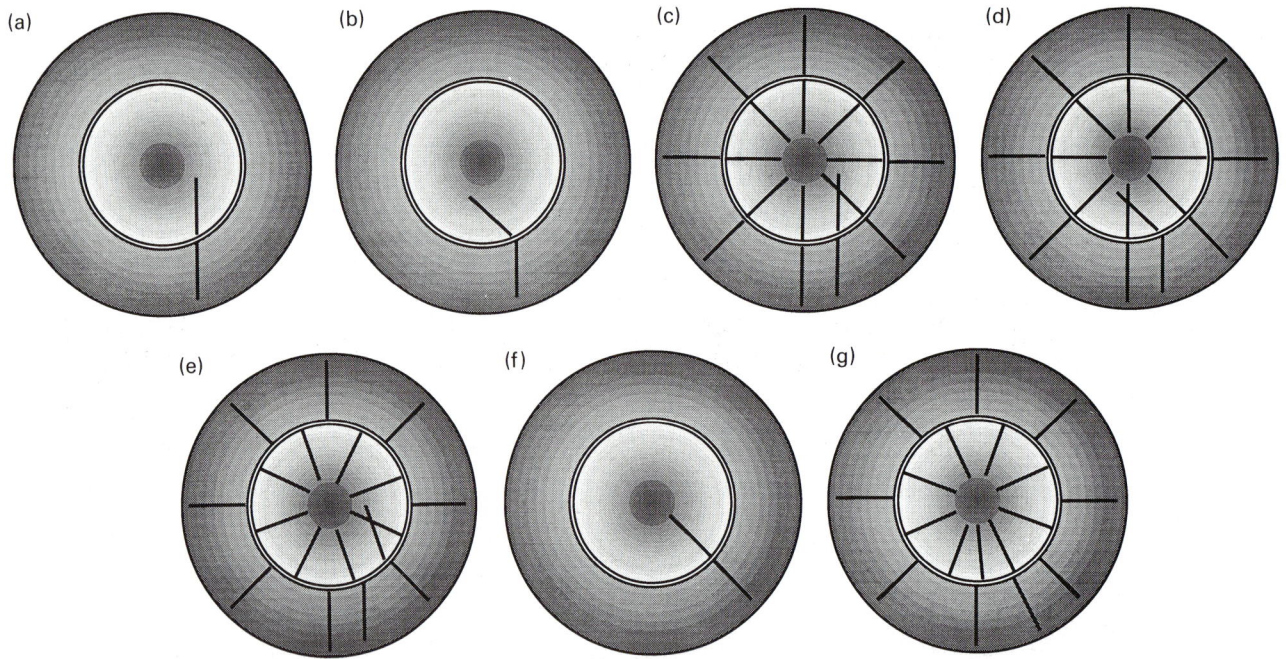

Fig. 10.46 The significance of making the reference mark tangential to the center rather than radial is illustrated in the following: (a) tangential mark; (b) if the tissue is inverted, the mark is dog-legged; (c) such a mark is especially important when operating on radial keratotomy cases; (d) tissue inverted; (e) tissue rotated; (f) there is no way to be sure this disk is inverted; (g) reference mark; reference mark; which one's the reference mark? Could the tissue be upside down? In a radial keratotomy case, a radial mark is especially confusing. With a proper mark, there's no confusion.

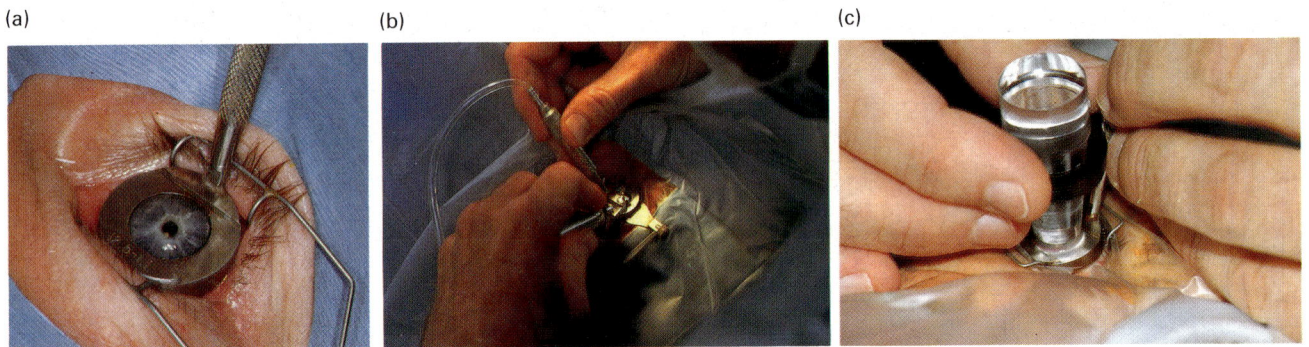

Fig. 10.47 (a) Make sure that there is plenty of clearance around the ring. The photo shows the correct position for the ring tubulature/handle. (b) The wrong ring handle position—below the eye. (c) The pre-surgical tonometer checks to insure complete pressurization of the globe.

dividual microkeratome as well as the experience and technique of the user. For example, some surgeons may consistently obtain sections 200 μm in thickness using a #25 plate, while others may get 280 μm with the same plate. It doesn't matter. The important thing is to be consistent in your technique.

Disk diameter

Always check the intra-ocular pressure with the tonometer before determining the resection diameter—at least for the first application of the ring

(Figure 10.47). The disk diameter will be suggested by the computer program typically used in this surgery. The author usually uses a 7.25 mm diameter disk for myopia and ignores the computer's suggestion. It will be necessary to try a few rings before the correct one is found. For a section having a diameter of 7.25 mm, a #8 ring should be tried first.

It is not enough merely to place the ring on the eye and actuate the vacuum pump—great pains must be taken when placing that first ring on the eye. Begin by making sure that the ring fits within the palpebral fissure without obstruction. Sometimes, in deep-set

(a)

(b)

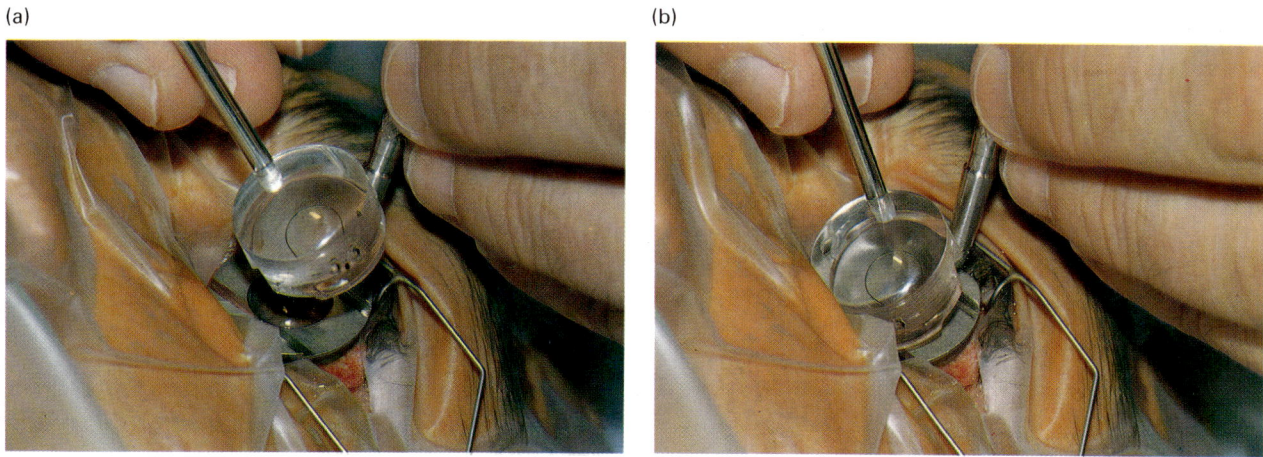

Fig. 10.48 (a) Angle the tonometer slightly and engage one edge against the lower ring guide. (b) Rotate the upper edge of the applanator down against the ring. This technique insures proper seating of the lens. It's easier than you might think to place the applanator lens askew in the ring guides, so take pains to insure that it is properly seated.

(a)

(b)

(c)

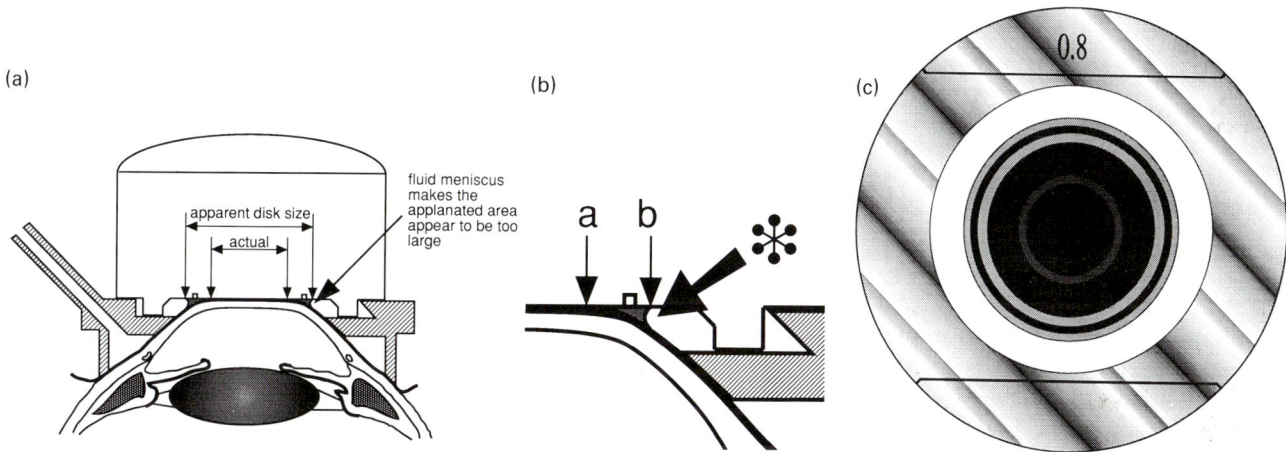

Fig. 10.49 (a–c) If the cornea is wet when the applanator is applied, the fluid meniscus will make the flattened area appear larger than it really is.

eyes, it will be necessary to proptose the eye somewhat by injecting more anesthetic. Be careful not to inject too much so as not to force the lids tightly against the eye. Center the ring carefully in relation to the pupil—a little exposed limbus is OK. Because the eye is not a perfect sphere it will tend to center itself when the vacuum is applied. Unfortunately, that center of equilibrium is seldom concentric with the optic axis, hence the eye will usually shift its position. Before applying the vacuum, therefore, grasp the conjunctiva firmly with a tissue forceps (such as a Bishop–Harmon) and anchor both hands on a firm base such as the brow or arm rest. Holding the eye and ring rigidly, apply the vacuum. Resist any tendency of the eye to de-center within the ring aperture. If it gets away from you, release the foot-switch immediately, re-position the ring and try again. Once you have satisfactory

centration, allow the vacuum sufficient time to seat the ring against the eye—10 to 15 seconds should do it. This maneuver will produce an indentation in the globe which will persist through the entire case, making centration of subsequent rings almost automatic. This is critical in keratomileusis-*in-situ* which requires two passes of the keratome and subsequently two ring changes.

With the vacuum on (Figure 10.48), check the intraocular pressure and disk diameter. If the applanated area is too small, select a lower-numbered ring and if too large, select a higher-numbered ring. Remember also to dry the cornea with a microsponge before making any measurements (Figure 10.49). If the readings seem difficult to obtain, place the lenses into sterile chilled water for a few minutes. Dry them carefully before placing on the cornea. A slight condensa-

(a)

(b)

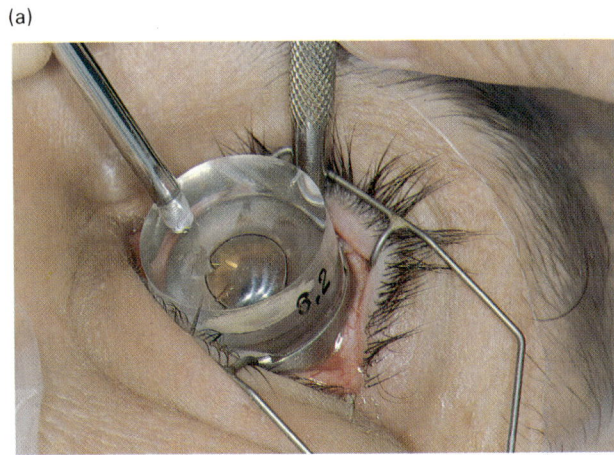

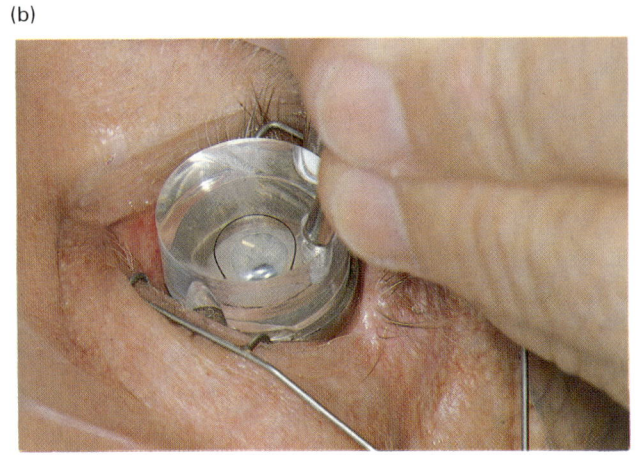

Fig. 10.50 (a) Cooling the applanators before use makes the contact zone easier to see. The applanated area lies just inside the reticle—the ring is the correct size for this case. (b) This ring is obviously too thick (high-number) for this case.

tion of moisture will occur outside the contact area when the applanator is placed against the patient's cornea, thereby facilitating the reading (Figure 10.50).

*Note:*The actual diameter of the resected disk will be about 0.2 mm larger than that applanated. This must be kept in mind to prevent a problem in hyperopic lamellar keratotomy where disk diameters are specified in tenths (see below).

A common mistake is not seating the applanator totally against the fixation ring. A less common mistake is mixing up applanators designed for different procedures or for different instruments. If you have a lathe or equipment from more than one manufacturer, make sure that all pieces are kept strictly isolated to avoid mix-and-match errors.

If the applanator is too large for the ring or if it is malpositioned, the applanated area will appear much smaller than normal and will tend to be displaced. Ordinarily such displacement can be corrected by sliding the applanator on the ring surface. If this is done and the applanation is still displaced (typically either up or down), the lens is not seated in the ring. Make certain that the applanator has not infiltrated from another set and replace it on the ring. Do not accept any measurement if unsure of the applanator. Remember—*measure twice, cut once*. Once the correct ring has been found you are ready to perform the keratectomy.

Making the section

Check to see that the microkeratome moves freely in the ring off the eye. If the keratome does not pass freely through the ring off the eye, it is certain not to do so on the eye. If the keratome hangs up in the ring during a resection, a disk of irregular thickness and shape is the inevitable result.

Position the ring back on the eye, making certain that it is centered in reference to the premarked central optical zone, and apply vacuum to the eye—check both the intra-ocular pressure and ring centration. When operating on the left eye, hold the ring with the right hand, tubulature at 12 o'clock, resting the hand on the patient's forehead—reverse hands for the right eye. Do not hold the ring with the tubulature at the 6 o'clock position—the cheek does not provide a solid base for support. Furthermore, the forearm of the holding hand will inevitably press on the patient's nose, obstructing the airway. The holding hand is also vulnerable to being hit from below, like from the anesthesiologist's or patient's hand trying to clear a breathing space. Rotate the ring handle temporally so that the nasal side of the ring is slightly higher than the temporal side (Figure 10.51). This will avoid the problem of the head striking the nose. Do not pull up

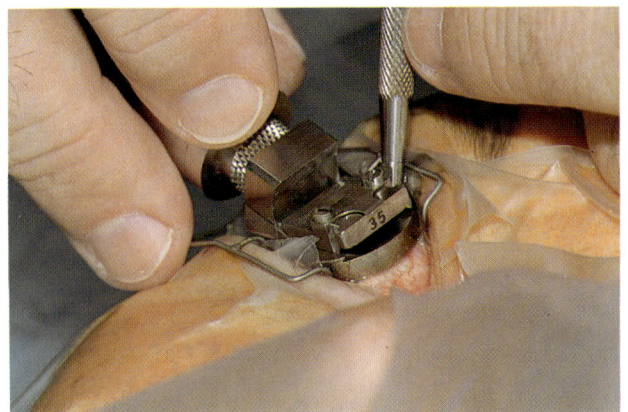

Fig. 10.51 In some patients the nose will interfere with complete excursion of the keratome head, resulting in an incomplete section. By rotating the ring temporally, the problem is avoided (see also Chapter 15).

(a)

(b)

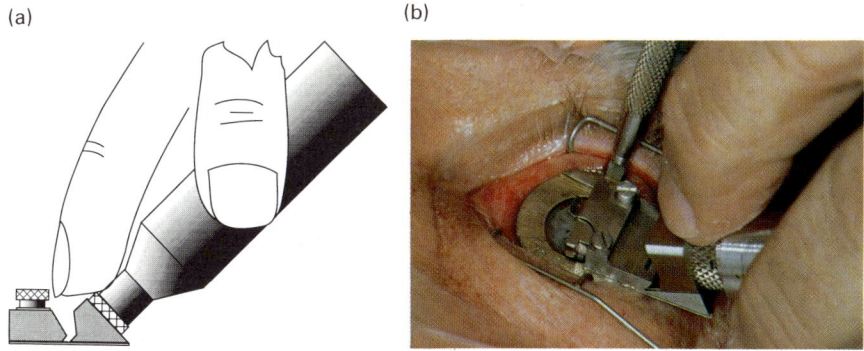

Fig. 10.52 (a and b) The correct way to hold the keratome. The instrument should be held securely but lightly. Do not force the microkeratome through the rings—let it glide through on its own. Movement of the keratome should be smooth and steady.

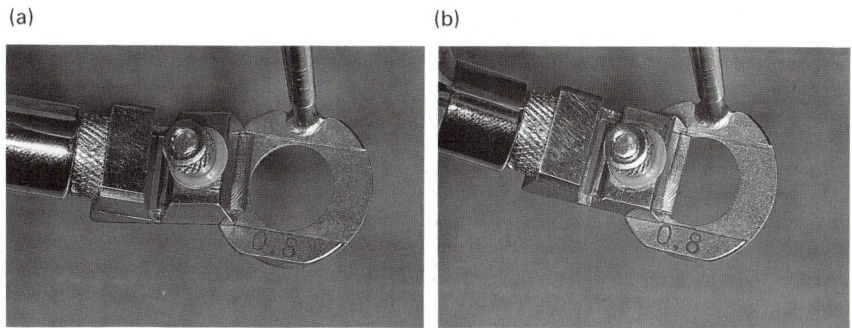

(a)

(b)

Fig. 10.53 (a and b) In double-dovetail guide rings, it helps to angle the head slightly to fit it into the guides.

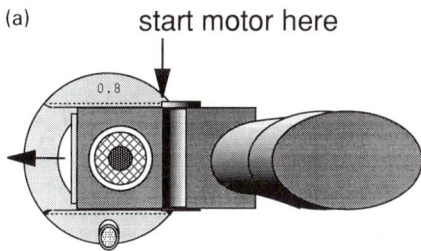

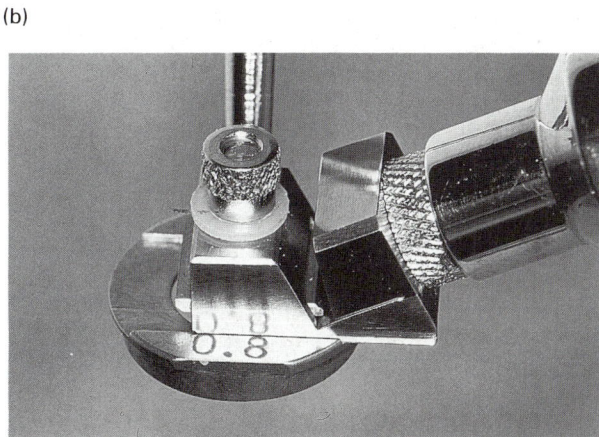

(a)

start motor here

(b)

Fig. 10.54 (a and b) The keratome is advanced until the leading edge of the blade corresponds with the temporal edge of the ring aperture. Start the motor at that point. Starting the motor too late can result in a flat-sided disk with a thin edge.

on the ring when performing this rotation—suction can be lost if this is done and it will always happen at the wrong moment. Neither should you press down on the ring, thereby pushing the eye back into the orbit. That maneuver is sure to decrease lid clearance, hindering passage of the head. The idea is to support or fixate the eye. Make sure your ring hand is planted firmly against the patient's brow.

Hold the instrument as shown in Figure 10.52 and engage the microkeratome in the ring guides. Make sure that both dovetails are engaged in double-dovetailed rings. That can be more easily accomplished

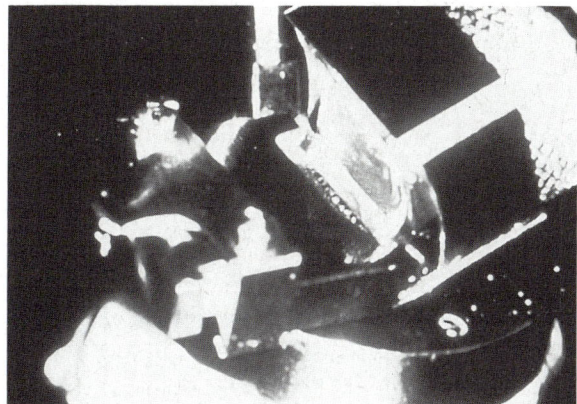

Fig. 10.55 The tissue disk issuing from the keratome feed slot. Watch the disk as it emerges from the keratome head. When it stops moving forward, the section is complete.

by angling the head slightly, as shown in Figure 10.53. Move the instrument nasally until the front blade edge is even with the temporal ring aperture (Figure 10.55). Wet the cornea with saline.

Does the blepharostat clear the ring?

Obstruction to free head passage through the ring can come from objects external to the ring itself. The end result is the same and is to be avoided at all costs. If the lid speculum is interfering, have the assistant grasp the upper and lower blades of the speculum with a hemostat to spread the lids. If that doesn't work, it may be necessary to do a canthotomy.

Depress the motor foot pedal and move the instrument nasally. The keratectomy is performed in a smooth, even manner at moderate speed. *Don't stop!* The translation across the ring should be smooth and even. A little BSS on the guides may help. *Do not use any silicone oil or any lubricant other than water!* It is vital that the movement be slow and even without any hesitation or stopping. It should take about 3 seconds (a count of one thousand one, one thousand two, one thousand three is about right). If the instrument moved freely before applying the ring to the eye, it should do so now. In the SCMD unit, the turbine sets

up a high-frequency vibration which tends to assist movement through the ring, almost floating it along.

The most common error made by novices is holding the microkeratome too rigidly. Your hand should just support the instrument and provide movement. Most right-handed people will find that left-eyed keratectomies seem to go better than right-eyed ones. This is because most people are not over-controlling the keratome with the left hand but are doing so with the right hand. Relax! Guide the instrument without any rotational force. Remember you only have to move the head about a quarter inch (0.6 cm) to complete the cut. The author recommends that the surgeon view the microkeratome through the microscope, watching the tissue disk as it feeds through the slot (Figure 10.55). By concentrating on the movement of the tissue you will inevitably relax. Furthermore, you can easily control the speed of the keratome by watching the feed rate: when the tissue stops moving out of the slot, the keratectomy is complete.

Do not stop the motor until the section is complete, however. When the blade edge meets the nasal side of the ring aperture, release the motor foot pedal and then the suction (Figure 10.56). *Do not release the vacuum* until the motor stops at the completion of the keratectomy. Remove both the ring and the microkeratome from the eye together (Figure 10.57). If any resistance is met, gently disengage the microkeratome by backing it up with the motor off. If you haven't stopped the motor too soon, all should be well. Disengage the microkeratome from the ring and set the ring aside. Place the special cover over the cornea (Figure 10.58). Remove the resected tissue with a fine-toothed forceps by gently teasing it out of the keratome head. To do this, turn the microkeratome over and pull the exposed tissue edge out on to the plate (Figures 10.59 and 10.60). If you try to pull it in the opposite direction, it could be cut. If it is bunched up behind the

(a)

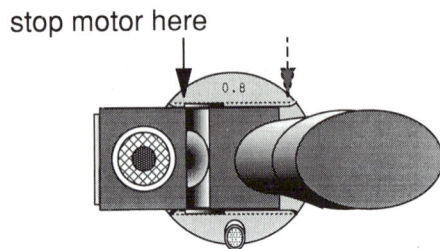

(b)

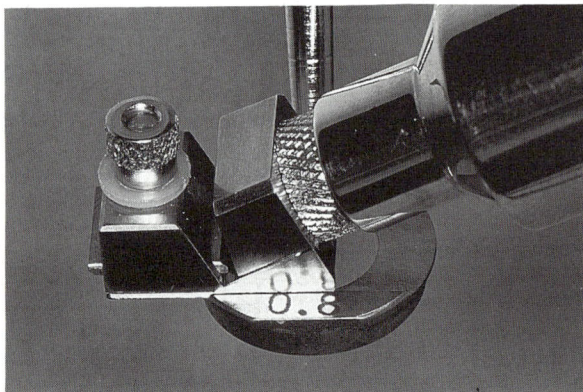

Fig. 10.56 (a and b) Stop the motor when the blade edge reaches the nasal side of the ring aperture or the tissue stops feeding through the slot.

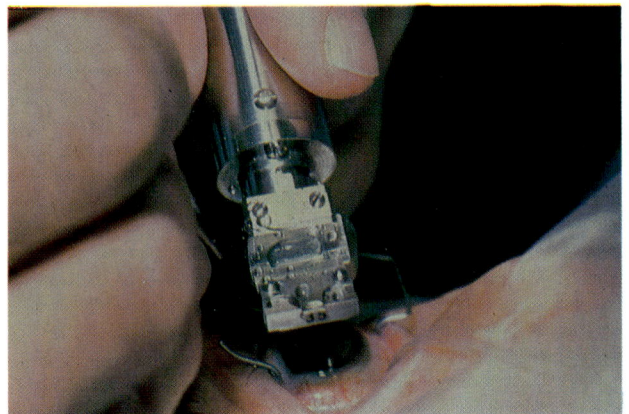

Fig. 10.57 The keratome and the ring are removed from the eye as a unit.

(a)

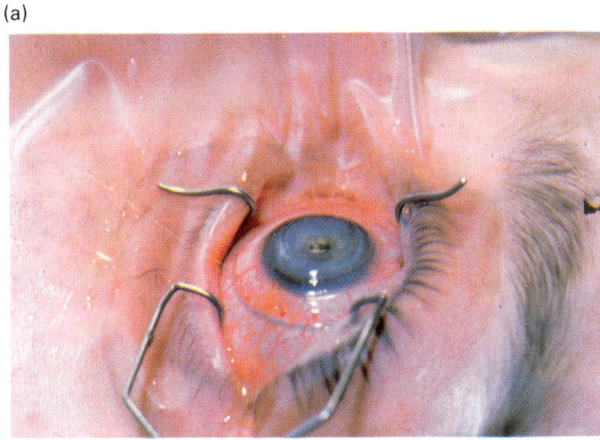

(b)

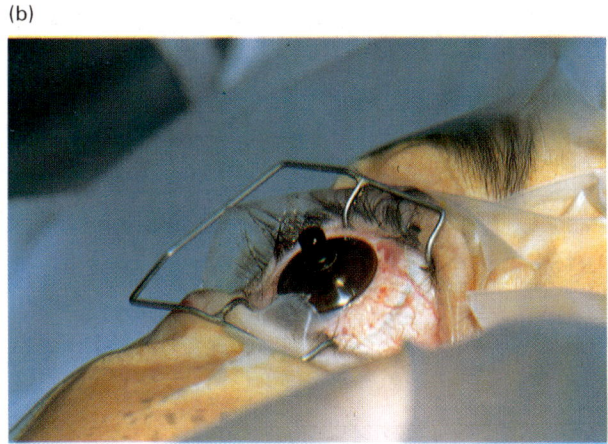

Fig. 10.58 (a) A completed keratectomy. Note the saddle depression from the ring. The appearance of this depression signals that adequate suction was obtained. Additionally, this saddle makes it easier to center the second pass in keratomileusis-*in-situ*. (b) Place the cover over the cornea as soon as possible.

(a)

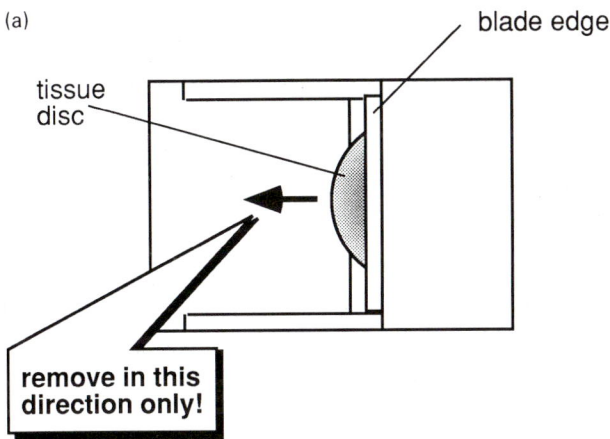

tissue disc

blade edge

remove in this direction only!

(b)

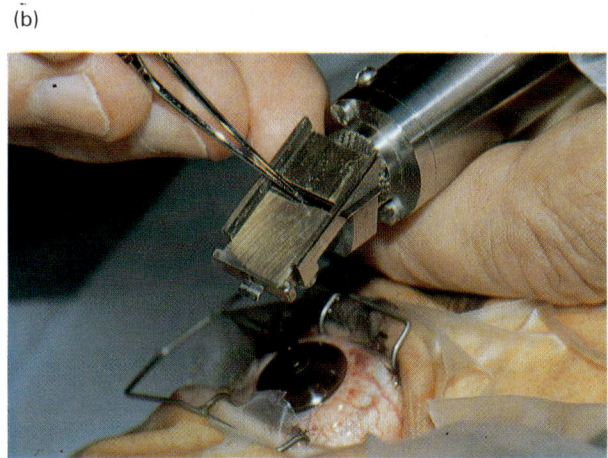

Fig. 10.59 (a,b) If an edge of tissue is protruding through the bottom of the keratome, remove the tissue by teasing it on to the blade, away from the blade edge. Do not pull it up through the feed slot.

(a)

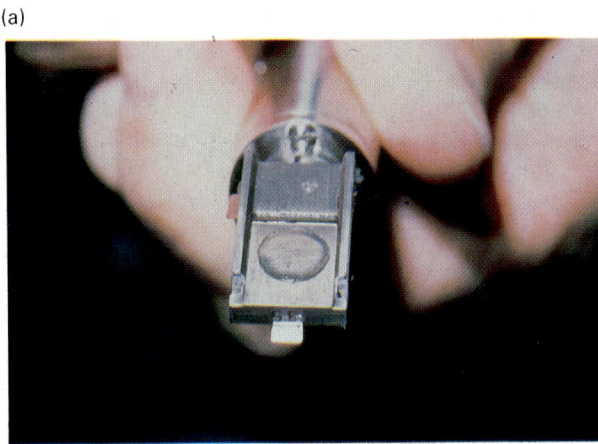

(b)

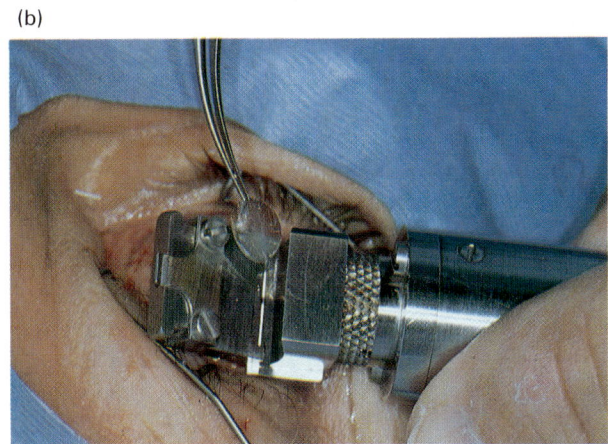

Fig. 10.60 (a) Examine the disk for defects while it is flattened out on the applanator plate. (b) A keratectomy disk on a radial keratotomy patient. Note that there is no fraying or splitting of the disk edges at the incisions.

(a)

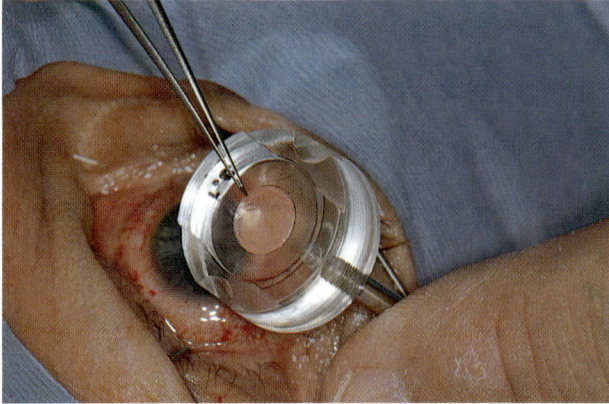

(b)

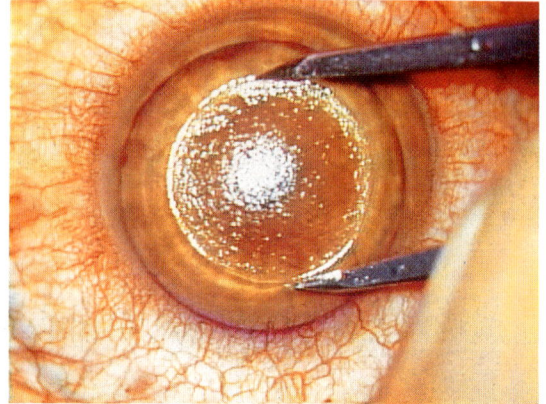

Fig. 10.61 (a) The diameter can be verified by placing the disk on to the applanator lens. This is a good way to inspect the tissue for defects under the microscope. (b) A caliper provides an alternate. Remove any lint or particles that you find.

(a)

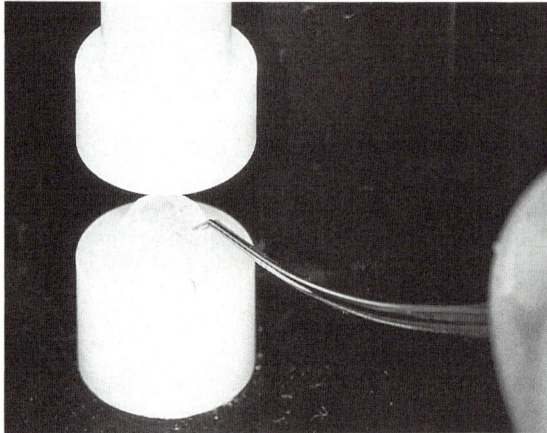

(b)

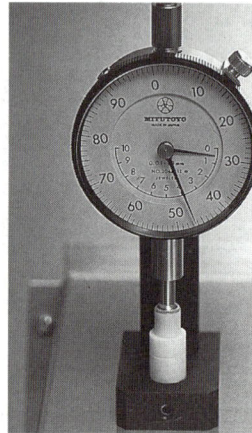

Fig. 10.62 (a,b) Transfer the disk to the tissue gauge and measure its thickness. This information is fed into the computer before and after cryo-preservation.

head and free of the blade, move it out with a closed forceps. Place it, epithelial side down, on to the applanator lens to check the diameter and the disk edge under the microscope (Figure 10.61).

Transfer the tissue to the sterile tissue gauge and measure the thickness—record this (Figure 10.62). Since this tissue is usually quite thick, gentle handling with a fine-toothed forceps will not damage it. Moisten both plates of the gauge before putting the tissue on the bottom plate, otherwise it's going to stick to the plastic and be hard to remove. Make sure that there are no folds or wrinkles in the tissue disk. Gently lower the upper anvil on to the tissue and take a reading. *Do not tap on the knob!*

Did you remember to zero the gauge before use?

It may be necessary to wet the disk to remove it from the gauge—don't force it! Place the tissue, epithelial side down, into the moist chamber and replace the chamber cover.

Always measure the disk thickness to be sure that you are getting the depth of section that you planned on. Most beginners will find that their initial sections are somewhat thinner than expected. This occurs because they are hurrying the keratectomy. On the other hand, if you go too slowly, you could enter the anterior chamber. This is particularly likely to happen if you stop moving the microkeratome halfway across.

Another cause for a thinner section can be too low an intra-ocular pressure prior to performing the resection. If the pressure is not high enough, insufficient elevation of the cornea into the ring occurs as well. With less pressure, the tissue also tends to flow away from the blade. Experienced keratotomists can compensate for this somewhat by slowing up the rate of translation, but this is not to be recommended.

Too slow a movement can lead to striations or ridges

in the section. This is more likely, however, to be caused by a too slow motor speed. The motor speed is fixed in the Steinway unit. It is adjustable in the SCMD unit and has been pre-set at the factory. That setting should be marked or recorded before you change it. If the motor speed is too slow, not only will the cut be uneven but it will also be too thin. Always check both the motor speed and intra-ocular pressure before starting the keratectomy. If your intra-ocular pressure is consistently lower than 65 mmHg (22 in of water on the vacuum gauge) and there is no apparent problem with the rings, i.e. they seem to be holding, then the system will need adjustment. This is not something that can easily be done by yourself—it should be done by the manufacturer.

The most likely problem with vacuum will be found in the periphery and not with the pump setting. The same is true with the motor speed. The speed of the motor has been carefully adjusted to produce full rpm with the loads expected under normal circumstances. If slowing occurs it will more likely be found to be due to binding introduced in the assembly of the micro-keratome. Motor speed problems are unlikely to be a problem, particularly with the gas turbine which generates considerable torque. In fact, the motor generates sufficient torque to overcome minor binding due to misalignment of the blade during head assembly. This condition can lead to spalling and the deposition of tiny metallic particles (spalls) on the resection bed or on the under-surface of the disk (see Chapter 15). The caveat is make sure that head assembly is correct and check for binding before using the instrument.

Check list for keratectomy

1 Turn on power supply.
2 Attach aspirator (suction) tube.
3 Check vacuum by occluding tube.
4 Release occlusion. Vacuum should drop to zero.
5 Inspect blade edge under microscope.
6 Assemble microkeratome head.
7 Insure blade movement.
8 Set plate.
9 Assemble motor handle.
10 Apply grease and attach head to handle.
11 Attach gas supply tubing to power unit.
12 Check performance of motor.
13 Test microkeratome in ring(s).
14 Mark central zone.
15 Place reference mark.
16 Place and center fixation ring.
17 Depress vacuum actuator switch.
18 Check adherence of ring.
19 Dry cornea.
20 Perform tonometry.

21 Check dimensions of applanation.
22 Moisten cornea.
23 Keratectomy—slow and even movement.
24 Release motor switch and vacuum switch—simultaneously.
25 Remove disk from microkeratome.

Additional steps are performed as required for the procedure at hand.

Pre-operative caveats

The cutting edge of the blade must be checked under the microscope. This can be done by checking the brightness; any irregularity in the shine of the edge means a nicked blade which must be replaced.

Once the microkeratome has been assembled, it must be tested in the rings to make sure that it slides freely, to insure a proper cut. Finally, it must be started for a few seconds to check if the blade is moving freely and the speed is correct.

Although, as a rule, there are usually no accidents or problems during the keratectomy, failure to heed each point can lead to difficulty. If you forget to check the blade, you can be sure that it will have a nick in it. If you forget to check the vacuum, it will fail at the worst possible moment. If you neglect to check for free movement of the microkeratome in the rings, it will bind halfway across. Check every point. It is a good idea to have an assistant read off each point as you go, waiting for your response before going on. If you do this in the early cases, it will be safe to resort to a printed check list later on.

The preceding discussion is valid for keratectomies done for lathing as well as for keratomileusis-*in-situ*, hyperopic lamellar keratotomy, keratophakia, or for laser keratomileusis. We will now move on to lathing of the tissue disk.

Lathing

Transfer the resected disk to the crucible containing the kitton green preservative solution (Figure 10.63). The author always places the tissue into the solution stromal (curved) side up. Make sure that the tissue is completely submerged, place the crucible in a safe place and start the timer. The computer will ask for the preserved thickness of the tissue. The author has been advised by Ruiz to enter the same value found for the unpreserved disk thickness—this is our standard practice. While the tissue is soaking in the kitton green, the new cutting radius, displacement, and angle α should be set and locked in.

After 1 min, a Barraquer lenticule spoon is used to retrieve the disk from the preserving solution. Figure 10.64 shows how the tissue disk is transferred to the delrin base, with the epithelial side against the base. A

(a)

(b)

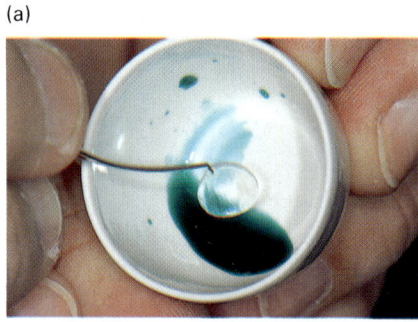

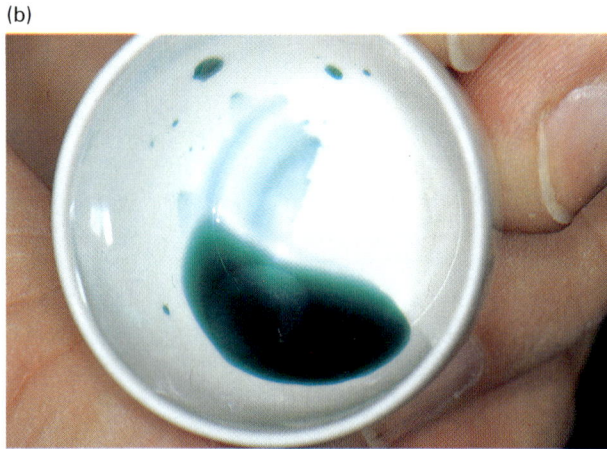

Fig. 10.63 (a) The disk is placed into a solution of kitton green for 1 min. (b) Make sure that the disk is completely submerged. It is easy to see the disk against the white background.

sable brush or a microsponge is used to draw off as much liquid as possible without disturbing the disk. Merely touching the bristles to the junction of the tissue and the base usually suffices.

Turn on the lathe motor to about 15 rpm or so (the disk should be turning slowly) and using the edge of the Barraquer spoon lightly touched to the disk edge, center the disk on the base (Figure 10.65). A little practice will make this an easy task. Stop the motor and re-set the freezing timer (it was used to time the preservation step). Press the HEAD button to start freezing the tissue and start the timer (Figure 10.66). Run the tool up close to, but not touching, the tissue. Start the tool freezing and the tissue slowly turning. Watch the tissue very carefully at this point. The tissue will change color as it freezes. As first it will turn a dark green and will appear granular (Figure 10.67). After about 45 seconds or so the tissue will undergo a sudden change. It will seem to recede or shrink back against the plastic base—it does, of course, indeed shrink at this point. At the same time its color will become a light white–green. Check the tool—it should be frozen by now and look it. Increase the lathe speed. You may now proceed to carve the tissue disk into a lenticule. One caveat—even if the tissue coloration changes early, do not begin lathing until 45 seconds, *minimum*, has elapsed.

Lathing continues until the displacement given by the computer program has been reached—typically

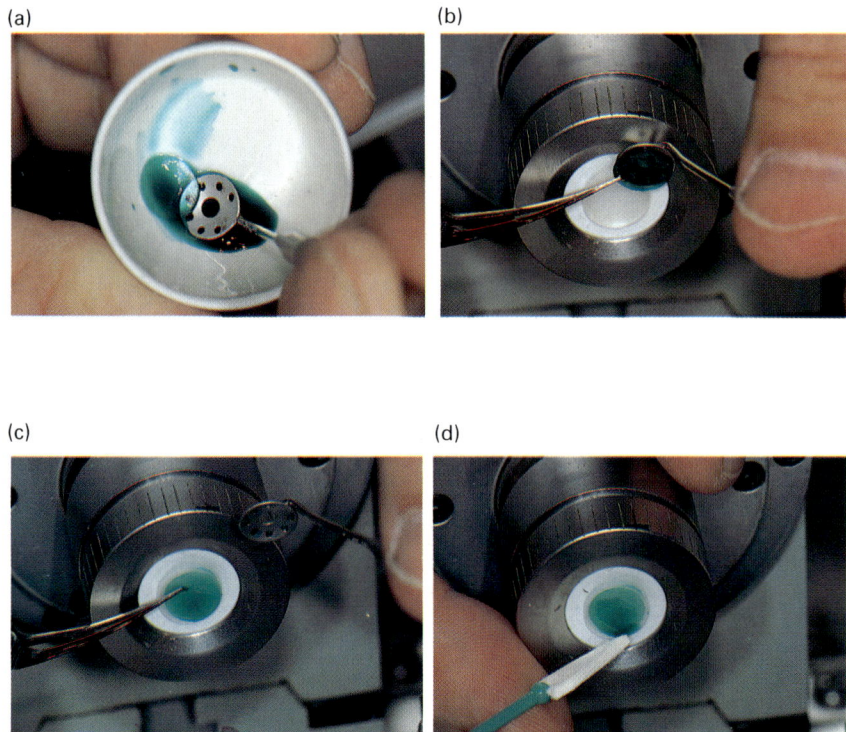

(a)

(b)

(c)

(d)

Fig. 10.64 (a) The tissue is removed from the preservative solution with a lenticule spoon. (b,c) A forceps or sable brush is used to *slide* the disk on to the Delrin base. Sliding the tissue serves to prevent air bubbles being trapped behind the disk. (d) A microsponge is gently touched to the junction of the disk edge and base. Capillary action will draw away most of the excess fluid.

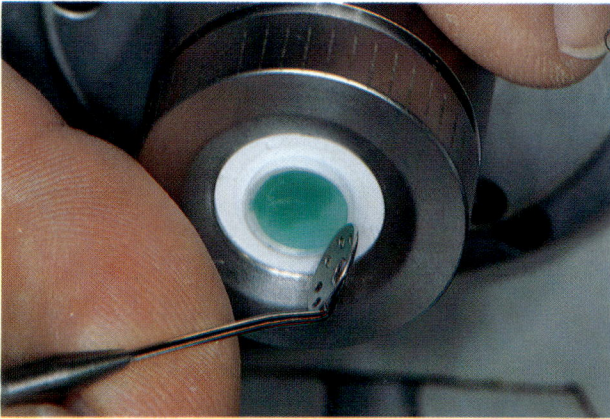

Fig. 10.65 The Barraquer spoon is used to center the disk while the lathe head is turning slowly.

the stop will prevent any advancement beyond that point. Make sure that each pass of the tool across the face of the tissue disk is smooth and even (Figure 10.68). A *dry* sable brush can be used to brush away shavings from the tool tip if they are obscuring your view. If this is a myopia case, this completes the lathing phase of the operation. If, however, this is a case of hyperopia, the cutting radius will have to be re-adjusted and the wing portion of the lenticule lathed (Figure 10.69).

When lathing is complete, turn off the gases and retract the tool to its fullest extent. Turn off the lathe motor and push in the locking knob to prevent rotation of the lathe spindle. The delrin base, tissue and all, is

removed from the lathe and plunged (tissue side up) into a bath of saline heated to body temperature. The author uses a special heater block which holds a container designed for this purpose. Stop the freezing timer and record the display.

The Barraquer spoon is now used to remove the lenticule from the thawing chamber and to transfer to the moist chamber (Figure 10.70). Remove excess liquid from the chamber with the sable brush, cap the chamber and place it in a secure spot. Lathing is complete; it is now time to clean the recipient bed.

Figure 10.71 shows the various lenticule configurations and the abbreviations used to label them (see Table 10.1). While not comprehensive, it is included as a guide to the topic in this and other treatises.

Clean-up

Remove the corneal cover and with a sable brush and copious irrigation, ''scrub'' the keratectomy bed. This scrubbing is just vigorous brushing to insure that any lint or epithelial cells are removed. Next dry the bed with a moistened microsponge. Do not use the cellulose sponges (such as Weck-Cel) for this purpose. They have a tendency to leave small particles behind. This drying step is to reveal any threads or small pieces of metal that may have come off the microkeratome and which were not dislodged by the irrigation or missed by the scrubbing. Remove these with a fine forceps and irrigate again. *Use high power!* Replace the cap.

Hold the moist chamber under the microscope and

(a) (b)

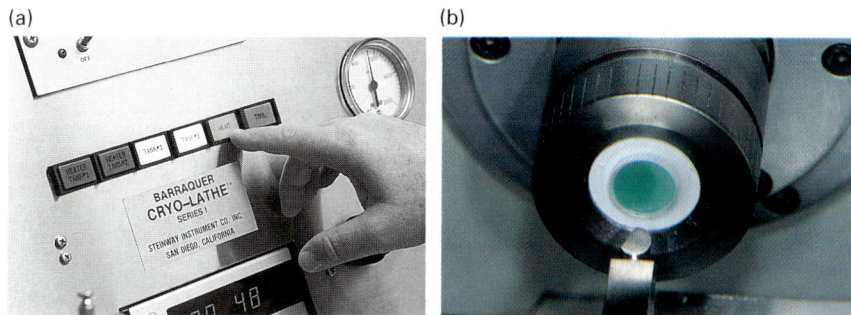

Fig. 10.66 (a) Start the head (and tissue) freezing first. The lathe head should be slowly revolving at this time. (b) Run the tool up close to, but not touching, the tissue and start the tool freezing.

(a) (b)

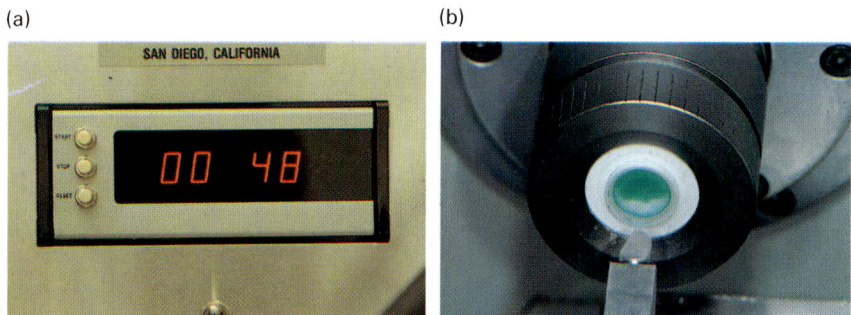

Fig. 10.67 (a) A sudden change in the appearance of the disk signals that freezing has occurred. (b) At least 45 seconds should elapse before starting the lathing process. This insures that complete freezing/shrinkage of the tissue has occurred.

(a)

(b)

(c)

(d)

(e)

(f)

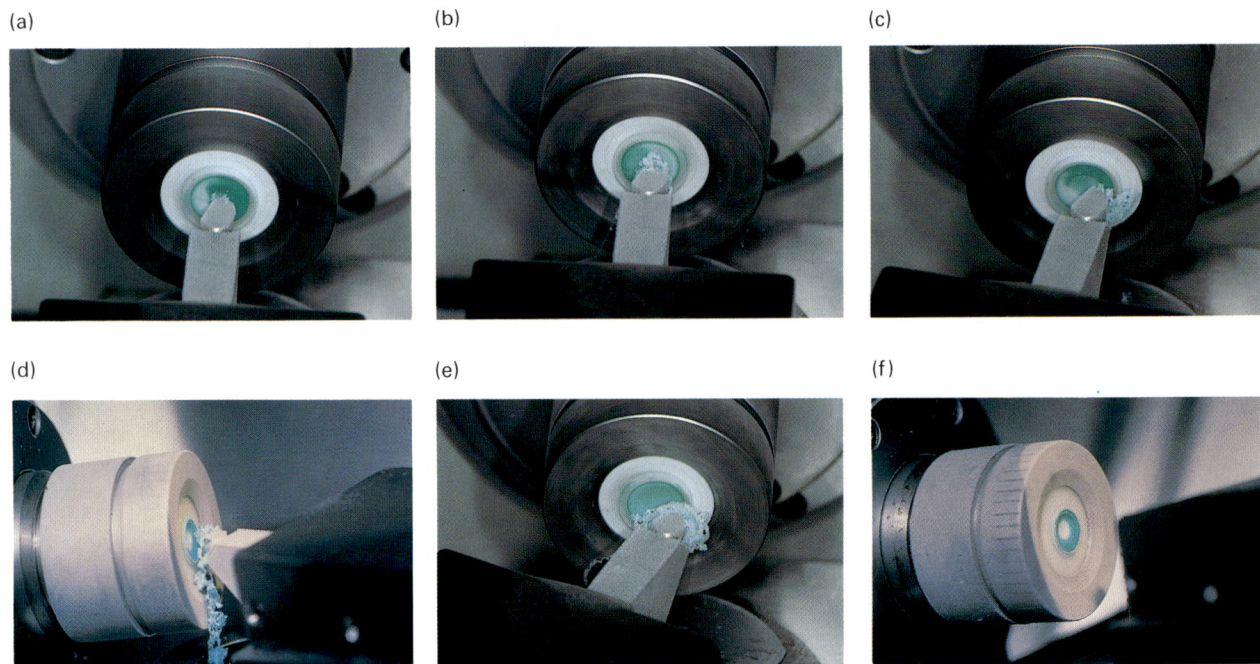

Fig. 10.68 (a–f) Lathing the disk. Advance the tool slowly, taking complete passes across the tissue surface before advancing further. Make the swing-through smooth and even. The finishing pass is made twice. Retract the head completely when lathing is complete.

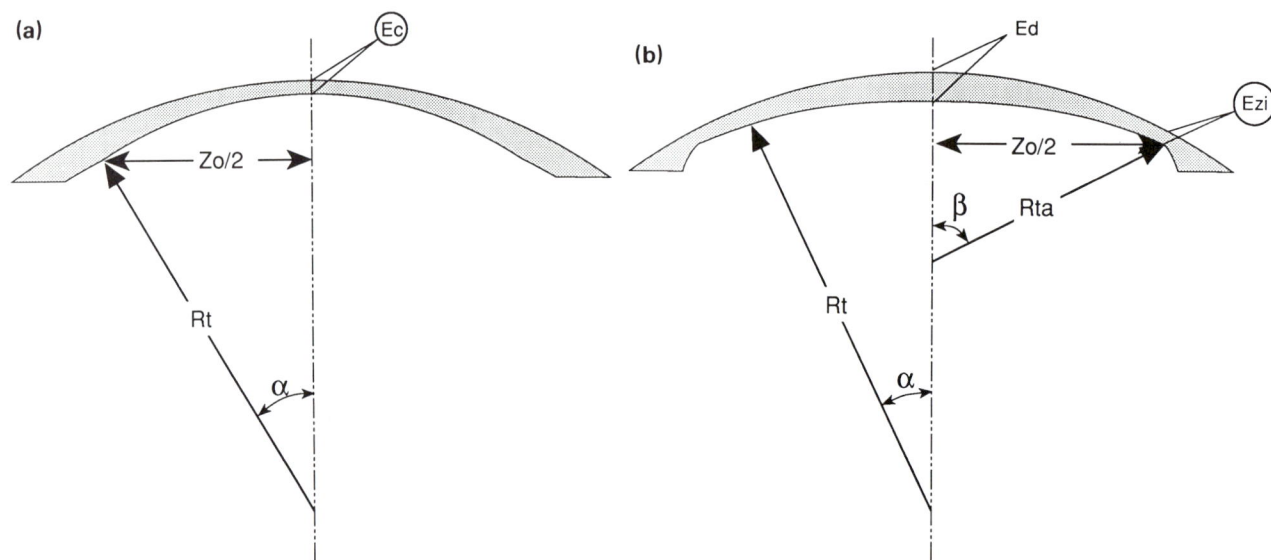

(a)

(b)

Fig. 10.69 (a) In cases of myopia, only one setting of the cutting radius and angle α is needed. The nature of the hyperopic lenticule shape is such that two separate settings of the cutting angle and radius are required (b).

remove the lid. *Very* gently irrigate and brush the under-surface of the resected disk (Figures 10.72 and 10.73). It may be necessary for your assistant to hold the chamber for you. If so, make sure that he or she is observing through the microscope at the same time. Do not perform the cleaning by resting the tissue on the cornea. To do so is to invite a visit from the "epithelium fairy."

Now remove the tissue from the chamber using the lenticule spoon or a fine-toothed (0.12 mm) Colibri

forceps. Be very gentle with the tissue at this point. Tissue for keratomileusis-*in-situ* is much thinner than that encountered in hyperopic lamellar keratotomy or in cryo-lathing and is easily torn—have a care. Here is where the lenticule spoon really pays for itself. Using a drop or two of BSS, float the tissue within the moist chamber so that it can be easily picked up by the spoon. If you are concerned about tearing or have a tendency to hold the tissue too firmly or don't have the spoon, try using a Pierse-Hoskins type of iris forceps.

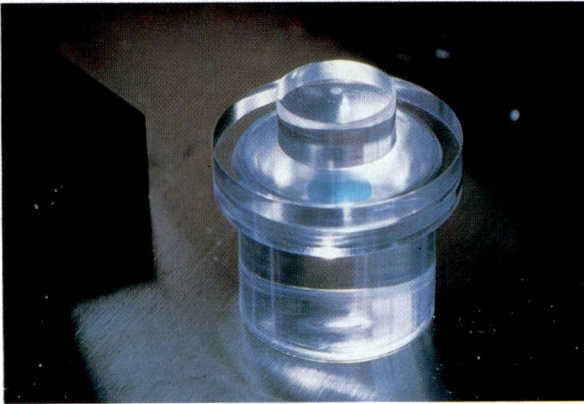

Fig. 10.70 The tissue is stored in the moist chamber while the resection bed is irrigated and debrided.

reference mark. It should line up exactly. If it doesn't and seems to join the corneal mark at an angle, you have placed the tissue on to the eye *upside down*. This is very easy to do with the thin keratomileusis-*in-situ* disk—the natural cupping seen with thicker sections and which aids in identifying the epithelial side is absent.

As mentioned in the discussion on hyperopic lamellar keratotomy, it can especially be troublesome in radial keratotomy cases with all the corneal scars (see below). That's why the type of mark illustrated above is recommended; it's difficult to confuse it with those scars. Once the tissue is aligned, touch a microsponge to the junction to soak up excess fluid. This also tends to "tack" the tissue down.

Suturing the corneal disk

At least three cardinal sutures of 10-0 nylon should be used (at 12, 6, and 9 o'clock) to hold the tissue in place and prevent rotation. Don't try to skimp with one or two. Even José Barraquer uses three sutures. So if the

Remove, or have your assistant remove, the corneal cover, wet the eye, and place the tissue *epithelial side up* into the keratectomy bed (Figure 10.74). Gently, using the sable brush and/or the edge of the forceps, rotate the tissue into alignment with the previously made

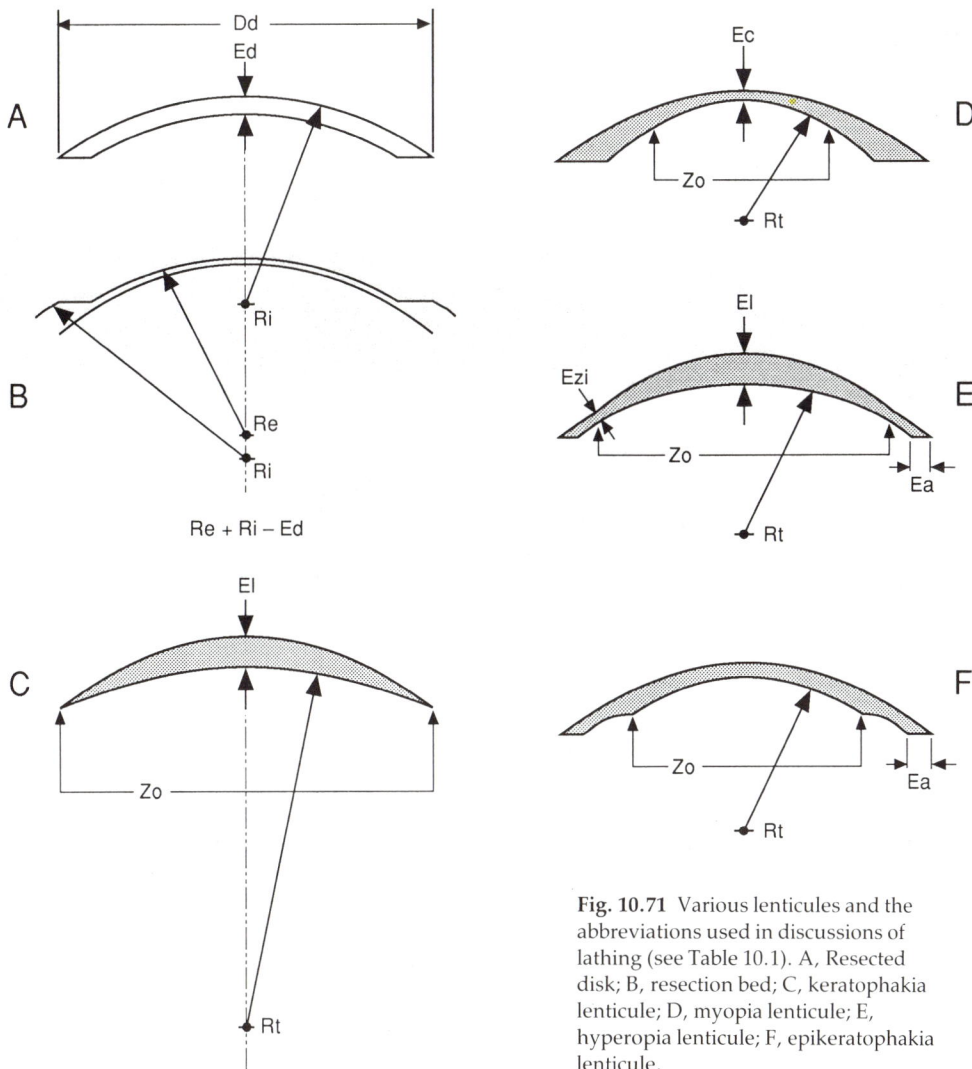

$$Re + Ri - Ed$$

Fig. 10.71 Various lenticules and the abbreviations used in discussions of lathing (see Table 10.1). A, Resected disk; B, resection bed; C, keratophakia lenticule; D, myopia lenticule; E, hyperopia lenticule; F, epikeratophakia lenticule.

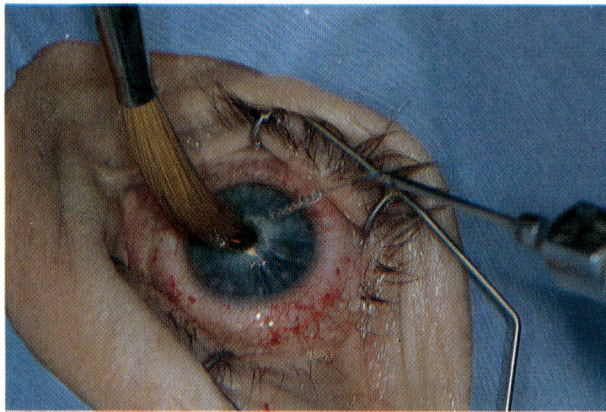

Fig. 10.72 Do not stint in the irrigation and brushing of the resection bed. Debris is easier to remove now before the lenticule is sutured in place.

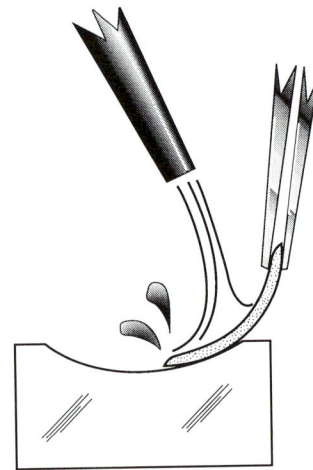

Fig. 10.73 Clean the under-side of the lenticule in the moist chamber. Do not rest the tissue on the cornea to do this. That technique is sure to implant epithelial cells into the interface. Direct a gentle stream of saline downward on to the disk, using a soft brush to dislodge any particulate matter.

(a)   (b)   (c)

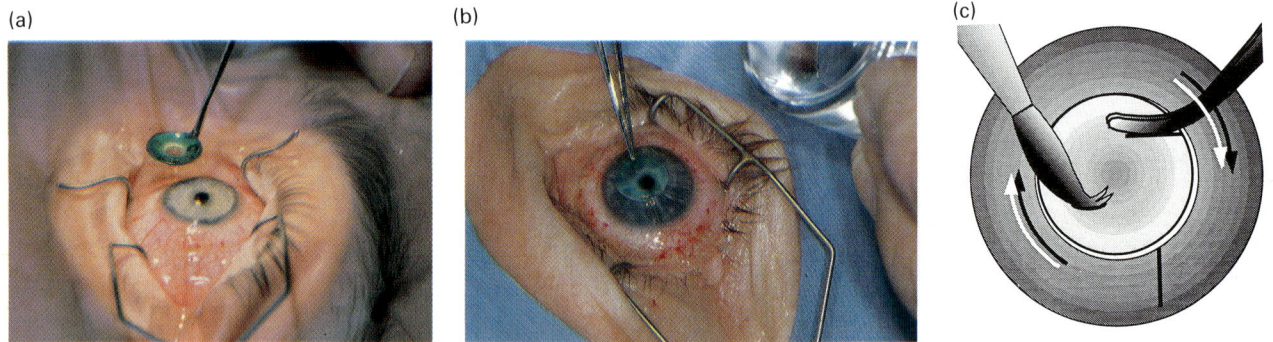

Fig. 10.74 (a) Transfer the lenticule to the eye with the tissue spoon. (b) Place it on to the resection bed. (c) Rotate the lenticule with brush and curved forceps. Align the reference mark. The disk and resection bed should be wet when performing this maneuver. Avoid sliding the disk over the edge of the resection bed to prevent seeding the interface with epithelial cells.

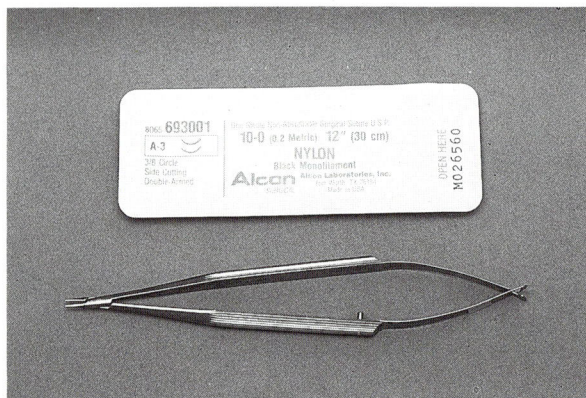

Fig. 10.75 The A-3 needle/nylon configuration by Alcon is the author's choice. A fine, straight needle holder may be easier to use by some surgeons.

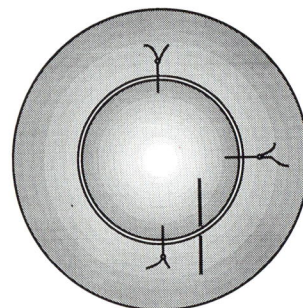

Fig. 10.76 Cardinal sutures. These sutures are for the purpose of preventing gross misalignment of the disk during placement of the running suture—do not tie them tightly. There should not be any furrows in the disk—this is not a keratoplasty! Place interrupted sutures at 12, 6, and 9 o'clock. Start at the 12 o'clock position; next do the 6 o'clock suture.

master does it, so should you. The Alcon A-3 (or CU-11) 10-0 nylon with spatulated (side-cutting) needle seems to work well in these cases (Figure 10.75). It should be cut in half, with one half used for the cardinals.

Begin suturing with the 12 o'clock cardinal (Figure 10.76). Grasp the upper edge of the tissue disk with either 0.12 mm corneal forceps or the double-pronged Hofman–Polack forceps (Katena K5-1566) or similar, being careful not to rotate the tissue. Place the first suture through the tissue sufficiently back from the disk edge to hold without tearing out. Bring the needle through and into the cornea at the edge of the resection bed and out. Tie it so as just to coapt the edges. Pull the knot to the limbal side and cut the ends long. The 6 o'clock suture should be placed next, again insuring that the disk is not displaced or rotated. It is not necessary to hold the tissue with forceps but it might be helpful for the first few cases to do so. Tie the suture so that little, if any, furrowing occurs in the disk. The last cardinal is then placed. In this case, counter-traction at 3 o'clock is needed to keep from displacing or tearing the disk. Again, tie the knot only tight enough to coapt the edge.

The placement of the eight-bite, anti-torque suture is not all that difficult if approached in a precise step-wise fashion. Begin suturing at the 3 o'clock position by passing the needle through the disk at 3 o'clock, approximately 1.0 mm from the edge. Angle it at 45° to the resection margin and pass the tip between the edges of the disk and resection bed (Figures 10.77 through 10.79).

Do not run the needle through the tissue at the bottom of the bed (Figure 10.80). In keratomileusis-*in-*

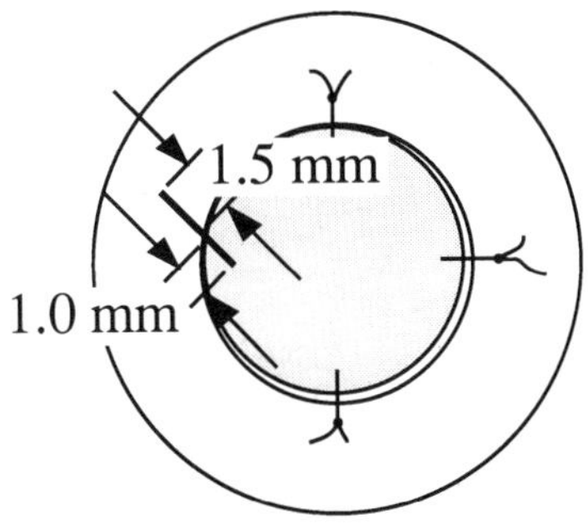

Fig. 10.78 Placement of suture bite. Try to keep the entry points on the disk as equidistant from the edge as possible. The exit points on the corneal sides are not as important.

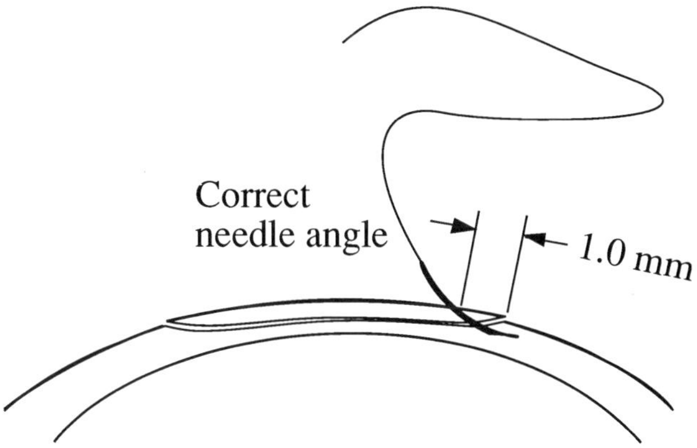

Fig. 10.79 Correct needle path. The needle should come out at the bottom edge of the disk and enter the corresponding portion of the resection edge without entering the bottom of the bed.

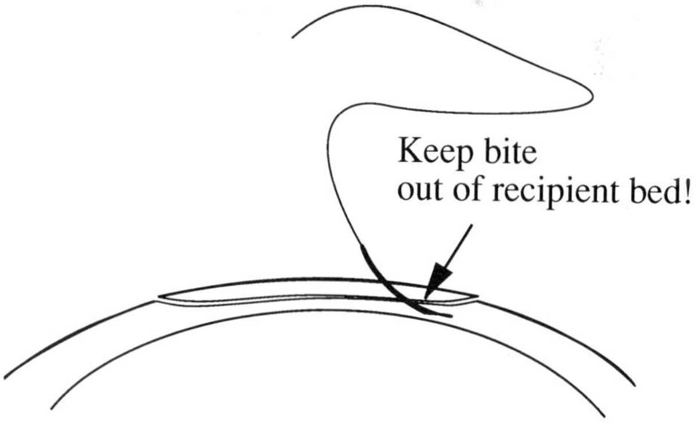

Fig. 10.80 Incorrect needle path. Avoid catching the tissue of the resection bed with your needle and suture. The tissue disk must be allowed to move and adjust itself freely over the resection surface to minimize astigmatism.

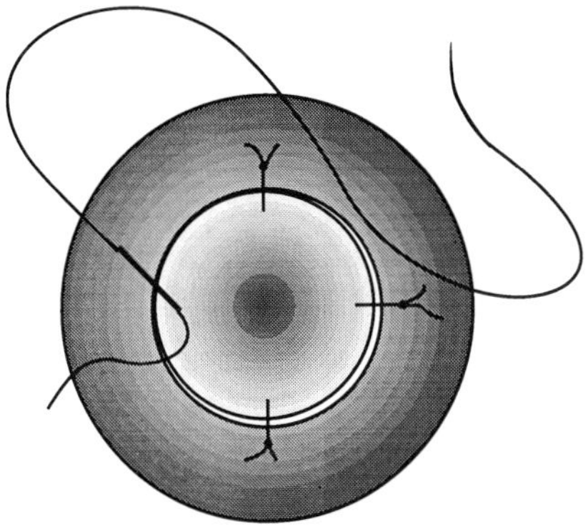

Fig. 10.77 First suture pass. Fixation at the limbus directly in line with the suture path provides good control over the procedure. The author tends to fixate behind the needle (on the opposite limbus), but some find it easier to fixate in front. When suturing the thin keratomileusis-*in-situ* disk, it is best to avoid handling it with forceps of any kind. It really isn't necessary at any rate. If the needle tip is angled down slightly and pressed against the disk, the needle will easily cut its way through the tissue without undue distortion or displacement of the disk itself.

situ it is useful to push straight back against the eye with the slanted needle tip rather than trying to sweep it through the disk edge. In this way the needle will penetrate the thin disk through and through without displacing it. Withdraw the tip sufficiently to make the limbal portion of the bite, entering at the bottom of the limbal edge and exiting about 1.5 mm from the edge

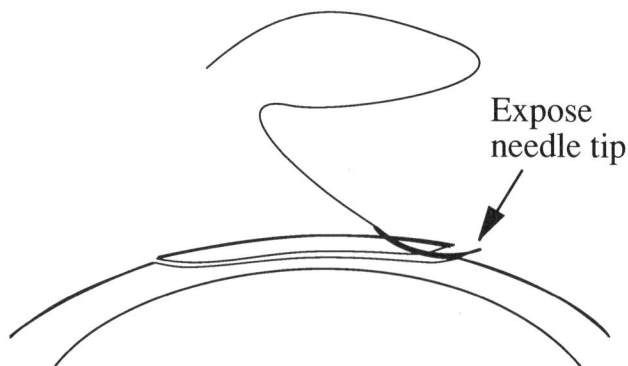

Fig. 10.81 Correct needle path. Note the track of the needle.

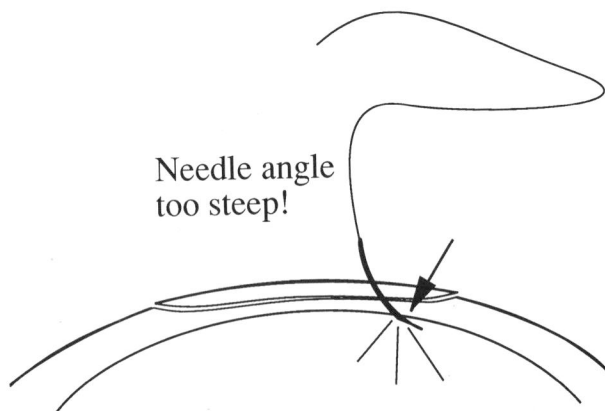

Fig. 10.82 Incorrect needle path. Shallow bites are the order of the day. Too great an angle of the suture tip practically insures that the needle will enter the AC. If aqueous appears, withdraw the needle and place it properly—no ill effects are likely in that event.

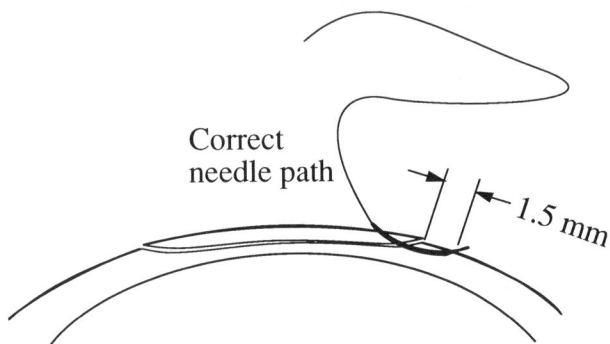

Fig. 10.83 Try to expose the needle tip. By exposing the tip of the needle each time while slightly raising up on the disk, the surgeon is assured that tissue at the bottom of the resection is not trapped.

(Figure 10.81). It helps to grasp the limbus with corneal-scleral forceps adjacent to the point the needle will exit. Do not push the forceps toward the needle holder. This will make the cornea bend upwards, causing the needle to plunge deeper, possibly entering

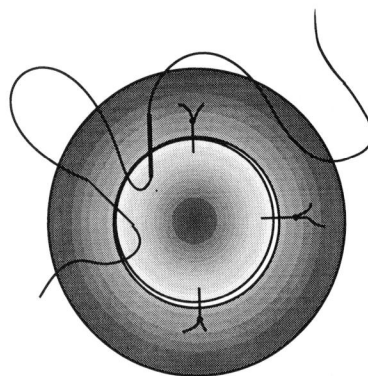

Fig. 10.84 Second suture pass. The next bite begins halfway between the 3 o'clock and 6 o'clock position and is angled so as to produce a 90° included angle with the external limb of the previous bite. Again withdraw the needle back from the edge to insure that none of the resection bed is included in the bite. The disk must be free to move within the resection bed.

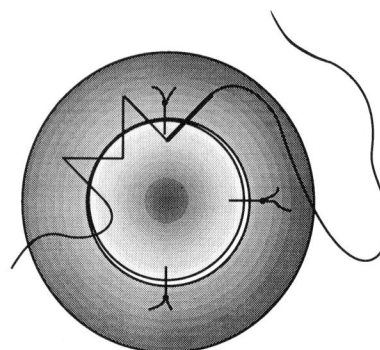

Fig. 10.85 Third suture limb. Begin the third bite at the 6 o'clock position, angling it at 45° in the same manner as the first. Draw up the slack so that the suture limbs lie flat and apposed to the corneal surface.

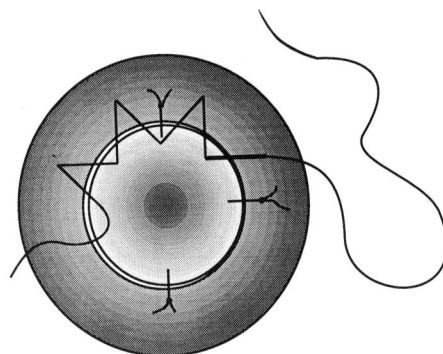

Fig. 10.86 Fourth suture pass. The fourth limb begins midway between the 6 and 9 o'clock positions and is directed at 180°. Again, take up the slack so that all the previously placed limbs are lying flat. Do not let the suture drag across the surface of the lenticule. Not only will this displace the lenticule itself, but it may tear off the epithelium. If you have displaced the lenticule, wet the area and gently, using the back of a curved forceps, move the tissue back into place. Pulling on the appropriate suture limb in the direction you wish the lenticule to move helps.

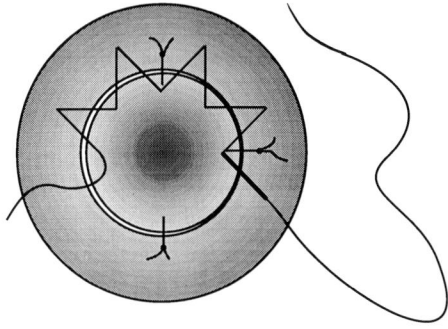

Fig. 10.87 Fifth suture pass. All of the previous limbs of the suture were placed backhand. For the next parts, reverse the needle and begin at the 9 o'clock position, positioning the needle to make the fifth bite at 45°.

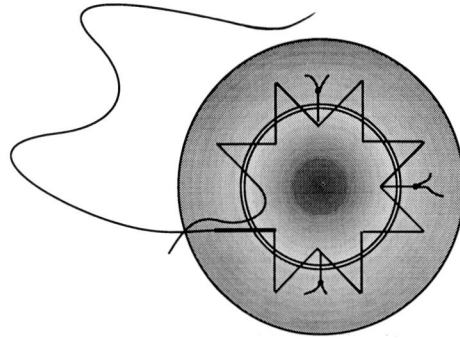

Fig. 10.88 Sixth suture pass. The sixth limb begins between the 9 and 12 o'clock positions and is directed toward the surgeon.

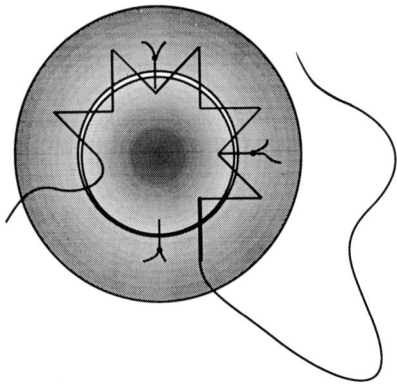

Fig. 10.89 Seventh suture pass. The seventh suture limb starts at 12 o'clock and again makes a 45° angulation to the tissue edge, making sure not to include the cardinal suture at that position.

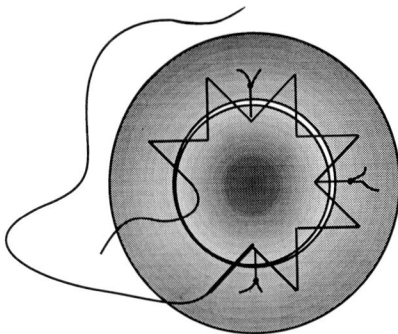

Fig. 10.90 Last suture pass. Finally the eighth bite enters the disk (lenticule) between the 12 and 3 o'clock positions and is directed horizontally. You are now ready to tie the knot.

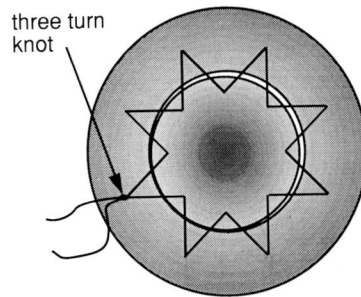

Fig. 10.91 First knot—three-turn surgeon's knot. When snugging up the first (three-throw) knot, hold the standing end on tension and aligned with the superficial limb as shown. Pull the other end of the suture down toward the limbus. This will crimp and lock the knot, keeping it from slipping.

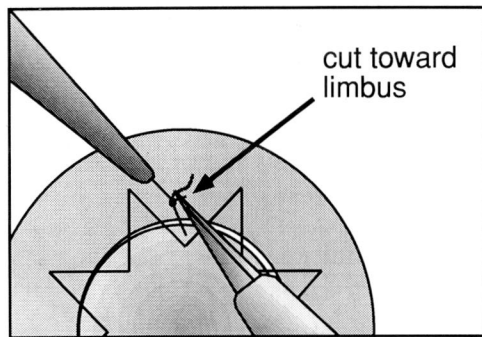

Fig. 10.92 Removing cardinal sutures. Cut and remove the cardinals carefully to avoid severing the running suture.

the anterior chamber (Figure 10.82). To prevent this, pick up the needle tip and expose it under the edge of the disk. Then place it flat on the recipient bed and pass it through the limbal side of the resection (Figure 10.83). Pull the excess suture through so as to leave about 1 in (2–3 cm) loose. Continue with the remaining seven passes (Figures 10.84 through 10.90).

The slack in the suture is drawn up and a three-throw or "surgeon's" knot is made, pulling the suture ends in such a way as to cause the knot to end up off the lenticule as close to the exit point on the limbus as possible (Figure 10.91). Snug up the suture sufficiently so that all limbs are straight and against the corneal surface. At this point the disk and bed are wetted with BSS to allow the disk to slide. Cut and remove all three cardinals, taking care not to cut the continuous suture

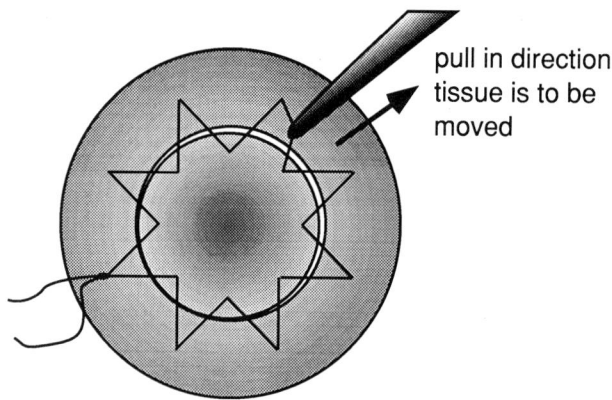

Fig. 10.93 Pull up gently on the suture limbs. Pull up all the slack in the running suture. If the disk is displaced, pulling on the suture limb in the direction you wish the tissue to move will cause it to slide over. Leave it slightly de-centered directly opposite and away from the knot.

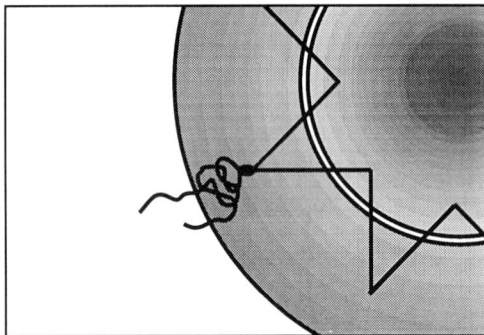

Fig. 10.94 Finish off the knot. Re-tighten the three-throw surgeon's knot and add a single throw. This maneuver will cause the disk to center itself. The next throw should be square to the one previous so as to lock the suture. The resultant knot should be tight and compact and will not slip.

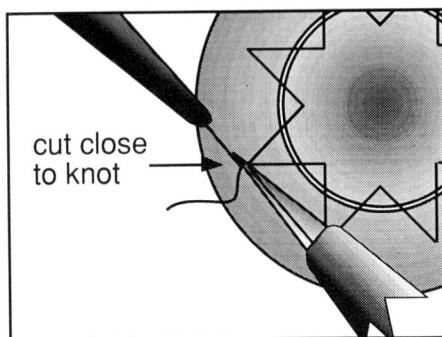

Fig. 10.95 Cut the knot flush. The suture should now be cut close to the knot, using a sharp, 15° razor knife. Lay the flat of the tip against the knot and cut the suture by pulling up on the ends, bending them over the blade edge. Do not pull too hard or the knot will also be cut.

(Figure 10.92). If the cardinals are removed before tying the knot, the lenticule will be dragged or displaced toward the knot.

Some displacement of the lenticule may occur even with the cardinals in place. In that event it must be re-centered within the resection bed. By pulling up gently

on the suture limbs toward the side you wish the lenticule to move, it will oblige by sliding in that direction (Figure 10.93). This maneuver may have to be done several times. Leave the lenticule slightly de-centered to the side *opposite* the knot. The lenticule should end up just touching the resection edge at 3 o'clock, leaving a gap between the lenticule and the edge everywhere else.

The loosened suture should be snugged up and a single throw added to the previous triple. To keep the knot from "traveling," hold the standing part of the suture on tension and pull the other limb down and away from the knot. The knot should not move and should be located at the exit point of the last bite and on the scleral side of the keratectomy incision. Do not tie the knot so snug as to produce furrows in the disk. The ideal is to tie the suture just tight enough so that it lies flat against the cornea and is not loose. Add another single-throw square to finish off (Figure 10.94).

Under magnification use a sharp razor knife to cut the suture ends on the knot. Direct the cutting edge away from the knot, angled slightly up. Hold the tip against the knot with the edge extending past the knot. Hold each loose end with a forceps and bring it up against the blade edge, bending the suture over the edge slightly. It doesn't take much tension to cut the suture. Repeat for the other suture end (Figure 10.95).

The next and final step is to bury the knot. This adds immeasurably to the patient's comfort but also reduces irritation and blinking which slow epithelial healing. Using two smooth tying forceps, grasp each of the exposed suture limbs as shown. With the left hand, pull the suture toward the knot while at the same time pulling away with the right hand. The knot will disappear into the suture tract handily (Figure 10.96). Do not pull the knot into the resection bed or into the disk. If it goes in too far, ease it in the other direction. It should lie just below the corneal surface on the scleral (limbal) side of the incision (Figure 10.97). Equalize the suture limbs if necessary.

Perform a sub-conjunctival injection of Garamycin and Decadron/Depomedrol. Apply an antibiotic/steroid drop (TobraDex) as well as a cycloplegic/mydriatic (such as 1% Cyclogyl) and a drop of anhydrous glycerine. Patch the eye with two cotton patches, a Fox eye shield and paper or other hypoallergenic tape.

Complications and problems encountered during this surgery will be covered in Chapter 15, under the section on intra-operative complications.

Post-operative care

The patch is worn overnight and it is recommended that it be replaced nightly (along with a shield) until

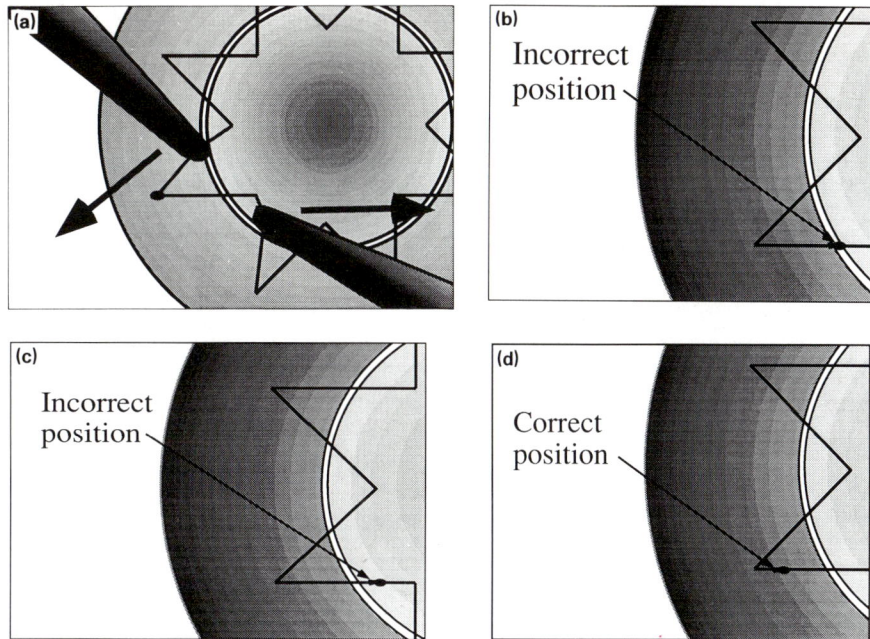

Fig. 10.96 Pull the knot below the surface. The knot must be buried to reduce patient discomfort and allow a smooth surface for re-epithelialization. Do this by pulling gently on the suture in the direction shown (a). The knot should disappear beneath the surface without difficulty. Do not neglect this step. (b) Often the knot is pulled in too far. Do not let it stay in the gap. Letting it stay in there provides a path for the epithelium to infiltrate the interface. (c) The knot cannot lie in the disk either. Leaving the knot in the disk can promote the same event as well as tissue erosion, especially through the thinner keratomileusis-*in-situ* lenticule. Neither of these occurrences is a good thing and should be avoided. (d) The correct position of the knot is just below the surface of the limbal cornea.

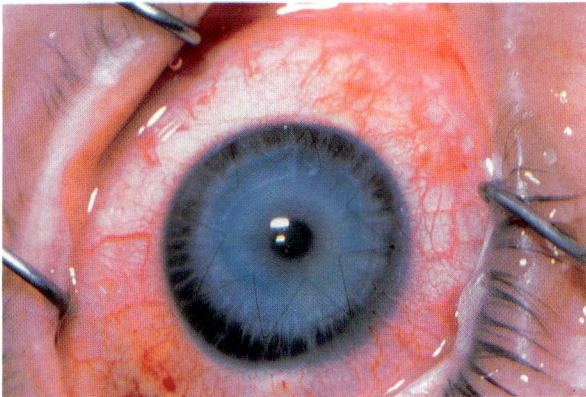

Fig. 10.97 The sutured lenticule. The suture limbs should indent the surface slightly but there should be no wrinkles in the tissue.

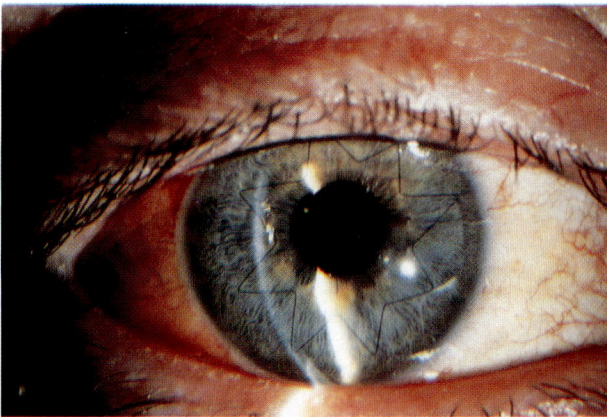

Fig. 10.98 MKM—48 hours post-surgery.

the sutures are removed. The patient is placed on FML and MURO-128 drops, three or four times daily until the sutures are removed—usually in 2 weeks.

Epithelialization will normally be complete within the next few days because freeze damage of the tissue has occurred (Figure 10.98). Except for the residual edema and sub-conjunctival hemorrhage from the fixation ring, the eyes will be essentially non-reactive. In fact most of the post-operative discomfort will come from the sub-conjunctival hemorrhage rather than the resection. The use of cycloplegics or strong analgesics for comfort is rarely necessary. When vision in the operated eye has returned to 20/40 or better, surgery on the fellow eye can be done. This could take several months (see section on results of lamellar refractive surgery, below).

The sutures are left in for 2 weeks (14 days). They can be easily removed at the slit-lamp with topical anesthesia. A 15° razor knife is used for this and is prepared by making a small right-angled bend in the tip as shown below. This small hook is used to pull up the exposed suture limb and then by turning the blade 90°, the suture is cut. The running suture is cut in the middle of a limb in at least four places (Figure 10.99). The loose ends are then grasped with smooth fine-tipped forceps (Kelman-McPherson, Katena K5-5030) and the suture pulled out *from the limbal side*. Do not pull toward the lenticule; it is very easy to pull it off the cornea at this stage. Patching after suture removal is not usually necessary but a drop of antibiotic/steroid is advised. Some patients will do much better if they are given artificial tear drops (Tears Natural II) to use for the next few weeks, as needed.

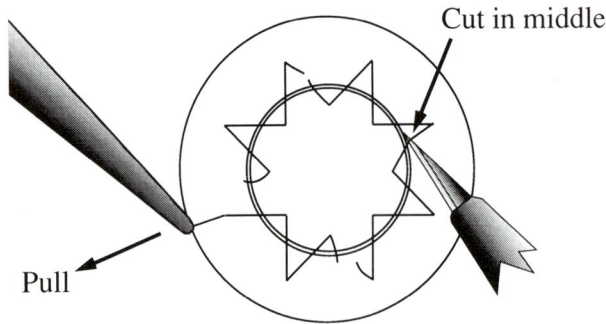

Fig. 10.99 Removing sutures. Cut the exposed limbs in at least four places using a razor knife. Lift up the severed limbs and pull the suture toward the limbus.

Variation in technique for homoplastic keratomileusis

In homoplastic keratomileusis, several points must be stressed to insure success. First of all, it is important to cut the donor lenticule first. There are several reasons for this, not the least of which is possible damage to the donor lenticule. The resection has to be as thick as possible—as much as 450–480 μm—not especially easy to accomplish. Some cheat by removing the plate from the keratome—a technique not to be recommended. Secondly, the disk has to be at least 0.3–0.5 mm smaller in diameter than the recipient bed to minimize the possibility of epithelial ingrowth. Epithelialization is typically slower than in autoplastic cases as well, which increases the chance for this complication—a situation which is compounded if the donor tissue tends to over-hang the recipient bed. Donor tissue varies in its response to the keratectomy, chiefly due to variations in water content. Preserved corneal buttons, especially those in Optisol, are less prone to variation, however. A typical disk for homoplastic keratomileusis should be cut to 7.0 mm for an original 7.2 mm resection. However, it may come off at 6.8 or 7.2 mm. It will be easier to resect the recipient disk to the required larger diameter, 7.2–7.5 mm, respectively, thus the surgeon has a better chance at getting it right.

Time on the lathe will be longer with homoplastic and hyperopic cases. During the lathing, the thick donor disk must be converted to a thinner, parallel-sided disk. Thus the displacement is set several times: twice in myopia cases—once for the thinning, and once for the optical carving—and three times for hyperopia. Figures 10.100 through 10.102 show post-operative keratomileusis cases.

Non-freeze lamellar techniques

Both theoretic and experiential considerations have triggered attempts to simplify the original Barraquer procedure and possibly eliminate the necessity for

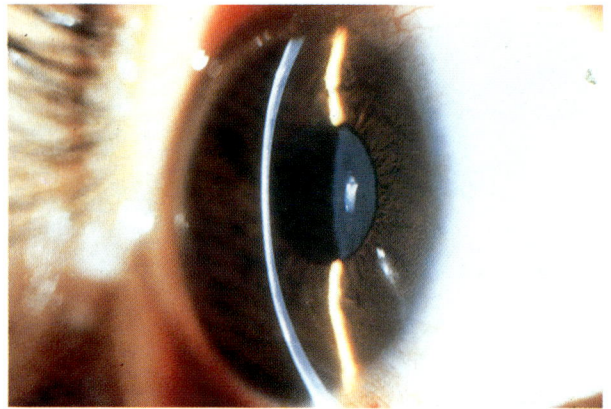

Fig. 10.100 Myopic keratomileusis. The Ec in this case was less than optimal. The correction was excellent but the transparency is poor—the patient will need a homoplastic procedure.

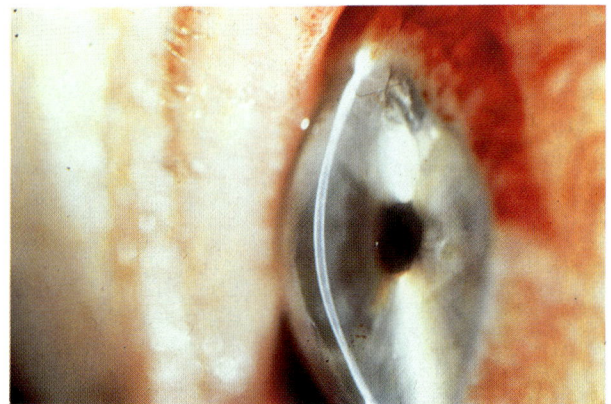

Fig. 10.101 Typical appearance of hyperopic keratomileusis.

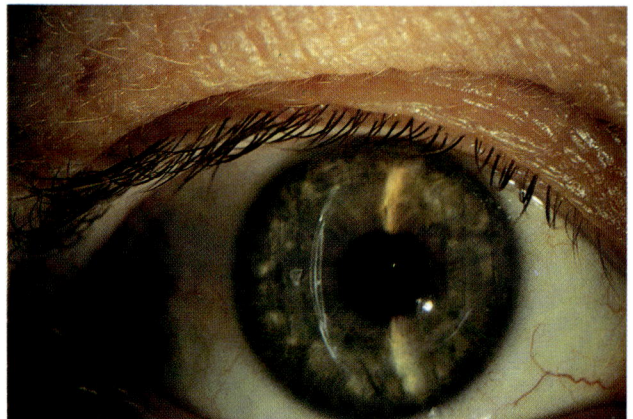

Fig. 10.102 Lathed MKM over an under-corrected radial keratotomy.

freezing the tissue. While the process of freezing enables a precise shaping of the resected disk, it none the less results in the death of the keratocytes and considerable edematous reaction. Both of these factors

(a)

(b)

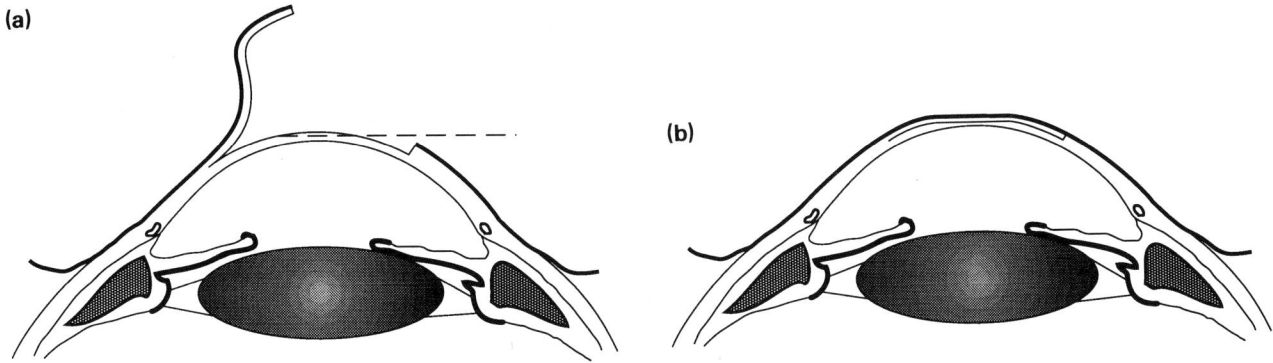

Fig. 10.103 (a and b) Barraquer's stromal resection. After dissecting the corneal cap, the keratome is used to remove the central disk.

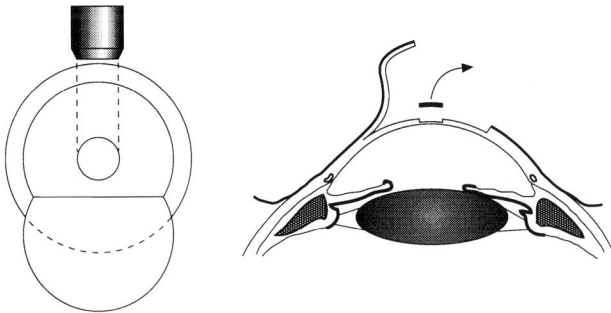

Fig. 10.104 Pureskin's modification of Krwawicz's central stromectomy.

concluded that freeze-lathing offered the best combination of accuracy and predictability.

Krwawicz followed Barraquer's work with his stromectomy cases in 1964 though he had attempted to modify the corneal curvature through other methods previously [4–6]. Pureskin modified Krwawicz's technique by using a trephine to demarcate the resection (Figure 10.104) [7]. Elstein and co-workers reported their work on rabbits in 1969 [8]. In 1985 Hoffmann and Jessen devised a method of stromectomy utilizing double suction rings and curvature templates called keratokyphosis (Figure 10.105) [9]. None of these latter techniques successfully answered the challenge presented by classic keratomileusis, however.

Barraquer–Krumeich–Swinger (BKS) technique

In 1977, Swinger and colleagues developed a simplified method of corneal re-shaping by resecting a section of cornea and then by inverting the resected tissue over a suction die, cutting away a central portion of the disk to flatten its center (Figures 10.106 through 10.109) [10]. This procedure had the advantage of not requiring freezing of the tissue but introduced a few problems of its own.

The first problem was that those who attempted the

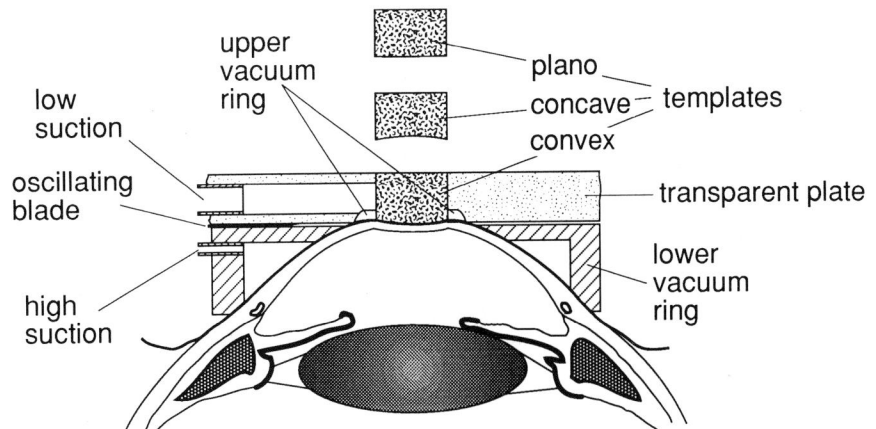

contribute to a prolonged post-operative recovery period and to certain of the complications seen, such as delayed epithelialization and ingrowth (see Chapter 4).

It is not surprising that Barraquer himself conducted the first experiments with non-freeze techniques. His most promising results came from his work with making an additional pass over the eye to remove a second thin section approximately 6.0 mm in diameter after partially removing the first resection (Figure 10.103) [3]. His attempts to affect the reduction of myopia by varying the thickness of the secondary section were not wholly successful, and he eventually

Fig. 10.105 Hoffmann and Jessen's keratokyphosis.

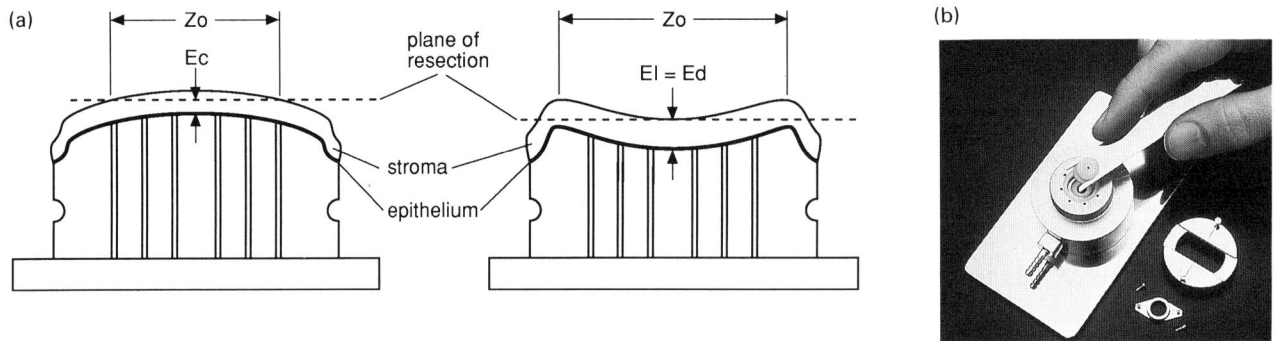

Fig. 10.106 Principle of the non-freeze, BKS technique. (a) Plastic vacuum fixation plates in varying curvatures are employed with the BKS unit. (b) A convex plate is used for myopia and a concave plate for hyperopia.

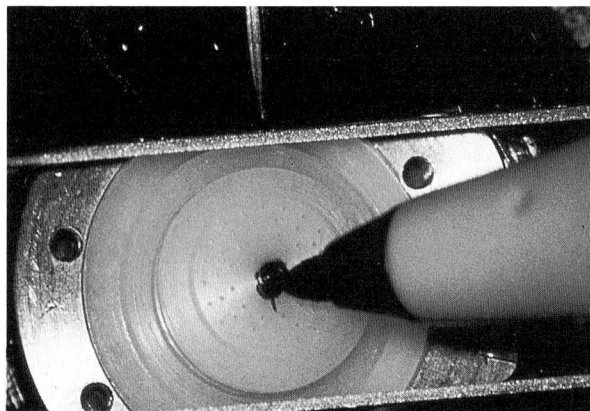

Fig. 10.107 A gentian violet pen is used to mark the center of the fixation plate.

operation were misled into believing that this method somehow simplified the procedure. This is because many thought that the lathing of the tissue was the toughest part of the operation, whereas, in reality, it is the keratectomy itself (the most difficult part of the operation to perform well) that is crucial to success in lamellar surgery. In addition, the technique specified a primary resection whose diameter was 9.0 mm—a size difficult to cut smoothly, especially of the thickness required—300–350 μm. This tissue disk had next to be draped, upside down, over one of several perforated suction dies of differing curvature, precisely centered and then secured with a serrated clamping ring which inevitably crushed the outermost portion of the disk. Vacuum was produced by a syringe which evacuated the chamber beneath the disk and a stopcock which, hopefully, held that vacuum until the case was complete. Thickness of the portion to be resected was controlled by either utilizing a plate similar to the original Barraquer microkeratome or by means of an adjustable guide ring (in later models). Resection diameter was controlled by die curvature which, by being fixed, was essentially a compromise.

While early success was reported in the laboratory, such success did not follow in the clinical studies [10,11]. Irregular astigmatism occurred in many cases, probably due to imperfect disk centering but also undoubtedly due to poor fixation which allowed the resected disk to move during the second cut. Another factor is the character of the corneal tissue itself. Bereft of the support of Bowman's layer (which it is when

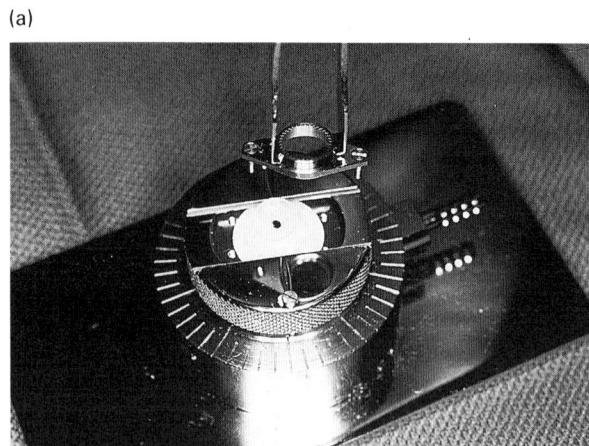

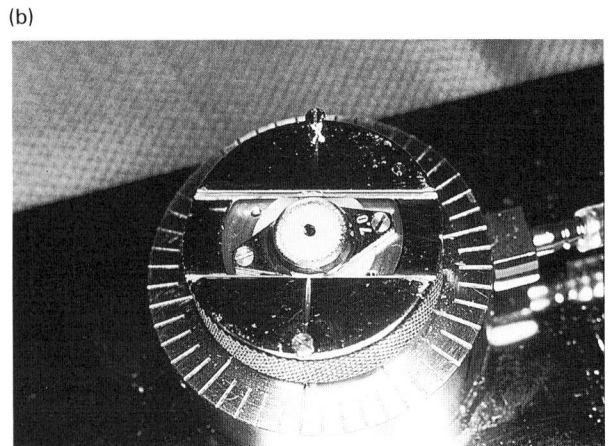

Fig. 10.108 The resected disk is centered over the fixation plate—epithelial side down (a) and clamped with the retainer plate (b).

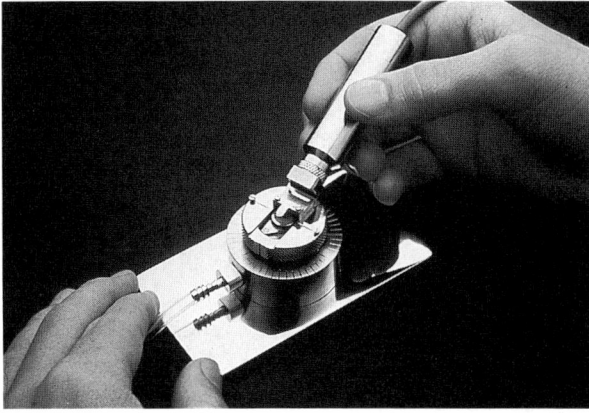

Fig. 10.109 A vacuum is drawn on the tissue via the side port. The guide ring is then adjusted by screwing it up or down, as with the Barraquer artificial anterior chamber. The keratectomy proceeds as usual.

inverted), the stroma takes on the consistency of jelly and tends to flow when pushed—as by the edge of a blade. This shearing of the surface introduces irregularity and elongation of the resection. Thus, what is supposed to be a circular resection actually turns out to be somewhat elliptic in shape. When such a section is laid against the cornea it tends to match the curvature of the recipient bed. Since the major and minor meridians of the resection have different chord lengths, astigmatism results, often of the irregular variety. Further, predictability was something to aspire to but was not realized sufficiently in clinical practice. Despite some suggestions and attempts to fabricate epikeratophakia lenticules by this method, few, if any, clinical cases are being performed in this country currently [12].

Hyperopic lamellar keratotomy

In classical myopic keratomileusis, one of the causes for loss of effect with the surgery is deep keratome sections. If the posterior corneal layers are thinner than 20% of the central corneal thickness, late, low-order corneal ectasia will occur producing a steepening of the central corneal curvature and an increase in the myopia. While reviewing cases of late loss of effect in MKM, Ruiz noted that the amount of ectasia or central steepening seemed to be related to the size of the disk removed by the keratome [13]. He experimented with rabbits and found that by making a section 80% of the central corneal thickness and varying the size of the disk removed, he could produce steepening of the cornea proportional to the disk size. No manipulation of the tissue other than the initial section was necessary. By simply replacing the tissue disk upon the eye and securing it with a running, anti-torque suture, up to 8.5 D of corneal steepening could be obtained. He applied this technique to human corneas

in December 1984. In early 1985, Bores was the first to perform this procedure in the USA [14]. These first cases were in radial keratotomy hyper-corrections; later, cases with "pure" hyperopia were operated.

The procedure, called a keratotomy because while tissue is removed it is immediately replaced, is relatively straightforward in its execution. The microkeratome head is fitted with a plate (or the plate adjusted with the setting screw) to obtain a resection thickness of 70% of the central ultrasonic pachymetry. The actual procedure is difficult to perform and requires great skill with the microkeratome—something only obtained through extensive practice and experience—but it can be learned. In retrospect, hyperopic lamellar keratotomy is somewhat more difficult to perform than keratomileusis-*in-situ* because the diameter and tissue thickness are critical to success (Figure 10.110). Stabilization can be assisted by the application of 5% saline drops three times daily for up to 3 weeks to reduce tissue edema.

Disk diameter and thickness are extremely important in this surgery. Sometimes the exact plate cannot be found (in fixed-plate keratomes) which matches the disk thickness needed and the closest size must be made to serve. Because of this limitation, the author had made a microkeratome head which could be adjusted continuously so as to provide a closer approximation of the resection depth required. This head is driven by a gas turbine motor which provides higher rpm and greater torque than the earlier models (see section on SCMD microkeratome head, above). This combination results in much smoother resections than before but inevitably compromises had to be made in the design.

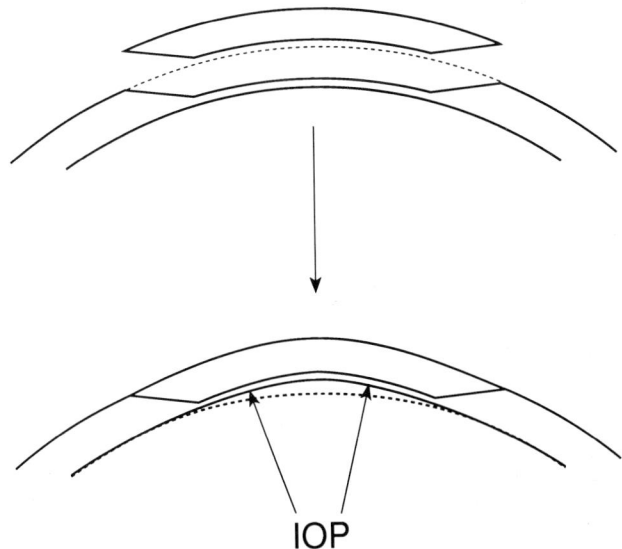

Fig. 10.110 Hyperopic lamellar keratotomy. This surgery works by allowing a controlled ectasis of the cornea to occur, therefore both disk thickness and diameter are critical. Only one section (deep) is made in this surgery.

Centration of the resection

Centration is accomplished as in classic keratomileusis (see above). Make sure that the reference scribe mark is tangential to the pupil or a 4.0 mm optical zone mark—not radial.

Plate setting

In hyperopic lamellar keratotomy, only one pass of the microkeratome across the cornea is required. Typically the section is made to 70% of the central corneal thickness, as measured by ultrasonic pachymetry. If necessary, refer to the section on pachymetry in Chapter 5. The disk thickness is determined by the following guidelines:

1 If the central corneal thickness is ≤0.52 mm, set the plate so as to obtain a section no thicker than 360 μm or 70% of the pachymetry.
2 If the corneal thickness is 0.53–0.60 mm, set the plate so as to obtain a section of 360–420 μm or 70% of the pachymetry.
3 If the thickness is >0.60 mm, set the plate so as to obtain a section of no greater than 450 μm.

For example, a patient has a central corneal thickness of 0.522 mm (522 μm). Set the plate so as to obtain a section of 360 μm. Typically, the sections taken with the SCMD adjustable keratome are some 60–80 μm thicker than the plate setting, but this will vary with the individual machine. Thus, in the example above, the actual plate setting would be 360 less 60–80 μm (i.e. 260–300 μm) depending on the characteristics of the particular head.

Disk thickness − keratome bias = plate setting

It follows, therefore, that each head must be calibrated individually. This can be done by making several sections at various settings, preferably using cadaver eyes. In doing so, be advised that the sections taken from these eyes will typically be 20 μm thicker than those from a living eye. If, then, a particular keratome is consistently cutting 70 μm more than the actual setting, the plate would be adjusted to 310 μm (70 − 20 = 50 μm). After sectioning the disk should measure 360 μm, which is the thickness desired.

In over-corrected radial keratotomy patients, the plate setting should be 10% less than that for an unoperated cornea. It has been found that radial keratotomy corneas pull up into the ring somewhat higher than do uncut corneas. This may be due to these corneas being somewhat more malleable than unincised corneas. In the example case, a disk thickness of 330 μm should be made. This would mean an actual plate setting of 280 μm using the head described.

In no instance should the section be less than

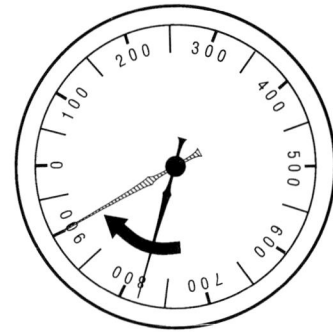

Fig. 10.111 Adjust the plate to the desired tissue thickness. Always adjust the setting so that the plate moves from thicker to thinner (i.e. open to closed), never vice versa. This prevents possible problems from the plate getting hung up. Note that the gauge is read in reverse. That is, 900 μm is really 100 μm, etc.

0.30 mm (300 μm). A cornea requiring a 250 μm section would have a central thickness of 380–400 μm, which is approaching that seen in keratoconus. Lamellar sections should probably not be done in cases of keratoconus except for the purpose of re-inforcing the cornea, in which case a wet epikeratophakia lenticule would be a better choice.

Because of the variability in resection thicknesses required, a fixed-plate keratome is not ideal for performing this surgery. The SCMD adjustable-plate microkeratome was designed especially for this surgery and is recommended, as is the Steinway automatic corneal shaper.

Plate setting with the SCMD unit

The operation of setting this keratome has been outlined in a previous section. Some points need emphasis, however. Most importantly, the plate setting must be done with the anvil as close as possible to the blade without touching it. While steadying the keratome with one hand, turn the plate adjustment screw until the indicator stops at the desired setting (Figure 10.111). Remember that this setting is the desired tissue thickness less the keratome overage or bias. To avoid confusion and possible error, the gauge can be set to account for the bias of a particular microkeratome. To do this, set the zero point as usual then, while the anvil is still resting on the blade, rotate the dial face clockwise until the needle indicates the amount of bias in the system. This is your new zero point—lock the gauge ring. Now when the plate is set at 100 μm, you will get 100 μm (Figure 10.112).

Remove your hands from the head and gauge ring for the final reading. Typically the indicator will have moved and now show another reading. In that case, make the corresponding adjustment to the plate until the desired setting is indicated when the microkeratome is hanging free.

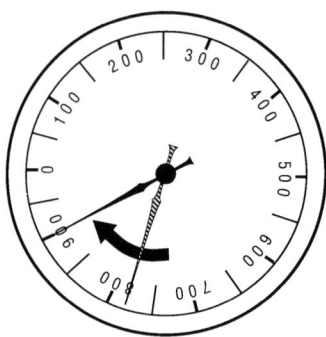

Fig. 10.112 Plate set to 100 μm disk thickness. Keep in mind that while the gauge setting indicates a plate setting of 100 μm, the resultant tissue disk is likely to measure somewhere around 170 μm. This is because the microkeratome typically cuts a thicker section than that set. The exact amount of overage (bias) that will occur is dependent on the specific instrument, requiring each one to be calibrated individually, but is usually on the order of 60–80 μm.

Now raise the anvil again and re-check the zero setting. If the zero point has shifted, be certain that the anvil is correctly positioned before re-setting the gauge. If anything has been changed, it will be necessary to re-set the plate. Once the setting is satisfactory, remove the head from the setting ring and apply a tiny amount of lubricant to the motor shaft and re-attach the keratome head to the turbine handle, making sure that it is screwed all the way in and is finger-tight.

Resection diameter

The diameter of the resection necessary is selected from Table 10.2 or from the computer program and the proper fixation ring selected. It will be necessary to try a few rings before the correct one is found. Since the sections in hyperopic lamellar keratotomy are much smaller in diameter than those for keratomileusis, it is suggested that a good size to begin with would be a #10—two steps higher than usually required. Always

Table 10.2 Nomogram for HLK

Hyperoia (D)	Diameter of disk (mm)
1.5	6.5
2.0	6.4
2.5	6.3
3.0	6.2
3.5	6.1
4.0	6.0
4.5	5.8
5.0	5.6
5.5	5.4
6.0	5.2
6.5	5.0
7.0	4.8
7.5	4.6

check the intra-ocular pressure with the tonometer before determining the resection diameter, at least for the first application of the ring. Remember also to dry the cornea with a microsponge before making any measurements.

Remember that the actual diameter of the resected disk will be about 0.2 mm *larger* than that applanated. If the table calls for a 6.2 mm disk, choose a ring that will produce an applanated area of 6.0 mm. It may not be possible to obtain an applanation that precise each time, however. You are advised, in that case, to cut a disk slightly *smaller* than required. For example, it is found that although the case calls for a resection diameter of 5.6 mm, one ring applanates to 5.8–6.0 mm and the next size up applanates to 5.2 mm. Choose the ring that produces the 5.2 applanation. It is better for the patient to end up slightly myopic than to remain hyperopic. There are sufficient applanators within the usual instrument set to be able to determine the exact size a ring applanates, so take the time to check. It doesn't take much time to be sure.

Making the section

Always check to see that the microkeratome moves freely in the ring before attempting to resect a disk. Put a drop or two of saline on the corneal surface and on the microkeratome head before starting. Don't, however, flood the eye. If the cornea is too wet, some unevenness of the section will result.

Make the section as described in the section on keratomileusis, above, and check the thickness with the tissue gauge. Put the resected disk into the moist chamber and clean up the resection bed. Remove the tissue from the chamber using the Barraquer lenticule spatula or a fine-toothed (0.12 mm) Colibri forceps. The tissue can be floated, epithelial side down, on to the spatula using a drop of BSS. Be very gentle with the tissue at this point. While it is less fragile than a lathe-cut lenticule, it can still be torn.

Rotate the tissue until its reference mark comes into alignment with the corneal mark. It should line up exactly. If it doesn't and seems to join the corneal mark at an angle, you have placed the tissue on to the eye upside down. This is a very rare occurrence with hyperopic lamellar keratotomy because of the disk thickness but can happen if you have not been paying attention. It can be especially troublesome to align the tissue in some radial keratotomy cases because of the radial corneal scars. That's why the tangential type of mark is recommended. It is difficult to confuse it with the radial keratotomy scars. If this is a problem with such cases, it may help to outline the reference mark by dabbing it with the skin-marking pencil, thus making the mark more prominent.

Suturing of the resected tissue back on to the cornea

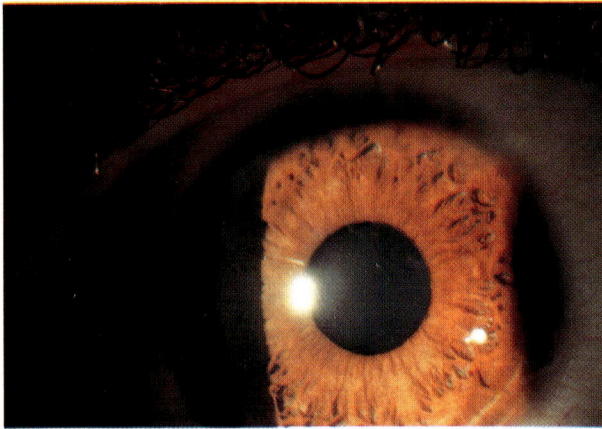

Fig. 10.113 Appearance of hyperopic lamellar keratotomy eye 6 months post-surgery.

is the same as in keratomileusis and is covered in the section on suturing the corneal disk, above. Figure 10.113 shows a post-operative hyperopic lamellar keratotomy case.

This technique is especially applicable to cases of radial keratotomy that have resulted in induced hyperopia. In these cases, resection of the corneal disk should not be attempted before 6, or preferably 8, months post radial keratotomy. At this time the cornea should be sufficiently stabilized and the incisions strong enough to allow a smooth resection. Sutures must be carefully placed so as not to open the incisions. Despite such care and the nature of the suturing pattern, which assists in preventing such occurrences, opening or fraying will occur at the extreme edges of the tissue disk in some cases. Such fraying has not produced unusual healing, nor has induced astigmatism been a hallmark in the cases of the author's experience (Figure 10.114).

Keratomileusis-*in-situ*

The first human cases of keratomileusis-*in-situ* were performed in Bogota, Colombia in May 1987. The anterior lamellar sections were secured, as in MKM, by the classic, running eight-point anti-torque suture. Epithelialization was generally complete within 24 hours. Useful vision was restored within days rather than the months usually seen in freeze-lathed cases. Encouraged by the results in these patients, Bores performed the first US cases of keratomileusis-*in-situ* in November 1987 on patients whose fellow eye had received classic, freeze-lathe surgery. All patients reported a more comfortable post-operative course and all remarked upon the rapidity of onset of clear vision. The results, however, were not identical to those initially reported by Ruiz (L.A. Ruiz, 1989, personal communication). The incidence of induced post-operative astigmatism was somewhat higher than that seen in classic MKM, for example, especially irregular astigmatism (see section on results, below).

Keratomileusis-*in-situ* differs from classic keratomileusis in that the corneal curvature change is made by the microkeratome and not the lathe. In order for this to work, two passes of the microkeratome must be made (Figure 10.115). This latter requirement is easier to accomplish than one might expect—it depends, really, upon the correct placement of the first ring. If the first ring is properly centered before suction is applied and the eye held until the ring is firmly seated, a saddle-shaped impression is made in the limbal sclera which makes placement of the ring for the second pass a snap.

Since both the thickness and the diameter of the first and second resections are different, two different rings and applanators must be used. An adjustable plate

(a)

(b)

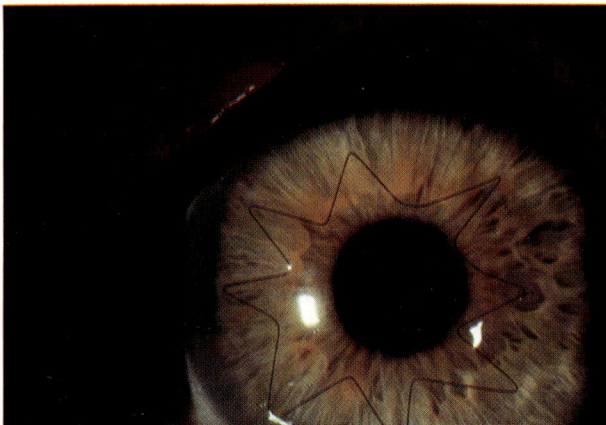

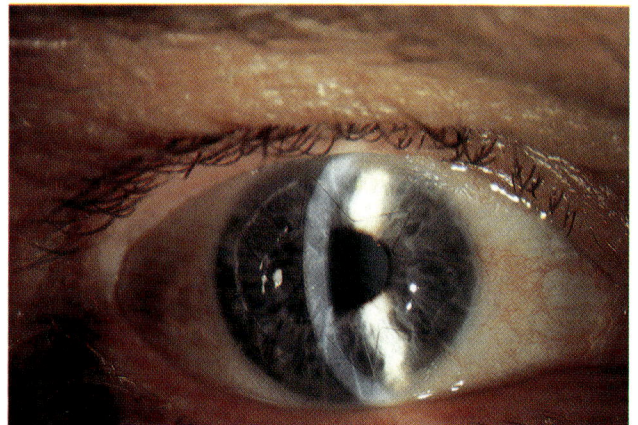

Fig. 10.114 Hyperopic lamellar keratotomy in over-corrected radial keratotomy. (a) 36 hours post-surgery in a four-incision case; (b) 7 days post-surgery. Note the smoothness of the surface.

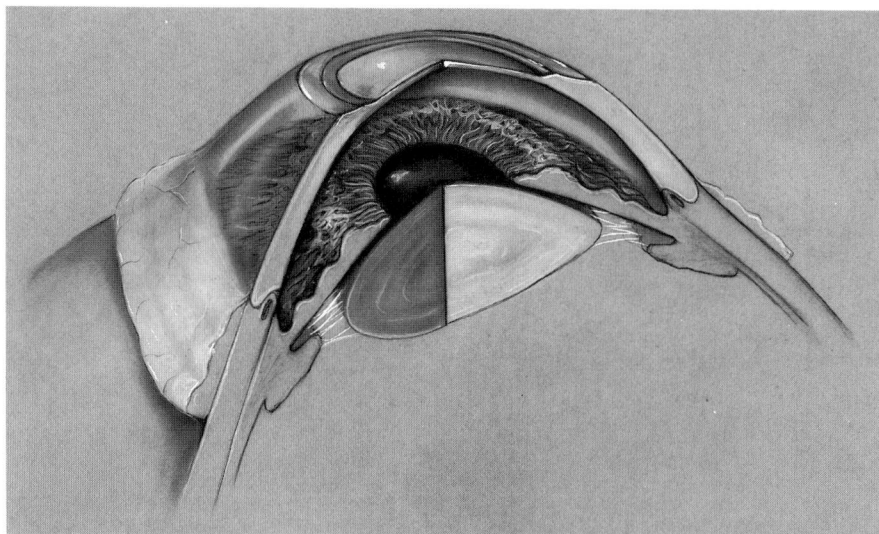

Fig. 10.115 Keratomileusis-*in-situ*. Note that two keratectomies are required.

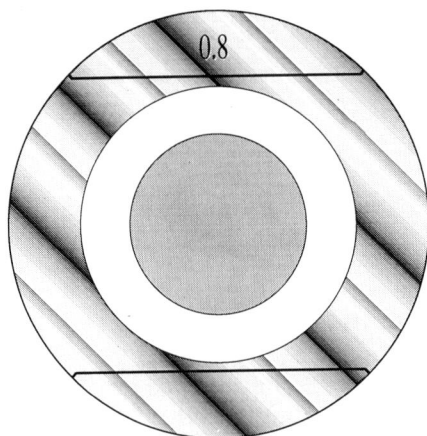

Fig. 10.116 First pass in keratomileusis-*in-situ*. The first section should be well-centered. This is the go–no go point. If this section is not well-centered, neither will the second one be. It would be better to suture the disk back on and try again after 4–6 months have elapsed in such an event. The resultant disk is very thin and fragile (110–140 µm), so handle it with great care.

keratome was designed for this surgery (see section on SCMD microkeratome head, above).

The first pass removes the corneal "cap" (Figure 10.116). This section is typically 0.13–0.15 mm (130–150 µm) in thickness and 7.25 mm in diameter. This disk is much thinner than those encountered in classic keratomileusis and requires special handling. The second pass removes a smaller diameter disk which can range from 0.05 to 0.15 mm (50–150 µm) in thickness and 3.5–5.0 mm in diameter.

Set the SCMD microkeratome plate as outlined under hyperopic lamellar keratotomy (or choose a fixed plate whose thickness accomplishes the same thing) so as to obtain a disk whose thickness will range from 130 to 150 µm. Assemble the head and handpiece and test the motor by depressing the foot pedal. Check the gas gauge on the SCMD unit to insure that the setting has not been changed. Set the entire handpiece assembly aside for the present.

Centration of the resection

Two passes means two different rings. The difficulty, at least theoretically, is marking the second pass exactly centered upon the first. This problem is more theoretic than actual—it all depends upon the centration of the first ring. In practice, this is easier to accomplish than you might expect, although care must be taken. Remember, it is not possible precisely to align the tissue on the lathe either. To insure exact centration, a special bullseye marker has been designed. This marker is described in more detail above (see section on instrumentation for keratomileusis, above). In kerotomileusis-*in-situ* it will be found that pre-marking the optic axis, as explained in the beginning of this chapter, will facilitate accurate centration. It is possible to accomplish this by using the constricted pupil as a guide, but doing it the first way takes very little extra time and is more accurate.

At first, it may be helpful to coat the marker with 1% tincture of brilliant green applied with a cotton bud (an alternative is to use a fresh gentian violet skin-marking pen: Katena K20–4500). This will produce a bright green, semi-indelible mark upon the corneal surface (Figure 10.117). If this is done, make sure that the alcohol has completely dried upon the marker before applying it to the cornea, or else the epithelium will be damaged and strip off. Do not place the mark, however, until the patient has been anesthetized or received the block, and only after a ring has been applied to the eye and the clearance checked.

Once the cornea has been marked, go about the business of choosing the proper fixation ring as usual, making sure that the aperture is concentrically aligned

(a)

(b)

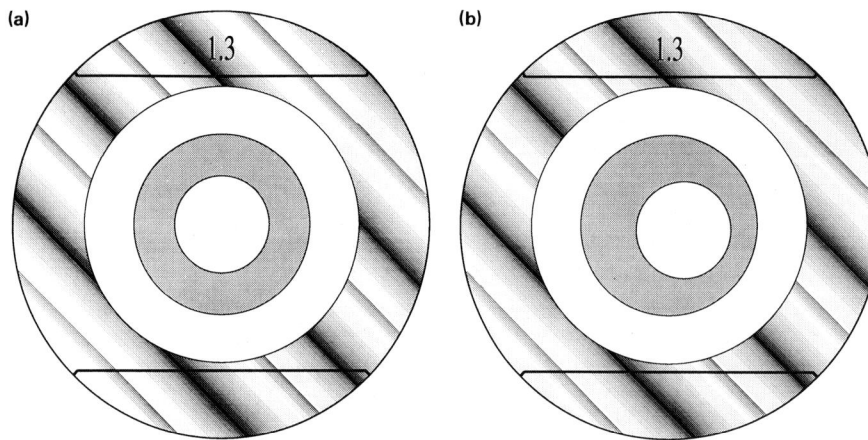

Fig. 10.117 (a) Properly centered second section. If the first section is well-centered, then, like the illustration, the second section should be likewise. (b) Off-centered second section. This should not happen but can if the surgeon does not pay attention to how the second ring is placed on the eye. The first ring makes an indentation on the eye into which the second ring should just about fall. You really have to work at it for the second ring to be out of position.

with the bullseye before applying suction. Use a ring of such a size as to produce a resection 7.25 mm in diameter (typically a #8 or 9). Position the ring, making certain that it is centered in reference to the pre-marked bullseye. Remember, the left hand fixates the right eye and vice versa. Once the proper ring has been selected and the disk size checked with the applanator, the keratectomy can be performed.

Transfer the tissue to the sterile gauge and measure the thickness of the first resection. Make sure to zero the instrument before use. *Do not tap on the knob!* The range of acceptable thickness of this first section is 0.10–0.15 mm (100–150 μm). The ideal section should measure 0.12–0.14 mm (120–140 μm). It may be necessary to wet the disk to remove it from the caliper—don't force it! Place the tissue, epithelial side down, into the moist chamber and replace the lid. Enter the thickness into the computer or otherwise record it. The computer program will tell you both the diameter and the thickness necessary for the second section or you can look it up on the supplied nomogram.

Select the correct applanator lens for the second section by choosing the diameter suggested by the computer or nomogram. The range of diameters for the second section will be from 3.5 to 5.0 mm. The most appropriate size will range from 4.0 to 4.7 mm (for myopia ≤5.50 D, use 4.7 mm; for myopia >5.50 D, use 3.7–4.2 mm). Once the resection diameter has been selected, the computer or nomogram will tell you what plate setting to select to obtain the proper thickness. Read the plate setting out loud so that your assistant can check you. He or she should repeat back the setting after looking at the computer screen or nomogram and tell you if there is a discrepancy.

SCMD adjustable head

Unscrew the head and place it into the gauging ring. Re-check the zero setting and make any appropriate adjustments. Next adjust the plate so as to produce a section of appropriate thickness. These second sections typically range from 60 to 90 μm in thickness. Re-assemble the head and handle. Adding additional lubricant is usually not required and should be avoided.

Second pass

Next select the second ring by consulting Table 10.3. Since the diameter of this section is smaller than the first, a higher-number ring must be used. Try a ring which is five sizes larger than the primary ring number, which in this example means a #13 (the first ring was a #8). Fit it carefully in place using the bullseye as a guide. Apply the vacuum but this time do not check the intra-ocular pressure. Check with the applanator for correct diameter (using the inner, smaller, reticle). Change rings as needed to obtain the desired diameter, although if you've chosen one as suggested this will usually not be necessary. Make sure that the cornea is dry before measuring.

Move the keratome a little slower than for the first section. The disk to be removed is smaller and thinner and resistance is less. There is a tendency to cut much faster than the primary section. This inevitably causes the second section to be much thinner than desired and is a major cause for under-correction. Remove the resected tissue from the microkeratome and place it on the applanator. Check the diameter. Next place the tissue into the gauge. This tissue section is extremely thin and very difficult to manage. Often the tissue will be frayed or splintered, in which case measurement is impossible. This seems to be more frequent with the slower, electrically powered heads, however. A drop of water on the tissue gauge anvil will facilitate flattening of the tissue. Remove excess fluid by touching the edge of the drop with a microsponge. Make sure that the tissue is absolutely flat and not folded or wrinkled. Let the upper anvil down gently and take a reading. *Do not tap on the knob!* Call out the reading and

Table 10.3 Ruiz KMIS nomogram

Myopia spherical equivalent (D)	Optical zone size							
	3.5	3.7	4.0	4.2	4.5	4.7	5.0	5.2
2.5	0.016	0.017	0.021	0.023	0.026	0.029	0.033	0.036
3.0	0.018	0.021	0.024	0.027	0.031	0.034	0.039	0.043
3.5	0.021	0.024	0.028	0.031	0.036	0.040	0.045	0.049
4.0	0.024	0.027	0.032	0.035	0.041	0.045	0.051	0.056
4.5	0.027	0.030	0.036	0.040	0.046	0.050	0.057	0.062
5.0	0.030	0.033	0.039	0.043	0.050	0.055	0.063	0.069
5.5	0.032	0.036	0.043	0.047	0.055	0.060	0.069	0.075
6.0	0.035	0.039	0.046	0.051	0.059	0.065	0.074	0.081
6.5	0.038	0.042	0.050	0.055	0.064	0.070	0.080	0.087
7.0	0.040	0.045	0.053	0.059	0.068	0.075	0.085	0.093
7.5	0.043	0.048	0.057	0.063	0.072	0.079	0.091	0.099
8.0	0.045	0.051	0.060	0.066	0.077	0.084	0.096	0.104
8.5	0.048	0.053	0.062	0.069	0.080	0.088	0.101	0.109
9.0	0.050	0.056	0.066	0.073	0.085	0.093	0.106	0.115
9.5	0.052	0.059	0.069	0.077	0.088	0.097	0.111	0.120
10.0	0.055	0.062	0.072	0.080	0.092	0.102	0.116	0.126
10.5	0.057	0.064	0.075	0.083	0.096	0.106	0.120	0.131
11.0	0.059	0.067	0.078	0.087	0.100	0.110	0.125	0.136
11.5	0.062	0.069	0.081	0.090	0.104	0.114	0.130	0.141
12.0	0.064	0.072	0.084	0.093	0.108	0.118	0.135	0.146
12.5	0.066	0.074	0.087	0.096	0.111	0.122	0.139	0.151
13.0	0.068	0.077	0.090	0.100	0.115	0.126	0.144	0.156
13.5	0.070	0.079	0.093	0.102	0.118	0.130	0.148	0.161
14.0	0.072	0.081	0.095	0.106	0.122	0.134	0.152	—
14.5	0.074	0.083	0.098	0.108	0.125	0.137	0.156	—
15.0	0.077	0.087	0.101	0.112	0.129	0.141	0.161	—
15.5	0.078	0.088	0.103	0.114	0.132	0.145	—	—
16.0	0.080	0.090	0.106	0.117	0.135	0.148	—	—
16.5	0.082	0.092	0.108	0.120	0.138	0.152	—	—
17.0	0.084	0.095	0.111	0.123	0.142	—	—	—
17.5	0.086	0.096	0.113	0.125	0.145	—	—	—
18.0	0.088	0.099	0.116	0.128	0.148	—	—	—
18.5	0.090	0.101	0.118	0.131	0.151	—	—	—
19.0	0.092	0.103	0.121	0.134	0.154	—	—	—
19.5	0.093	0.105	0.123	0.136	0.157	—	—	—
20.0	0.095	0.107	0.125	0.139	0.160	—	—	—
20.5	0.097	0.109	0.128	0.141	—	—	—	—
21.0	0.099	0.111	0.130	0.144	—	—	—	—
21.5	0.100	0.112	0.132	0.146	—	—	—	—
22.0	0.102	0.114	0.134	0.149	—	—	—	—
22.5	0.104	0.116	0.136	0.151	—	—	—	—
23.0	0.105	0.118	0.139	0.153	—	—	—	—
23.5	0.107	0.120	0.141	0.156	—	—	—	—
24.0	0.109	0.122	0.143	0.158	—	—	—	—
24.5	0.110	0.123	0.145	0.160	—	—	—	—
25.0	0.112	0.125	0.147	—	—	—	—	—
25.5	0.113	0.127	0.149	—	—	—	—	—
26.0	0.115	0.129	0.151	—	—	—	—	—
26.5	0.116	0.130	0.153	—	—	—	—	—
27.0	0.118	0.132	0.155	—	—	—	—	—
27.5	0.119	0.134	0.157	—	—	—	—	—
28.0	0.121	0.135	0.159	—	—	—	—	—
28.5	0.122	0.137	0.161	—	—	—	—	—
29.0	0.124	0.139	—	—	—	—	—	—
29.5	0.125	0.140	—	—	—	—	—	—
30.0	0.126	0.142	—	—	—	—	—	—
31.5	0.130	0.146	—	—	—	—	—	—
32.0	0.132	0.148	—	—	—	—	—	—

Plate setting in millimeters.

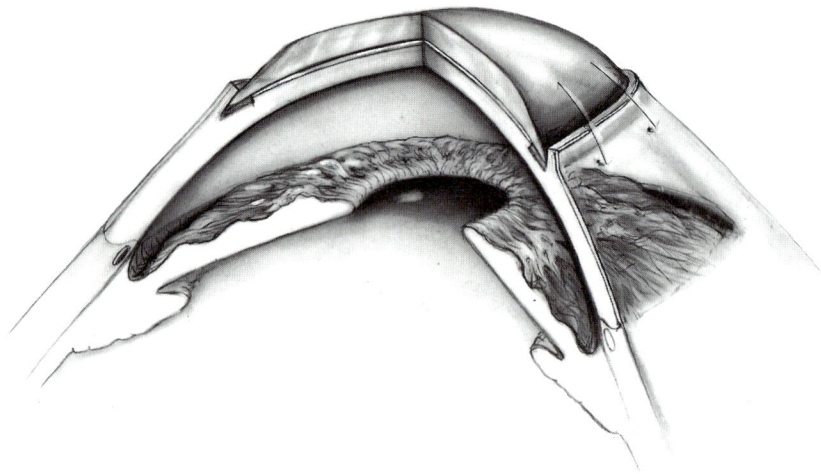

Fig. 10.118 Old-style epikeratophakia using an annular keratectomy and undermining. Note the wide gap required to be crossed by the epithelium.

enter it into the computer and the operative sheet. Did you make sure that the tissue gauge was still zeroed before-hand?

Post-operative care

A patch is worn overnight and it is recommended that it be replaced nightly (along with a shield) until the sutures are removed. The patient is placed on FML and MURO: 128 drops, three or four times daily until the sutures are removed—usually in 2 weeks.

Epithelialization will normally be complete by the next morning because freeze damage of the tissue has not occurred. Post-operative return of clear vision is much more rapid than in classic keratomileusis. Until vision in the operated eye has returned to 20/40 or better, however, it is best to delay surgery on the fellow eye. Suture removal follows in the same manner as for keratomileusis (see above).

Epikeratophakia

It seems a good idea that if keratomileusis works, why not suture the lenticule to the surface of the eye, producing thereby a "living" contact lens (Figure 10.118)? Why not indeed? Building on a concept first described by Ruiz, Werblin began experimenting with the concept of corneal tissue "appliqués" to correct ametropia [15–29]. This work was later expanded and refined by McDonald et al. [30]. The concept of attaching prelathed human tissue, which could be ordered up like a contact lens, to an eye to correct both near- and far-sightedness, was and is appealing (Figure 10.119) [31,32]. In a carefull constructed prospective study which underwent three or four changes in protocol during its life, considerable useful data emerged.

The technique found its first application in treating aphakia. While successful, considerable discrepancy between predicted and actual final refractive error was found. Epithelialization was prolonged and in some

(a)

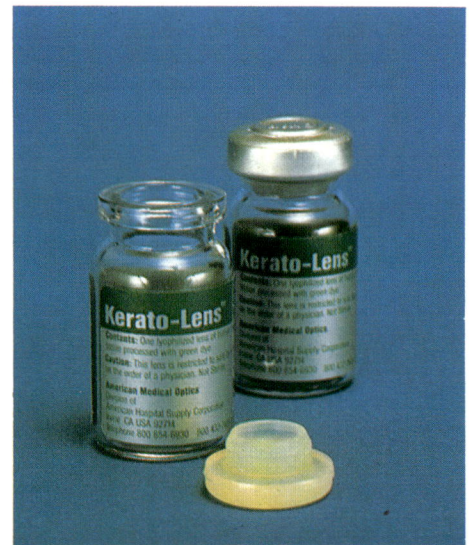

(b)

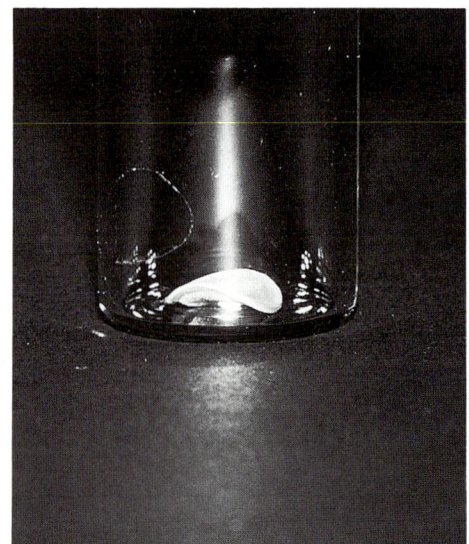

Fig. 10.119 (a and b) Kerato-Lens—lyophilized epi-lenticule (or "potato chip") as supplied by Alcon.

(a)

(b)

(c)

(d)

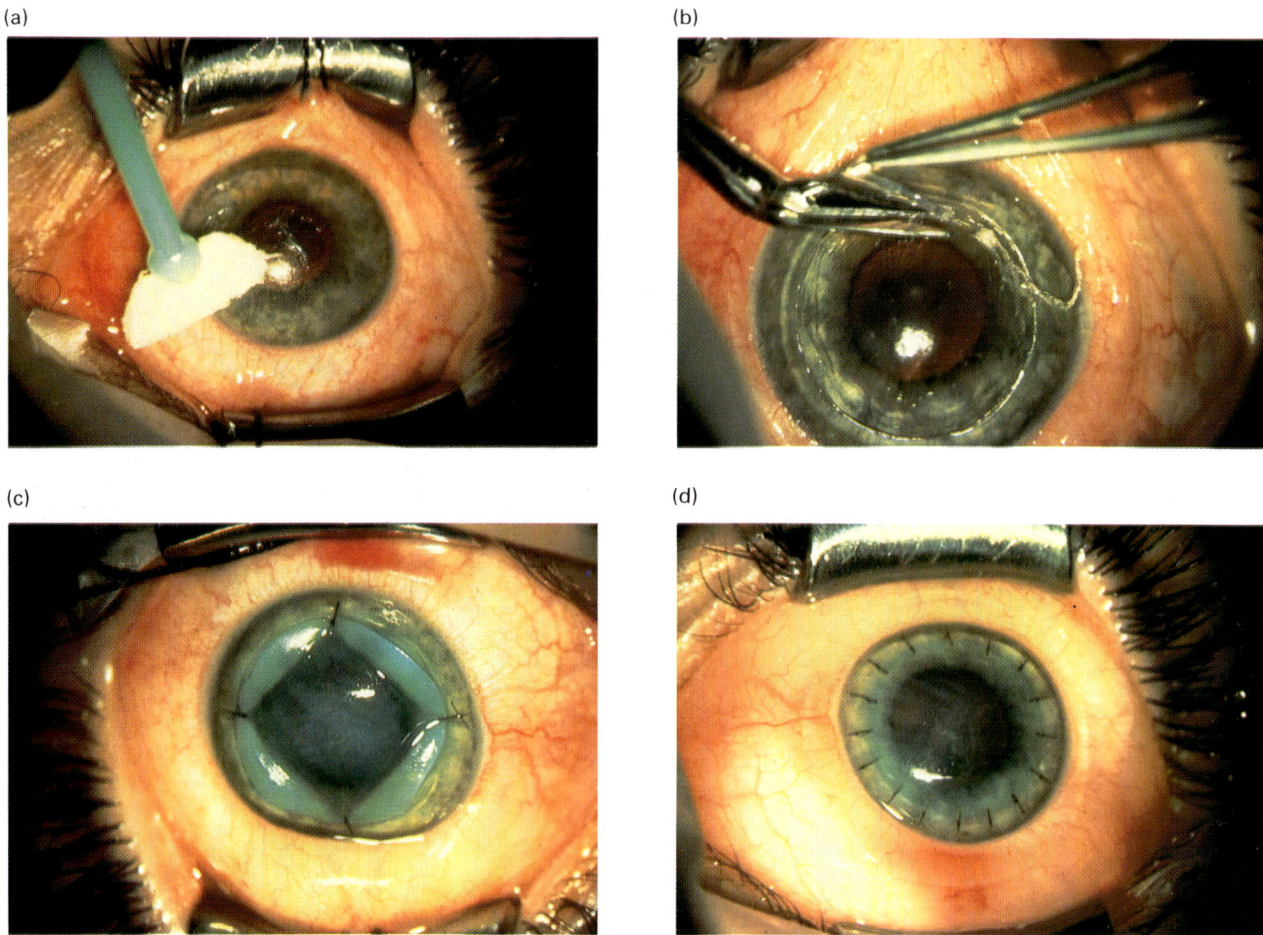

Fig. 10.120 (a) The epithelium is removed from the surface using a truncated WeckCel moistened with 10% cocaine (not alcohol). (b) Shallow trephination is followed by a scissors keratectomy. (c) The reconstituted epi-lenticule is secured by four cardinal sutures pulling the wing into the undermined cornea incision. (d) Sixteen interrupted sutures are used.

cases resulted in failure of the lenticule. While first described as reversible, in its original form the surgery resulted in both permanent corneal curvature changes and scarring. The results in myopic cases were worse and in some cases produced as much as ±17 D of variation from that predicted. This was reduced somewhat by a re-design of both the lenticule and the incision. However, the results so far do not justify its application in myopes of any degree, with the possible exception of those with keratoconus.

Early technique and results

The original methodology for epikeratophakia was to mark and cut a circle approximately 8.0 mm in diameter through Bowman's and partially into the corneal stroma, after first removing the epithelium in the center (Figure 10.120a,b). A wedge-shaped tissue annulus was then resected with scissors. The outer edge of the resection bed was then undermined to provide a pocket for the epi-graft's "wing." The lenticule was then tucked into the annular resection,

whereupon it was sutured in place with 16 interrupted 10-0 nylon sutures so placed as to draw the wing into the prepared pocket (Figure 10.120c,d).

Needless to say, the outcome of the surgery was subject to many variables, not the least of which was the inevitable variable tension applied to the epi-lenticule by the interrupted sutures. It was found that considerable difference in the ultimate correction depended upon the degree of suture tension applied, especially in myopic lenticules [33]. Then, too, postoperative astigmatism was hard to control, not only because of the sutures but also because of the irregularity in the hand-cut annular resection. The original technique was then changed to marking and cutting two concentric circles approximately 7.5 and 8.0 mm in diameter respectively through Bowman's. A wedge-shaped tissue annulus was then resected with scissors between the trephinations. This resulted in a more even annulus but missed the point—that a resection of tissue was occurring (Figure 10.121).

Epithelialization was delayed in most cases, sometimes as long as a week or more, for a number of

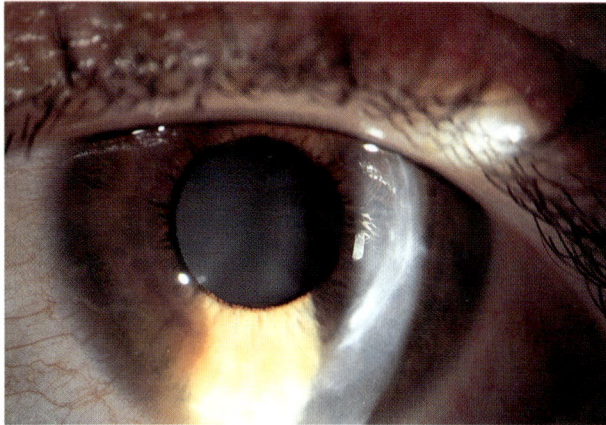

Fig. 10.121 Post-operative old-style epikeratophakia. Note the wide scar associated with the annular keratectomy.

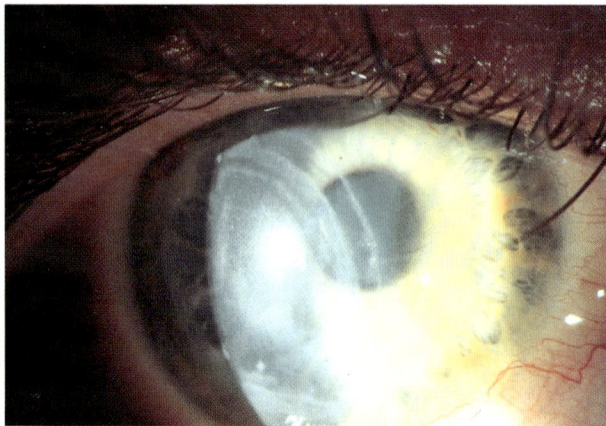

Fig. 10.122 Delayed re-epithelialization is often responsible for lenticular failure in these cases.

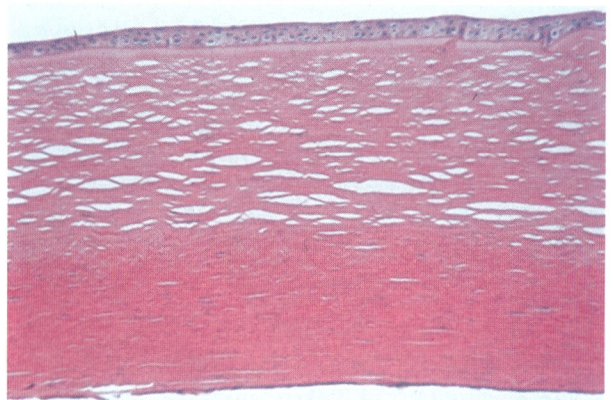

Fig. 10.123 Light microscopic appearance of an epi-lenticule applied 10 years before.

reasons. One of these was the necessity of the new cells to "jump the gap" created by the resected annulus. The problem was more prevalent in aphakic lenticules, probably because of their increased thickness. This delay would sometimes precipitate a reaction leading to loss of the lenticule, necessitating repeating or abandoning the procedure (Figure 10.122) [34]. None the less, once established, these lenticules are well-tolerated by the eye (Figure 10.123).

Wet epikeratophakia

By using freshly frozen and lathed tissue (so-called wet epi) and a slanted, circular corneal incision, coupled with the Barraquer anti-torque suture, the author has accomplished good results with this technique in cases of keratoconus (Figures 10.124 and 10.125). It is not possible, using current methods, to predict the post-operative refractive error in these cases, but most result in improvement of both unaided and aided

visual acuity, coupled by a strengthening of the central cornea. Sufficient time has not elapsed with these cases to determine long-term corneal stability, but results so far are promising (see below).

Another area which has shown encouraging results with epikeratophakia is in pediatric aphakia [35–37]. Here the outcome has been universally good and will probably continue to remain so. It is a reasonable alternative to the implantation of an intra-ocular lens in these cases. While good results have been reported in low hyperopia, other techniques—less traumatic and more predictable—have come on the scene [38]. Still, it has been used in radial keratotomy over-corrections with good results and could be a solution to high irregular astigmatism post radial keratotomy (Figures 10.126–10.128).

This procedure has been touted as reversible. Experience, however, has shown that while the procedure is certainly "re-doable"—that is, a lenticule can be removed and replaced—the term reversible does not apply. In the author's experience, once Bowman's layer has been severed in this way, permanent changes occur in the central corneal curvature—curiously enough, often in the direction of *flattening*. This effect has been shown experimentally by Gilbert and colleagues, when shallow trephinations of eye bank eyes were made [39]. This is an interesting finding in view of the results obtained by Gills with deep circular radial incisions and the effect of the hexagonal configuration [40].

Keratophakia—homo- and alloplastic

Keratophakia arose from a need which was not being adequately met at the time of its inception and predates keratomileusis for myopia. The condition of aphakia, while restoring sight, in many ways left the patient in worse condition than before the surgery.

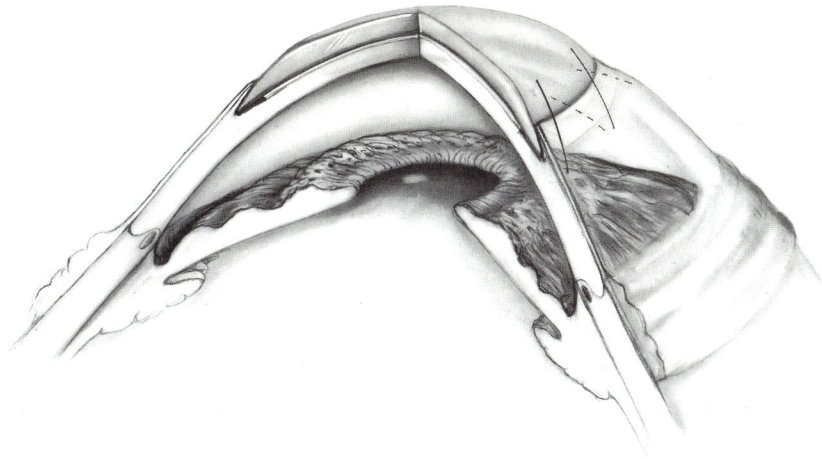

Fig. 10.124 The so-called wet-epi. Note the relatively smooth transition and small gap for the epithelium to bridge.

(a)

(b)

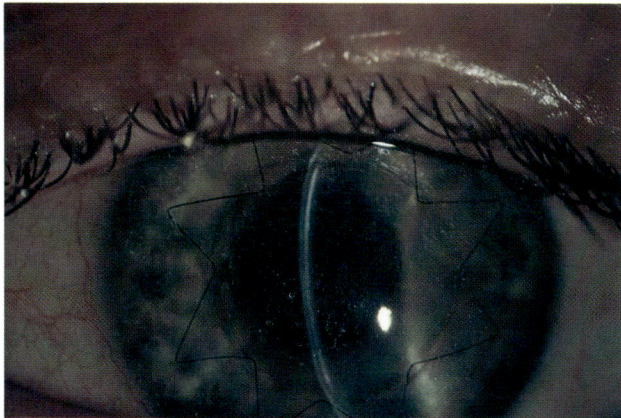

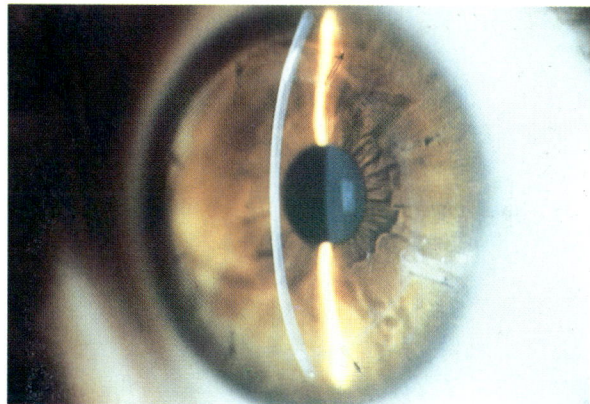

Fig. 10.125 (a) A wet-epi, 2 weeks post-surgery. (b) Myopic epi using the wet technique. Note the almost invisible keratectomy scar. Compare with Figure 10.121.

One can only speculate on the number of hip fractures resulting from the wearing of aphakic spectacles. Casey Wood's classic paper documenting his own experience with aphakia aptly describes the day-to-day existence of one with that condition; it should be required reading for all cataract surgeons. The procedure is designed for high hyperopia usually associated with cataract surgery. With the advent of intra-ocular lens implants, the need for this type of procedure has declined. However, it is still indicated in those patients in whom the introduction of the intra-ocular lens is contraindicated, such as severe diabetics. These contraindications—never absolute—are diminishing in number and variety, however.

Homoplastic keratophakia

In this surgery, thick sections of fresh or preserved donor corneal tissue are utilized (Figure 10.129). Furthermore, tissue not suitable for use as transplant material can be employed, including that which has

been cryo-preserved for prolonged periods [41,42]. This is fortunate in that no drain is placed upon the scanty transplant tissue supply. Fresh tissue needs to be desiccated a little before lathing; usually a blow dryer or a stream of anhydrous nitrogen is used.

Planned cases should have small-incision cataract extraction before the keratophakia procedure. Aphakic cases should have had an uneventful healing period of at least 6 months or more. The suction ring drives the intra-ocular pressure to at least 65 mmHg—sufficient to rupture an incompletely healed incision. What's more, the wound site must be smooth. Either an incompletely healed or non-smooth wound area can cause problems with maintaining suction. A break in suction during the keratectomy always results in an irregular section—both in thickness and in shape—which leads to induced astigmatism.

The lathing procedure is similar to that of keratomileusis except that the tissue is placed upon the base with the *convex side out* so that Bowman's layer is removed entirely (Figure 10.130). The lathing is done

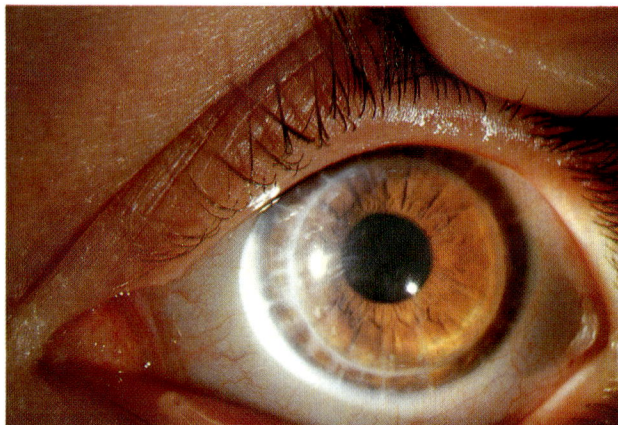

Fig. 10.126 Epi-lenticule over a radial keratotomy done for keratoconus 6 years before—1 year post-epi.

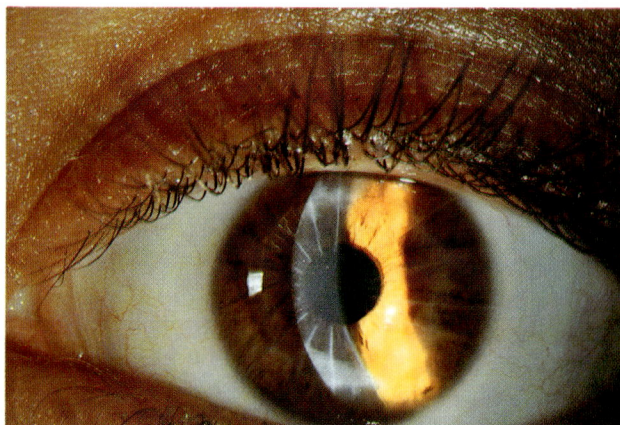

Fig. 10.127 An over-corrected radial keratotomy eye which underwent a lyophilized epi which subsequently failed. The post-epi corneal curvature *steepened* in this case—the usual reaction is to flatten.

(a)

(b)

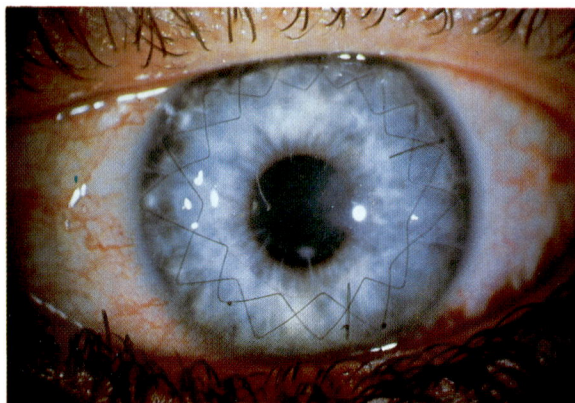

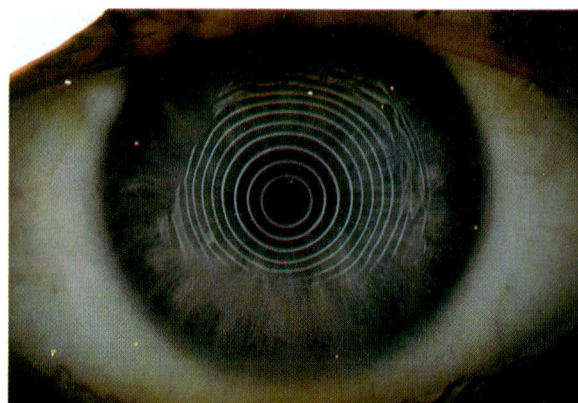

Fig. 10.128 (a) An epi-lenticule applied to a radial keratotomy over-correction—1 month post-epi. (b) Note the smooth circular photokeratoscopy mires. (Courtesy of S. Slade.)

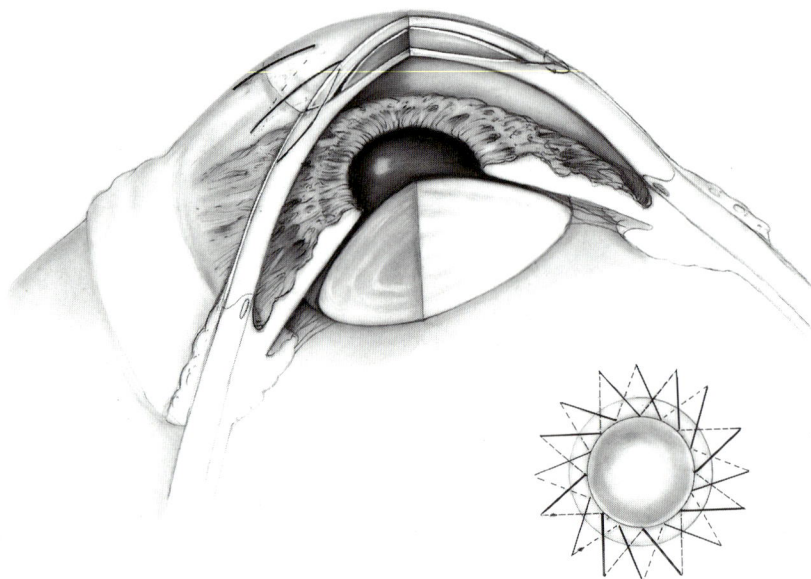

Fig. 10.129 The principle of keratophakia.

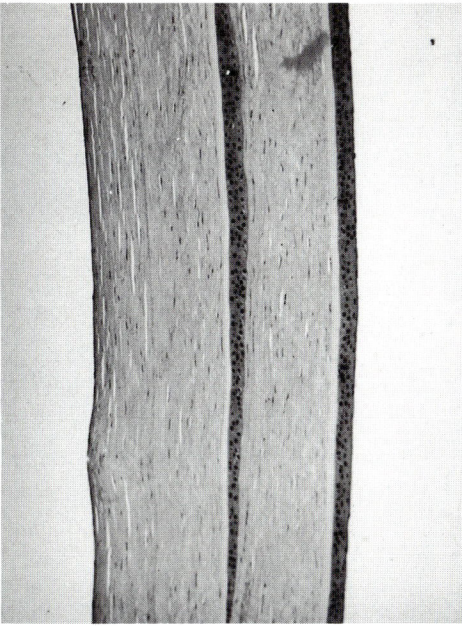

Fig. 10.130 An incorrectly lathed keratophakia lenticule. Note the presence of intact Bowman's and re-growth of epithelium. Note also the viable keratocytes within the lenticule.

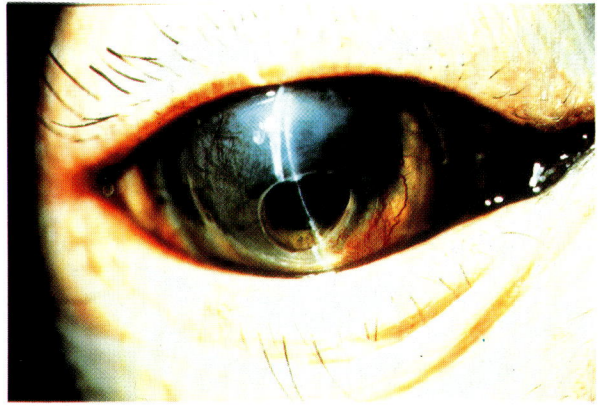

Fig. 10.132 Anterior stromal melting over a non-permeable intra-corneal lens. (Courtesy of B. McCarey.)

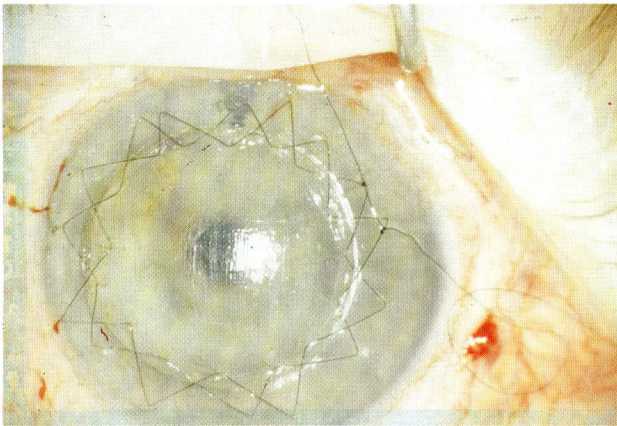

Fig. 10.131 Keratophakia.

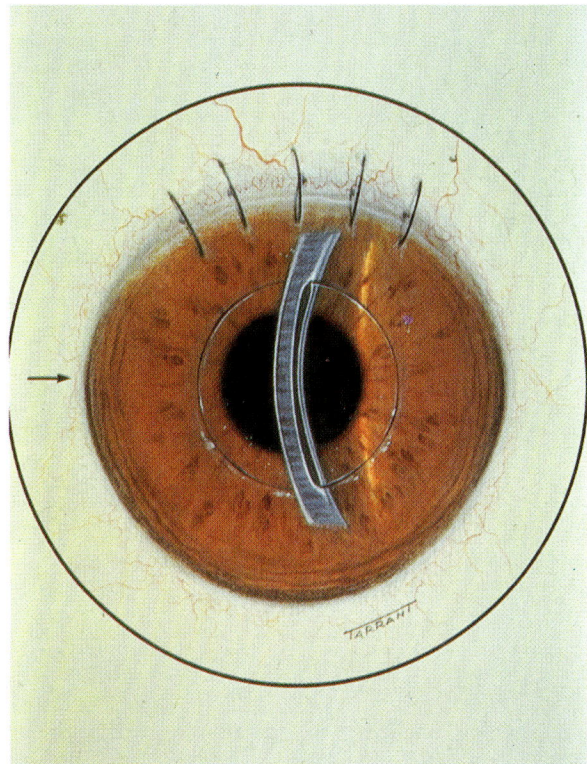

Fig. 10.133 Incorrect position for an intra-corneal lens; it should be more anterior than this drawing shows.

in a similar manner and is accomplished before the keratectomy is performed on the patient. In kerato-phakia the patient's resection is larger than in kerato-mileusis and the thickness is determined by the amount of refractive error to be corrected. There is a tendency to adjust the thickness (and consequently the diameter) to make it slightly thinner in higher cases to control the overall central corneal thickness. The lenticule is placed in the bed and the patient's tissue placed over it. Cardinal sutures are placed in four quadrants rather than three, as in keratomileusis. A double running non-torquing suture is then placed, providing 16 areas of support (Figure 10.131). The

cardinals are then removed and the eye treated as in keratomileusis.

Post-operative care is similar to that of keratomileusis except that the sutures are allowed to remain for a longer period of time. Recovery of vision is quite slow and a number of patients will never achieve the same level of corrected vision as pre-operatively. None the less, the technique is a valuable procedure in indicated cases. Theoretically, there is no upper limit to the amount of hyperopia that one can correct. However,

(a)

(b)

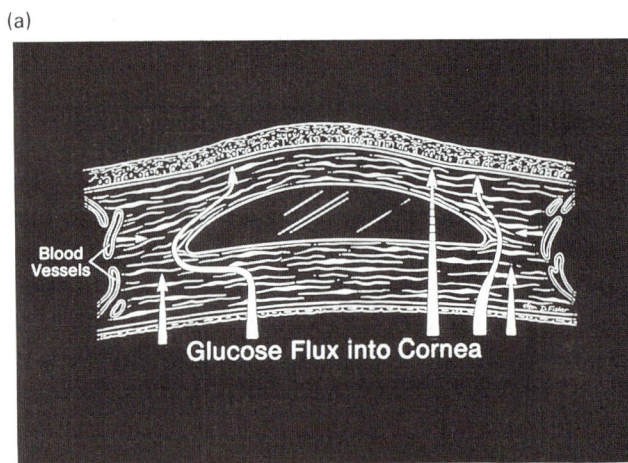

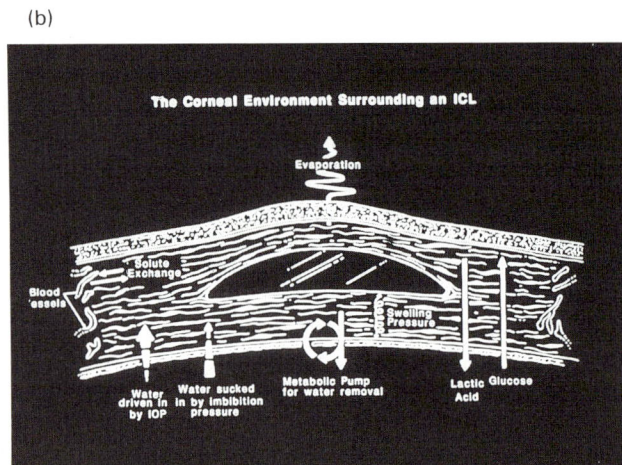

Fig. 10.134 (a) Glucose movement within the cornea; (b) the corneal environment surrounding an intra-corneal lens. (Courtesy of B. McCarey.)

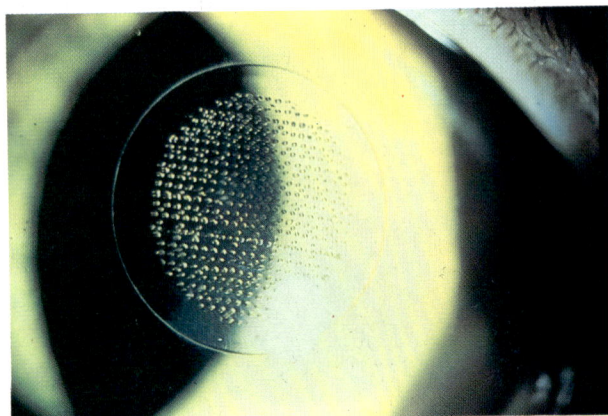

Fig. 10.135 Implanted fenestrated polysulfone intra-corneal lens. (Courtesy of R. Lindstrom.)

the considerations of corneal physiology and anatomy set an upper limit of 22 D with this surgery.

Alloplastic keratophakia

It is probably incorrect to group allopathic corneal stromal implants with homoplastic implants (kera-tophakia); allopathics should perhaps be called intra-corneal lenses. However, the principles are the same, even though the materials may differ. Barraquer's original work involved the correction of aphakia by the method of stromal implants. During the course of many years he tried many different materials, finding that human corneal tissue produced the best results [3,43–47]. The objections to the use of other materials were the same, with few variations, namely that they all interfered with corneal nutrition of either the anterior or posterior stroma or both (Figure 10.132). The course of trial was also the same: implantation was best done at the junction of the outer and middle thirds and eventually all materials (except human and later, hydrogel) needed to be fenestrated to improve corneal physiology—all eventually failed [48] (Figure 10.133). The problem with non-permeable intra-stromal implants is that they must live in harmony with a complex environment (Figure 10.134).

Choyce has experimented with allopathic corneal inlays for years [49–54]. He has reported trials with a material known as polysulfone [55]. This original work was expanded by Lane and others [56–62]. Original

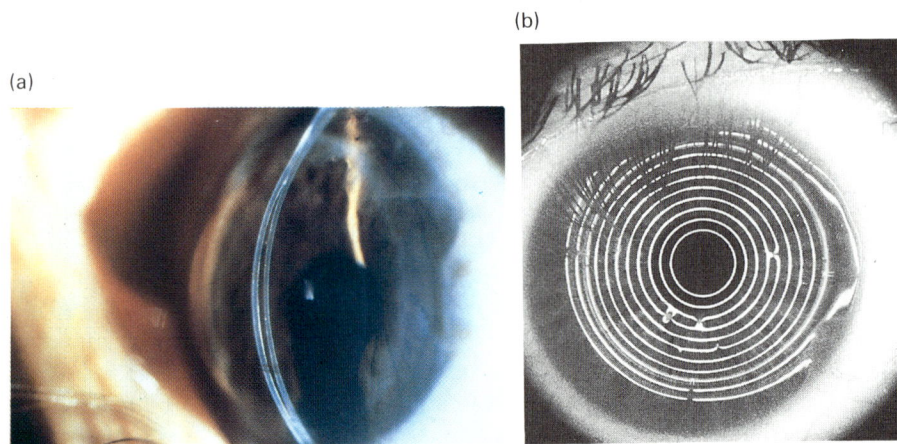

(a)

(b)

Fig. 10.136 (a) Implanted hydrogel intra-corneal lens at 2 months. (b) As this photokeratoscopy shows, the corneas are usually smooth.

(a)

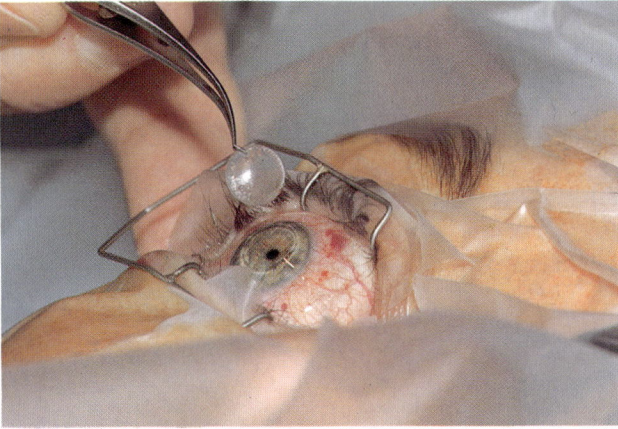

(b)

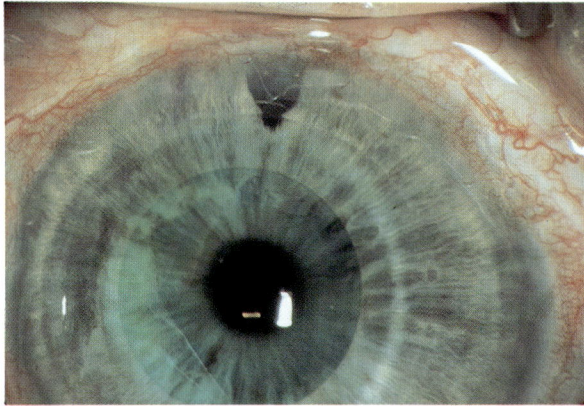

(c)

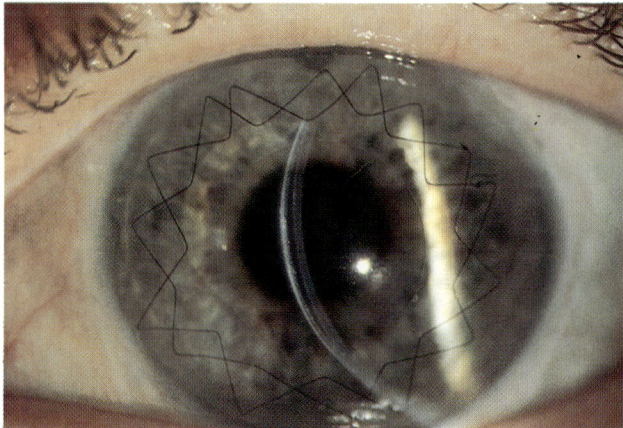

Fig. 10.137 (a) The corneal cap should be at least 8.0 mm in diameter. (b) The hydrogel intra-corneal lens has been dyed with kitton green for improved visibility. (c) The usual double running suture is used to secure the lenticule.

results, as in the past, have been reported as favorable. Significantly, the lenticules which began as solid have become fenestrated in the latest versions (Figure 10.135).

Werblin has reported greater success with the implantation of hydrogel materials within the corneal

stroma of animals, including non-human primates [63–70]. This study has recently been expanded to include human aphakes and the results in the first small group have been promising (Figure 10.136).

The technique, except for the lathing, is the same for alloplastic as for homoplastic keratophakia; the most difficult part is still the keratectomy (Figure 10.137).

There has been very little intolerance shown by the corneal stroma to the hydrophilic material in most cases. An unusual reaction to the material has occurred in the monkey model (Figure 10.138). This exact reaction has not been seen in human subjects. However, two human cases have shown small granular precipitates which lie on the intra-corneal lens and accumulate at its edge (Figure 10.139). In the author's case, these precipitates contributed to poor post-operative vision and the decision to remove the implant. Van Reij reported a bilateral case with poor visual acuity in one eye after a year; the patient responded with improved vision to explantation of the intra-corneal lens and implantation of a Worst Claw lens (Figure 10.140; G. van Reij, 1990, personal com-

(a)

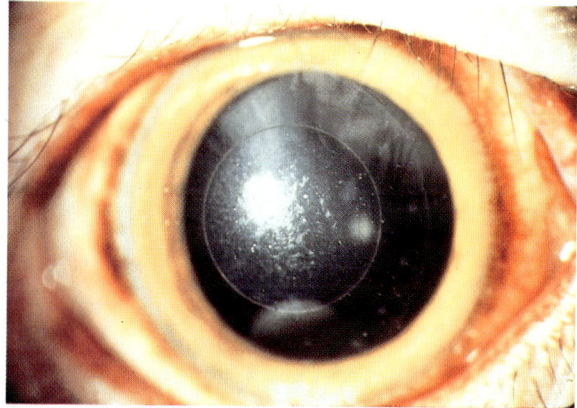

(b)

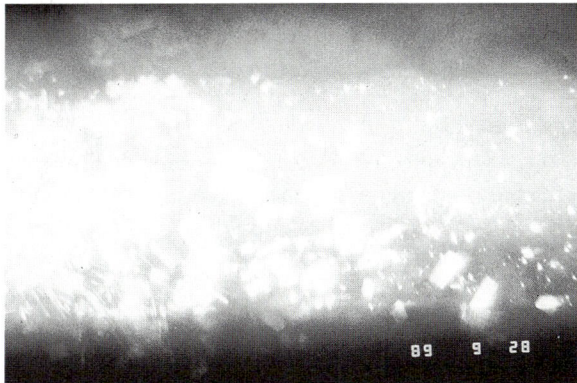

Fig. 10.138 (a and b) An unusual crystalline keratopathy occurring in a monkey with a hydrogel intra-corneal lens. (Courtesy of B. McCarey.)

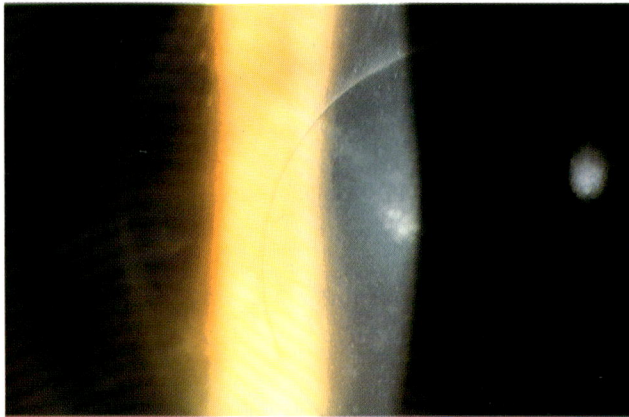

Fig. 10.139 Peculiar granulated material at the interface and edge of a hydrogel intra-corneal lens. (Courtesy of F. Price.)

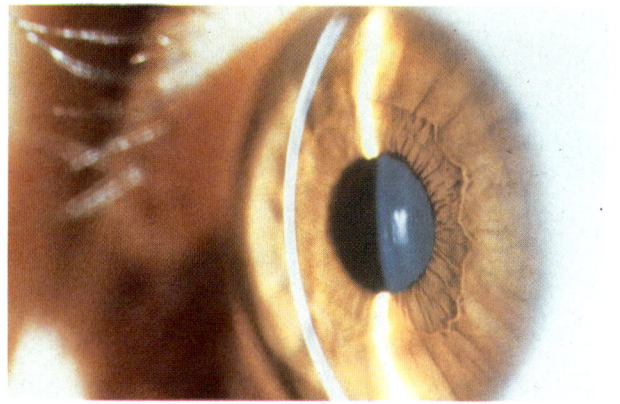

Fig. 10.141 MKM eye 18 years post-surgery.

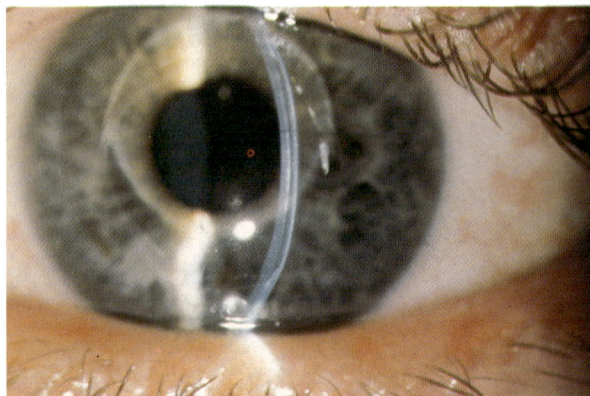

Fig. 10.140 Hydrogel-implanted eye with poor visual acuity at 1 year. (Courtesy of van Rij.)

munication). Time alone will tell whether this or any allopathic material can be implanted safely.

Impacting on this procedure is the diminishing need for this type of surgery due to improvement in both intra-ocular lens technology and implantation techniques. The hydrogel study has been suspended, not because of complications but for want of indications. Whether additional work in this area will continue is moot. The costs of such research continue to increase every year. Federal restrictions have only added to the bill. This fact, coupled with the short-sighted and litigious attitude of many Americans, stimulated by rabid consumerism and techno-terrorism, has encouraged manufacturers to do the initial and clinical trials out-of-country—if they do them at all.

Results of lamellar refractive surgery

MKM

Long-term stability of the correction and vision is excellent with this technique (Figure 10.141). The

Table 10.4 Details of hyperopic lamellar keratotomy Group 1 cases

Parameter	Values
Age	23–58 years
Range	+2.00 to +7.00 D
Total eyes	23
Iatrogenic (radial keratotomy over-corrections)	6
Natural	17

Table 10.5 Side-effects experienced by hyperopic lamellar keratotomy Group 1

Side-effect	n
Glare	0
Photophobia	0
Cells and flare	0
Delayed epithelialization	0

Table 10.6 Complications experienced by hyperopic lamellar keratotomy Group 1

Complication	n
Thin section	1
Thick section	1
Induced astigmatism	4
Irregular	0
Epithelial ingrowth	0
Over-correction >1 D	4
Under-correction >1 D	6

Table 10.7 Details of keratomileusis-*in-situ* Group 1 cases

Parameter	Values
Age	18–47 years
Range	−6.50 to −22.00 D
Total eyes	37

Table 10.8 Side-effects experienced by keratomileusis-*in-situ* Group 1

Side-effect	n
Glare	0
Photophobia	0
Cells and flare	0
Delayed epithelialization	0

Table 10.9 Complications experienced by keratomileusis-*in-situ* Group 1

Complication	n
Induced astigmatism >0.5 D	3
Irregular	2
Epithelialization	0
Under-correction >1 D	29
Over-correction >1 D	3

Table 10.10 Details of hyperopic lamellar keratotomy Group 2 cases

Parameter	Values
Age	20–47 years
Range	+2.00 to +7.00 D
Total eyes	17
Iatrogenic	3
Natural	14

Table 10.11 Side-effects experienced by hyperopic lamellar keratotomy Group 2

Side-effect	n
Glare	0
Photophobia	0
Cells and flare	0
Delayed epithelialization	0

Table 10.12 Complications experienced by hyperopic lamellar keratotomy Group 2

Complication	n
Induced astigmatism >0.5 D	4
Irregular	0
Epithelial ingrowth	1
Over-correction >1 D	1
Under-correction >1 D	6

Table 10.13 Details of keratomileusis-*in-situ* Group 2 cases

Parameter	Values
Age	18–47 years
Range	−6.50 to −26.00 D
Total eyes	22

Table 10.14 Side-effects experienced by keratomileusis-*in-situ* Group 2

Side-effect	n
Glare	0
Photophobia	0
Cells and flare	0
Delayed epithelialization	0

Table 10.15 Complications experienced by keratomileusis-*in-situ* Group 2. Eight cases of induced astigmatism out of 22 cases total is much higher than in classic MKM

Complication	n
Induced astigmatism >0.5 D	6
Irregular	2
Epithelialization	0
Under-correction >1 D	16
Over-correction >1 D	1

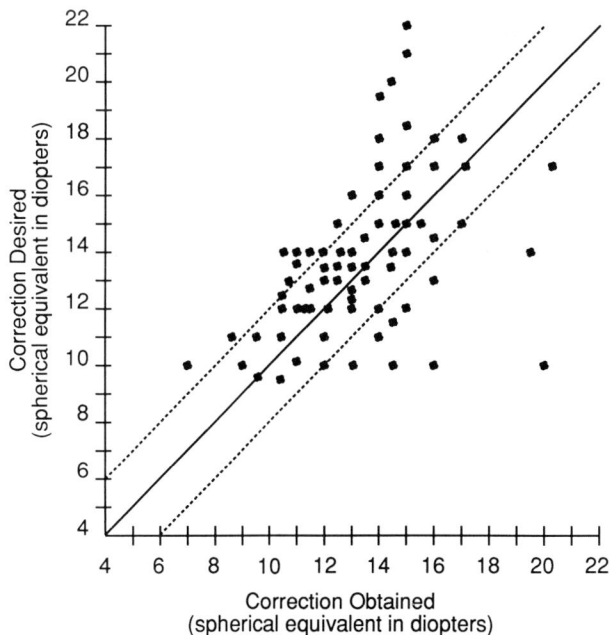

Fig. 10.142 Scattergram showing the author's results with classical MKM in 72 cases.

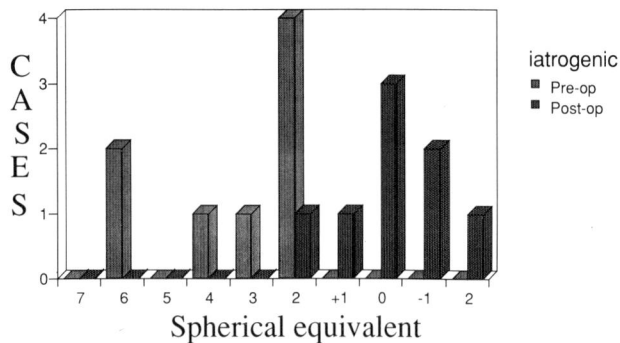

Fig. 10.143 Hyperopic lamellar keratotomy Group 1. The lighter shades represent the pre-operative conditions and the darker shades the post-operative conditions.

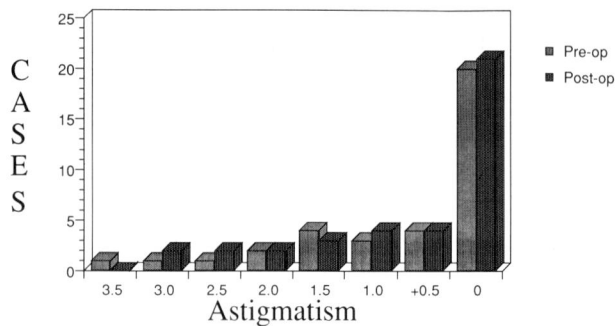

Fig. 10.144 Hyperopic lamellar keratotomy Group 1. The post-operative trend is toward less hyperopia.

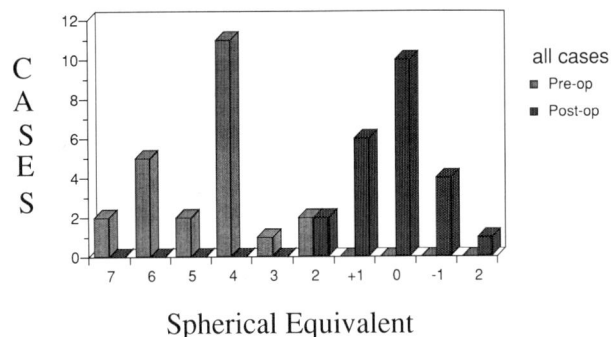

Fig. 10.145 Hyperopic lamellar keratotomy Group 1. Although the mean of the astigmatism has not changed, some regular astigmatism was induced by the surgery.

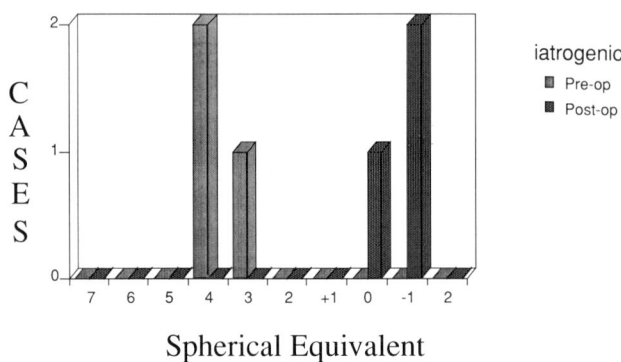

Fig. 10.146 Keratomileusis-*in-situ* Group 1. All cases showed a reduction in the myopia but not in a predictable manner.

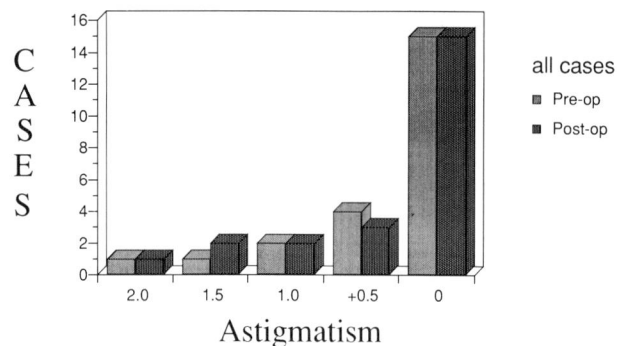

Fig. 10.147 Keratomileusis-*in-situ* Group 1. This graph masks the astigmatism—regular and irregular—induced by the procedure.

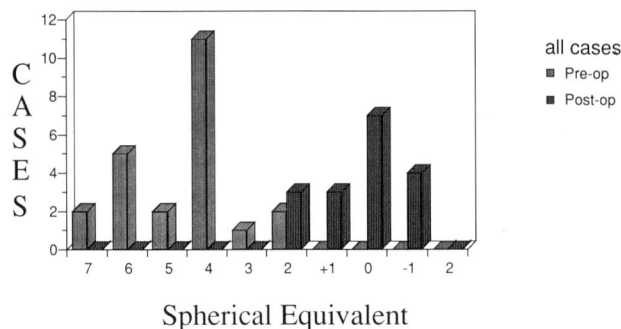

Fig. 10.148 Hyperopic lamellar keratotomy Group 2. Iatrogenic cases. Predictability was improved in this group.

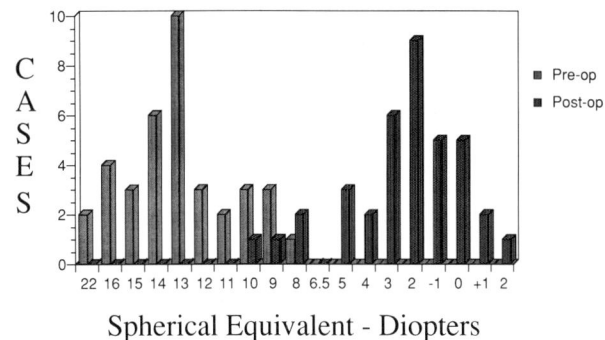

Fig. 10.149 Hyperopic lamellar keratotomy Group 2. Overall, the reduction in hyperopia was uniform.

author's experience with this procedure is somewhat small, not having become involved with lamellar procedures until late 1984. The results in the author's cases are summarized in Figure 10.142. Of the 72 cases in the author's series with follow-up greater than 1 year, six (8.3%) developed astigmatism greater than 1D post-operation. In all but one of these cases the astigmatism was myopic reflecting an undercorrection of the patient's myopia. In two cases the astigmatism was irregular and required that the surgery be repeated. Four of the regular and both of the irregular astigmatism

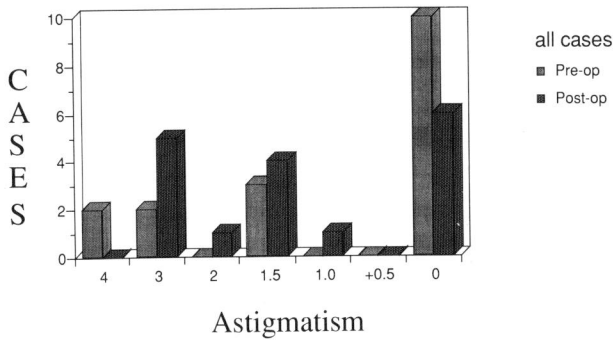

Fig. 10.150 Hyperopic lamellar keratotomy Group 2. The mean astigmatism is reduced in this series overall, but four cases of regular astigmatism were induced, off-setting the gain.

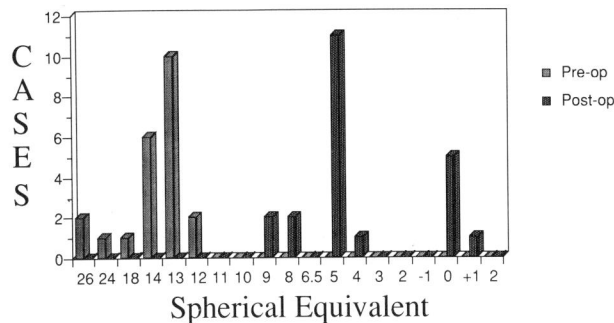

Fig. 10.151 Keratomileusis-*in-situ* Group 2. Many of the higher degrees of myopia were only partially corrected.

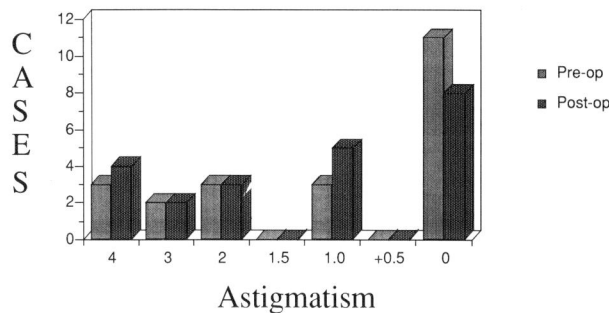

Fig. 10.152 Keratomileusis-*in-situ* Group 2. Again, the cases of induced astigmatism are masked by the statistic.

cases occurred in patients who experienced epithelial ingrowth or cysts. Forty (55.6%) of the cases were undercorrected of which 15 (20.8%) were undercorrected more than 2 D. Of these 15 cases, seven occurred in patients whose pre-operative myopia exceeded 17 D. In most cases radial keratotomy incisions were successful in reducing the undercorrections except in one case where very little additional flattening occurred. Twenty-five (34.7%) of the patients were over-corrected of which 10 (13.8%) were over-corrected in excess of 2 D. Most of the over-corrections in excess of 2 D received additional surgery (either HKM or

HLK) to correct the error. Using Barraquer's limit of accuracy of ±2 D, 46 (63.9%) cases fell within that limit. It would appear from this experience that the greatest accuracy of the calculation formulas lies with cases between 12 and 16 D of pre-operative myopia [71]. The low incidence of irregular healing as evidenced by the small number of cases of irregular astigmatism bares out the safety of this procedure. The side-effects and complications to be expected with this procedure are discussed in Chapter 15.

Hyperopic lamellar keratotomy and keratomileusis-*in-situ*

Discussion

The results of the author's first two series of patients, hyperopic lamellar keratotomy and keratomileusis-*in-situ*, are shown in Tables 10.4 through 10.15 and Figures 10.143 through 10.152. While the overall outcome has been satisfactory, there are unresolved problems with the surgery that must be addressed. The most important of these is the incidence of irregular astigmatism in cases of keratomileusis-*in-situ*. While the tables show good resultant spherical equivalents, they do not tell the whole story since they tend to mask the astigmatism induced by the surgery. The first figure represents the percentage of irregular astigmatism while the figure in parentheses is the total astigmatism induced within the group. While two out of 37 cases (Group I; Table 10.9) and two out of 22 (Group II; Table 10.15) may not seem like much, that 5% (8% total) and 9% (27% total) occurrence of as- tigmatism is considerably higher than in classic keratomileusis and incidences of irregular astigmatism approaching 22% have been reported elsewhere (F. Navarro, 1990, personal communication). The appearance of this astigmatism is undoubtedly related to alignment of the two resections with one another but is also associated with that relationship as regards the visual axis. While in classic keratomileusis a slight misalignment of the tissue disk center with the visual axis is tolerated, the problem is compounded if there is any misalignment of the sections themselves in addition.

This is due as well to the nature and size of the second resection. When these cases are refracted, the second resection is clearly seen as if it were a stromal implant. That is, the edge is quite discrete. This implies that the refractive surface has a strong curvature at that intersection. If the second section is small and is slightly de-centered, the distortion produced by this strong curvature is very perturbing to vision and may be reflected by distorted corneal mires. By definition this is irregular astigmatism. This further implies that the true optical zone is much smaller than the disk diameter and in cases wherein the diameter is 3.0 mm, the optical zone approaches 2.0 mm or less. Such a zone size admits of no leeway with respect to centration. That resection size plays a role is seen in the most recent series by the author in which the second, or refractive, section is made with a much larger diameter and with a thickness no less than 100 μm. In these cases (most with 6 months' follow-up), the incidence of irregular astigmatism approaches 3%—more in line with classic keratomileusis.

As stated earlier, when the corneal tissue is removed from its supporting base (Bowman's membrane), it becomes very unstable and has many of the characteristics of a gel. This property becomes more pronounced in thin sections. This is easily demonstrated when the tissue is gauged. It is possible to tease it into very thin sections which, of course, is reflected in variable thickness readings. Histologic examinations are not able to shed much light on the actual tissue thickness because of artifacts introduced during the preparation process. It is the author's contention, however, based on clinical experience, that tissue thickness is a factor in the appearance of irregular astigmatism and that results are shown to improve when the refractive (second) section is made no thinner than 100 μm.

The other problem is that of predictability. In keratomileusis-*in-situ* it is less than that of classic keratomileusis. In approximately half the cases, the resultant reduction in myopia is within ±1.00 D, whereas in the remainder—while the myopia was, in all cases, reduced—the discrepancy can be as great as 5.00 D. It is apparent that the Barraquer formula cannot be applied without modification in these cases. Ongoing work in this area has suggested some

changes which are currently being applied with some success. However, more time will be needed to ascertain the accuracy of the modified formula as well as the upper limit of correction that can reasonably be expected with this surgery.

In hyperopic lamellar keratotomy the predictability exceeds 80%, ±1.00 D, in cases ranging from 2.50 to 6.0 D. While the theoretic upper limit seems to be 7 or 8 D, such cases require extremely small resections (5.00 mm or less); these are extremely difficult to cut accurately and thickly enough to obtain sufficient correction. Also, the cases of induced astigmatism seem to cluster in the higher-diopter cases. There would appear to be a lower limit to the practical size of the disk resected. What that size is in actuality is not known at this time.

Conclusion

It is this author's opinion, based upon actual experience with this surgery and classic keratomileusis, as well as observation of the work of others, that the techniques of hyperopic lamellar keratotomy and keratomileusis-*in-situ* are potentially valuable additions to the refractive surgeon's armamentarium within their current limitations. Currently the author advises those who would apply this surgery to patients to limit such cases to hyperopia in the range of 2.50–5.00 D and to myopia in excess of 13.00 D. The lower limit of myopia is chosen to reduce the chance of overcorrection in this as yet unpredictable surgical procedure. Further, while hyperopic lamellar keratotomy is extremely useful in cases of radial keratotomy overreaction, such application should not be attempted

Table 10.16 Results of epikeratophakia in aphakia

Cases	Pre-operative			Post-operative		
	Spherical equivalent (D)	Mean unaided vision	Mean corrected vision	Spherical equivalent (D)	Mean unaided vision	Mean corrected vision
6	12–14	20/400	20/30	0–2	20/60	20/70
9	14–16	20/400	20/30	0–1.5	20/50	20/80
4	16–18	20/400	20/30	0–1	20/60	20/75

Table 10.17 Results of fresh epikeratophakia in keratoconus

Cases	Pre-operative			Post-operative		
	Spherical equivalent (D)	Mean unaided vision	Mean corrected vision	Spherical equivalent (D)	Mean unaided vision	Mean corrected vision
17	*	<20/400	20/30	+0.50 to −3.0	20/40	20/25

* rational refraction not possible

until or unless the surgeon possesses considerable skill both with the microkeratome and the suturing of thin tissue sections. Corneal transplant experience alone is not sufficient qualification for performing this surgery.

Epikeratophakia

The author has used both the freeze-dried "potato chip" lenticules as supplied by AMO and has made his own lenticules—wet epi. Fresh epi-lenticules sutured into slant-cut circular keratotomy with a non-torquing suture have proved to be most satisfactory in kerato-conus cases. The results of such application are summarized in Tables 10.16 and 10.17. As in keratomileusis, side-effects and complications of this surgery are discussed in Chapter 15.

Keratophakia

The author has performed both homoplastic and allopathic keratophakia procedures with indifferent results. The two cases of homoplastic keratophakia for aphakia resulted in improved vision (as opposed to spectacles) but were a long time in coming right. Epithelialization was prolonged (longer than 2 weeks in both cases) and vision remained below 20/100 for at least 6 months despite the apparent clarity of the lenticule. In neither case was irregular astigmatism present but low-grade regular astigmatism was $-2.25\,D$ in one case and $1.87\,D$ in the other—after 1 year. Both patients required spectacle correction, remaining moderately hyperopic ($+3.25 + 1.87 \times 97$ in one case; $+2.50 + 2.25 \times 165$ in the other) and had a best corrected vision of 20/40 and 20/50 respectively at 2 and 3 years post-operation.

The author has implanted one hydrogel intra-stromal lens as part of the AMO study. After 9 months, the patient's best corrected visual acuity is 20/80 with considerable ametropia: $-7.50 + 4.50 \times 88$. The overlying corneal tissue remains clear but there is a fine refractile, crystalline deposit on the lens itself and accumulated along its edge (see above). The lenticule will probably be removed if the vision and/or the deposit does not clear.

This is a good technique. The hydrogel material is the first of the implanted allopathic materials to retain clear corneas in all examples. The problems are indications and availability. The study has been suspended for reasons mentioned above and it is unlikely that the company will make lenses available on an "if come" basis.

References

1 Barraquer JI. Queratoplastica refractiva est. Inform Oftal (Inst Barraquer) 1949; 2:10.

2 Barraquer JI. Queratoplastia. Arch Soc Am Oftal Optom 1961; 3:147.

3 Barraquer JI. C. Clasification de las queratoplastias refractivas. II. Metodos que modifican la curva de una o ambas superficies corneales, variando la relacion entre ellas. In: *Queratomileusis y Queratofaquia*. Instituto Barraquer de America, Bogota, 1980.

4 Krwawicz T. Proby zmiany krzywizny rogowski droga doswiadczalnych operacji plastycznych. (Attempted modification of corneal curvature by means of experimental plastic surgery.) Klin Occna 1960; 30:229–236.

5 Krwawicz T. New plastic operation for correcting refractive error of aphakic eyes by changing corneal curvature: preliminary report. Br J Ophthalmol 1961; 45:59–63.

6 Krwawicz T. Lamellar corneal stromectomy. Am J Ophthalmol 1964; 57:828.

7 Pureskin NP. Oslablenie refraktsii glaza putem chastichnoi stromektomii rogovitsy v eksperimente (Weakening ocular refraction by means of partial stromectomy of cornea under experimental conditions.) Vestn Oftalmol 1967; 80:19–24.

8 Elstein JK, Sehgal VN, Kaplan MM, Katzin HM. Instrumentation and techniques for refractive keratoplasty. Am J Ophthalmol 1969; 68:282–291.

9 Hoffmann F, Jessen K. Keratokyphose zur optischen Korrektur der Aphakie. (Keratokyphosis for the optical correction of aphakia.) Fortschr Ophthalmol 1985; 82:86–87.

10 Swinger CA, Krumeich J, Cassiday D. Planar lamellar refractive keratoplasty. J Refract Surg 1986; 2:17–24.

11 Binder PS, Krumeich JH, Zavala EV. Laboratory evaluation of freeze vs non-freeze lamellar refractive keratoplasty. Arch Ophthalmol 1987; 105:1125–1128.

12 Krumeich JH, Swinger CA. Nonfreeze epikeratophakia for the correction of myopia. Am J Ophthalmol 1987; 103:397–403.

13 Ruiz LA. *Lamellar Keratectomy for Hyperopia*. Kerato Refractive Society, Dallas, 1987.

14 Bores LD. Hyperopic lamellar keratotomy (HLK). Postoperative results. Kerato Refractive Society Annual Meeting, Dallas, 1987.

15 Googe JM, Palkama KA, Werblin TP. The histology of epikeratophakia grafts. Invest Ophthalmol Visual Sci 1981; 20(suppl):8.

16 Werblin TP, Klyce SD. Epikeratophakia: the surgical correction of aphakia. I. Lathing of corneal tissue. Curr Eye Res 1981; 1:123–129.

17 Werblin TP, Kaufman HE. Epikeratophakia: the surgical correction of aphakia. II. Preliminary results in a non-human primate model. Curr Eye Res 1981; 1:131–137.

18 Morgan KS, Werblin TP, Asbell PA, Loupe DN, Friedlander MH, Kaufman HE. The use of epikeratophakia grafts in pediatric monocular aphakia. J Pediatr Ophthalmol Strabismus 1981; 18:23–29.

19 Werblin TP, Kaufman HE, Friedlander MH, Sehon KL, McDonald MB, Granet NS. A prospective study of the use of hyperopic epikeratophakia grafts for the correction of aphakia in adults. Ophthalmology 1981; 88:1137–1140.

20 Werblin TP, Kaufman HE, Friedlander MH, McDonald MB, Sehon KL. Epikeratophakia—the surgical correction of aphakia. Upd1981. Ophthalmology 1982; 89:916–920.

21 Asbell PA, Werblin TP, Loupe DN, Morgan KS, Kaufman HE. Secondary surgical procedures after epikeratophakia. Ophthalm Surg 1982; 13:555–557.

22 Berkowitz RA, McDonald MB, Werblin TP. Epikeratophakia for myopia. Invest Ophthalmol 1982; 22(suppl):201.

23 Kaufman HE, Werblin TP. Epikeratophakia for the treatment of keratoconus. Am J Ophthalmol 1982; 93:342–347.

24 Werblin TP. Epikeratophakia: techniques, complications, and

clinical results. Int Ophthalmol Clin 1983; 23:45–58.

25 Werblin TP. Epikeratophakia: a new treatment for corneal irregularity and keratoconus. W Va Med J 1983; 79:26–28.

26 Werblin TP, Blaydes JE. Epikeratophakia: existing limitations and future modifications. Aust J Ophthalmol 1983; 11:201–207.

27 Werblin TP, Blaydes JE, Kaufman HE. Epikeratophakia: the surgical correction of astigmatism—preliminary experimental results. CLAO J 1983; 9:61–63.

28 Yamaguchi T, Koenig S, Kimura T, Werblin T, McDonald M, Kaufman H. Histological study of epikeratophakia in primates. Ophthalm Surg 1984; 15:230–235.

29 Goodman GS, Peiffer RLJ, Werblin TP. Failed epikeratoplasty for keratoconus. Cornea 1986; 5:29–34.

30 McDonald MB, Koenig SB, Friedlander MH, Hamano T, Kaufman HE. Alloplastic epikeratophakia for the correction of aphakia. Ophthalm Surg 1983; 14:65–69.

31 Baumgartner SD, Zavala EY, Binder PS. A laboratory analysis of lyophilized epikeratophakia lenticules. Invest Ophthalmol Visual Sci 1985; 26(suppl):204.

32 Arffa RC, Busin M, Barron BA, McDonald MB, Kaufman HE. Epikeratophakia with commercially prepared tissue for the correction of aphakia in adults. Arch Ophthalmol 1986; 104:1467–1472.

33 McDonald MB, Kaufman HE, Aquavella JV et al. The nationwide study of epikeratophakia for myopia. Am J Ophthalmol 1987; 103:375–383.

34 Grossniklaus HE, Lass JH, Jacobs G, Margo CE, McAuliffe AM. Light microscopic and ultrastructural findings in failed epikeratoplasty. Refract Corneal Surg 1989; 5:296–301.

35 Hiles DA. Epikeratophakia—an alternative to glasses, contact lenses and intraocular lens for optical correction of aphakia in children. Trans Pa Acad Ophthalmol Otolaryngol 1986; 38:279–285.

36 Morgan KS, McDonald MB, Hiles DA et al. The nationwide study of epikeratophakia for aphakia in children. Am J Ophthalmol 1987; 103:366–374.

37 Morgan KS, McDonald MB, Hiles DA et al. The nationwide study of epikeratophakia for aphakia in older children. Ophthalmology 1988; 95:526–532.

38 Ehrlich MI, Nordan LT. Epikeratophakia for the treatment of hyperopia. J Cataract Refract Surg 1989; 15:661–666.

39 Gilbert ML, Roth AS, Friedlander MH. Corneal flattening by shallow circular trephination in human eye bank eyes. Refract Corneal Surg 1990; 6:113–116.

40 Gills J. Trephination in combination with radial keratotomy for myopia. In: *Radial Keratotomy*, R Schacher et al. (eds). LAL, Dennison, 1980.

41 Friedlander MH, Rich LF, Werblin TP, Kaufman HE, Granet N. Keratophakia using preserved lenticules. Ophthalmology 1980; 87:687–692.

42 Maguen K, Pinhas S, Verity SM. Keratophakia with lyophilized cornea lathed at room temperature: new techniques and experimental surgical results. Ophthalm Surg 1983; 14:759–762.

43 Swinger CA, Barraquer JI. Keratophakia and keratomileusis—clinical results. Ophthalmology 1981; 88:709–715.

44 Barraquer JI. Keratophakia for the correction of high hyperopia. J Cryosurg 1964; 1:39.

45 Barraquer J. Modification of refraction by means of intracorneal inclusions. Int Ophthalmol Clin 1966; 6:53.

46 Barraquer JI. Keratophakia. Trans Ophthalmol Soc UK 1972; 92:499–516.

47 Barraquer JI. Queratofaquia. In: *Cirugia Refractiva de la Cornea*, Istituto Barraquer de America, Bogota, Colombia, 1989.

48 Beekhuis WH, McCarey BE, van Rij G, Waring GO. Complications of hydrogel intracorneal lenses in monkeys. Arch Ophthalmol 1987; 105:116–122.

49 Choyce DP. Intra-cameral and intra-corneal implants. A decade of personal experience. Trans Ophthalmol Soc UK 1966; 86:507–525.

50 Choyce DP. Implants and the human body. Lancet 1968; 2:633.

51 Choyce DP. The present status of intra-cameral and intracorneal implants. Can J Ophthalmol 1968; 3:295–311.

52 Choyce DP. Perforating and non-perforating acrylic corneal implants, including the Choyce 2-piece perforating keratoprosthesis. Ophthalmol 1969; suppl:292–300.

53 Choyce DP. Sovremennoe sostoianie problemy implantatisii intraokuliarnykh linz i intrakornealnykh implantatov (The current status of the problem of implantation of intraocular lenses and intracorneal implants.) Vestn Oftalmol 1969; 82:27–38.

54 Choyce DP. Intra-corneal plastic implants. 2. Nurs Times 1970; 66:715–718.

55 Choyce DP. The correction of refractive errors with polysulfone corneal inlays. A new frontier to be explored? Trans Ophthalmol Soc UK 1985; 104:332–342.

56 Kirkness CM, Steele AD, Garner A. Polysulfone corneal inlays. Adverse reactions: a preliminary report. Trans Ophthalmol Soc UK 1985; 104:343–350.

57 Lane SS, Lindstrom RL, Williams PA, Lindstrom CW. Polysulfone intracorneal lenses. J Refract Surg 1985; 1:207–216.

58 Lane SS, Lindstrom RL, Cameron JD. Fenestrated intracorneal lenses. Ophthalmology 1987; 94(suppl):125.

59 Lindstrom RL, Lane SS, Cameron JD, Mindrup EA, Choyce DP. Intracorneal lenses. Trans New Orleans Acad Ophthalmol 1988; 279–296.

60 McCarey B, Lane S, Lindstrom R. Alloplastic corneal lenses. Int Ophthalmol Clin 1988; 28:155–164.

61 Lane S, Lindstrom R, Cameron J et al. Polysulfone corneal lenses. J Cataract Refract Surg 1986; 12:50–60.

62 Lane SS, Lindstrom RL. Polysulfone intracorneal lenses. Int Ophthalmol Clin 1991; 31:37–46.

63 Werblin TP, Blaydes JE, Fryczkowski A, Peiffer R. Refractive corneal surgery: the use of implantable alloplastic lens material. Aust J Ophthalmol 1983; 11:325–331.

64 Werblin TP, Blaydes JE, Fryczkowski AW, Peiffer R. Stability of hydrogel intracorneal implants in non-human primates. CLAO J 1983; 9:157–161.

65 Werblin TP, Fryczkowski AW, Peiffer RL. Myopic correction using alloplastic implants in non-human primates—a preliminary report. Ann Ophthalmol 1984; 16:1127–1130.

66 Werblin TP, Peiffer RL, Fryczkowski A. Myopic hydrogel keratophakia: preliminary report. Cornea 1984; 3:197–204.

67 Peiffer RL, Werblin TP, Fryczkowski AW. Pathology of corneal hydrogel alloplastic implants. Ophthalmology 1985; 92:1294–1304.

68 Werblin TP, Fryczkowski AW, Peiffer RL. Hydrogel keratophakia: measurement of intraocular pressure. CLAO J 1985; 11:354–357.

69 Werblin T, Patel A. Myopic hydrogel keratophakia. Improvements in lens design. Cornea 1987; 6:197–201.

70 Werblin TP, Peiffer RL, Patel AS. Synthetic keratophakia for the correction of aphakia. Ophthalmology 1987; 94:926–934.

71 Barraquer JI. *Cirugia Refractiva de la Cornea: Resultados*. Instituto Barraquer de America, Bogota, Columbia, 1989.

11
Laser Refractive Surgery

Be not the first to set the old aside,
Nor yet the last to leave the new untried.
[Alexander Pope]

The term laser is an acronym for *l*ight *a*mplification by *s*timulated *e*mission of *r*adiation—and may be the sexiest acronym in the human lexicon. It carries with it visions of Star Wars, connotations of unfettered power, and a mystique of benevolent utility. The very nuance of the term is that of something embodying everlasting welfare—"we don't know what it means but it sure *sounds* great!" It has been made the subject of unprecedented media hype and has acquired a reputation for accuracy and applicability—some of it justified, some not. Many see lasers as the Greek panacea—the universal cure, the ultimate liniment. Or the penultimate snake oil, since the term laser itself has been used to sell everything from trinkets to automobiles.

There is no question that such devices, through the beam of electromagnetic radiation that they emit, are extremely powerful things. They can, in an instant, vaporize the most refractory of substances. Heady stuff this, both to witness and to contemplate. It is, however, this very power that makes them extremely dangerous devices. Dangerous, not only in their manifest (as well as latent) power, but in their ability to fascinate, nay mesmerize, us—perhaps into applying them in ways that may prove to be more harmful than beneficial.

The author once made an unfortunate response to an interview question regarding the application of lasers to refractive surgery when he replied, somewhat tongue-in-cheek, that "lasers are the refractive surgical instrument of the future and are likely to be so for the next 10 years." This answer was not original; it was in fact a paraphrasing of something someone else had said about the same subject. It was, moreover, unfortunate because it was mistaken in some quarters as "sour grapes" and taken in others as a jest. The author's intent, however, was to point out that the routine use of lasers in refractive surgery is not *now* (however much some individuals and manufacturers would like it to be) and that considerable research and trial are ahead of us. Considering the power of the term laser to stimulate individuals' imaginations, the potential for harm if lasers are applied willy-nilly, is very great—and that is no joking matter.

Lest it be said that the author is somehow categorically opposed to the use of such devices in refractive surgery, he will go on record by stating that the potential of the laser for such use is high and some of the early work is promising despite certain disappointments. It is further averred that the author expects lasers will play an important, and possibly dominant, role in such surgery in the future. However, let the record also show that none of the early results reported justify the hype surrounding such application. The public as well as the ophthalmologist are ill-served by a self-serving media blitz. The question *cui bono*?

cannot yet be answered, the patient. The situation surrounding the laser in refractive surgery does not duplicate that of the introduction of radial keratotomy (RK) but it is ironic that RK is being held up as a standard for the results of laser surgery to emulate. It is even more ironic that many of the self-same individuals who, in the recent past, called for radical controls on RK, have decried controls being laid upon the lasers with which they have a closely held interest: an example of the NIH (not invented here) syndrome.

It is the purpose of this chapter, not to view lasers enigmatically but to shed some light (no pun intended) on these fascinating devices and their possible application in refractive surgery. To that end, we will outline the physical properties of the laser—what makes it go, as it were—and the effect of such amplified light, good and bad, upon living tissue. In addition, we will share with you some of the techniques currently being applied to the corneal surface to modulate its shape along with their results, as well as provide a glimpse of some laser technology still to come.

The beginning of lasers

Lasers evolved as an off-shoot of work on microwave amplifying devices called masers—another acronym, this time meaning *m*icrowave *a*mplification by *s*timulated *e*mission of *r*adiation. At first they were called optical masers because they amplified light in much the same way that masers amplified microwaves. Arthur L. Schawlow and C.H. Townes are given credit for the idea which they originally proposed in 1958, although similar concepts are said to have been under development in the Soviet Union at that time [1]. The first practical laser, using ruby, was built and operated in the USA in 1960 by Theodore H. Maiman (see below) [2]. This was followed in 1961 by the first continuous laser—again in the USA—by Ali Javan. In fact, the USA has led the way in laser research since that time with semiconductor lasers appearing in 1962 and liquid dye lasers in 1966 [3,4]. Various other types of gas, solid crystal, and tunable dye lasers have made their entrance upon the scientific stage in the ensuing years.

Fundamentals of laser mechanics

Lasers produce light, as do ordinary lamps, but lasers produce it with such intensity and spectral purity that laser light seems to have properties quite different from ordinary light. We seldom, however, notice the properties of light other than the visual. Even its heating effect, which is noticeable in direct sunlight (especially here in Arizona), is seldom appreciated under conditions of comfortable illumination. Therefore, the fact that certain types of coherent light can

burn holes through steel is cause for amazement even amongst the sophisticated. We have, all of us, been subject to He-Ne rapture* at one time in our careers. The reason for this seeming naiveté is that most of our interaction with light has been with its incoherent or anarchic form. If ever there was an example of "power through group action," that of laser light fits the bill. But all lasers are not created equal, they differ among themselves even more than ordinary light sources do. To understand the kinds of properties that lasers can have, and the properties that some lasers do have, we shall first look at how lasers operate and how they differ from all earlier sources of light.

Before the advent of lasers, essentially all light was generated by hot objects of one kind or another, whether it was the sun, a bonfire, a candle, a lantern or the filament in an incandescent lamp (see also Chapter 3). The light produced from such sources results from the discharge of energy which occurs when the electrons within the thermally excited atoms change state (Figure 11.1). An atom that is, for an instant, raised to some high energy level can drop back to a lower one, emitting the stored energy as a burst of light. If the energy released is large, the light quantum has a high frequency and a correspondingly short length. A smaller energy release corresponds to a longer wavelength and lower frequency.

The wavelengths emitted by any particular substance depend upon the energy levels of that substance. However, every substance has many energy levels as well, and so it is usual for sources to emit many, or even a continuous distribution of wavelengths of light. If a single pure color of light is needed, however, it can only be obtained by filtering out all the rest of the wavelengths. When that happens, usually there is not much power remaining in the narrow region of the desired wavelength. A laser, on the other hand, can emit all its power as a nearly pure single wavelength or frequency.

In ordinary light sources, the individual atoms radiate quite independently as they are excited. This has several consequences, one of which is that a light ray is as likely to emerge in one direction as in any other; and so the light is always emitted nearly equally in all directions. Such light is called incoherent light, for obvious reasons. Ordinary light sources are really not very powerful, although some of them appear very bright. Lasers, however, generate light that is highly coherent and hence very intense.

When two light waves arrive simultaneously at the

---

* This term was coined to describe the tendency of the ophthalmic surgeon who—so taken with the sight of posterior capsule being blasted to bits under the focus spot—keeps pushing the button on the YAG laser until all remnants of capsule have been totally vaporized.

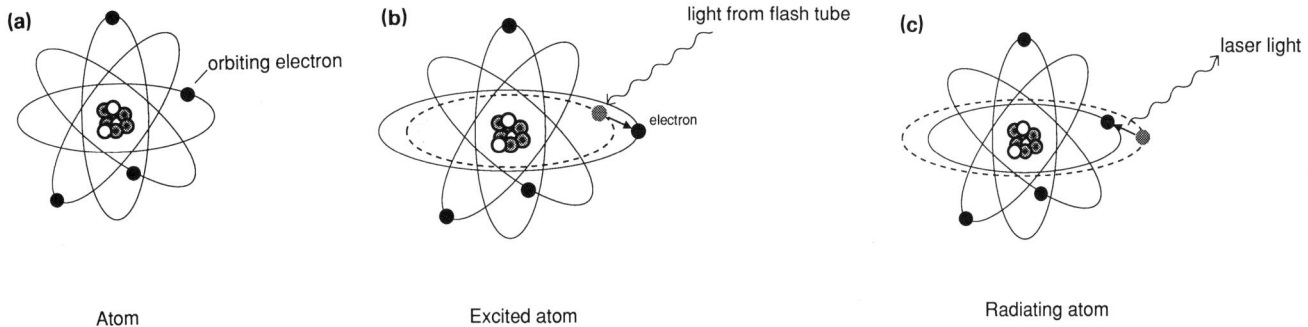

Fig. 11.1 (a) Typical atomic structure; (b) a photon striking an orbiting electron causes it to jump up one level; (c) when the electron spontaneously jumps back to its original level (decays), a photon is emitted.

same place they may add to or subtract from the resultant intensity. This phenomenon, called interference, has already been discussed in Chapter 3, and so will not be repeated here. However, as pointed ou. there, it is this very fact of interference that explains lasers, and that drives them. The essence of the laser is to stimulate the emission of light by encouraging constructive or additive interference. It does so because the many individual atoms are forced to emit in phase, instead of being allowed to emit randomly. This forcing is the process of stimulated emission of radiation, which was predicted theoretically by Einstein in 1917. If, during the brief interval that an atom is excited, a photon from a similar atom reaches it, the arriving photon will stimulate the excited atom to emit radiation. The induced radiation will have the same frequency, wavelength, and phase as the stimulating photon or wave. As the wave passes through a medium that contains many excited atoms, the resultant wave becomes amplified by this process of stimulated emission.

The reason why the laser is not found in nature (at least in our current singularity) is that the probability of spontaneous emission is usually so high in comparison with that of induced emission that the possibility of an electron staying in an excited level long enough to be induced to a lower level is slight. In the laser, electrons are raised into so-called meta-stable states—a population inversion is created. These states are of higher energy than the ground state but are restricted by the laws of quantum mechanics, so that the probability of spontaneous emission to the ground state is very low—the reverse of the normal situation. In fact, transitions to the ground state from these levels are forbidden (see also Chapter 3). Hence the term meta-stable—the atom is in an almost stable configuration. Because the probability of its spontaneously decaying to a lower level is so slight, the probability of induced emission is greater than the probability of spontaneous emission. All that is needed is a supply of photons of the proper wavelength to stimulate the atoms to emit coherent light.

Some substances can either absorb certain wavelengths or amplify them, depending on what fraction of their atoms is excited. If the medium is not excited and all the atoms are in their lower energy states, radiation can only be absorbed. If more than half the atoms are excited into the upper state, amplification exceeds absorption. This phenomenon never occurs for a system of atoms in equilibrium at any temperature, no matter how high, however—otherwise the universe and everything in it would have burnt to a crisp long ago (recall the ultraviolet catastrophe discussed in Chapter 3). Thermal agitation does excite atoms but always leaves more of them in the lower state than in the higher. If the temperature is sufficiently high, significant numbers of molecules will be found in upper levels. The distribution of atoms within these levels is described by Boltzman's distribution—a higher energy level always has fewer atoms populating it than a lower level. Fortunately, it turns out not to be too difficult to force or pump most of the atoms into an excited state—akin to beating a wasp's nest with a stick. Once excited, the atoms do not hold their energy for very long—usually for only a small fraction of a second (in contra-distinction to wasps)—before losing it by spontaneous or stimulated emission or in some other way. Thus, the amplifying stage, with more than half the atoms in the upper energy state, must be created and maintained by some kind of vigorous pumping.

A number of different ways have been found to accomplish this pumping, and they have been applied to many materials. It turns out that it is possible to obtain amplification by stimulated emission of radiation at wavelengths throughout the visible spectrum with some materials and far into the ultraviolet and infrared regions with others. Thus, if we have a coherent light wave, it can be amplified by stimulated emission. However, in almost all lasers, the amplification is used as part of the process of generating a coherent wave from atoms that are randomly excited. To do this, we must enclose the excited atoms in some suitable kind of resonator.

Masers

Masers utilized a metallic box called a cavity resonator that would store (or fit) just one particular microwave and no other. This box can be of a practical size since typical microwaves have a wavelength of 1.0 cm or so. If excited atoms or molecules that can emit this particular wavelength are put into the box, any radiation they emit will be stored within the resonator. This stored radiation (which is ricocheting around within the enclosure) then stimulates other atoms or molecules to emit their energy as radiation at the same wavelength and phase as the stored wave. Soon the stored wave is strong enough so that stimulated emission occurs before the atoms have any chance to emit spontaneously and then essentially all the radiation becomes coherent. A small amount of the radiation is allowed to leak out through a coupling hole to provide the maser's output, but enough is retained in the resonator at any given instant to continue the process as long as excited atoms or molecules are supplied.

Visible light, on the other hand, has a wavelength much shorter—by about some 20 000 times—than the centimeter-length radio waves, so it is not practical to build a resonator as small as the wavelength; and, even if it were, the box would not be large enough to hold many atoms. Therefore, the laser's resonator is made to a more convenient size, which can range in length from a millimeter to some meters, but is always many times larger than the wavelength of the light itself. Such a box, if it were constructed like the microwave cavity resonator, could sustain waves of almost any length, going in almost any direction, and would not select any waves to store and amplify and hence would be essentially useless for our purposes.

For these reasons a laser uses a resonator that has convenient dimensions but is of a special kind. It can be thought of as cavity (box) resonator with all of the box, except the two end walls, discarded. The laser structure is, therefore, typically a long rod or column of some active material, with mirrors at the ends of the column. This is a satisfactory resonator for any wave that travels along the long axis of the structure. Such a wave can zip back and forth between the mirrors, gaining energy by stimulating emission from the excited atoms as it goes. If one of the end mirrors has been made partly transparent, some of this stimulated light can leak out through it. This laser structure was first proposed by Schawlow and Townes in 1958 and is used in almost all examples of these devices.

Properties of laser light

From the structure of a typical laser, we can easily deduce the properties of laser light. The light emerging from a laser will be a highly directional beam, since a

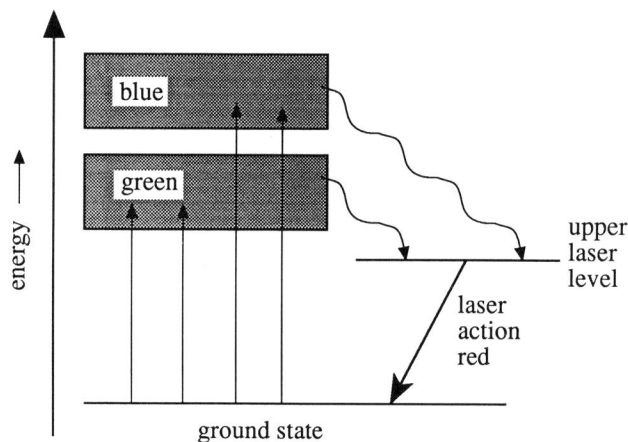

Fig. 11.2 Ruby laser meta-stable state.

wave can remain in the active medium long enough to be built up appreciably only if it is traveling along the axis of the resonator. Such a beam is intense because the atoms are stimulated to emit much faster than they ordinarily would. The beam of light is also usually monochromatic because the condition for amplification is satisfied only, or at least most strongly, at a single wavelength. Finally, the laser light beam is coherent because all the atoms are stimulated to emit in synchrony with the photons that are flailing about between the mirrors.

The first laser to be built and operated was constructed by T.H. Maiman in 1960, who used a solid rod of pink ruby (an aluminum oxide crystal containing 0.05% chromium ions in place of the equivalent number of aluminum ions). The chromium ions in ruby can absorb and be excited by either green or blue light, and these excited atoms quickly drop down to a resting meta-stable state (Figure 11.2). This meta-stable state has a lifetime of about 3 ms at room temperature, and atoms might accumulate for a while when the pumping light is first turned on. However, atoms in the meta-stable state can spontaneously emit red light at a wavelength of 694.3 nm. This is in the very deep red portion of the spectrum at a wavelength so long that the typical eye is only about 1/200th as sensitive to it as it is to green. However, the pumping process is so efficient and the intensity of the beam so high that the red beam can be easily seen when the laser is operating.

In this, as in many other solid-state lasers the mirrors are placed directly on the ends of the solid rod, which have been polished flat and parallel to each other. The exciting light is an intense flash from a xenon-arc lamp, much like those used in a photographer's strobe light. If enough light has been received from the pumping lamp during the few milliseconds that chromium ions remain in the meta-stable state, enough excited ions are accumulated so that amplification by stimulated emission begins. A laser beam is then set up and emerges through one of the partially silvered ends of the rod. Because a very bright lamp is required to produce enough excited atoms in the short time available, the first ruby laser (and many subsequent solid-state lasers) operated only in a short burst, lasting for about 0.5 ms. However, during this burst the power output is extremely large, being typically of the order of 1000–10 000 W and confined to a relatively narrow beam with a divergence of about 0.01 rad (0.5°).

The construction of a typical optically pumped solid crystalline laser is shown in Figure 11.3. The flash-lamps are placed close to the rod and surrounded by a reflector which concentrates the light on to the rod. This same structure can be used to produce different wavelengths and different power levels, depending on the individual materials used within the rod. Two of the other commonly used solid-state materials incorporate neodymium ions rather than chromium, in either suitably doped glass or a crystal of yttrium–aluminum–garnet (YAG). The neodymium ion lasers emit radiation in the near infrared at a wavelength of 1000 nm (1.06 µm). Both ruby and neodymium lasers produce radiation that can be transmitted through the transparent parts of the eye and so can be used in eye surgery, or can cause eye damage if carelessly applied. Some other types of lasers operate far into the infrared and produce light that is absorbed in the outer parts of the eye and thus are suitable for surface applications.

When the light from such a pulsed laser is focused with a lens, it produces a small spot of very high intensity. For example, if the focal length of the lens is f and the angular divergence of the laser is q, measured in radians (1 rad = 57.3°), the diameter of the spot at the focus is equal to fq. Its area is, therefore,

$$\frac{\pi f^2 q^2}{4}.$$

Thus, the power density in this focal spot is power divided by the area, that is,

$$\frac{4P}{f^2 q^2}.$$

As a typical example, if the laser delivers 1000 W during its brief flash, the divergence is 0.01 rad, and the focal length of the lens is 2 cm, then the power density is 3×10^6 W/cm^2. If this focus occurs in a transparent medium, there is negligible absorption and nothing noticeable happens. However, if the focus occurs on the surface of an opaque medium, the power may be absorbed to a very small depth and consequently in a very small volume. For example, an opaque material such as carbon will absorb the light at a distance of about 10.5 cm, and within the absorbing surface layer the power density would be, in the laser

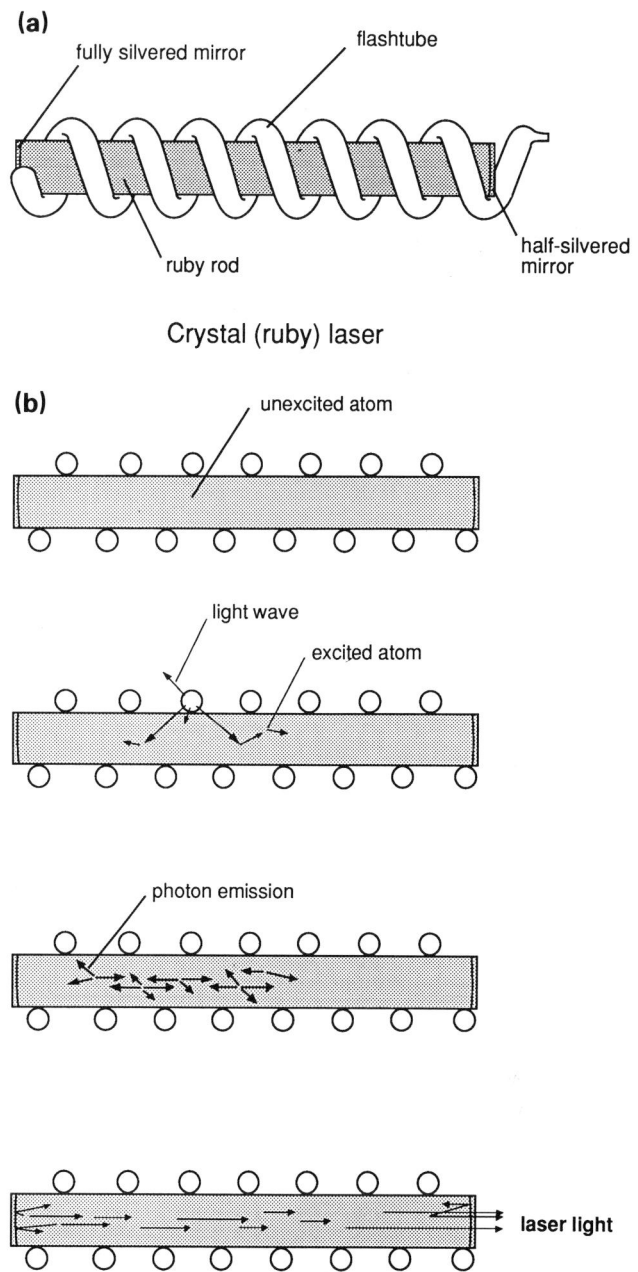

Fig. 11.3 Typical solid or crystalline (ruby) laser construction and action.

of our example, about 10^{11} W/cm^3. This is a very high value and the material would be immediately heated to incandescence and a portion of the surface would vaporize.

Few biologic materials are as opaque as that, however, and the effect of the laser is to heat a small portion of the tissue to some moderately high temperature. For example, when the laser is used in retinal surgery, the light traverses the clear parts of the eye with little absorption until it strikes the pigment epithelium of the retina, where it is absorbed and converted to heat. The degree of heating in this small focal spot can be controlled by adjusting the power of the laser or by defocusing the lens.

The pulse of light from most lasers does not deliver very much energy, but if the power is concentrated, so is the energy. It is the total energy delivered per unit volume that determines the heating effect of the absorbed beam. For example, it requires 1 cal or 4.18 J to heat 1 ml of water through 1°C. It requires 620 cal or about 2600 J/ml to heat water from room temperature to 100°C—to boil it. A typical small, pulsed ruby laser might deliver an energy of 0.025 J in a pulse lasting about 0.5 ms. With this as an example, if the laser light pulse is absorbed in a volume of 0.0001 ml, the energy density is 2500 J/ml, which is just sufficient to vaporize most of the water in the target volume. If it is absorbed in a larger volume, the temperature rise will be less, and there will be no boiling.

It is important to note that the effects of pulsed laser heating can be extremely localized. If one were to apply the heat slowly, much of it would be conducted away into surrounding material and would heat a larger volume than was desired. A short pulse, however, can produce its effects by heating the absorbing target so quickly that the event is over before the heat has had a chance to spread out appreciably. It is hard to get used to just how very rapid the laser heating can be. Perhaps it is best visualized by noting that the sudden heating can vaporize dark, light-absorbing ink off a sheet of paper without harming the paper underneath or even remove carbon ink from a rubber balloon without damaging the balloon, or even human skin when used to remove tattoos, or eye liner.

Since biologic tissues have characteristic wavelengths at which they absorb or do not absorb light, it would be desirable to be able to choose the wavelength for the purpose at hand. In principle, this can be done by choosing the right material, although there is no simple rule to say which material will work at which wavelength.

Solid lasers

The reason why solid laser materials are especially effective for pulsed operation is that they have a much higher density than a gas and so can have more active ions and store more energy to be released in the laser pulse. In the sort of laser that has been described, this pulse typically lasts about 0.5 ms or 500 μs. However, there is a method that permits the energy to be released in a much shorter and therefore much more intense pulse, typically millions of waves for some billionths of a second. This is the technique called Q-switching, whereby the quality factor of the resonator is altered during the pumping cycle. It can be visualized as shown in Figure 11.4, where one of the mirrors is removed from one end of the rod and a shutter is interposed between the mirror and the rod. Initially the shutter is closed as the flashlamp begins to pump light into the rod and thereby excite some of the active ions. After a short interval, enough ions are excited so that laser action would begin, except that the mirror is blocked and the laser action is incomplete. It is thus possible to go on exciting more ions without starting the laser action, so that a large number of ions can be accumulated in the excited state—a mechanism akin to that of a capacitor. Then the shutter is suddenly opened so that the laser action is complete and the energy is released in one giant short pulse—capacitor discharge (Figure 11.5).

There are a number of different ways of making the shutter. It can be a mechanical shutter. For instance, the mirror may rotate so that it is parallel to the other mirror for only a short interval. An electro-optical shutter, such as a liquid Kerr cell or a solid Pockels cell, may also be used. One of the simplest ways to provide Q-switching is to use a bleachable dye, either solid or liquid. For ruby, the dye might typically be some blue material such as cryptocyanine in solution contained in a glass cell of optical quality. This dye strongly absorbs the red light and prevents any spontaneous light emitted by a ruby rod from reaching the mirror. However, it is rather easily bleached, and when sufficient spontaneous ruby light has reached the dye cell, it bleaches sufficiently to let the red light pass to the mirror and the giant pulse begins. Q-switched lasers have delivered pulses as high as 1 billion watts, with a duration of perhaps 5–10 ns (billionths of a second). With some refinements, even shorter pulses, as short as 0.001 ns (1 ps), have been generated by a technique known as mode locking.

Mode locking

Despite the purity of the light produced by laser action, the nature of the process is such that inhomogeneity exists within the beam. Regardless that these inhomogeneities may be small, they are sufficient to degrade the quality of the beam. Thus, some method must be employed to improve beam quality. One method of doing this is through a process known as mode locking. Mode locking is a technique for producing periodic, high-power, short-duration laser pulses. It can be either active or passive in nature. Active mode locking uses a shutter mechanism which opens at regular intervals corresponding to the cavity round-trip time of one of the many laser modes—with an Nd:YAG such pulses are about 50 ps in duration. Any other modes are damped.

Passive mode locking is accomplished by using certain dyes whose absorption decreases with increasing irradiance. A dye is chosen with an absorp-

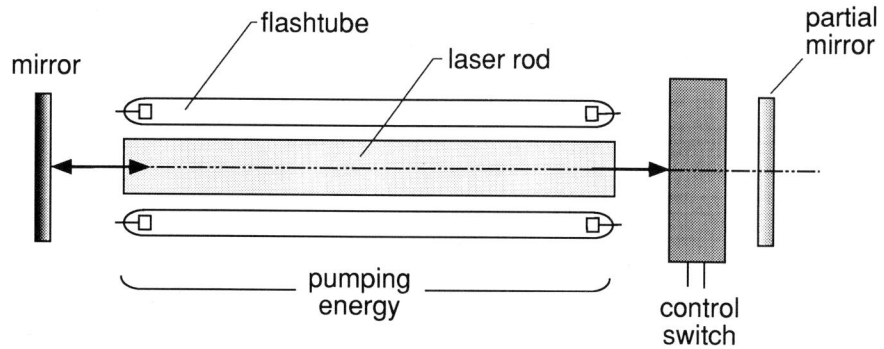

Fig. 11.4 Switched laser.

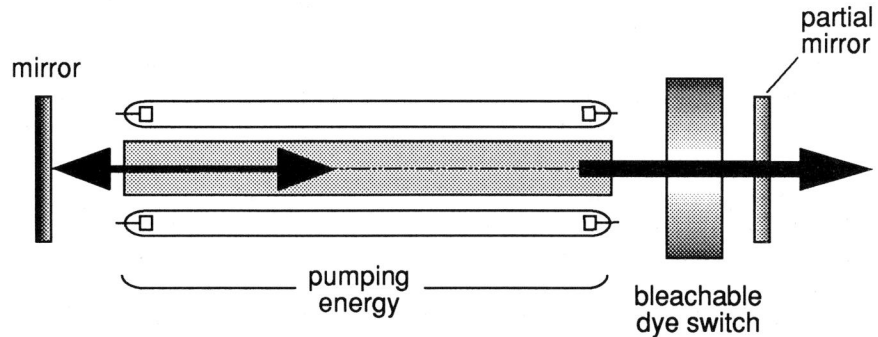

Fig. 11.5 Dye laser.

tion band at the lasing transition frequency. Such a dye (cryptocyanine, for example) is called a saturable absorber. At low light levels, the dye is opaque. As the number of excited molecules increases, a point is reached when the dye becomes transparent or bleached and a laser pulse is emitted (Figure 11.6). Initially, the laser medium emits spontaneous radiation which gives rise to incoherent fluctuations in the beam energy density. Some of these fluctuations may be amplified to such an extent that the peak part of the fluctuation is passed by the saturable absorber with little attenuation. The low-power parts of the fluctuation are more highly attenuated thus a high-power pulse can grow within the cavity, providing the dye has a short recovery period. Typically, when a saturable absorber is used to mode lock a laser, the laser is simultaneously Q-switched.

Q-switching [5]

Q-switching is another technique for obtaining short, intense bursts of oscillation from lasers. First it should be understood that the term Q is used to represent the quality factor of the laser resonating chamber. Q can be defined in general by the expression:

$$Q = \frac{2\pi \cdot \text{stored energy}}{\text{dissipated energy per cycle}}$$

or

$$Q = \frac{\text{resonant frequency}}{\text{linewidth}} = \frac{v}{\Delta v}$$

Single high-power pulses can be obtained by introducing time- or energy-dependent losses into the cavity. The effects of such losses can be interpreted in terms of spiking oscillations. If there is initially a very high loss in the laser cavity, the gain due to population inversion can reach a very high value, without laser oscillations occurring. The high loss prevents laser action while energy is being pumped into the excited state of the medium. If, when a large population inversion has been achieved, the cavity loss is suddenly reduced (i.e. the cavity Q is swiched to a high value), laser oscillations will suddenly commence. On Q-switching, the threshold gain decreases immediately (to the normal value associated with a cavity of high Q) while the actual gain remains high because of the large population inversion. Owing to the large difference between the actual and the threshold gain, laser action within the cavity builds up very rapidly and all of the available energy is emitted in a single large pulse. This quickly depopulates the upper lasing level to such an extent that the gain is reduced below threshold and the lasing action stops. The time variation of some of the laser parameters during Q-switching is shown schematically in Figure 11.7.

Q-switching dramatically increases the peak power obtainable from lasers. In the ordinary pulsed mode, the output of an insulating crystal laser such as the

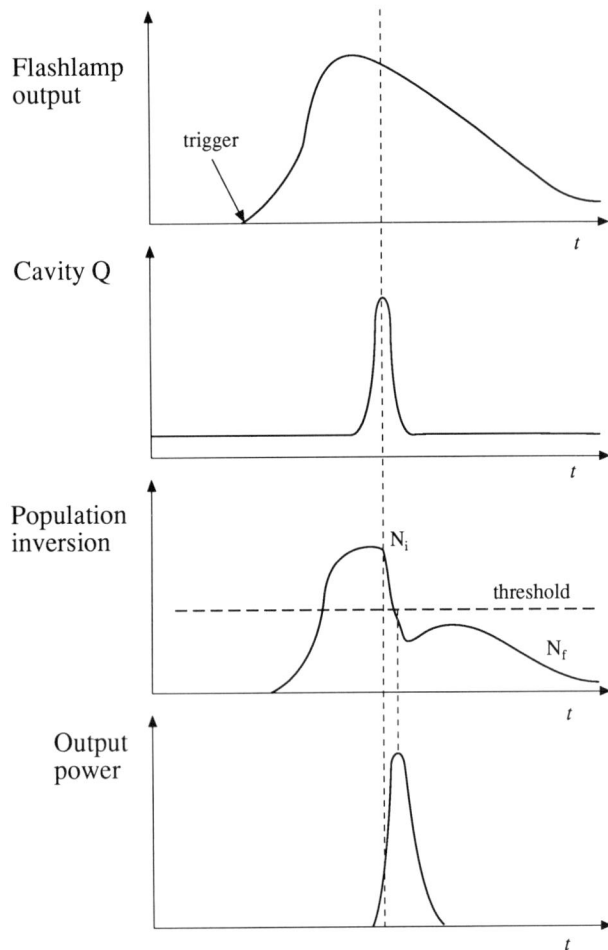

Fig. 11.6 Principle of Q-switching (from Wilson J, Hawkes JFB. *Optoelectronics, An Introduction.* Simon and Schuster, Cambridge, pp 227–230, 1989).

Nd:YAG consists of many random spikes of about 1 μs duration with a separation of about 1 μs; the length of the train of spikes depends principally on the duration of the exciting flashtube source, which may

be about 1 ms. Peak powers within the spikes are typically of the order of kilowatts. When the laser is Q-switched, however, the result is a single spike of great power, typically in the megawatt range, with a duration of 10–100 ns. It should be noted that, although there is a vast increase in the peak power of a Q-switched laser, the total energy emitted is less than in non-Q-switched operation owing to losses associated with the Q-switching mechanism. Q-switching is carried out by placing a closed shutter (i.e. the Q-switch) within the cavity, thereby effectively isolating the cavity from the laser medium. After the laser has been pumped, the shutter is opened, so restoring the Q of the cavity. A little thought reveals that there are two important requirements for effective Q-switching. These are:

1 The rate of pumping must be faster than the spontaneous decay rate of the upper lasting level, otherwise the upper level will empty more quickly than it can be filled so that a sufficiently large population inversion will not be achieved.

2 The Q-switch must switch rapidly in comparison to the buildup of laser oscillations, otherwise the latter will build up gradually and a longer pulse will be obtained, so reducing the peak power.

In practice, the Q-switch should operate in a time less than 1 ns.

Rotating mirror method

This method, which was the first to be used, involves rotating one of the mirrors at a very high angular velocity such that the optical losses are large except for the brief interval in each rotation cycle when the mirrors are very nearly parallel. Just before this point is reached a trigger mechanism initiates the flashlamp discharge to pump the laser. As the mirrors are not yet parallel, population inversion can build up without laser action starting. When the mirrors become parallel,

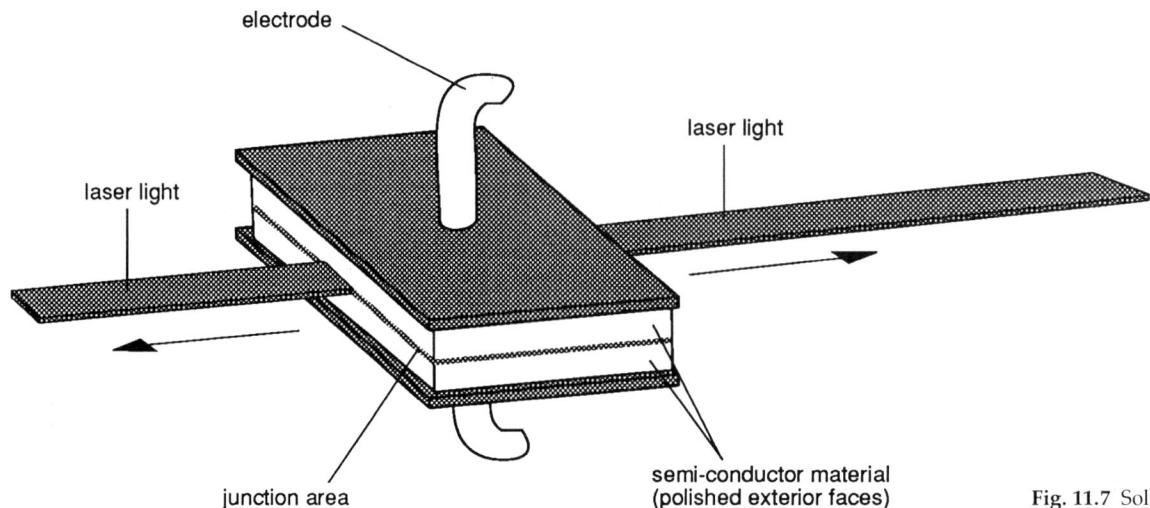

Fig. 11.7 Solid-state laser.

Q-switching occurs, allowing the Q-switched pulse to develop, as illustrated in Figure 11.6.

The repetition rate of laser firing is determined by control of the flashlamp and not by the speed of rotation of the mirror, which may be very high. If the laser fired every revolution, the repetition rate would be $\cong$ 1000 times per second, a rate which is prohibitive as excessive heating of the laser rod would occur. Although rotating mirror-type Q-switches are cheap, reliable, and rugged, the method suffers from the major disadvantage of being slow. This results in an inefficient production of Q-switched pulses with lower peak power than can be produced by other methods.

Electro-optic, magneto-optic and acousto-optic modulators can be used as fast Q-switches. If a Pockels cell (a doubly refractive crystal whose refractive state changes when an electrical current is applied; in a Kerr cell light produces the change), for example, is used and the laser output is not naturally polarized, then a polarizer must be placed in the cavity along with the electro-optic cell. A voltage is applied to the cell which converts the linearly polarized into circularly polarized light. The laser mirror reflects this light and in so doing reverses its direction of rotation so that on re-passing through the electro-optic cell it emerges as plane polarized light, but at 90° to its original direction of polarization. This light is therefore not transmitted by the polarizer and the cavity is switched off. When the voltage is reduced to zero, there is no rotation of the plane of polarization and Q-switching occurs. The change of voltage, which is synchronized with the pumping mechanism, can be accomplished in less than 10 ns and very effective Q-switching occurs. Alternative arrangements using Kerr cells and acousto-optic modulators are available. In the case of the acousto-optic modulator, an acoustic signal applied to the modulator deflects some of the beam out of the cavity, thereby creating a high loss. When the sound wave is shut off, Q-switching occurs as before. Acousto-optic devices are often used when the laser medium is continuously pumped and repetitively Q-switched, as is frequently the case with Nd:YAG and carbon dioxide lasers.

Passive Q-switching

Passive Q-switching may be accomplished by placing a saturable absorber (bleachable dye) in the cavity. At the beginning of the excitation the dye is opaque, thereby preventing laser action and allowing a larger population inversion to be achieved than would otherwise be the case. Passive Q-switching has the great advantage of being extremely simple to implement, involving nothing more than a dye in a suitable solvent held in a transparent cell. Suitable dyes include cryptocyanine for ruby lasers and sulfur hexafluoride

for carbon dioxide lasers. Lasers that use a saturable absorber for Q-switching are also mode-locked if the dye, once bleached, recovers in a short time compared with the duration of the mode-locked pulses (see section on mode locking, above).

Non-linear laser operation

With the giant pulse from a Q-switched laser, the effects of the light can no longer be considered as simple heat. The light is an electromagnetic wave and the electric field at the focus of these intense pulses can be as much as millions of volts per centimeter or even more. This electric field increases as the square root of the power density and is equal to 1 million V/cm at a power level of 10^{10} or 10 billion W/cm^2. At a power density much above this, and one that can easily be obtained by focusing a Q-switched laser, a spark breakdown can be obtained in open air. Moreover, many othewise transparent materials act in a manner referred to as non-linear at these power levels. The non-linearity refers to the relationship between the electric field and its immediate effect—the electric displacement. In a non-linear medium it is possible to generate true optical harmonics that have twice or three or more times the frequency of the incident light with correspondingly short wavelengths. Thus, a red light can be converted to ultraviolet, and under some circumstances a very large fraction of this light can be so converted. Intense high-frequency vibrations may be set up inside transparent media under some conditions. This is all very well except that this non-linear transformation may be into a frequency range that is more detrimental than useful. Case in point—193 nm ultraviolet. Some investigators have noted that tissue treated with this wavelength often glows with a visible blue color.

The explanation of non-linear effects lies in the way in which a beam of light propagates through a solid. The nuclei and associated electrons of the solid form electric dipoles. The electromagnetic radiation interacts with these dipoles causing them to oscillate which in turn causes the dipoles themselves to act as sources of electromagnetic radiation. If the amplitude of the vibration is small, the dipoles emit radiation of the same frequency as the inciting radiation. If this radiation is intense (irradiance increases), the relationship between this intensity increase and the induced dipole vibration becomes non-linear, resulting in the generation of harmonics of the original radiation. Thus frequency doubling or second harmonic generation (or higher) occurs.

Non-linear optics is a very large and complicated subject, and there are many possible phenomena that have been investigated in some simple materials, and are becoming reasonably well-understood, but that have not been much explored in biologic material. It is quite conceivable that such high-power lasers, emitting red light, could produce the chemical and biologic effects of ultraviolet light inside some material that the ultraviolet itself could not penetrate. Some chemical reactions that ordinarily require ultraviolet light have been demonstrated to be producible by intense red light. Lest anyone think that these effects are to be feared at all power levels, however, it must be pointed out that many of these effects have a threshold and they do not occur at all below this threshold power level. It seems fairly certain that at power levels of a kilowatt or so most of the effects observed in most materials can be understood simply as rapid heating effects, without specifically considering the electro-magnetic and non-linear phenomena.

The processes of non-linear optics can be used to generate new wavelengths from existing lasers. With care, relatively high conversion efficiencies can be obtained even at levels so low that non-linear effects in most materials are not ordinarily noticeable. Special non-linear materials such as lithium niobate and barium sodium niobate have been used to generate optical harmonics, producing green light from the infrared neodymium glass or garnet lasers. In this way, continuous or repetitively pulsed lasers with average powers of the order of 1 W in the green can be constructed. The non-linear material also makes it possible to construct tunable laser-type devices. Basically, these consist of some kind of a driving laser and a converter that converts the light to other desired wavelengths.

Gaseous lasers

One of the simplest kinds of lasers is that using a gas discharge of the sort common to a neon sign or a related electrical discharge at a different pressure and voltage condition. The gas-discharge laser consists of a long narrow tube, containing the gas or mixture of gases, with mirrors at the end of this column. No separate pumping lamp is needed. The first of these gas-discharge lasers pulsed a mixture of helium and neon gas (He–Ne), with about 10 times as much helium as neon. The combined effect of these two gases is strongly to excite a few particular levels in neon during the discharge, so that laser action can be obtained at several wavelengths in the infrared and visible regions. The exact wavelength is usually determined by coating the mirrors to be good reflectors for only a particular wavelength and not for other possible wave-lengths that the medium can amplify. Most often, these He–Ne lasers are operated in the visible orange-red region at a wavelength of 632.8 nm. He–Ne lasers are very commonly used as aiming beams for other laser systems as well as for other devices and purposes.

Small He–Ne lasers give power outputs of the order of 1 mW, which produces a small, bright-appearing spot on a white surface but is not intense enough to do much burning. For example, such a laser can be used to generate the coherent light beam used to measure an optical surface (see Chapter 6) or serve as a lecture pointer. A continuous beam of even 1 mW power has many other laboratory uses and demonstrates very easily the peculiar properties of coherent light. When the beam from a He–Ne laser or any other continuous visible laser illuminates a surface, the surface has an unusual characteristically grainy, sparkling appear-ance. This occurs because the light from the laser is coherent and any part of the wavefront can interfere with any other part of the wavefront constructively, adding up to a higher intensity, or destructively, pro-ducing a lower intensity. After the light is scattered by a rough surface, for instance a wall or a piece of paper, the waves from individual points spread out in all directions and overlap at many places in space and produce a three-dimensional interference pattern that the eye perceives. This complex interference pattern shifts when the eye is moved even slightly, so the surface appears to sparkle. However, if the *surface* is moving, even fairly slowly, the pattern is averaged out so that the graininess and sparkling disappear. The size of the sparkle pattern depends upon where the eye is focused, thus the pattern can be used as an indicator of the eye's focus.

He–Ne lasers can be built with power outputs as high as several hundred milliwatts, or even up to 1 W. However, it is usually easier to obtain such power levels from other gas-discharge lasers by means of higher currents, in narrower tubes and with lower pressures of gas. These lasers use such gases as argon, krypton, or xenon. The gas is ionized in the electrical discharge, and laser emission occurs from particular energy levels of ions. Krypton can produce a number of wavelengths from the red to the violet. Argon gas lasers can easily give 1 or more watts of green light at a wavelength of 488 nm. Argon lasers have been used for surgery of various kinds, because the focal spot is intense enough to produce rapid heating. Moreover, the wavelength of the argon laser is short enough and the power density in the absorbing region high enough to be strongly absorbed by hemoglobin so that the heating can be much more sharply localized. These gas lasers can also be pulsed either singly or repetitively, but their peak powers are usually not nearly as high as those from the solid-state lasers.

There are many other types of gas lasers that pro-duce light with wavelengths varying from the ultra-violet through the visible and infrared regions out even to the millimeter wavelength radio region. Most notable of these is the carbon dioxide laser, which operates in the infrared at a wavelength of 10.6 μm

(10 600 nm). This laser is relatively efficient, perhaps 30%, and can be made in large sizes.

Power outputs from several hundred to many thousand watts can be obtained in a well-directed beam. The carbon dioxide radiation is absorbed by almost every non-metallic material and can produce extremely intense heating and rapid burning, cutting, or drilling if high powers are used.

There are still other types of lasers, including optically pumped liquids. Some of these use solutions of organic dyes. Since many fluorescent dyes are known, it is possible to select one for any desired wavelength region in or near the visible portion of the spectrum. The output wavelength can even be controlled to some extent by varying the solvent or by mixing two dyes in different proportions. Fine control of the wavelength may require incorporating a prism or diffraction grating in the instrument to limit the wavelength distribution within the beam.

Semiconductor lasers

Semiconductor lasers have the appearance of a small transistor or rectifying diode but are made of materials such as gallium arsenide or indium antimonide (Figure 11.7). They can also be quite efficient, not requiring the pumping action of light but only an electric pulse, thus they are simpler to construct. Current solid-state diode lasers deliver 808 nm of laser light at various power levels. Most semiconductor lasers operate in the far red or infrared regions. However, semiconductor lasers are usually made only in small sizes; to obtain much power for more than a short instant requires that they be operated in arrays, using a considerable number of them. Some can be operated continuously, but most easily when they are cooled to temperatures well below room temperature. A typical single-diode laser operated at room temperature might give 10 000 pulses per second, each pulse lasting 1000 billionths of a second and having a peak power of about 10 W. The total energy in each pulse is thus about 1 millionth of a joule, and the average power over many pulses and intervals between them is about 0.001 W.

Clinical application of laser light

Lasers were used in ophthalmology almost as soon as they had become available. In 1961, Campbell and his group [6] began in New York and in 1962, fellow Kresge alumnus Chris Zweng [7] began in Palo Alto—both with a pulsed ruby laser. In 1966, L'Esperance and his group began their work with the argon laser in animals, carrying it into humans in 1968. Commercial argon lasers became available in 1971—the author purchased one of the first ones when he was director of the Laser and Fluorescein Angiography Clinic at

Table 11.1 The effective output wavelength of various lasers

Laser type	Wavelength (nm)
Excimer (F2)	157
Excimer (ArF)	193
Excimer (KrF)	248
Excimer (XeCl)	308
Helium–cadmium (He–Cd)	325
Nitrogen (N2)	327
Argon (Ar)	488/514.5
Krypton (Kr)	458/548/647
Copper vapor (Cu)	510.6/578.2
Rhodamine G	560–640
Gold vapor	627.8
Helium–neon (He–Ne)	632.8
Ruby	694.3
Gallium arsenide	905
Neodymium:YAG (Nd:YAG)	1064
Erbium	1228
Hydrogen fluoride (HF)	2900
Erbium:YAG (Er:YAG)	2900
Color center	2900
Raman	2900
Carbon dioxide	10600

Harper Hospital in Detroit. The year 1971 also saw the first work being done with the krypton and frequency-doubled Nd:YAG lasers at Harkness Eye Institute. In Detroit, Beckman was doing work with the carbon dioxide laser and in 1973, Krasnow performed the first laser trabeculectomy with a Q-switched ruby laser.

Medical laser applications are big business. Millions of dollars have been expended to produce instrumentation to meet (or stimulate) market demand. With the current interest in these devices to modify corneal curvature, the game has often been played with something less than the full spirit of fair play and occasionally divorced from the scientific spirit as well. However, the rapid technologic development continues despite the concern expressed that method patents issued to single persons and companies would discourage diverse corporate investment and hamper investigation by a broad range of researchers [8].

Tissue response to light energy

Before we get too heavily involved in the details of lasers and their application in ophthalmology we need to consider the effect of light energy on living tissue. Light, much like oxygen, can produce profound cellular changes—many of them in the "not good" category. Case in point—skin cancer, or less ominous (but more painful), sunburn. Mutagenesis, however, is only part of the spectrum of interactions between cells and light—some reactions are more subtle and not all are bad.

Currently, we have available laser systems that alter tissue using photochemical, photothermal, or photo-

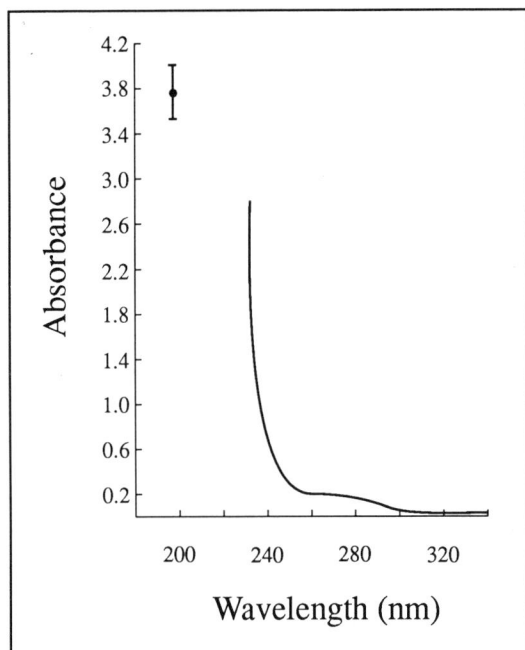

Fig. 11.8 Plot of absorbance versus wavelength in the far ultraviolet spectrum for bovine cornea. The point at 193 nm represents the average of laser transmission measurements made on eight different 32 μm thick samples. The error bar indicates 1 s.d. (from Puliafito CA, Steinert RF, Deutsch TF, Hillenkamp F, Dehm EJ, Adler CM. Excimer laser ablation of the cornea and lens. Experimental studies. Ophthalmology 1985; 92:741–748).

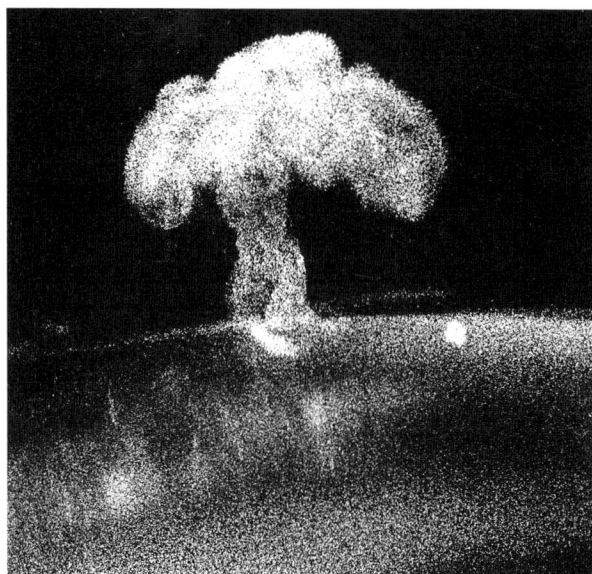

Fig. 11.9 Ablation plume during laser corneal photoablation at 193 nm (from Puliafito CA, Stern D, Krueger RR, Mandel ER. High-speed photography of excimer laser ablation of the cornea. Arch Ophthalmol 1987; 105(9):1255–9).

disruptive techniques. Photo-coagulation occurs when light energy is absorbed by the target tissue and converted to heat. The reaction can be anything from protein denaturization to carbonization to vaporization. Most ophthalmologists are familiar with the effects produced by the argon laser used to treat various forms of retinopathy and in laser trabeculectomy. There are newer laser tissue coagulators—among which are solid-state diode lasers—all providing energy in many forms. Dye lasers are available that have either continuous or pulsed output. Mid infrared solid-state crystal lasers deliver wavelengths anywhere from 1.96 μm (thulium:YAG) and 2.1 μm (holmium: YAG) to 3 μm (erbium:YAG)—all delivering useful wavelengths and energy fluxes.

The range of tunable systems is even wider. In addition, tunable lasers can deliver continuous output or pulsed energy, making them valuable for surgical tasks ranging from coagulation to controlled tissue ablation.

Excimer lasers, with pulsed output in the ultraviolet range, have a unique combination of properties that makes them suitable for corneal surgery at 193 nm as well as lens fragmentation and tissue drilling at 308 nm. These lasers operate through a singular process known as ablative photo-decomposition. Because organic materials have a strong absorbance for ultra-

violet radiation below 300 nm, this part of the light spectrum is very powerful in its ability to produce destructive effects within these tissues (Figure 11.8). Ultraviolet photons are highly energetic and can directly break chemical bonds—which is the key to their effectiveness, but also to their potential danger. Ultraviolet radiance breaks protein molecules into diatomic and triatomic fragments which, because of the tremendous energy transfer taking place, are blown clear of the illuminated area. These particles, by being blown away, take with them much of the surplus energy within the system and thus prevent more than minimal thermal damage to surrounding tissue (Figure 11.9).

The jury is still out on other forms of damage. Ultraviolet light is well-known to be both mutagenic and carcinogenic—we have mentioned skin cancer—its effects in the cornea are only now being examined [9–19]. Seiler's observation of secondary fluorescence of corneal tissue during excimer ablation is troubling [20], as is Clarke's finding of free radicals following laser angioplasty [21]. Nuss and co-workers concluded that 193 nm ultraviolet light has little if any mutagenic effect on corneal tissue [22]. However, effects such as cascading could elicit secondary ultraviolet wavelengths of a more deleterious nature [23].

Lasers currently under clinical evaluation and testing operate in ranges from the far ultraviolet to the mid infrared. Almost every wavelength region in the electromagnetic spectrum has a potential clinical application. Many factors, including variations in wavelength, continuous or pulsed delivery pattern, amount

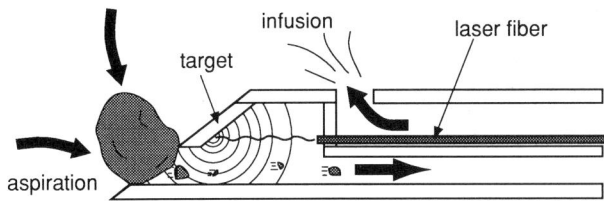

Fig. 11.10 Laser phakolysis.

of total energy out of total energy applied, and the delivery system of the laser light, will produce a wide range of clinical effects. Numerous studies examining these potential applications are legion; a few examples are listed here:

1 Researchers are injecting chromophores (indocyanine green) to enhance retinal vascular coagulation.
2 Successful filtering procedures are being done using pulsed laser light aimed gonioscopically into the angle, which has previously been saturated with methylene blue dye using iontophoresis. Absorption and ablation are sufficiently enhanced by the presence of the dye and the short laser pulses to produce a draining fistula.
3 Investigators seeking applications in general surgery have used light absorption by dye–fibrin mixtures stabilized in a viscous medium to seal blood vessels in animals and humans.
4 The corneal surface can be re-shaped to change its refracting properties through direct effect or through doping of the tissue with photo-reactive materials.
5 The laser might also possibly be used to remove cataracts (Figure 11.10).

Safety

Of course, new technical devices such as lasers also present us with moral, economic, and intellectual challenges. First, we must be mindful that lasers have unique hazards. As new wavelengths evolve, we must study not only unexpected effects of the laser light, but any other hazards associated with use of the instrument (see discussion above on ultraviolet lasers). Safety for the surgeon, surgical assistants, and any other operating room staff requires safety glasses tailored to the particular laser wavelength in use. The excimer is a typical example of a laser that introduces a new potential hazard. There is the small matter—with excimer lasers—of the extremely toxic fluorine gas used in these devices. Fluorine gas management is new in the clinical environment and requires special planning and laser design for safe use. Proper venting of the laser and the treatment room is essential—the toxicity of the gas is extremely high.

According to OSHA, delayed effects such as photo-retinitis, accelerated aging of biologic tissue, cataractogenesis, and carcinogenesis can result from laser exposure. Depending on the wavelength and exposure dose, these impairments can be irreversible. Laser side-effects can be initiated in three ways: thermally, photochemically, or both. They are thermally initiated in the infrared spectrum and photochemically initiated in the ultraviolet spectrum. In the visible blue end of the spectrum, both processes can begin. Factors that can contribute to undesirable effects include total exposure time, pulse duration, the various absorption spectra of different biologic systems, and wavelength. Regardless of the wavelength involved, there is a time-dependent and a wavelength-dependent effect. While exposure time determines the major risk factors for potential thermal damage from infrared laser light, wavelength still determines the relative penetration depth of the energy. Exposure time, by the rule of additivity, which applies to most photochemical damage mechanisms, a very low dose rate, or irradiance, may be potentially hazardous when accumulated over a full procedure. The safety limit for all ultraviolet lasers with wavelengths less than 310 nm, such as the argon fluoride or krypton fluoride, is probably at $3 \, mJ/cm^2$ per day.

Pulse duration

Short pulses allow very little time for heat flow, therefore depth of damage remains wavelength-dependent. But for continuous-wave lasers, such as the carbon dioxide, heat flow completely masks the selective absorption effects of the laser's very different penetration depths.

Absorption

During photoablation, the cornea absorbs 100 W of the energy from wavelengths shorter than 280 nm. It absorbs more than 90 W of photon energy when the wavelength increases to 300 nm, but about 1 photon in 50 reaches the lens. At 360 nm, the lens absorbs most photons.

Wavelength

Wavelengths much longer than 320 nm are not energetic enough to break bonds, and wavelengths shorter than 300 nm are absorbed by the cornea. So an acute cataract can result from only a narrow band of wavelengths. *In vitro* tests have shown that use of the 193 nm wave (excimer) is associated with very little evidence of mutagenesis or carcinogenesis. Both the penetration depth of the radiation and the absorption spectrum of the DNA in each cell determine how mutagenic a given wavelength of laser light will be, according to Seiler and colleagues [19]. In theory, they say, the penetration depth of laser radiation should be approximately one-half of a cell's diameter to enter the nucleus and to produce mutagenic effects. Seiler *et al.* further caution that even though we know that 193 nm is a very efficient wavelength for doing refractive and curative corneal ablation, we still have to keep in mind that while the risk of creating mutagenic effects is very small, it is not zero. The risk is also wavelength-dependent. The risk from 193 nm is 1000 to 10 000 times less than the risk from 248 nm radiation, for example [20].

Although reports on the mutagenicity of short-wave (193 nm) ultraviolet laser light are contradictory, no doubts exist as to the potential of 248 nm laser light to induce DNA repair mechanisms [19,20]. Light at 308 nm has a low threshold for the induction of cataract [25]. As secondary radiation (for reasons governed by physical laws in the longer wavelength range) is known to be emitted from the area of 193 nm laser light impact, a cataractogenic potential of far ultraviolet light cannot be completely excluded.

The Food and Drug Administration's biggest concern regarding excimer laser treatment of myopia was to rule out any association with excessive scarring, poor healing, or recurrent erosion despite the pre-clinical research used to establish the fluence levels and repetition rates. Although re-epithelialization has been shown to occur quickly after laser treatment and does not appear to be a problem, the mode of cell attachment is *not* wholly normal. For example, Bowman's layer does not re-form and is, instead, replaced by a pseudo-membrane. Endothelial injury has also been seen [26,27]. It is unlikely that this will prove to be a problem given the experience with RK. However, it must be remembered that the effects of light upon living tissue are insidious and incompletely understood. Two other questions have dominated the field of excimer laser ophthalmic surgery during the past several years:

1 Will the cornea heal transparently if the excimer laser is used to remove a portion of lamella that includes Bowman's layer?
2 Can refractive error be altered in a predictable manner by removing elements of Bowman's layer and stroma to a pre-determined configuration?

These questions have, at this writing, not been answered to general satisfaction. Corneal response and stability are also of concern. There may well be many similarities between laser wounding and diamond knife wounding, but Puliafito and co-workers suspect that there will probably be some surprises as we follow those patients receiving exposure to excimer laser for longer periods [28].

Excimer laser applications

High-power, pulsed ultraviolet laser light has been shown to etch precisely not only synthetic material

[29], but also biologic tissues, such as atherosclerotic lesions [30], hair and cartilage [31], and skin [32], and is also being considered for use in neurosurgery and angioplasty [33–35].

Depending upon which side of the fence you are standing on, the results of the current clinical excimer trials are either encouraging or discouraging. At this writing, the number of such patients is small, follow-up is limited, and questions about the safety and efficacy remain. The excimer has been used mostly as a refractive tool to date, specifically to correct myopia and astigmatism. Attempts have also been made to correct hyperopia, and there is considerable hype that some day the laser will be used to perform RK—which it may, but it has yet to achieve results that in any way surpass current methods.

Steve Trokel and the history of the excimer laser in ophthalmology*

Excimer lasers had their birth in 1975 when two physical chemists, Velazco and Setser, working at Kansas State University, noted that certain physical properties of the meta-stable states of rare gas atoms resembled those of the alkali metals [36]. They reported that they found a similarity of the chemical properties of meta-stable xenon atoms (Xe) to sodium and lithium in their ability to react with halogens (such as fluorine) to produce an unstable compound, Xe (fluorine, chlorine, etc.) [37–39]. The halogens fluorine and chlorine exist in a gaseous state under normal temperatures and are highly active. High pressure is necessary, however, because the so-called noble gases are a stand-offish lot whose atoms do not mix well with the madding crowd of other atoms—hence the name noble. However, under certain circumstances—such as high pressure—they are crowded together and they knock each other about sufficiently so as partially to ionize. In that state they can be induced to form unstable combinations with other atoms.

This noble gas–halogen compound rapidly dissociates to the ground state of the individual molecules with the release of an energetic ultraviolet photon—and therein lay the significance. Velazco and Setser inferred from this that the diatomic noble gas–halides were of special interest because "these bound-free emissions have considerable potential as ultraviolet laser systems for excitation of mixtures of Xenon (or other rare gases) and halogen containing compounds". Such a laser would have widespread application in the plastics industry as well as in designing and building of semiconductor systems. It has other intriguing

*The author is grateful to Steven Trokel, MD, for his gracious assistance and permission to use much of the material contained within this history, which is from his personal archives.

possibilities as well. All that was needed was a big enough stick to get the wasps moving.

A few months following their suggestion that this meta-stable compound could be used as the basis of a laser, four molecules, XeF, XeCl, XeBr, and KrF, were observed to undergo light amplification by stimulated emission when they were excited by an electron beam under proper conditions. Hoffman *et al.*, for example, in early 1976, observed laser action at "1933 Å" (193.3 nm) from the ArF molecule [40]. The energy source used to pump this laser was a 2 MeV electron beam with 6 kJ beam energy—a big stick indeed. This system was cumbersome, and of limited practical use for widespread experiments—linear accelerators are somewhat bulky. It was not until later that same year that sufficient experimentation showed that a more practical laser system could be constructed. Instead of requiring a linear accelerator to produce the electron beam, Burnham and Djeu demonstrated laser action with ArF in a relatively compact device using a transverse electric discharge akin to lightning [41]. The space required to house such a device was thus brought down from a building to room size.

Pre-ionized discharge had long been used in infrared molecular lasers, and Burnham's demonstration that the technology would work in the ultraviolet led to the development of practical ultraviolet lasers. Burnham and co-workers had used a modified Tachisto carbon dioxide laser for their work, so it was not surprising that Tachisto was the first company to market a laser designed to operate in the ultraviolet end of the spectrum. By the close of 1976, laser action had been demonstrated for the biologically important ultraviolet wavelengths from 193 nm using ArF to 351 nm using XeF.

As always, once something has been born, it is within human nature to christen it with a name. Nomenclature for these early ultraviolet lasers was mixed. The word excimer had been coined by Stevens and Hutton in 1960 as a contraction of excited dimer to describe an energized molecule with two identical components, hence it was a natural for this situation [42]. When analyzing the action of these lasers, it was thought that the argon molecule formed an excited dimer during the pre-ionization phase of its excitation. This was ultimately found not to be true, yet the term persisted. Alternative names have been used for these lasers and include rare gas–halide lasers, which describes the gas mixture in the cavity, and the name of the specific gas mixture, i.e. argon–fluoride laser, to describe a specific system. Another name was suggested when the actual lasing compound was recognized to be an excited complex molecule consisting of two different elements, the rare gas and the halide. Some workers suggested that this was best described as an excited molecular complex and the

word exciplex was coined to describe the lasers—but it does not "ring", if the truth be told. Excimer won through because it has the virtue of greater simplicity and the perversity of being first. The terms rare gas–halide and the specific gas lasing mixture continue to be used to describe these laser systems, nevertheless.

Subsequently, the potential medical and industrial applications of these new lasers were the subject of a meeting at the 1977 Optical Society of America. In the next few years, a great deal of discussion began appearing in the optical and electronic literature as well as in the press [43–46]. By 1978, both Tachisto and Lambda Physik (in Göttingen, Germany) were marketing excimer lasers for laboratory use.

Taboada and colleagues [47] were the first to investigate the ocular biological interactions of these new lasers. Tests were made on the response of rabbit epithelium to ArF exposures at the Laser Effects Branch of the Radiation Sciences Division at the USAF School of Aerospace Medicine. Taboada had considerable experience studying damage thresholds within the eye, having investigated the effects of mode-locked and Q-switched Nd:YAG laser pulses on ocular tissues in the past. ArF exposure on the rabbit cornea was noted to produce either opacification or fluorescein staining, which took the general shape of the laser beam distribution. In a subsequent study of the damage effects of 193 nm ArF on the eye, Taboada and Archibald reported the first studies of the interaction of this far ultraviolet light with the cornea, looking for damage similar to that produced by the ArF (248 nm) beam [48].

Steve Trokel, who had, at that time, considerable interest in lasers, especially Nd:YAG systems, was preparing a clinical monograph describing high-powered pulsed Nd:YAG lasers. He invited Taboada to contribute a chapter describing the effects of pulsed lasers on ocular tissues. Taboada accordingly sent him reprints of his published papers and a chapter for the monograph which included a more detailed description of the excimer laser–cornea interaction. Trokel's attention was immediately caught by a phrase Taboada used to describe the effect on the cornea of the ArF laser radiation at varying energy levels:

> At the higher levels, exposures of 27.5 mJ/cm² or greater, an immediate indentation of the corneal surface appeared taking the shape of the beam. One hour later, the surface indentation would "fill in."

Taboada postulated that the far ultraviolet light "was resonantly captured in random electromagnetic cavities formed by the microprojections of the anterior epithelial cell layer which may have caused a preferential temperature jump in this thin layer of tissue." That of course should have produced a swelling, not an indentation. His observation of an indentation

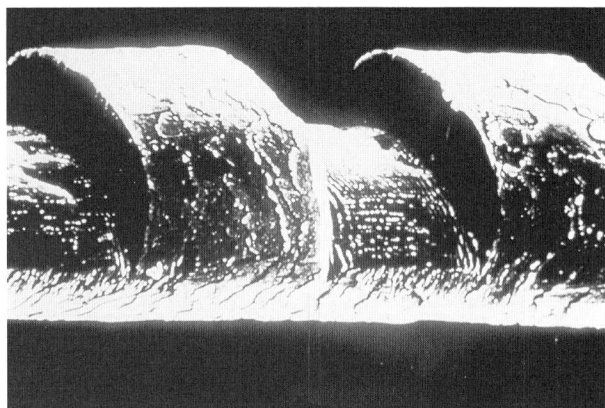

Fig. 11.11 Electron micrograph of grooves cut into a hair by an excimer laser.

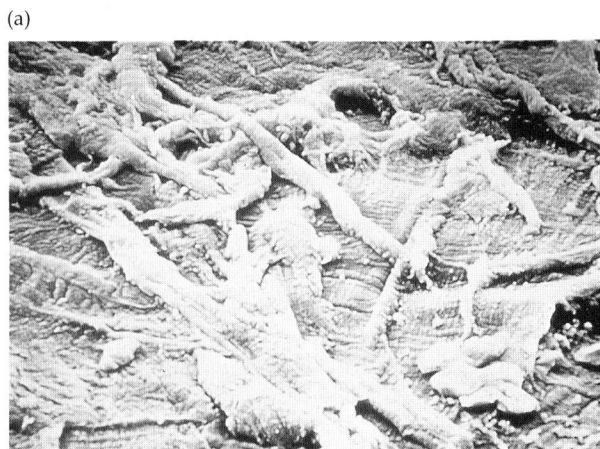

(a)

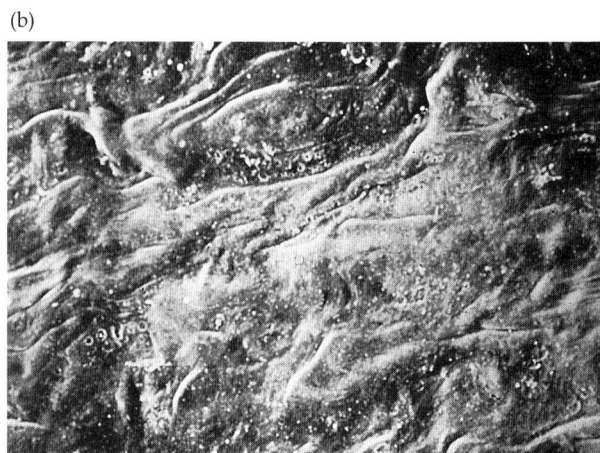

(b)

Fig. 11.12 Comparison of a corneal button cut with a trephine (a); and a laser (b).

suggested to Trokel that tissue was being *removed* not heated, and he sought access to an excimer laser to study this phenomenon and to verify his proposition. If his idea was correct, perhaps it would be possible to use this technology to perform more precise RK. It seemed that the technical limits of knife incision technology might be overcome by using a laser technique that would create a more predictable incision to follow the corneal curve. However, Trokel also considered the possibility that laser keratomileusis could be done by directly removing tissue from the corneal surface to modify its curve. This idea was seen as somewhat droll and was not greeted with enthusiasm. Accurate control of tissue removal to the standard of precision that would allow the cornea to heal with normal optical properties was considered somewhat far-fetched.

Only experimentation could confirm the surgical potential of these laser systems, and in the beginning of 1983, Trokel spent considerable time seeking access to an excimer laser. His efforts bore fruit when he was introduced to Rameesh Srinivasan, a photochemist working with the argon–fluoride excimer laser at IBM's TJ Watson Laboratories in New York.

Srinivasan showed Trokel his own studies in which he had described the ablation of plastics using 193 nm laser light. Srinivasan discussed the applications of this modality to other organic materials which included ablating fine grooves in a strand of human hair (Figure 11.11). Describing the effect of 193 nm light on plastic, Srinivasan wrote: "A threshold . . . for ablative photo-decomposition . . . was measured at 10 mJ/cm². Thus, one pulse at 16 mJ/cm² gave an etch mark that was clearly visible in reflection, whereas 50 pulses at 4 mJ/cm² pulse did not leave any etch mark" [49]. At this point, the possibility of optical fine-tuning of the corneal surface seemed at once less droll and more reasonable. Only further experimentation would show the utility of this method to cut clear cornea.

Following the first reports by Taboada and co-workers on the response of the corneal epithelium to ArF and KrF excimer laser pulses in 1981, Trokel and colleagues achieved a precise linear ablation of bovine (veal) cornea with 193 nm radiation [50].

The first eye done showed a crisply edged groove, made deeper in successive sections. Histologic analysis showed no collateral damage and a uniquely smooth ablated surface (Figure 11.12). Srinivasan's collaboration proved to be of enormous value. In particular, he was able to define the correct pulse rates and the minimal irradiances necessary to achieve the desired effect. Furthermore, his lasers were fully calibrated and their beam profiles had been carefully studied, allowing the achievement of particularly clean cuts. Homogeneity of the laser beam is paramount in accurate wide-surface ablation and in depth control—a problem still.

The results of these experiments and the essentials of the ArF excimer laser–cornea interaction were reported in 1983 [50]. The investigators demonstrated that they were able to remove a fraction of a micrometer of corneal tissue with each pulse of the laser

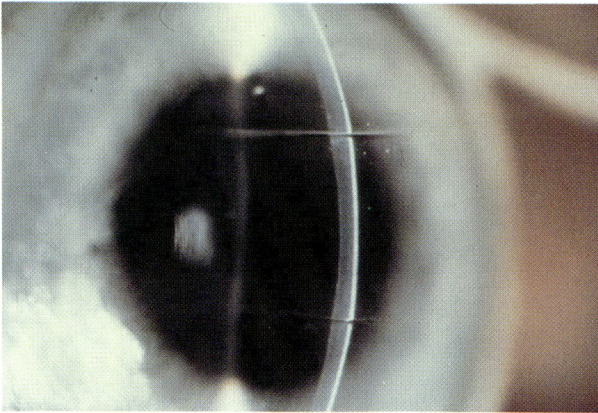

Fig. 11.13 T-cuts made in a human cornea with the excimer laser.

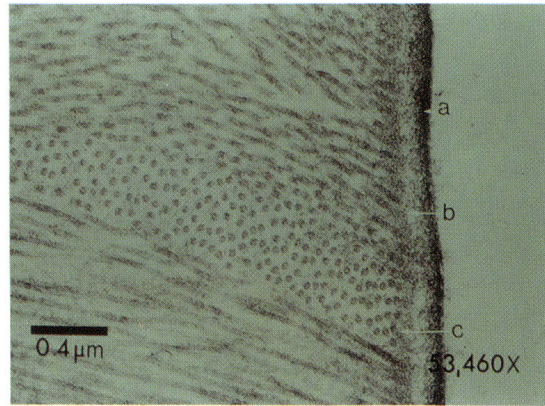

Fig. 11.14 High power electron micrograph of an excimer laser ablated surface. Three zones of structural abnormalities approximately 0.7 μm in thickness can be identified: (a) an outer densely staining region, (b) a middle lightly staining region; and (c) an inner region showing some increasing staining in an area where the fine structure of the collagen is partially preserved (from Puliafito CA, Steinert RF, Deutsch TF, Hillenkamp F, Dehm EJ, Adler CM. Excimer laser ablation of the cornea and lens. Experimental studies. Ophthalmology 1985; 92(6):741–748).

light; data showed a removal rate of about 0.25 μm of tissue per pulse. Further, the resulting surfaces were shown to be extremely uniform and smooth. On biomicroscopic examination and by light microscopy no damage to the adjacent stroma was observed. Electron microscopy revealed an extremely narrow three-banded zone (each band with 0.07 μm) of damage. Lastly, it was possible to control the shape and pattern of tissue removed by adjusting the distribution of the incident laser beam. Possible surgical applications of the ArF laser, both to cut slits in the cornea which would resemble an incision, and to remove large areas of tissue to produce a controlled laser lamellar keratectomy—laser keratomileusis—were discussed.

Trokel visited the Lambda Physik facility in mid 1983—immediately after the first series of experiments was completed—and they provided him with a model 102 excimer laser for his laboratory at Columbia, and they showed him how to obtain a 9 mm beam circle of sufficient fluence to ablate tissue. During this trip Trokel also visited Heroldsberg to discuss these early results with Reinhardt Thyzel, who was then owner of Meditec Laser Company—one of the first companies to produce a clinical Nd:YAG. Thyzel believed that this laser–cornea interaction would be *the* technique for producing an improved version of RK and he began development of a medical excimer laser project straight away.

Most of the emphasis at that time was in the application of the excimer to perform RK. There are obvious limitations to the RK technique, among them incision depth control—still an elusive problem, even for that marvel of human ingenuity, the laser. When Trokel showed slides of these first corneal tissue excisions, the impact was profound because we had all been accustomed to seeing laser interactions that produced extensive destruction of surrounding tissues [51]. The preservation of the tissue contours was remarkable and strengthened the premise that this modality could

be applied in a clinical setting (Figure 11.13). In planning experiments, the necessity for development of an effective delivery system quickly became apparent, as did the realization that this application would require support and help from industry. Furthermore, there were many questions about excimer laser functions and ultraviolet laser optics that required considerable technical expertise.

Earlier attempts had been made to alter the corneal refractive power by direct mechanical tissue ablation techniques [52,53]. However, a strong presumption that maintenance of Bowman's layer was essential to maintain epithelial integrity and thus stromal transparency existed [54]. As yet no one had been able to cut a completely smooth surface on a cornea, so the jury was still out.

One of the first experiments done with the new Lambda Physik laser was to remove a large 9 × 9 mm square of corneal stroma from a rabbit cornea. Neal Burstein, who was studying electric potentials across the corneal endothelium, showed that the treated cornea retained a normal electrical potential across its surface.

In the spring of 1984, Trokel and Marshall did a series of collaborative investigations. Using a crude delivery system they went on to study the texture of the ablated corneal surface (Figure 11.14), as well as the ultrastructural detail of each layer of the cornea. Animal corneas were exposed to the laser radiation in New York and immediately taken to London to Marshall's laboratory. In 1984, Trokel would produce lesions on rabbit and monkey corneas on Thursday mornings, pack the enucleated eyes in ice, and grab a

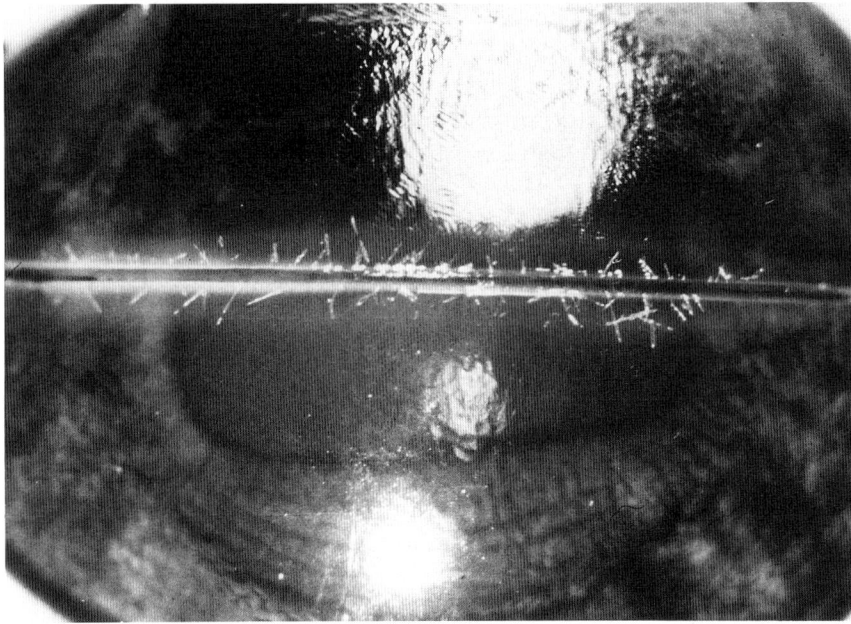

Fig. 11.15 Linear cracks extending laterally from a 249 nm ablated incision. These appear shortly above threshold and disappear at higher irradiances. They have been unique to 249 nm irradiated tissues (from Krueger RR, Trokel SL, Schubert HD. Interaction of ultraviolet laser light with the cornea. Invest Ophthalmol Visual Sci 1985; 26:1455–1464).

cab to Kennedy. He would arrive at Heathrow at 7:00 a.m., take the underground to Russell Square and walk the two blocks to Judd Street, where Marshall's laboratory was located. These studies were first done on rabbit corneas and then in monkey eyes, both acutely and after healing. Most impressive was the smoothness of the ablated area and the optical quality of the re-epithelialized healed surface [55–59].

Meanwhile, in New York, Ronald Krueger, an electrical engineer (then a medical student), helped Trokel investigate the nature of the laser–tissue interaction. They determined thresholds, ablation rates, healing patterns, and measured ablation parameters at all available excimer wavelengths (Figures 11.15 and 11.16) [60–62].

Particularly interesting were the results of studies in which Trokel's group created a fungal corneal ulcer and excised a large circular disk of tissue which healed the ulcer without producing corneal haze [63,64]. This gave impetus to the thought that the excimer, by virtue of its ability to produce extremely fine layered ablations with minimal tissue interaction, could be used therapeutically—perhaps even to excise scar tissue [65,66].

At the same time, Munnerlyn was at work deriving the quantitative relationships associated with removing corneal tissue. He had calculated that for a 4 mm optical zone, only 5 μm of tissue need be removed to reduce the corneal refractive power by 1 D. At Munnerlyn's urging, Trokel ablated a series of 3 mm circles in rabbit corneas to progressively increased depths. Several weeks after they had healed, only the eye with the deepest ablated zone showed any stromal haze; the others had healed without discernible

opacification by slit-lamp examination. These experiments gave Munnerlyn and others in the industry the impetus to proceed with the development of clinical excimer laser systems.

Munnerlyn wrote a paper using the results of these early animal studies to show the relationship of tissue removal to optical zone size to achieve a given optical effect. The formula states:

$$\text{depth of ablation} = \frac{\text{diopters of change}}{3} \times (\text{diameter of optical zone})^2$$

For an example with a 6 mm optical zone, 4 D of myopia is corrected with a 48 μm ablation depth [67]. Today a slightly smaller (5.5 mm) optical zone is used. With that zone size the ablation rate is 10 μm/D. Thus, in the example cited, 40 μm of tissue will be removed using 166 pulses at 5 Hz.

In this paper, he coined the term photorefractive keratectomy to describe this technique [68]. However, it took 4 more years before the paper was accepted for publication because it was deemed "too speculative and of no practical value."

Thus it was that, for a time, Steven Trokel's laboratory in New York continued to have the only excimer laser in the world dedicated exclusively to ophthalmic research. This situation changed abruptly, however, in mid 1985 when the interest in ophthalmic and refractive applications of this technology suddenly exploded, at the same time as the development of commercial interest in excimer laser systems. Attention then became diverted from the laboratory and directed more into the clinical arena.

(a)

(b)

(c)

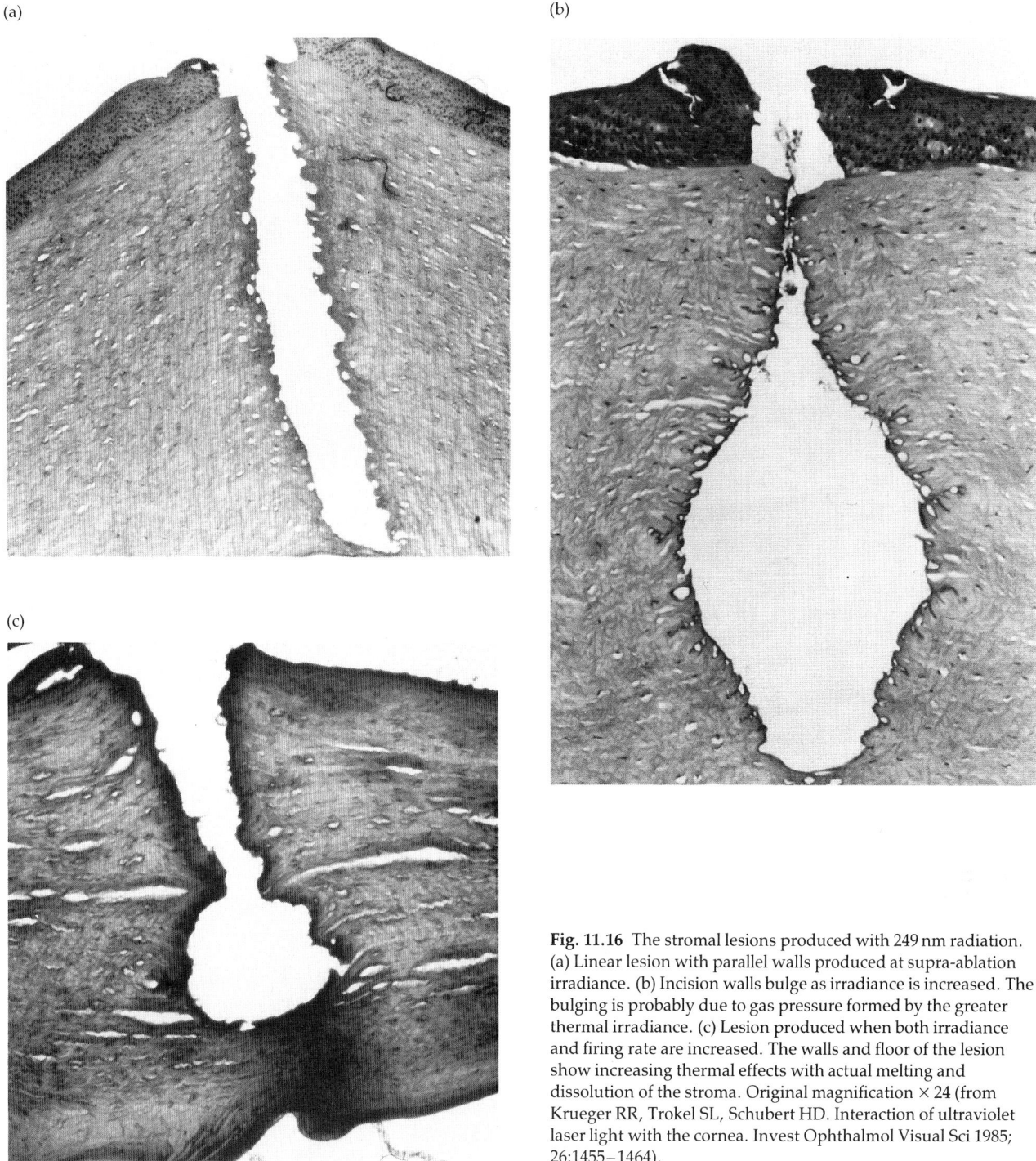

Fig. 11.16 The stromal lesions produced with 249 nm radiation. (a) Linear lesion with parallel walls produced at supra-ablation irradiance. (b) Incision walls bulge as irradiance is increased. The bulging is probably due to gas pressure formed by the greater thermal irradiance. (c) Lesion produced when both irradiance and firing rate are increased. The walls and floor of the lesion show increasing thermal effects with actual melting and dissolution of the stroma. Original magnification × 24 (from Krueger RR, Trokel SL, Schubert HD. Interaction of ultraviolet laser light with the cornea. Invest Ophthalmol Visual Sci 1985; 26:1455–1464).

Being able to ablate polymers in a precise way does not necessarily lead to clinical success. It is one thing to blitz the cornea in animal eyes. It is still another to do it in cadaver eyes or even blind human eyes—such exercises merely prove feasibility. And there is a large gap between feasibility and suitability—an idea is easier to conceive than to execute. Therefore, it should come as no surprise that the clinical application of this modality has some formidable hurdles to overcome

and it is by no means certain that such obstacles will fall.

Overview

The ability to cut precise sections with the argon fluoride excimer laser at a wavelength of 193 nm is based on the absorption mode of the high-energy far ultraviolet photons within the first few micro-meters of

(a)

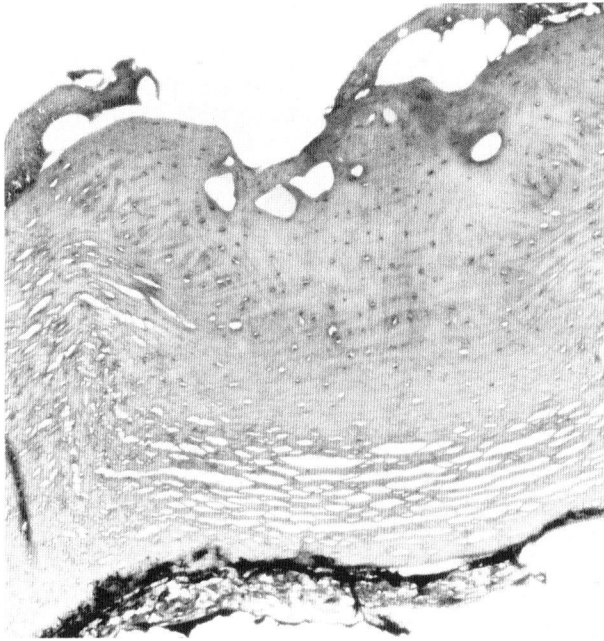

(b)

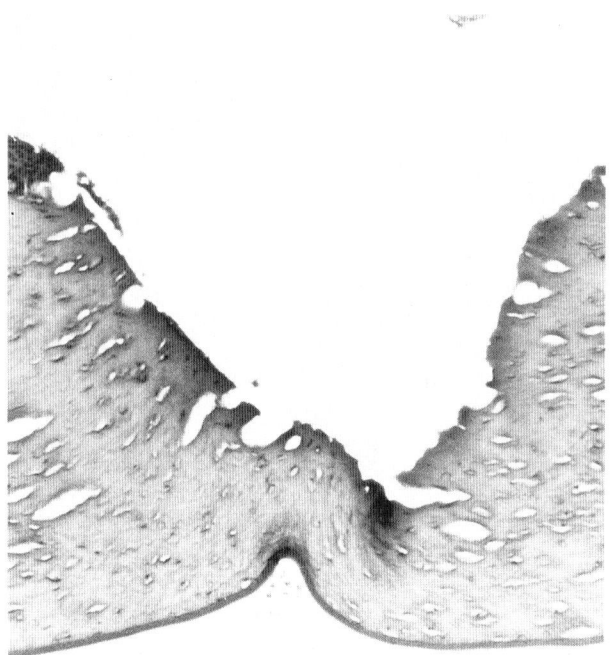

(c)

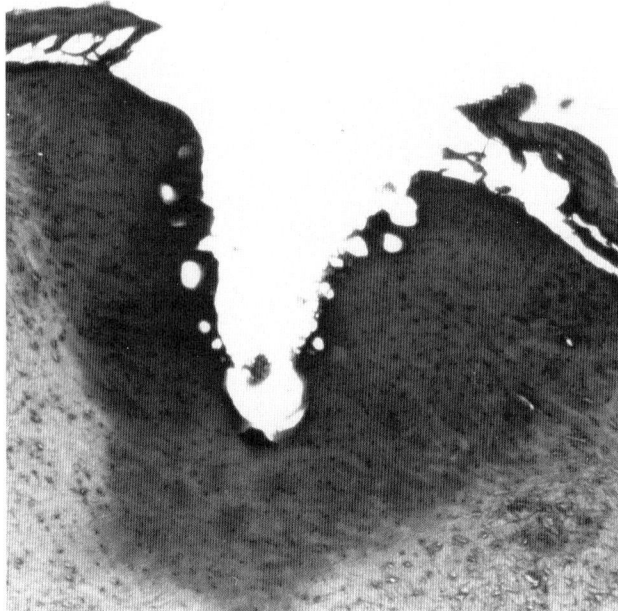

Fig. 11.17 Ultraviolet light (351 nm). (a) Extensive disorganization of the stroma below the ablation threshold. There is widespread heating and destruction of the corneal stroma. (b) A low firing rate above the ablation threshold shows tissue removal with local stromal changes. Gas bubbles can be seen extending into the stroma, and an obvious thermal interaction zone can be identified. (c) Both the firing rate and irradiance are higher and a broader thermal zone can be seen. Original magnification × 24 (from Krueger RR, Trokel SL, Schubert HD. Interaction of ultraviolet laser light with the cornea. Invest Ophthalmol Visual Sci 1985; 26:1455–1464).

the focal point. The ablated particles are ejected at supersonic speed, carrying most of the excess thermal energy with them, thereby producing corneal incisions with an adjacent zone of damage that is in the sub-micro-meter range (0.1–0.3 μm) [55,57,69–71]. Consequent corneal wounds appear to be sealed by a pseudo-membrane and keratocytes appear normal immediately adjacent to the ablation area [72]. In contrast, the use of longer wavelengths (KrF at 248 nm, XeCl at 308 nm, and XeF at 351 nm) always induced ragged incision edges and a comparatively broad zone of tissue damage (Figure 11.17) [61]. This is probably not a consequence only of the increased absorption length of these wavelengths in the cornea (as compared to 193 nm), but also of significant thermal loading [19,23]. Furthermore, the energy-absorbing target chromophore may play a role in the various mechanisms of photoablation [22]. Steinert found the threshold for ablation in a human eye at 193 nm to be 46 mJ/cm^2. For KrF (248 nm) it was 58 mJ/cm^2. At all exposures, it required a higher fluence for the 248 nm beam than for the 193 nm to obtain comparable results.

Applications

On the therapeutic side, experiments have centered primarily on treating superficial corneal pathology. Glaucoma filtration surgery and trephination of corneal transplants are also on the excimer wish list, although the latter may prove impractical.

The excimer has been used mostly as a refractive tool to date, specifically to correct myopia and astigmatism. Attempts have also been made to correct hyperopia, and there is considerable hype that some day the laser will be used to perform RK—which it may, but which it has yet to achieve in any way which surpasses current methods.

For refractive surgery with the excimer laser, three basic principles are currently being investigated:
1 Linear or arcuate excisions for the correction of myopia—laser radial keratectomy—and astigmatism—laser transverse or arcuate keratectomy.
2 The removal of tissue from the central, healthy cornea—laser keratomileusis.
3 The preparation of plano or powered lenticules for epikeratophakia.

Laser radial keratectomy

Laser radial keratectomy is following the approach that has been taken over the last decade with RK for the correction of myopia and astigmatism. Similar to synthetic polymers, the etch depth per pulse is dependent on laser fluence and plotting reveals a sigmoidal-shaped curve whose steep part shows an almost logarithmic relationship [60,73]. Inflection points in these plots correspond to the fluence levels for the most efficient ablation. In enucleated human eyes incision depth and flattening were found to correlate well with laser output. Up to 5.35 D of flattening was achieved [71]. As the pulse-to-pulse amplitude fluctuation is highly variable in all currently available excimer lasers (around 5–8%), ablation at the inflection points may be clinically undesirable, as small changes in laser output would significantly alter ablation rate [74]. Ablation at higher fluences may be preferable since there does not appear to be any increase in ultrastructural damage with fluences between 400 and 600 mJ/cm^2 per pulse: at these levels the etch depth plot has the smallest slope [67]. Other research groups have used the laser attached to a slit-lamp to perform *in vivo* radial keratectomies in experimental animals [75]. Lack of significant corneal inflammation with possibly weaker wound-healing response—as compared to

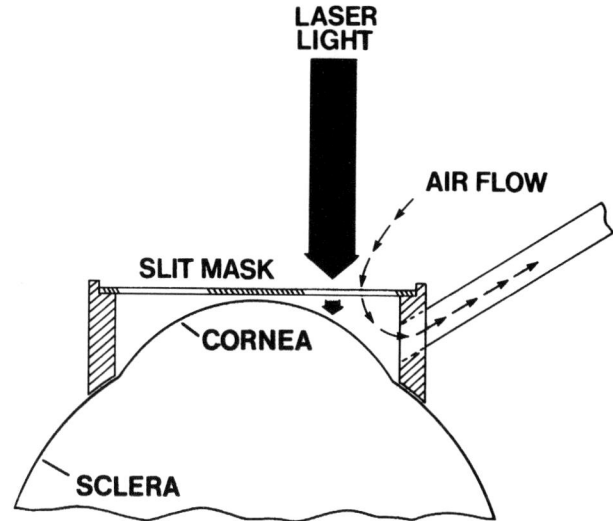

Fig. 11.18 Cross-section of typical ablation mask. (Courtesy of MediTec.)

thermokeratoplasty or diamond blade RK—is the hallmark of these laser incisions [76].

Theoretically there are several advantages of the excimer laser use for radial keratectomy. No direct contact with the cornea during the procedure is required, as with the diamond knife incisions, but is usual when a mask is used. This would allow a real-time monitoring of the progress during surgery by performing a continuous topographic analysis of the corneal contour (see the section on laser keratomileusis, below). The use of suitably shaped masks allows for simultaneous incisions with a high spatial accuracy and repeatability, thus eliminating some of the variables of conventional RK (Figures 11.18 through 11.20). With a repetition rate in the 20–50 Hz range ablation would only require a few seconds, thereby reducing variability caused by dehydration during conventional surgery [77].

It must be realized that while the laser can make a relatively atraumatic cut in the cornea—a cut that resembles that made by a saw—substance is removed, not cleaved (Figures 11.21 and 11.22). According to Steinert and Puliafito there are certain practical limits as to the narrowness of the kerf (minimum around 30 μm) that can be created by the laser [67]. Tissue fluid seeps into the space that is created during excision, thus narrowing it—a diamond knife only splits the tissue without removing it. The ablation depth per pulse is dependent not only on the hydration of the cornea, but also on the width of the groove [78].

Because the excimer laser produces an excision rather than an incision, the ingrowth of a broader epithelial plug might result in slower wound healing and thereby not only an increased or unpredictable

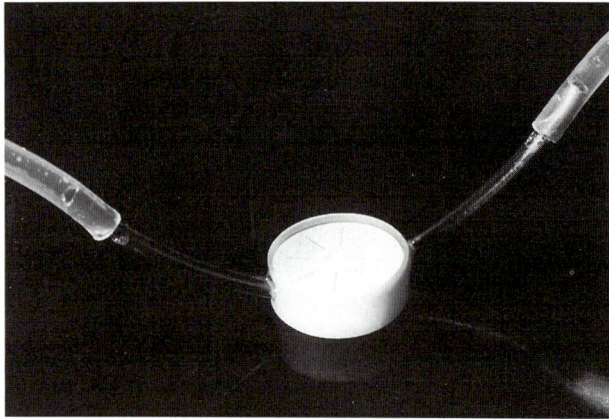

Fig. 11.19 Frontal view of an eight-incision corneal mask. (Courtesy of MediTec.)

(a)

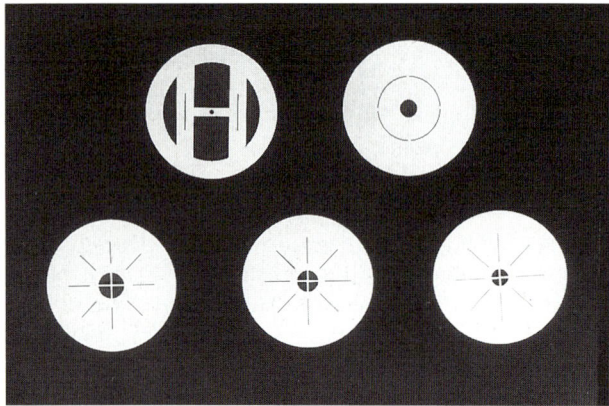

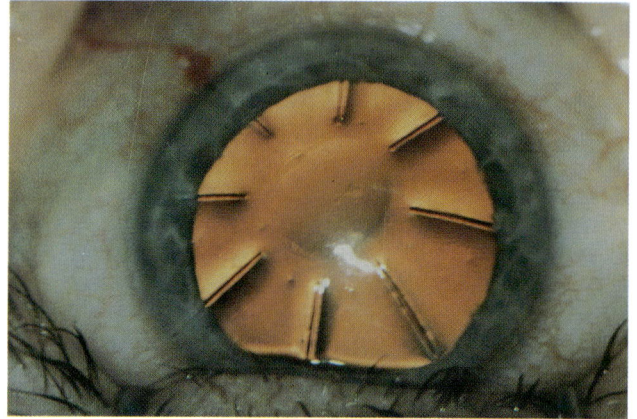

Fig. 11.20 Corneal masks for radial keratotomy, penetrating keratoplasty, and astigmatism. (Courtesy of MediTec.)

(b)

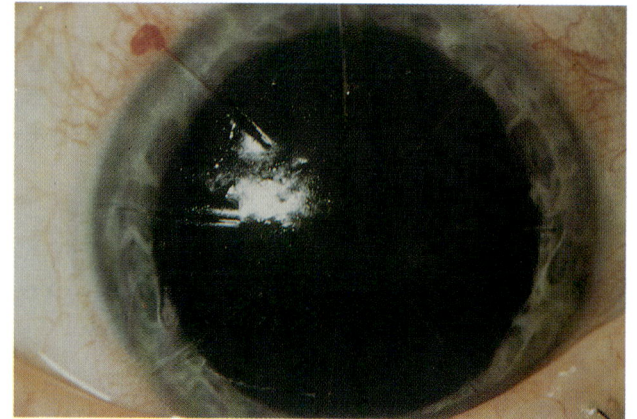

Fig. 11.21 Human eye with excimer laser RK immediately post-ablation. Incision length is 3.0 mm, incision width 70 μm, with an incision depth of 300 μm (60% of central corneal thickness). (Courtesy of MediTec.)

effect (compared to conventional RK), but also prolonged diurnal fluctuations and a diminished long-term stability of the achieved correction (Figures 11.23 and 11.24). Are wider scars less flexible and/or do they somehow convey more resistance to rupture than incisions? Not likely, thus while solving one problem (maybe), laser RK could possibly create others. Steinert suggests that wider scars might result in greater curvature change, especially if enhanced by pharmacological wound-healing agents [67]. However, studies to date of agents such as EGF have been disappointing—it is not possible to over-drive the system. Incision RK, with its smaller area scar, might actually respond better to such agents. Furthermore, comparisons of early steel knife data with those of smoother diamond knife results seem to indicate that the finer incisions of the diamond are accompanied by an improvement in outcome [79,80].

Several technical problems have to be solved prior to widespread clinical use. Although the total duration of

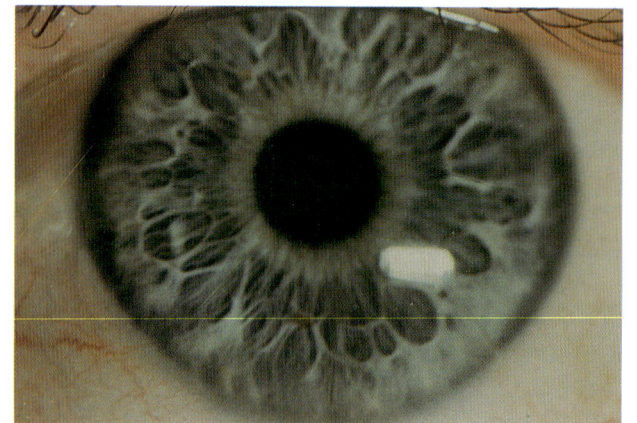

Fig. 11.22 The same eye 1 week post-operation. Diopter change + 2.0 D. (Courtesy of MediTec.)

surgery is comparatively short, immobilization of the eye and/or coupling of the laser beam to the cornea with protection of areas that should not be irradiated are mandatory. The use of a suction cup with evenly spaced slits ·and of coated contact lenses has been proposed [81–83].

Real-time monitoring of excision depth at present eludes technical means, although Stern and co-workers have described the femtosecond optical ranging of corneal incision depth with the use of a colliding pulse mode-locked ring dye laser [84]. A high rate of corneal perforation has been described by several groups, possibly caused by individual response variations in the patient's corneas [28].

Dehm and associates have shown changes to the endothelium following 90% incisions of the corneal depth with 193 nm laser light, similar to those seen after incisional RK. Higher-density exposures lead to a denudation of the endothelium under the ablation zone (Figure 11.25) [26,27,85]. Ablations with KrF (248 nm) revealed loss of cells and severe damage in the tissue surrounding the excisions. In addition, ultrastructural changes in Descemet's membrane have been reported, probably as a result of acoustico-mechanic shock waves or secondary radiation [86,87].

The excimer laser offers several potential technical advantages for RK but these advantages may not appreciably change either the results or post-operative course in the long run. Additionally, both the cost and sophistication of the equipment weigh heavily against the method becoming clinically viable—further investigation is needed.

Astigmatism and laser keratectomy

The excimer laser has also been used in a limited number of patients to correct astigmatism. Here the laser produces curved excisions that essentially mimic

(a)

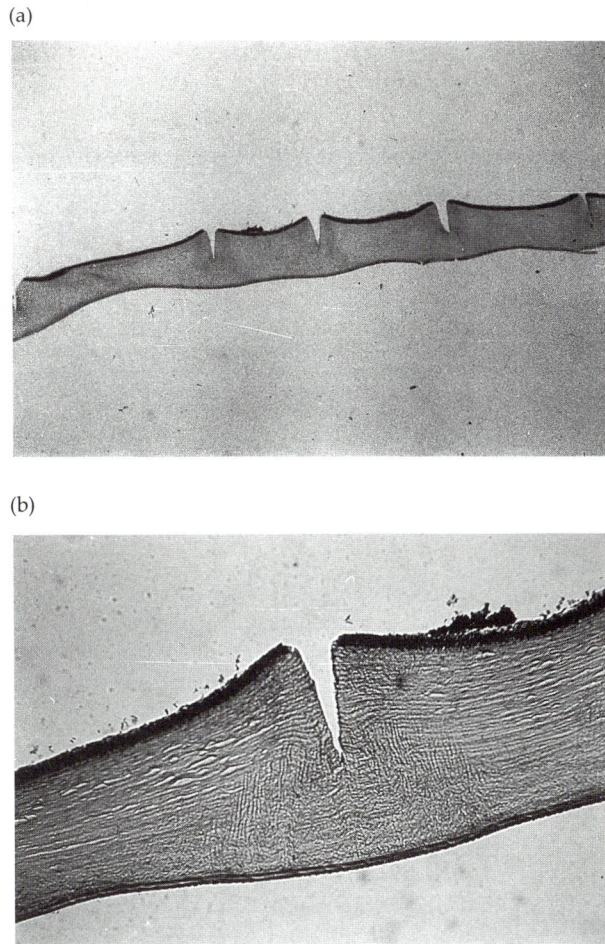

(b)

Fig. 11.23 Incision in rabbit cornea immediately post-application. (Courtesy of MediTec.)

the classic T-incisions made with a knife. A contact lens that has been coated with reflective material and contains small openings or slits is used to permit projection of the laser beam on to the appropriate

(a)

(b)

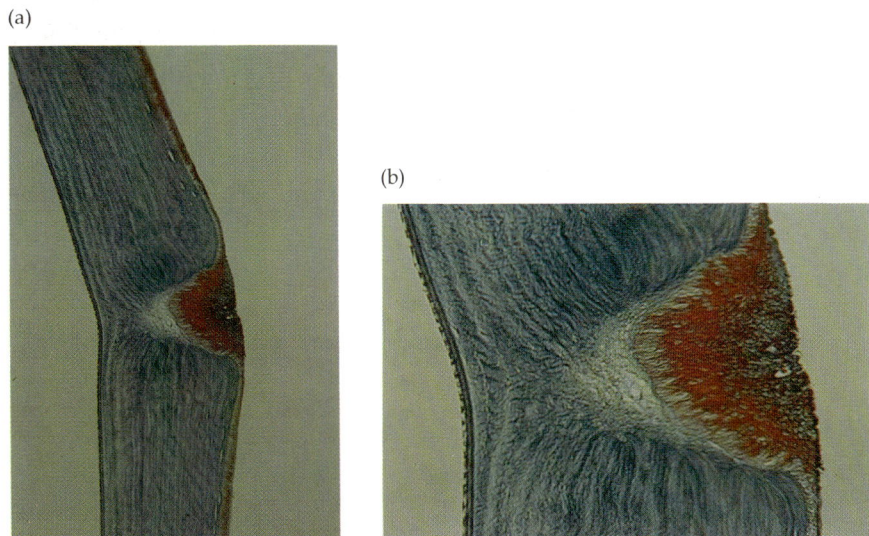

Fig. 11.24 Similar incision in rabbit cornea 2 months post-application. The epithelial plug is beginning to thin and new stroma is visible. (Courtesy of MediTec.)

(a)

(b)

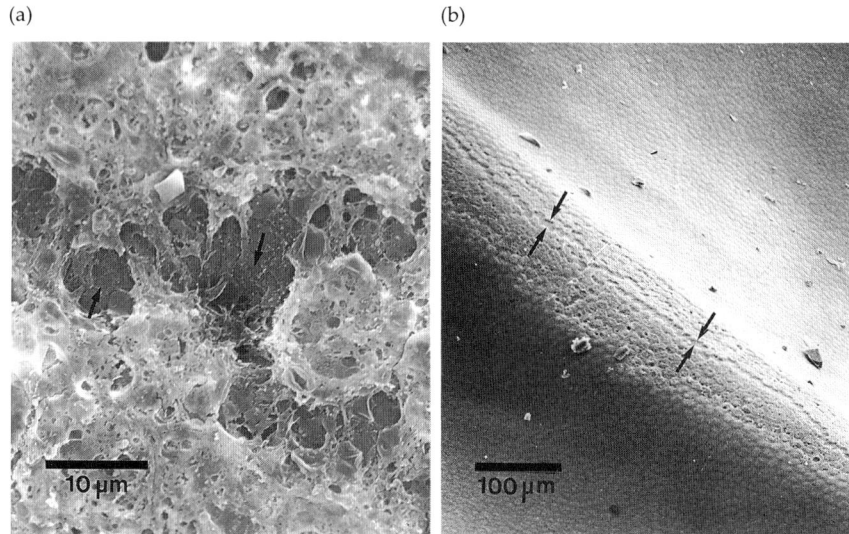

Fig. 11.25 (a) Endothelial surface ridge raised by ablation; (b) damaged endothelium following laser tissue ablation (from Dehm EJ, Puliafito CA, Adler CM. Endothelial injury in rabbits following excimer laser ablation at 193 and 248 nm. Arch Ophthalmol 1986; 104:1364–1368).

part of the cornea. Candidates enrolled in the initial phase of study were restricted to those with 3–5 D of astigmatism. It may be that the procedure can be used to correct greater amounts of astigmatism, but the clinical study has not been expanded to date (R.E. Fenzl, 1991, personal communication). According to Fenzl, the excimer has not only produced excellent results, but also provides increased predictability compared with conventional surgery. Fenzl claims that the depth predictability achievable with a knife is only 110–115 μm—but cites no evidence establishing that figure—whereas the accuracy that can be obtained with the laser is 14 μm. Follow-up extending to 18 months in patients enrolled in the initial clinical trial shows that the procedure is associated with stable results and no complications. Using the suction cup–slit technique, Seiler and co-workers have corrected corneal astigmatism of up to 4.16 D. Since small variations in excision depth—within 10%—cause large differences in the resulting astigmatic correction (±2.5 D), reproducibility and predictability depend mainly on the precise control of the ablation depth [78].

Attempts at treating astigmatism through elliptic ablation zones have also been undertaken [88,89].

Laser keratomileusis

By far the most serious test application of the excimer has been in laser keratomileusis, where it has been used in attempts to correct myopic errors through large-area ablation of the cornea. This type of refractive corneal surgery performed with the ArF excimer laser is based on the expectation that tissue can be removed with sub-micro-meter precision from the central corneal surface in such a gentle manner that the corneal epithelium heals over the ablated area without hyperplasia

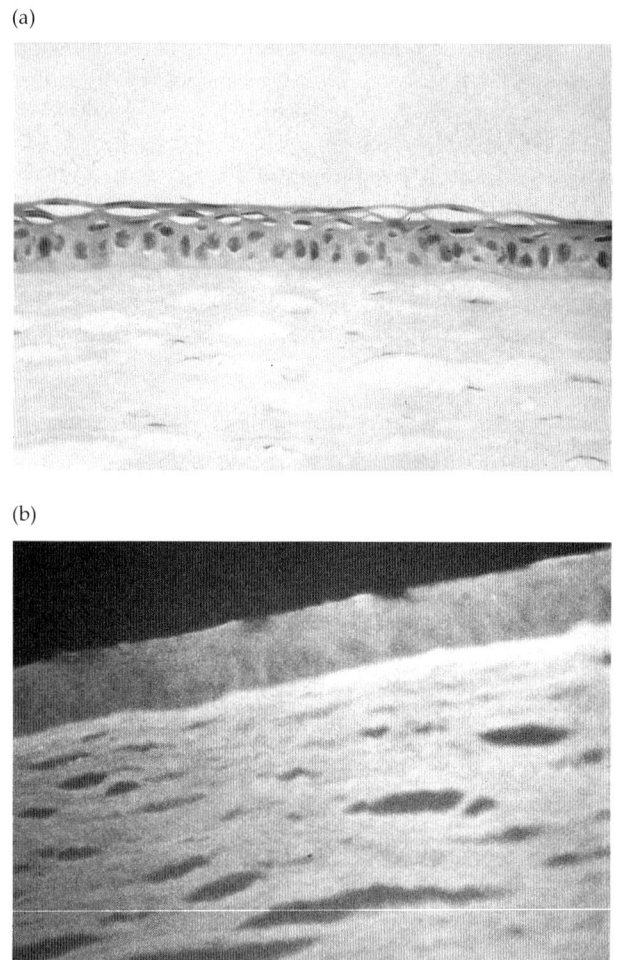

(a)

(b)

Fig. 11.26 Four weeks after a 2 D, 4.5 mm ablation. (a) Hematoxylin & eosin, original magnification × 475; (b) TEM, original magnification × 60 000. There is re-epithelialization with basement membrane complexes and hemidesmosomes (from Goodman GL, Trokel SL, Stark WJ, Munnerlyn CR, Green WR. Corneal healing following laser refractive keratectomy. Arch Ophthalmol 1989; 107:1799–1803.

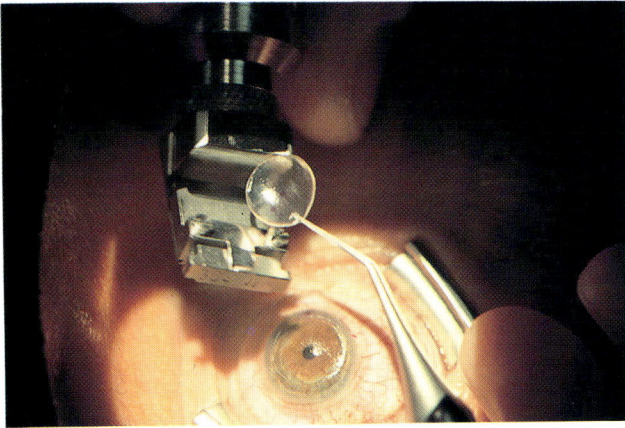

Fig. 11.27 Large keratectomy with the keratome. (Courtesy of S. Brint.)

(a)

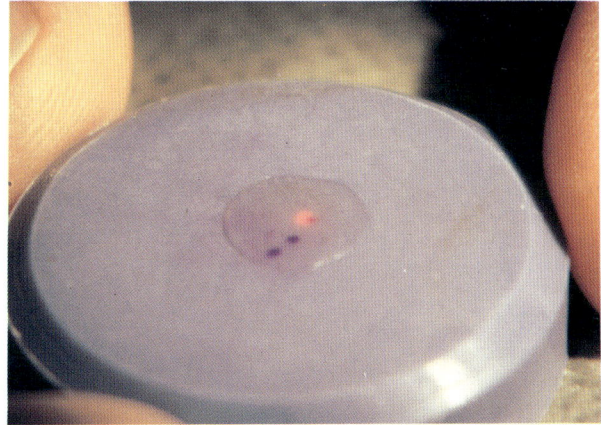

(b)

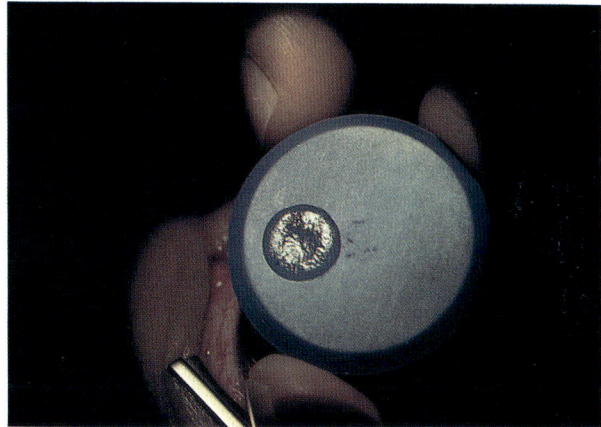

Fig. 11.28 (a) Ablation being performed. Centration is by inspection; (b) ablated tissue disk. (Courtesy of L. Buratto.)

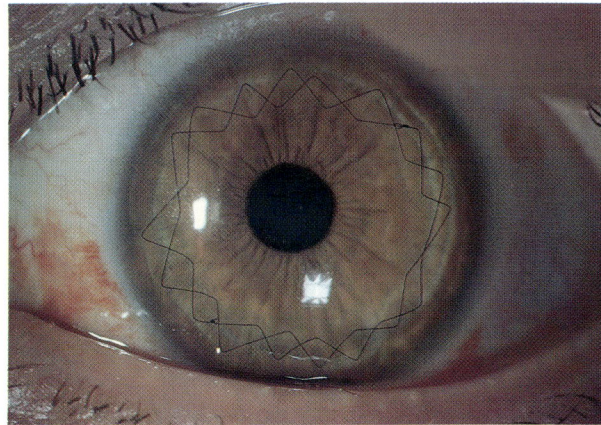

Fig. 11.29 Post-operative laser keratomileusis. (Courtesy of L. Buratto.)

and activation of significant repair mechanisms causing scarring—photoablative refractive keratectomy (Figure 11.26). The new anterior radius of curvature would thus achieve the desired optical correction in the same way as classical myopic and hyperopic keratomileusis, keratophakia, intra-stromal hydrogel implantation or epikeratophakia [90]. Initial experience with clinical use in partially and full-sighted humans has been reported as positive, but several important biologic issues require further study. These include the predictability of the procedure, its long-term stability, and the effect on corneal clarity and regularity.

Both Steven Brint at LSU and Lucio Buratto of Milan have performed laser keratomileusis (photo-keratomileusis) under a keratectomy with some success. Buratto has the longest experience. His technique and results are outlined below (L. Buratto, 1991, personal communication).

Thirty eyes of 22 patients underwent treatment. All patients had anisometropia that did not respond to glasses and/or contact lenses. All disks were resected with a #30 plate and had a diameter of 8.5 mm, reflecting the investigator's experience with the BKS unit used for the keratectomies (Figure 11.27). In freeze-lathing cases, the average disk diameter is 7.0–7.5 mm, In two cases the disk thickness was less than 240 mm, which created post-operative problems—which it would in classic MKM.

A Summit Technologies Excimed UV 200 excimer laser was used. The ablations were performed with a repitition rate of 10 Hz, a fluence of 180 mJ/cm^2, and an optical zone ranging from 3.5 to 4.5 mm. The resected disks were laid flat on a hard rubber base for the treatment (Figure 11.28). Post-operatively the patients were treated with topical tobramycin five times daily until the corneas had re-epithelialized, with dexamethasone five times daily added thereafter (Figure 11.29). Sutures were removed in 14 days.

The average pre-operative myopia was −17.875 ± 3.32 D. The mean residual refraction at 6 months was −2.126 ± 1.40 D. Intrastromal haze was observed in five cases (16.6%). Best corrected vision remained at

(a)

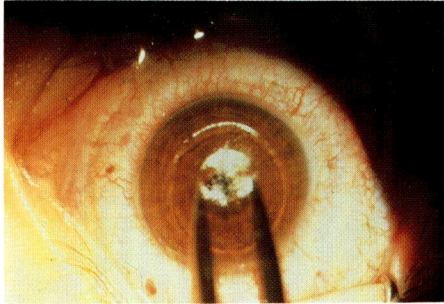

(b)

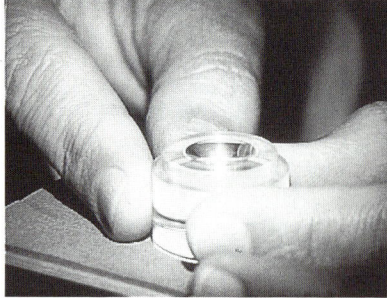

Fig. 11.30 (a) Note decentration of the ablated zone in this case of *in situ* laser ablation; (b) it is difficult to insure accurate centration when holding the tissue beneath the laser beam.

the pre-operative level in 74% of the cases, improved in 16%, and declined in 10%. Uncorrected vision was 20/50 or better in 10% and 20/100 in 83.3%. Astigmatism pre- and post-surgery was essentially the same, being 2.02 ± 1.04 D pre-surgery and 2.26 ± 1.09 D post-surgery. It should be noted—as pointed out in Chapter 10—that these figures can be misleading presented in this way. It is not known how many of this group actually lost astigmatism, how many gained, and in how many astigmatism was reversed. This caveat is underscored by the fact that Buratto reports that four of 30 (13.3%) developed irregular astigmatism. This is higher than the average in freeze-lathing. However, if we remove the two thin sections in which such distortion is inevitable, we are left with a 6% incidence of irregular astigmatism. This is more in line with freeze-lathing and is better than in keratomileusis-*in-situ* (see Chapter 10). Such astigmatism is usually related to decentration of the ablated zone within the resected disk and can be minimized with improvements in centration and beam delivery (Figure 11.30). Of this group, two were thin sections with subsequent wrinkling of Bowman's layer. This also happens in freeze-lathe cases when the central thickness is less than 0.10 mm post-lathing. Of these two cases, one required a homoplastic graft at 6 months due to extremely poor vision.

In the author's view, this application shows the most promise in terms of both results and predictability because it eliminates the freezing stage. However, the methodology currently pursued is likely to introduce error in the result, especially irregular astigmatism. The author has predicted that the incidence of irregular astigmatism with this technique under present circumstances will approach or exceed that of keratomileusis-*in-situ*—namely 16%—and for the same reasons, size and centration of the ablation zone.

Centration of the tissue to be shaped is critical. When a tissue disk is removed from the eye, all landmarks are lost. A properly resected disk does at least have the virtue of being round. If cut to a thickness of at least 300 μm (the same general thickness advocated

for freeze-lathing), distortion of the tissue will be minimal. The author recommends that a leaf be taken from Barraquer's book and that the tissue disk be placed within a perforated concave plastic base on a rotating table. The table can be precisely located on the laser beam axis. This table can be spun at a variable rate using the techniques outlined in Chapter 10 to center the wet disk while spinning. Once the disk is well-centered, a light vacuum can be drawn upon the disk via the tiny perforations in the base; this will hold it firmly in place. Excess fluid can be drawn off with a microsponge or blown off with a gentle stream of nitrogen. Ablation should be carried out while the disk is spinning to insure evenness of the ablation (see discussion, below). If this system cannot be implemented, the author predicts that a better result will obtain with *in situ* ablation than with the current method because centration will be somewhat better.

Discussion of laser applications in refractive surgery

To date, the excimer laser has been used to treat myopia in patients with pre-treatment spherical equivalents ranging from −2 to −12 D. Follow-up of the effect on refractive error has shown a reduction of myopia in most patients, with an initial hyperopic overshoot during the first month after treatment, a shift downward over the next 1–2 months due to stromal remodeling, and re-stabilization of the effect within 3–6 months after surgery. Emmetropia has been achieved in some patients who have undergone myopic keratomileusis, but serious under-corrections have also been observed.

The term dirty beam is widely used to describe ultraviolet lasers [74]. The output of the laser tube is not homogeneous, frequently showing hot spots (Figure 11.31) [91]. Furthermore, the pulse energy shows great variations between single pulses—more so in the low-energy range. The average pulse energy falls off as the number of pulses delivered increases. This fall-off depends upon the gas-filling status of the laser tube. Additionally, the laser-induced changes,

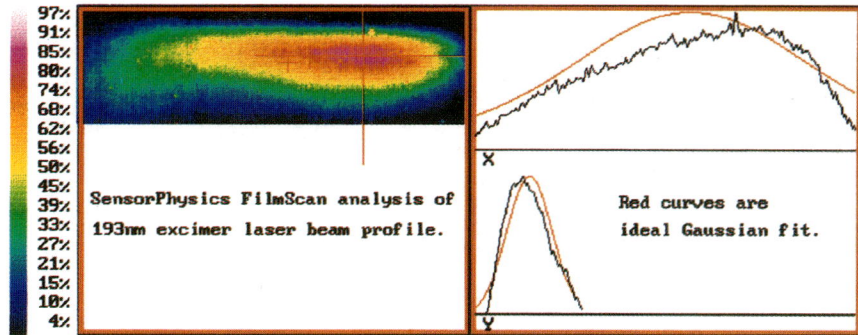

Fig. 11.31 Analysis of 193 nm excimer beam profile shows a maximized beam. (Courtesy of SenssorPhysics, Redwood City, CA—FilmScan Beam Analyzer.)

occurring within the delivery system itself as the laser is in use—even when multiple coated optical elements are used in the delivery system—add to the ambiguities [92]. This necessitates monitoring devices being integrated into the newer laser systems [93].

Quality of ablation not only depends on the homogeneity of the beam but also on the method of creating smooth transition zones between single pulses so as to avoid the creation of significant steps (Figure 11.32). A major effort is underway to improve the quality of the laser beam prior to ablation of biologic tissue. Circular and rectangular masks have been used for the treatment of myopia, hyperopia, and astigmatism. It has been acknowledged, however, that steps between the zones will still be created [93]. Moving slits, dynamic diaphragm imaging on the cornea, or constricting diaphragms, have all been proposed to smooth out this transition [94–96].

It will also be important to determine whether there is a superior delivery system. Use of an ablatable mask surface versus an iris disphragm may not make a difference clinically. The technique essentially uses the excimer laser to create an impression of a mask on the cornea. The mask is formed in the same shape as the lens tissue desired to be removed from the

cornea and ablates at the same rate as the cornea. The primary theoretic advantage is that it would offer optimal flexibility, since it replaces the moving pads or moving slit-beam of the laser with a mask customized to any desirable shape. However, a high-quality laser beam is necessary to produce uniform ablation of the mask, and while ablation of the mask image on to the cornea has been accomplished, it remains to be seen whether or not it is associated with a better refractive result—beam quality is not the excimer's strong suit. Various fluids have been studied for the same purpose [97].

There is still hope that by eliminating the above-mentioned variations in homogeneity and transition zones, the healing response of the cornea can be minimized. Epithelial–stromal interactions are probably important but have not been analyzed in detail. Adjustability seems theoretically possible as additional ablations can be performed; the potential risks of infection, additional scarring, and even increased variability remain unaltered, however.

In order to monitor accurately the progress of ablation, a keratoscope has been integrated into one system that is supposed to demonstrate corneal topography during surgery [93,98]. There are formidable obstacles to overcome to make such real-time surface monitoring a functional reality. Photokeratoscopy techniques are of insufficient sensitivity to be used for this purpose. The same can be said for raster-stereography. Holographic methods would serve but currently require too much computational time [99,100].

As Taylor and associates have emphasized the variability in response from one cornea to another despite reasonable uniform conditions of treatment, the individual biologic variation in wound healing appears to be the pivotal point of success or failure of laser keratomileusis [101]. This variability must necessarily result in unpredictability of the refractive outcome. Thus tissue response, implicated in RK variability, is not avoided by using the laser.

McDonald *et al.* noted that in their series of partially sighted patients treated with the excimer laser for

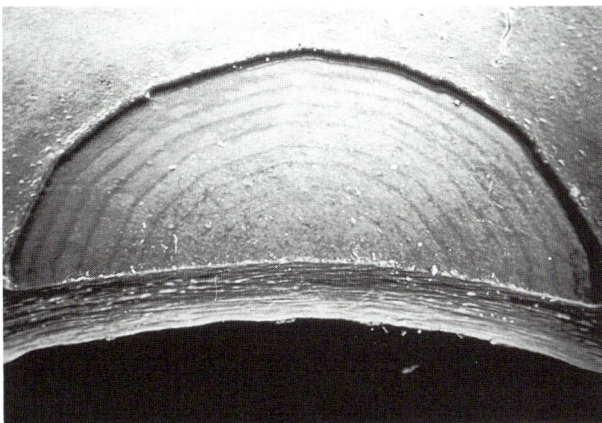

Fig. 11.32 Photoablated corneal surface.

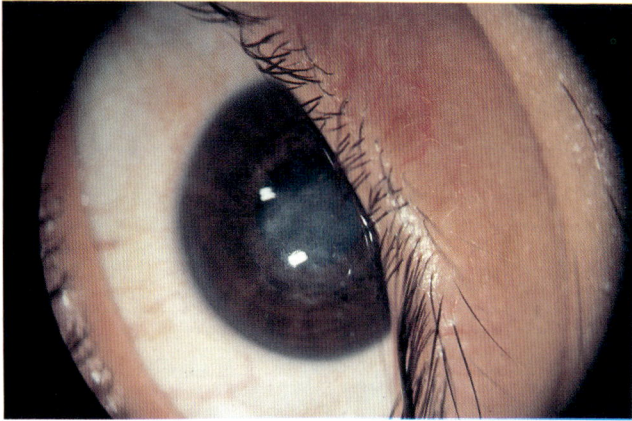

Fig. 11.33 Corneal haze following laser corneal photoablation.

myopic correction, serious under-correction primarily affected those individuals whose pre-operative refraction was greater than 5 D [102]. It was clear that patients who were high myopes did less well than those whose dioptric error was initially 5 D or less. Since the optimal range of myopia correction for RK is up to −5 D, such

results are not good enough to justify the use of laser in these cases. Keratometry studies in these cases have shown that, unlike other refractive procedures currently in use, large-area ablation with the excimer laser produces stable central flattening of the cornea and does not induce astigmatism in the vast majority of patients. However, the amount of induced astigmatism following RK is also less amongst experienced keratotomists. Reporting on a series of 21 sighted patients who underwent myopic ablation with the excimer laser, Deitz noted that only two of the 21 patients had an increase of astigmatism greater than 1 D (M.R. Deitz, 1991, personal communication).

A few years ago, excimer investigators had hoped that corneal tissue could be ablated without eliciting a response from the corneal stroma. But results from these studies now demonstrate that this is not true. Both in experimental animals and in the first series of patients, sub-epithelial scarring—a faint, reticular haze by slit-lamp microscopy—has persisted for many months (Figure 11.33) [59,101,103]. This fine haze has been noted in virtually all patients who have undergone laser keratomileusis, but at this writing it does

(a)

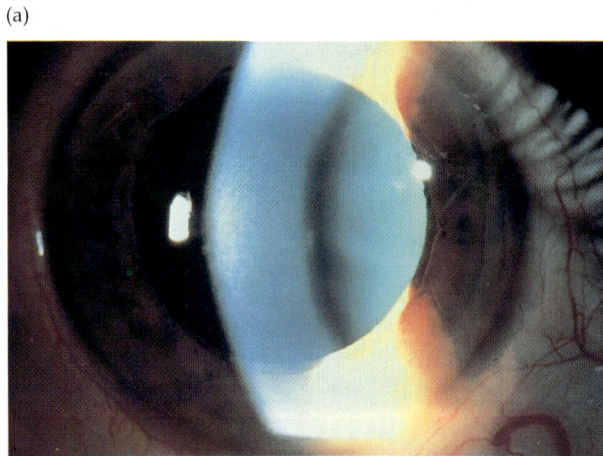

(b)

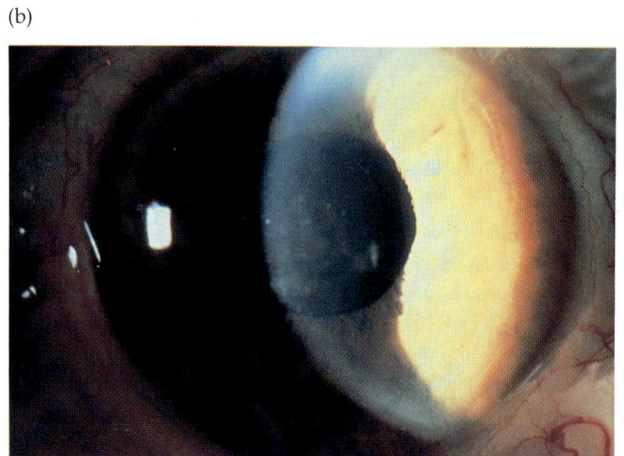

(c)

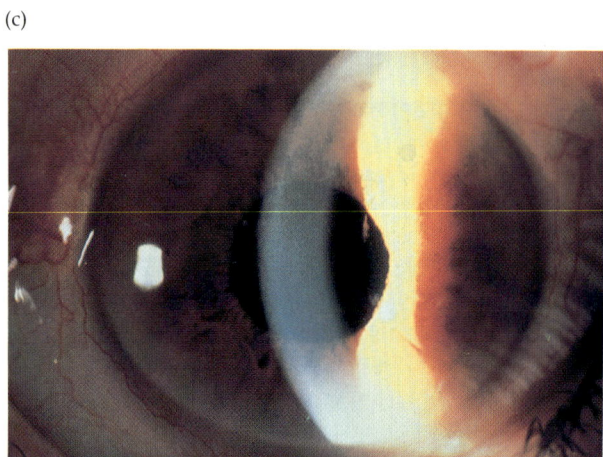

Fig. 11.34 Photoablative refractive keratectomy. (a) 1 month post-surgery; (b) 3 months post-surgery; (c) 9 months post-surgery.

(a)

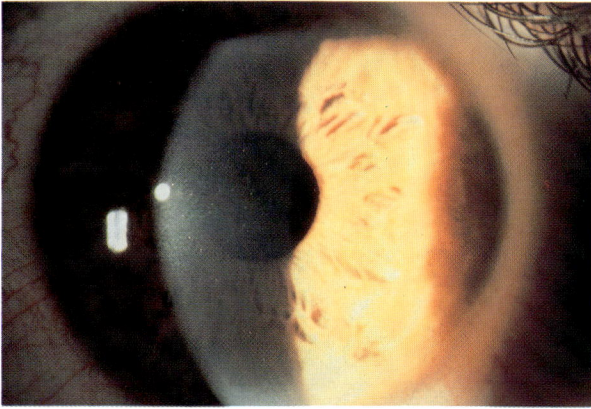

(b)

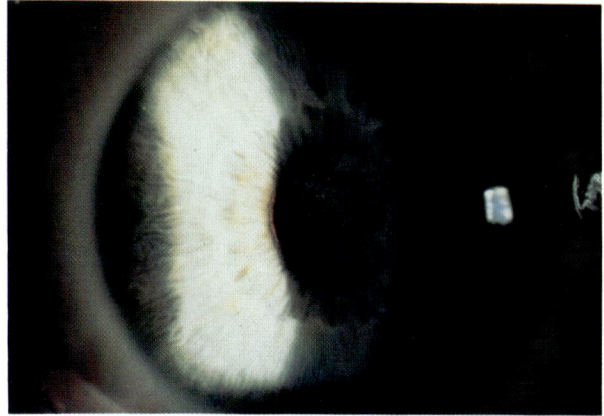

(c)

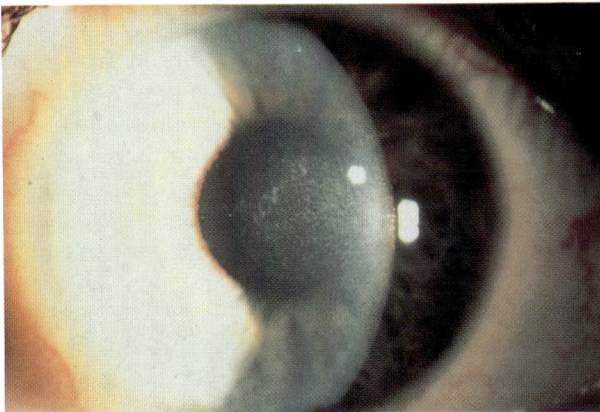

(d)

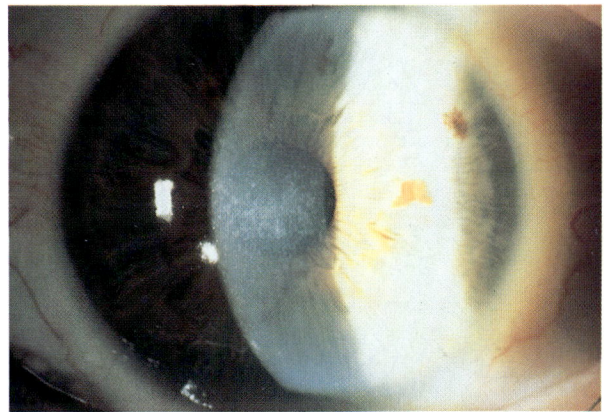

(e)

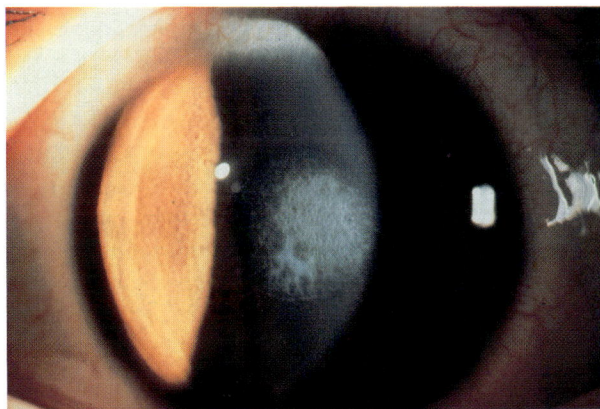

Fig. 11.35 Degrees of post-laser ablation haze: (a) none; (b) 1+; (c) 2+; (d) 3+; (e) 4+. Note the reticular nature of the scarring. (Courtesy of T. Seiler.)

not appear to pose a clinically significant problem. The haze develops a month or more after surgery and reaches a maximum at 3 or 4 months, following which it fades to the point where its detection by a trained observer becomes more difficult (Figures 11.34 and 11.35). Steroid drops may be useful for improving the quality of corneal clarity. In McDonald's series, mean corneal clarity was rated good among 10 partially

sighted patients who underwent laser keratomileusis and received only steroid treatment at ablation to decrease early iritis. However, when the post-operative treatment regimen was changed to include a tapering dose of topical steroids for 1 month, only trace amounts of haze could be detected among 19 sighted patients.

This change may well cause clinically significant light scattering and image degradation and thereby

(a)

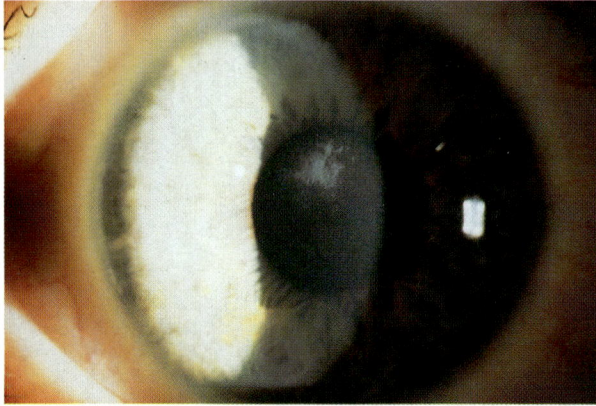

(b)

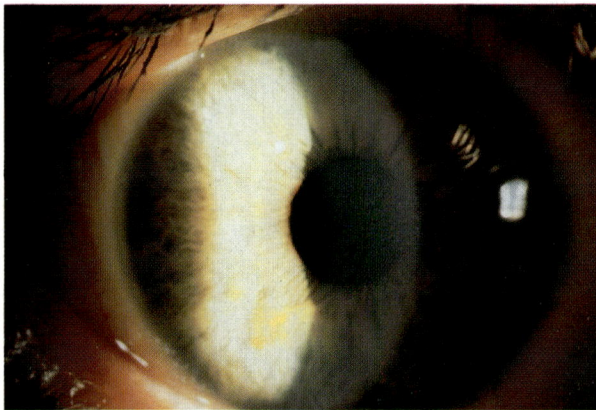

Fig. 11.36 (a) Area of post-laser scarring causing degraded vision; (b) same eye after additional laser energy was used to remove the scar. (Courtesy of T. Seiler.)

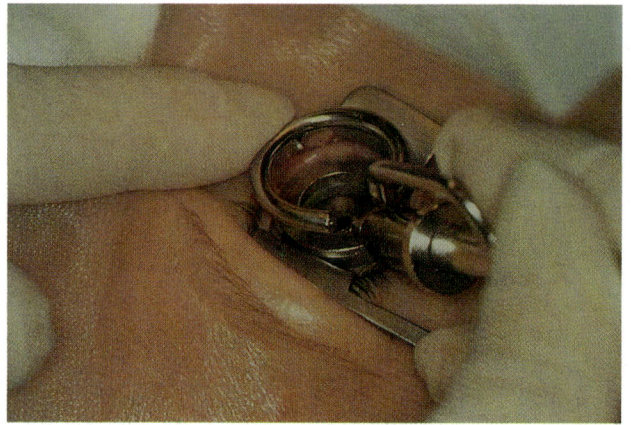

Fig. 11.37 New type of fixation ring with integral nitrogen purging system. (Courtesy of M. McDonald.)

render the procedure unacceptable for use on normal corneas for the correction of ametropia. In troublesome cases, additional laser energy can be used to remove the area of scarring (Figure 11.36). In contrast, others have claimed successful "anterior corneal sculpting" without scarring and stable dioptric correction in 20 out of 20 non-human primate eyes 12 months after surgery, as well as excellent dioptric correction (within 10%) and clear corneas in three blind human eyes [104]. On histology a proliferation of keratocytes in the area of ablation with secretion of new extra-cellular matrix, as well as hyperplasia of the epithelium was demonstrated, both adding up to a regression of corneal flattening that was initially achieved [67,98,105].

A lot of discussion has revolved around the issue of choosing an optical zone when performing laser keratomileusis. The depth of the procedure must be increased for a given dioptric change and ablation zone, but greater ablation depths are associated with greater biologic problems, including increased tendency toward haze and regression. Epithelial "gap-

filling" tends to reduce the correction in deeper ablations. Therefore, most protocols have established the use of optical zones that vary with the intended amount of correction in order to maintain constant depth. However, it must first be determined if smaller optical zones are consistent with good, clear vision or whether they result in loss of contrast sensitivity or glare disability. It has been the author's experience that smaller optical zones are attendant with increased post-operative problems, including glare and irregular astigmatism. This is especially true with techniques involving lamellar resections [106].

Another issue that needs to be resolved is whether there are systemic factors that can play a role in determining the success of the procedure. For example, Zabel and co-workers reported complete regression in one patient who was later found to be 2 weeks pregnant at the time of the laser surgery [107]. This particular patient had also previously failed epikeratophakia, and Zabel *et al.* question whether epikeratophakia might alter the corneal structure so that the response to refractive keratectomy may also be affected. Reactions such as the one described should not come as a surprise, however. Experienced contact lens practitioners as well as refractive surgeons often report the same or similar phenomena with pregnant patients. It has ever been the author's practice to recommend that such patients wait at least 3 months post-partum (or post-breast-feeding) before performing any refractive surgical procedure surgery, particularly RK. Such precautions should also be observed in patients either just going on or coming off birth control medication.

In addition to the biologic issues that remain in question, many technical issues regarding the use of laser keratomileusis need to be resolved. One of these issues concerns eye fixation and patient positioning. Although total ablation time to achieve significant cor-

(a)

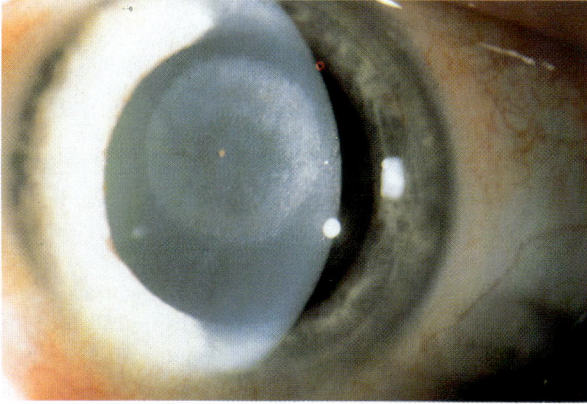

(b)

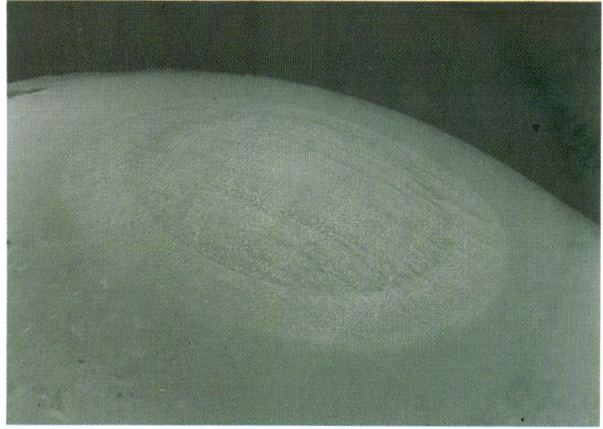

(c)

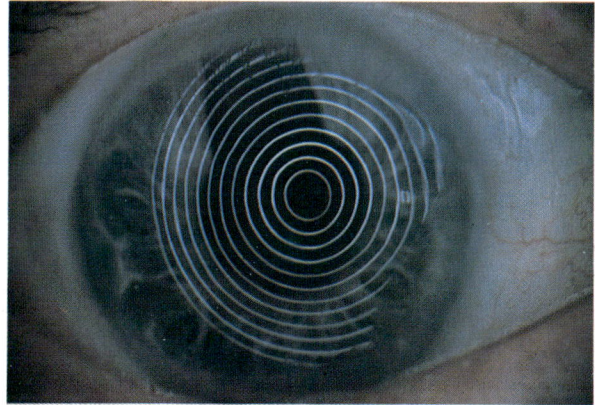

Fig. 11.38 (a) Typical appearance of hyperopic treatment area; (b) SEM of corneal surface after treatment for hyperopia; (c) post-operative topographical appearance after laser treatment. (Courtesy of T. Seiler.)

rection is short, spatial stability of the eye within micro-meters is mandatory and fixation of the globe by a suction ring has been used (Figure 11.37) [98]. Computerized optical tracking of the eye seems to offer some practical advantages—retro-bulbar anesthesia (for the placement of the suction ring) with all its attendant hazards in the myopic eye (see Chapter 15) could probably be eliminated. Technical limits of the method, however, have not been solved in a way to allow clinical use. However, adaptation of mirror—laser gun-sight optics may be feasible. The various laser systems available offer different methods for fixation, but it remains to be seen whether any of these is indeed the optimal approach.

Should the challenging problems of wound healing and radiation-mediated cell damage finally be solved, a computer simulation of laser keratomileusis—still in the early developmental stages—will help not only to understand but also to predict the final outcome of lamellar refractive corneal surgery [108]. Furthermore, there is ongoing work (still in the developmental phases) with intra-stromal ablation using frequency-doubled YAG lasers. Sort of keratophakia in reverse—instead of putting something in, we take something

out. Since no incision is necessary, Bowman's is not disturbed. The thought is appealing but some reflection is in order. If we hearken back to Puliafito's photographs of the ablation plumes and Trokel's of the expanded wound cavities from gas formation, we are led to ask the question: what happens to all the little bits? The gas and byproducts of the blast effect of photo-decompensative tissue ablation do not just get "beamed out" of the stroma—they have to go somewhere, or stay where they are. There is some question about the carcinogenic effect of such mono- and diatomic particles left *in situ*, not to mention the effect of rapidly expanding gases on tissue integrity.

Preparation of plano or powered lenticules for epikeratophakia

The method originally described by Barraquer for the shaping of donor tissue (applied in keratophakia and epikeratophakia) or of an anterior lamella from the patient's own cornea (for myopic and hyperopic keratomileusis) makes use of the cryo-lathe, a sophisticated device that causes cell death of all keratocytes during the procedure, unless cryoprotective measures

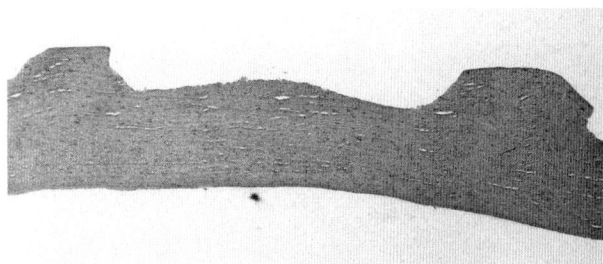

Fig. 11.39 Light micrograph demonstrates surface irregularity achieved using the excimer laser to perform a 50 μm deep ablation with the cornea partially masked by stainless steel screening. (Hematoxylin & eosin, original magnification × 40) (from Fasano AP, Moreira H, McDonnell PJ, Sinbawy A. Excimer laser smoothing of a reproducible model of anterior corneal surface irregularity. Ophthalmol 1991; 98:1782–1785).

are taken [109]. Despite this fact, histologic examination of keratomileusis lenticules has demonstrated the presence of living keratocytes, which presumably have infiltrated from the underlying stroma, postoperatively [110,111]. It has not been conclusively demonstrated that living keratocytes are necessary for the success of keratomileusis in any event. Still, there are some indications that non-destructive tissue-shaping could speed recovery in such cases and perhaps eliminate some of the complications seen with the freeze-lathing technique [112–114]. Lieurance and associates have demonstrated the shaping of unfrozen tissue using the excimer laser at 193 nm and recently the first successful plano lamellar transplants in the human eye have been reported by others [115].

(a)

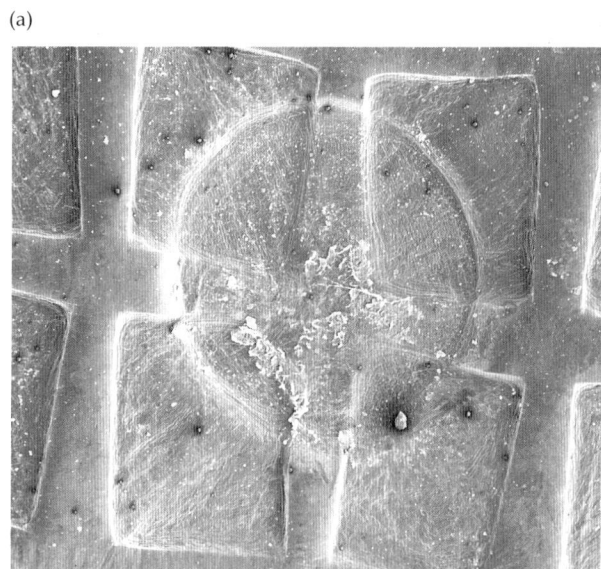

(b)

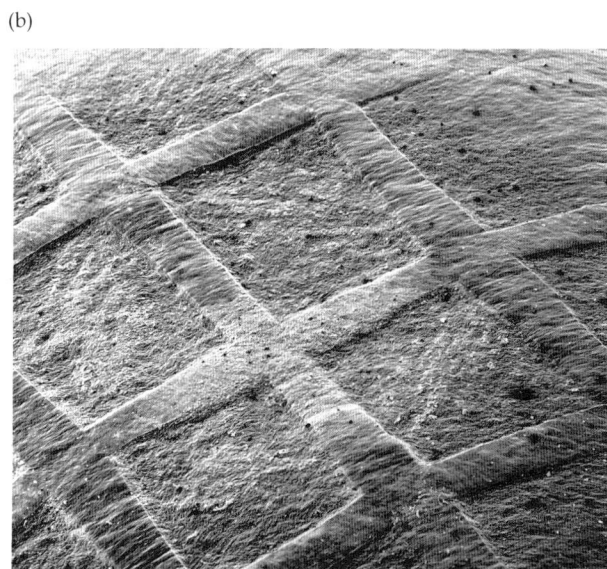

(c)

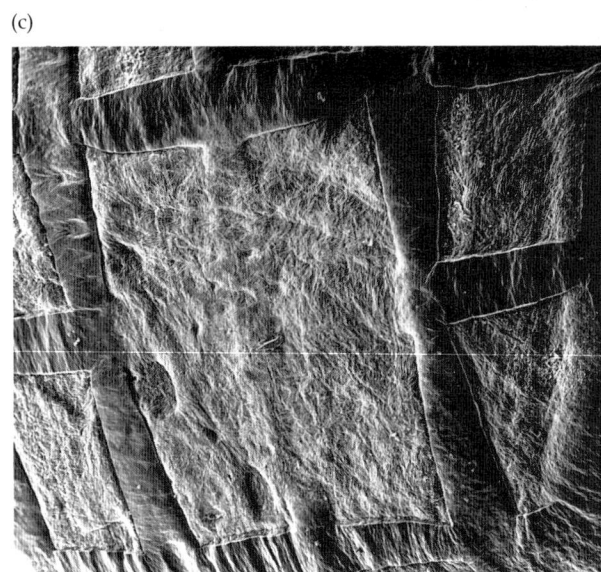

Fig. 11.40 SEM of irregular cornea re-ablated to a depth of 50 μm, using a repetition rate of 10 Hz, without application of fluid to the surface. (a) Depressions and elevated ridges persist (× 35). (b) SEM of similarly re-ablated cornea after application of fluid shows surface irregularity to be decreased relative to the original model (Fig. 11.39) and (a), above. Original magnification × 35. (c) SEM of cornea re-ablated as in (b) but with a reduced repetition rate of 2 Hz. Surface irregularity is minimal compared with the pre-ablation model and with (a) and (b), above. Original magnification × 35.

(a)

(b)

(c)

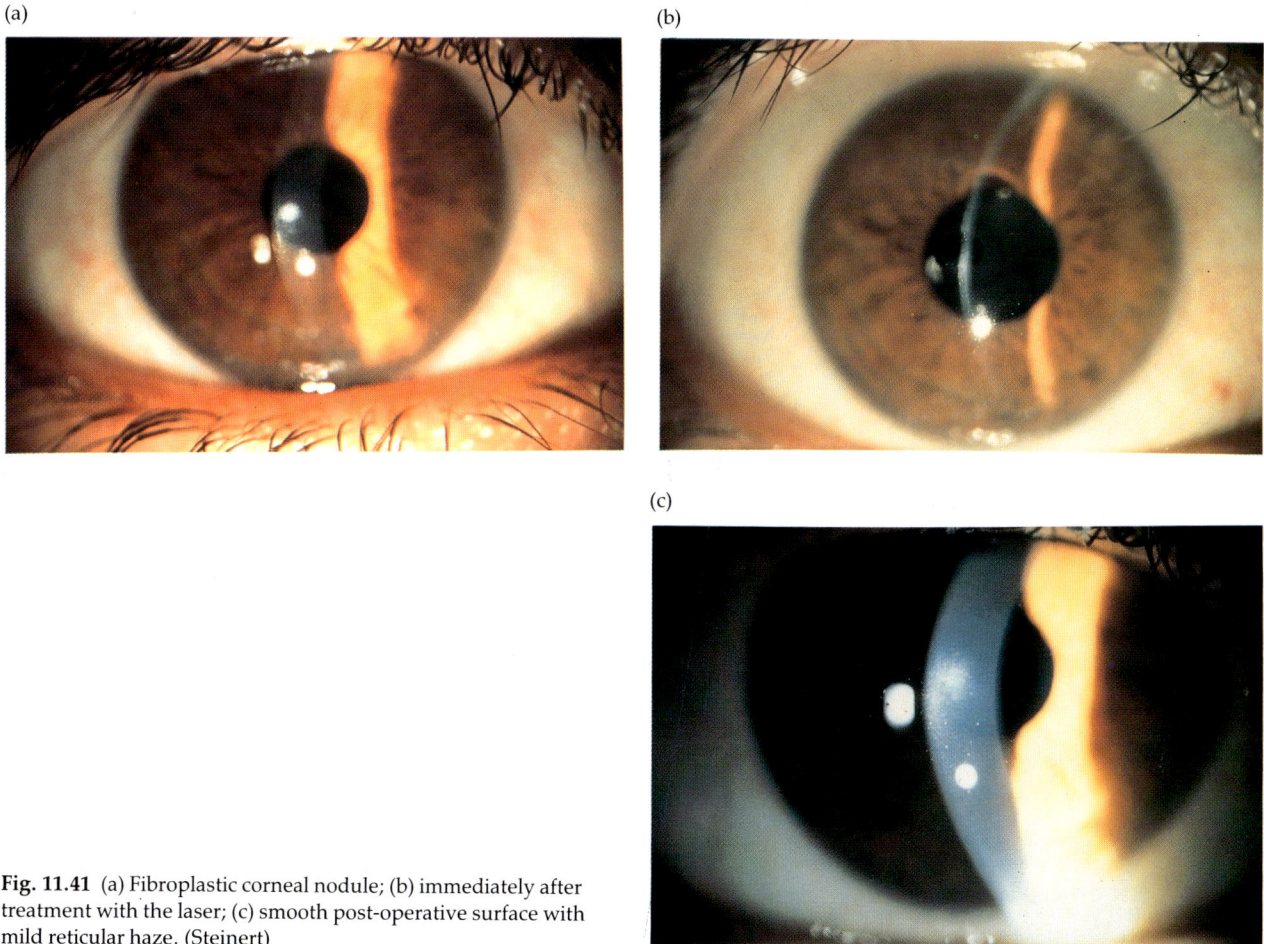

Fig. 11.41 (a) Fibroplastic corneal nodule; (b) immediately after treatment with the laser; (c) smooth post-operative surface with mild reticular haze. (Steinert)

Hyperopia

Less promising results have been obtained in limited experiments to correct hyperopia through photo-ablative means (Figure 11.38). It appears that these attempts have been unsuccessful because the ablation zone is filled in by remodeling of the epithelium, eliminating any effect of the excimer in the mid-periphery of the cornea. This phenomenon also seems to be an active factor in myopic patients as well. Gimbel has reported better results in a case of laser ablation over an epikeratophakia (H.V. Gimbel, 1991, personal communication). However, the physical conditions involving the onlay graft in epikeratophakia are not the same as those existing within an integrated structure like the corneal stroma and conclusions drawn from results in these cases should not be applied to the results of hyperopic laser ablations in general. Furthermore, patients have been treated with excimer for hyperopia in the past, and results similar to Gimbel's have been also been achieved, but these regressed after about 5 months.

Laser corneal therapeusis

One of the most exciting uses of such surface ablation is in superficial keratectomy, essentially planing off the roughened corneal surface to promote smoother epithelial re-growth. One of the questions that remains regarding superficial keratectomy using the excimer laser is whether there is an optimal laser strategy and surfacing agent. In current protocols, a methyl-cellulose-type preparation is first applied to level the surface of the cornea. This allows removal of the affected areas, or peaks, without injury to the healthy tissue found in the valleys. Fasano and his colleages reported on phototherapeutic keratectomy using a rabbit model (Figures 11.39 and 11.40). In a series of 30 monkeys followed for up to 18 months, Fantes and colleagues reported that type III collagen and keratin sulfate were found to be deposited in sufficient amounts that they actually filled in the ablated area to some degree [116]. There also appeared to be some biologic variability in the wound-healing response. This implies that it will not be possible to do an exact

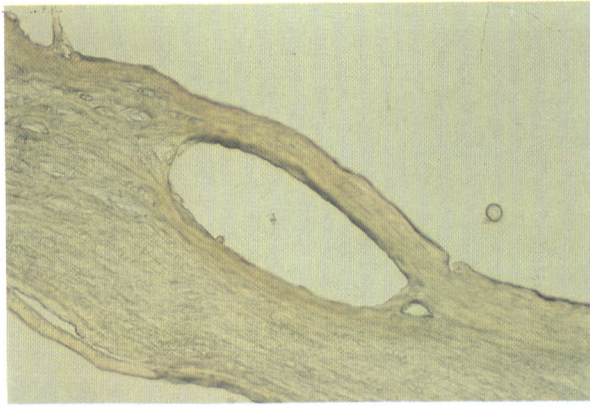

Fig. 11.42 Intrastromal corneal ablation performed using a frequency-doubled YAG system from Intelligent Laser Systems. (Courtesy of S. Brown.)

(a)

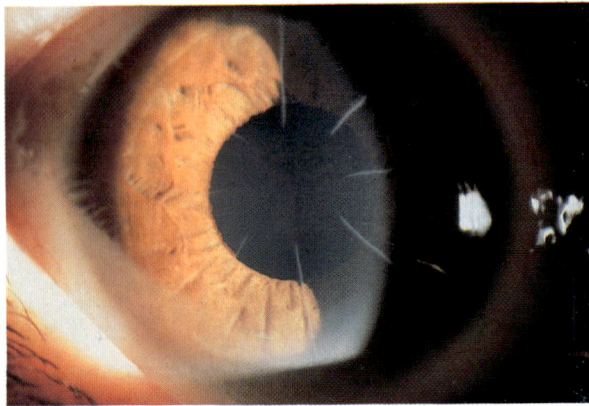

(b)

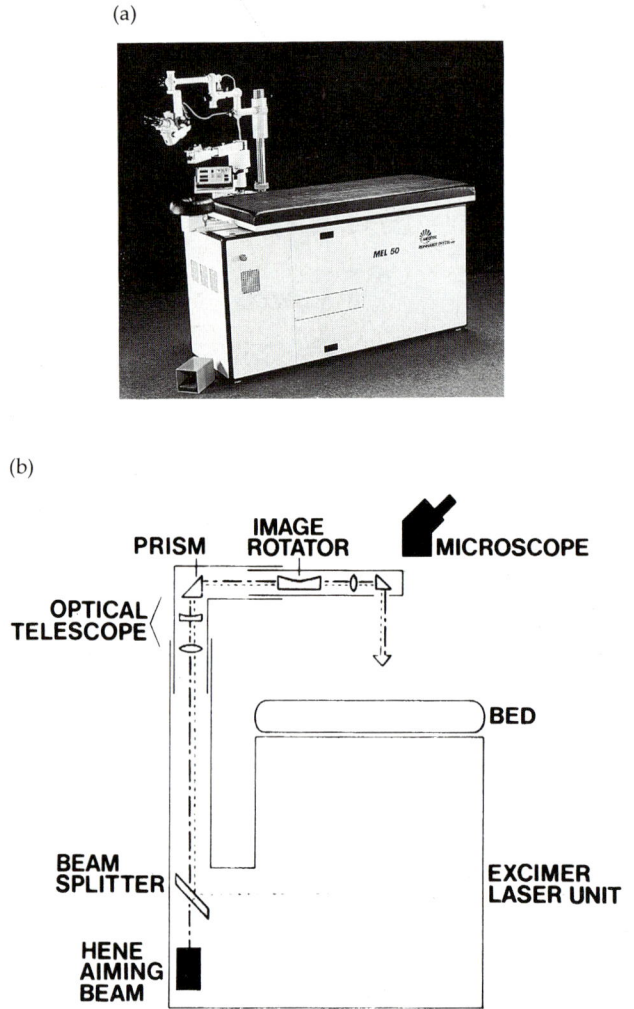

Fig. 11.43 An eight-incision RK patient 6 months post-laser ablation for under-correction. (Courtesy of T. Seiler.)

Fig. 11.44 Various laser delivery systems for refractive surgery. (a) The MediTec MEL 50 excimer laser; (b) schematic of the MEL beam delivery system. (Courtesy of MediTec.)

pre-treatment calculation of the amount of cornea to be ablated since it cannot be predicted how much tissue fill-in will occur. There can also be a regression of effect as a result of the wound-healing response. Topical corticosteroids, which reduce the fibroblast production of the new tissue, can modulate this to some extent, but they do not provide precise control. Still another effect is the development of glare. The scar tissue that is formed does not have the structure of normal corneal tissue. This is, of course, the precise circumstance with refractive ablation. In these cases, the small amount of persistent corneal haze still allows improved visual acuity above and beyond that of the previous condition, however. Nevertheless, the scarring is not very intense and can be lessened with the use of corticosteroids.

Steinert and Puliafito reported a case of a fibroplastic nodule at the apex in a case of keratoconus removed through excimer ablation [66]. Despite previous

surgical keratectomy, it had recurred over a few months (Figure 11.41). Using an energy level of 180 mJ/cm^2, a 1.0 mm zone, and a repetition rate of 10 Hz, 242 pulses were applied. Methylcellulose was applied to adjacent cornea to limit exposure damage. Contact lens tolerance returned to 8 hours post-treatment within 2 weeks of the treatment. The nodule has shown no signs of returning.

The future of laser refractive corneal surgery

Intensive research is now being performed on the application of the excimer and other types of lasers for refractive corneal surgery. Improvement of the current experimental and early clinical results—mainly as far as sub-epithelial scar formation is concerned—is mandatory for acceptance in widespread clinical use and could come from applying less laser energy (per volume of tissue) removed.

(a)

(b)

(c)

(d)

(e)

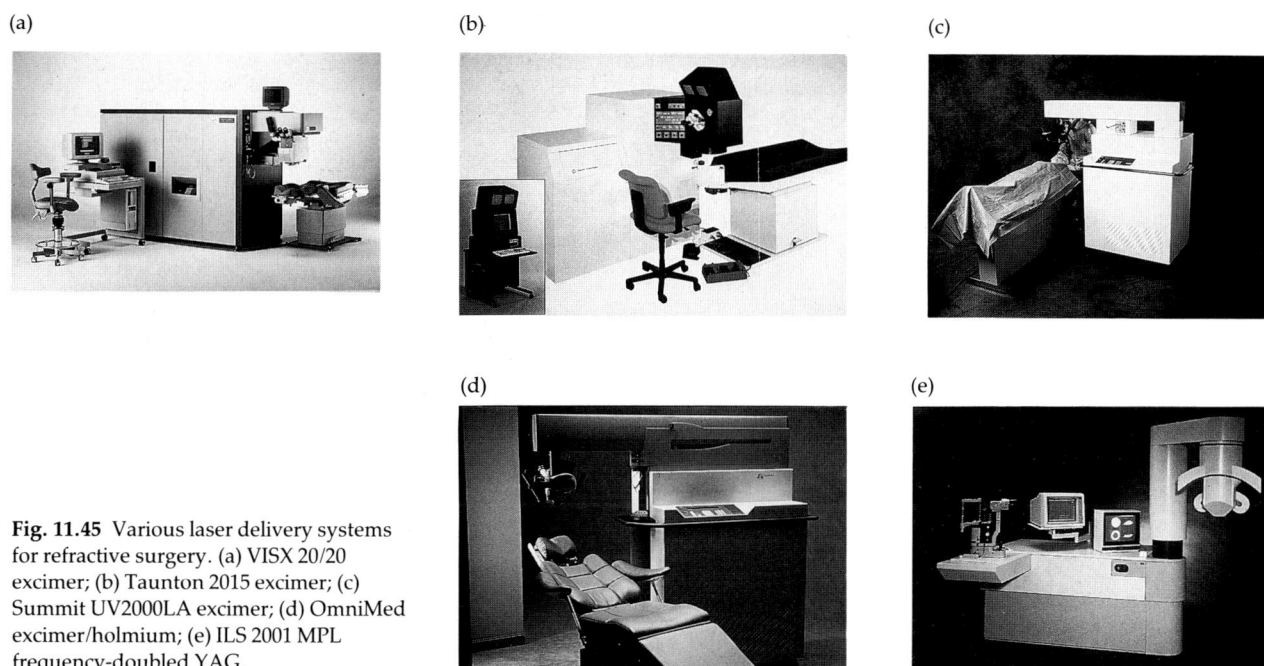

Fig. 11.45 Various laser delivery systems for refractive surgery. (a) VISX 20/20 excimer; (b) Taunton 2015 excimer; (c) Summit UV2000LA excimer; (d) OmniMed excimer/holmium; (e) ILS 2001 MPL frequency-doubled YAG.

There are some promising areas for exploration. First, the use of shorter excimer laser pulses now available (in the 300 fs versus the usual 10–20 ns range), as it has been shown that the etching behavior of PMMA could be significantly improved and that materials like Teflon and sodium chloride could he structured by controlled ablation for the first time [78]. Secondly, the use of biocompatible dopants (such as oxybuprocain or fluorescein) that would act as additional chromophores and can absorb photon energy at even higher wavelengths seems possible [73]. A similar mechanism has been described for a variety of synthetic polymers [117]. Both methods could help to reduce further the penetration depth of those photons of the ultraviolet laser pulse that do not etch away corneal layers (for lack of sufficient bond-breaking energy) but still may adversely affect and thereby stimulate stromal cells. Similarly in synthetic polymers chemical processes can occur even below the bottom of ablated areas [118]. Some of the problems could possibly be eliminated by tangential corneal ablation, as patented by Belgorod.

Ablation of tissue within the stroma itself, leaving the superficial layers (including Bowman's) intact may answer some of the objections to surface ablation (Figure 11.42). However, no one has, as yet, answered the additional question as to where the explosive bi-products are to go during this procedure (see the figure of laser plumes above). Additionally, there is no evidence that the cornea will achieve or retain an altered curvature after such treatment.

As the evaluation of potential ultraviolet-induced mutagenesis and cataractogenesis has not yet come to a definite conclusion, as detailed above, researchers have continued to evaluate the corneal ablation characteristics of laser sources emitting photons at higher wavelengths. In the visible range Troutman and co-workers [119] have reported on attempts to create an intra-lamellar stromectomy without affecting Bowman's layer of Descemet's membrane using a pumped dye laser system (at 595 nm) that creates an optical breakdown within the tissue [78]. Whether a non-disrupted Bowman's membrane allows for refractive changes similar to the effect found in RK remains to be investigated. Excisions made with picosecond and femtosecond lasers at 532 and 625 nm showed almost as little tissue damage as excisions made with excimer lasers at 193 nm [120].

Following previous work with the carbon dioxide laser (emitting at 10.6 mm) in the mid infrared spectrum (with the water molecules of the cornea strongly absorbing this radiation), newer attempts have investigated the potential use of the hydrogen fluoride laser (3.0 mm), a Raman-shifted Nd:YAG laser (2.80 and 2.92 mm) and an Er:YAG-laser (2.94 mm) for corneal surgery—water shows absorption peaks in this range as well [51,121,122].

The concept of laser adjustable synthetic epikeratoplasty (LASE) has recently been presented in order to avoid some of the problems inherent in direct laser ablation of the corneal surface. As the central host cornea is covered by the synthetic epikeratophakia lenticule that is to be shaped by the laser beam, the risk of irreversibly damaging the patient's optical zone is minimized. Stromal regeneration and scarring in the ablation zone do not occur and multiple ablations can be carried out, if the correction is unsatisfactory or changing over time. If necessary the lenticule could be replaced, as is sometimes the case in epikeratophakia. The stable attachment of the epithelium to the surface of the artificial lens—an indispensable requirement for LASE—has not yet been solved despite numerous attempts, however.

Another recent concept is the use of the excimer laser to treat an RK under-correction. This is especially of value in cases that have already received the maximum number of incisions. An even more exciting possibility is the use of the excimer laser in combination with conventional RK to correct higher degrees of myopia. A 10 D myope could have eight incisions to reduce his/her refractive error to 5 D with RK followed a few months later by excimer photoablation to remove the remaining ametropia—thus combining the best of both worlds (Figure 11.43).

There is no doubt that laser corneal surgery still holds great challenges, but also promises for investigators and corneal surgeons. As the techniques rapidly progress the hope increases that in the not too distant future many ametropic patients may benefit from simple outpatient laser surgery (Figures 11.44 and 11.45).

References

1 Schawlow AL, Townes CH. Infrared and optical masers. Phys Rev 1940, 1958; 112.
2 Maiman TH. Stimulated optical radiation in ruby masers. Nature 1960; 187:493.
3 Siegman AE. *Introduction to Masers and Lasers*. McGraw-Hill, New York, 1971.
4 Wilson J, Hawkes JFB. *Lasers: Principles and Applications*. Prentice-Hall, New York, 1987.
5 Wilson J, Hawkes JFB. Optoelectronics, An Introduction. Simon and Schuster, Cambridge, 1989.
6 Kapany NS, Peppers NA, Zweng HC, Flocks M. Retinal photocoagulation by laser. Nature 1963; 199:146.
7 Koester CJ, Snitzer E, Campbell CJ, Rittler MC. Experimental laser retina coagulator. J Opt Soc Am 1962; 52:607.
8 McDonald MB. Future of R&D jeopardized. J Refract Surg 1987; 3:207.
9 Chilbert MA, Peak MJ, Peak JG, Pellin MJ, Gruen DM, Williams GA. Effects of intensity and fluence upon DNA single-strand breaks induced by excimer laser radiation. Photochem Photobiol 1988; 47:523–525.
10 Ediger MN. Excimer-laser-induced fluorescence of rabbit cornea: radiometric measurement through the cornea. Lasers Surg Med 1991; 11:93–98.
11 Gebhart E, Lang GK, Tittelbach H, Rau D, Naumann GO. [Chromosome mutagenicity of a 193 nm Excimer laser.] Fortschr Ophthalmol 1990; 87:229–233.
12 Green HA, Margolis R, Boll J, Kochevar IE, Parrish JA, Oseroff AR. Unscheduled DNA synthesis in human skin after in vitro ultraviolet-excimer laser ablation. J Invest Dermatol 1987; 89:201–204.
13 Green H, Boll J, Parrish JA, Kochevar IE, Oseroff AR. Cytotoxicity and mutagenicity of low intensity, 248 and 193 nm excimer laser radiation in mammalian cells. Cancer Res 1987; 47:410–413.
14 Kochevar IE. Cytotoxicity and mutagenicity of excimer laser radiation. Lasers Surg Med 1989; 9:440–445.
15 Kochevar IE, Buckley LA. Photochemistry of DNA using 193 nm excimer laser radiation. Photochem Photobiol 1990; 51:527–532.
16 Kochevar IE, Walsh AA, Green HA, Sherwood M, Shih AG, Sutherland BM. DNA damage induced by 193-nm radiation in mammalian cells. Cancer Res 1991; 51:288–293.
17 Matchette LS, Waynant RW, Royston DD, Hitchins VM, Elespuru RK. Induction of lambda prophage near the site of focused UV laser radiation. Photochem Photobiol 1989; 49: 161–167.
18 Rimoldi D, Miller AC, Freeman SE, Samid D. DNA damage in cultured human skin fibroblasts exposed to excimer laser radiation. J Invest Dermatol 1991; 96:898–902.
19 Seiler T, Bende T, Winckler K, Wollensak J. Side effects in excimer corneal surgery. DNA damage as a result of 193 nm excimer laser radiation. Graefes Arch Clin Exp Ophthalmol 1988; 226:273–276.
20 Bende T, Seiler T, Wollensak J. [Superficial ablation of the cornea using the excimer laser (193 nm).] Fortschr Ophthalmol 1989; 86:589–591.
21 Clarke RH, Nakagawa K, Isner JM. The production of short-lived free radicals accompanying laser photoablation of cardiovascular tissue. Free Radic Biol Med 1988; 4:209–213.
22 Nuss RC, Puliafito CA, Dehm E. Unscheduled DNA synthesis following excimer laser ablation of the cornea in vivo. Invest Ophthalmol Visual Sci 1987; 28:287–294.
23 Bende T, Seiler T, Wollensak J. Side effects in excimer corneal surgery. Corneal thermal gradients. Graefes Arch Clin Exp Ophthalmol 1988; 226:277–280.
24 Trentacoste J, Thompson K, Parrish RK, Hajek A, Berman MR, Ganjei P. Mutagenic potential of a 193-nm excimer laser on fibroblasts in tissue culture. Ophthalmology 1987; 94:125–129.
25 Zigman S. Light damage to the lens. In: *Clinical Light Damage to the Eye*, D Miller (ed). Springer-Verlag, New York, 1987.
26 Dehm EJ, Puliafito CA, Adler CM. Endothelial injury in rabbits following excimer laser ablation at 193 and 248 nm. Arch Ophthalmol 1986; 104:1364–1368.
27 Dehm EJ, Puliafito CA, Adler CM, Steinert RF. Corneal endothelial injury in rabbits following excimer laser ablation at 193 and 248 nm. Arch Ophthalmol 1986; 104:1364–1368.
28 Puliafito CA, Wong K, Steinert RF. Quantitative and ultrastructural studies of excimer laser ablation of the cornea at 193 and 248 nanometers. Lasers Surg Med 1987; 7:155–159.
29 Srinivasan R, Mayne-Banton R. Self developing photoetching of poly (ethyleneterephthalate) films by far-ultraviolet excimer laser radiation. Appl Phys Lett 1981; 41:576–578.
30 Linsker R, Srinivasan R, Wynne JJ, Alonso DR. Far-ultraviolet laser ablation of atherosclerotic lesions. Laser Surg Med 1984; 4:201–206.
31 Srinivasan R, Wynne JJ, Blum SE. Far-ultraviolet photoetching of organic materials. Laser Focus 1983; 19:62–66.
32 Lane RJ, Linsker R, Wynne JJ, Torres A, Geronemus RG. Ultraviolet-laser ablation of skin. Arch Dermatol 1985; 121: 609–617.
33 Lane RJ, Wynne JJ. Medical applications of excimer lasers. Lasers Appl 1984; 3:59–62.
34 Grundfest WS, Litvack F. Forrester JS. Laser ablation of human atherosclerotic plaque without adjacent tissue injury. J Am Coll Cardiol 1985; 5:929–933.
35 Muller D, Svrluga R. Excimer lasers offer promise in surgical applications. Laser Focus 1985; 21:71–81.
36 Velasco JE, Setser DW. Bound-free emission spectra of diatomic xenon halides. J Chem Phys 1975; 62:1990–1991.
37 Searles SK, Hart GA. Appl Phys Lett 1975; 27:243.
38 Ewing JJ, Brau CA. Appl Phys Lett 1975; 27:350.

39 Brau CA, Ewing JJ. Appl Phys Lett 1975; 27:435.

40 Hoffman JM, Hays AK, Tisone GC. High-power UV noble-gas-halide lasers. Appl Phys Lett 1976; 28:538–539.

41 Burnham R, Djeu N. Ultraviolet-preionized discharge-pumped lasers in XeF, KrF, and ArF. Appl Phys Lett 1976; 29:707–709.

42 Stevens B, Hutton E. Radiative lifetime of the pyrene dimer and the possible role of excited dimers in energy transfer processes. Nature 1960; 186:1045–1046.

43 Eden J, Burnham R, Champagne LF, Donohue T, Djeu N. Visible and UV lasers: problems and promises. Inst Electr Electronic Eng 1979; 16:50.

44 Huestis DL. The excimer age: lasing with the new breed. Optical Spectra 1979; 13:51.

45 Rhodes CK. *Excimer Lasers: Topics in Applied Physics.* Springer Verlag, New York, 1979.

46 Ruderman W. Excimer laser in photochemistry. Laser Focus 1979; 15:68.

47 Taboada J, Mikesell GW, Reed RD. Response of the corneal epithelium to KrF excimer laser pulses. Health Phys 1981; 40:677–683.

48 Taboada J, Archibald CJ. An extreme sensitivity in the corneal epithelium to far-UV ArF excimer laser pulses. Proc Sci Progr Aero Med Assoc, San Antonio, Texas, 1981.

49 Srinivasan R. Kinetics of the ablative photodecomposition of organic polymers in the far-ultraviolet (193-nm). J Vac Sci Tech 1983; 4:923–926.

50 Trokel SL, Srinivasan R, Braren B. Excimer laser surgery of the cornea. Am J Ophthalmol 1983; 96:710–715.

51 Keates RH, Pedrotti LS, Weichel H, Possel WH. Carbon dioxide laser beam control for corneal surgery. Ophthalmic Surg 1981; 12:117–122.

52 Olson RJ, Kaufman HE, Rheinstrom SD. Reshaping the cat corneal anterior surface using high speed diamond fraise. Ophthalmic Surg 1980; 11:784–786.

53 Mueller FO, O'Neal P. Some experiments on corneal grinding. Exp Eye Res 1980; 6:42–47.

54 Barraquer JI. Bases de la keratomileusis. Excerpta Medica International Congress Series 1963; 148:85.

55 Marshall WJ, Trokel SL, Rothery S, Schubert H. An ultrastructural study of corneal incisions induced by an excimer laser at 193 nm. Ophthalmology 1985; 92:749–758.

56 Marshall WJ, Trokel SL, Rothery S. Photoablation reprofiling of the cornea using an excimer laser photorefractive keratectomy. Lasers Ophthalmology 1986; 1:21–48.

57 Marshall WJ, Trokel SL, Rothery S, Krueger RR. A comparative study of corneal incisions induced by diamond and steel knives and two ultraviolet radiations from an excimer laser. Br J Ophthalmol 1986; 70:482–501.

58 Kerr-Muir MG, Trokel SL, Marshall J, Rothery S. Ultrastructural comparison of conventional surgical and argon fluoride excimer laser keratectomy. Am J Ophthalmol 1987; 103:448–453.

59 Marshall WJ, Trokel SL, Rothery S. Long-term healing of the central cornea after photorefractive keratectomy using an excimer laser. Ophthalmology 1988; 95:1411–1421.

60 Krueger RR, Trokel SL. Quantitation of corneal ablation by ultraviolet laser light. Arch Ophthalmol 1985; 103:1741–1742.

61 Krueger RR, Trokel SL, Schubert HD. Interaction of ultraviolet laser light with the cornea. Invest Ophthalmol Visual Sci 1985; 26:1455–1464.

62 Trokel SL. The cornea and ultraviolet laser light. In: *Laser in der Ophthalmologie*, Enke Verlag, Stuttgart, 1988.

63 Serdarevic O, Darrell RW, Krueger RR, Trokel SL. Excimer laser therapy for experimental Candida keratitis. Am J Ophthalmol 1985; 99:534–538.

64 Serdarevic O, Darrell R, Krueger R, Trokel SL. Le laser ultraviolet dans le traitement des keratomycoses. [The ultraviolet laser in the treatment of keratomycoses.] Bull Mem Soc Fr Ophtalmol 1986; 97:227–228.

65 Jacques SL, McAuliffe DJ, Blank IH, Parrish JA. Controlled removal of human stratum corneum by pulsed laser. J Invest Dermatol 1987; 88:88–93.

66 Steinert RF, Puliafito CA. Excimer laser phototherapeutic keratectomy for a corneal nodule. Refract Corneal Surg 1990; 6:352.

67 Steinert RF, Puliafito CA. Laser corneal surgery. Int Ophthalmol Clin 1988; 28:150–154.

68 Munnerlyn CR, Koons SJ, Marshall J. Photorefractive keratectomy: a technique for laser refractive surgery. J Cataract Refract Surg 1988; 14:46–52.

69 Puliafito CA, Stern D, Krueger RR, Mandel ER. High-speed photography of excimer laser ablation of the cornea. Arch Ophthalmol 1987; 105:1255–1259.

70 Aron-Rosa DS, Boerner CF, Bath P et al. Corneal wound healing after excimer laser keratotomy in a human eye. Am J Ophthalmol 1987; 103:454–464.

71 Cotliar AM, Schubert HD, Mandel ER, Trokel SL. Excimer laser radial keratotomy. Ophthalmol 1985; 92:206–208.

72 Serdarevic ON, Hanna K, Gribomont AC, Savoldelli M, Renard G, Pouliquen Y. Excimer laser trephination in penetrating keratoplasty. Morphologic features and wound healing. Ophthalmol 1988; 95:493–505.

73 Husinsky W, Mitterer S, Grabner G. Photoablation by UV and visible laser radiation of native and doped biological tissues. Appl Physics 1989; 49:463–467.

74 Kermani O, Koort HJ, Roth E, Dardenne MU. Mass spectroscopic analysis of excimer laser ablated material from human corneal tissue. J Cataract Refract Surg 1988; 14:638–641.

75 Steinert RF, Puliafito CA. Corneal incisions with excimer laser. In: *Refractive Corneal Surgery*, R Hofman and JJ Salz (eds). Slack, Thorofare, 1986.

76 Binder PS. What we have learned about corneal wound healing from refractive surgery (Barraquer lecture). Refract Corneal Surg 1989; 5:98–120.

77 Villasenor RA, Salz J, Steel D, Krasnow M. Changes in corneal thickness during radial keratotomy. Ophthalmic Surg 1981; 12:341–342.

78 Grabner G. The future for excimer-laser in refractive corneal surgery. Eur J Impl Refract Surg 1990; 2:135–140.

79 Deitz MR, Sanders DR, Raanan MG. A consecutive series (1982–1985) of radial keratotomies performed with the diamond blade. Am J Ophthalmol 1987; 103:417–422.

80 Bores L. Historical review and clinical results of radial keratotomy. Int Ophthalmol Clin 1983; 23:93–118.

81 Schroder E, Dardenne MU, Neuhann T, Tenner A. An ophthalmic excimer laser for corneal surgery. Am J Ophthalmol 1987; 103:472–473.

82 Seiler T, Bende T, Wollensak J, Trokel SL. Excimer laser keratectomy for correction of astigmatism. Am J Ophthalmol 1988; 105:117–124.

83 Seiler T, Bende T, Willensak J. Klinische Aspekte der Laserchirurgie der Hornhaut. In: *Laser in der Ophthalmologie*, J Wollensak (ed). Enke Verlag, Stuttgart, 1988.

84 Stern D, Lin WZ, Puliafito CA, Fujimoto JG. Femtosecond optical ranging of corneal incision depth. Invest Ophthalmol Visual Sci 1989; 30:99–104.

85 Berns MW, Liaw LH, Oliva A, Andrews JJ, Rasmussen RE, Kimel S. An acute light and electron microscopic study of ultraviolet 193-nm excimer laser corneal incisions. Ophthalmol 1988; 95:1422–1433.

86 Burstein N, Gaster R, Binder PS. Wound healing after excimer laser photoablation in the rabbit. SPIE 1988; 98:57–64.

87 Gaster RN, Binder PS, Coalwell K, Berns M, McCord RC, Burstein NL. Corneal surface ablation by 193 nm excimer laser and wound healing in rabbits. Invest Ophthalmol Visual Sci 1989; 30:90–98.

88 Lang GK, Naumann GO, Koch JW. A new elliptical excision for corneal transplantation using an excimer laser. Arch Ophthalmol 1990; 108:914–915.

89 Lang GK, Schroeder E, Koch JW, Yanoff M, Naumann GO. Excimer laser keratoplasty. Part 2: Elliptical keratoplasty. Ophthalmic Surg 1989; 20:342–346.

90 Brightbill FS. *Corneal Surgery*. C.V. Mosby, St Louis, 1986.

91 Kahlert HJ, Sowada U, Basting D. Excimer Laserstrahlen quellen für ophthalmologische Anwendungen. In: *Laser in der Ophthalmologie*, J Wollensak (ed). Enke Verlag, Stuttgart, 1988.

92 Bende T, Matallana M, Seiler T. [Calibration of the 193 nm excimer laser beam.] Biomed Tech (Berlin) 1990; 3:14–15.

93 L'Esperance FJ, Warner JW, Telfair WB, Yoder PJ, Martin CA. Excimer laser instrumentation and technique for human corneal surgery. Arch Ophthalmol 1989; 107:131–139.

94 Hanna K, Chastang JC, Pouliquen Y, Renard G, Asfar L, Waring GO. A rotating slit delivery system for excimer laser refractive keratoplasty. Am J Ophthalmol 1987; 103.

95 Arneodo J, Azema A, Botineau J, Crozafon P, Mayolini P, Moulin G. Corneal optical zone reshaping by excimer laser light photoablation (PKM method). In: *Laser Technology in Ophthalmology*, J Marshall, H Kugler, D Ghedini (eds). Amsterdam, 1988.

96 Missotten L, Boving R, François G, Coutteel C. Experimental excimer laser keratomileusis. Bull Soc Belge Ophthalmol 1986; 220:103–120.

97 Kornmehl EW, Steinert RF, Puliafito CA. A comparative study of masking fluids for excimer laser phototherapeutic keratectomy. Arch Ophthalmol 1991; 109:860–863.

98 L'Esperance FA, Taylor DM, Warner JW. Human excimer laser keratectomy: short-term histopathology. J Refract Surg 1988; 4:118–124.

99 Bores L. Corneal topography—the dark side of the moon. Soc Photo Inst Eng Proceedings (SPIE), Los Angeles, 1991.

100 Gross GW, Baker P, Bores LD. Corneal topography via two wavelength holography. Soc Photo Inst Eng, 1985.

101 Taylor DM, L'Esperance FAJ, Del Pero RA et al. Human excimer laser lamellar keratectomy. A clinical study. Ophthalmol 1989; 96:654–664.

102 McDonald MB, Frantz JM, Klyce SD et al. Central photorefractive keratectomy for myopia. The blind eye study. Arch Ophthalmol 1990; 108:799–808.

103 Aron-Rosa D, Carre F, Cassiani P et al. Keratorefractive surgery with the excimer laser. Am J Ophthalmol 1985; 100:741–742.

104 McDonald MB. The future direction of refractive surgery.

105 Tuft S, Marshall J, Rothery S. Stromal remodeling following photorefractive keratectomy lasers. Ophthalmol 1987; 1:177–183.

106 Barraquer JI. Keratomileusis. Int Surg 1967; 48:103–117.

107 Zabel RW, Sher NA, Ostrov CS, Parker P, Lindstrom RL. Myopic excimer laser keratectomy: a preliminary report. Refract Corneal Surg 1990; 6:329–334.

108 Hanna KD, Jouve FE, Bercovier MH, Waring GO. Computer simulation of lamellar keratectomy and laser myopic keratomileusis. J Refract Surg 1988; 4:222–231.

109 Lee TJ, Wan WL, Kash RL. Keratocyte survival following a controlled rate freeze. Invest Ophthalmol Visual Sci 1985; 26:1210–1215.

110 Zavala EV, Binder PS, Deg JK. Refractive keratoplasty. Lathing and cryopreservation. CLAO J 1985; 11:155–162.

111 Binder PS, Krumeich JH, Zavala EV. Laboratory evaluation of freeze vs non-freeze lamellar refractive keratoplasty. Arch Ophthalmol 1987; 105:1125–1128.

112 Bores LD. Shortened recovery from keratoplasty and epikeratoplasty. Arch Ophthalmol 1989; 107:167.

113 Bores LD. Mechanical modulation of the corneal surface. Int Clin Ophthalmol 1991; 31:25–36.

114 Zavala EY, Binder PS, Rock M. Light and electron microscopy of nine failed epikeratoplasty for keratoconus cases. Ophthalmol 1990; 97:137.

115 Gabay S, Slomovic A, Jares T. Excimer Laser-processed donor corneal lenticules for lamellar keratoplasty. Am J Ophthalmol 1989; 107:47–51.

116 Fantes F, Hanna KD, Waring GO et al. Wound healing after excimer laser keratomileusis (photorefractive keratectomy) in monkeys. Arch Ophthalmol 1990; 108:665–675.

117 Srinivasan R, Braren B. Ultraviolet laser ablation and etching of polymethylmethacrylate sensitized with an organic dopant. Appl Physics 1988; 45:289–292.

118 Srinivasan R. Ablation of polymer and biological tissue by ultraviolet lasers. Science 1986; 234:559–565.

119 Troutman RC, Veronneau TS, Jakobiec FA, Krebs W. A new laser for collagen wounding in corneal and strabismus surgery: a preliminary report. Trans Am Ophthalmol Soc 1986; 84:117–132.

120 Stern D, Schoenlein RW, Puliafito CA, Dobi ET, Birngruber R, Fujimoto JG. Corneal ablation by nanosecond, picosecond, and femtosecond lasers at 532 and 625 nm. Arch Ophthalmol 1989; 107:587–592.

121 Keates RH, Levy SN, Fried S, Morris JR. Carbon dioxide laser use in wound sealing and epikeratophakia. J Cataract Refract Surg 1987; 13:290–295.

122 Codere F, Brownstein S, Garwood JL, Dresner SC. Carbon dioxide laser treatment of the conjunctiva and the cornea. Ophthalmol 1988; 95:37–45.

Refract Corneal Surg 1988; 3:158–167.

12

Clear Lens Extraction for Myopia

Things done well, and with a care,
exempt themselves from fear.
[Henry VIII]

History of clear lens extraction

We have already alluded to the initial suggestion of Boerhaave in 1708 in which he proposed clear lens removal for high myopia (see Chapter 2) [1]. It is commonly believed that it took nearly 200 years before this idea was implemented in the work of Fukala and Vacher. It has usually been assumed that the technique was introduced *de novo* by Fukala in 1889. This, however, is clearly not the case, since Vacher published in close proximity to Fukala. Scholars may argue about who—Fukala or Vacher—should receive primacy for clear lens extraction for myopia but the argument is moot considering the evidence of history. Vacher particularly would like to give credit to a fellow countryman—the Abbé Desmonceaux—and bask in reflected glory as the re-discoverer of the method [2]. Vacher states:

> The myopia operation, ie: the extraction of a clear lens, is now a century old and was invented by a Frenchman, the Abbé Desmonceaux; all honor belongs to him . . . Just as the extraction of a cataract is the invention of a Frenchman [here he is probably referring to Jacques Daviel], so is the extraction of a clear lens for curing high myopia the idea of a Frenchman and should be called the Desmonceaux operation . . . I congratulate myself that I have contributed to the rehabilitation of an operation of French origin; it is the merit of the ophthalmologist Desmonceaux to have announced its advantages and to have performed it regularly as of 1776.

There's a serious flaw in that reckoning, however. The Abbé (in his own words, "because of lack of courage") did not operate and was an indifferent physician by all accounts; in fact he may have referred such cases to Janin (see below).

Janin reported in detail the case of an elderly woman who had been myopic since childhood such that she could only read at a distance of 2½ in (approx. 6 cm); she developed a cataract when she was 70 and had an extraction performed by Janin in 1769. After the operation the patient could see much better at distance than before the cataract had developed—she could read at a distance of 15–16 in (38–40 cm) without glasses [3].

Otto argues, persuasively, that Janin's true purpose was to correct the myopia *per se*, not just remove the cataract [4–6]. The author is inclined to agree with him after reading Janin's published descriptions. It's clear that Janin intended to operate for the myopia. He stresses the necessity of operating on young patients, that the myopia has to be high and that "the clear lens is best for most favorable surgical results." It appears likely that the self-effacing Abbé referred such cases to Janin whom he describes as *"occuliste le plus*

431

experimenté.'' Whatever the circumstances, clear lens extraction was precisely described in 1713 by Heister 27 years *before* Desmonceaux and Janin, in any event [7].

Albrecht von Haller, himself a myope, in his famous and generally well-known work *Elementa Physiologiae*, states:

> The myope can be improved . . . by extracting or couching the clear lens thereby decreasing considerably the refractive power of the eye [8].

Von Haller did not perform surgery either, saying that he was more likely to do harm than good. He was, instead, a philosopher, a physician, a poet, and a writer whose book was, during the 18th century, quoted by nearly every medical author writing at the time. Haller, in no manner an intellectual thief, further writes that he got the idea from a monograph by Woolhouse (*De cataracte et glaucome* [9]) and also writes in his *Bibliothek Chirurgische*:

> Joseph Higgs, Chirurg. Birminghamensis, a practical essay on the cure of venereal, scorbutic, arthritic, leprous, scrophulous and cancerous disorders. In a method entirely new. London 1745. *The myopia was cured by couching the lens.*

The following paragraph from Higgs' book (page 37) is of interest:

> Some years ago I proposed to Dr. Desaguliers a method for relieving nearsighted persons, by depressing the crystalline humour, as in couching; inasmuch as, when that medium is removed, one of a less density will succeed, which will supply the place of glasses. But the experiment I have never as yet tried.

Desmonceaux (1734–1806) published his *Traité des maladies des yeux et des oreilles, considerées sous le rapport des quatre âges de la vie de l'homme* (Treatise on the disease of the eye and the ear, considered in correlation with the four ages of man) in 1786. In it he wrote:

> Myopes with a far point at 2–3″ are very unhappy because they see what is at their feet very indistinctly; they are not suitable for performing any work. Therefore I recommend to extract the lens while these patients are still young. This will decrease the extension of the cornea and sharpen the image of objects. This I have shown in a small monograph of 1776: this operation is less dangerous than a cataract extraction. The lens which is still clear will easily be extracted after the capsule has been opened. This method to help myopes of high degree was heretofore unknown as it developed from the cataract extraction. It will only be of use to those who have to work (II, page 140) [10].

Since Desmonceaux did no surgery whatsoever, this advice has the flavor of: ''Go right ahead, I'll hold your coat.'' He goes on:

> The cataract is not the only indication to perform a corneal incision. It may be indicated for severe myopes as we assume that the cause of this disease is a too voluminous lens. I have observed this operation often and it was often successful. Every lens in whichever condition it may be can easily be extracted. The high myope will obtain a true advantage from this operation and will improve his vision considerably (I, page 406).

The mystery is, who did he watch do it often? Probably Janin, with whom he maintained a correspondence but we do not know with certainty. The monograph referred to above, *Letters et observations . . . sur la vue enfants naissants* (Paris, 1775) contains the following sentences on page 5:

> This surgical procedure seems to be new but it can be successful and will nearly always be successful when performed by the skillful hands of Baron Wenzel. He has proven this several times and he has been most charitable when operating on poor patients who come to me for help [11].

It is not clear who if anyone may have performed this procedure *often* (specifically to reduce myopia) following these suggestions, despite Desmonceaux's observations. It is highly likely, however, that *someone* did in view of Desmonceaux's comments to the effect that a Baron Wenzel had done so. In any case the reference is probably to Wenzel Sr since Jr wrote his thesis in 1779. Hirschberg notes that Wenzel Jr does not mention this procedure in either his *Traité de la Cataract* (Paris, 1786) or his *Manual d'Oculistique* (Paris, 1808). Hirschberg tends to favor von Haller for primacy in precisely describing the operation. Notwithstanding, it's likely that von Haller would have been the first to deny this—he credits the original idea to Woolhouse [9]. Here Hirschberg does what, unfortunately, he frequently does—step out of scholarly mien. He obviously dislikes Woolhouse but is ambivalent, naming him a charlatan from one side of his pen and a brilliant surgeon out of the other. He then goes on to damn Woolhouse further with faint praise [10].

Richter mentions cataract extraction for myopia but is cautiously ambivalent:

> The only method would be the extraction or couching of a lens; but this procedure is, even in patients with the highest degree of myopia, of little benefit as it may lead to complete loss of vision . . . but should one not attempt in a case of severe myopia to couch or extract the lens in order to decrease the refractive power of the eye? (III, pages 489–496) [12].

Beer is more forthright but still cautious:

> Is it not possible to help a patient with an extremely severe myopia by extracting the lens? The success of a cataract extraction in patients who

before the cataract had a high myopia would speak for such an approach; no other patient has such a good vision after the operation than the myope. His vision improves after the cataract operation to an extent that he could not imagine. What is, however, the success rate of this operation? Especially when we extract a clear lens? It is possible that the myopic patient who sees quite clearly all the instruments which approach his eye becomes apprehensive and resistant. Would this not make the final result more uncertain than in a usual cataract extraction? Is it not difficult to extract a lens that has not become opaque? Somebody who has never tried it can really not evaluate it. It does, however, seem worthwhile to try this procedure at least on one eye of highly myopic patients (II, page 659) [13].

Hirschberg insists, despite what appears to be strong evidence that such surgery was indeed carried out, that no such operation was performed up until the latter 19th century. Yet he says in the same section that in 1858, Weber and Mooren cautiously attempted it. Although he promises to discuss it "later," this author is unable to discover where Hirschberg's "later" is. That he is clearly opposed to such surgery is evident in his stating flatly: "During the 18th century mankind was still spared the scourge of the myopia operations" (page 341) [10].

The first *unambiguous* reports of actual cases of clear lens extraction for myopia were apparently made by Fukala in 1889, and history will not be harmed by assigning the credit to him [14], rather than Vacher who has the aroma of a "wanna-be," or, if the reader is of a fairer mien, to both Fukala and Janin. However, as Darwin stated: "in science the credit goes to the man who convinces the world, not to the man to whom the idea occurs."

Modern clear lens extraction

It would be a mistake to assume that clear lens extraction for myopia is merely a matter of removing the lens itself. Eyes that are candidates for this surgery are high myopes, with all that term implies. They are long, they are thin-walled, and they are prone to developing glaucoma and retinal detachments as well. Many of them will already have poor visual acuity either secondary to posterior pole changes or to the inevitable minification of images. As many as 22% will not have binocular vision [15]. The visual field is likely to be restricted with scotomas and night blindness. Color vision may also be impaired.

Merely plucking out the lens—whether it is done intra-capsularly or, preferably, with phakoemulsification—will destabilize the eye sufficiently to invite either of the major complications mentioned. Glaucoma is

one thing but a detachment in a high myope is bad news. It is the consensus among those of us who perform this surgery that the implantation of an intra-ocular lens—even one with no power—is, therefore, a must. The placement of a posterior chamber lens, whether "in-the-bag" or in the sulcus serves to stabilize the eye by preventing the vitreous from moving forward. Detachments appear to occur less often under those circumstances; getting the correctly powered lens is the problem.

Intra-capsular cataract extraction (ICCE) carries with it a high incidence of retinal detachment—1–3% as opposed to 0.005–0.01% in unoperated eyes [16–20]. In myopes this incidence increased to 6% [21]. The incidence of this complication following extra-capsular cataract extraction (ECCE) has been decidedly reduced—1.4–1.7% in the general population—it is probably less with an implant. The data for myopic ECCE procedures are somewhat blurred, however. Praeger, using phakoemulsification and standard ECCE techniques, reported an incidence of 18 (6.5%) retinal detachments in 278 cases, which is high. Among those 18 eyes, 11 (15.5% of all cases) had experienced loss of vitreous (out of a total of 14 such cases) [22]. Another way to look at these figures is to state that this series had a 78.5% incidence of retinal detachment in myopic eyes experiencing vitreous loss during cataract surgery and 61.1% of the detachment cases followed vitreous loss. The whole idea of ECCE is to avoid vitreous loss, however, which is more easily managed with phakoemulsification, especially will small incisions. Verzella, in a series of 1047 cases of myopic clear lens extraction, reported an incidence of only eight (1%) retinal detachments using just this technique [23].

The patient selected for clear lens extraction requires more of a workup than the normal "run-through" for routine cataract extraction. Besides the usual A-scan biometry, intra-ocular pressure, and K-readings, the author adds a B-scan, gonioscopy, indirect ophthalmoscopy, retinal photography, an Ishihara color perception examination, and an Amsler grid and fluorescein angiography—the latter if there are some posterior fundus indications.

This situation is a natural for a small incision with capsulorhexis and flexible or narrow optic lens procedures, primarily because of wound size. Standard ECCE procedures are *not* recommended. One reason for advocating the first approach is the higher skill levels required for small incision procedures, purely and simply stated. As the incision gets smaller, both in the sclera and in the capsule, the margin for operator error gets smaller as well. Working in the bag to remove the lens material keeps trauma of the anterior chamber structures to a minimum. Additionally it forces the surgeon to work slowly and carefully and pay attention to the eye.

The other reason is that capsule rupture is more likely to occur in high myopes with nuclear expression techniques. These typically require large incisions which are inherently destabilizing for the eye. The larger incision takes longer to heal and, in my experience, so do ECCE eyes generally. These patients are also prone to be steroid responders so the less time they are on anti-inflammatories the better (see also Chapter 13). Clear lens extraction is a viable option for the high myope despite the potential hazards. Modern techniques can reduce the morbidity considerably.

Sutureless lens surgery

Since Kelman first introduced phakoemulsification in 1965 and extracted a cataract through a small opening, surgeons have looked forward to the day when visual rehabilitation could be accomplished through that same small incision. It wasn't until the late 1980s, when reliable foldable lenses made out of silicone material became available for general use, that ophthalmologists could begin to accomplish this dream. With the use of small-incision lenses, surgery could be carried out through a 4 mm incision or smaller and visual recovery decreased from the usual time of 6–12 weeks to as early as 1–2 days, with a stable refraction in 7–14 days. In early 1990, McFarland discovered a patient whose single suture became untied the day after surgery. There was neither a leak nor a shallowing of the anterior chamber despite the obvious loss of support from the absent suture. Many surgeons became intrigued with this phenomenon and felt that the size, shape, and configuration of the scleral incision, as well as its distance from the surgical limbus, were important factors in obtaining a water-tight seal.

The author is grateful for the following contribution by Paul Ernest—a noteworthy pioneer in small-incision, sutureless, lens surgery.

When I began performing sutureless surgery in February of 1990, it was my feeling that the key factor in watertight wounds was not the size, shape, or configuration of the scleral incision, but the creation of an internal corneal lip incision which acts as a one-way valve.

Technique

A one-third to one-half depth scleral incision is made 1–2 mm posterior to the surgical limbus, 4 mm in width, with a #64 Beaver blade. Using an angled #66 Beaver blade, starting at the lateral margin, a dissection is carried forward towards the surgical limbus and into clear cornea approximately 1 mm beyond the capillary arcade. The same blade is used to widen the tunnel and

corneal incision to a full 4 mm without entering the chamber (Figure 12.1).

A 15° razor knife is used to make a counter-puncture at 3 o'clock, following which a 3.2 mm, angled keratome blade is passed into the scleral tunnel to the end of the corneal dissection. The keratome blade is passed slowly into the anterior chamber so as to insure a linear incision. The blade is then removed, viscoelastic instilled in the anterior chamber, a blunt-tipped keratome blade is substituted, and the internal incision widened to 4 mm. The purpose of the blunt-tipped keratome blade is to protect against a false passage through the already-made corneal incision. Upon completion of the internal wound, standard capsulorhexis is performed. The nucleus of the cataract is emulsified within the posterior capsule using a central debulking technique and rotation of the peripheral nuclear rim, which is removed in segments (Figures 12.2 through 12.5).

Author's note: the method of Ernest is preferred to remove the nucleus. In Ernest's technique great care is taken to insure that the nucleus is freely mobilized within the lens before proceeding. If, as someone once said, the genius is in the details, then the success of phakoemulsification (especially though a long tunnel incision) lies in careful preparation of the hard nuclear material for extraction. Insuring that the nucleus is free within the epi-nucleus allows extraction without excess movement of the probe tip and the attendant danger of irrigation sleeve obstruction and chamber collapse. During extraction, the epi-nuclear material provides an additional cushioning effect to prevent capsular damage.

Viscoelastic is introduced into the anterior chamber, completely filling it. A 15° phako tip is then used to groove the nucleus to a depth of 1.5 times the diameter of the probe. A cyclodialysis spatula through the side port assists the phako probe in rotating the nucleus to produce the cross-shaped groove (Figure 12.6). A Dodick nuclear cracking forceps is then introduced into the anterior chamber and the nucleus split, using the forceps to rotate the nucleus twice—cracking each quadrant in turn (Figure 12.7a). Additional viscoelastic is instilled into the chamber and the nuclear fragments are removed piecemeal (Figure 12.7b). Figure 12.8 compares the phako energy required with sculpting and cracking (a), and (b) the mean endothelial cell counts (pre- and post-operative) in each method.

Upon removal of all cortical material using an automated I&A handpiece, viscoelastic is re-instilled into the anterior chamber. A three-piece, AMO silicone lens is folded in a McDonald forceps (Model 2), the support loops tucked into the crease and the lens passed through the scleral

(a)

(b)

(c)

(d)

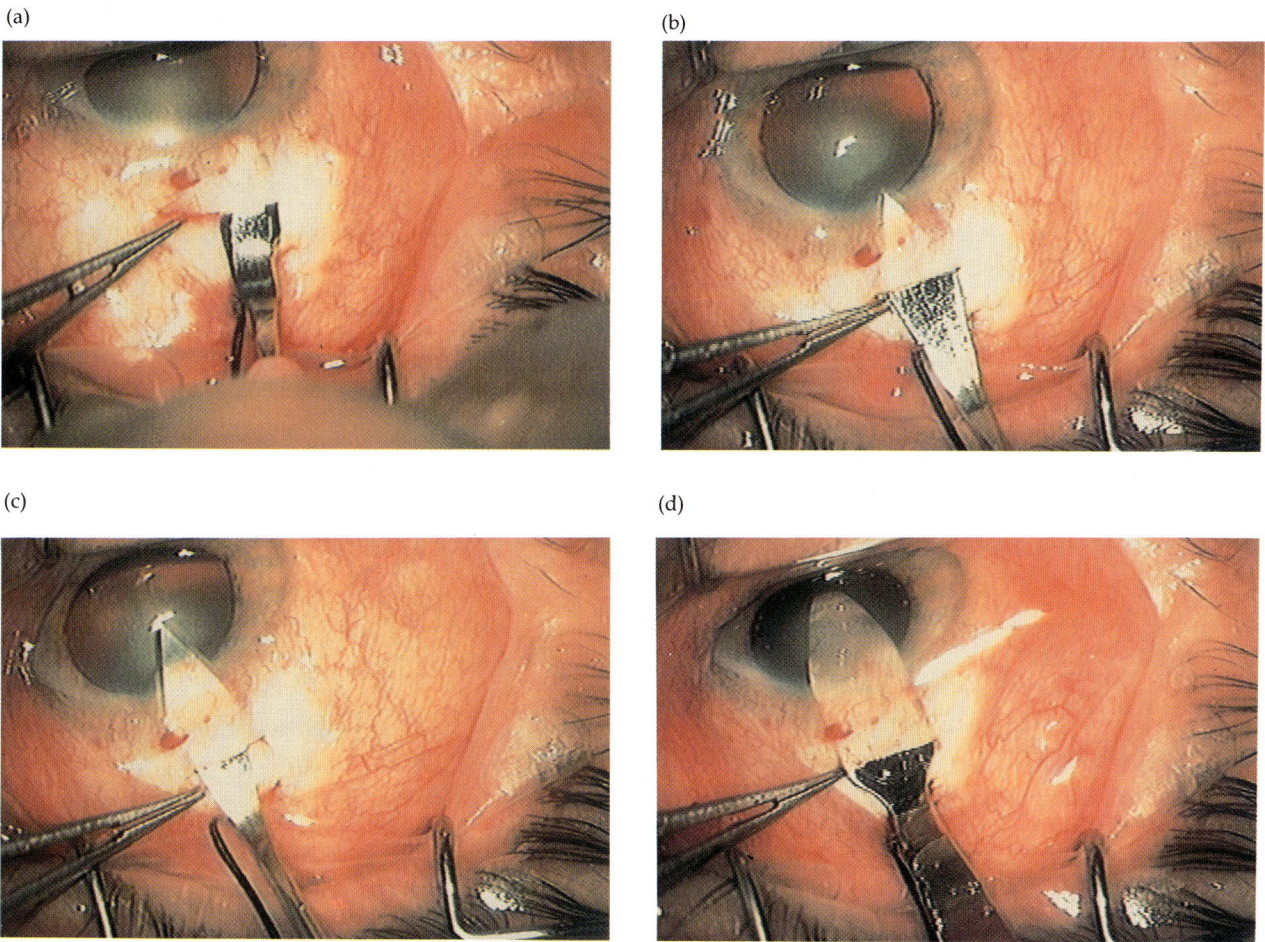

Fig. 12.1 Ernest's method of sutureless cataract surgery adapted by the author. (a) 4 mm tunnel incision is made beginning 2 mm from the limbus; (b) a phakotome is then introduced into the tunnel; and (c) then enters the anterior chamber approximately 1.5 mm in clear cornea; (d) a blunt-tipped, bevel-down keratome completes the incision. (Courtesy of P. Ernest.)

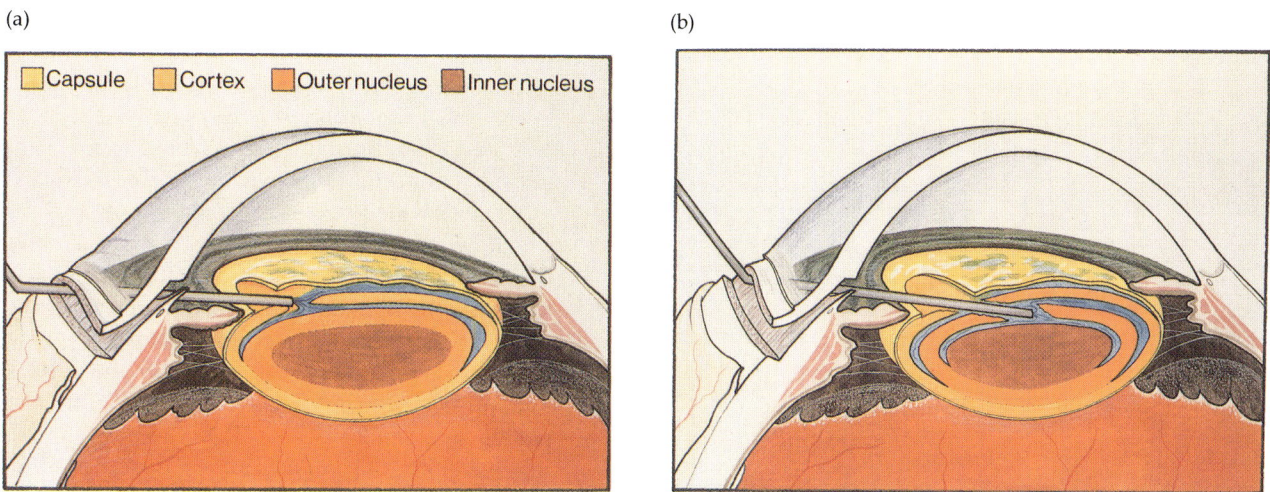

(a)

(b)

Capsule   Cortex   Outer nucleus   Inner nucleus

Fig. 12.2 (a) A small opening or capsulorhexis is made and hydrodissection of the nucleus is performed; (b) hydrodelineation of the nucleus follows. (Courtesy of J. Singer.)

(a)

(b)

(c)

(d)

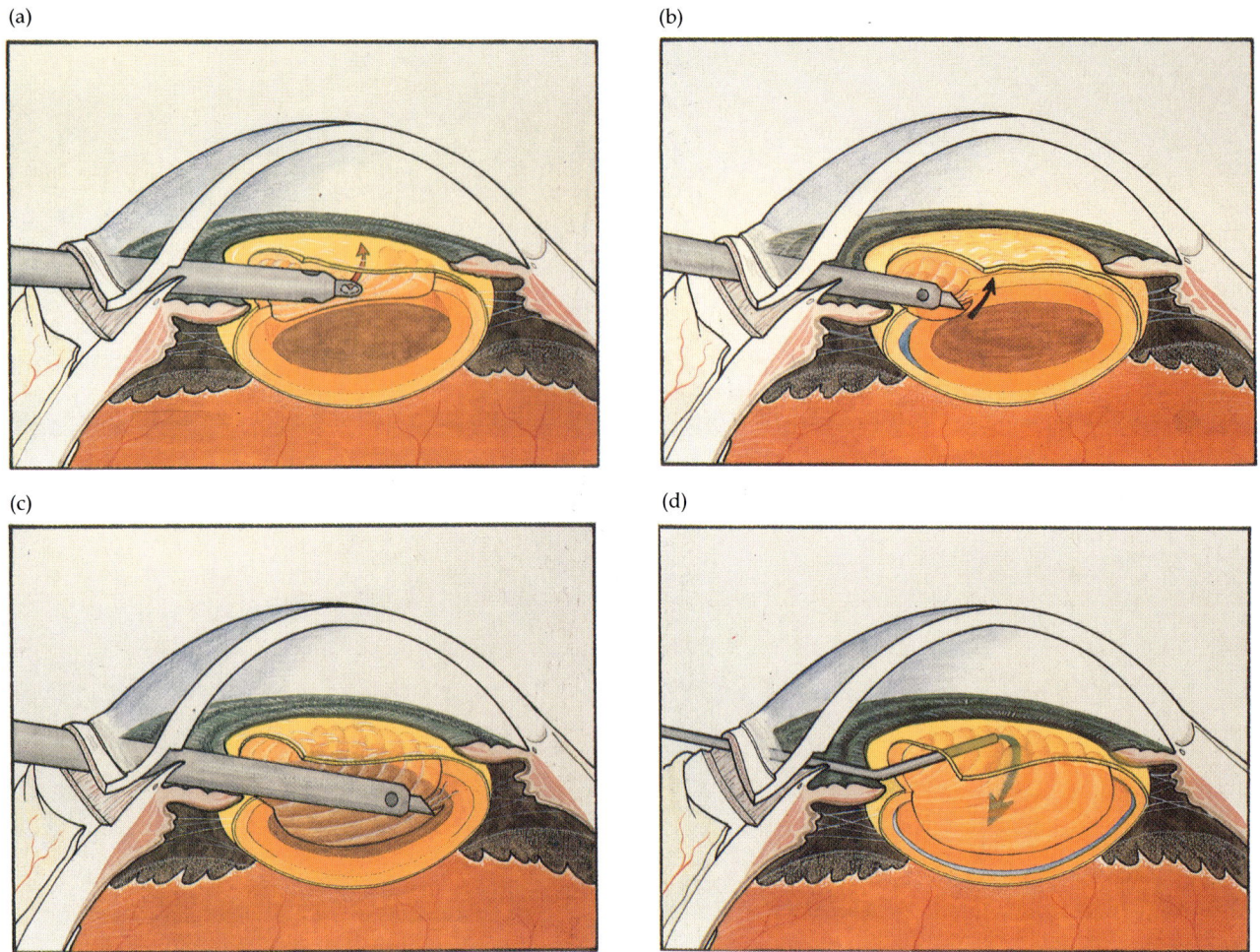

Fig. 12.3 (a and b) Thinning of the anterior cortex/nucleus is followed by (c,d) debulking of the central nucleus. (Courtesy of J. Singer.)

tunnel into the anterior chamber. Special care is taken to insure that the leading as well as the trailing edge of the lens does not engage Descemet's membrane. Once the lens is

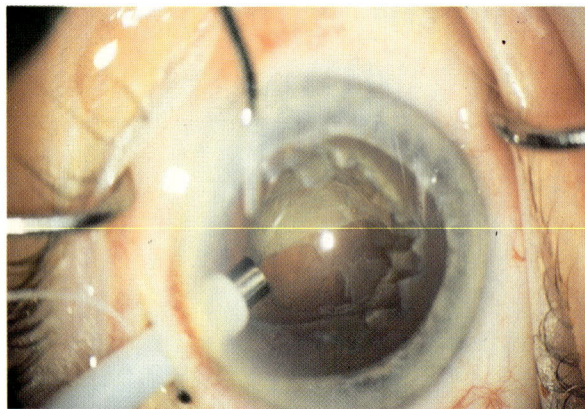

Fig. 12.4 Further dissection of the posterior nucleus is accomplished.

completely inside the anterior chamber, the forceps is rotated, directing the folded loops against the posterior capsule. The lens is opened in a two-stage manner, first releasing the loops and then the optic of the lens. The two-step release is important to prevent a sudden explosive movement which can tear the posterior capsule.

Following its insertion, the lens is rotated within the capsular bag both to insure centration and also to free up the remaining cortical material at the 12 o'clock position. Any residual cortex left at 12 o'clock is removed at this time employing the implant as a protective barrier against tearing the posterior capsule. Viscoelastic is carefully removed from the anterior chamber using the I&A unit. The implant is rotated and tapped posteriorly (balotted) with the I&A tip to cause any trapped viscoelastic to extrude from behind the implant.

The wound is tested, both at high and low

(a)

(b)

(c)

(d)

(e)

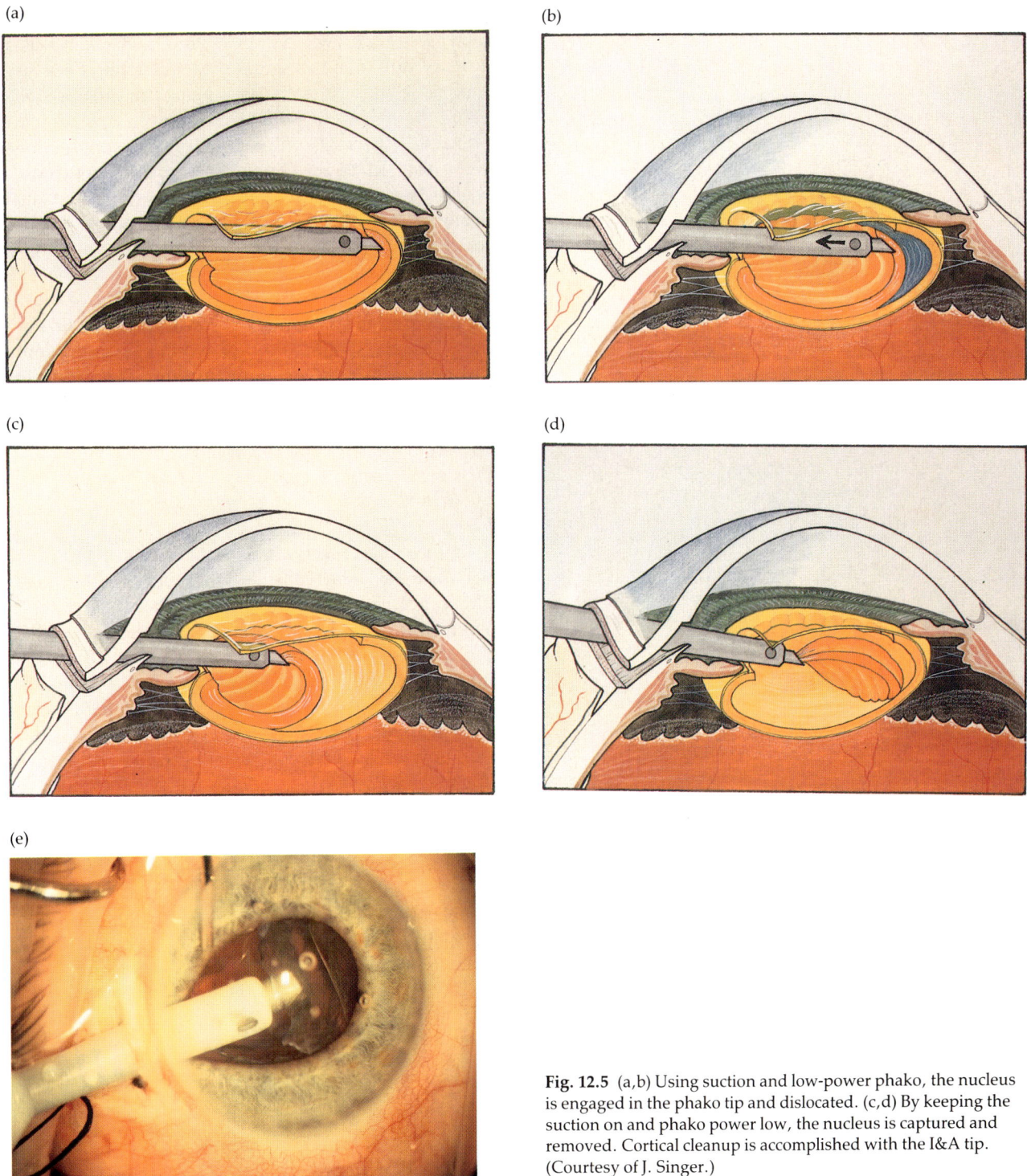

Fig. 12.5 (a,b) Using suction and low-power phako, the nucleus is engaged in the phako tip and dislocated. (c,d) By keeping the suction on and phako power low, the nucleus is captured and removed. Cortical cleanup is accomplished with the I&A tip. (Courtesy of J. Singer.)

pressure, to be sure that no leakage of fluid occurs. Fluid is then removed from the anterior chamber via the counter-puncture to insure that the eye is soft post-operatively. Conjunctiva is closed over the wound using light cautery. Subtenon's injection of a steroid (such as DepoMedrol and an antibiotic (such as Garamycin) follows.

Results

In 1500 consecutive cases no shallowing of the anterior chamber or hyphemas occurred. No delayed filtering blebs were seen. Gonioscopy of the superior angle revealed no signs of peripheral anterior synechiae. Occasional patients experienced an increase in intra-ocular pressure after surgery due to the tightness of the corneal lip incision and the presence of residual

(a)

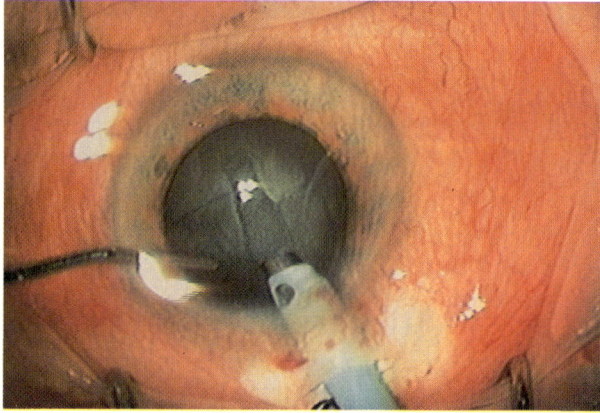

(b)

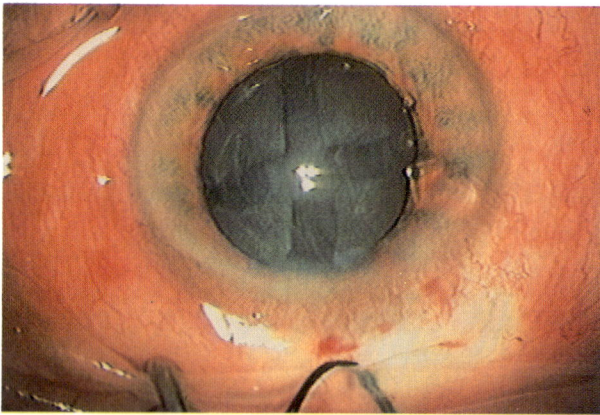

Fig. 12.6 The nucleus is grooved to 1.5× the phako tip diameter (a) using a cyclodialysis spatula through a side port to help rotate the nucleus into position (b). (Courtesy of P. Ernest.)

viscoelastic. This was successfully treated (in extreme cases) with a sterile paracentesis through the previously made counter-puncture incision. Figure 12.9 shows the incidence of induced astigmatism following

this technique using vector analysis. There was no increase in corneal astigmatism on the day after surgery due to any residual corneal edema. Recovery time is equal to previously made tunnel incisions using the horizontal stitch closure advocated by John Shepard. Patients without surgical complications were able to receive their final prescriptive lenses within 14 days. Figure 12.10 show the resulting visual acuities following four different wound closure methods.

No limitation of patient activity or protective eye wear was necessary, either during daylight or nighttime hours, and patients were able to rub their eyes after surgery without fear of wound leaks. Patients on anti-coagulants including aspirin, Persantin and Coumadin were able to maintain a full dose of medication, including the day of surgery, without any risk of hyphema—due to the construction of the corneal lip incision. Patients were advised of an increased risk of peri-ocular and sub-conjunctival hemorrhaging, however.

Reduced visualization of the 12 o'clock nuclear cortical material occurred due to infolding of the cornea. This problem was reduced by enlarging the wound to 4 mm prior to performing phakoemulsification. If the corneal incision was carried beyond 1.5 mm, an increase in hydration of the stroma would obscure visualization of the superior cortical remnants. Any corneal hydration that did occur resolved within 48 hours. An occasional small flap-like dehiscence of Descemet's was seen. This usually happened in patients receiving high-diopter silicone lenses prior to the use of the McDonald forceps, which gives much better compression of these thicker implants. In lens powers in excess of 21 D, an SI20 silicone lens could be used taking advantage of its increased refractive index. The new SI30 lens may eliminate explosive release and endothelial rubbing entirely.

(a)

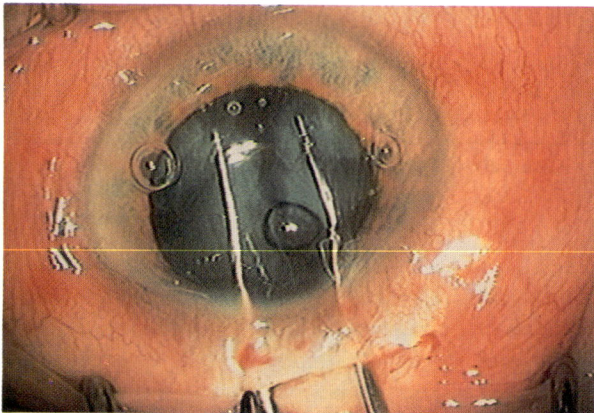

(b)

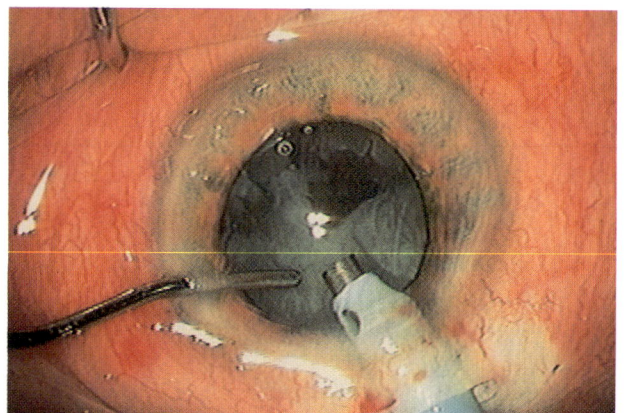

Fig. 12.7 A Dodick nuclear cracker is used to split the nucleus into four pieces (a) which are then extracted piecemeal (b). (Courtesy of P. Ernest.)

(a)

MEAN PHACO ENERGY

(joules)

9624 — Sculpting
8351 — Cracking

(a)

UNCORRECTED VISUAL ACUITY AT DAY 1

scVA 20/40 OR BETTER

13% No lip; x-stitch
39% No lip; horiz. stitch
35% 1.5mm lip; horiz. stitch
28% 1.5mm lip; sutureless

(b)

MEAN ENDOTHELIAL CELL COUNTS (cells/mm²)

Mean count (cells/mm²)

■ Preop ■ Postop

Sculpting: 2003 (Preop), 1601 (Postop)
Cracking: 1986 (Preop), 1509 (Postop)

(b)

CORRECTED VISUAL ACUITY AT WEEKS 2-3

scVA 20/40 OR BETTER

82% No lip; x-stitch
92% No lip; horiz. stitch
91% 1.5mm lip; horiz. stitch
95% 1.5mm lip; sutureless

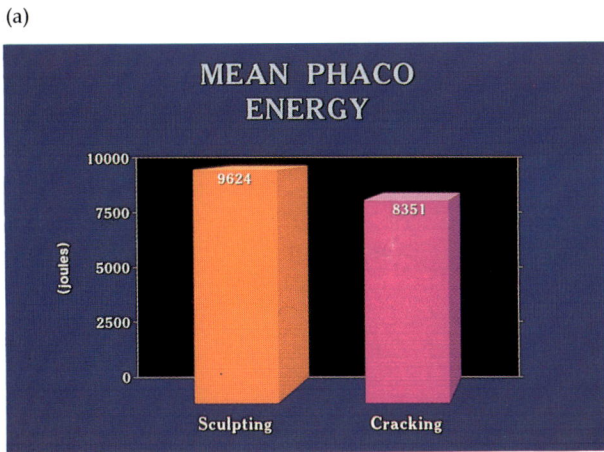

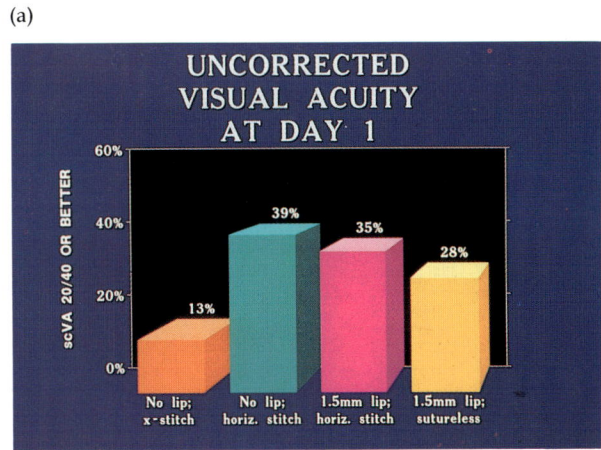

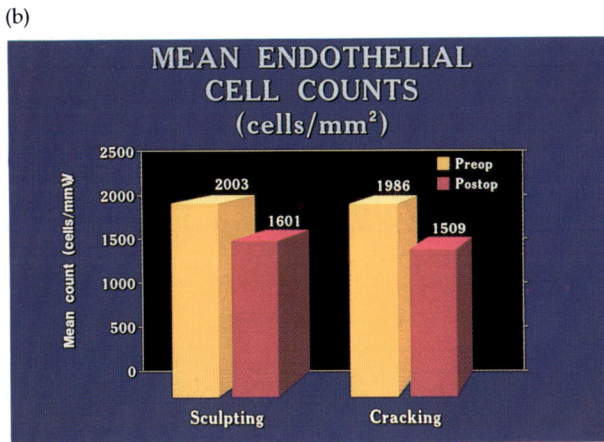

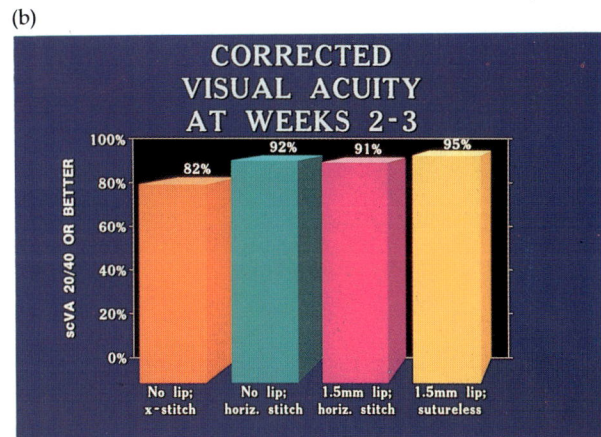

Fig. 12.8 (a,b) Phako energy required and endothelial cell counts in both the nuclear sculpting and cracking techniques.

Fig. 12.10 Visual acuities following four different wound closure techniques. The slight decrease in vision at 1 day for sutureless surgery is attributed to the small amount of corneal edema which occurs at the wound site. (Courtesy of P. Ernest.)

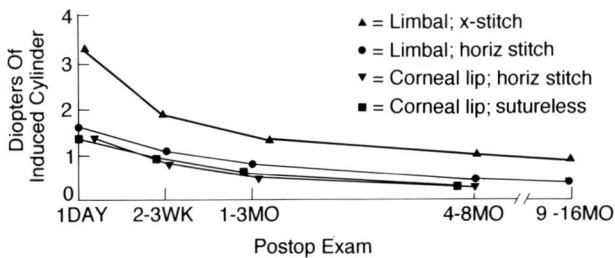

Diopters Of Induced Cylinder

▲ = Limbal; x-stitch
● = Limbal; horiz stitch
▼ = Corneal lip; horiz stitch
■ = Corneal lip; sutureless

Postop Exam: 1DAY 2-3WK 1-3MO 4-8MO 9-16MO

Fig. 12.9 Induced astigmatism following sutureless lens surgery. (Courtesy of P. Ernest.)

Experimental verification of sutureless wound strength

Using a corneal lip incision, it is possible to construct a sutureless wound that is three-step in nature and that is stronger than the standard two-step incisions closed with sutures (Figures 12.11 through 12.13). A series of incisions were made in human cadaver eyes using the corneal lip incision as well as standard incisions of 4, 5, 7, and 12 mm in length, closed with interrupted 10-0 nylon sutures. A transducer attached to a 23-gauge needle was inserted into the eye at the 6 o'clock position. A needle puncture incision was made through cornea at 3 o'clock and balanced salt was injected into the anterior chamber. The intra-ocular pressure was carefully measured and any change in wound integrity was observed: It was found that even at pressures exceeding 400 mmHg, the corneal lip incision did not show any leakage or change in its shape. However, at 200–400 mmHg, in all sutured wounds with vertical closure and running 10-0 nylon sutures, the wounds ruptured, sutures broke, and chambers collapsed. Even 5 and 7 mm incisions closed with horizontal and infinity sutures demonstrated leaks at 400 mmHg.

It is easy to see how such a valve-like wound (as advocated by Ernest) would tend to remain sealed with increased intra-ocular pressure. However, some authors have suggested that such wounds may increase the risk of ocular infection through external forces

(a)

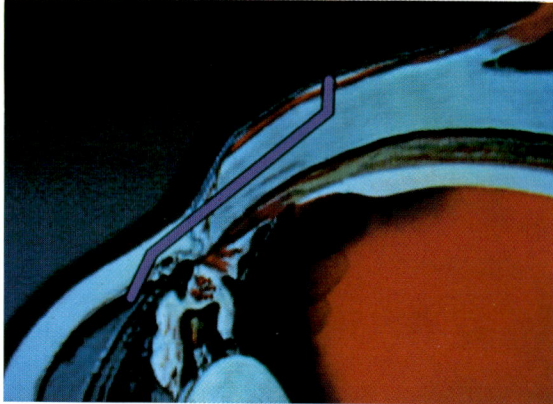

(b)

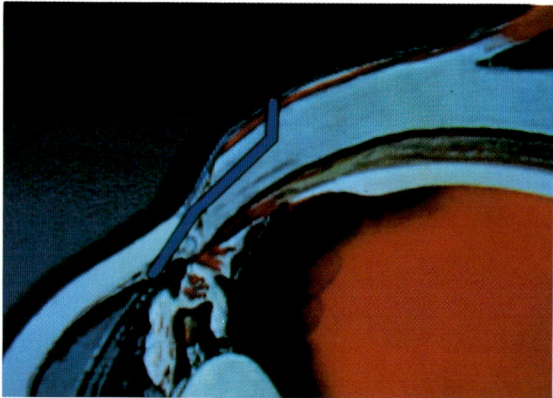

Fig. 12.11 (a) The three-step incision of sutureless surgery; (b) the standard two-step incision. (Courtesy of P. Ernest.)

(a)

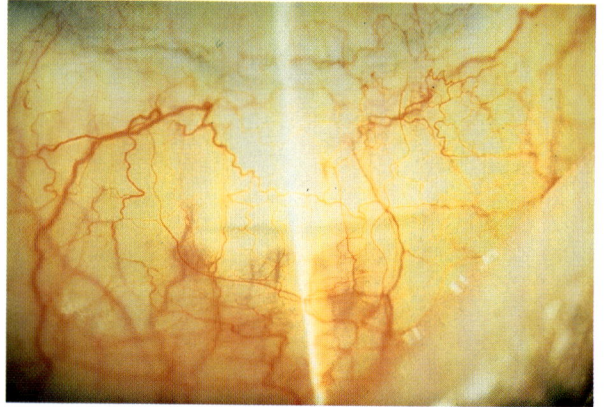

(b)

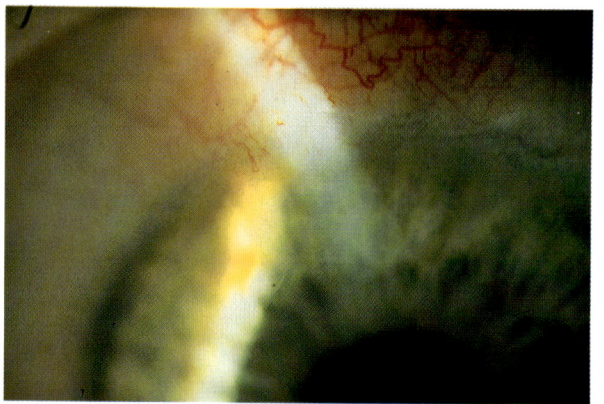

Fig. 12.12 (a) The scleral portion of the wound; (b) the corneal portion.

[24,25]. To test how such a wound would withstand direct external pressure, Ernest and his colleagues devised an additional study with cadaver eyes [26]. Ten different wound types were tested. The results are summarized in Figure 12.14. The data supported the following conclusions:

1 4 mm incisions with 1.5 mm internal corneal lips withstood external pressures of up to 525 psi, for initial intra-ocular pressures of 10–25 mmHg.

2 Other wounds (larger or with shorter lips) leaked and did not withstand external forces as well when initial intra-ocular pressure was lower.

One patient with a sutureless incision received a blow from a golf ball (driven from a distance of 150 m) to his operated eye 9 days post-surgery. The impact was sufficient to knock the patient almost unconscious but the eye remained intact with no sign of any wound dehiscence. Conversely, two patients, 6–12 months after cataract surgery using the planned extra-capsular technique and interrupted suture closure, suffered

falls with trauma to the operated eye. In both cases the cataract wound ruptured with expulsion of the intra-ocular lens, iris, and vitreous (Figure 12.15).

Fyodorov has a group of 94 patients with follow-up ranging from 2 to 6 years, in which clear lens extraction has been performed (Table 12.1; S.N. Fyodorov, 1991, personal communication). In 72% of the cases, best corrected visual acuity was 0.5 or greater. Pre-operative treatment included scleroplasty and retinal photocoagulation. The incidence of retinal detachment in this group was <2%. This points up the importance of careful surgical technique as well as dealing with the myopic eye as a pathologic entity.

Franco Verzella has the largest experience with this technique to date and his data are impressive (Figures 12.16 through 12.20). The author's experience follows (Table 12.2). The author has not had any cases of retinal detachment in his small series, whereas Verzella reported only three (0.66%), a truly impressive result.

(a)

(b)

(c)

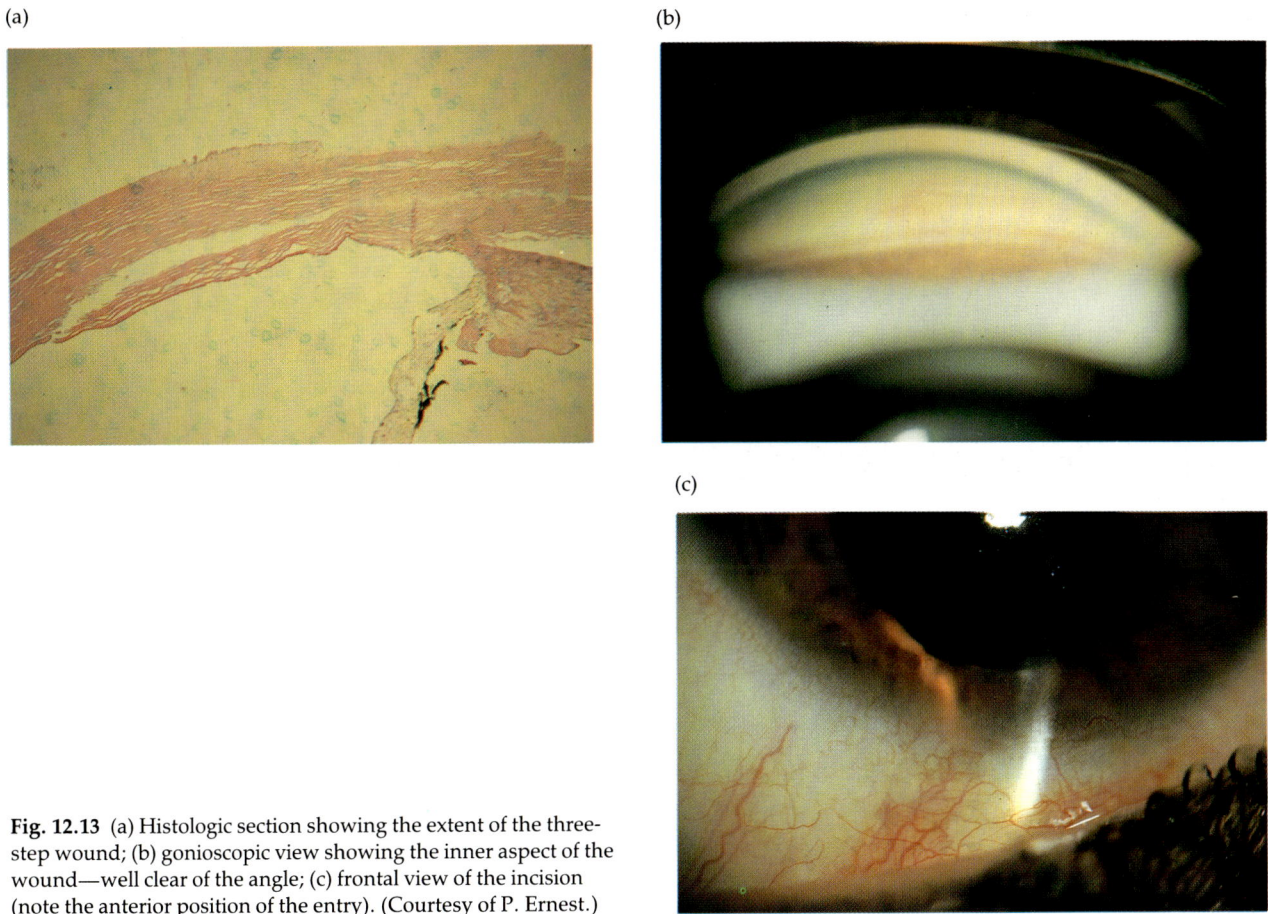

Fig. 12.13 (a) Histologic section showing the extent of the three-step wound; (b) gonioscopic view showing the inner aspect of the wound—well clear of the angle; (c) frontal view of the incision (note the anterior position of the entry). (Courtesy of P. Ernest.)

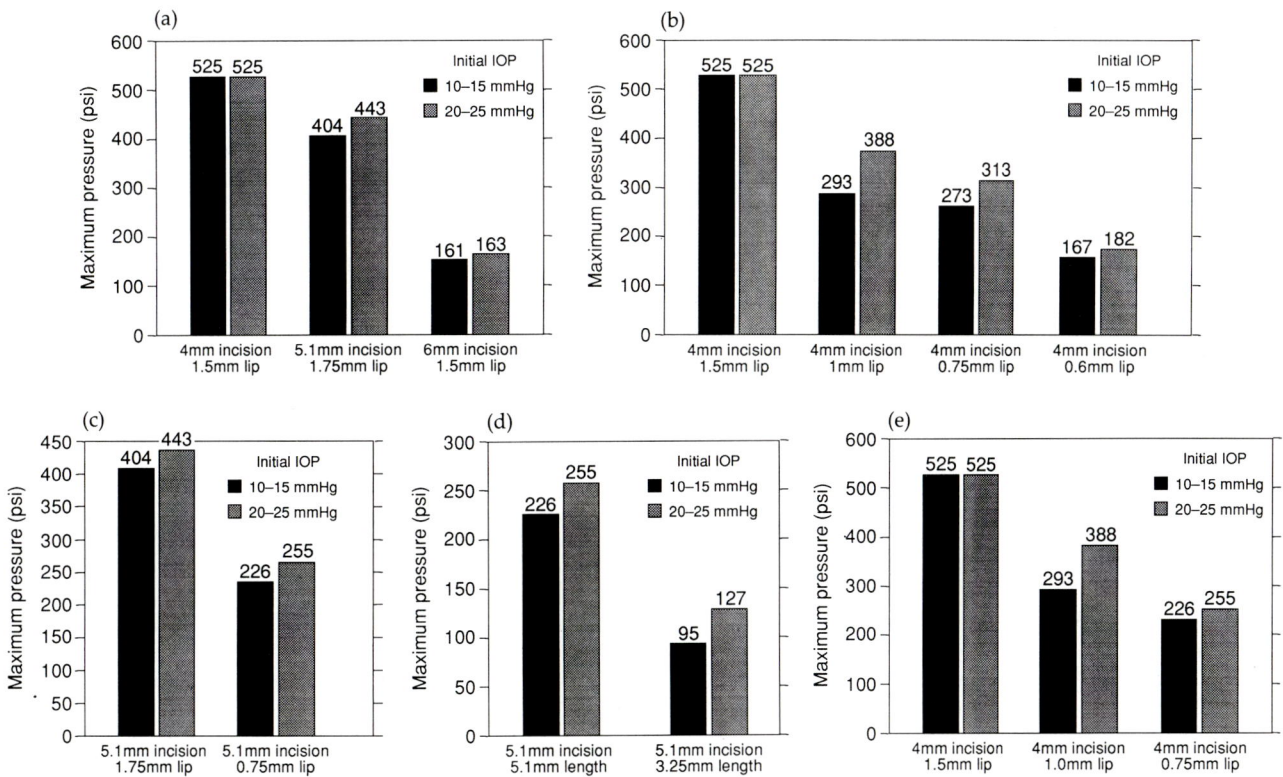

Fig. 12.14 Wound strength as a function of (a) incision width, (b,c) size of internal lip, (d) width/length ratio, (e) varied initial intra-ocular pressure. (Courtesy of P. Ernest.)

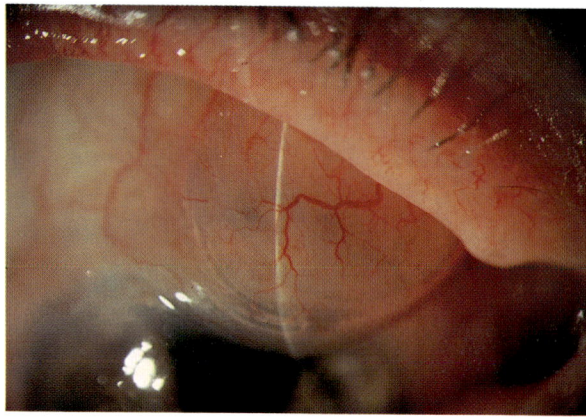

Fig. 12.15 A subconjunctival posterior chamber IOL following blunt trauma in an eye having had a planned ECCE surgery with sutures. (Courtesy of P. Ernest.)

Table 12.1 Clear lens extraction for myopia

Variable	Value
Number of patients	94
Age range	18–56 years
Refraction range	15–34 D
Mean pre-operative vision	
Uncorrected	0.02
Corrected	0.0–0.6
Mean post-operative vision	
Uncorrected	0.40
Corrected	0.16–1.00

Phakic anterior chamber lens implantation

We learn wisdom from failure much more than success; we often discover what will do, by finding out what will not do; and probably he who has never made a mistake never made a discovery. [Samuel Smiles]

Tadini and Casaamata

Ask the average ophthalmologist who Sir Harold Ridley is and you'll get a knowing smile. Ask the same ophthalmologist who Alessandro Tadini and Giovanni Virgilio Casaamata were and the smile disappears. Which is a pity, since these gentlemen anteceded Mr Ridley by some 200 years, albeit not successfully. This is not to take anything away from Sir Harold Ridley. He, after all, did something about it while Tadini only made the suggestion and Casaamata carried it out, half-heartedly.

Not much is known of Casaamata and even less of Tadini. Most of what we do know about the latter is through the memoirs of that notorious rake, Casanova. Casaamata was an ophthalmologist of Italian birth, who at the time of the event alluded to, was court physician to Friedrich III (later the Polish King August II), Elector of Saxony. It is curious that despite that obviously honorable position, Hirschberg dismisses him as a mere itinerant surgeon and deigns to give him a mere 13 lines in his *History of Ophthalmology* [11]. During this period Casaamata established one of the

HIGH MYOPIA: CATARACT EXTRACAPSULAR EXTRACTION

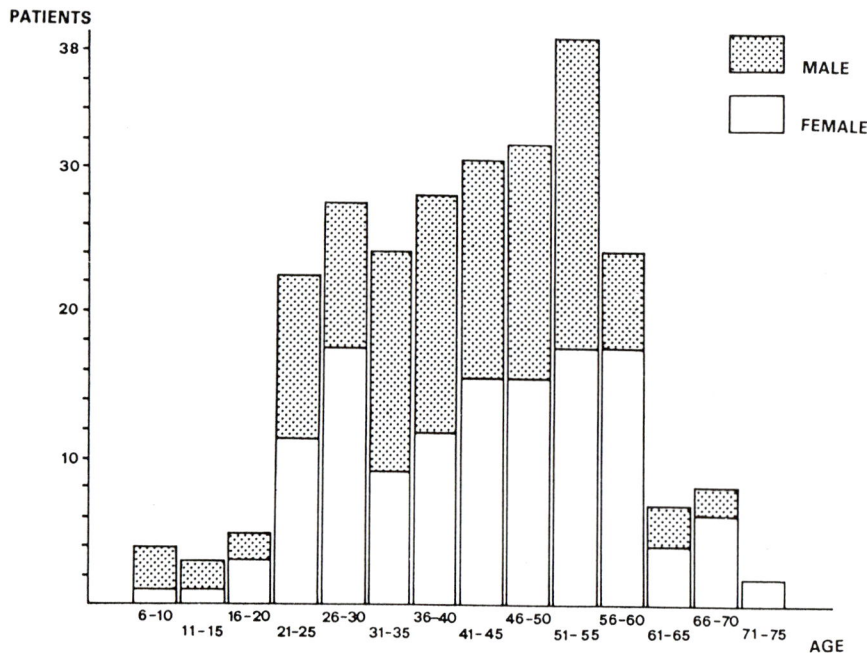

Fig. 12.16 Sex and age distribution of 458 eyes followed for 6 years. Range 6–71 years; 89% 21–60 years. (Courtesy of F. Verzella.)

Eyes

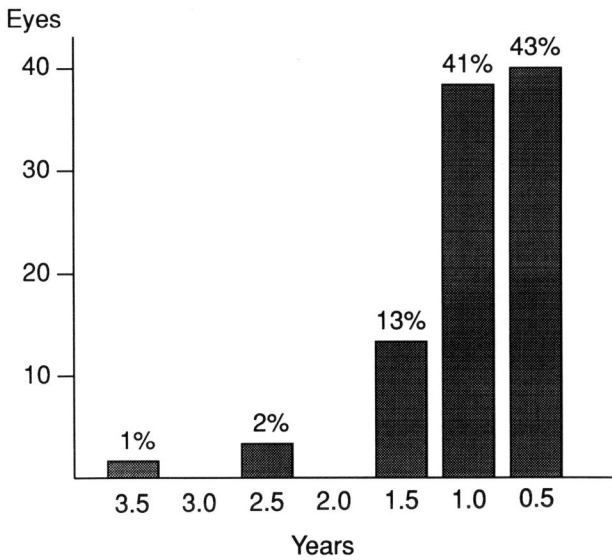

Fig. 12.17 Interval between lens extraction and posterior capsulotomy. (Courtesy of F. Verzella.)

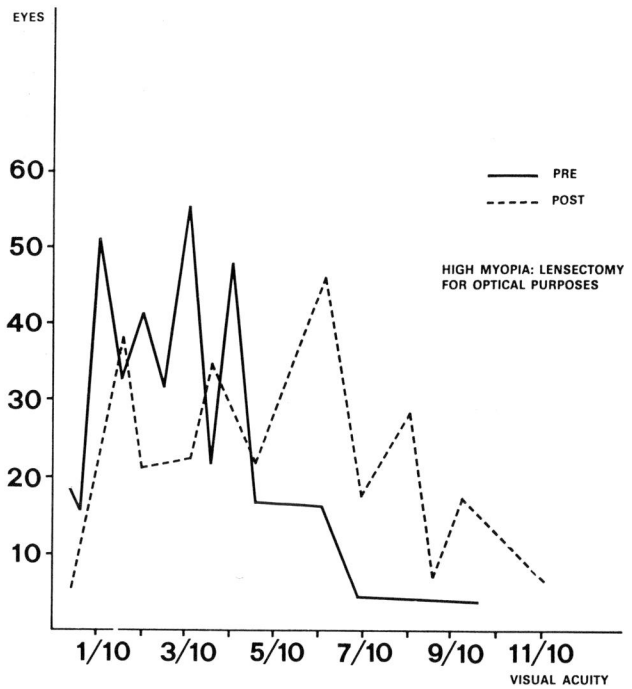

EYES

PRE

POST

HIGH MYOPIA: LENSECTOMY FOR OPTICAL PURPOSES

VISUAL ACUITY

Fig. 12.18 Best corrected visual acuity before and after clear lens extraction. Pre-operative range 0.04–0.95; post-operative range 0.04–1.2. (Courtesy of F. Verzella.)

first eye hospitals in Germany. While he did travel extensively to operate, this was the custom of the time. His permanent residence was Dresden. Casaamata obviously deserves more than the few lines Hirschberg gives him. For one thing, he was well-trained. For another, he established in 1782 what is probably the very first eye hospital—in his home. Beer, in his *Bibliotheca Ophthalmica*, describes him as an innovative

and talented surgeon who had an unusual method of operating—he sat on the table and the patient occupied the chair (actually three chairs were used: one for the patient and one each for Casaamata's feet).

No EYES

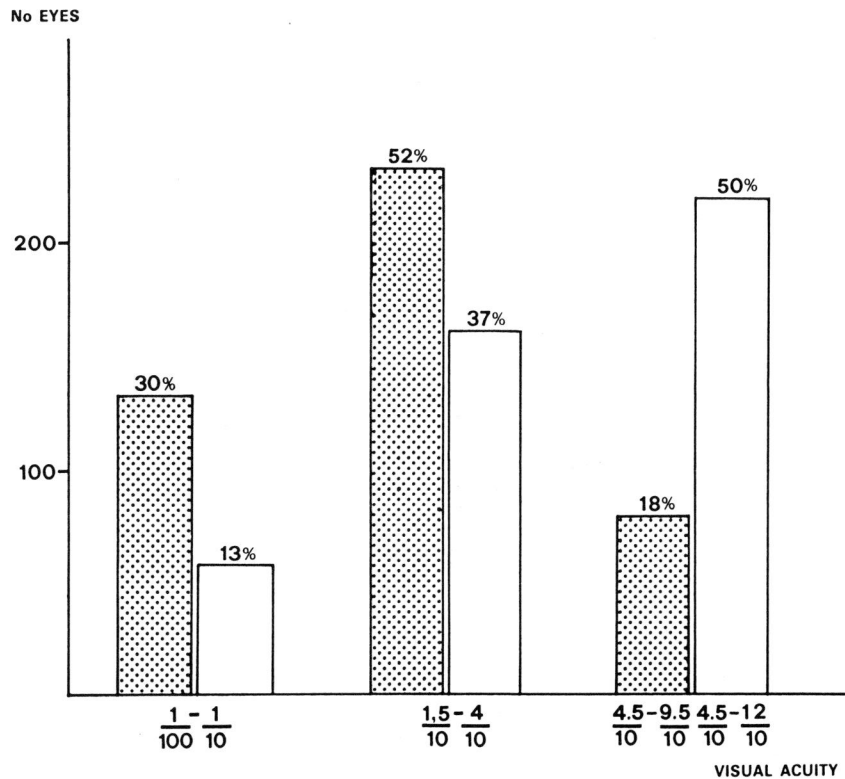

VISUAL ACUITY

Fig. 12.19 Comparison of pre- and post-operative vision by vision groups. For example, 30% of the patients had a best corrected pre-operative vision between 0.01 and 0.1, whereas only 13% were in that group post-surgery. (Courtesy of F. Verzella.)

No EYES

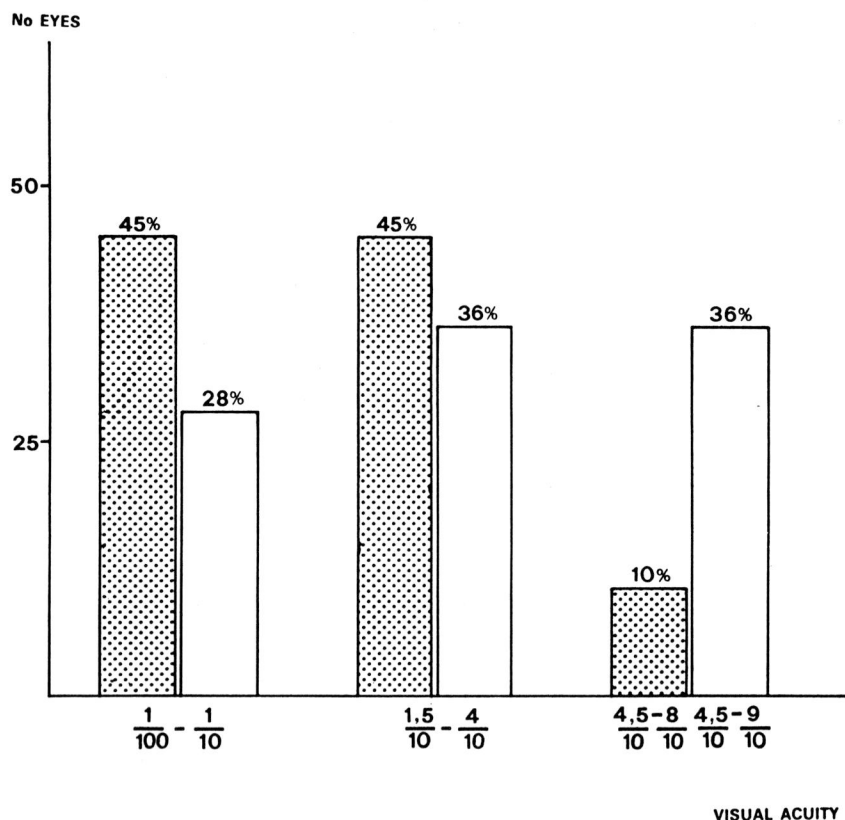

VISUAL ACUITY

Fig. 12.20 The same comparison made with patients giving evidence of myopic maculopathy. (Courtesy of F. Verzella.)

Table 12.2 Results of clear lens extraction in the author's small series

Variable	Value
Number of patients	37
Age range	28–58 years
Refraction range	9–21 D
Mean pre-operative vision	
Uncorrected	0.1–0.5
Corrected	0.5–1.0
Mean post-operative vision	
Uncorrected	0.4–1.0
Corrected	0.5–1.0

Beer mentions that Casaamata once substituted a glass lens for the extracted one but gave no details [27].

A contemporary, Dr Rudolph Schiferli, had also published a small handbook entitled *Theoretisch-praktische Abhandlung über den grauen Starr* (A theoretical and practical dissertation on cataract) in 1797. He observed and wrote about the techniques of many surgeons of his day. Within the chapter "Post-operative treatment" of this handbook he writes:

Casaamata made the attempt to insert a glass lens through the operative wound and under the cornea. He found that this lens could not take the place of the original because it fell to the bottom of the eye.* But one has another way to replace the

loss of the lens and this is the best and common one: they are namely, convex lenses worn before the operated eye, as spectacles [28].

Nevertheless, further investigation reveals that this idea was not original to Casaamata. It seems to have come from another Italian citizen, Tadini.

Of Tadini little is known except that he was one of that singular class of physician known as the itinerant ophthalmologist. Most of these were indifferent surgeons at best and charlatans at worse. Tadini may well have been both—he certainly thought well of himself. Of course, so did Giacomo Casanova. His memoirs, none the less, contain more than just an inventory of his amorous conquests; he included an abundance of historical information including medical anecdotes [29]. He had met both Boerhaave and von Haller and writes jocularly about another eye physician of his acquaintance—Alessandro Tadini—whom he had met twice.

The first of these meetings was in Warsaw, Poland. There he was asked to mediate in a dispute between the vagabond Tadini and an established surgeon of the city whom Tadini had labeled a dunce after the failure

*He therefore decided that the idea had no merit. This attitude prevails today as a corollary to the NIH (not invented here) syndrome. That is, "we can't (or didn't) do it, therefore nobody can."

of the latter to remove a lady's cataract completely. Casanova writes:

> I was, with the greatest pleasure, ready to listen to the two hostile doctors. The old one was German, though he spoke French relatively well. He attacked Tadini in Latin but the latter interrupted him immediately, by saying, the lady (who was also present) has to be able to understand what they were saying. Obviously Tadini didn't understand a word of Latin. The German eye doctor tried to reason with him. He said: "It is true that the incising of the cataract gives both the patient and the surgeon the certainty that the cataract will not return; but that surgery is less safe and puts the patient in danger of going blind when losing the irreplaceable crystalline lens."
>
> Whereupon Tadini committed the stupidity of pulling out a small box containing small glass balls resembling the crystalline. [The human lens was often called the crystalline in the older literature. It is still referred to as that even today in some cultures.] "What is that supposed to mean?" said the old surgeon. "I", said Tadini, "possess the skill to insert these glass lenses through the cornea." At this the old surgeon laughed so hard and long that the lady couldn't help but join in. I would have liked to have laughed as well, but was embarrassed to be taken for an ignoramus and kept still. Tadini undoubtedly thought that my silence was a rebuke to the German and hoped to bring on a thunderstorm when he turned to me.
>
> I answered: "Since you wish to know my opinion, I'll tell you. There is a very big difference between a tooth and the crystalline of the eye and you are wrong to suppose that one could fit a glass lens into the eye between the cornea and retina like pulling out an old tooth and replacing it with a false one. Sir, I have never fitted a person with a false tooth which is possible; but surely an artificial crystalline is not" [29].

Tadini left the meeting in disgrace. The old professor published an article in the *Warsaw News* ridiculing Tadini and managed to persuade his cronies on the faculty to insist that Tadini take an examination in his professed *métier*. Tadini responded by attacking the professor physically and had to flee the city.

Casanova met Tadini again in Barcelona where the former was incarcerated for his philandering. It seems that Tadini had arrived in town without credentials. Refusing to submit to an examination (in Latin) prior to setting up shop, he was inducted into the army instanter and assigned a job more suited to his talents—that of a jailer. At the end of their meeting Casanova asked:

> "So, what did you do with those glass lenses?"
>
> "After Warsaw, I gave them up, though I am sure they would have been a success."
>
> "It seems that he had never really tried them."

Thus Casaamata is established as the first to attempt to insert a pseudophakos. It is unlikely, though, that Tadini had ever met Casaamata; they moved in somewhat different circles. Casaamata could certainly not have read the memoirs of Casanova since these were published in 1818, 20 years after Casanova's death and 11 years after his own. It is possible that the Warsaw episode mentioned above came to Casaamata's attention in his role as court physician. There is, however, another simpler explanation. In those days Dresden was one of the most opulent capitals of Europe. The Elector was, as were so many other nobles, a patron of the arts and drew many talented people to his court. Among these were the actress Gianetta Casanova, the mother of Giacomo, and his younger brothers Francesco and Giambattista, who were painters. From 1785 Casanova himself served as the librarian of the Count Waldstein, in Dux (not far away) where he wrote his memoirs. There was plenty of opportunity for him to visit his family at the Saxon court where he undoubtedly told and retold the story of the "ridiculous" Italian ophthalmologist and his glass lenses.

Angle-supported lenses for myopia

Angle-supported lenses have been used following cataract surgery for years with more or less success; the more modern versions are considerably safer than the older models such as the Strampelli and the Danheim. It should not be thought, however, that it is the rigid lenses alone that have produced the complications reported. The Danheim (and later the Leiske) lenses have had their share of iridocyclitis, hyphema, glaucoma, and corneal decompensation. Because of this fact it cannot be said that the concept of an angle-supported myopic implant has been proved [30]. On the contrary, experience with lenses of that type has shown just the opposite—in phakic eyes.

Notwithstanding the opinion of some, the story of implantation of intra-ocular lenses into the phakic eye to treat myopia has a disastrous history. Strampelli implanted examples of his own design in 1953 with indifferent results [31]. The most notorious example, however, is that of Joaquin Barraquer's experience in 1959 [32]. Iridocyclitis, recurrent hyphema, secondary glaucoma, and corneal decompensation necessitated removal of most of the lenses implanted. While some blame can be laid to the fact that the surgery was performed with loupe magnification only, the lenses used were principally the cause of the corneal and anterior chamber problems encountered. That these complications were chiefly lens-caused is clearly shown by Drews who examined a group of 162 such

(a)

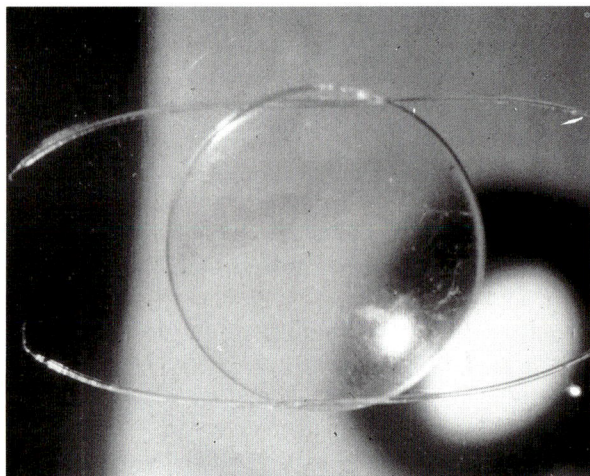

(b)

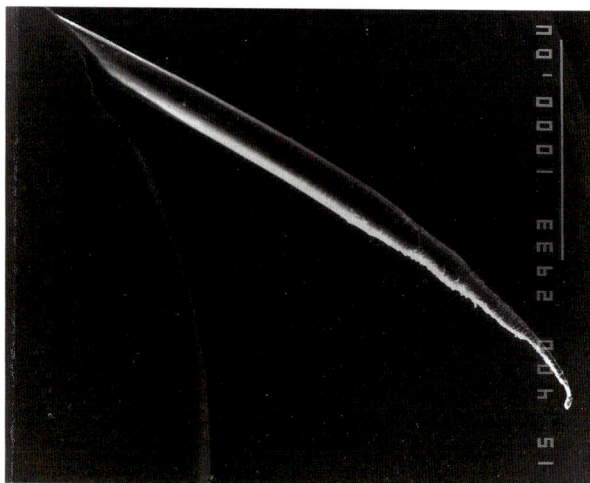

Fig. 12.21 Dannheim lenses from the Barraquer series. (a) This minus lens shows typical loss of the loop ends. (b) SEM confirms the loss due to biodegradation (from Drews RC. The Barraquer experience with intraocular lenses. *Ophthalmology* 1982; 89: 386–393.

intra-ocular lenses, some of which had been removed from phakic myopes (Figure 12.21) [33].

That the current crop of lenses are considerably better in both design and fabrication than their

predecessors is not in dispute. That these same lenses are likewise more suited for implantation into the phakic eye is a question whose resolution is not as yet complete. Still, some work is ongoing to test this premise, some using silicone-type construction and others PMMA. The most noteworthy of the latter is the Worst–Fechner iris claw lens (see below).

Georges Baikoff has been one of the leading exponents of angle-supported intra-ocular lenses to correct myopia. He recently reported on a series of 163 myopic implants of a multiflex-design PMMA minus lens with 2 years follow-up (Table 12.3). In almost 3% of the cases the implant required removal primarily for power error within the first 2 post-operative days. Rotation of the lenses (due to small size) was seen in 4% of the cases. All of these lenses were reported to have stabilized in their new positions, however. This phenomenon has been reported in ACLs for aphakia and almost always requires removal sometime in the post-operative course. Although one case is reported to have developed a cataract subsequent to the intra-ocular lens implant, cases in which some opacification of the lens preceded the surgery have not shown progression of those changes (Figures 12.22 through 23) [30,34].

Progressive endothelial cell loss following implantation of angle-supported intra-ocular lenses has been

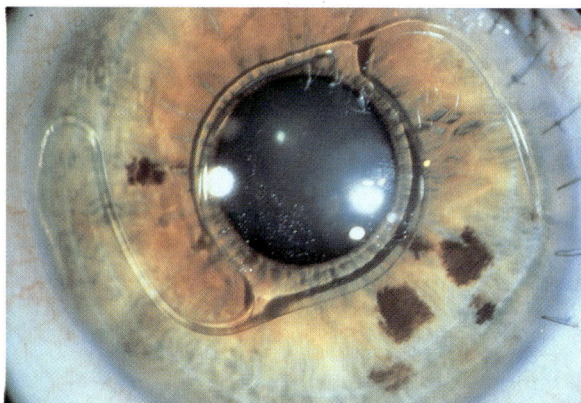

Fig. 12.22 ACL lens in a phakic eye for myopia. (Courtesy of G. Baikoff.)

Table 12.3 Visual results following phakic anterior intra-ocular lens implantation for myopia

	Pre-operative visual acuity	Day 1–2	Day 15–30	2–3 months	5–6 months
Myopia (D)*	−14.94 ± 4.68 (154)	−0.17 ± 1.25 (94)	−0.04 ± 1.33 (115)	−0.17 ± 1.11 (118)	−0.22 ± 1.08 (74)
Best corrected visual acuity†	0.47 ± 0.26 (163)	0.52 ± 0.23 (108)	0.61 ± 0.23 (127)	0.64 ± 0.25 (128)	0.62 ± 0.26 (92)

* Numbers in parentheses represent number of eyes.
† Snellen ratios (e.g. 0.5 = 20/40).

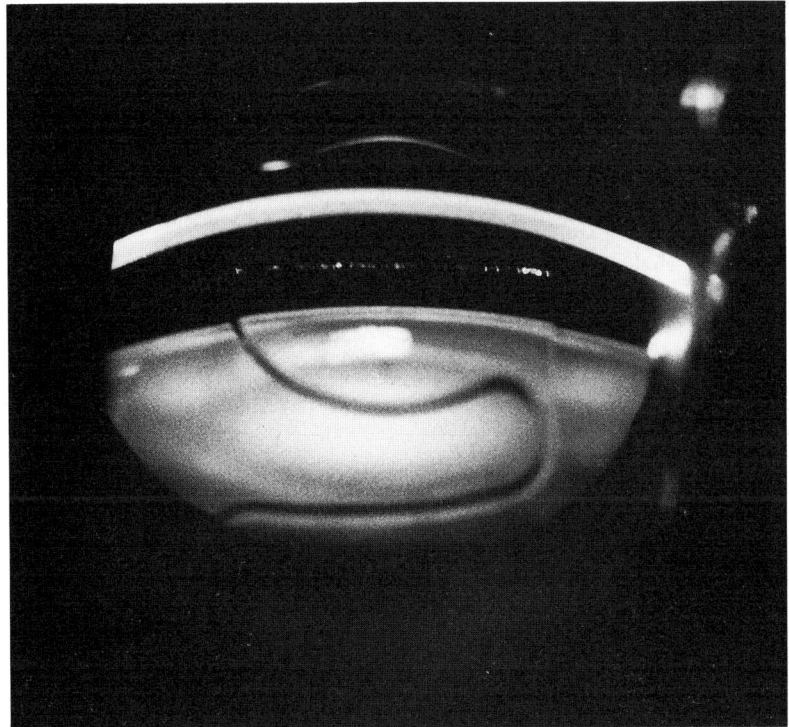

Fig. 12.23 This slit-lamp photo shows the space between the lens and the endothelium. (Courtesy of G. Baikoff.)

(a)

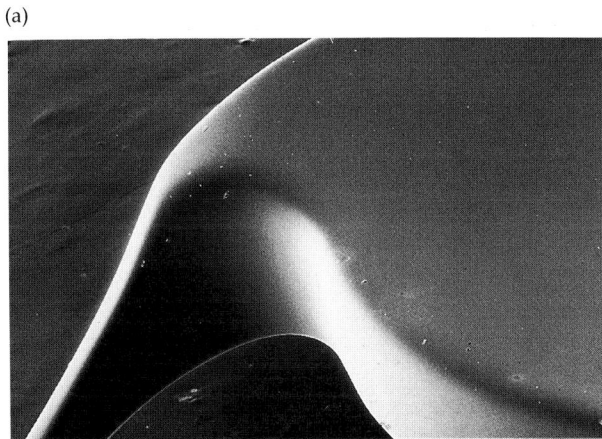

(b)

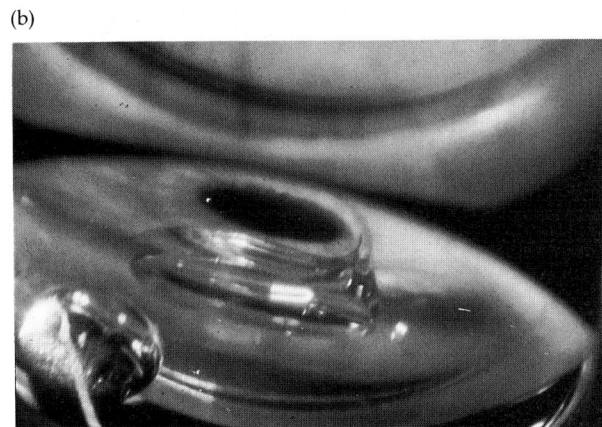

Fig. 12.24 (a) The smoothness of finish of the lens used by Baikoff is evident in this photo. (b) Gonioscopic view of first-generation implant. (Courtesy of G. Baikoff.)

reported elsewhere [35]. Baikoff reports no evidence of endothelial cell loss at 1 year. However, that study was retrospective. thus no proper baseline has been established from which to measure cell loss. How many cells were lost at the time of surgery, for instance? Sargoussi and Lesure, none the less, reported substantial endothelial damage at the footplates of the implant (Figure 12.27) [34]. These lenses are being implanted in the United States under investigative protocol (Figure 12.28).

Worst–Fechner biconcave iris claw lens

This lens has had a good track record in aphakic eyes—some 40 000 have been implanted since 1979

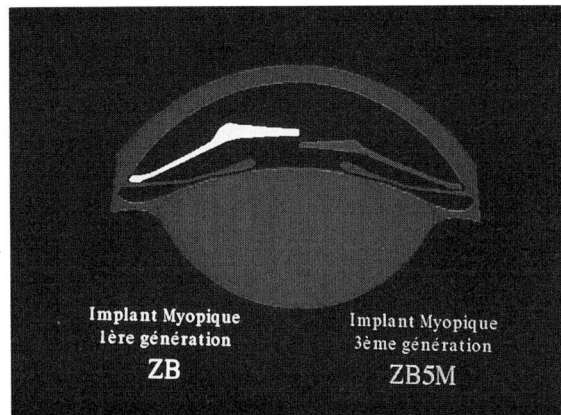

Fig. 12.25 The design change between the first and third generation of lenses. (Courtesy of G. Baikoff.)

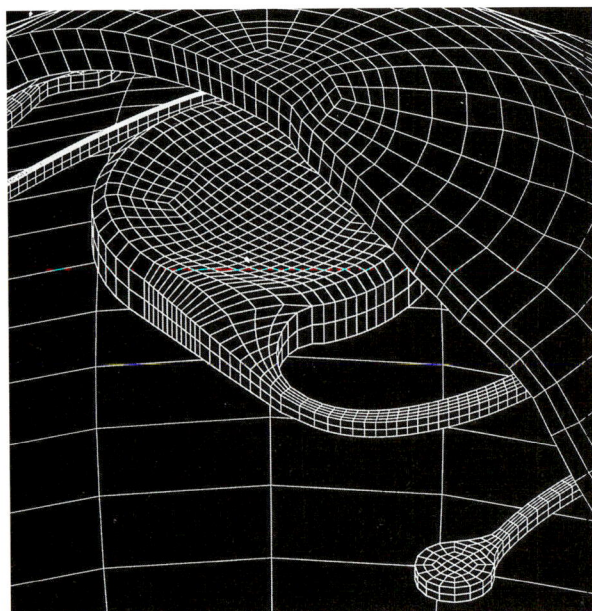

Fig. 12.26 Computer-simulated study of the functioning of a myopia-correcting implant within the eye. (Courtesy of Hanna.)

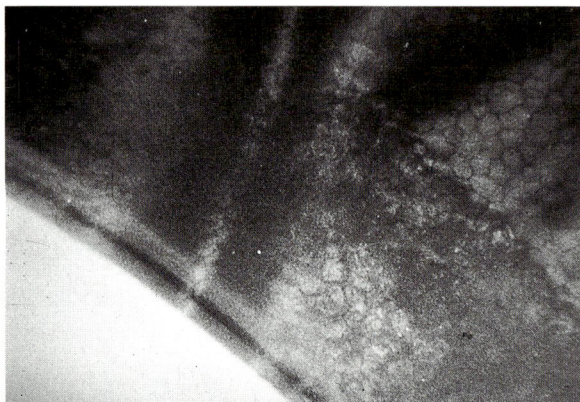

Fig. 12.27 Endothelial damage secondary to angle-supported lens (from Sargoussi *et al.*)

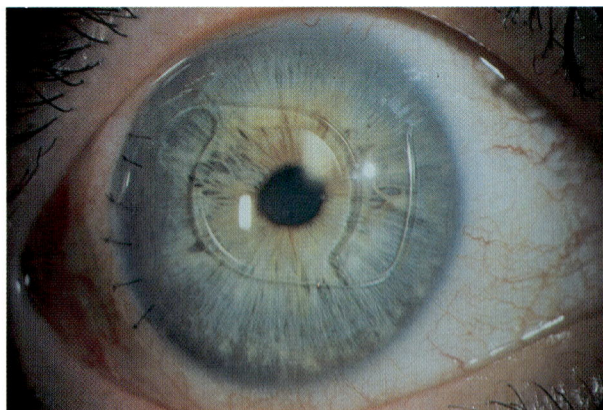

Fig. 12.28 First such lens to be inserted in the USA. (Courtesy of H. Kaufman.).

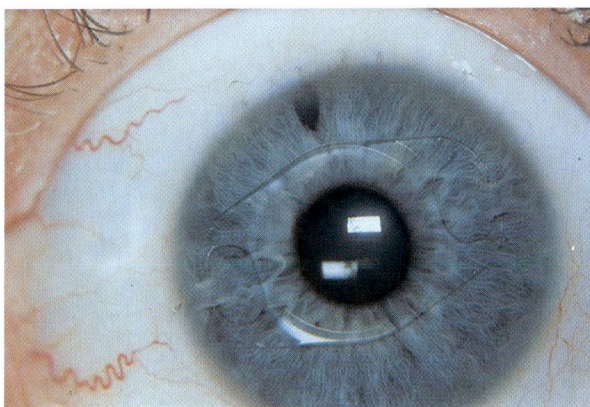

Fig. 12.29 Worst–Fechner claw lens. (Courtesy of G. van Rij.)

[36]. Some fewer of these lenses have been implanted in phakic eyes, chiefly by Fechner, since the first one in 1980 [37]. Worst and Fechner changed the lens to a biconcave design in 1986 (available from Ophtec, the Netherlands) [38]. Figures 12.29 through 12.31 demonstrate the method of implanting this lens. Some of the results obtained are shown in Table 12.4. The essential points are:

1 The anterior chamber has to be filled with viscoelastic.
2 Make a small nasal incision before making the larger temporal one.
3 Make a peripheral iridectomy to avoid pupillary block.
4 Use traction sutures or a Flieringa ring.

Silicone posterior chamber (epi-lenticular) lenses for myopia

The use of semi-elastic silicone material to construct intra-ocular lenses is not new. Ruedemann reported on a series of such lenses implanted in rabbits—a project begun in 1975 (Figure 12.33) [39]. Little if any reaction was noted in these notoriously reactive eyes. Shortly after this experience, Ruedemann inserted at least two such lenses into humans in the author's presence, in late 1976. Both were angle-supported and one of these was placed through a small opening (the previous incision having been partially sutured closed) and the lens unrolled in the AC with a spatula. Ruedemann commented at the time that the elasticity of the silicone material lent itself to this kind of implantation but that the problem was making it stiff enough. This problem has since been solved and the relative non-reactivity of the material is remarkable. The other point in its favour is the low specific gravity in aqueous. This means less inertia to damage delicate ocular structures during the nearly constant ocular movement. The author has noted in a study of PMMA, iris-fixated lenses, that lens

(a)

(b)

(c)

(d)

(e)

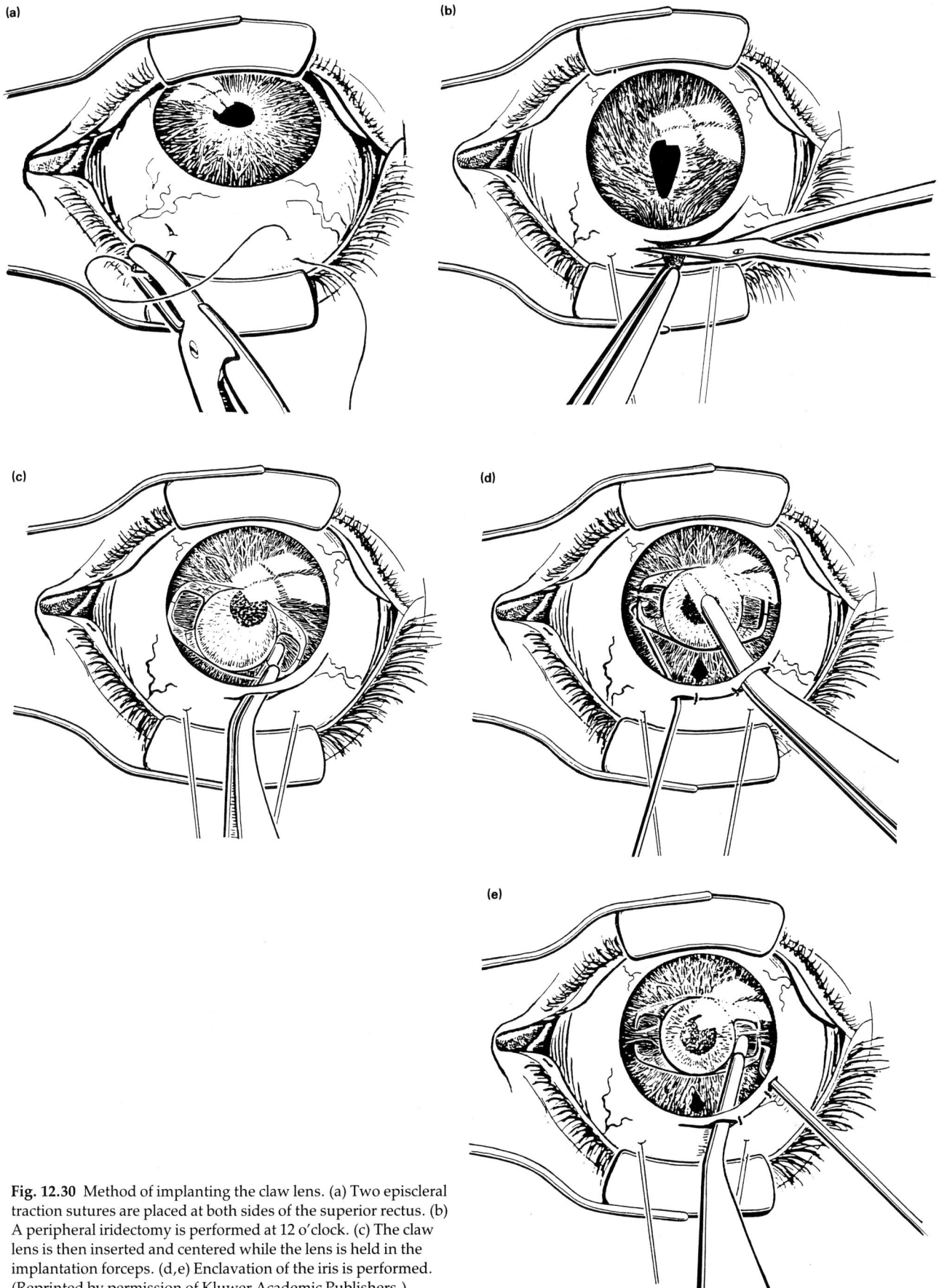

Fig. 12.30 Method of implanting the claw lens. (a) Two episcleral traction sutures are placed at both sides of the superior rectus. (b) A peripheral iridectomy is performed at 12 o'clock. (c) The claw lens is then inserted and centered while the lens is held in the implantation forceps. (d,e) Enclavation of the iris is performed. (Reprinted by permission of Kluwer Academic Publishers.)

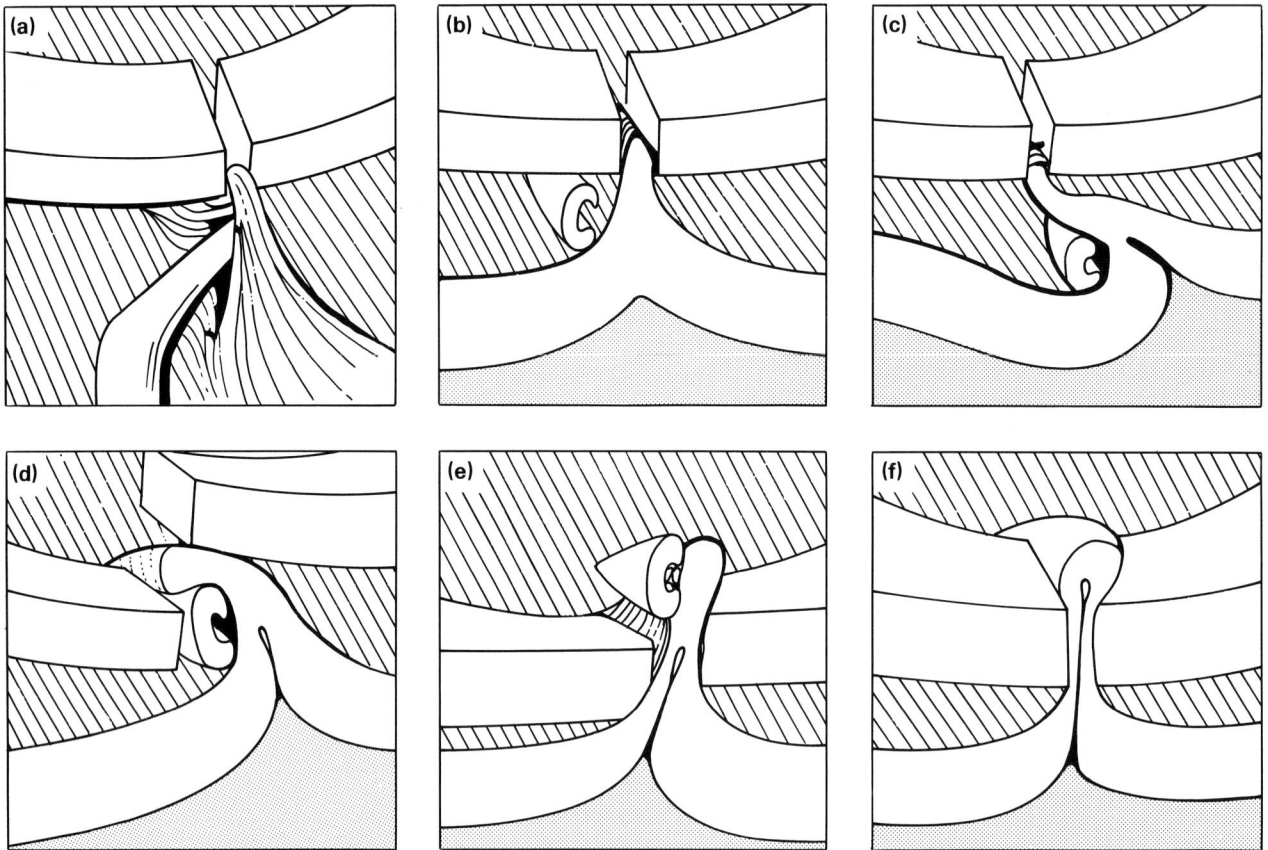

Fig. 12.31 The technique of enclavation. (a) The iris is looped up under the lens; (b) the "knuckle" of iris is pressed up into the haptic, engaging it; (c) the spatula is dropped down to pick up more iris; (d) the lens is supported with another tool while the spatula and iris are pressed up into the split haptic; (e,f) the iris is trapped within the haptic. (Reprinted by permission of Kluwer Academic Publishers.)

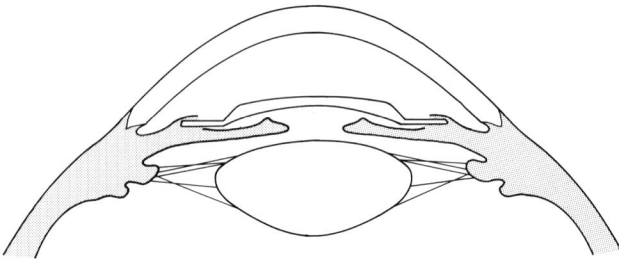

Fig. 12.32 Position of the claw lens within the AC. (Reprinted by permission of Kluwer Academic Publishers.)

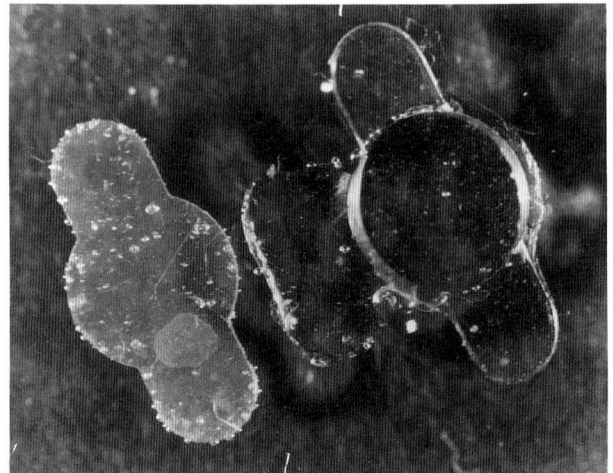

Fig. 12.33 Ruedemann's flexible silicone intra-ocular lenses.

weight—both in air and in aqueous—was related to the frequency of post-operative complications [40].

Fyodorov has proposed and tested a silicone, collar-button-type lens in a number of myopes [41]. Implantation of this particular lens has been fraught with difficulty [41]. Additionally, monocular diplopia has been reported at night and opacification of the natural lens has resulted in some cases [42]. In 1990, Fyodorov and his group began implanting a newly designed lens of a more elastic nature (Figure 12.34). The lens is of one-piece design with a slightly narrower haptic and a

5.5–6.0 mm optic which does not protrude through the pupillary opening. The lens is somewhat easier to implant, not requiring viscoelastic. A 1-year follow-up of 43 highly myopic eyes has been satisfactory with uncorrected visual acuity ranging from 0.5 to 1.0 and no serious or vision-threatening complications

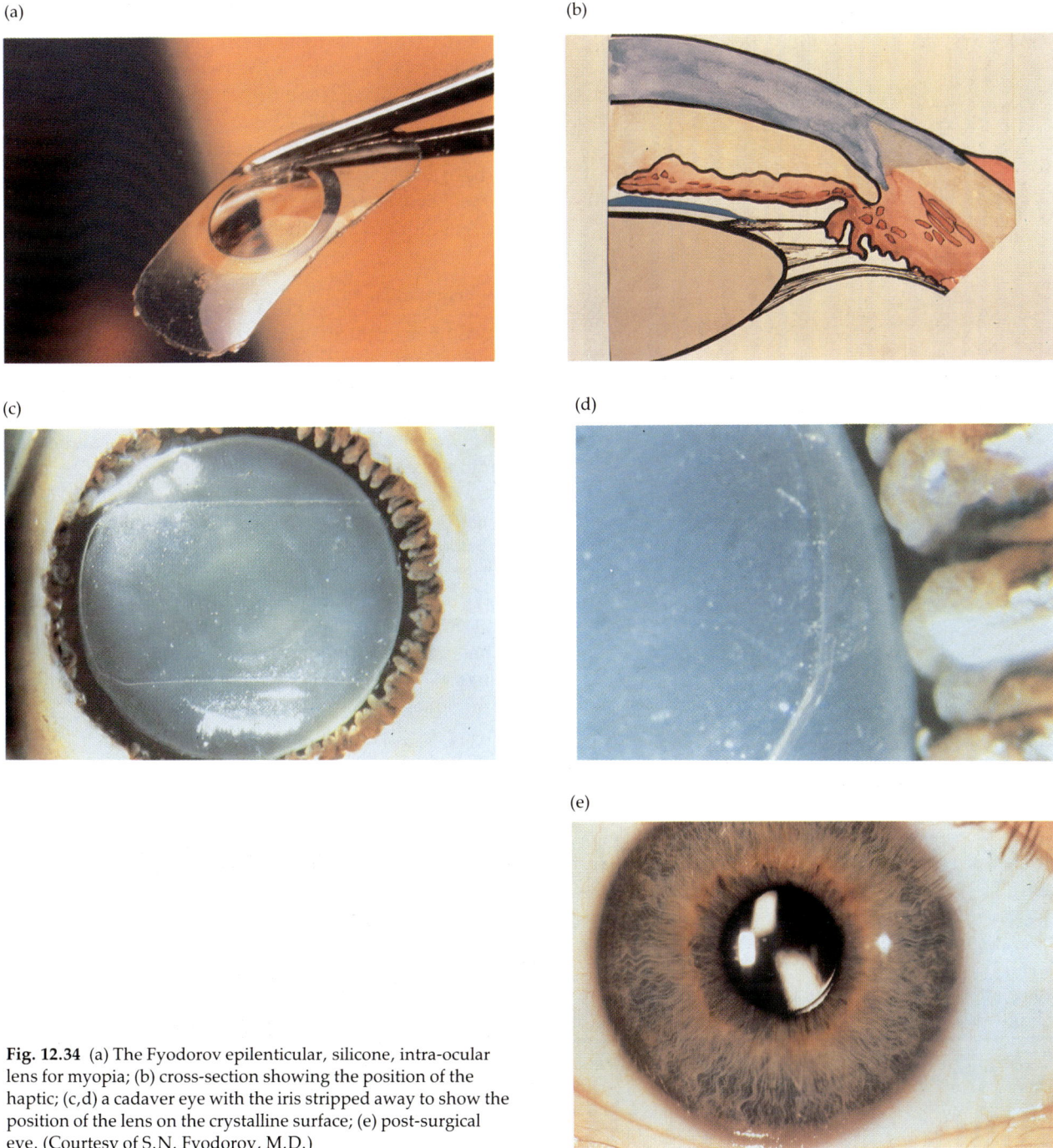

Fig. 12.34 (a) The Fyodorov epilenticular, silicone, intra-ocular lens for myopia; (b) cross-section showing the position of the haptic; (c,d) a cadaver eye with the iris stripped away to show the position of the lens on the crystalline surface; (e) post-surgical eye. (Courtesy of S.N. Fyodorov, M.D.)

(S.N. Fyodorov, personal communication). Recently Fyodorov and his group began the implantation of a similar lens made from highly polymerized collagen material (Figure 12.35).

Lens implantation for age-related macular degeneration

While the implantation of lens to treat a medical problem may not seem like refractive surgery, the author has chosen to include it because the ultimate effect is to change—dramatically—the refractive workings of the eye. Unlike cataract surgery which merely replaces a cloudy element, the implantation of a catadioptric lens, much like an anterior chamber phakos for myopia, changes the entire optical character of the eye.

Age-related macular degeneration (ARMD) is the leading cause of visual loss in adults age 60 years and older [43,44]. After age 60, the incidence increases to 28% of the adult population between ages 75 and 85.

(a)

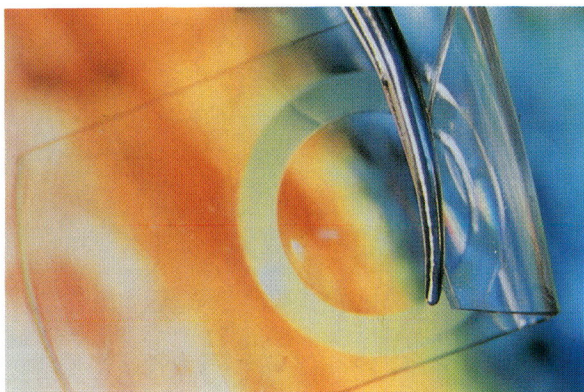

(b)

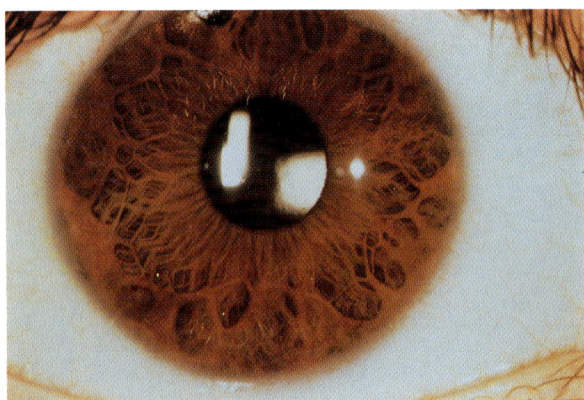

Fig. 12.35 (a) The Fyodorov collagen implant for myopia; (b) post-implant eye (Fyodorov).

Two clinical types of ARMD are recognized: the dry or atrophic form, making up 90% of cases, and the neovascular or wet form. Visual loss in the dry form is mild and slowly progressive but is severe in the wet type. Soft drusen seem to be associated with the onset of ARMD while the more discrete hard type do not. There is a 14.5% cumulative risk over 5 years that patients with bilateral soft drusen will develop macular neo-vascularization [45–48].

Until fairly recently, the treatment for wet ARMD has been the laser when possible. Short of transplanting the macula, the only treatment for the dry type has been vitamin and zinc therapy.

Low-vision aids

According to the Snellen chart, 20/20 visual acuity is normal; thus, anything less than this is, by definition, sub-normal. For practical purposes, however, ophthalmologists consider loss of visual acuity in the range of 20/50 to 20/80 to be a serious handicap. Reading becomes difficult when visual acuity is less than 20/70 and low-vision aids are prescribed for patients with this acuity if it has not responded to conventional therapy, such as cataract surgery. Although a variety of low-vision aids are available, all are based on the same principle: increasing retinal image size through magnification of the object.

The magnification power of a given vision aid is defined as the ratio of image size to object size. For the eye, the magnifying power is one for an object 25 cm from the eye. This value is logically assigned because the average eye can focus to a distance of 25 cm (4 D of accommodation).

Two types of low-vision aids are currently in use: telescopes and convex lenses. Telescopes have a two-lens system in which one lens produces an image near the eye and the other lens focuses the image on the retina. Convex lenses simply bring into focus objects that are closer than 25 cm to the eye. For example, an

Table 12.4 Results of clear lens extraction in eight myopes (from Worst JG, van der Veen G, Los LI. Refractive surgery for high myopia. The Worst–Fechner biconcave iris claw lens. Doc Ophthalmol 1990; 75:335–341)

Patient no/eye	Sex (M/F)	Age (years)	Intra-ocular lens (D)	Spherical equivalent		Visual acuity		Follow-up (months)
				Pre-op.	Post-op.	Pre-op.	Post-op.	
1 OD	M	21	−15.00	−18.00	−2.00	0.4	0.5	22
OS			−15.00	−18.00	−3.00	0.4	0.5	15
2 OD	M	35	−14.00	−14.00	0.50	0.3	0.5	14
OS			−14.00	−11.50	0.00	0.15	0.5	13
3 OD	M	57	−15.00	−15.00	0.50	0.4	0.5	9
OS			−16.00	−16.00	−0.50	0.5	0.6	8
4 OD	M	42	−17.00	−12.00	−1.00	0.4	0.4	1
OS			−13.00	−14.00	0.00	0.4	0.4	1
5 OD	F	35	−10.00	−10.00	0.00	0.3	1.25	3
OS			−9.00	−9.00	0.00	0.4	0.8	3
6 OD	M	56	−19.00	−18.50	0.00	0.25	0.4	2
OS			−19.00	−18.00	0.00	0.5	0.4	0.25
7 OD	M	35	−9.00	−8.00	0.00	1.0	1.25	3
8 OD	M	30	−14.00	−13.50	1.50	0.4	0.5	3
OS			−14.00	−13.50	2.00	0.6	0.8	0.25

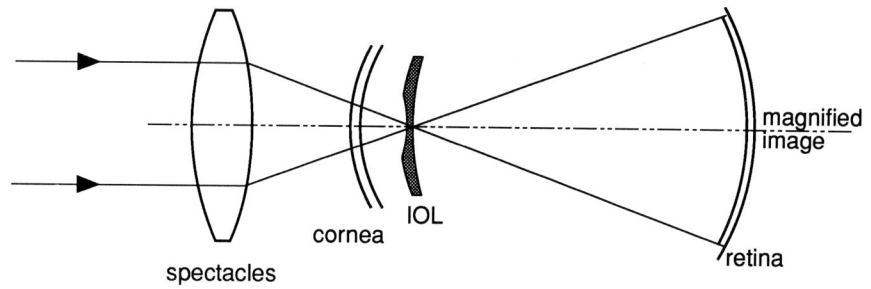

Fig. 12.36 Schematic of the Donn–Koester intra-ocular lens producing a Galilean telescope when a plus lens is placed before the eye (from Peyman G, Koziol J. Age-related macular degeneration and its management. J Cataract Refract Surg 1988; 14:421–430).

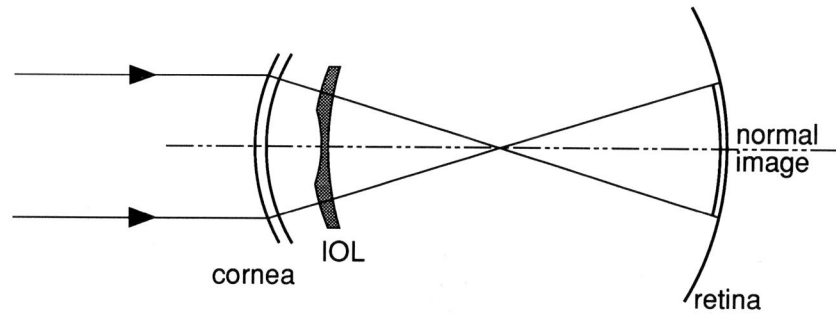

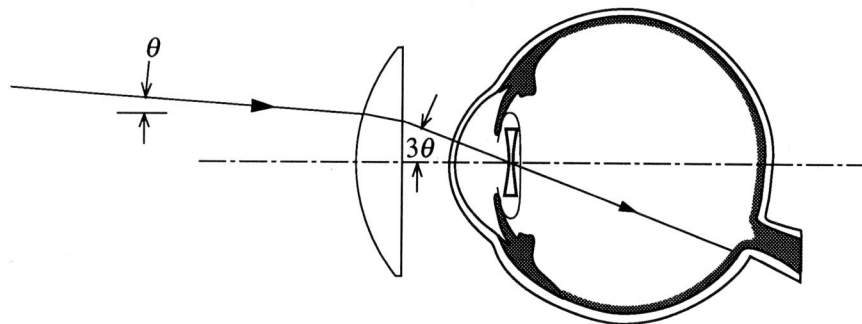

Fig. 12.37 Schematic of a ray passing through the plus (peripheral) portion of the Koziol–Peyman lens. Note the normal image size produced on the retina (from Peyman G, Koziol J. Age-related macular degeneration and its management. J Cataract Refract Surg 1988; 14:421–430).

Fig. 12.38 Schematic of a ray passing through the central (minus) part of the same lens, forming a Galilean telescope when a plus lens in placed before the eye. Note the magnified image size produced on the retina (from Peyman G, Koziol J. Age-related macular degeneration and its management. J Cataract Refract Surg 1988; 14: 421–430).

object held 6.25 cm from the eye would require 16 D of accommodation (100 cm divided by 6.25 cm) to bring this object into focus to produce 16/4, or four times, magnification.

Telescopes

Both Galilean and astronomical telescopic systems have been used as low-vision aids. Both models use a converging lens as the objective lens to create an image close to the eye. The astronomic telescope then uses a plus-lens ocular separated from the plus objective lens by a distance equal to the *sum* of their focal lengths (see Chapter 3). The image is inverted, however, and requires a prism to put the image upright. In the Galilean telescope, a minus ocular is separated from the plus objective lens by the *difference* in the absolute values of their focal lengths. This places an upright image formed by the objective lens at the focal point of the ocular.

The advantage of telescopes is their long working

distance. When telescopes are used as low-vision aids, close work can be brought into focus without bringing the material close to the eye. The image, instead of the object, is focused near the eye, and this image is then seen through the ocular of the telescope. The disadvantage of the telescope is the restricted field of view—4–10°. This makes walking or reading difficult.

Convex lenses

With a convex lens, the size of the retinal image increases as the object is brought nearer the eye. An object at 8.25 cm produces a retinal image four times greater than at 25 cm and requires a 16 D (100 cm/ 6.25 cm) lens to focus the image on to the retina. Because the rays are parallel when they emerge from the magnifying lens, the eye can be any distance behind the magnifier. However, the distance of the lens to the object must always be at the focal length, thus the patient will need to move closer to a magnifying lens to take advantage of the wider field of view.

(a)

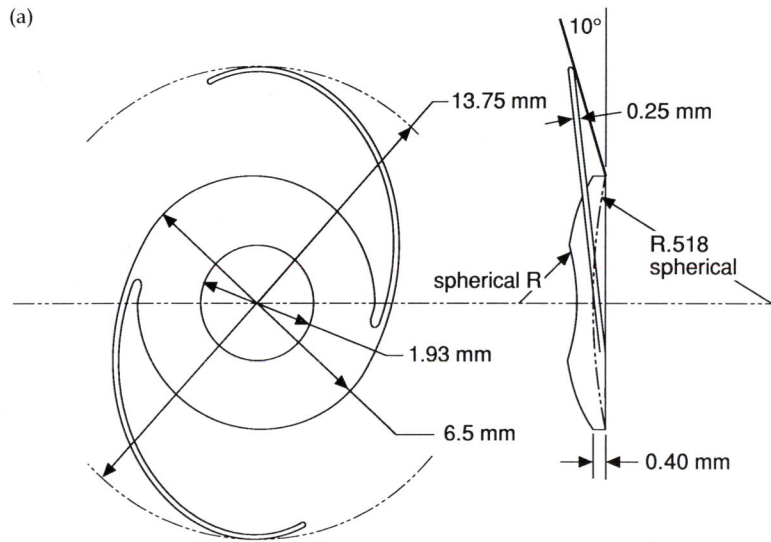

(b)

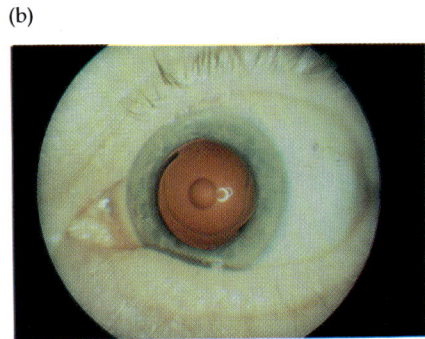

Fig. 12.39 (a) Schematic of the bioptic AMD-100B implant. (b) Photo of the implanted lens (from Willis TR, Portney V. Preliminary evaluation of the Koziol–Peyman teledioptric system for age-related macular degeneration. Eur J Implant Refract Surg 1989; 1:271–276).

(b)

(a)

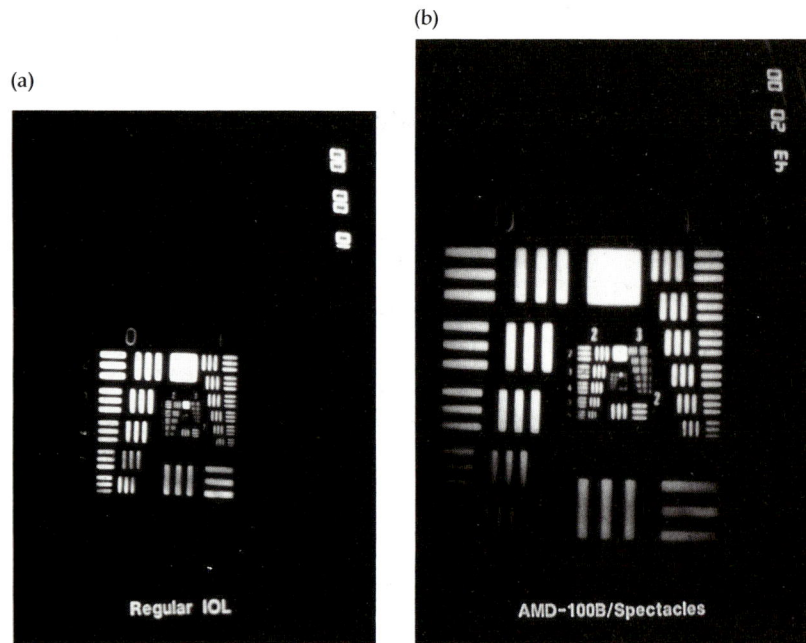

Fig. 12.40 (a) Resolution of a standard intra-ocular lens. (b) Resolution of the AMD-100B lens with spectacles. (Courtesy of American Medical Optics.)

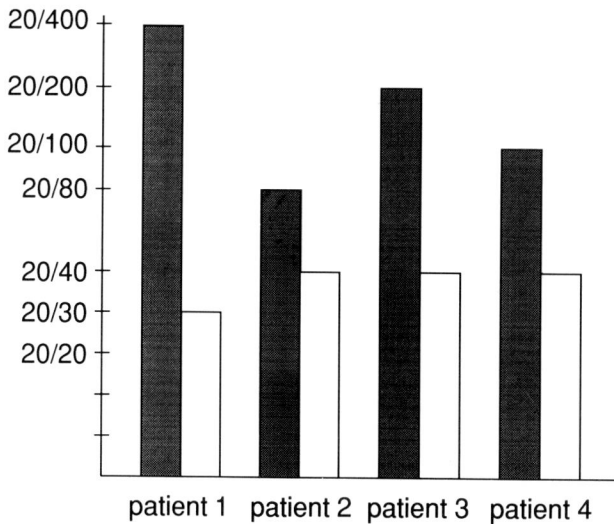

Fig. 12.41 Visual acuity in four subjects before and after implantation of the AMD-100B intra-ocular lens and fitting with dual-element spectacles. Near vision assessed in patients 2–4, and far vision in patient 1. (Courtesy of Willis.)

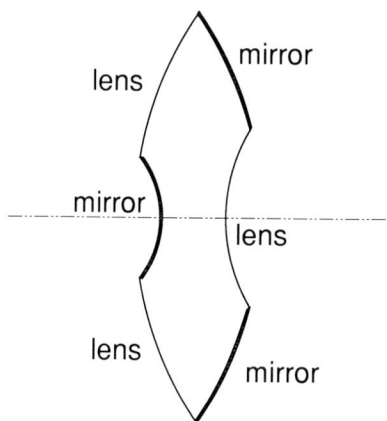

Fig. 12.42 Cross-section of a catadioptric lens with a mirrored surface. (Courtesy of Willis.)

Historical background

Choyce [49], and later Donn and Koester [50], proposed using a high-minus intra-ocular lens (Figure 12.36) as the ocular of a Galilean telescope in 1984. A high-plus spectacle lens would then be the objective lens. The advantage of this system is the enlarged visual field that results as the ocular lens of the telescope is placed within the eye. Donn and Koester calculated that a three-power telescope produced with this system would yield a visual field of 37° or three times the visual field of a conventional telescope. Furthermore, the field of vision and the amount of magnification obtained can be changed by adjusting the power and vertex distance of the spectacles without altering the implant.

This system has several serious disadvantages, however. First, without spectacle lenses, the implanted eye has an uncorrected hyperopia of 60 + D. In addition, when plus-lens spectacles are used, a magnified image is produced on the retina, but peripheral vision is substantially reduced. The magnified image will not fuse with the image in the fellow eye, so that eye must be occluded when using magnification.

Teledioptric and catadioptric intra-ocular lenses

To eliminate the disadvantages of external telescopes or high-minus intra-ocular lenses, two new intra-ocular lenses have been designed by Peyman and Koziol [51]. The Koziol–Peyman teledioptric lens has a one-piece optic with both plus and minus portions (Figures 12.37 through 39). The plus portion provides normal phakic vision, a full visual field, and preserves any pre-existing central vision. The high-minus (center) part of the lens acts as the ocular of a Galilean telescope when used with high-plus spectacles. A patient can then use special glasses whenever a magnified image is needed, as for reading, or remove them when a full field is required, as for walking. The visual field is approximately 80°—large enough to permit normal ambulation even with a magnified field of view. The currently produced lens has a very high resolution (Figures 12.40 and 41).

The catadioptric lens (Figure 12.42) uses mirrored surfaces to produce a magnified image without an external spectacle lens.

References

1 Boerhaave H. *Prælectiones publicæ, de Morbis Oculorum*. Haller (ed), Göttingen, 1746.
2 Vacher L. An operation for myopia. Annales d'Oculistique 1896; CXVI:8, 19.
3 Janin. *Mémoires et observations anatomiques, physiologiques et physiques sur l'oeil*. Paris, 1772.
4 Otto F. I. Beobachtungen uber hochgradige Kurzsichtigen und ihre operative Behandlung. [Observations of high myopia and its surgical treatment. I.] Arch Ophthalmol 1898; XLIII:324–328.
5 Otto F. II. Beobachtungen uber hochgradige Kurzsichtigen und ihre operative Behandlung. [Observations of high myopia and its surgical treatment. II.] Arch Ophthalmol 1898; XLVII:242–248.
6 Otto F. Berichtigung der sogenannten Richstellung des Herrn Dr. Fukala zu meiner Abhandlung uber Behandlung hochgradiger Kurzsichtigkeit. Albrecht Graefes Arch Ophthalmol 1898; XLVII:224–228.
7 Heister L. *A General System of Surgery in Three Parts*. London, 1759.
8 von Haller A. *Elementa Physiologiae Corporis Humani*. Lausanne, 1763.
9 Woolhouse W. *De Cataract et Glaucome*. Paris, 1717.

10 Desmonceaux A. *Traité des maladies des yeux et des oreilles, considerées sous le rapport des quatre âges de la vie de l'homme.* [Treatise on the diseases of the eye and the ear, considered in correlation with the four ages of man.] Paris, 1786.

11 Hirschberg J. The renaissance of ophthalmology in the eighteenth century, part 1. vol 3. In: *The History of Ophthalmology*, F Blodi (ed). Wayenborgh Verlag, Bonn, 1982.

12 Richter AG. *Chirurgische Bibliothek.* 1790.

13 Beer J. *Augenkrankheiten.* 1799.

14 Fukala V. [Operative Behandlung der hochstgradigen Myopie durch Aphakie.] Surgical treatment of high degrees of myopia through aphakia. Graefes Arch Ophthalmol 1890; 36:230–244.

15 Verzella F. Microsurgery of the lens in high myopia for optical purposes. J Am Intraocul Implant Soc 1985; 11:65.

16 Muller H, Papastylianos S. 3000 Kataraktextraktionen: Komplikationen und Ergebnisse. [3000 cataract extractions: complications and results.] Klin Monatsbl Augenheilked 1968; 152:476–487.

17 Liu CH. Cryoextraction on high myopes: an evaluation of 32 eyes. Ann Ophthalmol 1973; 5:1251–1254.

18 Mickiewicz L, Balmuchanow A. Krioekstrakcja zacmy u osob krotkowzrocynch. [Cataract extraction in myopic patients.] Klin Oczna 1974; 44:141–145.

19 Edmund J, Seedorff HH. Retinal detachment in the aphakic eye. Acta Ophthalmol (Copenh) 1974; 52:323–333.

20 Jaffe NS, Clayman HM, Jaffe MS. Retinal detachment in myopic eyes after intracapsular and extracapsular cataract extraction. Am J Ophthalmol 1984; 97:48–52.

21 Clayman HM, Jaffe NS, Light DS, Jaffe MS, Cassady JC. Intraocular lenses, axial length, and retinal detachment. Am J Ophthalmol 1981; 92:778–780.

22 Praeger D. Five years' follow-up in the surgical management of cataracts in high myopia treated with the Kelman phacoemulsification technique. Ophthalmology 1979; 86: 2024–2033.

23 Verzella F. *High Myopia: Microsurgical Extracapsular Extraction of the Lens for Optical Purposes.* Lens Editions, Keratorefractive Society, Chicago, 1983.

24 Hessburg TP, Maxwell DP, Diamond JG. Endophthalmitis associated with sutureless cataract surgery [letter]. Arch Ophthalmol 1991; 109.

25 Stonecipher KG, Parmley VC, Jensen H, Rowsey JJ. Infectious endophthalmitis following sutureless cataract surgery. Arch Ophthalmol 1991; 109:1562–1563.

26 Ernest PH, Kiessling LA, Lavery KT. The effect of external pressure on sutureless cataract wounds. J Cataract Refract Surg (in press).

27 Beer J. *Bibliotheca Ophthalmica.* 1799.

28 Schiferli RA. Theoretisch-praktische Abhandlung über den grauen Starr. [A theoretical and practical dissertation on cataract.] In: *Zur Geschichte der intraocularen Korrektur der Aphakia*, W Munchow (ed). Gabler, Jena, 1797.

29 Casanova G. *History of my Life.* 1818.

30 Baikoff G. Phakic anterior chamber intraocular lenses. Int Ophthalmol Clin 1991; 31:75–86.

31 Strampelli B. Sopportabilita di lenti acriliche in camera anteriore nella afachia e nei vizi di refrazione. Atti Soc Oftal Lomb 1953; 8:292.

32 Barraquer J. Anterior chamber plastic lenses. Results and conclusions from 5 year's experience. Trans Ophthalmol Soc (UK) 1959; 79:393–424.

33 Drews RC. The Barraquer experience with intraocular lenses. Ophthalmology 1982; 89:386–393.

34 Baikoff G. The refractive IOL in a phakic eye. Ophthalmic Pract 1991; 9:58–61.

35 Ellingson FT. The uveitis-glaucoma-hyphema syndrome associated with the mark VIII anterior chamber lens implant. J Am Intraocul Implant Soc 1978; 4:50–53.

36 Worst JG, van der Veen G, Los LI. Refractive surgery for high myopia. The Worst-Fechner biconcave iris claw lens. Doc Ophthalmol 1990; 75:335–341.

37 Fechner PU. Die Irisklauene-Linse. Klin Monatstbl Augenheilkd 1987; 191:26–29.

38 Fechner PU, van der Heijde GL, Worst JG. Intraokulare Linse zur Myopiekorrektion des phaken Auges. [Intraocular lens for the correction of myopia of the phakic eye.] Klin Monatsbl Augenheilkd 1988; 193:29–34.

39 Ruedemann ADJ. Silicone intraocular implants in rabbits. Trans Am Acad Ophthalmol Otolaryngol 1977; 75:436–455.

40 Bores LD. *Sputnik Lenses and Unreasonable Facsimiles Thereof.* American Intraocular Implant Society, Los Angeles, 1979.

41 Fyodorov SN, Zuev VK, Tumanian ER. Intraokuliarnaia korrektsiia miopii vysokoi stepeni. [Intraocular correction of high-degree myopia.] Vestn Oftalmol 1988; 104:14–16.

42 Fyodorov SN, Zuev VK, Aznavayev VM. Intraokuliarnaia korrektsiia miopii vysokoi stepeni zadnekamernmi otritsatelimi linzami. [Intraocular correction of high myopia with negative posterior chamber lens.] Oftalmochirugia 1991; 3:57–58.

43 Leibowitz HM, Krueger DE, Maunder LR *et al.* The Framingham Eye Study monograph: an ophthalmological and epidemiological study of cataract, glaucoma, diabetic retinopathy, macular degeneration, and visual acuity in a general population of 2631 adults, 1973–1975. Surv Ophthalmol 1980; 24 (suppl):335–610.

44 Klein BE, Klein R. Cataracts and macular degeneration in older Americans. Arch Ophthalmol 1982; 100:571–573.

45 Folk JC. Senile macular degeneration. Primary Care 1982; 9:793–799.

46 Sarks SH, Van DD, Maxwell L, Killingsworth M. Softening of drusen and subretinal neovascularization. Trans Ophthalmol Soc UK 1980; 100:414–422.

47 Strahlman ER, Fine SL, Hillis A. The second eye of patients with senile macular degeneration. Arch Ophthalmol 1983; 101:1191–1193.

48 Smiddy WE, Fine SL. Prognosis of patients with bilateral macular drusen. Ophthalmology 1984; 91:271–277.

49 Choyce DP. Galilean telescope using the anterior chamber lens as eyepiece. 156–161, HK Leivia, London, 1964.

50 Donn A, Koester CJ. An ocular telephoto system designed to improve vision in macular disease. CLAO J 1986; 12:81–85.

51 Peyman G, Koziol J. Age-related macular degeneration and its management. J Cataract Refract Surg 1988; 14:421–430.

13
Scleral
Re-inforcement

Somebody said that it couldn't be done
But he with a chuckle replied
That maybe it couldn't, but he would be one
Who wouldn't say so till he'd tried.
[Edgar A. Guest]

Despite the reluctance of some individuals in the contemporary medical community to accept myopia as a disease or affliction, as it once had been in the past, the fact remains that it is the fifth or sixth leading cause of blindness in the world today—which, if one gives it a moment's thought, is remarkable for a process considered a non-disease. Additionally there appears to be very little, if anything, that can be done to prevent it and even less to treat it—other than surgery—once established.

It should be clear by now (see Chapter 2) that occupational or environmental factors play a role in the evolution of myopia, however small that role may be. If that is true, then alteration of these factors should have some effect on either eliminating or at least slowing the progressive myopic process. Depending upon whose philosophy one adopts, such treatment can range from chemical to mechanic [1,2]. For example, some investigators believe that excess accommodation contributes to the observed progression of the myopic state [3,4].

McCollim conducted a unique experiment wherein pressure was applied to the globe of the eye by artificially induced contracture of the superior oblique muscles [5]. One of the two effects produced was 5 D of myopia; the other was dual vision which took years to subside, even after the pressure was released. It was surmised that the pressure, transmitted through the sclera to the vitreous, forced the vitreous against the back of the lens, flattening the periphery but not the axial (central) region, resulting in a high degree of negative spherical aberration, combined with increased accommodation. The author concluded that this suggests that accommodation can be actuated by contraction of the extra-ocular muscles. He further noted that when the lens is allowed to relax after a long period of accommodation, the return to the unaccommodated state is extremely slow, indicating that a significant factor in the etiology of myopia is repeated long periods of accommodation in which periods of rest are insufficient to allow the lens to return completely to the unaccommodated state. Thus the elastic memory of the natural lens is somehow impaired.

The Soviets (among others) have attempted to interfere with the myopic process by prescribing low plus glasses for *skolniki* (school children) along with base-in prism. There are some rather severe problems associated with conducting such studies and despite study design flaws, the Soviets have claimed that this mode of treatment has reduced the number of cases of progressive myopia in their series [6].

Other investigators have posited that this progression in myopia occurs through elevation of the intraocular pressure (IOP), which has been shown to occur during accommodation [7,8]. Fledelius demonstrated the strong myopigenic effect of elevated IOP in young eyes suffering from traumatic secondary glaucoma [9]. Another study reported significantly greater axial changes in the affected eye of children with monocular congenital glaucoma. This elongation was beyond that which could be attributed to normal growth. Successful surgery in these cases produced an early decrease in mean axial length of 0.8 mm [10]. There is a tendency for a higher mean IOP in myopes in any event [4,11–13]. Tomlinson and Phillips found that in patients aged 18–27, the average IOP was highest in myopia (15.49 ± 2.85 mmHg), and lowest in hyperopia (13.91 ± 2.28 mmHg). They found a strong correlation between applanation and both axial length and refraction [14]. Accordingly, anti-glaucomatous medications have been prescribed in an effort to keep the IOP below certain levels and hopefully prevent progression of the myopia. Unfortunately, the drugs employed carry with them sufficient hazard to make their use in children problematic, and the side-effects—not to mention lack of compliance—have proved to be troublesome. Furthermore, the results of such usage have been equivocal. Despite the pressure-lowering effects of pilocarpine, the induced accommodation caused by the drug may itself stimulate myopia, making its use for this purpose illogical. Still, some feel that it is reasonable to keep the IOP in high myopes below 20 mmHg [15]. None the less, the subject of ocular hypertension is still in flux. Perkins suggests that while the myopic eye is significantly more at risk of developing glaucoma, it is less likely to have ocular hypertension [16]. It should be noted in addition that the myope is more likely to be a steroid responder, which has considerable significance in refractive surgery (see also Chapter 9). Podos and colleagues tested a number of myopic patients and found that 88% of the cases in their series responded to steroid administration with IOPs in excess of 20 mmHg or more; in 29% of these the IOP exceeded 31 mmHg [17]. Amba and associates have suggested a genetic linkage between glaucoma and myopia [18,19].

Surgical techniques to produce ocular hypotension such as repeated paracentesis [20,21], iridectomy [22], sclerotomy [22,23], cyclodialysis [24], and myotomy or recession of the extra-ocular muscles [25], have all failed to yield impressive results and all seem to have a low benefit:risk ratio, and hence are not recommended.

A few simpler techniques that were intended to improve the circulation of the eye or strengthen the sclera are noted here, more for historical completeness than for any other reason. Among these are such treatments as the use of mild ocular compresses [26] and compression of the eye into the orbit [27,28]. This latter regimen appears to increase IOP, an event of no particular benefit and of some potential harm to the myopic eye (see the discussion on glaucoma, above). Massage of the eyes has also been suggested [29–31] as well as, more recently, ultrasound [32,33]. There is no scientific evidence, however, that any of these measures has been effectual in reducing or halting the progression of myopia.

Regardless of such claims and the "feelings" of practitioners as to the effect of certain factors on myopic progression, the medical treatment of myopia is, on balance, not a part of standard medical care—thus the progress of the affliction is left to chance. For the most part, this element of chance typically leads to an eventual stabilization of the growth of the eye in most, but unfortunately not all, myopes. This stabilization may not come, however, until the eye is severely myopic and showing all the signs and symptoms of pathologic myopia along with serious reduction in vision or worse. In these cases, the incidence of retinal detachment is high and the risk of total visual loss significant. Rarely, stabilization does not occur at all, eventually leading to total blindness—*malignant* myopia.* Additionally, staphylomatous eyes present unique impediments to normal visual acuity, visual field, binocularity, and stereopsis. They are also prone to premature cataract formation, glaucoma, and retinal detachment.

Pathology

The pathology of the ametropic (usually myopic) eye has been described in more detail elsewhere [15] and therein it was noted that posterior scleral elongation and thinning (posterior staphyloma) are the hallmark of severe as well as pathologic myopia. The basic pathology of high myopia is the gradual enlargement and elongation of the entire globe (Figure 13.1). The tunics of the eye (sclera, choroid, and retina) become stretched. The sclera in pathologic myopia is underdeveloped in both quantity and quality. The scarce and thin scleral fibers in the high myope can no longer support the globe sufficiently. Serious architectural abnormalities can be seen in the fiber bundle arrangement. The bundles themselves show disorganization. Electron microscopy shows the collagen fibrils to be of smaller diameter, and abnormal forms of these fibrils can also be observed. The ectasia of the thin posterior sclera, notably in the area of the staphyloma, tends to be progressive, especially during the first three decades of life. This ectasia is accompanied by an increasing incidence of degenerative changes in the fundus. The eye enlarges posteriorly, losing its spherical shape as it does so. The choroid becomes consequently thinner; its vessels become sclerotic and attenuated, resulting in decreased circulation. This enlargement does not progress at a uniform rate and

* It seems remarkable that a "non-disease" can become malignant.

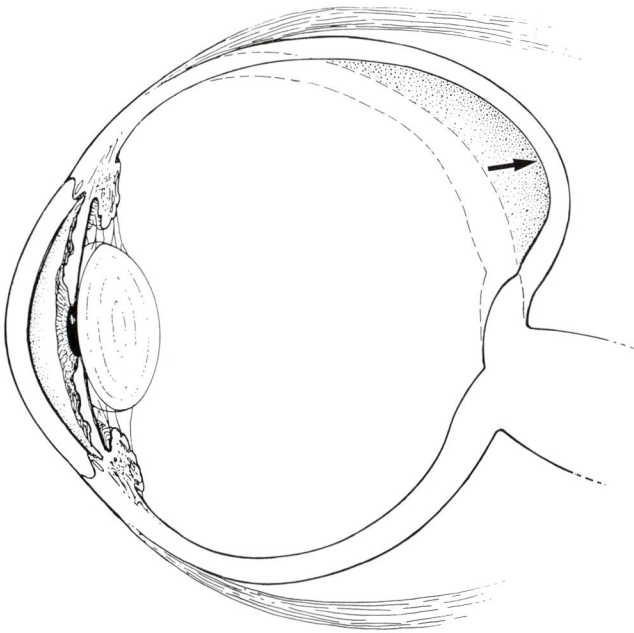

Fig. 13.1 Localized staphyloma characteristic of moderate to low high myopia.

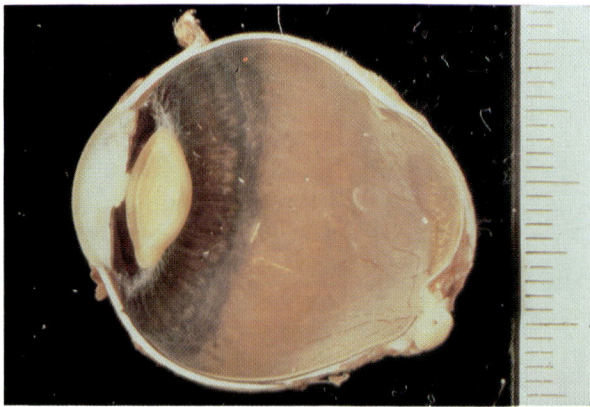

Fig. 13.2 Autopsy specimen clearly demonstrating a staphyloma and general enlargement of the globe associated with progressive myopia. (Courtesy of A. Momose.)

may ultimately result in localized staphyloma formation (Figure 13.2).

Hence, staphylomata can occur in any portion of the globe. They may appear at the equator or anterior to it, especially in highly myopic eyes that have developed retinal tears, holes, or retinal detachments. These staphylomata may make the placement of an encircling silicone band or segmental silicone explant extremely difficult because of the thin underlying sclera. Erosion of such explants into the vitreous is not unknown.

Von Ammon first suggested congenital weakness of the posterior sclera as causative [34]. He described an area of localized ectasia in the embryonic eye which

he termed the protuberantia scleralis. This area is contiguous to the optic nerve and it was thought to be caused by an embryonic opening of the sclera on the cerebral side. Normally closed at birth, this defect could produce staphylomata in the absence of normal development. Sondermann, studying fetal eyes, also found a scleral ectasia which developed at the fourth month of gestation and which gradually diminished as the embryo matured [35–37]. Such a fetal sclerectasis posterioris has not been corroborated by other investigators, however.

Grading changes for staphylomata formation in highly myopic eyes have been developed by Curtin and others [15]. However, these grading systems have involved the changes which can occur in all areas of the myopic eye. A system for specifically grading the progression of posterior macular staphylomata has long been needed. Such a grading system is presented here courtesy of Frank Thompson, MD, in which posterior temporal and macular staphylomata are divided into two types and 10 grades (Figure 13.3 and Table 13.1).

In many cases staphylomata develop on the nasal side of the optic nerve posterior to the equator. These staphylomata usually do not cause severe visual loss since they are not within the central visual axis. Those posterior staphylomata which develop in highly myopic eyes and involve the macula usually begin in the inferior temporal quadrant, anterior to the retinal arcades around the macula, and then progress into the macular area. They may be seen with indirect ophthalmoscopy as pale yellow areas with prominent choroidal vessels (Figure 13.4). Their appearance in the inferior temporal quadrant accompanies the characteristic development of peripheral retinal paving-stone degeneration in the anterior inferior temporal quadrant (Figure 13.5). Both this paving-stone degeneration and the staphylomata are frequently located near the inferior temporal vortex vein and the insertion of the inferior oblique. This may be due to torsional effects from the insertion of the inferior oblique, leading to further weakening of the already thinned scleral and choroidal tissues.

As the staphyloma progresses from the inferior temporal quadrant to involve the central macular and foveal area, the sclera between the disk and macula may become so weakened that an apparent tilting of the optic nerve occurs. This can sometimes be mistaken for neurologic disease when in reality the patient simply may have staphylomatous changes.

As the posterior staphyloma enlarges over the macular area, the choroidal tissue becomes thinned and pale yellow in appearance (Figure 13.6). Eventually breaks in Bruch's membrane or lacquer cracks may invest the macula. As these breaks evolve, encroaching vessels from the underlying choroid can lead to the

TYPE II - MACULAR STAPHYLOMAS

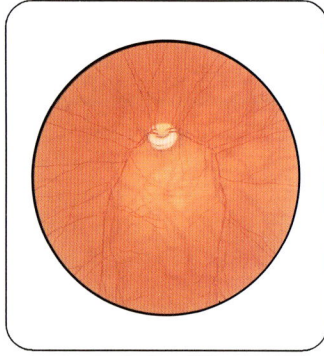

GRADE I

Macula staphyloma with thinning of R.P.E., contained within arcades and with possible breaks in R.P.E.

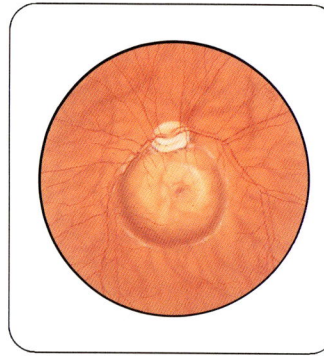

GRADE II

Macular staphyloma contained within arcades with atrophy of R.P.E. and choroid. CAT scan and B-scan reveals "nipple effect".

TYPE I - INFERIOR TEMPORAL STAPHYLOMAS

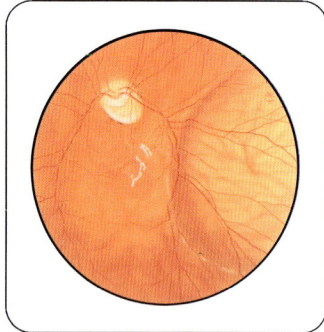

GRADE I

Minimal inferior staphyloma with thinning of R.P.E., not involving macula. Inferior to arcades.

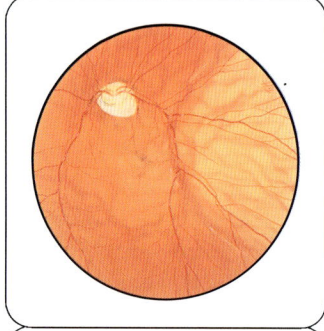

GRADE II

More defined staphyloma with increased thinning of R.P.E., encroaching inside arcades, but not yet involving macula.

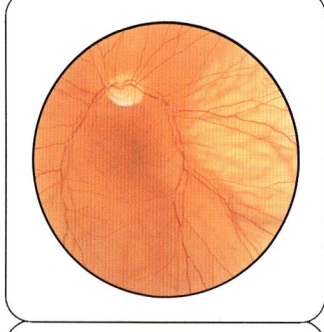

GRADE III

Definite staphyloma with thin R.P.E. involving macula.

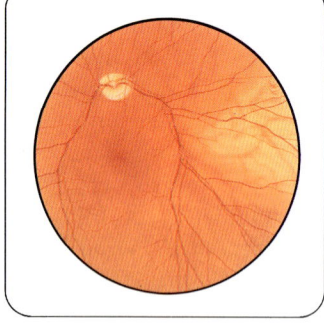

GRADE IV

Definite staphyloma involving macula with breaks in R.P.E. and / or possible "lacquer cracks".

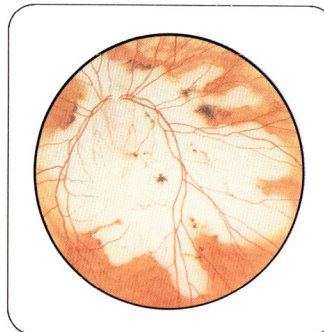

GRADE V

Definite staphyloma involving macula with small atrophic areas in R.P.E. and choroid.

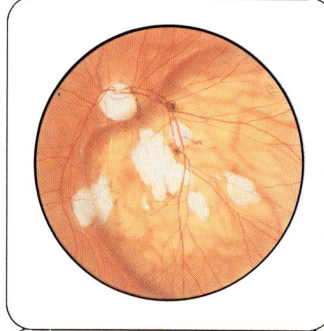

GRADE VI

Definite staphyloma involving macula with breaks in R.P.E., neovascular membrane, or Fuch's spot.

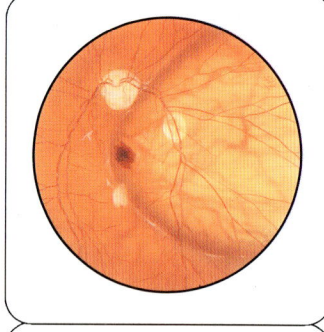

GRADE VII

Sharply defined staphyloma with large atrophic areas of R.P.E., choroid, and retinal ("white out") with sharply sloping staphyloma.

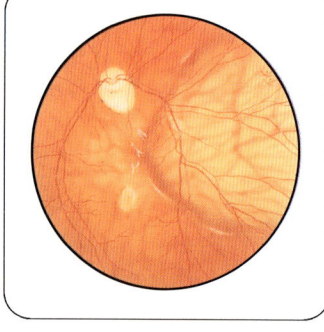

GRADE VIII

Complete loss of R.P.E., choroid, and retinal atrophy damage over posterior pole.

Fig. 13.3 Thompson's classification of myopic staphylomata (from Thompson FB. Scleral reinforcement. In: *Myopia Surgery. Anterior and Posterior Segments*, FB Thompson (ed). Macmillan, New York, 1990.

Table 13.1 Grading system for temporal staphyloma in high myopia. Adapted from Thompson FB. Scleral reinforcement. In: *Myopia Surgery. Anterior and Posterior Segments*, FB Thompson (ed). Macmillan, New York, 1990

	Type I—Inferior temporal staphylomata
Grade I	Minimal staphyloma, inferior to arcades, with thinning of RPE not involving macula
Grade II	More defined staphyloma encroaching within arcades, with increased thinning of RPE. No involvement of macula
Grade III	Well-defined staphyloma with thin RPE involving macula
Grade IV	Well-defined staphyloma involving macula with breaks in RPE and/or "lacquer cracks"
Grade V	Well-defined staphyloma involving macula with small atrophic areas in RPE and choroid
Grade VI	Well-defined staphyloma involving macula with breaks in RPE and associated neo-vascular membrane or "Fuch's spot"
Grade VII	Sharply defined staphyloma with large atrophic areas of RPE, choroid and retina
Grade VIII	Sharply sloping staphyloma. Complete loss of of RPE and choroid, and retinal atrophy over entire posterior pole—"white-out" phenomenon
	Type II—Macular staphylomata
Grade I	Macular staphyloma with thinning of RPE contained within the vascular arcades. Possible breaks in RPE
Grade II	Macular staphyloma contained within the vascular arcades with atrophy of RPE and choroid. Computed tomography scan and B-scans reveal "nipple" effect

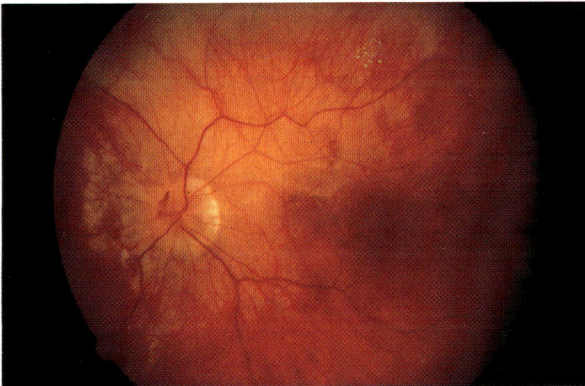

Fig. 13.4 Staphyloma beginning to involve the disk.

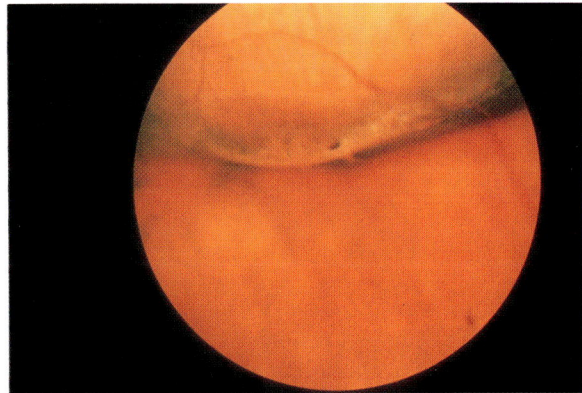

Fig. 13.5 Paving-stone degeneration with retinal hole.

formation of a neo-vascular membrane adjacent to or actually involving the capillary free zone of the fovea (Figure 13.7). Once the neo-vascular membrane develops, macular or peri-macular hemorrhages may occur. These may progress into Fuch's spots with consequent retinal gliosis and chorioretinal atrophy. If these hemorrhages develop in the foveal area, the visual acuity loss may be sudden and permanent.

After the development of lacquer cracks and hemorrhages, chorioretinal atrophy progresses until, at the end stage, the entire posterior pole of the eye becomes devoid of choriocapillaris, retinal pigment epithelium, lamina vitrea, and outer retinal elements. The posterior pole subsequently takes on a characteristic white-out appearance (Figure 13.8).

Retinal degeneration is accompanied by degradation of the vitreous. This can lead to peripheral holes and tears with subsequent detachment of the retina (Figure 13.9).

The degree of myopia is responsible for two separate clinical pictures. Those patients with higher degrees of myopia tend to develop more acute retinal and visual changes at a younger age. In contrast, those with a lower degree of myopia tend to present as older

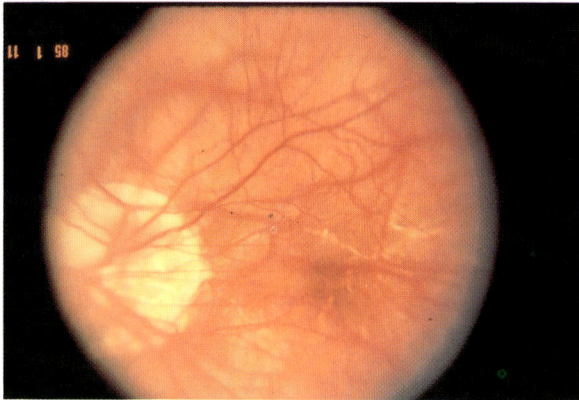

(b)

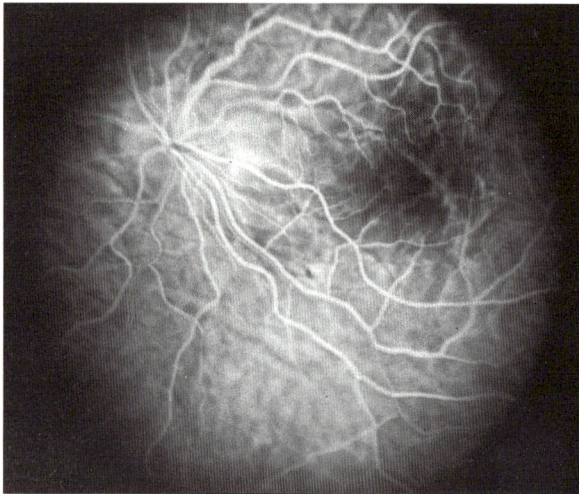

Fig. 13.6 (a) Lacquer cracks developing in macular area; (b) fluorescein angiogram showing lacquer cracks. (Courtesy of F. Thompson.)

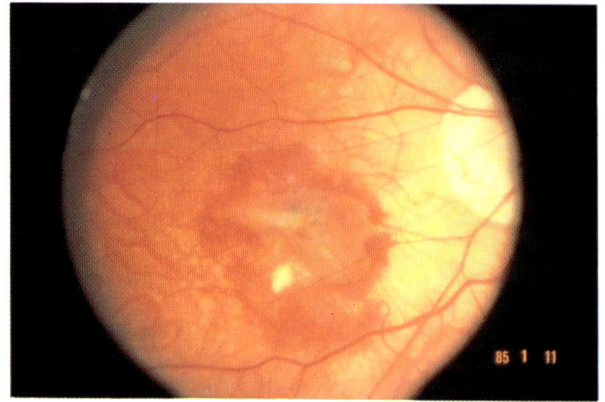

Fig. 13.7 Fuch's spot associated with sub-retinal neo-vascularization and gliosis.

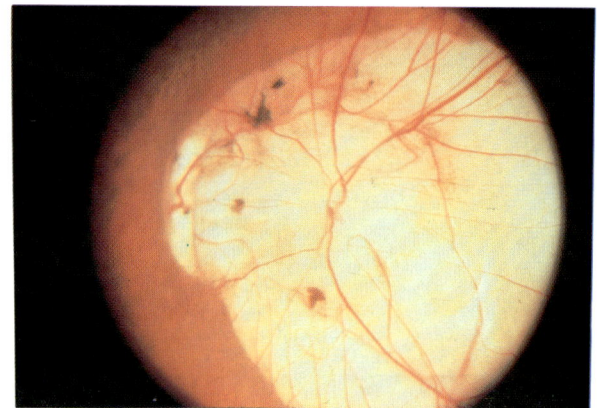

Fig. 13.8 Retinal white-out in advanced progressive myopic degeneration.

patients in whom the visual loss is more subtle and of slower onset. These patients have suffered the gradual destruction of the chorioretinal tissue at a much lower level of myopia but over a longer period of time.

Those patients who range in age from 70 to 90 years old (with as little as 4.0–8.0 D of myopia) can suffer deterioration of the chorioretinal tissue over smaller posterior staphylomata. It is unusual but not rare to see younger patients with central staphylomata at lower levels of myopia (4.0–6.0 D). No studies demonstrate the reason why the posterior scleral fibers are more prone to the formation of central staphylomata in these particular patients. Speculation associates this with other systemic problems, such as a deterioration of elastic collagenous material in other parts of the body (see also Chapter 2). Scleral reinforcement surgery is an attempt to support these macular staphylomata with some type of grafting material.

History of scleral re-inforcement surgery

This posterior staphyloma formation in high myopia remains a therapeutic challenge despite the fact that the condition was identified and described anatomically almost 200 years ago by Scarpa in 1801 [38]. In 1856, von Arlt [39] showed that increases in axial length and myopia were related to staphylomata involving the posterior pole of the eye. The observation, however, was not correlated with pathologic myopia until the work of von Ammon [40], von Graefe [41] and von Jaeger [42], later in the 19th century. Speculation about re-inforcement of the eye began even then.

Scleral augmentation has a sound scientific basis and such re-inforcement of the posterior sclera early in the course of the disease is a sound therapeutic goal. This has been amply demonstrated in animal models as well as clinically in a large number of case reports describing the use of patch grafts of homologous fascia lata or sclera for anterior scleral disease [43–45]. In his discussion of surgery for refractive errors, Rubin noted

(a)

(b)

(c)

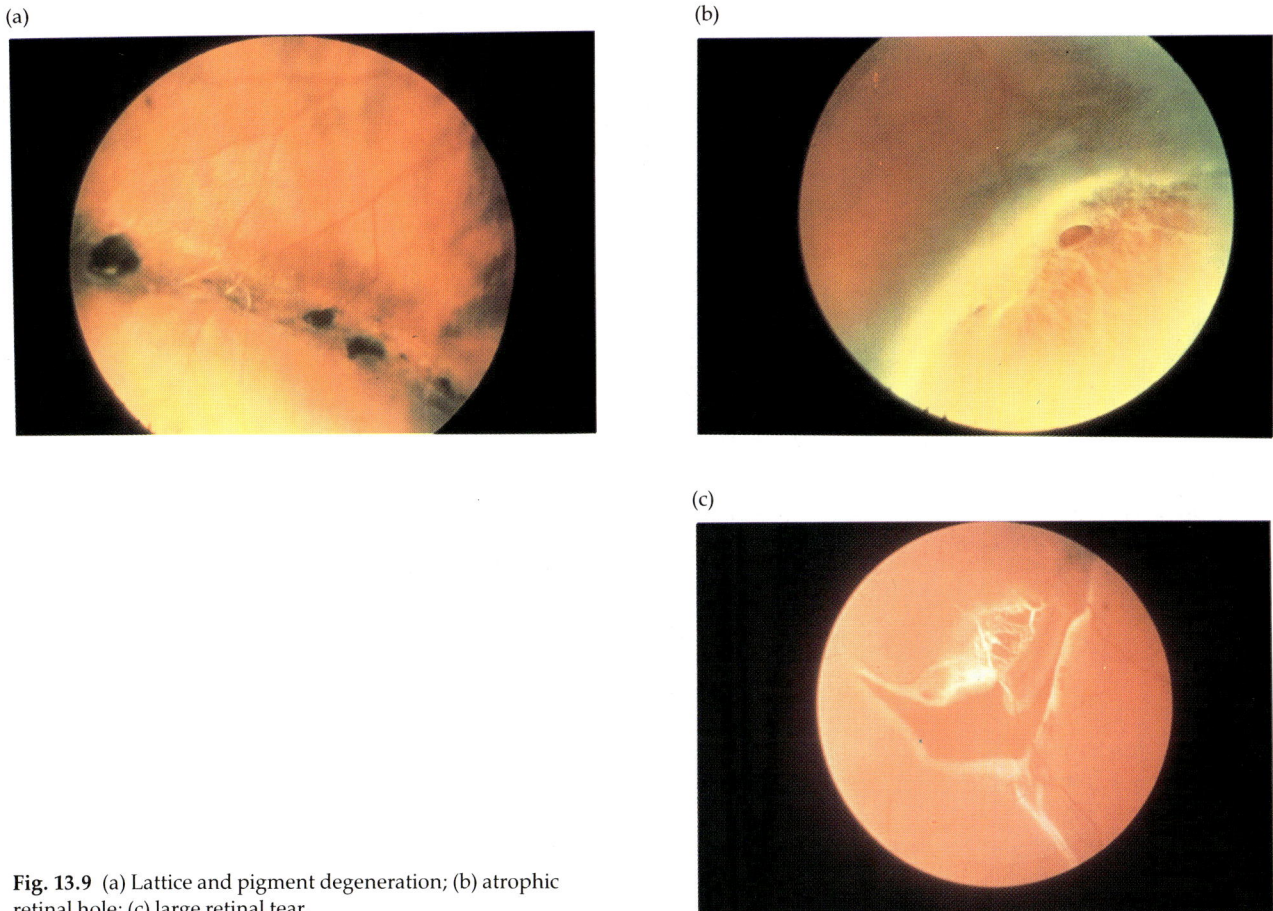

Fig. 13.9 (a) Lattice and pigment degeneration; (b) atrophic retinal hole; (c) large retinal tear.

that scleral reinforcement "is probably the only one of all the surgical techniques [for myopia] which attempts to correct a cause, rather than an effect" [46].

Various modalities to treat the sclera in myopia have been reported in the early literature—most aimed at modifying the axial length—the first by Muller in 1903, wherein he described a method of shortening the eyeball by resecting a ring of sclera at the equator [47].

Overlying grafts of dense collagenous tissues can give added support to the sclera. While surgical treatment for the strengthening of the back of the eye and re-inforcement of the posterior staphyloma in highly myopic eyes had been discussed in the early medical literature for many years, the first scientific report appeared in the Russian literature in the 1930s when Shevelev published a paper on the use of fascia lata to support the posterior sclera in dogs [48]. No further articles on the subject appeared until 1954 when Malbran reported on the use of peri-scleral explants in 21 human cases [49]. Scleral resection was also performed in seven (33%) of these patients. Malbran's object was to support the posterior sclera, preferably early in the course of high myopia, with the purpose of preventing further expansion of the posterior segment. Malbran's original series used homologous fascia lata,

although he had earlier experimented with equine and human tendon.

A number of different collagenous tissues have been used for re-inforcement in a variety of ways. Most investigators in the USA have used homologous sclera in the form of a belt or cinch placed vertically over the posterior pole, under the inferior and superior oblique muscles and sutured to the anterior sclera. Borley and Snyder first used the technique in the USA as a separate procedure as well as in combination with scleral resection [50]. The nine cases presented in their pioneering study combined a scleral homograft with lamellar scleral resection to shorten the axial length of the eye and included penetrating diathermy to treat areas of peripheral degeneration and retinal holes. This combination approach reduced the amount of near-sighted correction but unfortunately induced significant complications which included retinal detachment. Consequently the combination technique was abandoned.

Miller and Borley subsequently reported two large follow-up series summarizing surgeries in which scleral re-inforcement alone was performed. An occasional patient in this group underwent additional scleral resection, however. This approach appeared to be

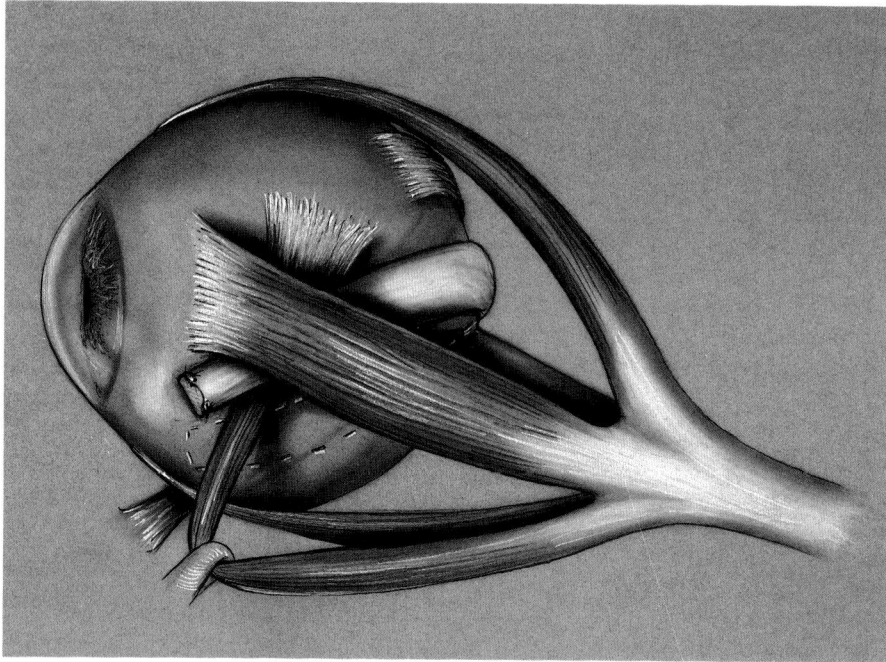

Fig. 13.10 Simplified technique for scleral re-inforcement as described by Snyder and Thompson (see text).

effective in halting the progress of the posterior staphyloma and the pathology of degenerative myopia in those cases [51,52].

The indications for surgery in these patients included rapid progression of childhood myopia, retinal detachment in the highly myopic eye, and visual loss in degenerative adult myopia. In reviewing the case reports in all these studies, it appears that the primary indication for surgery in the majority of patients has been deterioration of central vision in adults with myopia.

The procedures of Borley, Snyder, and Miller involved the detachment of the extra-ocular muscles—primarily the lateral rectus muscle—for better visualization of the posterior pole. They also placed the scleral strip *under* the superior oblique muscle. These two aspects of the surgery, however, increased the possibility of muscle imbalance and anterior segment complications.

In 1972, Snyder and Thompson described a simplified treatment for scleral re-inforcement (Figure 13.10 [53]; F.B. Thompson, 1990, personal communication). They placed the strip *over* the superior oblique muscle without removing any of the extra-ocular muscles using an Arruga spoon to provide visualization of the posterior pole. Cryotherapy, instead of thermal cautery, was used to treat the peripheral retinal degeneration and holes. This approach eliminated many of the complications noted with this procedure, as previously reported. This simplified technique, involving placement of the strip over the superior oblique, could, theoretically, prevent the proper apposition of the graft to host sclera [15]. None the less, experience

with the single-strip method and post-operative follow-up to 20 years has shown that there has been excellent adherence of the strip to the host sclera in all cases observed (F.B. Thompson, 1990, personal communication).

Curtin, in 1961, described the use of homologous scleral support of the posterior segment in young patients [54]. Miller published his experience with the procedure in 1974 in cases uncomplicated by retinal detachment [55]. In 1978 Thompson gave an account of nearly 200 cases of scleral re-inforcement using human sclera and the simplified technique [56]. The indications were a myopia of 10 D or more, decreasing vision, the presence of a posterior staphyloma, and incipient or established macular degenerative changes. In the majority of adults with degenerative myopia surgically treated, such surgery has been found to produce stabilization of the myopia and improvement in vision has been obtained.

Mechanism of action

It is difficult to explain the manner in which this improvement in vision is achieved. Malbran, at the outset, clearly indicated that "this therapeutic method does not pretend to be a panacea for the myopic alterations of the posterior segment of the eye" [49]. Myopic degenerative changes at the macula are basically abiotrophic but can be either ischemic or neo-vascular in nature. The mere physical support of the ectatic sclera has no known beneficial effect upon any of these pathogenic processes—the pathologic process is not reversed. It is likely that the strain upon the retina, choroid, and sclera at the posterior pole is reduced by the addition of an explant—the thicker the wall, the less the strain imparted by a given stress—in accordance with Laplace's formula. Laplace's formula refers to pressure within a hollow sphere: internal pressure is transmitted to the wall as a force that produces tangential, and therefore circumferential, stress. Factors modifying this effect are the radius of curvature of the sphere and the wall thickness, thus: $S = pr/2t$, where S = stress in g/mm^2, p = intrasphere pressure in g/mm^2, r = radius of curvature in mm, and t = wall thickness, also in mm. This is a phenomenon known to every child with a balloon. It takes more force to start blowing up the balloon than it does to continue blowing it up. Furthermore, once blown up and then allowed to empty, the balloon is easier to blow up the next time—the wall is weaker.

However, for peri-scleral re-inforcement to have any effect it seems logical to institute early application of such explants before ischemic and neo-vascular changes cause irreparable loss of retinal cells. In view of this, scleral re-inforcement has been recommended only as a preventive measure, to be used early on in the course of progressive pathologic myopia and before the advanced stages of posterior staphyloma development [57].

All current techniques for scleral re-inforcement attempt to arrest the deterioration resulting from the pathology occurring in highly myopic eyes with posterior staphylomata. Our discussion herein will limit itself to an elaboration of the simplified Snyder–Thompson technique using harvested human scleral explants.

Graft shapes

There are three basic graft shapes (Figure 13.11): cruciate with four arms extending anteriorly, Y-shaped

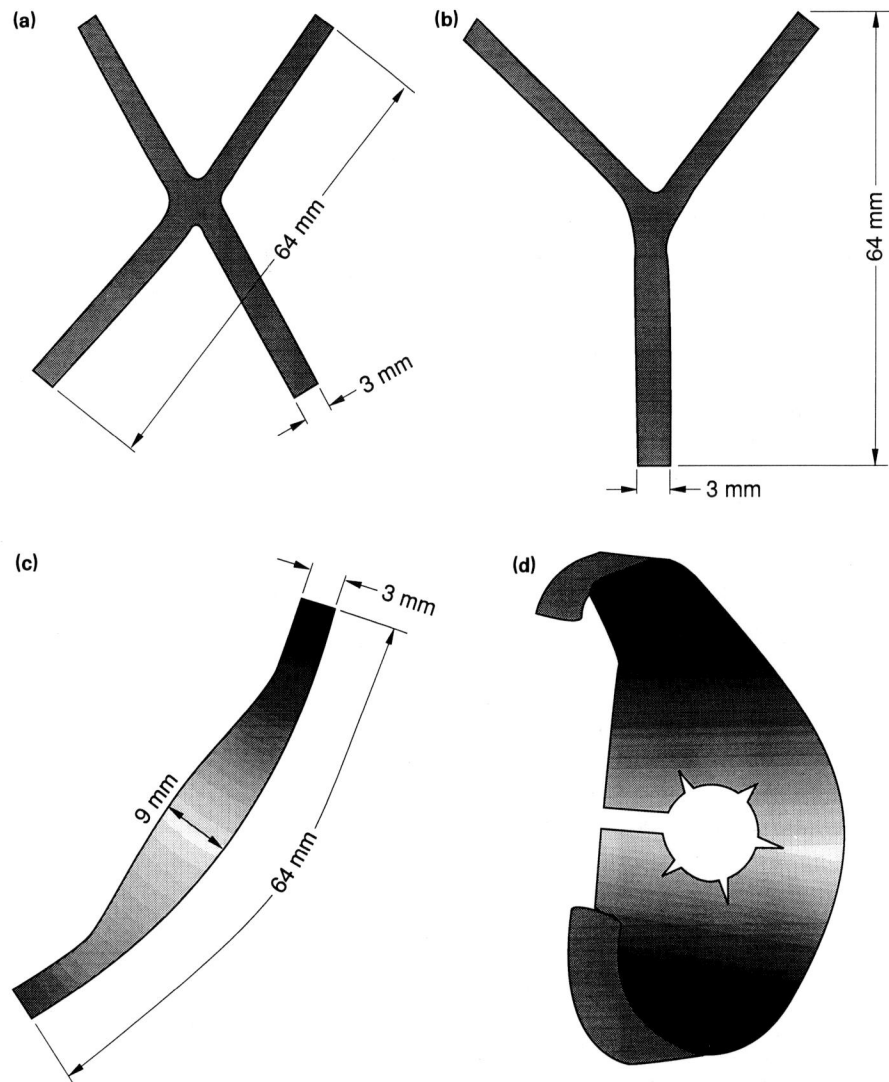

Fig. 13.11 The four explant shapes: (a) cruciate; (b) Y-shaped; (c) single strip; (d) calotte (skull cap) graft.

(placed both vertically and horizontally), and the single strip anchored anteriorly on the nasal side of the superior and inferior rectus muscles. The single strip is held in place over the posterior pole both by the optic nerve and by the posterior insertion of the inferior oblique muscle. A fourth type, the calotte, is used by few.

Curtin has used the cruciate type of explant with the ends of the graft sutured anterior to both sides of the superior and inferior rectus muscles. This type of graft tends to ride very close to the optic nerve and the ciliary arteries, increasing the likelihood of optic nerve impingement and posterior ischemia. This danger, coupled with the more difficult placement of this type of graft, has persuaded the author to favor the Snyder–Thompson procedure in his few cases. The use of this cruciate-shaped explant was further described by Curtin and Whitmore in a follow-up of some of their earlier surgeries [58]. Their report of cases from 5 to 16 years (median 8 years) of follow-up indicated that only 10 of 23 patients (44%) failed to show significant progression of myopia post-operatively. Additionally, only two of nine of these eyes failed to demonstrate increased axial lengths after surgery. This increase was nearly the same as that seen in the fellow, unoperated eye that was used as a control. The stabilization of refraction seen in these patients could as well be ascribed to the natural course of the disease as to any specific effect of the peri-scleral graft. The increase in axial length, it appears, was adequately compensated for by changes in total refractive power of the eye. In contrast to these unimpressive results, the effects of scleral re-inforcement surgery in Eastern European studies could hardly be better [59–63]. Alberth and colleagues, for example, reported a 7-year experience with 400 patients who had undergone fascia lata peri-scleral re-inforcement along with laser photo-coagulation [64]. The degree of myopia was decreased by a mean value of 3.0 D in 90%, while the visual acuity improved by a mean value of 0.15 in 70% of the patients treated. No retinal detachments or other serious complications were reported in this series.

Hanczye used a Y-shaped graft positioned both horizontally and vertically and has published the most extensive series of articles on this subject [65]. He used the meridional circumligation technique of Starkiewicz in which a horizontal autologous fascia lata graft was placed over the posterior sclera at the macula in 44 patients, the majority of whom were under 20 years of age [66,67]. An improvement in vision was usually noted, together with an average reduction in myopia of 1.5 D. A reduction in ocular axial diameter, averaging 1.5 mm, was also obtained. In 40% of patients a significant increase in visual fields was also noted along with the disappearance of isolated scotomata.

There was deterioration of the field in 13%, however. In this series a reduction in the ocular tension was also found post-operatively. Again, no serious complications were observed.

Nesterov and co-workers have also contributed extensively to the literature on this subject [68–70]. In a more recent report they summarize the results of 756 scleral re-inforcement procedures in which horizontally oriented autologous fascia lata was used [71]. They obtained a reduction in myopia that ranged from 0.5 to 8 D in 86% of these eyes. The axial length decreased an average of 1.47 ± 0.51 mm. Long-term follow-up (mean 6.8 years) in 244 eyes found that these earlier results were stable. Complications included compression of the optic nerve in one case and compression of vortex veins with choroidal hemorrhage in five cases.

The striking differences in results between these studies of Hanczye and Nesterov and those reported by Curtin are difficult to reconcile. The surgical techniques in general are similar—the skill of the surgeon is, of course, an important variable. It would appear, however, that the principal difference rests in the snugness with which the graft has been applied to the sclera. In the Eastern European technique considerable traction appears to have been placed upon the graft. This was deliberately not done in the cases reported by Curtin because rabbit studies had indicated that shrinkage of the peri-scleral graft ensued post-operatively [43]. However, Curtin's cases were almost all children in whom there can be a general enlargement of the globe despite the flattening of the posterior staphyloma. In these cases the criteron for success was refraction. Furthermore, there are theoretic arguments that can be made against the efficacy of overlying grafts of the macular region in posterior staphyloma development.

The most common type of staphyloma, that of the posterior pole, type I, originates nasal to the optic nerve and involves the macular area by expansion. If effective prevention of staphyloma formation is to be achieved, this nasal area must also be re-inforced [57]. This has been done in two clinical studies with encouraging early results. Zarkova and Negoda [72] in Russia and Whitwell [73] in Britain have contributed two large studies, each comprising over 40 patients, in which a calotte of homologous sclera was placed about the optic nerve. There can be little question that this approach is a distinct improvement in the re-inforcement effect of the surgery but this improvement is obtained at a greater risk of vascular accidents, as evidenced by the inadvertent occlusion of the superotemporal vortex vein in two patients in the British study. This resulted in intra-ocular hemorrhage and blindness. Additionally, whether placed horizontally or vertically, the Y-shaped graft may press on the optic nerve at the junctions of the arm of the Y, resulting in optic nerve atrophy.

Momose has reported a number of cases using Y-shaped grafts associated with lens extraction [74]. He noted the occurrence of secondary glaucoma and one case of optic atrophy among the 50 eyes in which he used the Y-shaped explant. Because of the increased risk of complications, Momose no longer uses this type of explant, preferring instead to use the single-strip type of support in his last 2000 cases (A. Momose, 1990, personal communication).

Most ophthalmic surgeons, particularly those in the USA, currently use the single-strip support technique whether using fascia lata, lyophilized dura, or sclera. The single strip offers the easiest method for placement, along with the widest area of support over the macula—the main objective of the operation. This approach significantly reduces the incidence of optic nerve impingement. No cases of optic atrophy or damage have been reported using this technique to date (F.B. Thompson, 1990, personal communication).

Curtin correctly points out that the single scleral strip has the disadvantage of only re-inforcing the macular staphyloma and does not prevent development of staphylomata in other areas (B.J. Curtin, 1990, personal communication). It should be noted, however, that macular staphylomata are the ones associated with the most profound and permanent visual loss—most of the visual elements required for fine vision, including reading and driving, are contained in this area. For this reason the sole compelling indication for a posterior scleral graft is the developing presence of a macular staphyloma.

Materials

There is much work that has yet to be done with both materials and techniques. Other grafts using different shapes and materials may someday prevent the development of staphylomata in other areas of the globe. A future technique may not only protect the central visual elements but at the same time prevent stretching and elongation of the entire eye.

In the 60 years since Shevelev's paper, a variety of dense collagenous materials have been employed for the re-inforcement of the posterior staphyloma. These materials range from fascia lata to lyophilized dura to human donor sclera. Homologous human donor sclera is mainly used for the re-inforcing material, particularly by US surgeons, partly because of its ready availability. In addition, sclera is easy to work with and does not tend to develop folds posteriorly, as is the case with other materials. When properly removed from the donor eye, sclera conforms to the contour

of the host eye more readily than any of the other reported materials. Furthermore, it is strong and holds sutures well.

In other parts of the world alternative materials are often used. Human sclera is avoided because of cultural, religious, or technical reasons. Momose in Japan published an optimistic report on over 2000 cases of scleral re-inforcement using lyophilized (freeze-dried) dura for posterior support (Figure 13.12) [75]. In 1984, Nesterov and co-workers [71] reported on the use of fascia lata in 756 operations while Fyodorov in Moscow uses human donor sclera in his scleral explant patients (S.N. Fyodorov, 1990, personal communication). However, one of the problems with fascia lata is that it requires a second surgical procedure on the patient to harvest the tissue. This prolongs the surgery and affords no opportunity for the preservation or sterilization of the harvested material.

The use of equine or porcine tendon has been proposed but not effected. To date, a single strip of homologous human sclera appears to offer the best support with the fewest complications of all the biologic materials.

As for allopathic materials, silicone and nylon are not recommended. The sclera of the highly myopic patient is extremely thin. Any pressure from these highly elastic materials can erode the underlying tissue, as has been noted after their use in retinal detachment surgery on both myopic and non-myopic patients.

The ideal material would be one that is firm, yet has the correct amount of flexibility and elasticity. A suitable artificial material would also eliminate the need for harvesting human tissue, insure proper and complete sterilization, be readily available and would not compress the underlying sclera. Such a material is polytetrafluorethylene, commercially available under the trade name Gore-Tex. This material was originally employed as a fabric but has been used for years by vascular surgeons in repairing aortic grafts. It offers promise as a material which can be easily obtained, sterilized, and stored and also provides some give without too much stretch. The experience with it is minimal at this time but some patients have recently undergone scleral re-inforcement surgery with this material in the USA (F.B. Thompson, 1990, personal communication).

Preparing the graft

A whole frozen donor eye is the source of scleral grafts—two such strips can be cut from each globe. When the donor eyes have been obtained, they should immediately be frozen. The strips should be cut

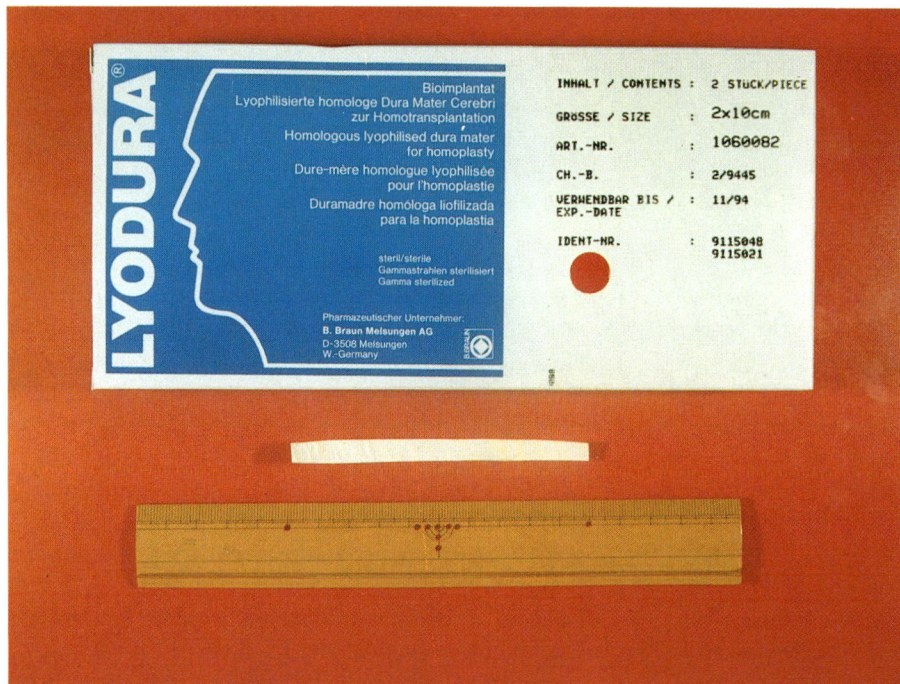

Fig. 13.12 Momose uses lyophilized human dura for his explants.

from them within 1–2 weeks after freezing to avoid potential explant weakening resulting from deterioration of the donor sclera. The globes must remain frozen all during this time. Because the eyes of a high myope are much larger than average, the prepared scleral strip must include sufficient corneal tissue so that the explant is long enough to reach around the entire circumference of the host eye. If corneal tissue is not included, the graft may be too short, making placement of the strip much more difficult, if not impossible. The sclera of highly myopic eyes should not be used for grafting because it is too thin and does not offer adequate support over the affected area. Since it is impossible to know the refractive status of most donor eyes, some globes will necessarily be found to be unsuitable during harvesting.

The strips are removed under sterile conditions. The instruments used are a methylene blue marking pen, a Bard-Parker knife with a #15 blade, rat-toothed forceps, sterile cotton-tipped applicators, sterile 4 × 4 gauze patches, and a Wescott-type scissors.

To make handling easier, the globes are only partially thawed before removing them from the storage containers. The optic nerve is cut flush with the sclera, and excess orbital fat and connective tissue removed. The donor globe is positioned so that the superior rectus muscle is up. The areas to be cut are marked using the methylene blue marking pen (Figure 13.13). The first mark is placed at the limbus carried posteriorly just adjacent to the optic nerve and brought in a curvilinear path to the opposite limbus nasal to the insertion of the inferior rectus. Two other dotted marks are made parallel to the original marks so as to delineate the path to be cut. The strip that incorporates the optic nerve is made slightly wider posteriorly.

An incision is made tangentially across the cornea in line with the center mark. Grasping the incision with a toothed forceps and using the Wescott-type scissors, the surgeon cuts along the initial middle dotted line circumferentially. The incision is continued around the eye until the globe is separated into two halves. The lines are again followed posteriorly and circumferentially until two scleral strips are obtained. The resultant strips should be in the shape of a boomerang, though not so abruptly curved. The resected strips should be at least 8 mm wide at their center, but may be as narrow as 3–4 mm at the ends. The length of the strip as measured along the curve should be at least 60 mm.

At this point, the surgeon uses the cotton-tipped applicators to roll up and remove the retinal and choroidal tissue from the inner side of each strip. Excess pigmented tissue is completely removed by scraping with the blunt side of the Bard-Parker knife. It is not necessary, nor is it desirable to depigment the sclera with iodine (as in eviscerations) in preparing these strips. Surplus Tenon's capsule and connective tissue on the external side of the strip, if any, should be removed.

The strips are stored submersed in a solution con-

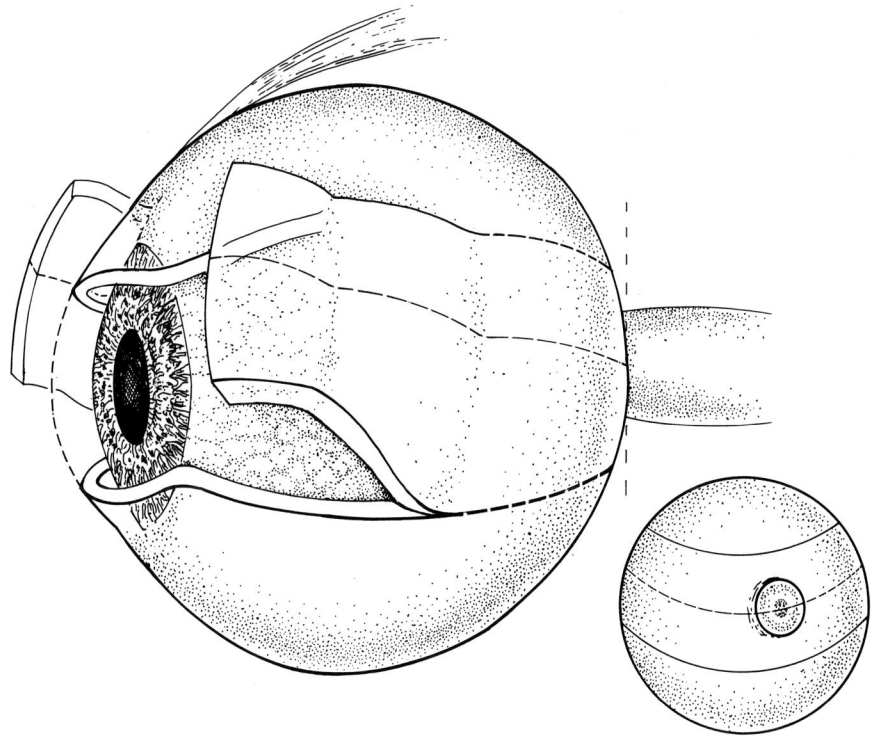

Fig. 13.13 Method for harvesting scleral explants.

sisting of two-thirds saline and one-third Neosporin (polymyxin B sulfate–neomycin sulfate–bacitracin zinc) within test tubes fitted with rubber stoppers or caps. An air pocket is left at the top of the tube to allow for expansion of the solution when it is frozen. The stopper is sealed and an adhesive label is placed on one side of the test tube. Each tube is marked with the date of harvesting, the length of the strip, and other pertinent details (e.g. the strip is slightly short, a little thin, more curved than normal). The test tubes are supported vertically in a test tube rack placed in a freezer and kept until surgery. Theoretically, as long as the strips are kept continuously frozen, they should remain viable. Thompson prefers to use them within 1 year of the date of freezing, however (F.B. Thompson, 1990, personal communication).

Patient selection

The primary candidate for surgery is a patient who has progressive posterior staphyloma on the temporal side of the optic nerve involving the macula. This condition can occur in any patient from 2 to 80 years of age and from −4.00 to −40.00 D of myopia. Indications for surgery are myopia greater than 7 D with:
1 Decreasing best corrected vision.
2 Documented increasing axial length (more than 1.0 mm of axial length progression per year for 2–3 years).

3 Progressive macular changes on fluorescein angiography.
4 Indirect ophthalmoscopy indicating a posterior staphyloma (evidence of thinning of the retinal pigment epithelium posteriorly).

Pruett correctly points out that there is a trend toward recommending refractive surgery for young patients with high degrees of progressive myopia [76]. Although many can benefit from certain procedures, staphylomatous eyes present unique impediments to normal visual acuity, visual field, binocularity, and stereopsis. They are also prone to premature cataract formation, glaucoma, and retinal detachment. An initially good surgical result can be utterly negated by continued scleral expansion along with posterior retinal degeneration. A review of these limitations should be included in discussions with patients considering refractive surgery.

Many patients will present with already well-developed staphylomata, angiographic evidence of chorioretinal atrophy or "lacquer cracks" and axial lengths measuring over 29–30 mm. In these cases, scleral re-inforcement should be considered without waiting for further changes. If possible, surgery should be performed prior to the development of a sub-retinal neo-vascular membrane so as to reduce the risk of bleeding during the operation. While preventing further enlargement of the staphyloma, scleral re-inforcement surgery does not always prevent additional progression of an existing sub-retinal neo-vascular network with its subsequent hemorrhage and visual loss.

If initial fluorescein angiography reveals a sub-retinal neo-vascular network and the membrane is at least 20 µm outside the capillary free zone, adjunctive laser therapy may be indicated. The laser, however, is contraindicated in the presence of sub-retinal neo-vascular membranes in the central foveal area. Current techniques of laser therapy have not been particularly successful in the treatment of membranes, even outside the capillary free zone. The membranes frequently re-form in any event and treatment of neo-vascularization may itself produce further bleeding.

Preventive therapy is always controversial. For example, laser therapy is presently being performed much earlier in patients with diabetic retinopathy to prevent the changes seen in the later stages of the disease. However, if scleral re-inforcement is as effective and safe as some believe it to be, then it may make sense to perform prophylactic surgery on highly myopic patients who fit the above criteria. This will prevent them from developing the complications resulting from the advanced stages of the disease.

There is a increasing number of geriatric patients being seen in western society and an increasing longevity projected for the future. Because of this, we may anticipate seeing more elderly patients who develop posterior staphylomata along with the typical changes of pathologic myopia at much lower levels of myopia than has been seen in the past. If these patients have either a non-dilated funduscopic examination or are examined without an indirect ophthalmoscope they may be misdiagnosed as having age-related macular degeneration (ARMD). It is imperative that these older myopic patients undergo indirect ophthalmoscopy for detection of any late staphyloma formation.

The practitioner must then make a differential diagnosis between the much more commonly seen ARMD and the late cases of myopic degeneration. Some aging patients will not develop the central pigment clumping, gliosis, and deterioration seen in late wet ARMD. Instead they will present with a progressive atrophy of Bruch's membrane, the pigment epithelium, and the retina and choroid over the posterior pole. Finally they may exhibit the typical "white-out" appearance seen in the high degrees of myopia in younger age groups. To add to the matter, the differential diagnosis between myopic degeneration and dry ARMD is frequently a difficult one (Figure 13.14).

Scleral re-inforcement should be seriously considered in some of these older patients. This is particularly appropriate for those who have lost central vision in one eye because of increased staphyloma formation and deterioration of the retinal elements, but maintain some reasonable level of visual acuity in the remaining

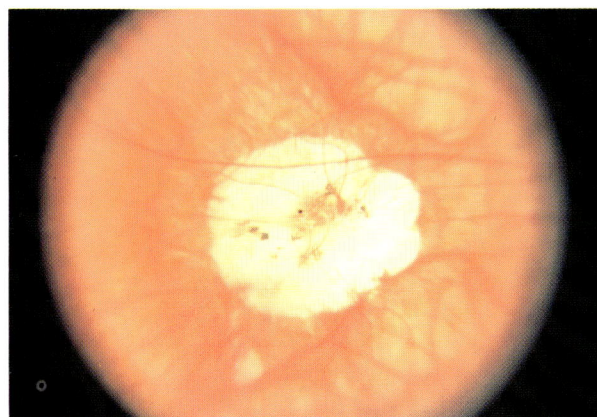

Fig. 13.14 Myopic degeneration is often difficult to distinguish from ARMD.

eye. Surgery may be the only recourse for preservation of vision in these cases.

Patient examination—pre-operative and post-operative

Highly myopic patients undergo a thorough eye examination which includes a complete ocular and medical history. In the younger patient particular attention is paid to recent or precipitous changes in the patient's refraction. For all patients, the examiner checks for recent decrease in the best corrected visual acuity. This is followed by near/distance visual acuity, a glare test, careful dilated slit-lamp examination, refraction, and measurement of IOP. Slit-lamp examination of the younger patient may reveal posterior sub-capsular cataracts.

Indirect ophthalmoscopy is particularly useful for observing posterior staphylomatous changes. Those beginning in the inferior temporal quadrant should be carefully documented. In addition, the peripheral fundus is inspected as the younger patient is much more likely to exhibit lattice degeneration and peripheral retinal breaks, holes, or tears. In the highly myopic patient, the examiner should carefully inspect the inferior temporal peripheral retina for paving-stone degeneration. While the indirect ophthalmoscopic view moves from the periphery toward the posterior pole of the eye, a sudden edge or drop-off, indicating a staphyloma, can easily be seen.

Computerized visual fields are performed and are especially useful in these cases. Many of these patients will be found to have central scotomata because of the previously described pathology. Static, computerized perimetry makes repeat comparison studies much easier and enhances their value in earlier detection of advancing changes.

Fluorescein angiography establishes the degree of loss of posterior pigment epithelium and the amount of choroidal and retinal deterioration. This technique is useful for delineating lacquer cracks and early development of sub-retinal neo-vascular membranes.

The examiner performs A-scan measurement of the axial length over both the macula and the deepest portion of the eye. The macular measurement and the greatest length of the eye may not necessarily coincide since posterior staphylomata are frequently off center, particularly in the early stages.

Axial lengths must be carefully measured by an experienced ophthalmic technician as the presence of staphylomata in many cases makes precise measurements extremely difficult. Since the slope of the posterior staphylomata may be rather sharply delineated, variations in the axial length are frequently encountered. The technician must be sure to read the longest part of the eye. A combination of fluorescein angiography and axial length measurements offers the most accurate diagnosis in the highly myopic patient.

B-scan ultrasonic measurements of the eye are not very good for following the progress of staphylomata. It is frequently difficult to get a clear static picture for subsequent evaluation and comparison. However, the so-called Z or isometric examination mode may be invaluable in locating staphylomata accurately for subsequent A-scan measurement.

As yet, there is no standardized measurement of scleral re-inforcement surgery results. Because the disease progresses slowly, follow-up needs to be done for a number of years to demonstrate long-term stabilization. There are problems and drawbacks with all of the measurements mentioned above, both as pre-operative indicators for surgery and as post-operative evaluations of results.

Refraction is not useful for following the progress of myopic staphylomata because factors other than staphyloma enlargement may influence refractive error. Many highly myopic, middle-aged patients tend to develop cataracts, lenticular swelling, and changes in refractive error from induced myopia. This can occasionally add −5 to −6D of myopia. If these patients undergo cataract removal (eventually becoming aphakic or pseudophakic), the refraction can change drastically, rendering difficult pre-operative and post-operative comparisons. In other cases, especially in children, the entire eye size may enlarge slightly to increase the refractive error though no posterior staphyloma may develop. After surgery younger patients can have an increase in axial length (and therefore myopia), even though the macular staphyloma may have been stabilized. This auto-adjustment in total refractive error may occur in adults as well.

Computed tomography or magnetic resonance imaging scans of the globe are often helpful, although cumbersome and expensive. Many patients are reluctant to repeat the scans because of this. Computer scans do, however, provide excellent imaging confirmation of scleral strip placement and can establish temporal strip integrity as well (Figure 13.15). Such a loss of integrity should always be suspected when advancing axial length is seen post-operatively.

Visual acuity measurements are somewhat subjective for both patient and examiner. Similarly, fluorescein angiography requires some subjectivity in determining further deterioration. Since fluorescein angiography requires an injection, many patients are reluctant to have it repeated at frequent intervals. Not a few patients will experience nausea and/or other unpleasant side-effects. Some can even develop a reaction to the fluorescein dye, which fortunately, although uncomfortable, is not usually serious. Anaphylactic-like reactions have, however, been reported.

Ultrasound measurements of axial length seem the most objective method of measuring the efficacy of the procedure. Often ultrasound is the only frequently repeatable diagnostic technique acceptable to the patient. As mentioned above, A-scan measurements of the length of the eye are difficult in patients with sharply sloping staphylomata. Only a practiced technician familiar with the highly myopic eye can obtain an accurate and reproducible axial length measurement.

Increase in axial length is not always a hallmark of progressive staphyloma, however. Younger patients may exhibit a growth of the entire axial length of the eye, even though the scleral re-inforcement procedure has stopped the progression of the macular portion of the staphyloma. Such growth may not even be suspected as there is often a compensatory adjustment in other refractive components (emmetropization), as noted in Chapter 2.

Pre-operative preparation

The patients are started on Tobrex (tobramycin 0.3%) antibiotic drops 2 days prior to surgery. The operative eyes are dilated with 10% Neo-Synephrine (phenylephrine hydrochloride), 1% Mydriacyl (tropicamide), and 1% atropine drops instilled every 10 minutes four times, beginning 1 hour prior to surgery. It is recommended that the lashes be clipped before surgery and the eyelids carefully scrubbed with half-strength Betadide (povidone-iodide *solution* (not preparation) for 2–3 minutes. Betadine preparation contains soap which can damage the corneal epithelium and irritate ocular tissue.

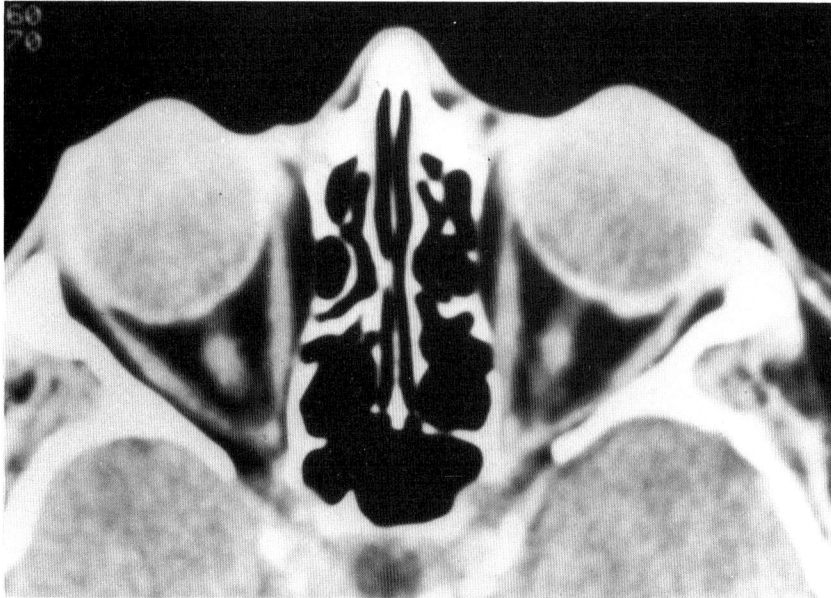

Fig. 13.15 Computed tomography scan showing scleral explant in one eye near the optic nerve. (Courtesy of F. Thompson.)

Surgical technique

The following description is provided courtesy of Frank Thompson: The surgery is preferably performed under general anesthesia. Retro-bulbar or peri-bulbar anesthesia is not recommended because the accompanying edema frequently distorts the periocular tissue posteriorly, making placement of the scleral strip difficult. Additionally, these patients occasionally have areas of scleral ectasia or anterior staphylomata. Because of the thin globe, there is a possibility of ocular perforation, either anteriorly or posteriorly. If local anesthesia is necessary, the surgeon should use a blunted, 25-gauge, Atkinson-type retro-bulbar needle to administer it with the patient looking down (toward) the needle. This will swing the thinner posterior pole of the eye up and away from the needle tip (see also Chapter 11 for more details of this technique).

A conjunctival incision is made in the supero temporal quadrant, approximately 4–5 mm posterior to the limbus. A fornix-based incision is preferred to a limbal incision because it allows more exposure of the posterior pole. In addition, later cataract surgery is less difficult because the limbal-based flap leaves the surgical limbus undisturbed.

The incision is extended into both the supero temporal and infero-temporal quadrants, leaving a small amount of conjunctival tissue overlying the medial rectus muscle. Since highly myopic eyes are very large, the extra-ocular muscles may also be attenuated, therefore care must be taken when making the conjunctival incisions so as not to sever or damage these muscles.

The underlying Tenon's capsule is incised and the sclera exposed. In younger patients this capsule is usually very thick, very vascular, and difficult to manipulate. In contrast, older patients may have subconjunctival tissue that is extremely thin and atrophic. In any event bleeding must be completely controlled with wet-field cautery to insure good visualization.

The superior, lateral, and inferior rectus muscles are isolated using muscle hooks. Care must be taken that the check ligaments and adhesions to the overlying conjunctiva and underlying sclera are stripped. Traction sutures of 4–0 black silk are placed beneath these muscles (Figure 13.16) and their ends secured with alligator clamps.

The traction sutures around the inferior rectus and lateral rectus muscles are grasped and the eye rotated *medially*. A muscle hook is passed parallel to the globe, hugging the sclera in the infero-temporal quadrant. The tip of the hook is then rotated outward and anteriorly to isolate the inferior oblique. Using a combination of blunt and sharp dissection, the inferior oblique is separated from the orbital septum and connective tissue surrounding the muscle—the orbital septum itself should not be incised. If orbital fat is allowed to come forward, later visualization will be more difficult.

Take care during this step that all fibers of the inferior oblique muscle are brought forward. The muscle may occasionally divide into two parts and sometimes there are muscle fibers which tightly hug the globe posteriorly. These must be brought forward as well, taking care not to tear them. Since the explant must be placed posterior to all the fibers of the posterior insertion of the inferior oblique muscle (insuring that

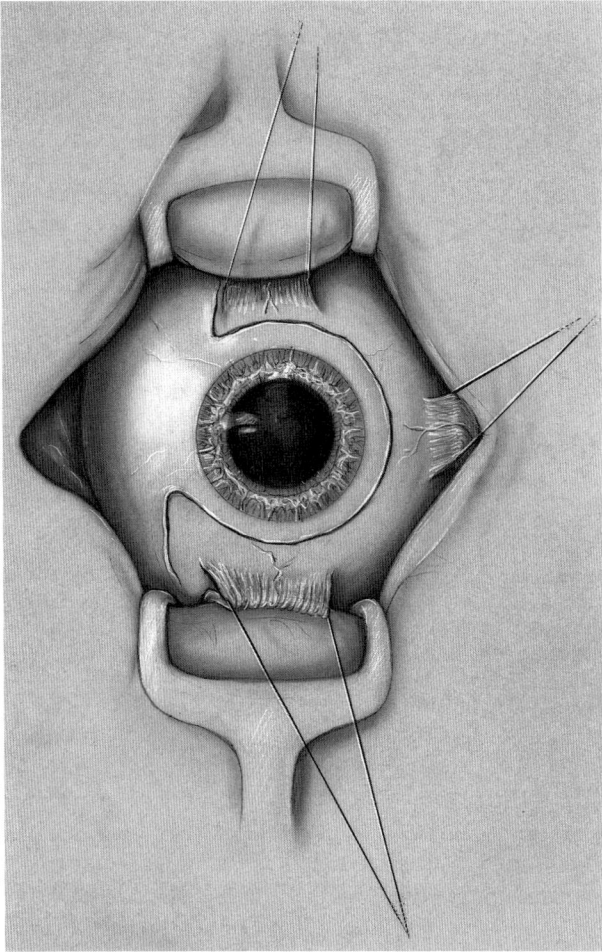

Fig. 13.16 The superior, inferior, and lateral recti are isolated.

the strip will not ride too far forward, be positioned accurately over the posterior pole and be held firmly in place), no muscle fibers can be missed. Repeat surgery may be necessary if the explant splits the anterior and posterior fibers of this muscle. In that event, the explant will inevitably shift anteriorly and create a bothersome muscle imbalance.

Once all fibers of the inferior oblique have been carefully isolated, an additional traction suture of 4–0 black silk is placed around this muscle. Next, passed posteriorly beneath both the superior and inferior rectus, a muscle hook is carefully used to strip away any adhesions extending from the muscles to the globe. The hook is passed gently under the lateral rectus muscle with the eye rotated medially. The adherent fibers are gradually stripped away until the hook can be pushed no further. At this point, the instrument should lie against the fat pad surrounding the optic nerve. There are important blood vessels in this area so gentleness is the order of the day. These adhesions will occasionally resist the hook sufficiently

that cutting with scissors will be required. If the patient has a pre-operative sub-retinal neo-vascular membrane, extreme care must be taken to prevent rupturing this membrane and causing subsequent macular bleeding. This can occur through too vigorous manipulation of the globe—remember the sclera is very thin in this area. The surgeon can easily visualize any posterior adhesive fibers with an Arruga spoon.

After the muscles are isolated and traction sutures placed around them, the periphery of the retina is inspected with the indirect ophthalmoscope and scleral depression is gently performed. Keep in mind always that the myopic sclera is abnormal and thin. The surgeon must work carefully to avoid tearing the vortex vein. Any atrophic holes or retinal tears can be treated cryosurgically under direct visualization with the indirect ophthalmoscope. The infero-nasal and infero-temporal quadrant are the most common sites for retinal tears, holes, and paving-stone degeneration. This is in contrast to the moderately myopic patient who demonstrates a tendency for retinal tears and holes in the supero-temporal quadrant.

The scleral strip, which has previously been thawed and soaked in an antibiotic solution, is now examined. The surgeon excises any excess connective tissue remaining on the strip and shapes it with the scalpel. The inner portion of the scleral strip is placed against the sclera of the host eye, *beneath* both the superior and lateral rectus muscles (Figure 13.17). As the inferior oblique muscle is pulled forward, the surgeon, using forceps, draws the strip through the opening made by tenting up the muscle. When the muscle is released, the posterior fibers of the inferior oblique will drag the strip backward toward the optic nerve (Figure 13.18). The scleral strip is then tucked under the inferior rectus muscle. The strip is then sutured to the sclera in the superior temporal quadrant, just posterior and nasal to the insertion of the superior rectus and at a 45° angle to the muscle insertion. The superior oblique muscle need not be isolated, however; the strip can be placed over the superior oblique without risking complication (Figure 13.19).

The traction suture around the inferior oblique muscle is now cut and removed, allowing this muscle to retract. The strip is then secured superiorly with two sutures of 5.0 collagen, Vicril (synthetic adsorbable polyglactin 910), or nylon.

With the *left hand*, the assistant grasps the end of the strip (in the inferior nasal quadrant) with a toothed forceps (such as a Bishop–Harmon). The traction suture around the lateral rectus muscle is held with the assistant's *right hand*—this suture is used to rotate the eye medially.

Using an Arruga spoon to visualize the posterior pole of the eye, the surgeon pulls the posterior conjunctiva

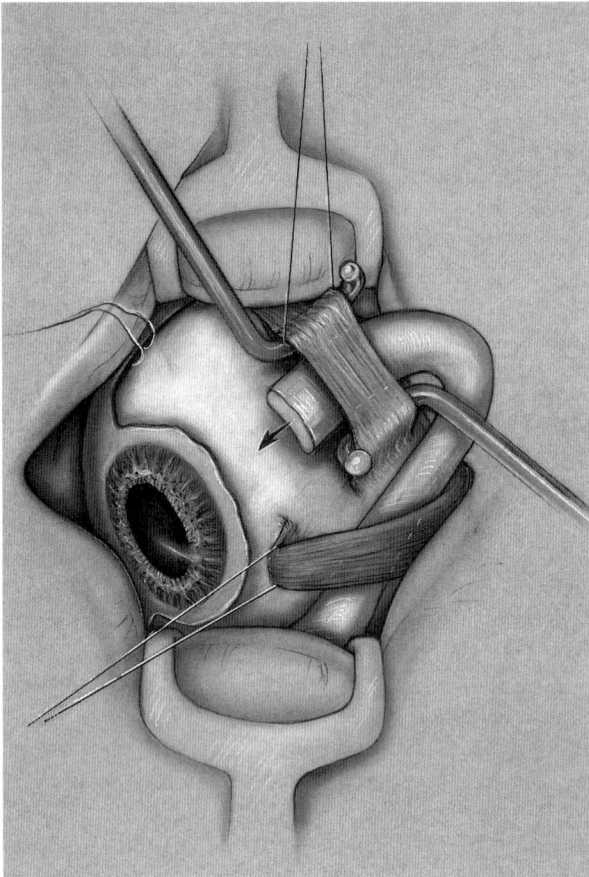

Fig. 13.17 Placement of the strip beneath the superior and lateral recti.

anteriorly. The strip is placed over the posterior pole either with a fine, smooth forceps or with a custom-designed, curved repositioning instrument (Figure 13.20b). In the first step, the assistant pulls on the

lateral rectus insertion to rotate the eye medially for greater exposure over the posterior pole. If the strip is too long and too loose posteriorly, the scleral graft is pulled forward in the inferior nasal quadrant and the excess trimmed away.

As the Arruga spoon is shifted from just superior to just inferior to the lateral rectus muscle, the scleral strip is checked to insure that it is positioned correctly over the posterior pole. In this maneuver, only the very anterior edge of the strip should be seen. In the inferior temporal quadrant the strip should be clearly located posterior to the insertion of the posterior fibers of the inferior oblique. The surgeon will need to inspect this region several times to insure proper placement of the strip. In some older patients, the inferior oblique is very flaccid and may not contract sufficiently. In this case the anesthesiologist will need to administer intravenous succinylcholine chloride to cause contracture of the extra-ocular muscles.

The traction suture around the lateral rectus is released by the assistant and the eye rotated superiorly. The explant is allowed to lie naturally against the globe in the inferior temporal quadrant. Often the strip will be seen to be too long, necessitating further excision of any excess. The strip is then sutured (with one suture of 5-0 collagen or Vicril) at a 45° angle just nasal and posterior to the insertion of the inferior rectus muscle (Figure 13.2). The needle is placed through the sclera slightly anterior to the position where the strip has been lying against the sclera. This insures that that some tension will be placed on the explant and that it is tight posteriorly when the suture is tied.

With the Arruga spoon. the surgeon once again examines the posterior pole, superior and inferior to the lateral rectus muscle. If the strip is tending to slide

(a)

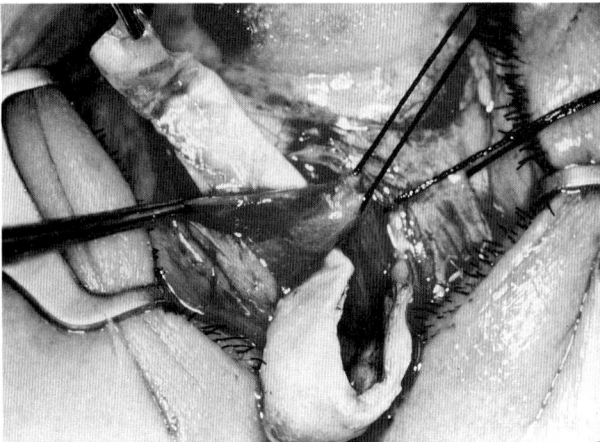

(b)

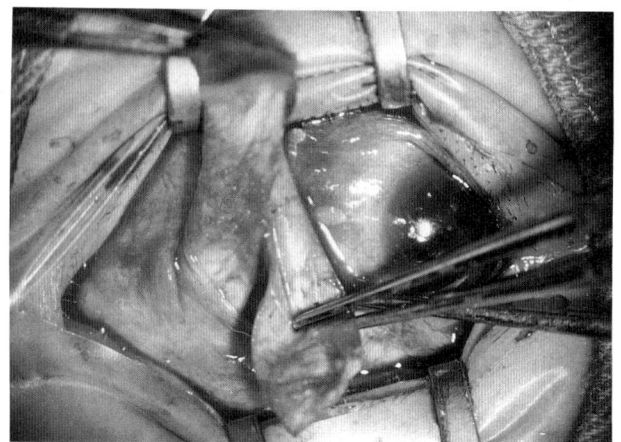

Fig. 13.18 (a) The strip is drawn under the isolated inferior oblique. (b) If the strip is long enough, crossing the ends over the medial rectus lightly helps seat the posterior part. (Courtesy of A. Momose.)

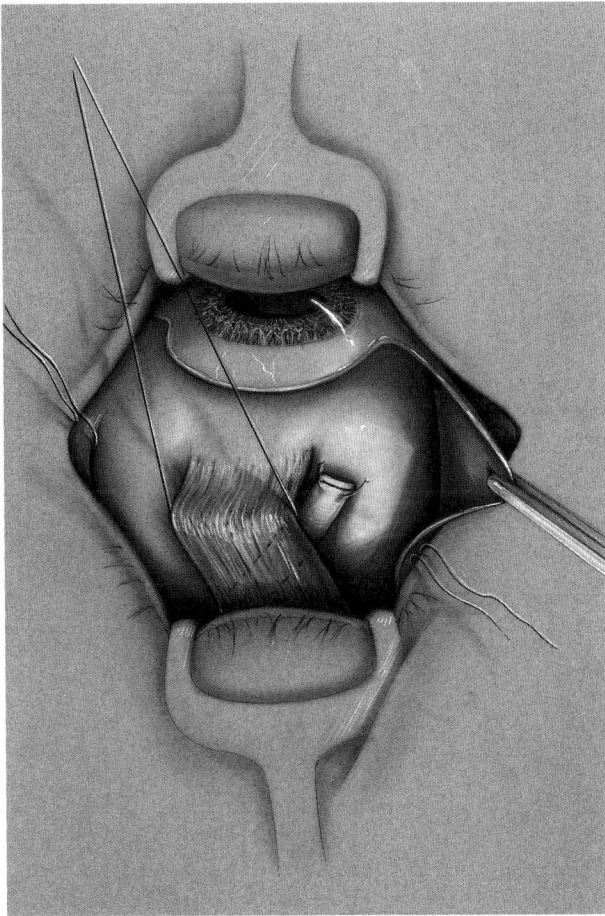

Fig. 13.19 The strip is passed beneath the superior rectus and over the superior oblique and sutured to the globe.

forward, it may be necessary to re-position it over the posterior pole. This is easier once the strip has been secured with a suture inferiorly. If the strip is still not fitting snugly against the sclera, the inferior suture can be removed. After an additional portion of the excess strip is excised, it can be re-sutured to the sclera in the manner previously described. The surgeon may need to perform this re-suturing several times to achieve proper placement and tension of the scleral strip over the posterior pole. Again, only the anterior edge of the strip should be visible during maximum nasal rotation of the globe once its proper placement is assured. An extra suture is then placed through the strip in the inferior nasal quadrant (Figure 13.22).

The fundus is again inspected with the indirect ophthalmoscope. Occasionally, a slight indentation over the posterior pole can be seen but this may not appear until several months after the surgery. The surgeon inspects the optic nerve head, and central retinal artery and vein to make sure that the scleral strip has not compromised the blood supply to the optic nerve and retina. The macula is inspected for

hemorrhage which can occur as a result of manipulation during the surgery, particularly in those cases where a sub-retinal neo-vascular membrane is present.

The IOP is checked with a Schiøtz tonometer. If the strip has been placed tightly over the posterior pole, the IOP may be elevated. Sometimes a partial temporary occlusion of the vortex veins may elevate the IOP as well. In these cases, intravenous mannitol 20% may be administered by the anesthesiologist to soften the eye.

The surgeon should make a final inspection of the posterior pole and scleral strip with the Arruga spoon. Once the strip is confirmed to be in position, the traction sutures around the extra-ocular muscles are removed. A small amount of Garamycin (gentamicin sulfate) is irrigated posteriorly. The conjunctival incision is closed with a running suture of 6.0 plain gut or 8.0 Vicril. Gentamicin sulfate is injected sub-conjunctivally along with 1.0 ml of Celestone (betamethasone sodium).

Normally a canthotomy is not necessary in performing scleral re-inforcement. However, in some oriental eyes or in eyes with very small palpebral fissures, it may be necessary to perform a lateral canthotomy to insure adequate visualization over the posterior pole. If this has been done, the canthotomy is closed routinely. The lid speculum is removed and Cortisporin (polymyxin B sulfate–bacitracin zinc–neomycin sulfate–hydrocortisone) ointment is instilled in the cul-de-sac. Benzoin is placed along the skin of the forehead and cheek; Elastoplast is applied over several eye patches as a pressure dressing.

Post-operative care

The patient remains in the hospital overnight for observation because there may be symptoms of pain, nausea, and vomiting similar to that experienced after retinal detachment surgery. Additionally, 8 mg of Decadron (dexamethasone sodium phosphate) *push* is administered intravenously immediately post-operatively and repeated 6 hours later. A final 8 mg dose is infected the morning following the surgery. That morning the dressing is changed and the eye is inspected. There is usually a considerable amount of chemosis and lid edema despite the administration of the steroids—patching with ointment is repeated until this chemosis subsides and the lids close normally.

If 1% atropine or 5% homatropine drops were given pre-operatively, the pupil should be dilated sufficiently for the fundus to be inspected the day following surgery. It is not crucial if the indentation from the scleral strip cannot be seen, however. Often some degree of choroidal edema or hemorrhage is present, particularly in the inferior temporal quadrant, although there have been no occurrences of vitreous

(a)

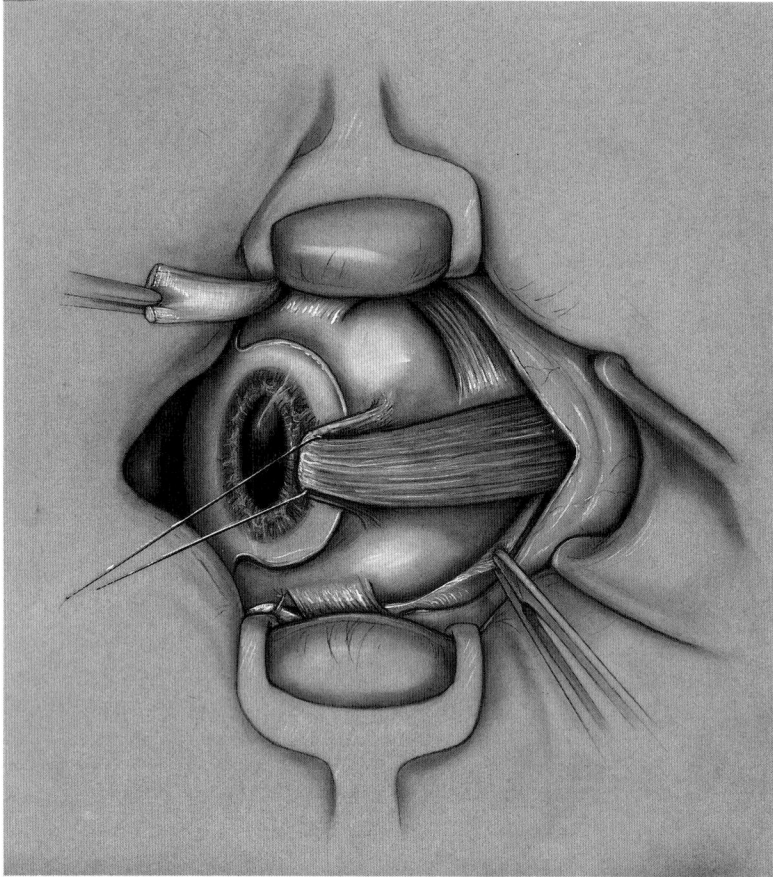

(b)

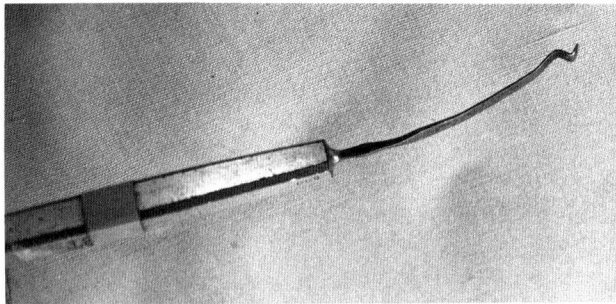

Fig. 13.20 The strip is positioned over the posterior pole with forceps (a) or with a specially bent iris spatula (b).

hemorrhage reported following the surgery at this writing.

Steroid ointment is again instilled and the eye re-patched with a pressure dressing. The eye remains patched for 2–3 days following surgery depending on the degree of chemosis, lid edema, and discomfort.

The patient is examined again at 3 days, 1 week, 3–4 weeks, and then as indicated. Depending on the degree of chemosis and inflammation around the eye, the patient is prescribed 15–20 mg of oral prednisone to be continued in a tapered dosage for 2–3 weeks post-operatively. The dosage of prednisone may be changed depending on the degree of post-operative inflammation and choroidal edema and/or hemorrhage. Choroidal edema usually resolves 4–5 weeks following the surgery.

When the patch is discontinued the patient is placed on steroid and antibiotic drops q.i.d. The antibiotic drops are continued for a week post-operatively while the steroid drops continue for 3–5 weeks following surgery.

A moderate degree of pain may persist for 2–3 days post-operatively. The patient can resume normal activities within 1 week from the date of surgery.

(a)

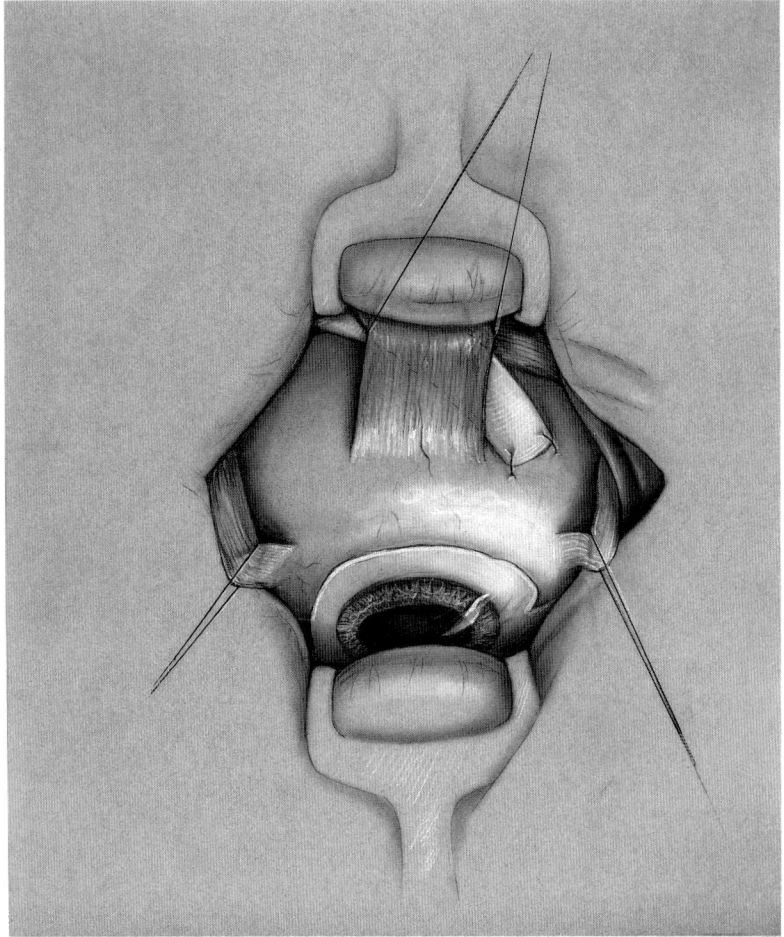

(b)

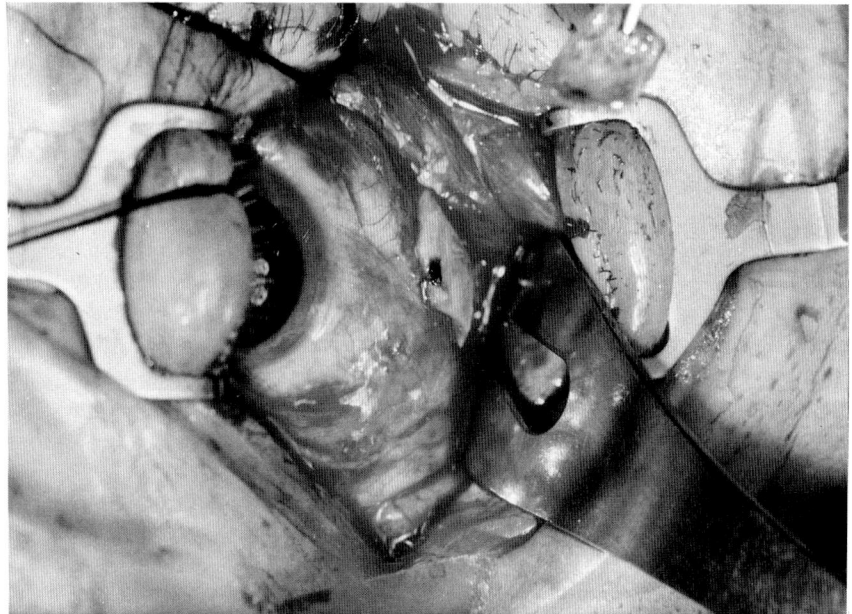

Fig. 13.21 (a and b) When the strip is correctly positioned, it is sutured just nasal, posterior to the insertion of the inferior rectus.

(a)

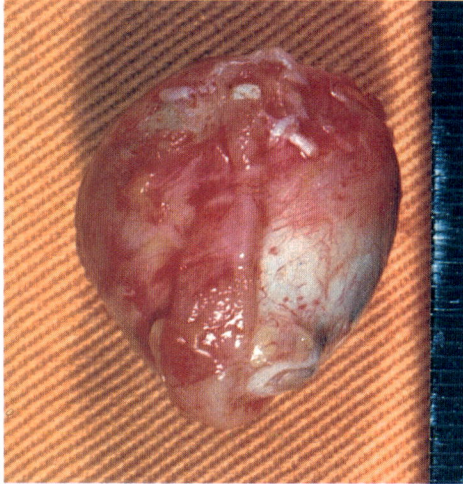

(b)

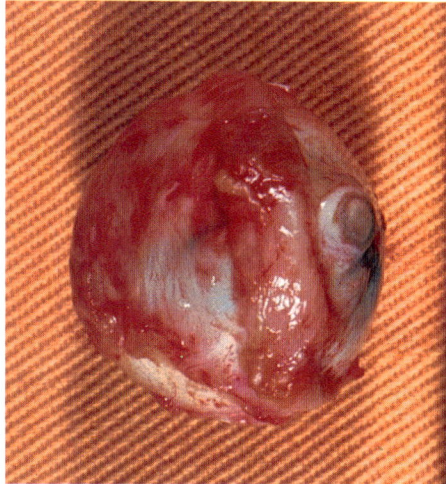

(c)

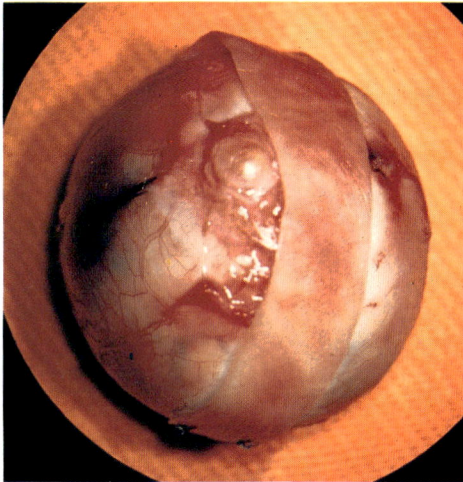

Fig. 13.22 (a–c) The proper positioning of the strip demonstrated on an enucleated eye. (Courtesy of A. Momose.)

Beginning 4–5 days post-operatively, the patient begins eye exercises consisting of looking as far as possible in the eight cardinal directions without moving the head. This may be quite uncomfortable for the first few days because the extra-ocular muscles are inflamed. The exercises are to be done for 1 min three times a day, for 3–4 weeks. These exercises help prevent later adhesions and muscle imbalance. Because of conjunctival irritation and chemosis, contact lens wearers must be cautioned not to wear their contacts on the operated eye for at least 2–3 weeks following surgery. The patient should have spectacles to wear. If not, he or she must be certain before the surgery that he or she can function with a monocular contact lens.

Refraction and A-scan measurements can be made 6–8 weeks following surgery and are repeated at periodic intervals. This technique provides the most objective assessment of staphyloma stabilization or flattening (Figure 13.23).

If surgery on both eyes is indicated, the second is operated on 2–3 months after surgery on the fellow eye, providing stabilization has occurred before proceeding.

If there is any question about subsequent placement, relocation or viability of the explant, computer scans (computed tomography or magnetic resonance imaging) can be of assistance. A computer scan provides clear imaging of the strip posteriorly. The graft's location and thickness can be easily seen. Because scans are expensive and tedious to the patient, they are indicated only in those cases where there is doubt about the placement or durability of the strip.

Complications

The discussion of complications which follows is taken from Thompson's study of 264 eyes (Table 13.2). The long-term complication rate for scleral re-inforcement has been low using the single-strip approach. Short-

(a)

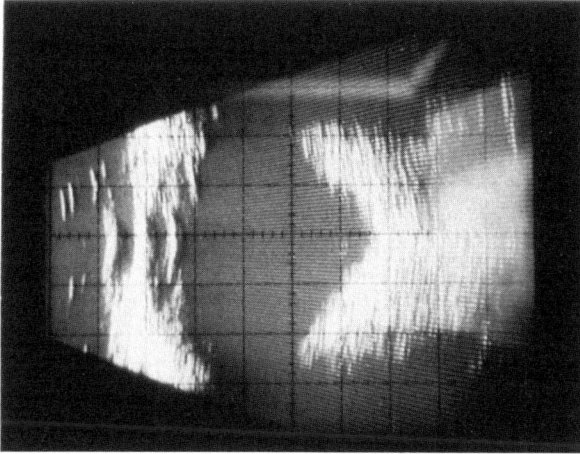

(b)

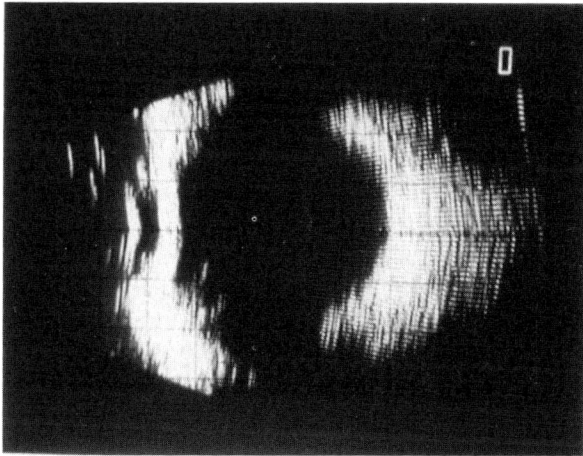

Fig. 13.23 B-scan of an eye before (a) and after (b) scleral re-inforcement, demonstrating the flattening of the posterior pole.

Table 13.2 Complications in 264 scleral reinforcements followed from 6 months to 18 years of age. Adapted from Thompson FB. Scleral reinforcement. In: *Myopia Surgery. Anterior and Posterior Segments*, FB Thompson (ed). Macmillan, New York, 1990

Complication	Eyes
Choroidal edema or hemorrhage (resolved without therapy)	10
Corneal dellen (resolved within 6 weeks)	2
Chemosis	264
Retinal detachment	2
Optic atrophy	0

term complications of marked chemosis and conjunctival injection occur almost without exception, and in all series. These are benign and quickly subside, although the chemosis may persist for 2–3 weeks. In some patients with small palpebral fissures, the conjunctiva may protrude between the lids during the first week.

There has been a 3–4% incidence of post-operative choroidal edema or hemorrhage, usually in the inferior temporal quadrant. This is probably secondary to compression of the inferior vortex vein by the strip, resulting in choroidal congestion.

In some cases damage to the vortex vein may occur during the surgery itself because the exit of the vein is very close to the area where the inferior oblique is isolated. This is especially true for some oriental eyes that have narrow palpebral fissures. In these cases, the surgeon may have difficulty visualizing the exit of the vein while isolating the inferior oblique, and damage

to the vein can result. These cases have resolved with systemic steroid therapy and have shown no incidence of retinal or vitreous hemorrhage. There are no cases of post-operative infection or instances where the strip has had to be removed.

A few patients will have transient motility problems following the surgery, but these normally resolve within 2–4 weeks. There is a low incidence of such problems because the extra-ocular muscles are not removed during the surgery and the superior oblique muscle is left untouched. The muscle exercises begun 4–5 days following the procedure have most likely contributed to the good result.

The only long-term problems involved two patients with pre-existing muscle imbalances. Both had pre-operative exophoria and hypertropia which had been corrected with prisms. These patients experienced a mild increase in their exophoria and hypertropia which required additional prismatic correction. Such patients should be warned that such problems may worsen following surgery.

Several instances of small corneal dellen have occurred in the temporal limbal margin anterior to the insertion of the lateral rectus muscle. This probably reflects temporary interference with the circulation of the anterior segment. It should also be noted that the surface of the anterior globe has been greatly disturbed and tearing will not be normal during the first few weeks. All such case cleared within 4–6 weeks of ocular lubricant therapy.

Two cases of retinal detachment are reported in Thompson's series. One of these presented at 10 years post-surgery and the other at 7 years. These were not deemed complications of the re-inforcement surgery itself, however. Both occurred as a consequence to the later development of lattice degeneration and of retinal tears and holes not present at the time of surgery. An 8% incidence of retinal detachment following scleral surgery is less than that reported for such complications occurring amongst high myopes at large.

The few published reports of optic nerve damage

following scleral re-inforcement have all used Y-shaped or a cruciate graft instead of the single scleral strip. Using either a Y or cruciate-shaped graft can lead to the graft pulling too tightly against the optic nerve which may then occlude the posterior ciliary vessels. The competence of the short and long posterior ciliary vessels and of the vortex veins must always be respected. The use of a horizontal band of donor sclera that fits closely about the optic nerve produced serious complications in one small series because of circulatory decompensation [77].

There have been no cases of optic nerve damage or optic atrophy among Thompson's cases. This can be explained by the fact that a large cushion of fat and connective tissue surrounds the optic nerve at its exit from the globe, protecting the nerve head. Furthermore, the single scleral strip does not press tightly enough against the optic nerve to cause permanent damage.

Theoretically, IOP could be elevated long enough post-operatively to occlude the central retinal artery. This can be a potential problem for the older patient with poor arterial circulation. Because of this, the surgical team should carefully monitor IOP before, during, and immediately after surgery. This monitoring is especially important for the eye with a tight orbit. In this case, retro-orbital bleeding can significantly increase pressure on the posterior vessels and nerve.

Results

All scleral re-inforcements included in Thompson's series were performed on patients who had deteriorating vision, fluorescein angiographic evidence of pathology, and increasing axial length. Among the 264 scleral reinforcements, 16 eyes were lost to follow-up.

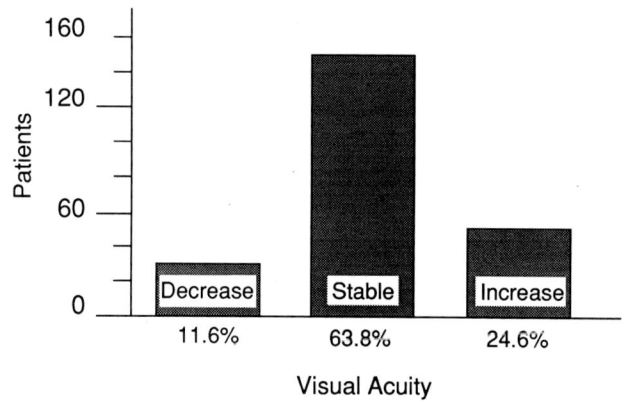

Fig. 13.24 Effect of scleral re-inforcement on the visual acuity in Thompson's series.

Figure 13.24 shows the visual acuity results of 224 patients with an average follow-up of 5.63 years. A decrease in acuity was defined as a loss of two Snellen lines on the visual chart. The findings show 26 (11.6%) of the patients had a decrease in acuity while 198 (88.4%) either stabilized or showed improved acuity. Of these 198, 143 (63.8%) were stable and 55 (24.6%) had improved vision.

The frequency distribution seen in Figure 13.25 has an abscissa representing the number of lines of acuity change. The curve is skewed to the right, indicating an influencing factor toward improved acuity in these patients. This is contrary to the usual, natural course in pathologic myopes. Among those who had preoperative and post-operative fluorescein angiography, approximately 90% exhibited stabilized angiographic changes.

The data provided in Figure 13.26 summarize the changes in axial length of a group of 77 patients with

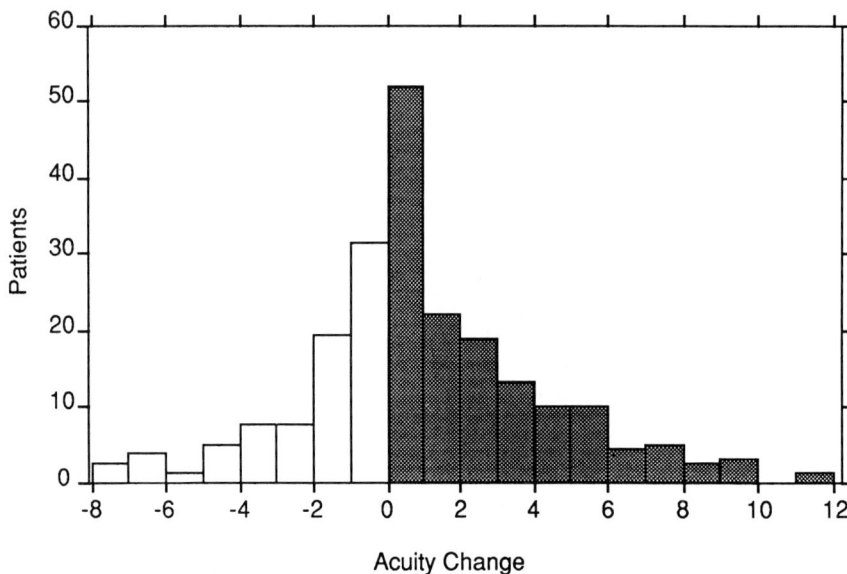

Fig. 13.25 Distribution of the visual acuity changes in this group.

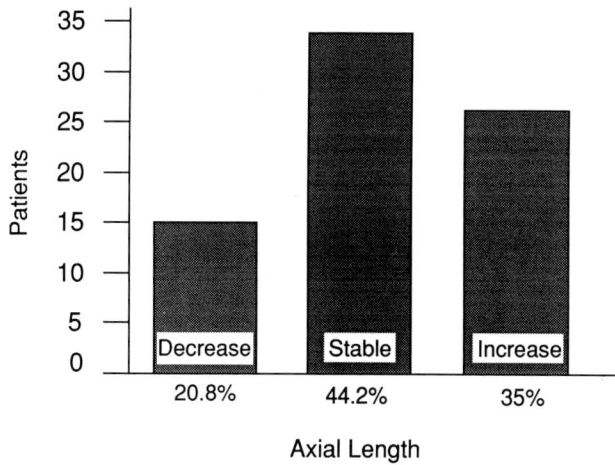

Fig. 13.26 The effect of scleral re-inforcement on the axial length of 77 patients in Thompson's series.

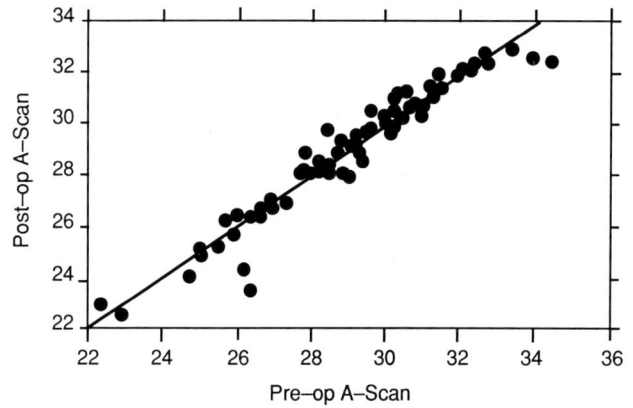

Fig. 13.28 Linear regression of pre-operative versus post-operative axial lengths in 77 patients.

an average follow-up of 3.54 years. The criterion for judging an eye to have changed in length was the repeatable measurement of a change of 0.3 mm or greater. This represents the smallest change which can reasonably be expected to be discriminated ultrasonically as an indication of lengthening or shortening of the eye.

At this level of statistical significance of 0.3 mm the results showed an increase in axial length in 16 (20.8%) out of 77 eyes. Stability or decrease in axial length was found in 61 (79.2%) eyes.

The frequency distribution of axial length changes presented in Figure 13.27 uses axial length change as the abscissa. The skew to the left indicates a force for stabilization or decrease in axial length which is equal to or greater than the force for elongation in the majority of eyes followed. Again this is contrary to the expected findings in any group of highly myopic eyes left to evolve naturally.

A scatterplot showing a linear regression of pre- and post-operative measurements is presented in

Figure 13.28. The efficacy of scleral re-inforcement surgery provided to the eye is suggested by the simple regression line slope of 0.976. In the author's two cases, both eyes retained stable axial lengths, as measured by A-scan and refraction.

Discussion

High myopia, defined as greater than $-8.00\,D$, is diagnosed in 3–5% of all myopic patients. The condition is the fourth to seventh leading cause of blindness, depending on the geographic area surveyed. High myopia is the seventh leading cause of blindness in the USA [15]. The incidence of myopic blindness increased from 0.1% in children under 5 years of age to 0.6% in the aged in Kahn and Moorhead's study [78]. The sharpest increase was noted to occur in the middle of the fifth decade. This, unfortunately, coincides with that period of life in which the talents and productivity of those affected are at a maximum, as well as with that time at which there is a peak in financial responsibility; thus, the impact of this blindness upon the family is particularly severe.

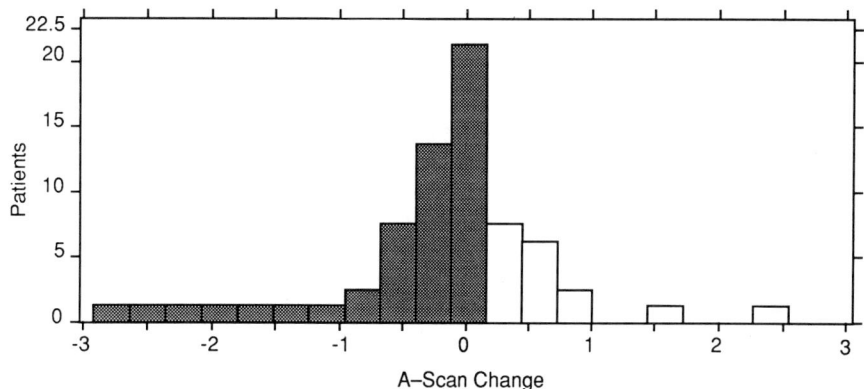

Fig. 13.27 Distribution of the effect on axial length.

In some areas of the world high myopia is much more common than it is in the USA. There appears to be a high concentration of high myopia in northern Italy and Sicily, for example. The data from the UK are of particular note because of Sorsby's interest in myopia [79]. In an early survey of blindness in England and Wales, he found myopia to be the second most frequent cause of blindness in persons between the ages of 30 and 49 years. In the next age-group (50–69 years) it ranked second only to cataract. Certain areas in Asia, such as China and Japan, report a prevalence of this condition in 15–20% of the population. In some Japanese prefectures, high myopia and its complications are the most common cause of blindness recorded. In China and Japan, ophthalmologists attribute high myopia among students (in their late teens to early 20s) to the intensive study of small printed characters. However, this has not been substantiated by formal study.

The prevalence of ametropia also varies with age. The typical incidence of myopia at age 6 months is 4–6%. The overall incidence of myopia amongst school children ranges from 4% in ages 4–14 in England to 25% in the same age group in Japan. In the USA, the large HANES study examined the incidence of myopia among youths aged 12–17 and found that the incidence rose from 29.3% at age 12 to 33.2% at age 17 (see also Chapter 2) [80].

The principal cause of permanent blindness from high myopia is the development of posterior staphylomata with subsequent choroidal and retinal deterioration. In highly myopic eyes, staphylomata occur in areas nasal and temporal to the optic nerve, and occasionally postero-temporal and antero-temporal.

Scleral re-inforcement offers the only treatment for the posterior staphyloma which destroys the retinal pigment epithelium, choroid, and retinal tissue in these highly myopic patients. The aims of this treatment are to:

1 Stop progression of the disease process.
2 Maintain and/or improve vision (especially in younger patients).
3 Reduce staphyloma formation.
4 Reduce or stop further macular damage.

The results reported in Thompson's 264 patients over a 20-year period are good, whether measured by visual acuity, fluorescein angiographic changes, or axial length measurements. All of the data show the treatment to be effective in a high percentage of cases. Also, the complication rate is low. There have been no serious vision-threatening complications either during the surgery or in the immediate post-operative period.

Despite the good results reported in the series of Thompson [56], Miller [81], Borley [82], and Snyder [83], scleral re-inforcement remains a controversial and ignored treatment in the USA. Scleral re-inforcement is performed on a much more frequent basis by Fyodorov (6000 cases) and Krasnov in the former Soviet Union, Momose in Japan, Brian and Hollows [84,85] in Australia, and Hanczye et al. [86] in Poland, among others.

Acceptance of scleral re-inforcement in the USA has been slow, partly because of unfamiliarity with the procedure and the scarcity of published clinical studies in the USA. Curtin's earlier series of scleral re-inforcements using the cruciate graft approach has recently been re-evaluated. Using refraction as the method of measurement, the authors reported discouraging long-term results in these patients. Several of these patients were adolescent, however, and younger patients can yield an inaccurate measurement of staphyloma stabilization. Yet, despite his disappointing analysis of the results, Curtin states that scleral re-inforcement is the only rational method presently available for treating macular staphylomata [15].

Acquiring and storing sclera presents difficulties, especially to those doing a relatively small number of these cases per year. Additionally, human sclera varies in quality depending on the donor eye from which it was obtained. The search for an adequate artificial material as a replacement of sclera for re-inforcement until recently has been disappointing. Kaufman has suggested Gore-Tex as a possible replacement for human sclera (H.E. Kaufman, 1990, personal communication). If a synthetic material provides a satisfactory substitute, it could be sterilized and stored without freezing. The synthetic strips could be a standard size, length, and thickness and, with this in mind, a template has been developed to insure uniformity (F.B. Thompson, 1990, personal communication).

Until now, other materials have been more difficult than human sclera either to work with or place in situ. Artificial materials such as silastic or silicone bands are unsatisfactory because these materials erode the already thin sclera under the band or strip. When re-operating for retinal detachment even in normal eyes, it is not uncommon to see that the sclera is thinned under a silicone sponge or band. This could be devastating to the existing thin sclera over the posterior pole of the myopic eye. Gore-Tex may avoid this problem, since it is more flexible than silicone.

American ophthalmologists seem to be reluctant to accept the efficacy of scleral re-inforcement until there is a prospective controlled study. Scleral re-inforcement has been performed over 6000 times in the former Soviet Union by Fyodorov's team (S.N. Fyodorov, 1990, personal communication). Momose in Japan has performed between 1000 and 2000 scleral reinforcements, most of them using a similar single-strip technique (A. Momose, 1990, personal communication). The extensiveness of the follow-up of these international series is unknown, but published results are similar to American studies.

Although the type of measurements and criteria used to determine efficacy can vary from surgeon to surgeon, the results seem to indicate prevention of further visual loss from myopic degeneration. A universal protocol needs to be established to measure the success and complication rate for this surgery.

In the USA, a multi-centered investigation, being developed by Thompson, the LSU Eye Center in New Orleans, and Retinal Associates in Boston, proposes to conduct a randomized study of scleral re-inforcement. Surgery would be performed on one eye and compared to the contralateral eye to evaluate long-term results. Gore-Tex and other artificial materials would be compared to human sclera. The study would be designed to follow patients for a period of 5–10 years. It will involve a long-term control study with strict criteria of pre- and post-operative measurements to evaluate the effectiveness of scleral re-inforcement surgery. This study should finally settle the 60-year-old question about the value of scleral re-inforcement.

While there may be controversy over this methodology or whether our current techniques are effective over the long haul, the fact remains that scleral re-inforcement remains the only rational method of increasing scleral resistance in eyes with progressive myopia and posterior staphyloma formation. Patients will continue to suffer further damage to their retinas and posterior circulation from progression of their pathologic myopia in the absence of a mode of re-inforcing their "blown-out" scleras. While waiting for the control study, ophthalmic surgeons may want to seriously consider implementing scleral re-inforcement therapy for highly myopic patients, since there is currently no effective or alternative treatment. The option is watchful waiting and sympathy, neither of which is of much benefit to the patient and of even less effect on the pathology.

References

1 Algan B. [The treatment of progressive malignant myopia with magnesium chelates of flavones. Apropos of 400 cases.] Bull Soc Belge Ophtalmol 1981; 192:103–112.
2 Smelovaskii AS, Golychev VN, Khomullo GV. Ob ispol'zovanii kal'tsitonina pri progressiruiushchei blizorukosti. [Use of calcitonin in progressive myopia.] Vestn Oftalmol 1988; 104:45–47.
3 Armaly M, Burian H. Changes in the tonogram during accommodation. Arch Ophthalmol 1958; 60:60.
4 Abdulla MI, Hamdi M. Applanation ocular tension in myopia and emmetropia. Br J Ophthalmol 1970; 54:122–125.
5 McCollim RJ. On the nature of myopia and the mechanism of accommodation. Med Hypotheses 1989; 28:197–211.
6 Bubolts L, Medvetskaia G. Opyt organizatsii pionerskikh lagerei sanatornogo tipa dlia detei s blizorukost'iu na baze obshcheozdorovitel'nykh lagerei i rezul'taty lecheniia v nikh. [Experience in organizing sanatorium-type pioneer camps for children with myopia based on general health-improvement camps and the results of their treatment.] Vestn Oftalmol 1980; 2:69–71.
7 Diaz-Dominguez D. Mas sobre miopia e hipertension ocular. Arch Soc Oftalmol Hisp-Am 1966; 26:935.
8 Diaz-Dominguez D, Montero Marchena J. Miopia media y tension ocular. Arch Soc Oftalmol Hisp-Am 1966; 26:241.
9 Fledelius HC. Distensibility of the young eye. Doc Ophthalmol 1981; 28:117.
10 Tarkkanen A, Uusitalo R, Mianowicz J. Ultrasonic biometry in congenital glaucoma. Acta Ophthalmol (Copenh) 1983; 61:618.
11 Kamali K, Hamdi M. Relation between applanation tonometry and errors of refraction. Ain Shams Med J 1969; 20:235.
12 Burton EW. Progressive myopia: a possible etiologic factor. Trans Am Ophthalmol Soc 1942; 40:340.
13 Bedrossian EH. Progressive myopia with glaucoma. Am J Ophthalmol 1952; 35:485.
14 Tomlinson A, Phillips CI. Applanation tension and axial length of the eyeball. Br J Ophthalmol 1970; 54:548–553.
15 Curtin BJ. *The Myopias. Basic Science and Clinical Management*. Harper & Row, New York, 1985.
16 Perkins ES. Morbidity from myopia. Sight Sav Rev 1979; 49:11–19.
17 Podos SM, Becker B, Morton WR. High myopia and primary open-angle glaucoma. Am J Ophthalmol 1966; 62:1038–1043.
18 Amba SK, Jain IS, Gupta SD. Topical corticosteroid and intraocular pressure in high myopia: I. Study of pressure response. Ind J Ophthalmol 1973; 21:102.
19 Jain IS, Amba SK, Gupta SD. Topical corticosteroid and intraocular pressure in high myopia: II. Study of pressure response to age, dioptric power, degenerative changes in the eye and scleral rigidity. Ind J Ophthalmol 1973; 21:108.
20 Grunert K. Verhutung und Behandlung der Kurzsichtigkeit und ihrer Folgeerscheinungen. Klin Monatsbl Augenheilkd 1928; 81:521.
21 Landolt E. *The Refraction and Accommodation of the Eye*. Young J. Pentland, Edinburgh, 1886.
22 Dransart H. Traitement du décollement de la rétine et de la myopie progressive par l'iridectomie, la sclérotomie et la pilocarpine. Ann Oculist (Paris) 1884; 92:30.
23 Holth S. Neue operative Behandlung der Netzhautablosung und der hochgradiger Myopie. Ber Zusammenkunft Dtsch Ophthalmol Ges 1911; 37:293.
24 Freide R. A modified cyclodialysis and its use in the treatment of juvenile progressive malignant myopia. Ophthalmologica 1959; 137:282.
25 Harlan GC. Rapidly progressive myopia permanently checked by division of the external rectus. Trans Am Ophthalmol Soc 1885; 4:24.
26 Donders FC. *On the Anomalies of Accommodation and Refraction of the Eye*, WD Moore (transl). The Hatton Press, London, 1864.
27 Bourdeaux. Le traitment des myopies extremes. Bull Soc Ophthalmol Fr 1914; 31:670.
28 Ivashina AI, Mikhailova GD, Balashova NV, Ioffe DI, Nikitin IM: Vazokompressiia glaza pri progressiruiushchei blizorukosti i kontrol' za ee effektivnost'iu (predvaritet'noe soobshchenie). [Ocular vasocompression in progressive myopia and the follow-up of its efficacy (preliminary report).] Vestn Oftalmol 1988; 104:31–34.
29 Bates WH. *The Bates Method for Better Eye Sight without Glasses*.

Henry Holt, New York, 1943.

30 Dianoux. Myopie et myotiques. Clin Ophthalmol 1912; 18:68.

31 Domec M. Massage. Pression. Myotiques. Myopie. Arch Ophthalmol 1912; 32:391.

32 Yamamoto Y. Hand ophthalmic supersonic therapeutic instrument. Jpn J Clin Ophthalmol 1963; 17:295.

33 Yamamoto Y. Ultrasonic treatment of acquired myopia. Ganka 1964; 6:935.

34 von Ammon FA. Die Entwickelungsgeschicte des menschlichen Auges. Albrecht Graefes Arch Ophthamol 1858; 4:1.

35 Sondermann R. Beitrag zur Frage der Myopie-genese. Klin Monatstbl Augenheilkd 1950; 117:573.

36 Sondermann R. Zur Frage der Myopiaprophylaxe. Klin Monatstbl Augenheilkd 1951; 119:178.

37 Sondermann R. Beitrag zur Genese und Prophylaxe der Myopie. Ber Zusammenkunft Dtsch Ophthalmol Ges 1951; 56:96.

38 Scarpa AA. *A Treatise on the Principal Diseases of the Eye*. J. Bregg, London, 1818.

39 von Arlt CF. *Ueber die Ursachsen und die Entsehung der Kurzichtigkeit*. Wilhelm Braumuller, Vienna, 1856.

40 von Ammon FA. Uber die angebornen Spaltungen in der Iris, Chorioidea und Retina des Menschlichen Auges. [About congenital colobomas of the iris, choroid and retina in the human eye.] Ophthalmologie 1831; 1:55.

41 von Graefe A. Zwei Sektionbefunde von Scleratio-Chronivites posterior und Bermerbegen uber diese Krankeit. Arch Ophthalmol 1854; 1:390.

42 von Jaeger E. *Beitrage zur Pathologie das Auges*. Kaiserlich-Konigliche, Hof-und Staatsdruckerei Vienna, 1870.

43 Curtin BJ. Surgical support of the posterior sclera, Part I, Experimental results. Am J Ophthalmol 1960; 49:1341.

44 Johnson WA. Transplantation of homografts of sclera on eye of dog, including volume determination: experimental study. Thesis, 1961.

45 Johnson WA, Henderson JW, Parkhill EM. Transplantation of homografts of sclera. Am J Ophthalmol 1962; 54:1019.

46 Rubin ML. Surgical procedures available for influencing refractive error. In: *Refractive Anomalies of the Eye*, US Government Printing Office, Washington, 1966.

47 Muller. Eine neue operative Behandlung der Netzhaut abhebung. Klin Monatstbl Augenheilk 1903; 41:459.

48 Shevelev MM. Operation against high myopia and sclerectasia with the aid of transplantation of fascia lata on thinned sclera. Russian Ophthalmol J 1930; 11:107.

49 Malbran J. Una nueva orientacion quirurgica contra la miopia. Arch Soc Oftalmol Hisp-Am 1954; 14:1167.

50 Borley WE, Snyder AA. Surgical treatment of high myopia. Trans Am Acad Ophthalmol Otolaryngol 1958; 62:791.

51 Miller WW, Borley WE. Surgical treatment of degenerative myopia. Trans Pac Coast Otoophthalmol Soc 1963; 44: 155–171.

52 Miller WW, Borley WE. Surgical treatment of degenerative myopia. Am J Ophthalmol 1964; 57:796.

53 Snyder AA, Thompson FB. A simplified technique for surgical treatment of degenerative myopia. Am J Ophthalmol 1972; 74:273–277.

54 Curtin BJ. Surgical support of the posterior sclera, Part II, clinical results. Am J Ophthalmol 1961; 52:853.

55 Miller WW. Surgical treatment of degenerative myopia: scleral reinforcement. Trans Am Acad Ophthalmol Otolaryngol 1974; 78:896.

56 Thompson FB. A simplified scleral reinforcement technique. Am J Ophthalmol 1978; 86:782.

57 Curtin BJ. The natural history of posterior staphyloma development. Doc Ophthalmol 1981; 28:207.

58 Curtin BJ, Whitmore W. Long-term results of scleral reinforcement surgery. Am J Ophthalmol 1987; 103:544.

59 Andrzejewska W. Further therapeutic results in progressive myopia by means of meridional cicumligation. Klin Oczna 1972; 42:263.

60 Belyaev VS. Some possibilities of treatment of high progressive myopia. In *Proceedings of the Third All-Russian Congress of Ophthalmologists*. Tipographia Vashnil, Moscow, 1975.

61 Belyaev VS, Ilyina TS. Late results of scleroplasty in surgical treatment of progressive myopia. Eye Ear Nose Throat Mon 1975; 54:109–112.

62 Eroschevskii TI, Panfilov NI. Meridional'noe ukruplenie sklery shirokoi fastsiei bedrapri progressiruiushchei blizorukosti. [Meridional reinforcement of the sclera with femoral fascia lata in progressive myopia.] Vestn Oftalmol 1970; 2:19–23.

63 Panfilov NI, IuV S. Otdalennye rezul'taty operatsii meridional'nogo ukrepleniia sklery skirokoi fastesiei bedra pri progressiruiushchei blizorukosti. [Remote results of the operation of meridional fixation of the sclera with broad fascia of the hip in progressive myopia.] Oftalmol Zh 1974; 29: 130–133.

64 Alberth B, Nagy Z, Berta A. Combined surgical procedure for the prevention of blindness caused by progressive high myopia. Acta Chir Hung 1988; 29:3–13.

65 Hanczye P. Surgical treatment of progressive high myopia: I. age of patients, observation, time and visual acuity. Klin Oczna 1972; 42:269.

66 Starkiewicz W. Meridional circumligation: a new method of surgical treatment of progressive myopia. Klin Oczna 1965; 35:363.

67 Starkiewicz W, Markiewicz-Jablonska E. Pierwsze wyniki leczenia postepujacej krotkowzrocznosci za pomoca circumligatio meridionalis. [First results in the treatment of progressive myopia by means of circumligatio meridionalis.] Klin Oczna 1967; 37:831–838.

68 Nesterov AP, Libenson NB. Ukreplenie sklery shirokoi fastsiei bedra pri progressiruiushchei blizorukosti. [Stengthening of the sclera with the broad fascia of the hip in progressive myopia.] Vestn Oftalmol 1967; 80:15–19.

69 Nesterov AP, Libenson NB. Strengthening the sclera with a strip of fascia lata in progressive myopia. Br J Ophthalmol 1970; 54:46–50.

70 Nesterov AP, Libenson NB, Svirin AV. Early and late results of fascia lata transplantation in high myopia. Br J Ophthalmol 1976; 60:271–272.

71 Nesterov AP, Svirin AV, Antipova OA. Scleral reinforcement. J Ocular Ther Surg 1984; 3:255.

72 Zarkova MV, Negoda VI. Grafting of homologous sclera in progressive myopia. Vestn Oftalmol 1970; 49:16.

73 Whitwell J. Scleral reinforcement in degenerative myopia. Trans Ophthalmol Soc UK 1971; 91:79–86.

74 Momose A. Posterior scleral support operation combined with extraction of lens in high myopia, two stage operation. Excerpta Medica 1979; 2/450:1232.

75 Momose A. Surgical correction of myopia. J Korean Ophthalmol 1983; 24:717.

76 Pruett RC. Refractive surgery: psychophysical considerations in progressive myopia. Ann Acad Med Singapore 1989; 18: 131–135.

77 Barraquer T, Barraquer JI. Nueva orientacion terapeutica en la miopia progresiva. Arch Soc Oftal Hisp-Am 1956; 16:137.

78 Kahn H, Moorhead U. *Statistics on Blindness in the Model Reporting Area*. US Government Printing Office, Washington, 1970.

79 Sorsby A. The incidence and causes of blindness: an international survey. Br J Ophthalmol 1950; 34 (suppl):13–14.

80 Sperduto R, Seigel D, Roberts J, Rowland M. Prevalence of

myopia in the United States. Arch Ophthalmol 1983; 10: 405–407.

81 Miller WW, Borley WE. Surgical treatment of degenerative myopia. Trans Pac Coast Otoophthalmol Soc 1963; 44:155–171.

82 Borley WE, Snyder AA. Surgical treatment of high myopia. Trans Am Acad Ophthalmol Otolaryngol 1958; 62:791.

83 Snyder AA, Thompson FB. A simplified technique for surgical treatment of degenerative myopia. Am J Ophthalmol 1972; 74:273–277.

84 Brian GR, Hollows FC. Sling markers in scleral reinforcement surgery. Ophthalmic Surg 1988; 19:647–648.

85 Coroneo MT, Beaumont JT, Hollows FC. Scleral reinforcement in the treatment of pathologic myopia. Aust NZ J Ophthalmol 1988; 16:317–320.

86 Hanczye P, Uher M, Koziorowska M. Circumligatio meridionalis. Uwagi dotyczace techniki operacyjnej oraz powikLan drugiego etapu operacji. [Meridional circumligation. Observations on the surgical method and the complications in the second stage of the operation.] Klin Oczna 1982; 84:325–327.

14

Surgery for Hyperopia

We have come to rely upon a comfortable time lag of fifty years or a century intervening between the perception that something ought to be done and a serious attempt to do so.
[H.G. Wells]

Refractive surgery is about myopia and astigmatism, or so it seems. In a review of extant literature, less than 10% of the articles dealing with the surgical treatment of ametropia—excluding aphakia—are about hyperopia. Although the first spectacles were prescribed in 1290 for hyperopia (actually for presbyopia) not myopia, it wasn't until almost 300 years later than myopes had some relief from their affliction in the form of glasses.

Perhaps it is because myopes need a correction most of the time or perhaps it's because there are more of them [1–3]. Whatever the reason, myopia has received the lion's share of attention. Yet a significant number of the world's population (almost 50% in most countries) are hyperopic *de novo*, not to mention those cases iatrogenically produced through one means or another. Grosvenor maintains that hyperopia represents a significant impediment to the learning process [4]. Evidence exists connecting it with behavioral problems as well as low academic standing amongst elementary school children (see Chapter 2).

While simple procedures for myopia abound, those for hyperopia are, however, like they said in the *Wizard of Oz*, a horse of a different color. Radial keratotomy for myopia is a cinch compared to the problem of hyperopia. Here the challenge is to induce steepening of the central cornea, instead of merely flattening it—not a simple matter. Flattening is practically automatic with relaxing incisions—the intra-ocular pressure does the job for you—not so steepening.

Hexagonal keratotomy

Various means have been employed in the surgical management of hyperopia ranging from the keratophakia of Barraquer to the thermokeratoplasty of Fyodorov, with varying claims of success. This section is about one of these methods—hexagonal keratotomy.

In 1979, Yamashita, building upon the work of Sato [5] and the experience of Gills [6], experimented with closed-ended incisional configurations in rabbits. He found the optimum configuration to be that of six incisions arranged and connected in the shape of a hexagon. By varying the diameter of the hexagon he was able to induce an increase in the central corneal curvature proportional to the size of the hex, the mean change being 2.20 D. These cases were first presented at the Keratorefractive Society in 1983 and he suggested that this technique might be a practical way to eliminate radial keratotomy over-corrections [7–10]. Encouraged by this work, Mendez applied the technique to human corneas the same year. By varying the size of the hexagon from 7.5 to 4.5 mm, up to 4 D of hyperopia could be reduced. Mendez found that a

6.0 mm hex resulted in a reduction in hyperopia of 1.50 D. A mean of 2.0 ± 0.75 D of correction resulted with a 5.5 mm hex, and 3.0 ± 0.75 D with a 5.0 mm hex. The corneas remained fairly stable and Mendez states that the overall patient complaints were less than with radial keratotomy (A. Mendez, 1991, personal communication). However, others reported that in some cases extreme gaping of the incisions occurred with resultant marsupialization and instability as well as astigmatism. In at least one case, severe central corneal edema with subsequent sloughing of tissue occurred necessitating a penetrating keratoplasty. Predictability is fair and no account is taken of sex, age, or corneal elasticity in establishing the hex size—unlike radial keratotomy.

The mechanism is simply that of complete relaxation of the corneal cap. This allows the natural elasticity of the cornea and the intra-ocular pressure to increase the arc height of the apex (Figure 14.1).

In an effort to eliminate some of the post-operative complications, several authors have advocated variations in the incision pattern ranging from open hexagons to overlapping apices [11].

Technique

Patients selected for this surgery should have no more than 3 D of hyperopia (Jensen advocates no more than 5 D) and range in age from 30 to 75 years. Workup is that typical for any refractive surgical procedure (see Chapter 6).

As in radial keratotomy, the effect of this procedure can be varied by using different size optical zones. A 5 mm optical clear zone, for example, will correct an average of 2.83 D, a 5.5 mm zone an average of 2.00 D, and a 6 mm zone will correct an average of 1.50 D of hyperopia. The best results are obtained when the hexagon is perfectly symmetric with uniform incision depths equal to no more than 85% of the corneal thickness—at the diameter of the hex. However, the apices of the hexagonal should not intersect, so as to avoid excess corneal wound swelling, wound spreading, and epithelial inclusions. The incisions must be regular and the depths of the cuts consistently deep to minimize astigmatism. However, post-operative astigmatism of 1–4 D can be inadvertently induced by this surgery. Jensen advocates T-cuts appropriate for the amount of astigmatism in that event and states that such an event is rather common (R.P. Jensen, 1991, personal communication).

Pre-operative sedation is given as for radial keratotomy patients (see Chapter 8). The unoperateds eye is covered with a Fox shield and the operated eye is prepped with Betadine solution. A wire lid speculum is used to hold the lids. As in radial keratotomy, the patient is then asked to fixate upon the microscope

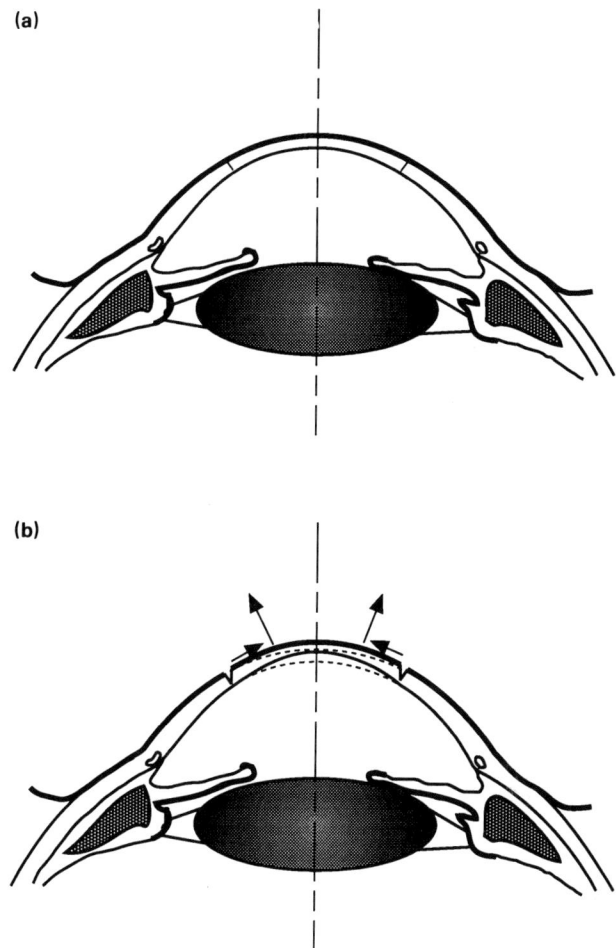

(a)

(b)

Fig. 14.1 Mechanism of hexagonal keratotomy. (a) The incisions weaken the corneal stroma cutting off all connection with the periphery. (b) The incisions gape, shortening the chord length. That plus the intra-ocular pressure increases the arc height.

light filament, whereupon the fixation point is marked with a blunt instrument taking care to compensate for any parallax errors that may exist in the microscope system. The hexagonal optical clear zone is then marked concentric to the optic axis—*not to the pupil*. It is helpful to coat the marker with 1% brilliant green (make sure it dries completely on the marker) or gentian violet (skin-marking pencil) to guide the blade.

The blade used is a Bores 35° LeCut double-edge diamond in a Katena handle, set to 85% of the average corneal thickness at the edge of the hex (see Chapter 8 for details on blade setting). The eye is fixated with a Bores wide fixation forceps (K5-3280) to provide complete control of ocular movement. The incisions are made with the vertical blade edge just inside the apex (Figures 14.2 through 14.6). The incision stops just short of the next apex and is withdrawn. All six incisions are made in this manner. The author has found that less post-operative astigmatism occurs if the beginning of each incision is back-cut (with the vertical

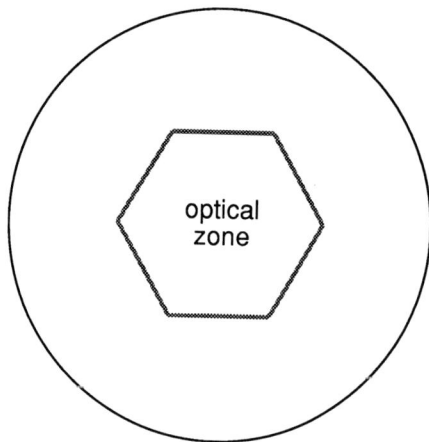

Fig. 14.2 An optical zone marker is a must with this surgery.

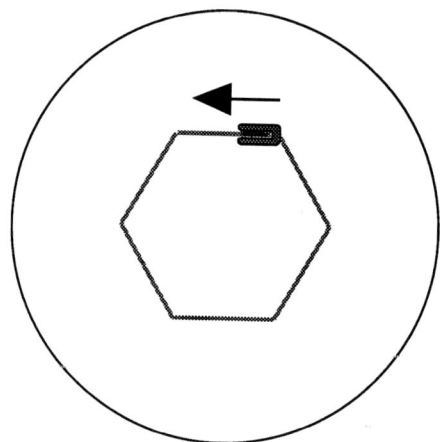

Fig. 14.4 Straddle the mark and move the blade along the mark, cutting with the vertical edge.

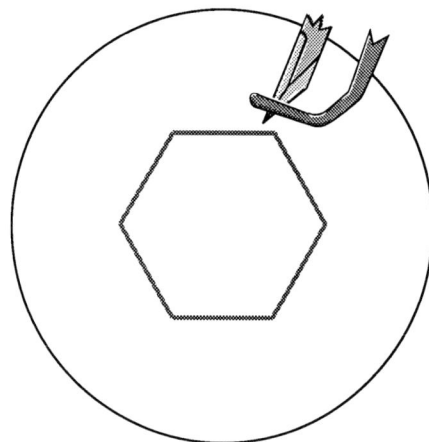

Fig. 14.3 Insert the tip of the blade just inside the apex along one side of the hex.

in the appropriate axis to treat astigmatism during the case, the author prefers to perform this operation at a later date [11]. The author has found that healing in hexagonal keratotomy is not as smoothly regular as in radial keratotomy and astigmatism often pops up in a wholly unexpected place in the first month or two. All incisions are gently irrigated with BSS at the conclusion of the case and a drop of antibiotic–steroid medication instilled.

Because of the tendency of the incisions to gape, all patients are double-patched and instructed to leave the patch on until their return visit the next morning. This is in contrast to patients undergoing radial keratotomy who typically remove their patch in 1–2 hours.

Results

The author's limited experiences with this particular technique were not encouraging and are based on a series of 22 patients ranging in age from 34 to 46, equally divided between males and females. Longest

edge) to insure even incision length throughout (Figure 14.7). It is a good idea always to make the incisions in the same sequence and back-cut each one as well. Although some authors will add a T-cut inside the hex

(a)

(b)

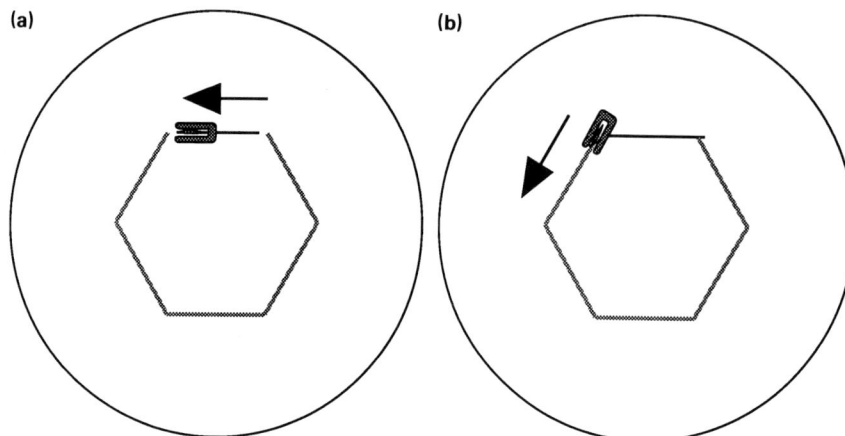

Fig. 14.5 (a,b) Stop just short of the apex. Remove the knife and cut the next limb of the hexagon.

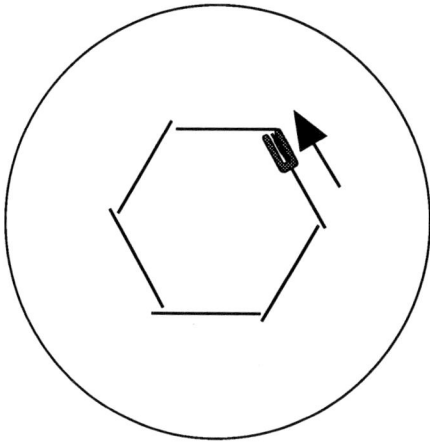

Fig. 14.6 Continue until all six sides are cut. Note that each side overlaps the end of the preceding one.

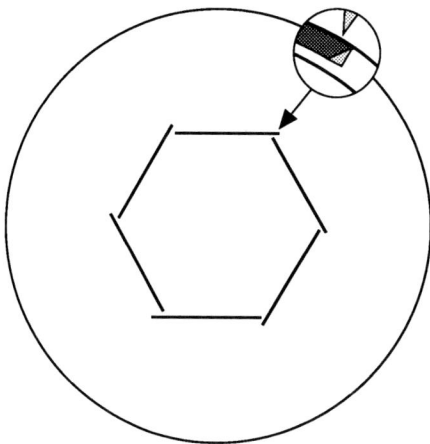

Fig. 14.7 Back-cut the beginning of each incision to remove the slanted entry.

follow-up is 6 years. Pre-operative hyperopia ranged from +2 to +6 D with a mean of +3.25 D and with no more than 0.50 D of astigmatism. While mean correction was 1.87 ± 0.75 D, the actual correction varied from 0.62 to 5.25 D, and did not correlate with the size of the hex. However, the least variation occurred with cases under +3 D using a larger pattern diameter. Furthermore, the incidence of induced astigmatism was high—45%—and in one case reached +3.5 D. The results in this small series should be compared with those of Jensen, who seems to have the largest experience with this procedure to date [12]. The differences are undoubtedly due to varying experience between the two surgeons as well as technique. The author is unable, however, to match the reported good results of Jensen and has chosen to suspend performance of this procedure in moderate to high hyperopia. However, because the hexes can be larger and the incisions can be slightly shallower, application of this technique to

reduce the effect of presbyopia is still entertained. In those cases, usually only one eye is operated to produce monovision.

The author has found that healing in HK is not as smoothly regular as in RK and astigmatism often pops up in a wholly unexpected place in the first month or two. Six of the author's cases showed profound destabilization of the central cornea and required suturing of the incisions (see below). These cases demonstrated a healing pattern and astigmatism similar to that seen after PKP. The author's patients typically complain more of discomfort with this procedure than with RK although the reason for this apparent increase in pain is not apparent since most cases epithelialize overnight. Fluctuation of vision is on a par with RK and vision rapidly clears post-operatively. Glare complaints are about equal in intensity to those noted with RK but it is the author's experience that residual astigmatism, either induced or congenital, is difficult to anticipate. For this reason the author prefers to deal with induced astigmatism after the fact—months after.

Jensen seems to have the largest experience with this procedure to date and he has reported his results recently [11]. Unfortunately, no conclusions can be drawn from the information as presented. Considering the nature of this procedure and its apparent ability to correct reasonable amounts of hyperopia it seems curious that nothing else has appeared in the literature *vis-à-vis* hexagonal keratotomy from individuals claiming to have done large numbers of these cases. To the date of this writing, only eight articles and one letter have been published on this technique—one of these was to report a ruptured globe.

Side-effects and complications

There is not much different about the sequelae of this procedure that does not occur with other incisional techniques—save one. This one unique attribute is the tendency for these incisions to gape—and with a vengeance. While this tendency is, to be sure, related to incision depth (and is occasionally seen in long T-cuts), it occurs even with optimum incision depth in hexagonal keratotomy. While this propensity has been lessened somewhat by not joining the apices of the incision pattern, it still occurs. Therein lies the source of what the author refers to as the jack-in-the-box effect (the sudden popping up of astigmatism) as well as some cases of severe corneal instability—not seen in radial keratotomy or lamellar cases.

The author has six cases of hexagonal keratotomy in which moderate-depth incisions were made with joined apices and whose hexagons were all 6.0 mm. Every one of these cases had severe central corneal instability requiring suturing—in one case very like a corneal transplant. This instability lasted, in one form

(a)

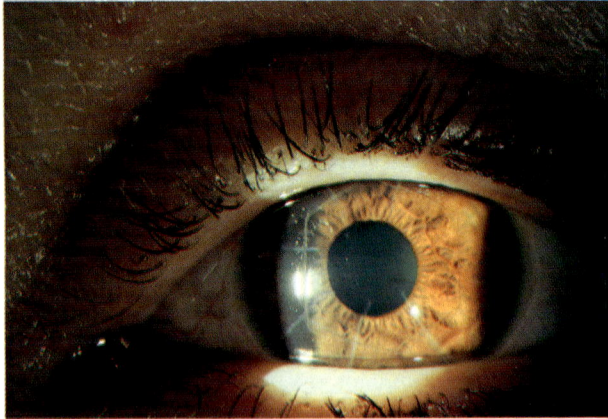

(b)

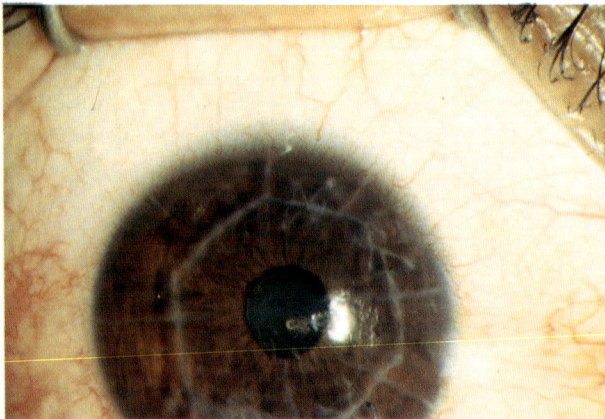

Fig. 14.8 (a) Hexagonal over radial keratotomy. Note the fairly clean intersection of the sides of the hex with the radials (see text). (b) Another case: note the sutures.

or another, for at least 5 years in each case. Despite repeated removal and/or addition of sutures, each one of these cases demonstrated variable astigmatism (sometimes reaching as high as 7 D) and all required contact lenses, which were both a joy to fit and to wear. Eventually they all came right—thankfully. While this is an indictment against joining up of the incisions, some few of this same phenomenon have occurred with the newer technique, albeit chiefly with smaller diameter patterns. Other refractive surgeons using this technique have experienced much the same thing in a few cases, especially in cases of over-corrected radial keratotomy (Figure 14.8). Even waiting for at least 6 months before adding the hex over the radial keratotomy radials has not saved patients from the problems of instability and high astigmatism. Seemingly perfect cases eventually decline into episodes of unstable astigmatism (Figure 14.9).

The moral of this story is that while this methodology might well be useful, some caution in its appli-

cation is required. Good-quality sapphire or diamond blades are a must, as is using a proper incision marker—this procedure should not be done free-hand. Wide (limbal–limbal) fixation is also necessary. Patients will require a more detailed informed consent before proceeding. The author has limited its application to low-level presbyopes and not at all to over-corrected radial keratotomy patients. The author's X-suture technique in mild cases and hyperopic lamellar keratotomy in high cases are recommended instead.

Arcuate incisions for hyperopic astigmatism

Alejandro Arciniegas and co-workers have devised a method for treating both mixed and simple hyperopic astigmatism by using arcuate incisions. Photokeratography demonstrates the elliptic nature of concentric zones in astigmatism and the circular nature of such zones in spherical surfaces (Figures 14.10 and 14.11). The aim of all astigmatic surgery is to convert these elliptic zones to circular ones (Figure 14.12). Arciniegas' work with rabbits has shown that arcuate incisions have three types of action depending upon the separation of the incisions:

1 Small zones (2–4 mm)—the clear zone steepens in both meridians.
2 Intermediate zones (5–7 mm)—the zone becomes flatter in the meridian of the incisions and steeper in the opposite meridian.
3 Large zone (8–9 mm)—the zone becomes flatter in the meridian of the incisions but the opposite meridian shows only a small amount of steepening.

Arciniegas maintains that the effect in large zones is due to the fact that no deepening of the anterior chamber occurs (Figure 14.13). On the other hand, smaller zones cause such a deepening effect (Figure

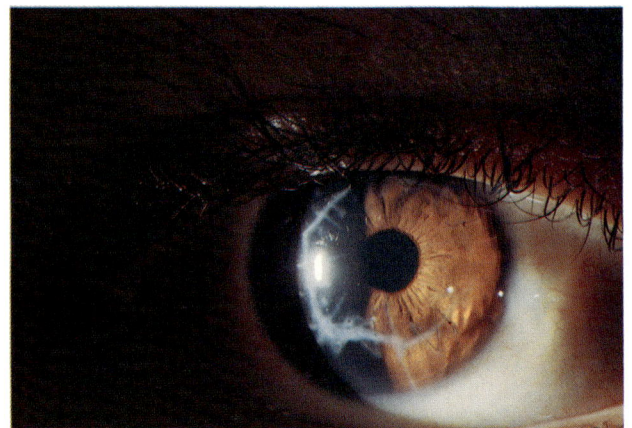

Fig. 14.9 A "run-of-the-mill" hexagonal keratotomy over RK. This patient eventually needed sutures.

(a)

(b)

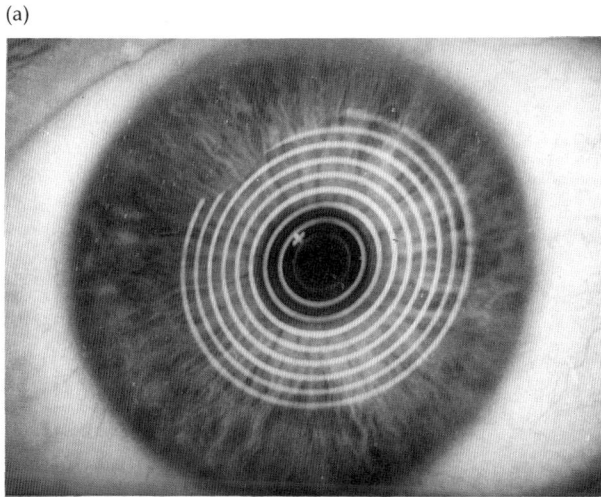

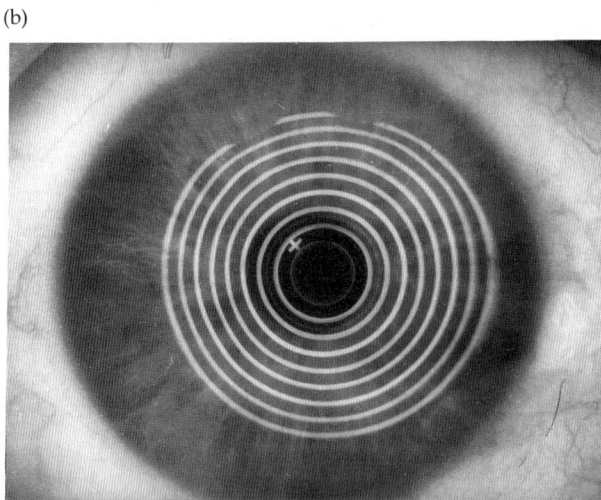

Fig. 14.10 (a) Typical elliptic pattern of an astigmatic cornea; (b) spherical pattern.

Fig. 14.11 Astigmatic corneas demonstrate an elliptic cap with a major and minor meridian.

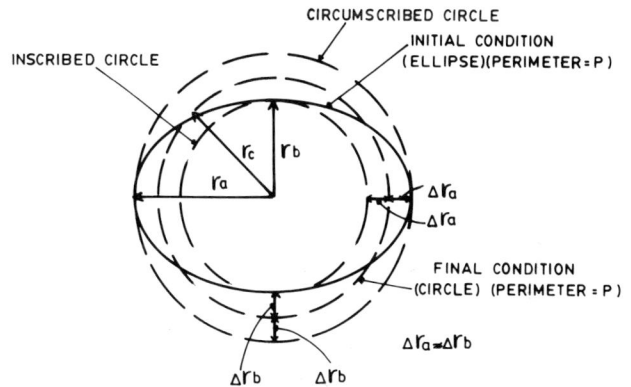

Fig. 14.12 The aim of astigmatic surgery is to convert this elliptic cap to a spherical one.

14.14). Two case reports in humans are illustrated here, in which changes in anterior chamber depth are shown by ultrasound (Figures 14.15 and 14.16).

These are intriguing data and are in contrast to this author's findings that relaxing incisions have no effect on axial length as measured by ultrasound. Further work will have to be done and it must be kept in mind that small increases in pressure on the probe during A-scan measurements can lead to changes in axial length measurement. This material is included here as speculative only.

Spiral or helicoid relaxing incisions

Arciniegas and co-workers also have been conducting a series of investigations to demonstrate the effect of different incisional configurations on hyperopia and myopia, with and without astigmatism (see also

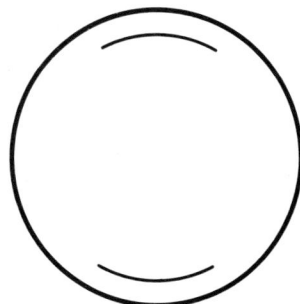

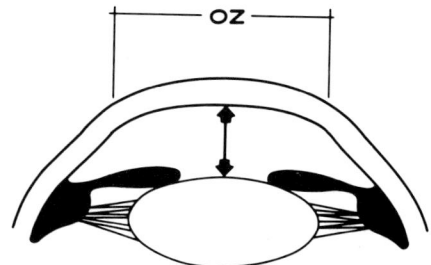

Fig. 14.13 Chamber deepening does not occur when the optical zone is near the limbus.

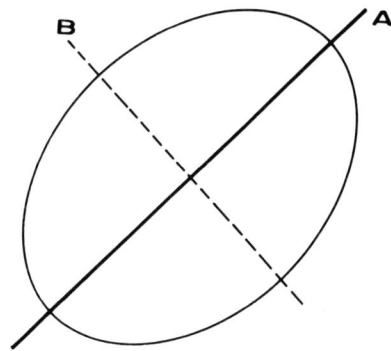

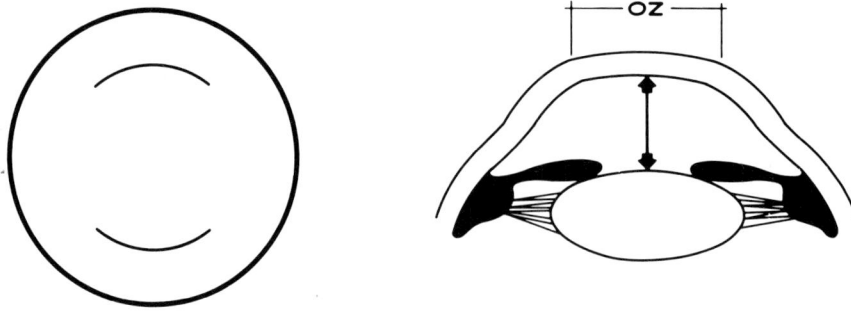

Fig. 14.14 As the optical zone becomes smaller, the anterior chamber theoretically becomes deeper.

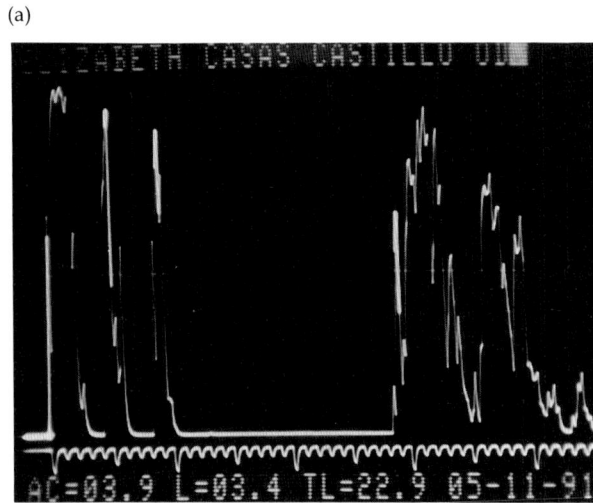

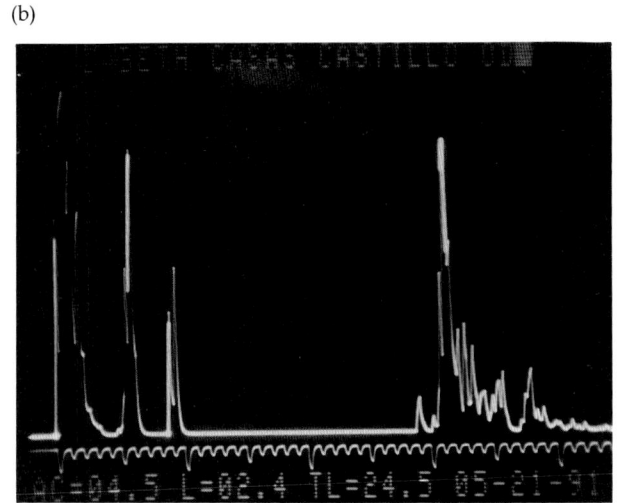

(a)

(b)

Fig. 14.15 Case 1. (a) Pre-operative ultrasound; (b) post-operative A-scan.

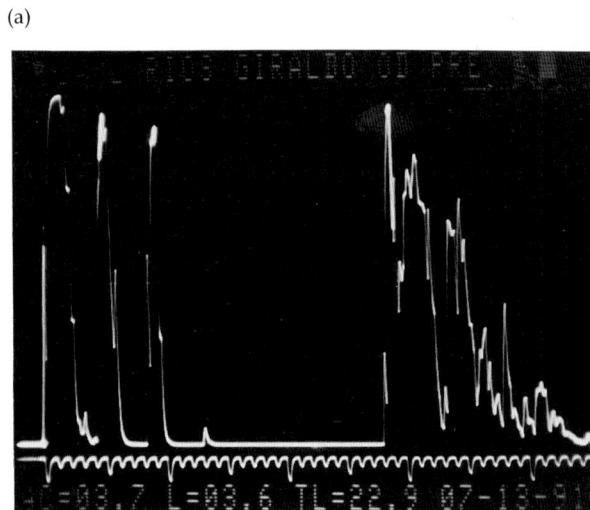

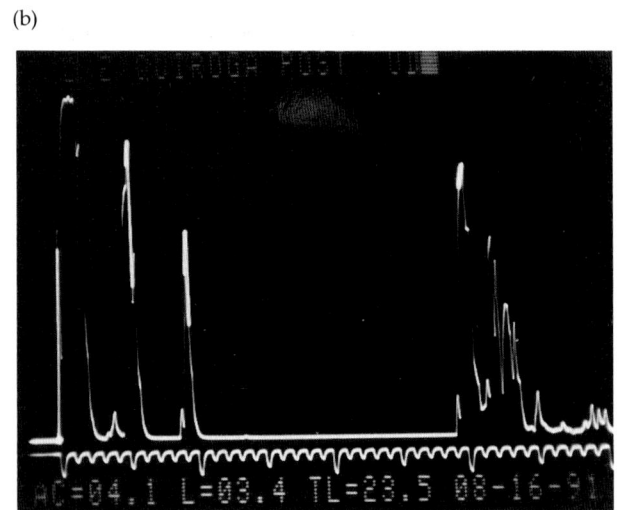

(a)

(b)

Fig. 14.16 Case 2. (a) Pre-operative ultrasound; (b) post-operative A-scan.

Chapter 9). This work involves using relaxing incisions to reduce hyperopia. The mechanism of action is attributed to a helical displacement of the corneal surface and a change in anterior chamber depth (Figure 14.17). It is presented as speculative only and not as a finished or recommended method of correcting hyperopia.

The current study involved 170 rabbit eyes using

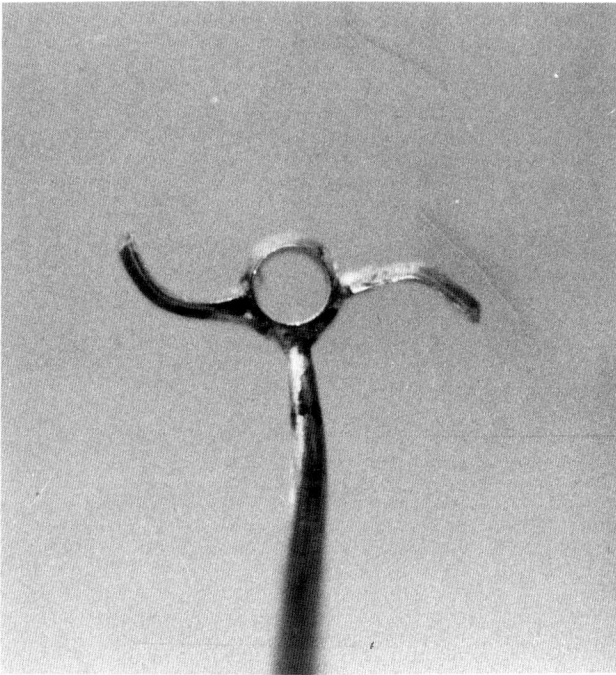

Fig. 14.17 Special helical marker for making the incisions.

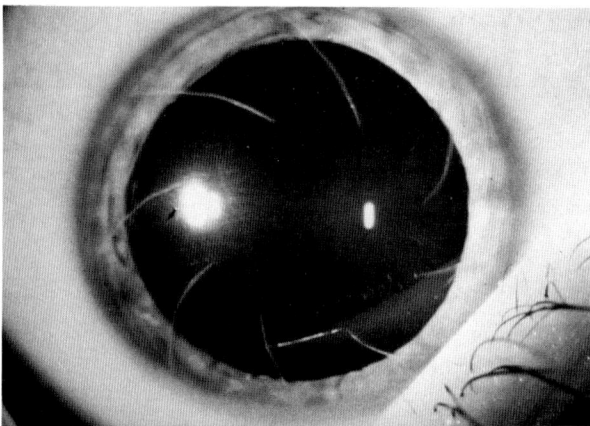

Fig. 14.18 Human cornea showing the incisions.

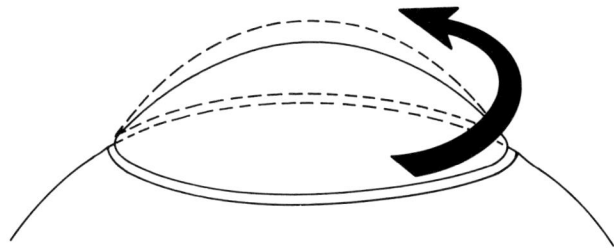

Fig. 14.19 The mechanism of action is a twisting movement of the cornea leading to an increase in the anterior chamber depth.

(a)

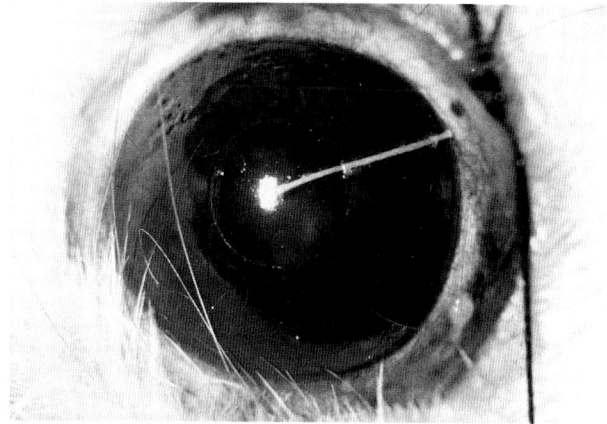

(b)

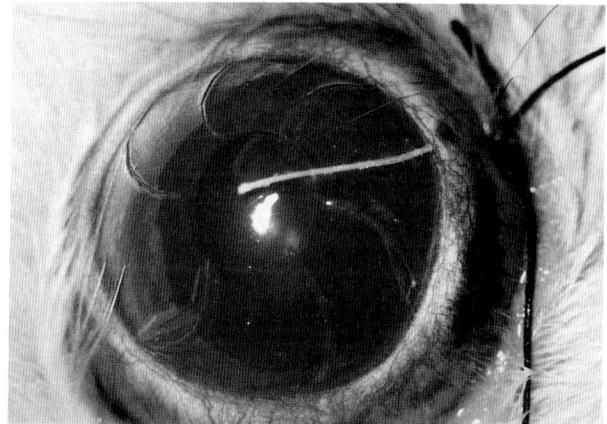

Fig. 14.20 The effect is illustrated using a length of suture on a rabbit cornea. (a) Pre-operative; (b) post-operative.

spiral-shaped incisions and optical zones varying from 3 to 7 mm. Incision depth was expressed as a percentage of the central corneal thickness as measured by ultrasonic pachymetry and was taken as 90%. Blade settings were set with a metal gauge under microscopic control. Figures 14.18–14.21 demonstrate both the method and the results of this experiment.

The author has been unable to demonstrate any changes in either axial length or anterior chamber depth following non-penetrating relaxing incisions of any variety. Schachar has shown temporary *shallowing* of the anterior chamber following thermokeratoplasty, but this finding was accompanied by a transient reduction in intra-ocular pressure after the procedure [12].

Thermokeratoplasty

Keratoconus differs from other forms of ametropia/astigmatism in that the cornea is indisputably abnormal, suffering from a thinning and an anterior protrusion that often produces a high degree of myopia with associated visual distortion. Fitting of contact lenses is a challenge and corneal transplantation, while highly successful, does not eliminate

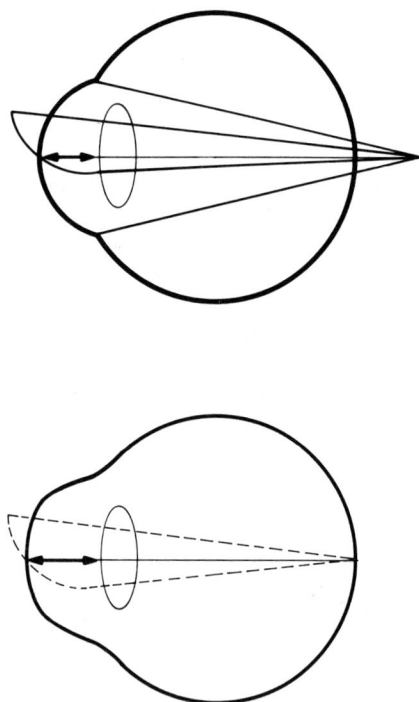

Fig. 14.21 The net effect of increasing the depth of the anterior chamber is to shorten the focal distance.

astigmatism and almost all patients will continue to wear contacts after surgery. Therefore, it makes sense to delay keratoplasty until vision is no longer satisfactorily served by appliances.

The procedure of flattening the cornea by surface application of heat is not a new idea, having been employed in the last century (see Chapter 9). It was revived with new technology to facilitate contact lens fitting and to reduce the need for, or at least delay, corneal transplantation. The early report of success in 59 eyes observed for 2 months to 2 years was followed by observations of inadequate visual improvement in the majority of cases, and the procedure fell into disuse in the USA, although it is in active use in Japan, where donor tissue for corneal transplantation is scarce and religious prohibitions an obstacle [13–16].

In 1981 Fyodorov and his group expanded on the earlier work of Gudechkov by applying radial, partial punctiform burns to the peripheral cornea for hyperopia—thermokeratoplasty. Some investigators in the USA have reported success in treating hyperopia with this technique as well [17–20]. Applied with a specially designed, computer-controlled probe, these partial-thickness burns were initially said to have corrected up to 5 D of hyperopia.

The pattern of the burns is similar to radial keratotomy in that the lesions are placed in a radial pattern (for spherical hyperopia) up to a pre-marked central optical zone diameter. Only the peripheral

(a)

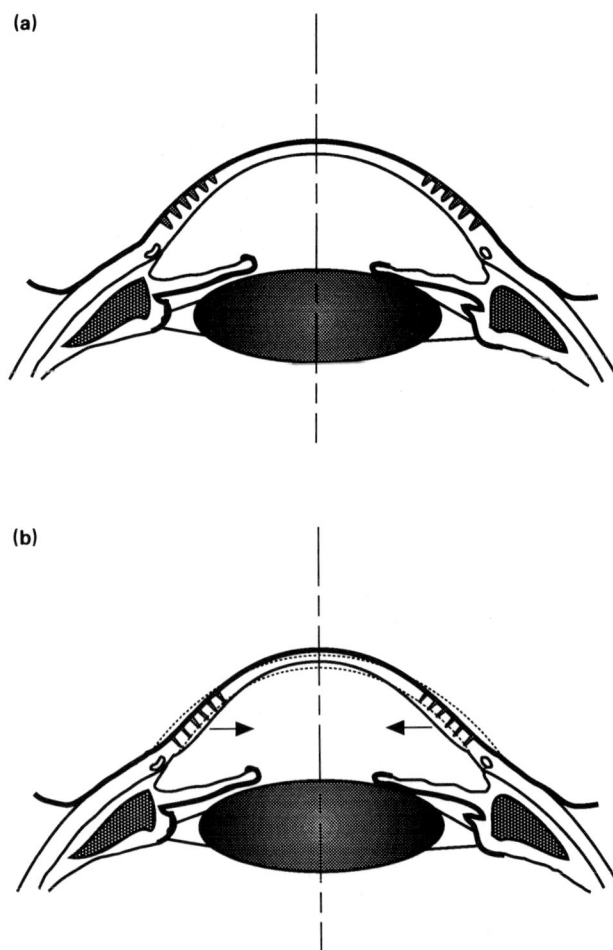

(b)

Fig. 14.22 Mechanism of thermokeratoplasty. (a) A series of deep punctate burns is made in the corneal periphery. (b) Shrinkage of the periphery occurs with concomitant increase in the central corneal curvature. This increase in arc height may also be accompanied by an increase in the depth of the anterior chamber, quite apart from that contributed by the steepening arc.

cornea is treated and the effect is titrated by varying the diameter of the optical zone and the number of radials. Unlike radial keratotomy, the burns flatten the corneal periphery in the area they are placed and steepen the central cornea, thereby reducing or eliminating hyperopia (Figures 14.22–14.31).

The procedure is usually performed on an outpatient basis under peri-bulbar anesthesia, although at least one author uses 4% topical Xylocaine [12]. The maximum temperature at the tip of the heat probe is 600°C, and each application lasts no more than 0.4 second. At the point of application, the coagulation zone reaches and penetrates through 90% of the corneal depth. The number of radial burn meridians ranges from eight to 14, while the size of the optical zone varies from 5 to 8 mm. The heat probe is applied in a series of burns along the meridian from the central optical zone to the corneal periphery. Before surgery, the effect of the

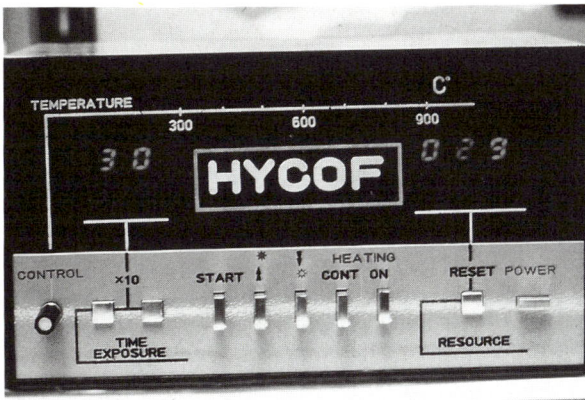

Fig. 14.23 Power unit for the thermokeratoplasty of Fyodorov.

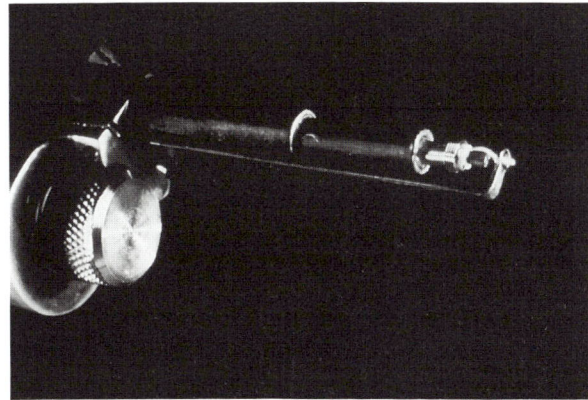

Fig. 14.24 Applications are with a computer-driven handpiece and guarded tip.

(a)

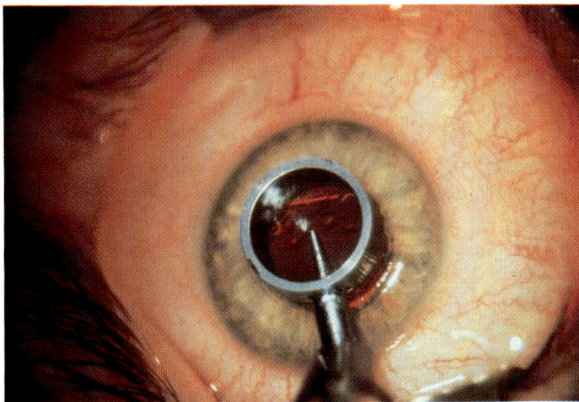

(b)

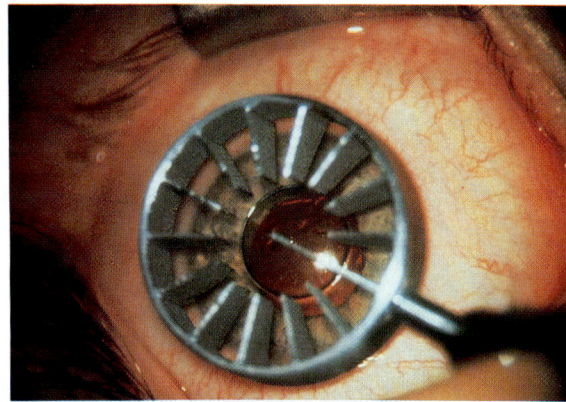

(c)

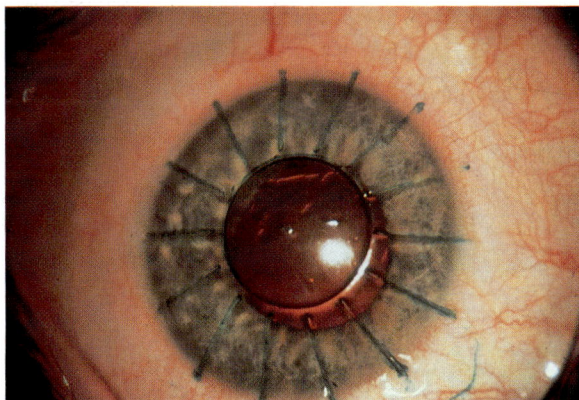

(d)

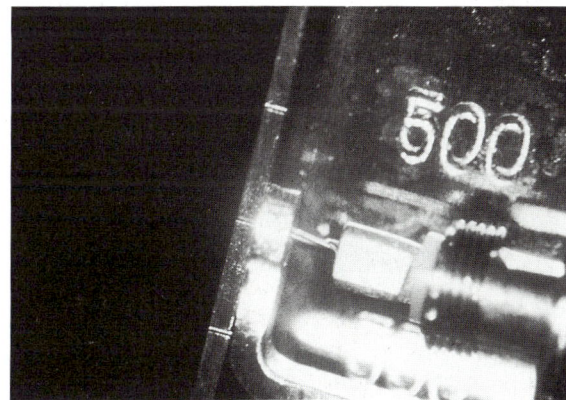

Fig. 14.25 (a) The central optical clear zone is marked; (b,c) followed by the radial application pattern; (d) tip is pre-set to the required depth using a standard RK knife gauge. (Courtesy of R. Marmer.)

procedure is calculated with the help of a computer software program that takes into account a number of variables, including the individual optical and anatomic characteristics of each eye, as well as the age of the patient.

Subsequent reports have not been as enthusiastic and results have been mixed [21,22]. The effect is variable and not well-controlled and seems to decline over time, with some cases reverting entirely. Scars can still be seen as long as 4 years later and recurrent

(a)
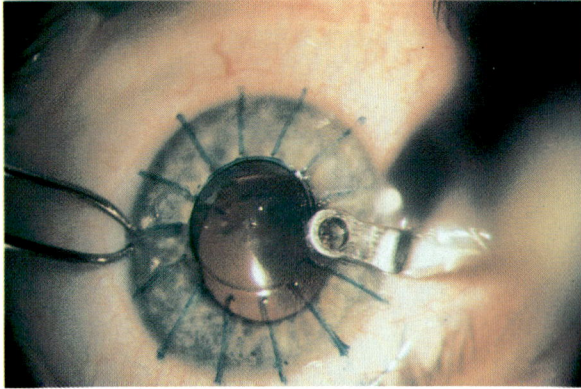

(b)
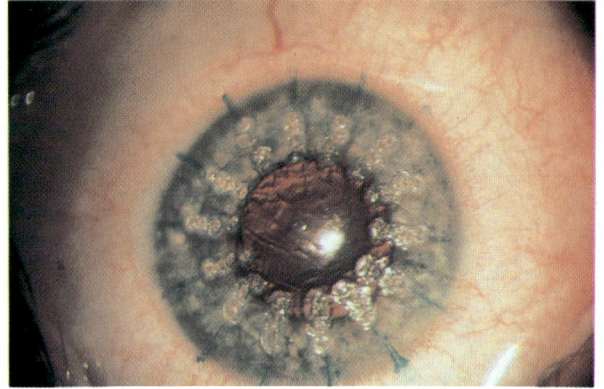

(c)
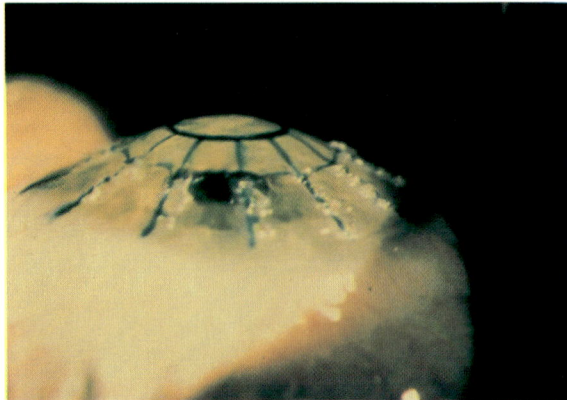

Fig. 14.26 (a) Three to four applications are made along each radial, starting at the optical clear zone; (b) completed treatment; (c) side view of treated cornea. Note the evident steepening of the central cornea.

(a)
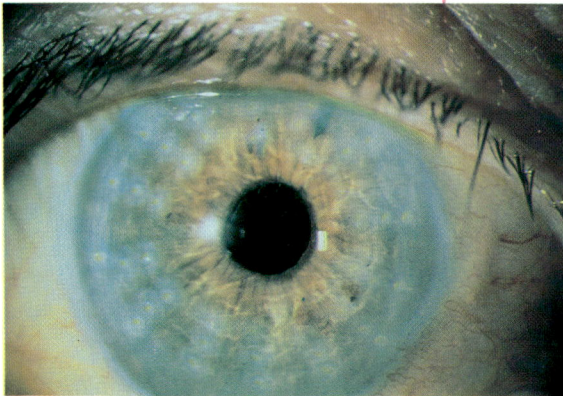

(b)
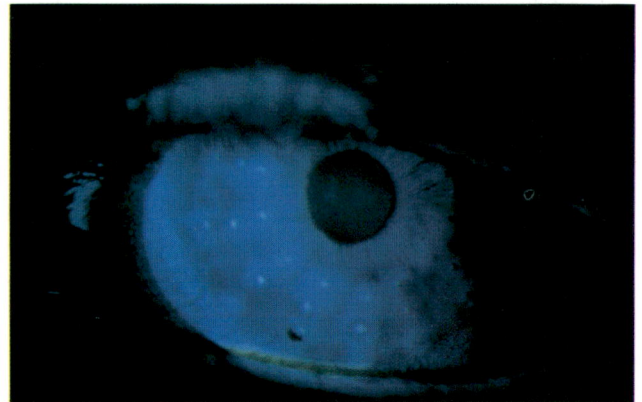

Fig. 14.27 (a) Thermokeratoplasty at 1 week; (b) note the pooling of fluorescein dye in the treatment sites.

erosions have been reported. Many of the previous practitioners have stopped performing this procedure (W. Ellis; Personal communication, 1991).

Reports from Fyodorov's group have been uniformly good with little or no regression noted [23]. In 197 eyes of 137 patients followed for a period of 5–7 years and reported by Fedchenko, the refraction had stabilized at 1 year. The mean refractive change in patients with pre-operative hyperopia ranging from 1 to 3 D was 1.6 D. Mean pre-operative unaided vision was 20/70.

At 1 year it had improved to 20/40 and at 5 years dropped to 20/50. In patients whose hyperopia ranged from 3.25 to 6.00 D, the average change was 3.3 D decreasing to 1.63 D at 5 years. In higher hyperopes, ranging from 6.25 to 9.00 D, the average decrease in refraction at 1 year was 4.93 D regressing to 3.75 D at 5 years. Unaided visual acuity at 5 years had improved from 20/250 to 20/70.

In 75% of all the cases treated at the Moscow center, the reported error of the predicted effect did

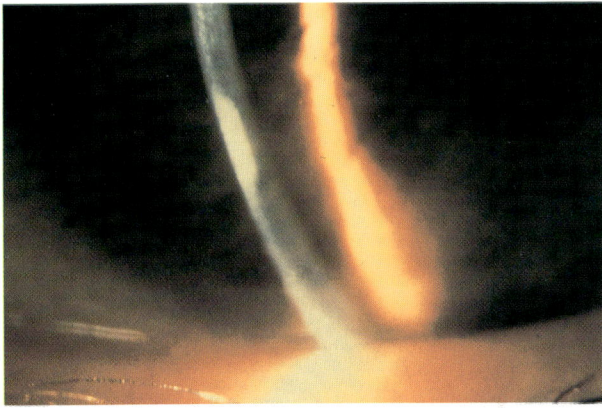

Fig. 14.28 Note the width and depth of scars.

not exceed 1 D. Average loss of corneal endothelial cells did not exceed 2.5%, and no inflammatory or degenerative changes were noted. At 1 year, bio-microscopy could still detect a slight cloudy and clinically insignificant opacification in the area where the probe had been applied.

The discrepancy between these results and those of some American investigators is difficult to explain and parallels the situation in scleral reinforcement surgery (see Chapter 13). However, a review of the scatter plots based upon the Russian data and reported by Neumann and co-workers shows a somewhat less optimistic result [24]. It should be noted that few, if any, patients in that series were completely corrected, nor were all included—data were patchy. Additionally, step-wise regression analysis of the available data showed no correlation of pre-operative factors with outcome. While 70.8% of the pre-operative hyperopia had been decreased at 1 year, only 40% were corrected to less than 1 D of emmetropia in that time.

Based upon what this author has seen of these patients, Neumann's report (and that of others), as well as the degree of corneal damage induced, it is the author's suggestion that there are, perhaps, less

(a)

(b)

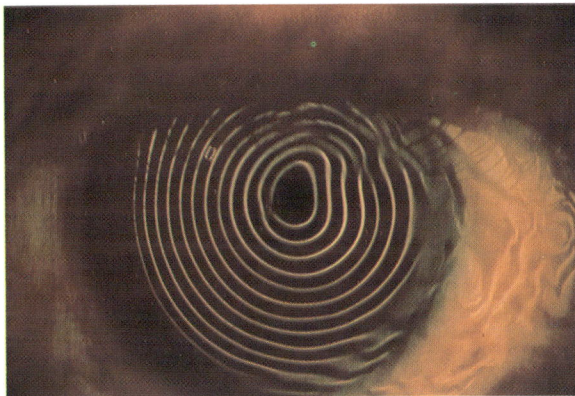 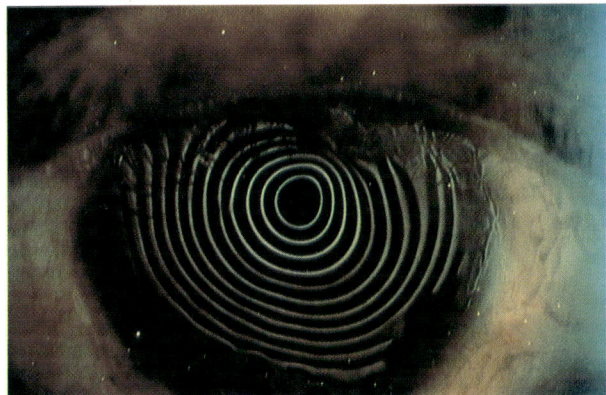

Fig. 14.29 Irregular astigmatism. (a) Pre-application; (b) post-application.

(a)

(b)

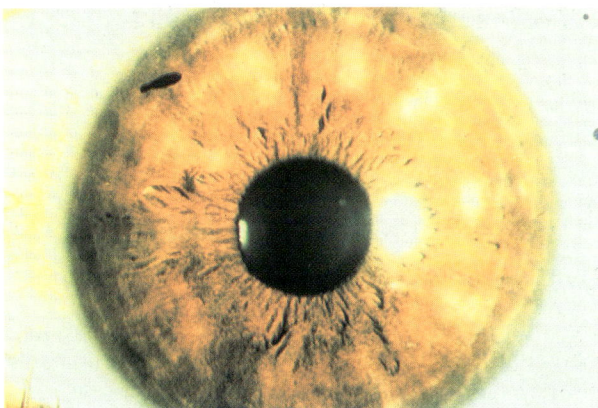 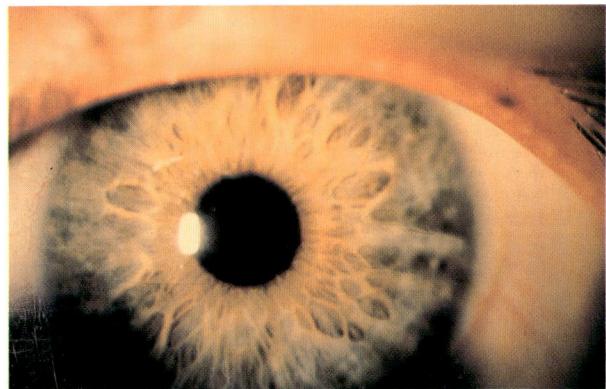

Fig. 14.30 Treated eye (a) at 6 months; and (b) at 2 years.

(a)

(b)

(c)

(d)

(e)

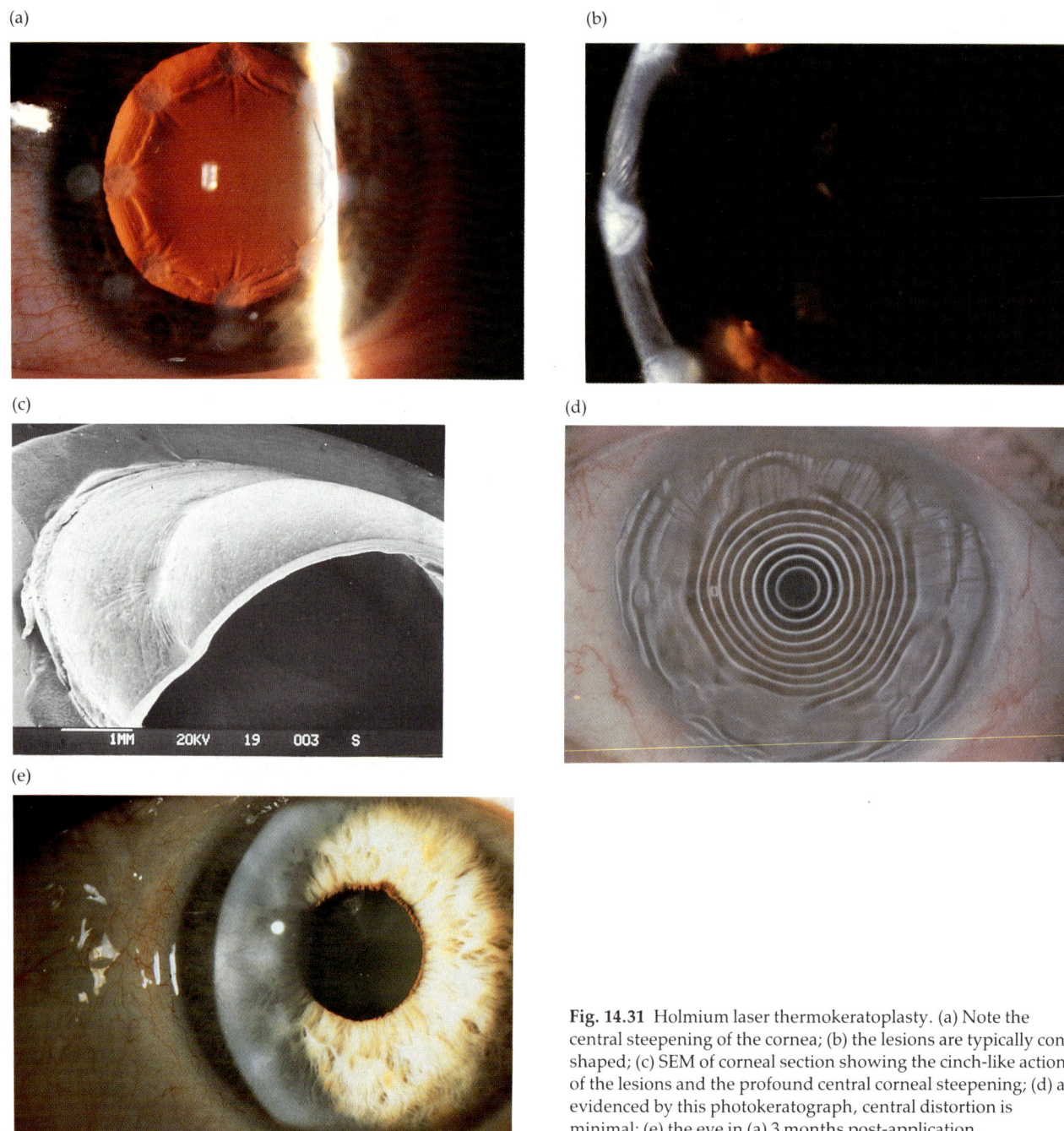

Fig. 14.31 Holmium laser thermokeratoplasty. (a) Note the central steepening of the cornea; (b) the lesions are typically cone shaped; (c) SEM of corneal section showing the cinch-like action of the lesions and the profound central corneal steepening; (d) as evidenced by this photokeratograph, central distortion is minimal; (e) the eye in (a) 3 months post-application.

sanguinary ways to correct hyperopia, particularly radial keratotomy over-corrections.

Holmium laser thermokeratoplasty

In an effort to control the amount and extent of stromal thermal damage and thus quantify the procedure, Seiler has employed the holmium laser to make the burns [30]. Figure 14.32 illustrates the effect of this application. Predictability still remains elusive. The striking thing to note is the extremely localized extent of the corneal burns and the apparent smoothness of the central changes. Whether the effect will remain stable over time or, like all previous attempts to use heat, gradually diminish over time, remains to be seen.

Over-corrections from radial keratotomy

This properly falls under the category of complications following radial keratotomy surgery and is discussed in Chapter 15.

Other methods of treating hyperopia—such as hyperopic keratomileusis (and other lamellar procedures), as well as laser keratomileusis—are discussed in their respective chapters.

References

1 Tassman I. Frequency of the various kinds of refractive errors. Am J Ophthalmol 1932; 15:1044.

2 Tenner AS. Refraction in school children: 4800 refractions tabulated according to age, sex and nationality. NY Med J 1915; 102:611.

3 Stenstrom S. Untersuchungen uber die Variation und Kovariation der optischen Elemente des menschlichen Auges. Acta Ophthalmol 1946; (suppl) 26:7.

4 Grosvenor T. The neglected hyperope. Am J Optom 1971; 48:376–382.

5 Sato T. Correspondence, a reply on surgical correction of myopia. Am J Ophthalmol 1954; 36:280–282.

6 Gills J. Trephination in combination with radial keratotomy for myopia. In: *Radial Keratotomy*, R Schacher *et al.* (eds). LAL, Dennison, 1980.

7 Gaster R, Yamashita T. Circumferential keratotomy to reduce hyperopia in rabbits. Invest Ophthalmol 1983; 24:149.

8 Yamashita T, Gaster R. *Experimental Hyperopia Correction.* Parts I and II. Keratorefractive Society, Chicago, 1983.

9 Yamashita T. *Hexagonal Incision to reduce RK Overcorrection. Experimental Study.* Keratorefractive Society, Atlanta, 1984.

10 Yamashita T, Schneider M, Fuerst D, Pearce W. Hexagonal keratotomy reduces hyperopia after radial keratotomy in rabbits. J Refract Surg 1986; 2:261–264.

11 Jensen R. Hexagonal keratotomy: clinical experience with 483 eyes. In: *Refractive Surgery*, M Friedlander (ed). Little, Brown, Boston, 1991.

12 Schachar RA. Radial thermokeratoplasty. Int Ophthalmol Clin 1991; 31:47–57.

13 Gasset AR, Shaw EL, Kaufman HE, Itol M, Sakimoto T, Ishii Y. Thermokeratoplasty. Trans Am Acad Ophthalmol Otolaryngol 1973; 77:441–454.

14 Gasset AR, Kaufman HE. Thermokeratoplasty in the treatment of keratoconus. Am J Ophthalmol 1975; 79:226–232.

15 Mandelberg A, Rao G, Aquavella J. Penetrating keratoplasty following thermokeratoplasty. Ophthalmol 1980; 87:750.

16 Keates RH, Dingle J. Thermokeratoplasty for keratoconus. Ophthalmic Surg 1975; 6:89–92.

17 McDonnell PJ, Neumann AC, Sanders DR, Salz JJ. Radial thermokeratoplasty for hyperopia (opinion). Refract Corneal Surg 1989; 5:50–54.

18 McDonnel PJ. Radial thermokeratoplasty for hyperopia. I. The need for prompt prospective investigation. Refract Corneal Surg 1989; 5:50–52.

19 Neumann AC, Sanders DR, Salz JJ. Radial thermokeratoplasty for hyperopia: encouraging results from early laboratory and human trials. Refract Corneal Surg 1989; 5:55–59.

20 Neumann A, Sanders D, Salz J, Bessinger D, Raanan M, Van der Karr M. Effect of thermokeratoplasty on corneal curvature. J Cataract Refract Surg 1990; 16:727–731.

21 Feldman ST, Ellis W, Frucht-Pery J, Chayet A, Brown SI. Regression of effect following radial thermokeratoplasty in humans. Refract Corneal Surg 1989; 5:288–291.

22 Feldman ST, Ellis W, Frucht-Pery J, Chayet A, Brown SI. Experimental radial thermokeratoplasty in rabbits. Arch Ophthalmol 1990; 108:997–1000.

23 Fedchenko OT. Infrakeratoplasty for the treatment of hyperopia. Ninth International Congress of Eye Research, Helsinki, Finland, 1990.

24 Neumann AC, Fyodorov SN, Sanders DR. Radial thermokeratoplasty for the correction of hyperopia. Refract Corneal Surg 1990; 6:404–412.

15

Side-effects and Complications of Refractive Surgery

Life is just one damned thing after another.
[Frank Ward O'Malley]

All surgical procedures, regardless how benign or "safe," carry with them certain side-effects and complications. Refractive surgery is, of course, no exception. Side-effects, for the purposes of this discussion, are defined as the usual, or expected, sequelae of a surgical procedure that disappear with time and with minimal or no treatment. These effects are usually self-limiting but for the time that they are present can create severe problems for the patient and may, subsequently, have to be dealt with by the surgeon.

Complications are unexpected, and/or deleterious, side-effects that require medical or surgical intervention and which may leave permanent effects. These effects, while fortunately quite rare, are usually those associated with any eye surgery and are dealt with in the same manner. Some are unique to this surgery and must be dealt with uniquely.

We will begin our discussion with radial keratotomy (RK) because the side-effects and complications occurring with this surgery encompass problems encountered with almost all other forms of refractive surgery. We will then follow with a section on those peculiar problems associated with lamellar corneal surgery. Problems unique to a specific procedure will be detailed either in a separate section or can be found within the chapter or section dealing with the specific modality. We will not cover in depth those complications which are seen during or following cataract surgery—these have been more than amply discussed in the various textbooks on the subject. The reader is referred to these for edification.

Radial keratotomy (relaxing incisions)

Side-effects: intra-operative

Epithelial stripping

In approximately 6% of cases in the author's experience, stripping of the epithelium in one or more areas will occur when making incisions. This phenomenon is more likely to occur after using topical anesthetics such as cocaine or 4% tetracaine but can also occur after use of buffered 0.5% tetracaine or proparacaine. In almost all cases, these same patients will have given a history of extreme intolerance to contact lenses or foreshortened wearing time—even with soft lenses. In a few cases the entire epithelial surface ripples when touched. In some of these same cases large, quadrantic sections of tissue have stripped off the corneal surface. The incidence of this side-effect was almost double during the time the corneas were kept wet during the surgery and seems to be caused by swelling of the epithelial cells in response to anoxia.

Generally speaking, small triangular areas of stripping (called concordes when first encountered because

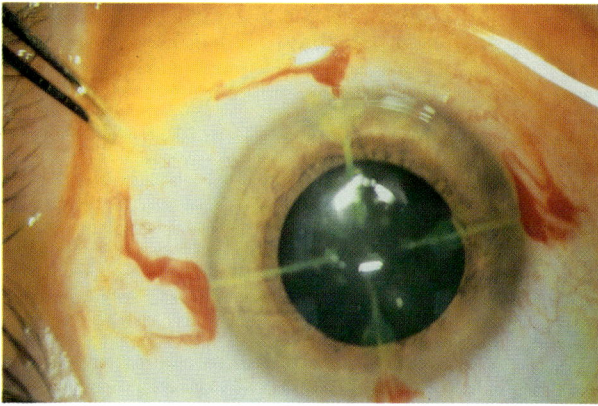

Fig. 15.1 Epithelial stripping—so-called concordes.

remove as much *peripheral* epithelium as you can before proceeding. Do not take off the central epithelium or you will lose your optical zone mark. Naturally, if this is a case of stepped incisions you will not be able to do this. The author has not found it necessary to change the blade setting in these cases to compensate for any possible change in corneal thickness, even when the stripping is extensive.

At the close of the surgery remove any loose tags of epithelium to insure smooth edges and then gently irrigate the interior of the incisions. Replacing the epithelial tags has not, in this author's experience, increased anything but the patient's post-operative discomfort. A pressure patch may increase patient comfort during the first 12–24 hours but it may become necessary to remove it before then—2–4 hours is usually sufficient. These patients normally require more or stronger post-operative analgesics.

Side-effects: post-operative

Glare

The most common side-effect and one that occurs in most RK patients is glare. Glare dazzle is produced by the corneal scars, and is especially noted at night when the pupil will dilate to 5–6 mm, exposing the ends of the incisions, making night driving difficult and sometimes impossible (Figure 15.3). A related side-effect is *photophobia*. Glare is usually self-limiting, beginning to diminish at 3–4 months, and is gone for the most part within the year. The PERK study noted that glare as measured by the Miller–Nadler glare tester was not significantly different at 1 year post-surgery as compared to the pre-operative measurements [1].

In general the best treatment for glare is to take steps to minimize it by careful pre-operative planning. The proper combination of incision number and optical zone size should be chosen from the computer-

of their resemblance to that aircraft in overhead view) occur along the incision line, with the apex of the triangle directed away from the direction of incision (Figure 15.1). They are more frequently encountered, even in dry cases, with dull blades and/or incompletely cleaned or poorly polished footplates. They can also occur if the knife handle is tipped forward and pressure applied to the front of the footplate, causing it to "dig in" (Figure 15.2).

This phenomenon can be minimized by using supersharp blades such as the XTAL sapphire in handles with highly polished footplates; by keeping the cornea dry; and by using only enough pressure on the knife to keep the footplate in contact with the corneal surface. The appearance of a prominent "motorboat wake" with the newer knifes is an indication of too much pressure and/or a dull blade.

When stripping occurs, gently wipe away the loose tissue from the cornea with a moistened microsponge, taking care not to make it worse. Clean debris away from the blade and off the bottom of the footplate. If it appears that more tissue is going to come away,

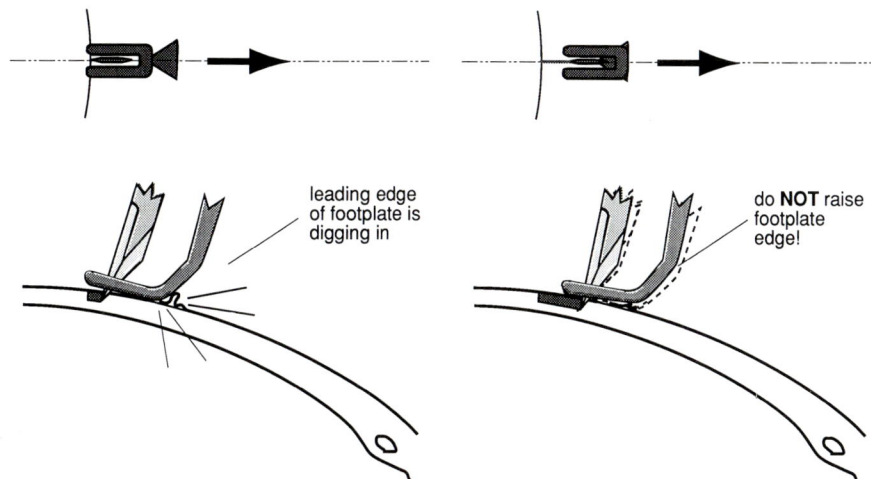

Fig. 15.2 Cause of concordes and the wrong way to deal with them.

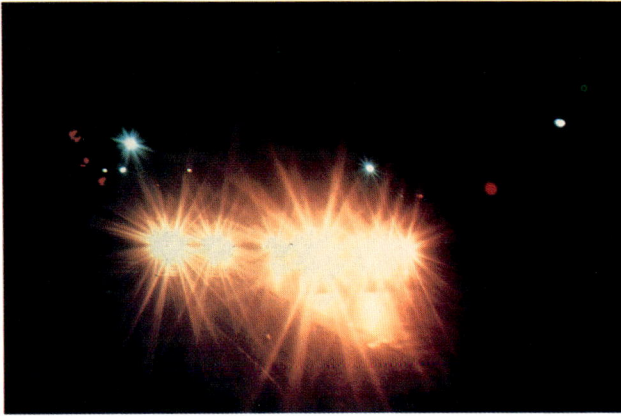

Fig. 15.3 Typical post-RK glare.

generated surgical table. Choose the largest zone with the least number of incisions, even if it means having to use multiple steps or re-deepening to achieve the correction desired.

The use of the newer, ultra-thin, ultra-sharp blades will produce extremely fine incisions and scars, further reducing the amount of glare. Also newer techniques in deepening incisions and re-operations have reduced the severity and longevity of the symptoms.

The treatment of glare can take many forms, with the main object that of diminishing its effect upon the patient. It is not possible totally to eliminate glare and patients vary in their response both to glare and its treatment. Some patients never complain at all. Pre-operative testing with a device such as the Miller–Nadler glare tester, while alerting the surgeon to a possible problem, has not proved useful in screening out patients with increased glare sensitivity. It is not unheard of for patients to complain of less glare post-operatively and show this in their test results. Some glare is associated with residual myopia or against-the-rule astigmatism and can be treated by simply fitting temporary spectacles.

Commercially available absorptive lenses will reduce the amount of visible light reaching the retina and may reduce some of these symptoms. The following may be of value:

1 Anti-reflective coatings, typically consisting of an ultra-thin layer of magnesium fluoride, create light wave interference, thus reducing reflected light. This will improve the optical performance of any spectacle lens and may reduce the multiple image reflections caused by oncoming headlights and other point sources of light.

2 Tinted spectacles are popular with the public for reduction in glare, although their effectiveness in the treatment of glare may be minimal. In the truly light-sensitive (or photophobic) individual, a dense pink tint allowing approximately 52% light transmission (cruxite C) may be of value. Neutral gray tints are available in densities as dark as 12% transmission. These absorb as much as 98% of ultraviolet along with infrared, and do not distort colors. If a significant reduction of light intensity during the day is required, these are a satisfactory lens. Green tints may be similarly used, but do not reproduce colors as well. Brown tints may also be of value, have some cosmetic appeal, and do slightly enhance contrast. They, however, cause color distortion. Yellow tinted spectacles absorb 100% of ultraviolet, transmit infrared, and about 83% of the visible spectrum. They tend to absorb heavily in the blue region and, therefore, reduce haze and enhance contrast slightly.

3 Polaroid sunglasses, alone or in combination with dense neutral gray coating, are of value in reducing total incident light as well as eliminating annoying surface reflections such as occur on water or snow. Such lenses are particularly effective in treating both glare and photophobia.

4 Photochromic lenses darken when exposed directly to ultraviolet light and lighten when ultraviolet light is withdrawn. In those patients exposed to particularly bright sunlight on snow or water, a combination of photochromic glass and a Polaroid filter, as found in the photopolar glasses, may be helpful.

5 Special lenses such as the NOIR are available which will absorb varying proportions of the visible spectrum and a majority of ultraviolet and infrared.

Topical pilocarpine in dilute strength (0.25–0.50%) may also be used to reduce glare dazzle symptoms through pupillary miosis. However, such use is of limited value and some patients will experience brow ache or difficulty in reading.

Often patients will complain of glare at night when what they are really experiencing is an enlarged blur circle resulting from the natural shift toward myopia experienced late in the day. In these cases, the problem might be eliminated by fitting the patient with spectacles to be worn only when driving at night. Sometimes repeat surgery may be necessary.

Photophobia

Photophobia is a short-lived side-effect, usually lasting no more than 14 days. It is associated with corneal edema and diminishes as the edema subsides. It usually does not require any treatment. For those patients with extreme photophobia, temporary spectacles of the type described above can be utilized. The post-operative use of low-concentration steroid drops during the first 2 weeks seems to diminish this side-effect.

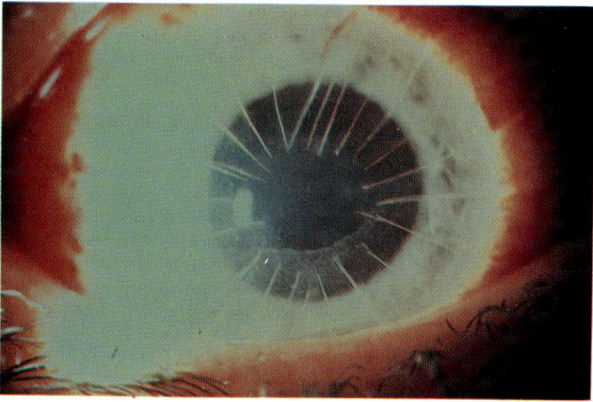

Fig. 15.4 Typical corneal edema seen during the wet surgery era. Note that the edema is present only in the incision areas.

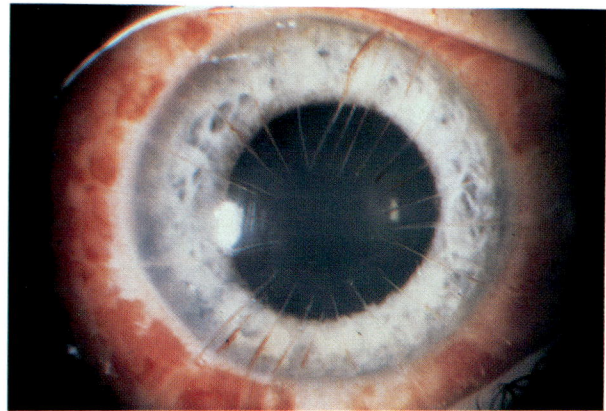

Fig. 15.5 Same cornea at 24 hours post-surgery. These two figures are also representative of the sub-conjunctival hemorrhaging accompanying incisions that extend across the limbus.

The author has personal knowledge of at least one RK case which came to penetrating keratoplasty because of glare.

Corneal edema

Corneal edema is seen in 93% of patients in the immediate post-operative period (Figures 15.4 and 15.5). It usually extends from the bottom of the incisions anteriorly, spares the area within the optical zone, and is usually of mild degree. Greater edema is most often seen in cases which have had 12 or more incisions and in those cases in which the incisions have been stepped or otherwise re-deepened or manipulated. It will also occur in those cases in which the cornea has been kept wet, or which have received excess irrigation of the incisions following the surgery [2]. The use of hypertonic saline solutions has been suggested (and tried by some investigators) but has not proved to be of much help. The use of such treatment is quite uncomfortable for the patient and of questionable value. Generally the edema subsides rapidly without treatment and is completely gone within 2 weeks.

Punctate keratopathy

Punctate staining of the cornea along the incisions is seen in all cases in the immediate post-operative period. The staining pattern is linear and begins to disperse at 48–72 hours. Some clusters of punctate staining areas can be seen grouped near the inner ends of the incisions for as long as 14 days (Figures 15.6 and 15.7). Persistent punctate (non-dispersed) is associated with tearing, increased photophobia, a foreign body sensation and is self-limiting (see also the section on recurrent corneal erosion, below).

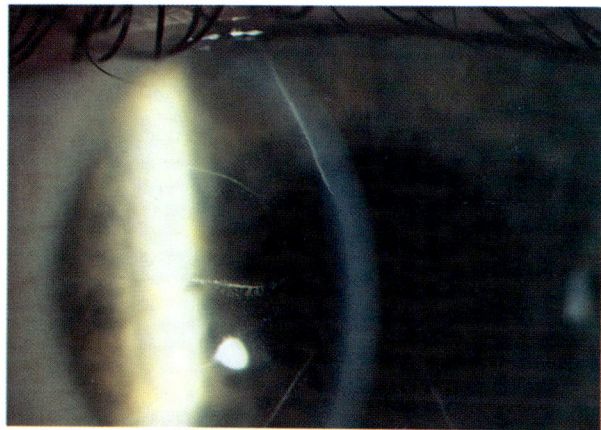

Fig. 15.6 Typical punctate epithelial disturbance seen in RK cases during the initial post-operative period.

Ghost images

In some patients there is a complaint of ghost images or, rarely, discrete monocular diplopia. Usually the patient describes images as having an associated secondary image, best described as similar to an out-of-convergence television picture. Occasionally these secondary images will be sufficiently separate to produce frank diplopia. In all occurrences of this phenomenon, vertical folds in Descemet's membrane can be faintly seen within the optical zone (Figure 15.8). These are more prominent in cases of diplopia and are closer to the optic center (Figure 15.9). Circumferential folds can also be found between the incisions outside the primary optical zone. If these are prominent they may add to the complaint of glare. The circular folds spread centrifugally and usually disappear by 4 months. Upon their disappearance, the

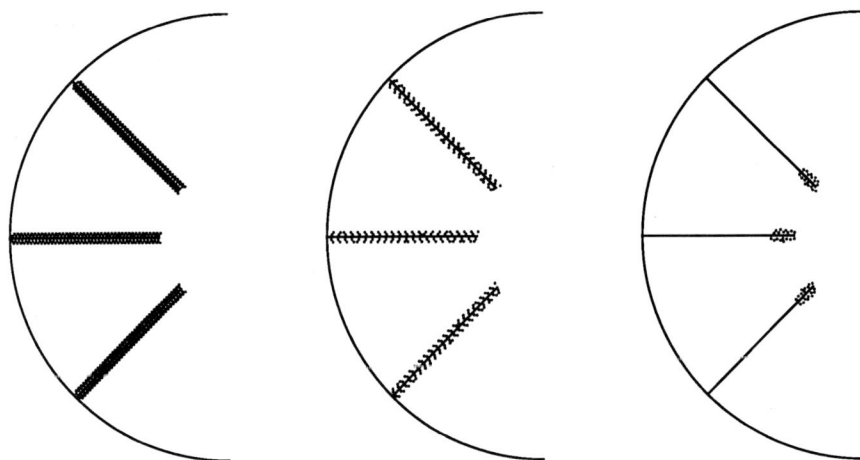

Fig. 15.7 Post-operative punctate staining pattern. Confluent punctate staining is seen in the first 24 hours. The density of the punctate pattern becomes less as time goes on, ending as clumping around the central portions of the incisions at 60 hours.

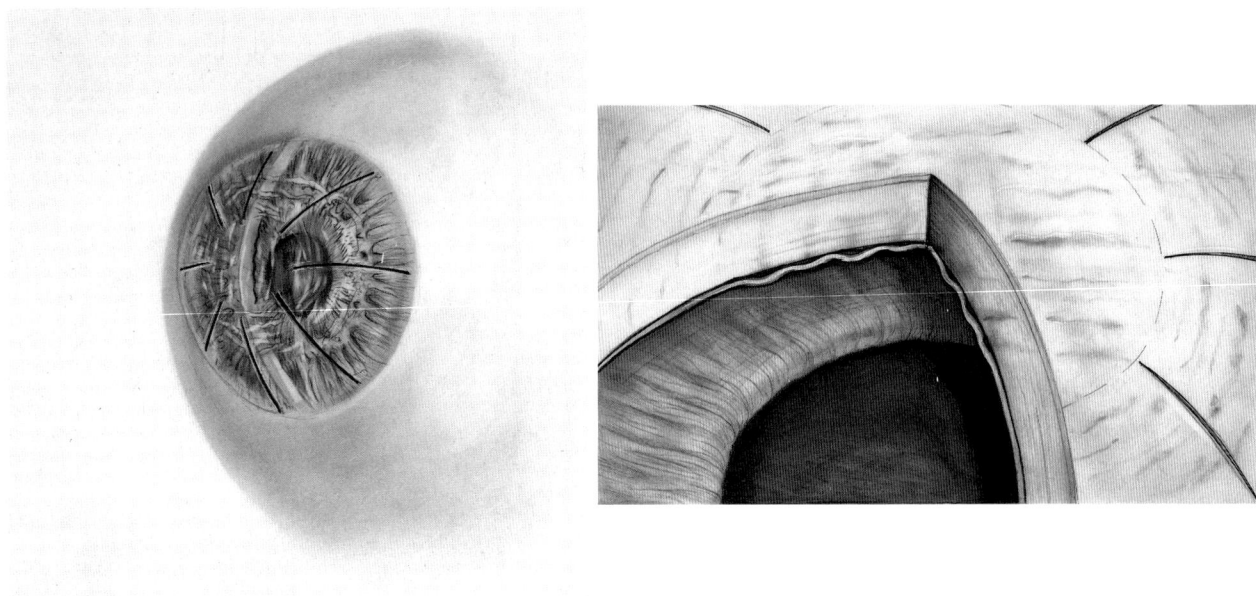

Fig. 15.8 Descemet's folds near the optic center.

vertical folds also leave, taking the diplopia with them. Contrary to the case with glare, correcting any residual myopia may make the symptoms worse. The problem is compounded by the presence of against-the-rule astigmatism, either pre-existing or iatrogenic. In the latter case, the symptoms may diminish as the astigmatism "perambulates" or disappears.

Binocular diplopia

This symptom will usually occur between surgeries as a result of anisometropia. Treatment is surgery of the fellow eye. Transitory binocular diplopia may occur shortly after surgery in young individuals. This may be as a result of over-convergence associated with over-accommodation. No cases of persistent binocular diplopia following this surgery have been reported to date.

Perambulating astigmatism

In those cases with pre-existing astigmatism or in "spectacle sphere" cases with corneal astigmatism and occasionally in purely spherical cases, induced regular astigmatism may be seen post-operatively. The axis of this astigmatism will change from day to day toward

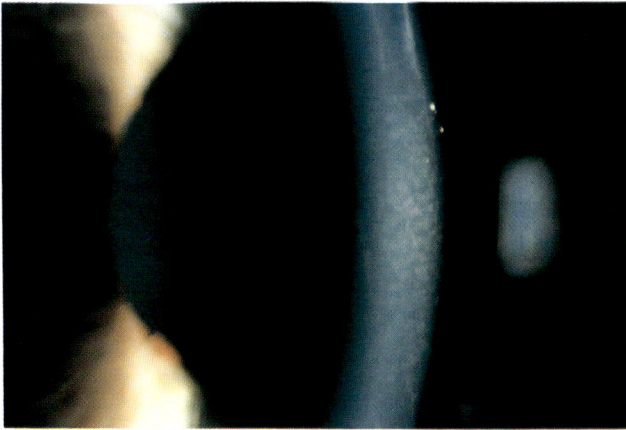

Fig. 15.9 Distribution of folds in Descemet's following RK surgery.

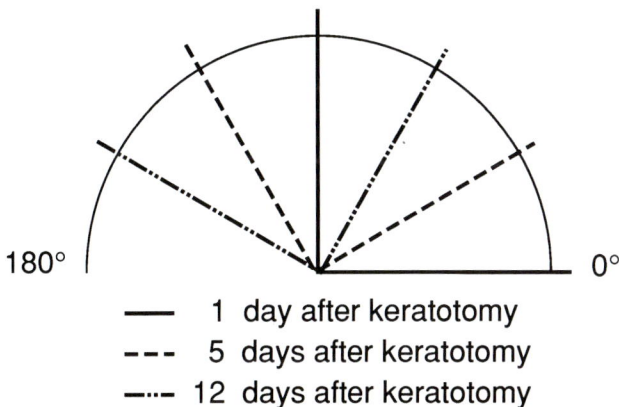

—— 1 day after keratotomy
- - - 5 days after keratotomy
—·—· 12 days after keratotomy

Fig. 15.10 Perambulating or wandering astigmatism following RK.

with-the-rule but may change course willy-nilly, hence its name: perambulating (or wandering) astigmatism (Figure 15.10). By itself it is a transient problem and in operated astigmatism cases is a good prognostic sign. Associated with residual myopia, it accounts for much of the fluctuation seen in these cases. It may aggravate other side-effects, notably glare and ghost images. Unless severe, treatment is not recommended and of little use since the situation is rapidly changing. Furthermore, re-operating astigmatism under these circumstances is highly dangerous (see also Chapter 9).

Asthenopia

Certain patients, particularly those in their early 30s, will complain of some difficulty with tired eyes or intermittent blurring while reading. These symptoms are generally seen in cases of pre-operative myopia greater than 4D. These patients may have normal near points of accommodation upon initial testing both pre-

operatively and post-operatively but tire upon repeated testing. Consequently, these patients will be unable to perform close work or to read comfortably for a time. The treatment is reassurance—reading glasses are not recommended—unless in the presbyopic age range. The problem can be likened to that of a short-distance runner suddenly being expected to run 10 km or more. These patients have not been called upon to utilize their accommodation fully until now—some "getting into shape" is what's required. Recall (Chapter 2) that the accommodative effort is increased in contact lens-wearing myopes [3].

Premature presbyopia

This is actually a misnomer. A better term perhaps would be unmasked presbyopia. True premature presbyopia has not been reported following this surgery—the lens is not being altered by the surgery, the cornea is. Causing the confusion has been the complaint by some patients that they can no longer read without their glasses as they had been accustomed to before the surgery. Careful questioning usually reveals that these same patients were not able to read comfortably before the surgery while wearing their distant correction either—especially if they are contact lens wearers. In fact some of these same patients were able to read only slightly better without their glasses than with them. It is not unusual to have to fit a myope with bifocals sooner than a hyperope.

It should also be borne in mind that many myopes experience some degree of asthenopia for near when wearing contact lenses (see Chapter 2). Such patients should be warned that after a successful RK procedure (or for that matter *any* procedure for myopia) some difficulty with near vision—particularly reading—may be experienced.

Interestingly, some patients who were previously unable to read comfortably while wearing a distant correction are able to read after having their myopia fully corrected by the surgery. This could be as a result of a multi-focal condition of the cornea occurring after surgery [4,5]. The author reported a series of cases in which the cause for the seeming loss of presbyopia appeared to be pseudo-accommodation wherein the pliable post-RK cornea was flexed by the ciliary muscles [6]. Helmholtz demonstrated that the corneal curvature *does* change slightly in the normal during accommodation—the incised cornea could be more susceptible to this effect [7]. The author's findings are summarized in Figures 15.11–15.14.

Treatment consists of reassurance of the patient and having him or her review the informed consent tape. Fitting of a proper reading spectacle may also be necessary. Most patients accept the situation with

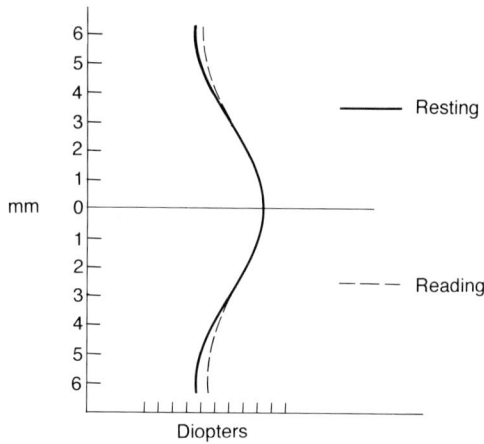

Fig. 15.11 Pre-operative central corneal curvature—distance and near.

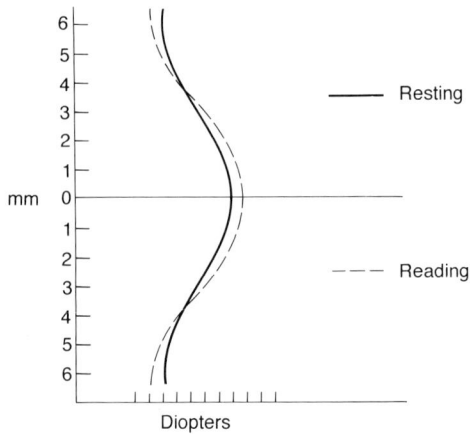

Fig. 15.12 Post-operative central corneal curvature—distance and near.

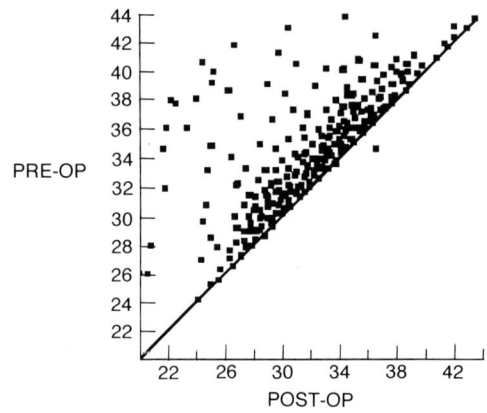

Fig. 15.13 Scattergram of near point of accommodation—pre- and post-operation.

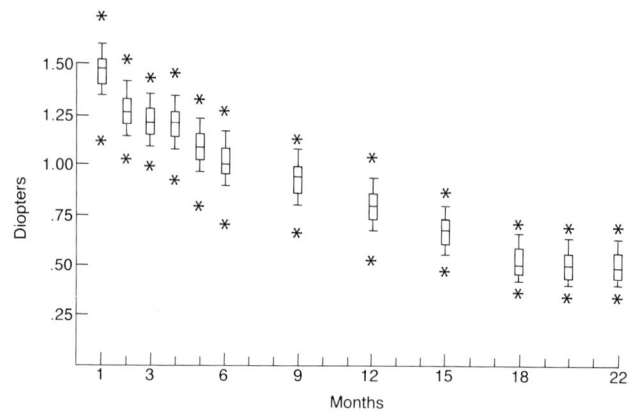

Fig. 15.14 Degree of pseudo-accommodation demonstrated over time.

good grace, saying that half a loaf is better than none. While not a preventive, proper informed consent (perhaps in the form of a video tape) will go a long way to soften the blow.

Fluctuation of vision

More than 80% of all RK patients will experience some degree of fluctuating vision throughout the day for the first 4–6 months. This phenomenon is infrequently seen in eight-incision cases and is undoubtedly related to the diurnal variation in intra-ocular pressure seen in the human eye [8]. Other factors, such as splinting of the malleable cornea by the lids during the night, may be a factor as well. Corneal edema occurring during the night has been suggested as an underlying cause [9]. This has not been borne out by repeated ultrasonic thickness measurements carried out on randomly selected patients at different hours of the day, although such changes in thickness have been seen in patients

with severe epithelial disease. While the cornea is increased in thickness post-operatively to some degree, no significant changes in this thickness have been found to occur diurnally (see the section on undercorrection, below).

Some studies have suggested that corneal shape changes due to diurnal pressure fluctuation are not a factor, by demonstrating no significant corneal curvature changes through the day [10–12]. In a series of patients examined by the author in 1979 over a period of 3 months, applanation pressures were measured on both the operated and the unoperated eye at varying times of the day, including late evening and early morning. In addition, ophthalmometry was performed on each eye. It was found that it was possible to detect small changes in the central corneal curvature by this method. While not conclusive because of the inherent inaccuracies within the method of measurement and the smallness of the changes, these changes were, nevertheless, significant in their own right. In every case in which the visual acuity was affected, the K-readings were measurably different in the operated eye as opposed to those in the non-operated eye for a given time period. In those patients, for example, who stated that their vision was better in the morning as opposed to the afternoon, the central corneas were uniformly flatter centrally in the morning than in the control eye (see the section on being there, below). This observation was well demonstrated by Deitz and associates [13] in a series of patients in whom the intra-ocular pressure was increased by use of topical steroids and has been corroborated by Fyodorov [14] as well as Feldman and co-workers [8].

The Bates effect [15] or phenomenon has not been suggested as a possible causative agent but may well play a part because the corneas of these patients are extremely malleable. It has been observed that many patients demonstrate good unaided post-operative visual acuity, despite their having a residual myopia which ordinarily would drop the vision to 20/100 or less. If the lids are held away from the eye in these same patients their vision falls to the expected levels. It is possible that varying degrees of orbicularis spasm or lid pressure exerted during the day (with more in the morning when fresh) produce varying amounts of flattening and hence varying acuity.

This side-effect, like glare, is self-limiting but may not go away completely for a number of years [16]. Large fluctuations—those inclined to induce patient complaints—last for a much shorter time and usually subside by 4–6 months. The fitting of a hard contact lens to reduce the fluctuation has been tried with limited success. These patients are often lens-intolerant in the first place. Further, an exact corneal curvature measurement, required in hard lens fitting, is not often possible during this period. The fitting of a soft contact lens for the same purpose is not recommended before 8 weeks because of the danger of neo-vascularization of the incisions. Since the lens is extremely flexible, its effect upon the variation in vision is small but some patients notice a diminution of visual variation.

Treatment is "tincture of time" and reassurance. The fitting of any visual appliance for this purpose before 12 weeks is an exercise in futility and in any case unnecessary unless there is significant residual myopia and/or astigmatism. In those cases the patient should be told that he/she may require additional changes somewhere down the line.

Upper lid edema

Approximately 16% of patients who have corneal abrasions demonstrate edema of the upper lid within 24 hours. The incidence of this side-effect after RK is approximately the same, and no special significance is placed on its occurrence. It lasts, for the most part,

only for a few days and rarely becomes severe enough to produce complaints. On those occasions, cool compresses and aspirin analgesia suffice. Tylenol (acetaminophen) does not seem to be as effective.

Increased color saturation

Along with the reduction of the myopia and/or astigmatism, this is one of the pleasant side-effects of this surgery and was first described by the author in 1979. It is experienced as an increase in the brightness and density of color in objects. Vision is described as "less pastel" in nature. The patients rarely complain of this and all exclaim about it. One such patient described it like Dorothy walking out into the land of Oz, hence its more popular name, "the Wizard of Oz phenomenon."

Spatial displacement

This side-effect is a psychologic reaction which occurs most often in patients who have had successful surgery in one—usually the non-dominant—eye. They describe scenes as if they were viewing them from one side (usually the operated side) and slightly above their actual position. Usually very transitory, disappearing when the second eye has been operated, it occasionally occurs even then. Sometimes the displaced feeling is sufficiently strong as to produce vertigo. Vertiginous patients may need medication. Fortunately, the phenomenon occurs very rarely and produces no lasting effects.

Complications—intra-operative

Divots (see also section on epithelial stripping, above)

This complication is universally seen as a consequence of incisions being made with a dull blade or the back side of any blade (Figure 15.15). These will still occur if an attempt is made to make incisions with the back of a single-edged blade. They are transverse tears through Bowman's membrane. The triangles point in the direction of the incision, are smaller than the concordes and result in permanent scarring which may increase both the intensity and persistence of glare (Figures 15.16 and 15.17). There is no effective treatment other than symptomatic (see section on glare, above). The solution is prevention by using sharp, double-edged blades for the surgery.

Corneal perforation

There are two types of perforation—micro, in which only the very tip of the blade has entered the anterior chamber, and macro, in which the opening is a frank

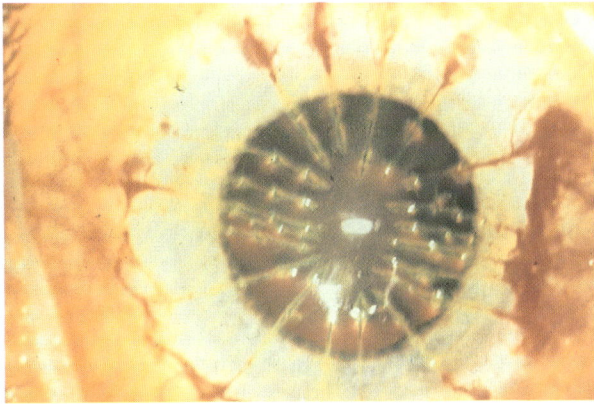

Fig. 15.15 Divots or tears in the corneal stroma—secondary to a poor blade.

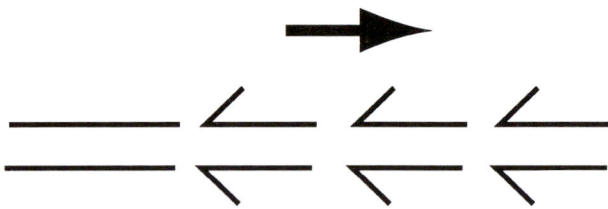

Fig. 15.16 Tears are angled away from the direction of blade travel.

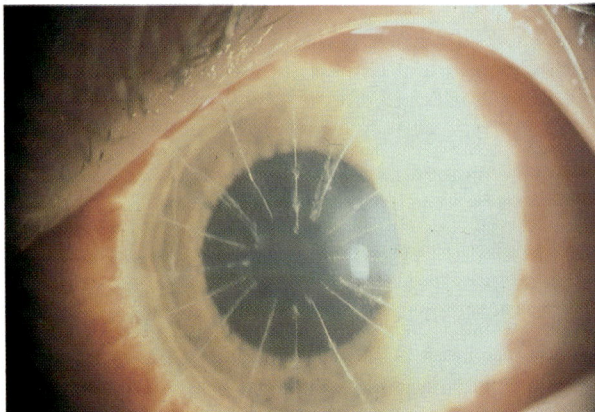

Fig. 15.17 Irregular scarring from transverse tears in Bowman's can increase the problem with glare.

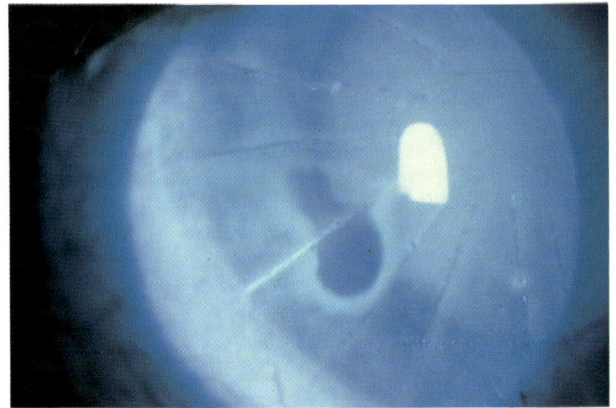

Fig. 15.18 Positive Seidel's sign, indicating an active leak—the sign of a micro-perforation.

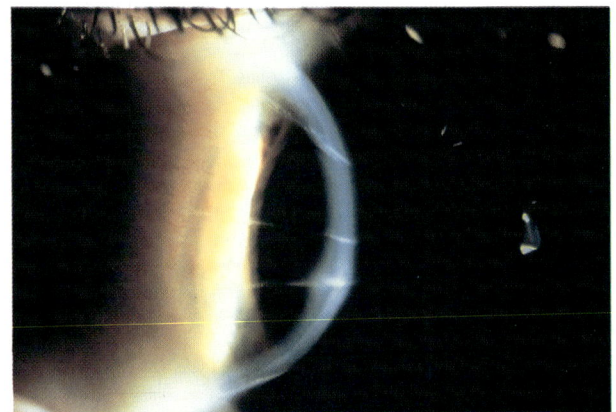

Fig. 15.19 Self-sealed leak—hallmark of a micro-perforation.

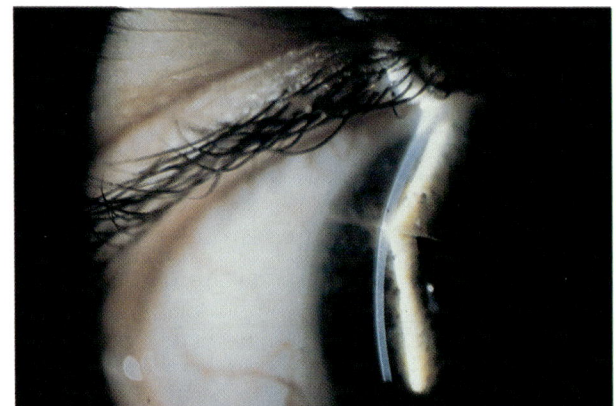

Fig. 15.20 Adherent leukoma—macro-perforation.

incision involving the anterior chamber (Figures 15.18 through 15.21). The latter occurs either because the incision is being made too rapidly when a thin spot or "dimple" is encountered or the micro-perforation went unnoticed and the incision was extended. These may occur initially at the edge of the optical zone with the first entry of the blade, in which case the blade was obviously set too long, or anywhere along an incision. The more likely spot for the latter event will be in the infero-temporal quadrant where such dimples are frequently encountered (Figure 15.22). The most

common place along the incision for this to occur is at the mid periphery, especially at the beginning of the second stepped incision in a multi-stepped incision case.

The incidence of surgical invasion of the anterior chamber in RK has been reported to vary from 6 to

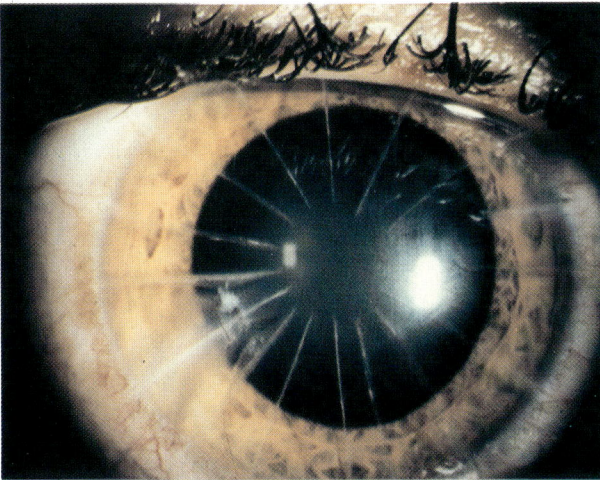

Fig. 15.21 Repaired macro-perforation. Note spreading of adjacent incisions.

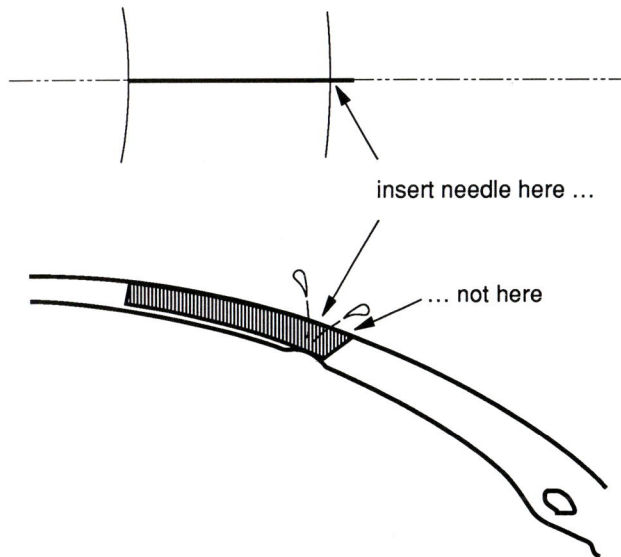

insert needle here ...

... not here

Fig. 15.23 Suture is placed before the end of the incision.

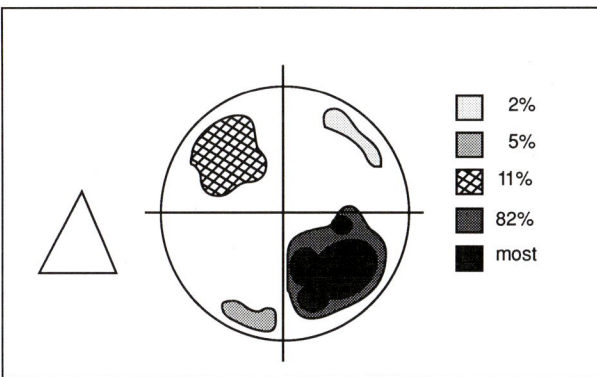

Fig. 15.22 Distribution of corneal "dimples" or thin areas.

33% [17]. The author has found the incidence to vary depending upon the blade used, the position on the learning curve for that blade the case was performed with, and the degree of myopia present. The highest incidence of penetration in the author's series occurred with the use of Sputnik steel blades about 1 month after beginning the use of ultrasonic pachymetry. This was 23% and occurred because of the practice of over-setting the blade 10–15% in each case. It could also have been due to an erroneous setting for the speed of sound through the cornea. When the author switched to the use of the sapphire blade the incidence dipped to 8% after only a few months of trial and error adjustment of the blade depth to obtain the optimum settings.

Do not be quick to envy the surgeon whose reported perforation rate is low without examining his or her technique and results. It is a small thing to obtain a zero incidence of micro-perforation—simply set the blade too shallow. There are those who advocate just such an approach (L. Kogan, 1985, personal communi-

cation). The problem with perforations is not the perforation itself, but the failure to accord sufficient significance to the puncture—it is a potentially serious invasion of the body's defenses. A small percentage of micro-perforations, however, is acceptable as an indication that the blade depth is close to optimum. The surgery works best with deep incisions and each surgeon should make the deepest incisions possible without incurring too great an incidence of perforation. In this author's opinion, an 8–10% incidence of micro-perforation is an acceptable incidence for the average surgeon. For the expert it could be slightly higher.

Unless the perforation has occurred at the beginning of a multi-step 16-incision case, it is not necessary to abandon the case providing that the leak can be stopped or has occurred after the initial incisions have been made (in a stepped procedure) and the surgeon is using an ultra-sharp crystalline blade. At the first sign of a perforation—which in most cases will be the sudden appearance of aqueous just behind the blade—the blade should be removed from the cornea immediately to prevent extension of the perforation. Sometimes a micro-perforation will show itself by a bead of aqueous appearing in one incision during the incising of another part of the cornea.

Perforations occurring while making the initial incisions should be sutured. Nylon 10–0 on a "fish-hook" needle is placed approximately 0.5 mm *behind* the end of the incision (toward the optic center). This is done because the leading edge of the incision is slanted backward from the surface of the incision (Figure 15.23). One suture is sufficient if placed very deep or above Descemet's. Complete the remainder of the incisions, leaving the sutured one until last. Perform all tag removal and free-hand re-deepening (if the chamber is not flat and the pupil is not dilated) before removing the suture. Do not leave the suture in place and do not cut it with your RK blade. Leaving the suture in place will cause gaping of adjacent incisions and is likely to result in the formation of irregular astigmatism (Figure 15.21).

In cases of micro-perforation, pressure-patching overnight is usually enough to allow the perforation to seal and the leak to stop (Figure 15.19). In most cases, the anterior chamber is of normal depth and absolutely quiet the following day. In those eyes that show a positive Seidel's (leakage demonstrated after topical fluorescein), repeat patching will solve the problem in the majority of instances. The author has had to resort to usage of a "bandage" contact lens in the face of persistent leak twice, and sutures once, in over 15 years' experience with this surgery.

A macro-perforation will announce itself by a sudden gush of aqueous and collapse of the anterior chamber (Figure 15.20). More than one suture may be needed to close such an incision. In rare cases such sutures may have to be left in place after the surgery. However, it is not recommended that they be left longer than 1 week. They should then be removed one at a time, allowing any subsequent leak to seal before removing another one. In no case should less than 24 hours elapse between removals.

Once the primary incisions have been made in a stepped case, the remaining portions of the incisions can be completed with the newer crystalline blades with confidence that the incisions will be of adequate depth. This is not true of steel blades or the older diamond blades.

Most of these perforations will seal off spontaneously, with a deep chamber forming within the first 24 hours. Attempting to re-inflate the anterior chamber using BSS or Healon (or other viscoelastic) is not recommended for the reason that there is a risk of introducing contamination. Further, there is a good possibility that this manipulation may cause the wound to leak even more. In addition, the risk of injuring internal structures is increased as well as the possibility of creating an epithelial downgrowth (Figures 15.24 and 15.25). If the leak is bad enough to require re-filling the anterior chamber, it is time to abort the case and possibly introduce sutures. Most of these perforation spots heal without excessive scarring. However, an occasional small area of sub-endothelial fibrosis may be seen (Figure 15.26). This process is, fortunately, self-limiting and only rarely interferes with vision.

This complication can be minimized by careful ultrasonic pachymetric mapping of the cornea; using ultra-sharp blades that plunge and cut to a known setting; and precise blade-setting. Gauges used to set blades

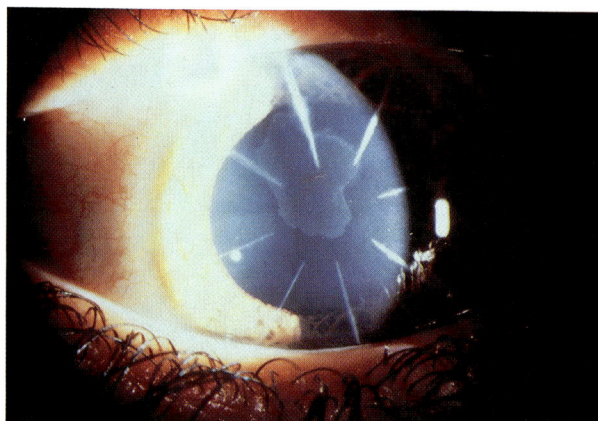

Fig. 15.24 Epithelial downgrowth following a micro-perforation. (Courtesy of P. Binder.)

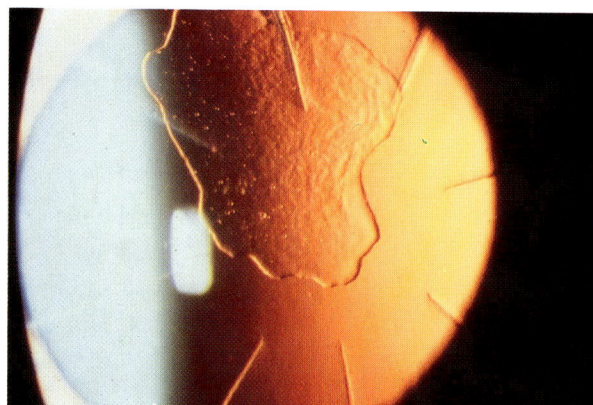

Fig. 15.25 Closer view of an epithelial downgrowth. The patient responded to cryotherapy of the lesion. (Courtesy of P. Binder.)

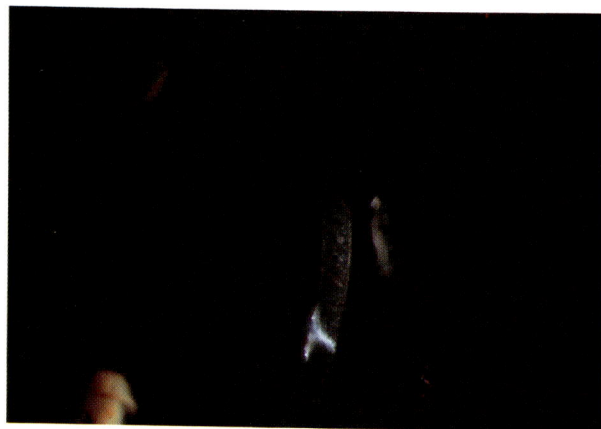

Fig. 15.26 Fibrous proliferation under Descemet's is sometimes seen after a micro-perforation.

should be checked with known standards to calibrate each one individually. An optical or shadowgraph gauge (such as the DGH-800) will help to reduce the incidence of such perforations.

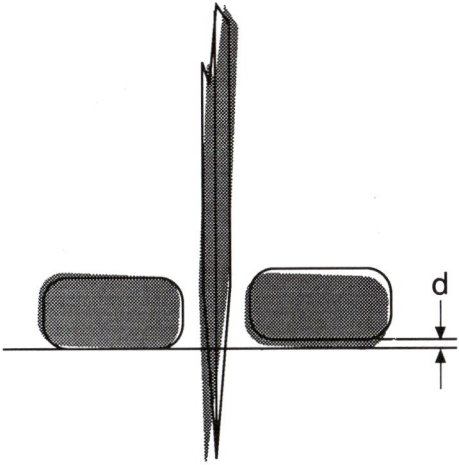

Fig. 15.27 An angled footplate can cause oblique incisions which in turn increase scarring and glare. The shaded figure represents the proper configuration.

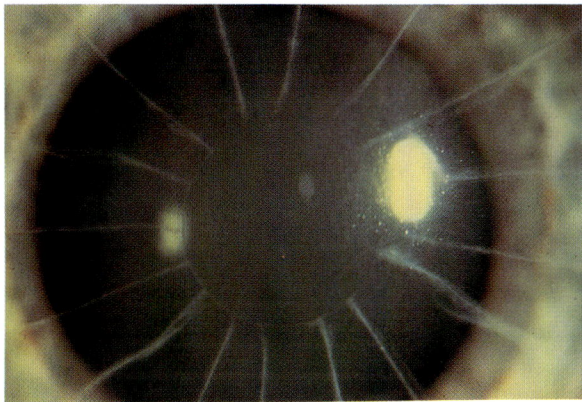

Fig. 15.29 Not only are the incisions irregular in this case, but so is the optical zone.

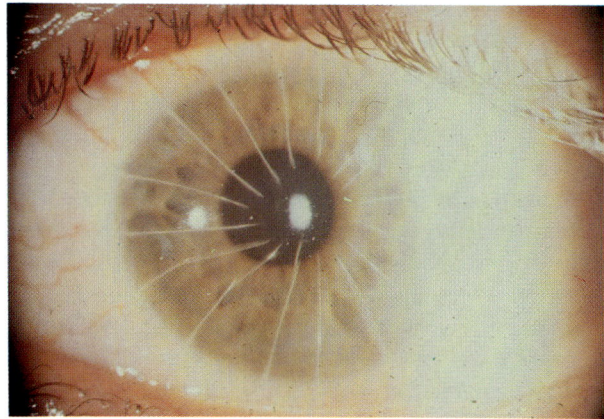

Fig. 15.28 Irregular and oblique incisions.

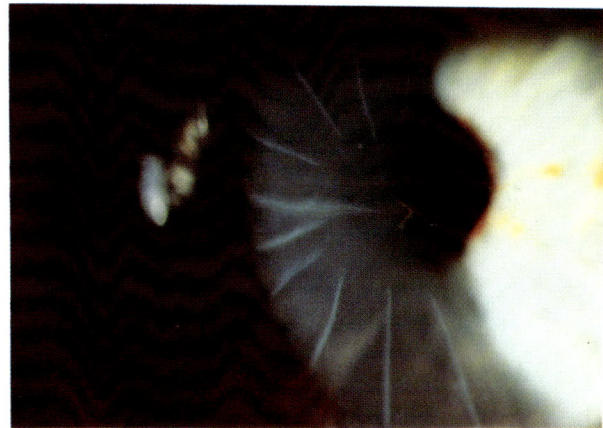

Fig. 15.30 Incisions made from the limbus have a tendency to wander as they approach the center. Sometimes they will join another incision or extend into the optical zone.

It is recommended that all patients in whom perforations have occurred be started on oral broad-spectrum antibiotics such as cephalosporin for a period of 5–7 days (see section on infection, below). If the chamber has been widely opened or if influx of fluid has occurred or is suspected (such as by seeing blood in the anterior chamber), it is advised that a sub-tenon injection of gentamicin (or equivalent) be done on the operating table at the close of the case.

Incision abnormalities

These complications are a manifestation of surgeon error and can generally be avoided. Incision abnormalities include obliquely incised cuts caused by failure to control the perpendicularity of the blade. Despite wider footplates this is still a problem, especially in soft eyes. Irregular incisions or ''doglegs'' are a result of blades being moved too slowly through tissue, sudden patient movement, loss of fixation, torquing of the eye due to incomplete fixation, oblique fixation, or blade handle footplates that are too short, too narrow, or offset (Figures 15.27 through 15.29). The sharper the blade, the less forgiving of slight lateral or torquing movements it will be. These irregularities are more unsightly than harmful but the causation can lead to confluent incisions. Confluent or joined incisions can occur while making parallel cuts. If care is not taken and/or a dull blade is used, one or more of the incisions can run into the adjacent ones (Figure 15.30). Oblique fixation is the most common cause for this because it permits the eye to rotate and the incision to drift sideways. When this occurs the travel of the blade has to be adjusted to curve the blade path away from the adjacent incision. If they do become joined, the short incision has to be re-cut so as to extend it to the limbus. There is a possibility of developing astigmatism due to irregular healing in these cases. In small zone cases, less than precise placement of the blade at the edge of the optical zone may join incisions. This can also occur when using the limbus-to-center (Russian) incision technique. There is no recovery from this. Occasionally the very tip of the tissue triangle that results retracts or gets dissolved in the healing process, producing a depressed scarred area and permanent glare.

Separated incisions or tissue "stalagmites" can occur during stepping of incisions. This is caused by imprecise placement of the blade at the beginning of the secondary incision. These errors prevent the complete outward movement of the cornea in this area; consequently the tissue is flatter here. Subtle irregular astigmatism results with degradation of best visual acuity, with or without correction. This complication can be prevented by using ultra-sharp blades, precision blade implantation, a light touch on the cornea, and proper fixation (see also Chapter 8).

Invasion of the optical clear zone is a much more serious complication which can result in increase in glare at the least, and frank loss of vision at the most. There are two ways in which the visual center can be compromised in this surgery. The first, and by far the most common, is decentration of the optical zone.

Optical zone decentration

Decentration of the optical clear zone is clearly a result of surgeon error. This can occur through inattention, failure to obtain cooperation by the patient, or marking concentrically to the pupil. By following a few simple rules (outlined in the section on technique in Chapter 8), this complication can be avoided. Displacement of the optical clear zone by inaccurate or careless marking of either the visual axis, the clear zone or both can lead to incisions in the clear zone or even across the visual axis. In cases of astigmatism, decentration of the optical clear zone will lead inevitably to irregular astigmatism. When in doubt that the patient is cooperating in fixating on the microscope light, have him or her look down, right, left, up, and then back at the light. Turn the microscope light way down if necessary and dim the room lights so as to be able to see the light reflex. Obey the old surgical adage: When in doubt—don't!

There is no treatment for this error other than symptomatic. The author has no knowledge of any case requiring keratoplasty for this specific reason.

Invasion of the optic axis or optical clear zone

This complication is almost exclusively confined to the Russian or centripetal incision technique and is always caused by surgeon error (Figure 15.31). Cutting from limbus to center is a hazardous undertaking at all times. The patient has only to look toward the blade to cause it to move into the optical zone. A dull blade will

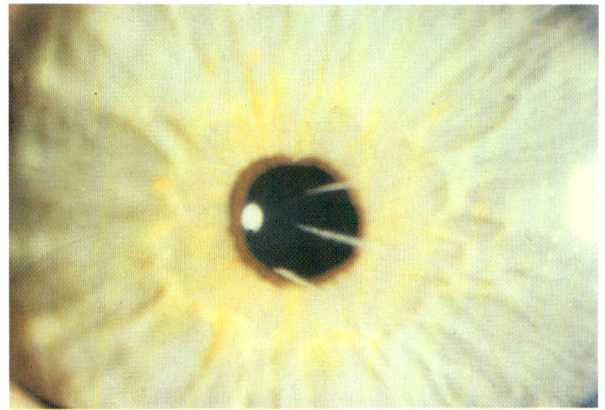

Fig. 15.31 Decentered optical zone.

contribute to this complication as well by making the speed of the cut difficult to control. Precise control and timing are necessary in order to stop the blade exactly on the edge of the clear zone. If the surgeon is inexperienced and/or the blade is dull, it is very likely that blade movement will cease before the edge of the clear zone is reached. If movement of the blade stops before reaching the edge of the clear zone, it will take more force to get it moving again than it did to keep it moving. In this event, entry into the clear zone is enhanced. This difficulty is enhanced further if the cornea is soft. Sometimes the force is sufficiently disproportionate that the blade "jumps" forward and enters the clear zone before it can be controlled or stopped.

This same scenario can be seen when backing up a double-edged blade to deepen the incision at the primary optical zone. It is less likely in that situation because Bowman's has already been incised and therefore tissue resistance will be markedly less. Still, care must be taken to prevent a disaster.

Consequently, with the centripetal or Russian technique, is not possible to have a precise optical zone margin and for the same reason [18]. Fixation must be behind the knife and the blade must be exquisitely sharp to perform this method safely. With certain blades, the setting must be modified to prevent perforating into the AC. All in all it is an unsafe and unsatisfactory methodology best reserved for redeepening of shallow incisions after the fact and only in experienced hands (see also the section on dealing with high myopia in Chapter 8).

Such an event can be prevented in a number of ways. Firstly, the surgeon should have considerable experience with RK before attempting limbus-to-center incisions. Next, the blade used for this type of incision must be very sharp. A sharp blade is more controllable and easier to start or stop. However, in a soft cornea, transverse folds can occur which can impede forward

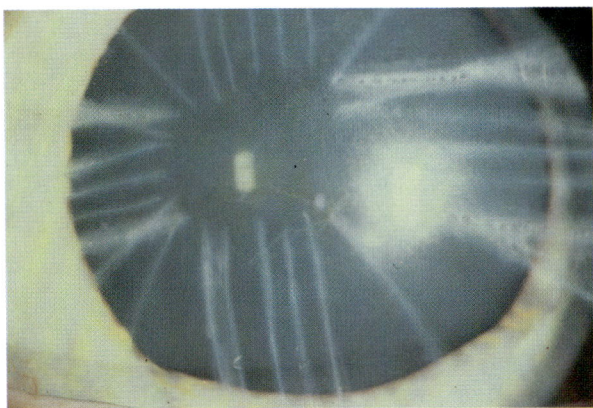

Fig. 15.32 Results of choosing the wrong initial astigmatic axis.

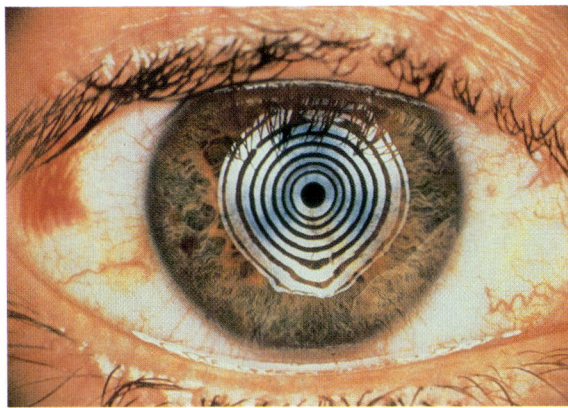

Fig. 15.33 Irregular astigmatism following RK. (Courtesy of A. Neumann.)

progress of the knife footplate. In this event, fixation *behind* the blade at the limbus will give the surgeon more control and may cause the folds to flatten.

Complications—post-operative

Astigmatism

The incidence of induced irregular astigmatism following RK is, fortunately, quite rare [19,20]. When it is seen its cause can usually be traced to a problem with the incisions, as described above. Regular astigmatism that remains after surgery is most often a result of an incomplete correction or residual myopia either through failure to correct for the astigmatic portion or ignoring it. While it is true that up to 1.50 D of astigmatism may disappear after operating for the sphere alone in 16-incision cases, this is not true for incisions less than 16 in number. The rule of thumb for the author is to compensate for the astigmatism when that component equals or exceeds 20% of the spherical myopia and/or when the astigmatism is against-the-rule (see also Chapter 9). Patients will tolerate surprisingly large values of with-the-rule astigmatism post-operatively. It is the author's considered opinion that a small residual with-the-rule astigmatism is not a bad thing and may actually improve the patient's visual perception.

One common cause of induced regular astigmatism is making astigmatism incisions in the wrong axis (Figure 15.32). This has happened to experienced surgeons as well as neophytes. It is a very real danger and the risk of this happening should not be minimized. This can occur due to misunderstanding of the principles of astigmatic correction and confusion of the axis with the meridian. All practitioners are advised to map out the incisional configuration well before, and not during, the day of surgery. If changes are believed to be required at the time of surgery, be sure that such

a change is absolutely correct before proceeding. If still confused or if any doubt exists—*do not do the case*. In fact, a good watchword for this surgery is, when in doubt—don't!

Use an optical device such as an eyepiece reticle or surgical protractor to mark the plus axis with the marker designed for this purpose. Before making the first incision, double-check the axis, preferably with one of your knowledgeable staff. When in doubt—bail out.

In cases of irregular astigmatism the cause of the irregularity must be addressed directly (Figure 15.33). If the problem is due to shallow incisions or some other incisional problem, and if the case is less than 1 month after the original surgery, the offending incision should be deepened, or the tag removed, or lengthened (or whatever) immediately. If more than 1 month has elapsed since the surgery, then the surgeon is advised to wait a minimum of 4–6 months to re-operate—preferably the latter. Sutures or intra-incisional debris should be removed immediately and the epithelium allowed to heal completely before proceeding. In unusual cases it may be necessary to perform additional incisions to relax or further modify the corneal shape to relieve the irregularity. Corneal topography is helpful here. In these cases the full waiting time of 6 months should be allowed to elapse before further surgery is done. It should be apparent that the timing of any additional surgery is predicated on stability of the cornea. If change is still occurring, then further waiting is mandatory.

It may be necessary to curette and suture tightly the incisions in the axis of greatest flattening in order to reduce the chord length, thereby steepening the corneal curvature (Figure 15.34). This is especially helpful in cases involving T (transverse) incisions (see also the section on over-correction, below).

The correction of induced irregular astigmatism is

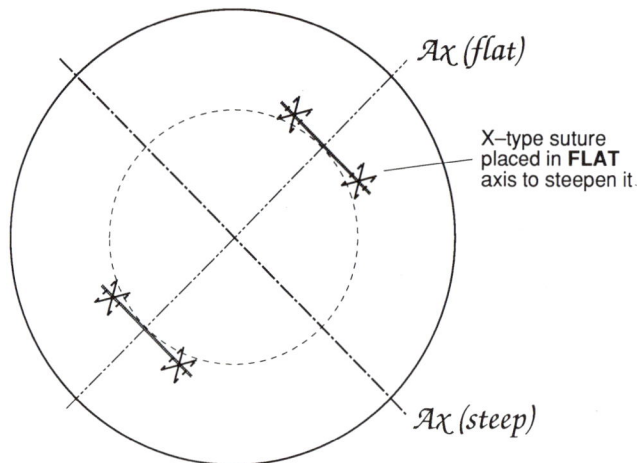

Ax (flat)

X–type suture placed in **FLAT** axis to steepen it.

Ax (steep)

Fig. 15.34 Correcting an over-corrected T-cut with sutures.

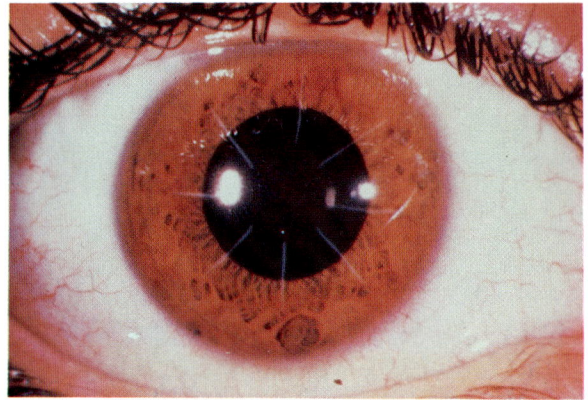

Fig. 15.35 Very short RK incisions. More than 20 incisions can produce the same effect—under-correction.

Correct Recut Technique

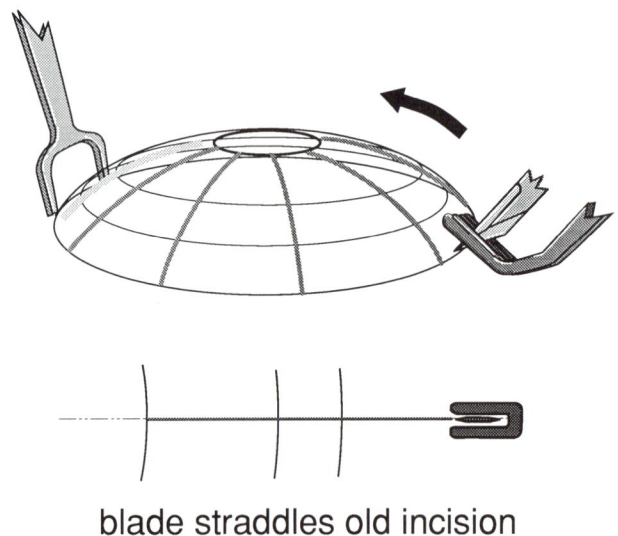

blade straddles old incision

Fig. 15.36 An incision is re-cut from the limbus to the center.

a specialized problem requiring tailored approaches based upon extensive experience. The less experienced surgeon is advised to seek consultation in all such cases.

While waiting for the cornea to stabilize or as an alternative to further surgery it may be advisable to fit a hard or gas-permeable contact lens. The usual rules apply. However, such a fitting should be delayed until 6–8 weeks have elapsed. This delay will minimize any tendency toward developing neo-vascularization.

Residual or induced regular myopic astigmatism can be treated as outlined in the section on under-corrections (see below). The best treatment is, as always, prevention by careful pre-operative evaluation and planning and the use of ultra-sharp blades set at maximum depth with careful blade placement and incision control.

Under-corrections (residual myopia)

Despite the best planning, some cases will end up with residual myopia. In the majority of these cases the cause will be incisions that are too shallow, too few, or too short (Figure 15.35), or optical zone too big [21,22]. All of these problems can be solved for the most part by correcting the deficiencies. Timing is the essence, however, in these corrective efforts.

Generally speaking, shallow incisions should be re-cut and deepened within the first month of the initial surgery. If not done within the first 30 days, then the deepening should be delayed for at least 4 months—waiting at least 6 months is better. When deepening incisions, the straight or vertical-edged blade should be used and the incisions deepened starting at the limbus and moving toward the center, using the previous incision as a guideline. Doubled incisions, with infolding of epithelium, can occur when trying to

re-cut incisions from the center to the periphery. As Figures 15.36 and 15.37 illustrate, it is not possible to keep the blade within the old incision track unless the incision is made from the limbus to center. The knife footplate straddles the old incision—the surgeon uses it as a guide. Figures 15.38 through 15.40 show the aftermath of incorrect technique. These types of incisions are notoriously unstable.

No more than eight incisions should be deepened at any one sitting. The eye becomes soft very quickly—thus there is a tendency for the blade to wander when approaching the center (Figures 15.41 and 15.42). Corneal pachymetry must be repeated because the cornea is always somewhat thicker post-operatively for some months—possibly a year or more (Figure 15.43) ([14], L.D. Bores, 1991, unpublished data). Mapping

Incorrect Recut Technique

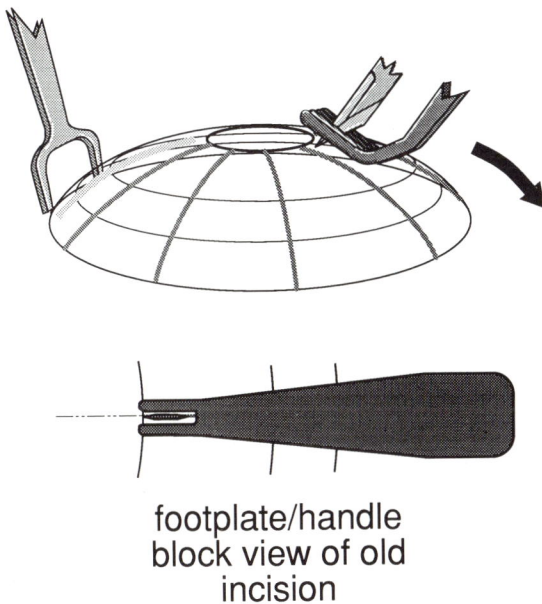

footplate/handle
block view of old
incision

Fig. 15.37 Attempting to re-cut from the center results in blade wander—the old incision is obscured by the knife handle.

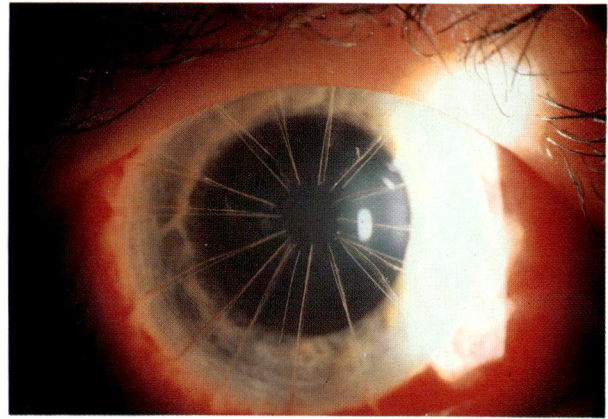

Fig. 15.38 Doubled incision—best case.

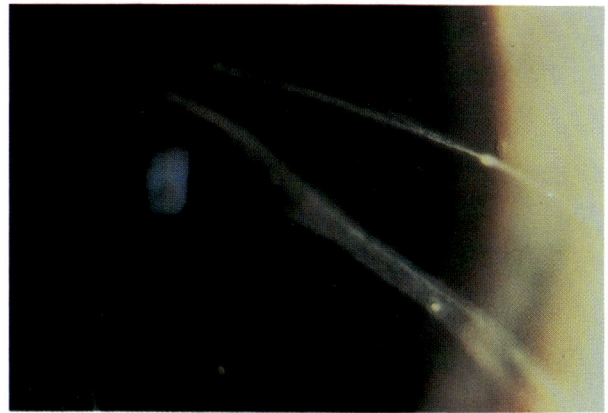

Fig. 15.39 Doubled incision—worst case.

can be done again between the previous incisions but it is usually enough to get the central pachymetry, adding the increase to the original pre-operative readings.

The decision to add incisions should be delayed until the corneas have become stabilized (around 4–6 months). The patient should then be re-examined and the parameters re-calculated using the pre-operative K-readings. This holds for astigmatic as well as spherical cases. Expect a correction of between 80 and 90% of the residual myopia and/or astigmatism.

When fitting spectacles, it is wise to wait a minimum of 2 weeks before doing so. There will be a small percentage of patients who will require a change of lenses within 6 months. Contact lens fitting should be delayed for at least 6 weeks for hard lenses and 8 weeks for soft lenses (including extended wear). There is an increased risk in developing neo-vascularization if soft lenses are fitted before that time.

Over-correction (induced hyperopia)

The author reported an incidence of post-operative hyperopia of less than 1% in a series of patients [23]. This phenomenon is more likely to occur in patients over 40 years of age with myopia less than 3 D [24–26]. It is also more likely to occur with cases calculated using nomograms that do not take age or scleral rigidity into consideration. It is not unusual, even in

well-calculated cases using regression formulae, for patients in this group to show an initial over-correction lasting upwards of 3–4 weeks. Deitz [24,27] and Waring [28] have noted that a certain percentage of patients undergoing RK have shown a progression of effect, some of whom have shifted to the hyperopic side—others have also reported a sporadic incidence of this complication [29]. The author has a few patients within his practice that have also shown a shift to the hyperopic side after 4 years post-RK but it is less than the 30% reported by Deitz and Waring. As a matter of fact, some of this so-called progression may be a result of a normal fluctuation in K-readings seen in normal, unoperated patients. Tables 15.1 through 15.4 and Figures 15.44–15.48 illustrate this phenomenon.

This problem is difficult to recover from, although if the hyperopia is less than 1 D it may well be lost eventually through a process called emmetropization (Figures 15.49 and 15.50). Any hyperopia greater than 1 D and lasting more than 6–8 weeks is likely to remain and poses a problem, especially for older patients. The administration of steroid drops (such as 1% Pred-

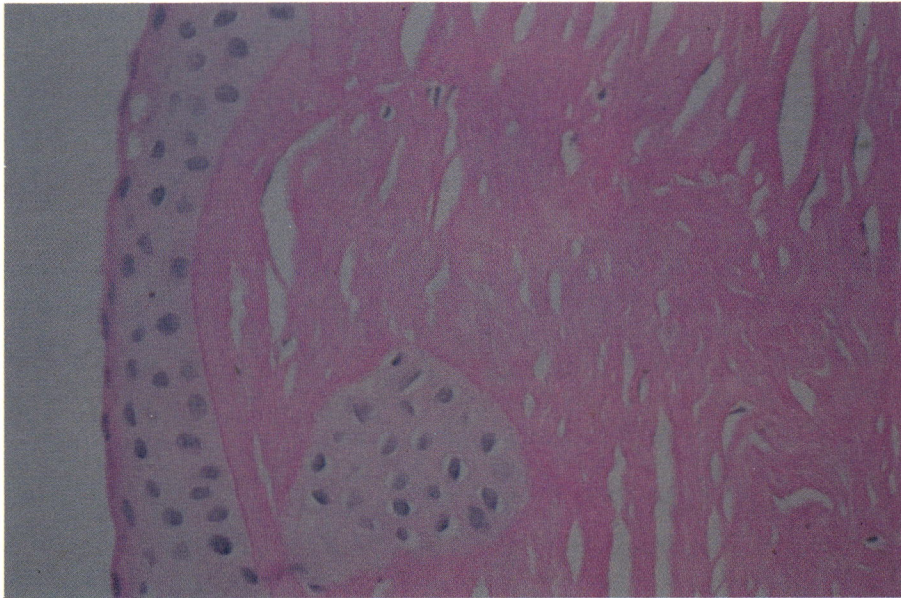

Fig. 15.40 Epithelium "plowed under" the stroma. (Courtesy of P. Binder.)

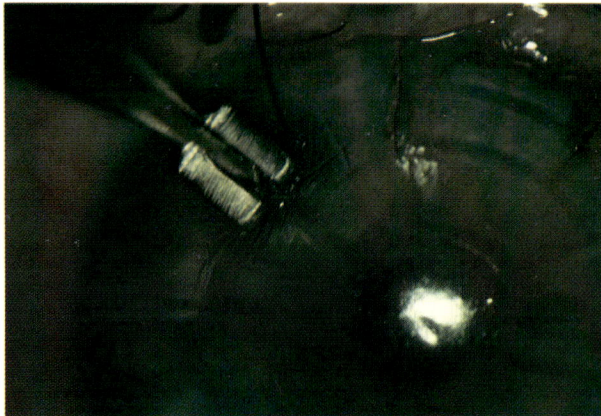

Fig. 15.41 The eye gets soft quickly in repeat operations. Note the wrinkles or furrows ahead of the footplate.

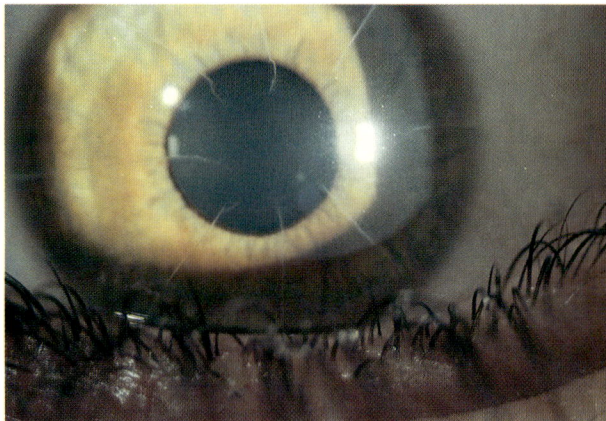

pre-op	520μ
5 days post–op	+80μ
3 months	+60μ
6 months	+40μ
1 year	+40μ

mean central pachymetry in 324 eyes

Fig. 15.43 Corneal thickness increases after RK surgery.

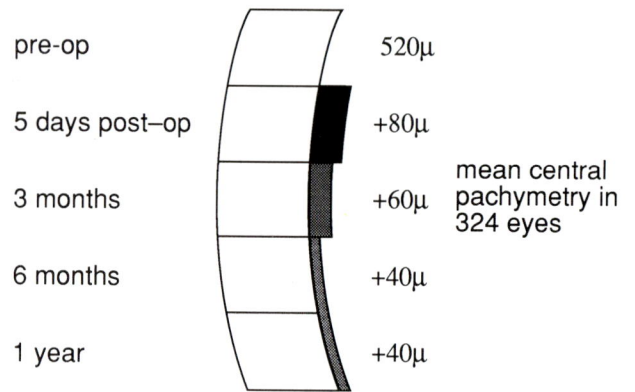

Fig. 15.42 Incisions tend to wander near the center.

Forte) q.i.d. for a period of weeks starting at about 8 weeks has, in some cases, reduced the over-correction by as much as 1 D.

In the past it had been recommended that deep incisions, beginning at 9 mm and extending across the limbus approximately 1.0 mm, be made so as to cause central steepening of the cornea (as demonstrated experimentally; J.J. Rowsey, 1988, personal communication). The author has performed this procedure on two eyes with good results. After 34 months of follow-up, each eye has retained approximately 1 D of steepening. However, the end result is not in any way predictable and additional experience with this method by the author and others has not supported the initial optimism. Additionally, there is a real danger of inflicting serious damage to the angle structures.

The use of anti-glaucomatous medication, such as β-

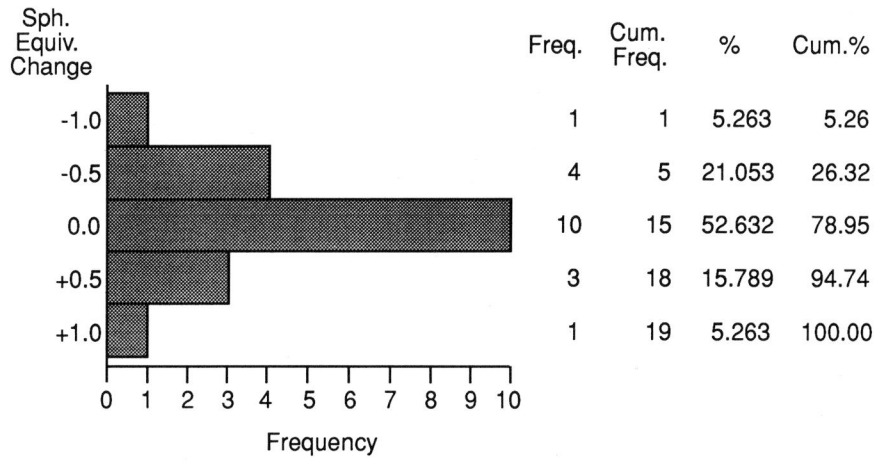

Sph. Equiv. Change	Freq.	Cum. Freq.	%	Cum.%
-1.0	1	1	5.263	5.26
-0.5	4	5	21.053	26.32
0.0	10	15	52.632	78.95
+0.5	3	18	15.789	94.74
+1.0	1	19	5.263	100.00

Fig. 15.44 Change in spherical equivalent in RK cases over 3 years. (Courtesy of S. Grandon.)

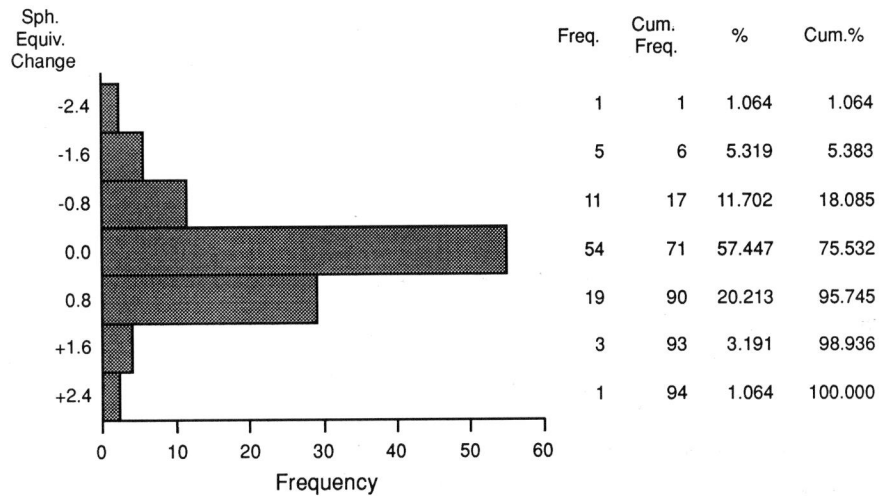

Sph. Equiv. Change	Freq.	Cum. Freq.	%	Cum.%
-2.4	1	1	1.064	1.064
-1.6	5	6	5.319	5.383
-0.8	11	17	11.702	18.085
0.0	54	71	57.447	75.532
0.8	19	90	20.213	95.745
+1.6	3	93	3.191	98.936
+2.4	1	94	1.064	100.000

Fig. 15.45 Change in spherical equivalent in control (no surgery) cases over 3 years. (Courtesy of S. Grandon.)

Table 15.1 Pre-operative patient statistics in Grandon's study

	Mean	s.d.	Min	Max
Age (years)	34/42	9.59	17	64
Spherical equivalent	−4.58	1.89	−1.12	−13.13
Corneal diameter	11.86	0.49	10.50	13.50
Axial length	25.00	1.01	22.40	28.20
Mean keratometry	44.23	1.45	40.44	47.81

Total number of patients, 335; number of male patients, 136 (40.6%); number of female patients, 199 (59.4%).

Table 15.2 Surgical technique used in Grandon's study

Variable	Value
Topical anesthetic	4.0% Xylocaine
Clear zone size range	3–6 mm
Knife used	Diamond set to 90–100% + 30 μm thinnest pachymetry
Incisions made	8
Re-deepening done in high myopic cases	
Post-operative antibiotics	12 days
Topical steroids	0–6 weeks
Timoptic gtts used in some cases	

Table 15.3 Mean changes in spherical equivalent in Grandon's study

	RK cases			Control cases		
Year	n	Mean	s.d.	n	Mean	s.d.
1	212	−0.12 D	0.68			
2	90	+0.64 D	0.64	94	+0.011 D	0.411
3	19	−0.13 D	0.47	94	+0.016 D	0.724

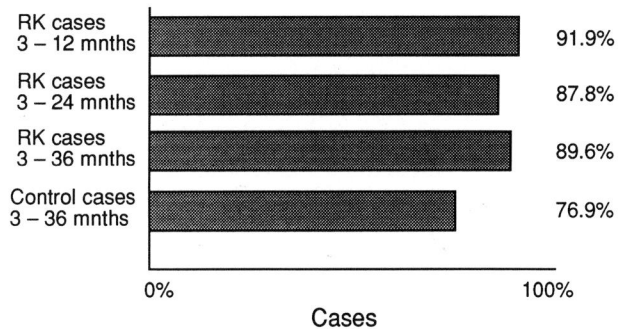

RK cases 3 – 12 mnths	91.9%
RK cases 3 – 24 mnths	87.8%
RK cases 3 – 36 mnths	89.6%
Control cases 3 – 36 mnths	76.9%

Fig. 15.46 Comparison of spherical equivalent changes in both groups. (Courtesy of S. Grandon.)

Table 15.4 Conclusions of the Grandon study

Variation in RK patients does occur over time, but not more than
the control group
There is no predominant hyperopic shift in the cases over time
The vast majority of cases remain stable over time
Statistical analysis of changes in myopia over time indicates that
pre-operative myopia may be a contributing factor

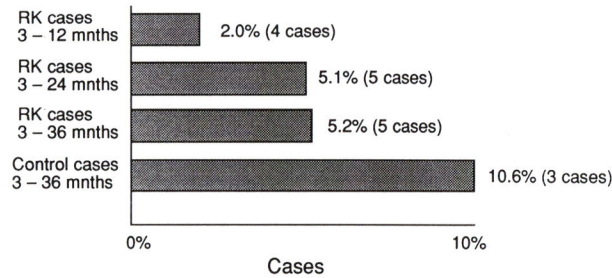

RK cases 3 – 12 mnths	2.0% (4 cases)
RK cases 3 – 24 mnths	5.1% (5 cases)
RK cases 3 – 36 mnths	5.2% (5 cases)
Control cases 3 – 36 mnths	10.6% (3 cases)

Cases

Fig. 15.47 Hyperopic shifts in both groups. (Courtesy of S. Grandon.)

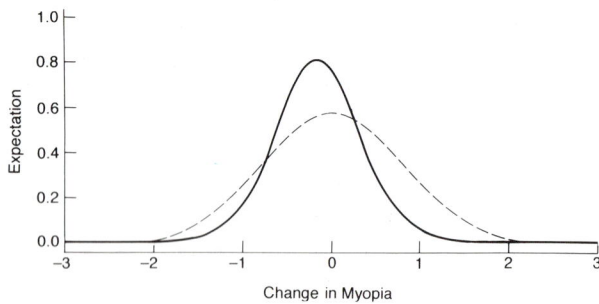

Fig. 15.48 Mean changes in spherical equivalent. (Courtesy of S. Grandon.)

Refraction Dynamics
3.0 D myopia — 12 eyes

Refraction	Observation Period (in years)						
	1/12	0.5	1	2	3	4	4.5
– 1.0 D	2	1	—	—	—	—	—
– 0.5 D	1	2	2	1	2	2	2
0	4	6	9	10	10	10	10
+ 1.0 D	3	3	1	—	—	—	—
+ 2.0 D	2	—	—	—	—	—	—

Fig. 15.49 Emmetropization in 12 eyes. (Courtesy of S.N. Fyodorov.)

blockers, has proved to be of some value in reducing
over-corrections of up to 2 D. It may be necessary to
continue the use of such therapy for as long as a year.
Even then, some cases have been reported in which
the hyperopia has returned upon discontinuing the

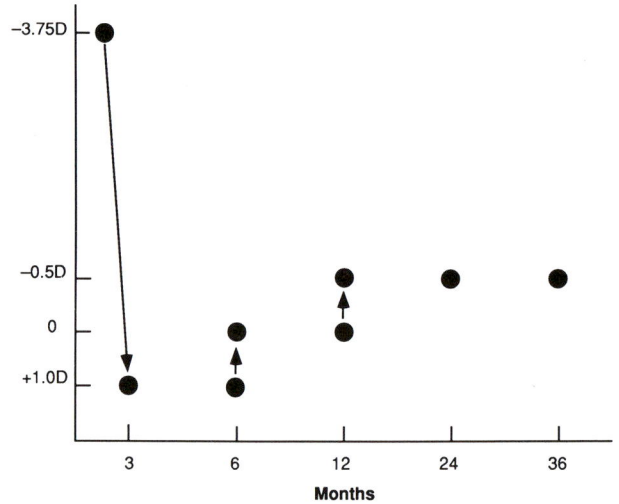

Fig. 15.50 Typical emmetropization pattern. (Courtesy of S.N. Fyodorov.)

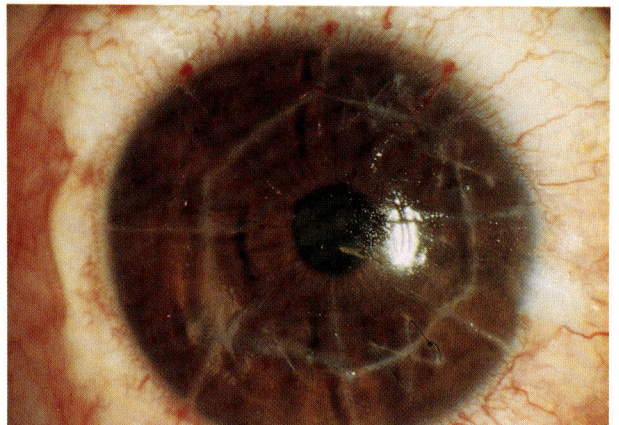

Fig. 15.51 Hexagonal procedure over RK. Despite a delay of
8 months between procedures the incision junctions
required suturing to reduce fluctuation of vision and
gross over-correction (too much myopia).

medication. Furthermore, not all normal subjects will
respond to beta-blockers with a reduction in intra-
ocular pressure. Such response as there is will be
variable. However, if there are no contraindications, it
may be worth trying.

Hexagonal incisions (HK) have been advocated for
over-corrections of up to 4 D of hyperopia [30,31].
The author has used a hexagonal pattern of 6 mm in
diameter for hyperopia of up to 1.75 D. While recovery
of vision is rapid it is often unstable. In these cases it is
necessary that the hex sides join or cross the radials. In
such cases, the objectionable gaping which usually
accompanies small-diameter hexes is often seen, requiring suturing (Figure 15.51). Splitting of the junction of the transverse and radial incisions has occurred
even after 1 year. Consequently, a minimum of 6
months (preferably more) should elapse before these

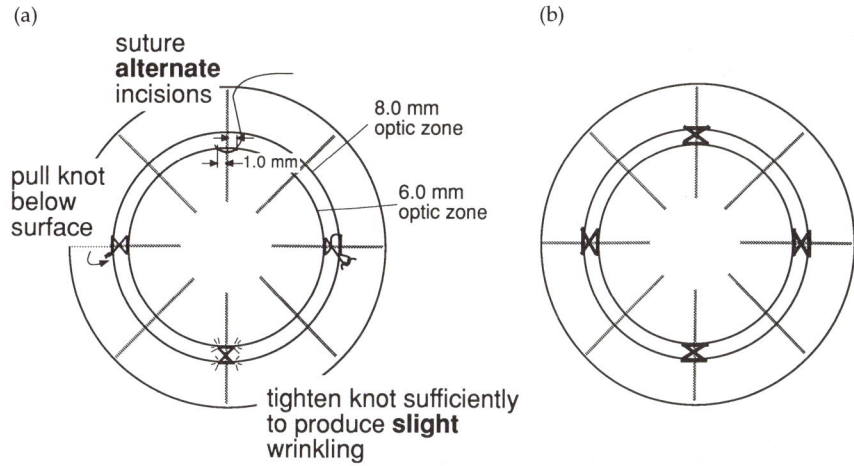

Fig. 15.52 (a and b) X-type sutures are placed symmetrically to steepen the cornea, thereby reducing induced hyperopia.

incisions are made to avoid gaping at the interstices. However, despite initial and favorable reports of the hexagonal procedure over RK, the author does not recommend that this technique be used in RK over-responders (see Chapter 14).

Likewise, the author does not recommend the use of thermokeratoplasty advocated by Schacher [32]. Placing the burns in the RK incisions results in a variable outcome often associated with induced astigmatism. This occurs because denaturation of the scar tissue does not appear to be a uniform process and scarring is often much greater than anticipated. Placing the burns between radial incisions often leads to splitting or widening of the adjacent incisions. Such splitting or widening also results in unpredictable astigmatism, sometimes of the irregular variety.

Recently the author has employed the method of hyperopic lamellar keratotomy, performed with the Barraquer microkeratome to correct induced hyperopia. By making a section of at least 80% in depth and by varying the diameter of the disk of tissue excised, hyperopia of up to 6 D has been predictably

reversed. The procedure has the advantage that the cornea has not been materially weakened, as is the case in hexagonal keratotomy. A non-torquing, 14-point suture is emplaced at the time of surgery and is removed within 7–14 days. The incidence of induced astigmatism is low. Since no freezing or lathing is involved, visual recovery is rapid (see Chapter 10 for a detailed description of this technique).

In cases of reversal of the astigmatism where the axis has rotated 90°, other methods must be used. This complication is mostly seen in cases where trapezoidal keratotomy (Ruiz procedure) has been used. Invariably, the T-incisions are found to be too long or gape during healing, producing wide, soft scars. The recommended approach is to strip out the old scar and suture it tightly closed with one or two X-type sutures of 10-0 nylon (Figure 15.52a). The sutures must be placed symmetrically, one on each side of the optic center—otherwise gaping may occur in the unsutured T-cut. The sutures close the gap and reduce the chord length, consequently increasing corneal steepening in that meridian.

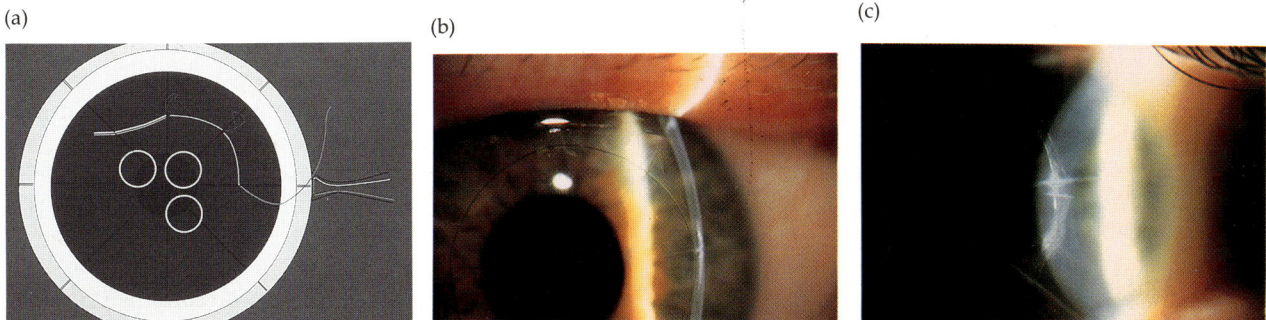

Fig. 15.53 (a) Method of placing the purse string suture. (b) Suture in place in a human cornea. (c) Cheese-wiring is inevitable as the suture ligature takes a natural curved position within the stroma. (Courtesy of Robert Hoffman.)

Such sutures placed at the ends of long T-cuts effectively shorten them and can reduce coupling and, at least theoretically, flatten the opposite meridian. The author prefers not to rely on theory and suggests employing the clinically proven method of suturing the incision in the flat meridian as described above, one pair at a time.

The same basic procedure can be employed to correct spherical over-corrections. In these cases, three or four X-type sutures of 10-0 nylon (Ethicon CUM-5 or similar) are symmetrically placed across the radial incision. These are placed between a 6 and 8 mm optical zone mark made on the cornea in the usual fashion and the knots pulled below the corneal surface (Figure 15.52b). The sutures are tightened sufficiently to produce very slight striations to appear around the suture. These are best seen if the cornea is dry. An over-correction of mild degree is the norm. This reverts within 7–10 days. Sometimes it is necessary to remove and replace sutures that are too tight or loose. These can be removed in 9–12 months but if the patient is comfortable the author leaves them in.

Starling and Hoffman have advocated the use of purse string intrastromal sutures as a way of reducing induced hyperopia (Figure 15.53a,b) [33]. Such a suture is technically difficult to place and inevitably results in some "cheese-wiring" with resultant loss of effect and induced scarring (Figure 15.53c). While no cases of erosion of this suture into the anterior chamber have as yet been reported, the possibility of such a complication exists, particularly if the suture is drawn too tightly.

As always, the best treatment of any complication is prevention. Educated guesswork and making surgical decisions using tables based on one or two preoperative parameters is not the best way to optimize this surgery for each patient. Only the use of computer programs employing algorithms derived from regressive analysis of actual cases can be relied upon to correlate the numerous parameters required for the successful outcome of this surgery.

Neo-vascularization

The author was the first to report the occurrence of this complication following the use of a soft contact lens immediately after surgery to stabilize the cornea (Figure 15.54) [34]. These cases are evidenced by vessels running along incisions in the superficial part of the scar [18]. Typically the encroachment is no more than 1 mm central to the capillary arcade. However, one case has occurred in which the vessels reached the edge of the optical zone (Figure 15.55; S.N. Fyodorov, 1990, personal communication). There have been few reported cases of neo-vascularization after RK except those associated with early contact

lens wearing [2]. With the exception of the one case reported by Fyodorov, all have responded to removal of the lenses and the application of topical steroids. All patients have eventually been able to wear contact lenses on a limited basis (W. Myers, 1988, personal communication).

Neo-vascularization is not inherent in the procedure of RK even in cases where incisions crossed the limbus. Except for some conjunctival "peaks" (Figures 15.56 and 15.57), in the absence of some inciting factor, neo-vascularization does not occur. The author has performed RK in two cases of superior limbic pannus after performing superficial keratectomies of the pannus. The pannus has not recurred nor has there been any evidence of new vessel growth in the area.

Infection

Fortunately this is a rare problem, possibly because we have tended to be cautious in our follow-up, placing all patients on antibiotic drops following the surgery and covering, with oral antibiotics (in some cases sub-Tenon's injection), those patients in whom perforations have occurred. It is also a rare happening undoubtedly because we are dealing with young healthy eyes whose tear complex is alive and well. Still the occasional infection does occur and ranges from small areas of epithelialitis to frank endophthalmitis. In 1982, Gelender and associates reported a case of endophthalmitis immediately following RK in a patient in whom a perforation into the anterior chamber had occurred and who had not been placed on antibiotics [35]. Fortunately that eye was saved by timely intervention with antibiotics and eventually a vitrectomy-lensectomy. At last report this eye had recovered a corrected visual acuity of 20/30.

Another patient was not so fortunate, developing an endophthalmitis 24 hours after surgery. Despite timely intervention, the eye was lost—surely not an expected sequela. Another patient developed a corneal infection approximately 1 month post-RK following a hairbrush injury. This infection went on to become a frank endophthalmitis without subsequent loss of the eye.

Deep intra-stromal keratitis was reported in three cases by Nirankari and colleagues, in 1983 (Figure 15.58) [36]. One of these cases was later shown to have had a history of previous herpetic keratitis. All of these eyes sustained a profound loss of vision (<20/200) associated with the onset of central stromal clouding some 3–4 months post-RK. All cases eventually responded to topical steroid therapy over an 8–10-week period with no recurrence reported to date. For this reason, any eye in which previous herpes keratitis has been documented or suspected is not considered a candidate for this surgery [37,38].

Several cases of localized disease seemingly limited

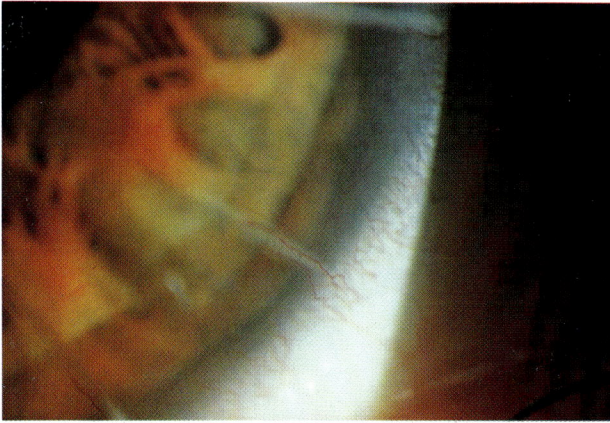

Fig. 15.54 First case of neo-vascularization reported after RK.

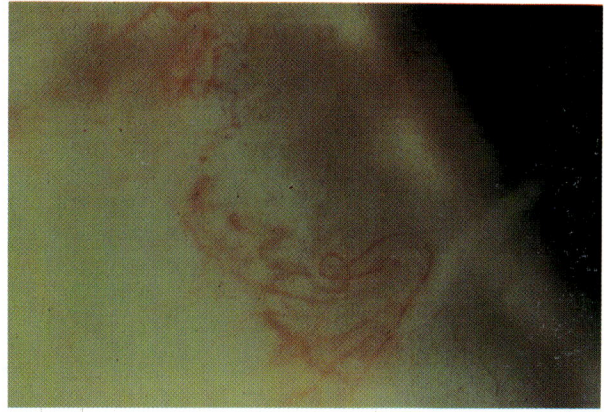

Fig. 15.57 Pseudo-pterygium after RK.

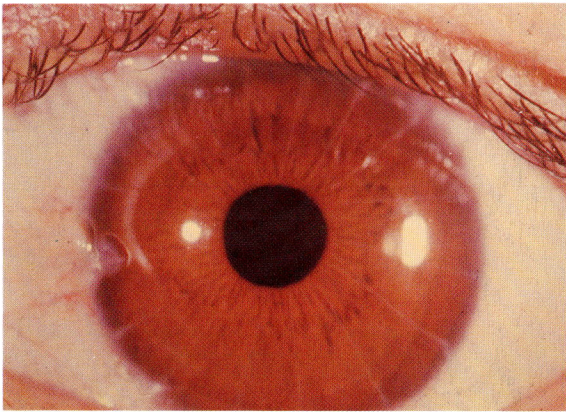

Fig. 15.55 Another, more advanced, case of neo-vascularization.

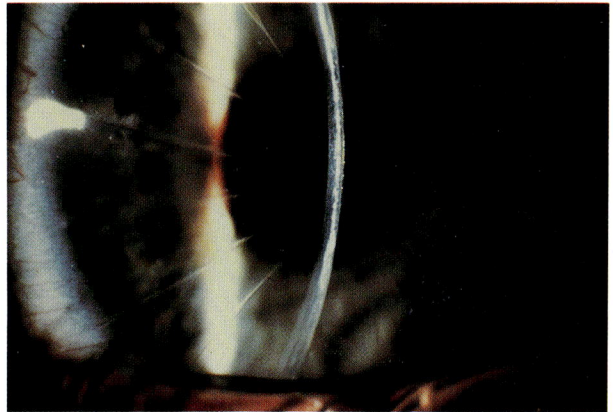

Fig. 15.58 Stromal reaction following RK in a patient with history of herpes keratitis. (Courtesy of M. Dietz.)

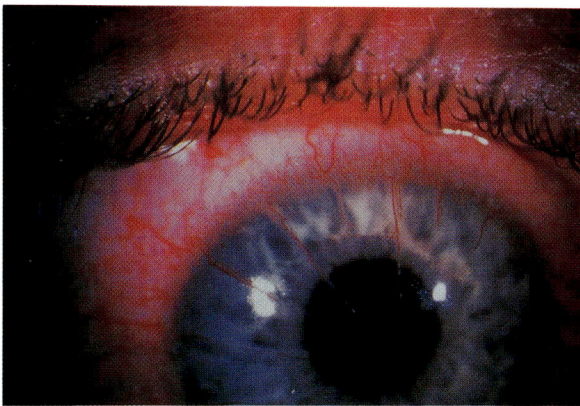

Fig. 15.56 Corneal limbal ''peak'' appearing when incisions cross the limbus.

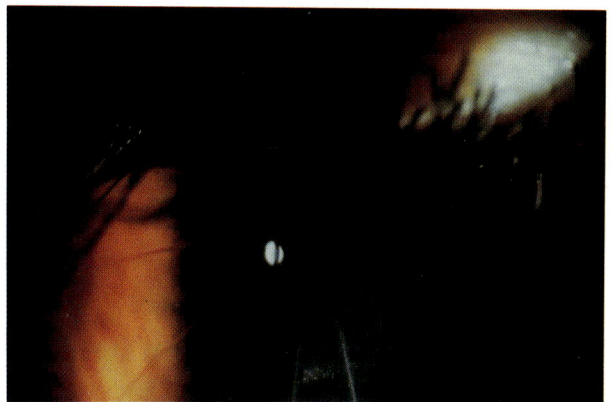

Fig. 15.59 Epithelial reaction at optical zone mark post-RK.

to the epithelium have been seen. Some of these occur as persistent optical clear zone marks, implying that the marker has either damaged the basement membrane or implanted some foreign substance (Figure 15.59). Other times the inflammatory process lies

between the incisions and filaments may develop (Figure 15.60).

Fyodorov and Durnev have reported a case of staphylococcal corneal ulcer occurring in an incision following a re-operation (Figure 15.61) [39]. This

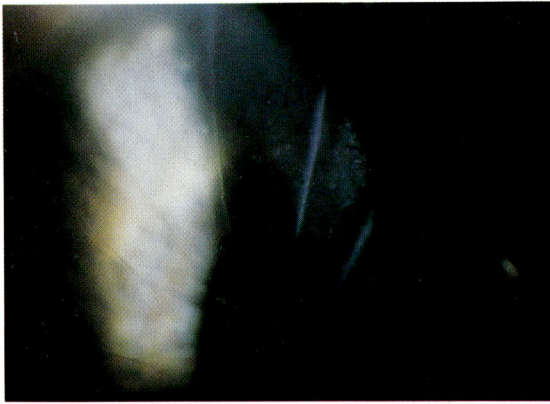

Fig. 15.60 Epithelialitis with a filament following RK.

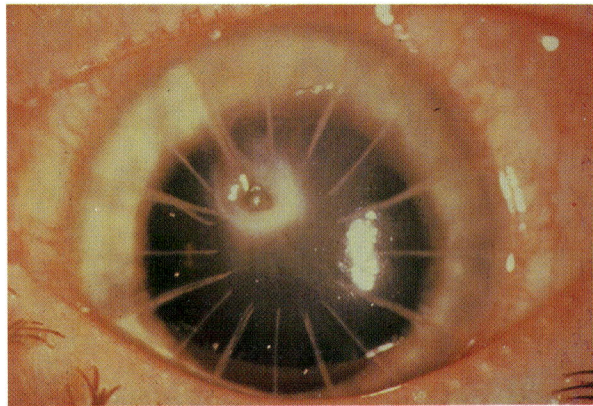

Fig. 15.61 Staphylococcal corneal ulcer.

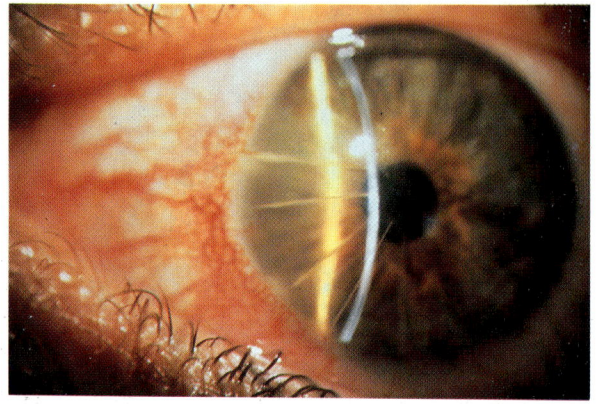

Fig. 15.62 Sterile keratitis surrounding an RK incision (from Geggel H. Delayed sterile keratitis following radial keratotomy requiring corneal transplantation for visual rehabilitation. Refract Corneal Surg 1990; 6:55–58).

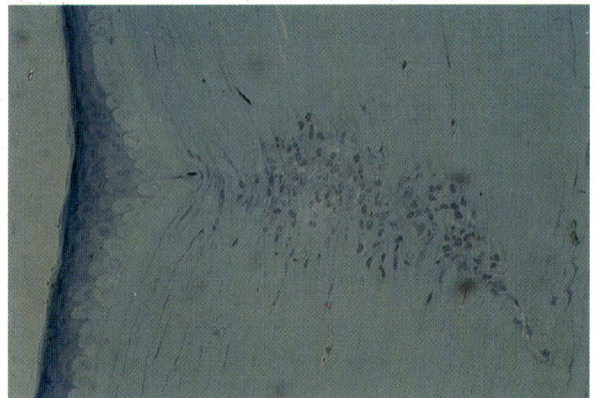

Fig. 15.63 Histologic section of incision area. (Courtesy of H. Geggel.)

patient responded to antibiotics and debridement but was left with a wide scar, causing increased glare. No astigmatism resulted and the visual acuity was said to have returned to 20/25.

Iritis beyond a few cells with a trace of cells is unusual in this surgery but of course hypopyon has been reported in the presence of corneal ulcers.

The PERK study has reported on two cases of post-operative intra-corneal abscesses, occurring some 2 years after the initial surgery. All eventually responded to conventional therapy as well [40–42]. Geggel reported a case of sterile keratitis which eventually required a penetrating keratoplasty (Figures 15.62 through 15.65). The author has also seen one case in which an intra-incisional abscess formed approximately 3 years post-RK. Topical antibiotics cleared the infection within 3 days on Ciloxan (topical ciprofloxacin; Figures 15.65 and 15.66). Since then two other cases have appeared, one occurring at 5 years, and the other at 7 years post-surgery (Figures 15.68 and 15.69). This can also occur in other forms of relaxing incisions (Figure 15.70).

It is obvious, since the majority of these cases involve the incisions initially, that the scar formed after

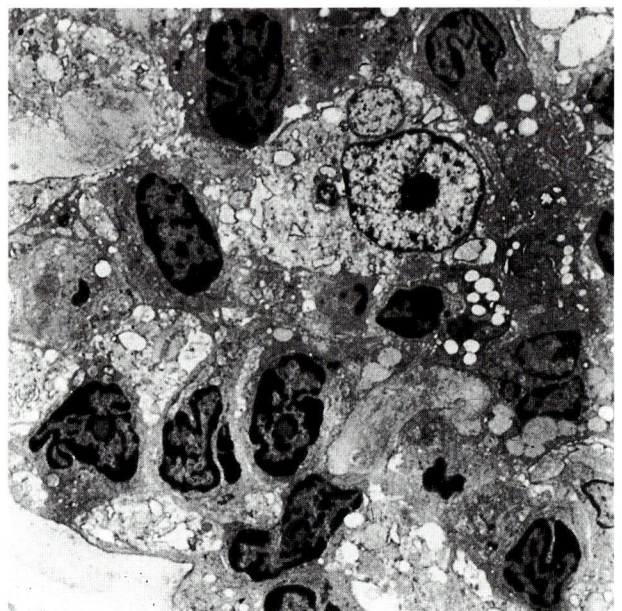

Fig. 15.64 Microscopic smear of the exudate. Note the absence of micro-organisms. (Courtesy of H. Geggel.)

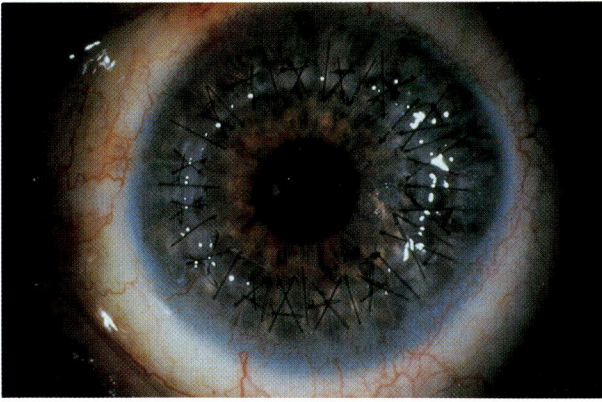

Fig. 15.65 Keratoplasty following a case of sterile keratitis. Note the use of X-type sutures to prevent incisions opening. (Courtesy of H. Geggel.)

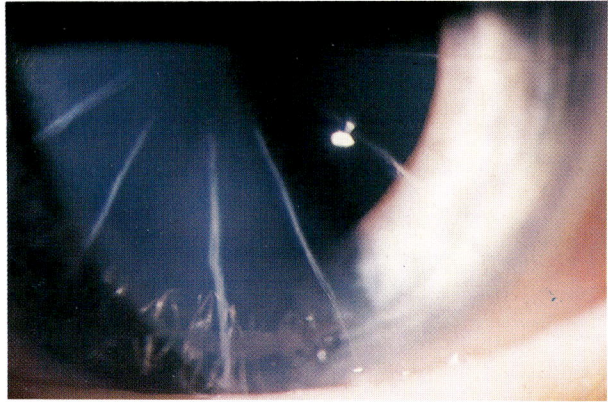

Fig. 15.68 Bacterial keratitis occurring 7 years after RK.

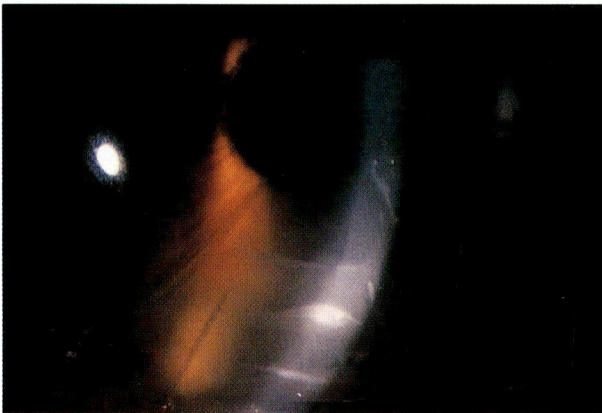

Fig. 15.66 Bacterial keratitis occurring 3 years after RK.

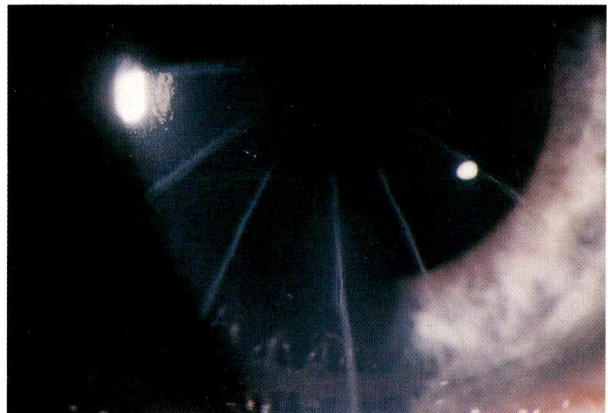

Fig. 15.69 Same case after 48 hours of treatment with ciprofloxacin.

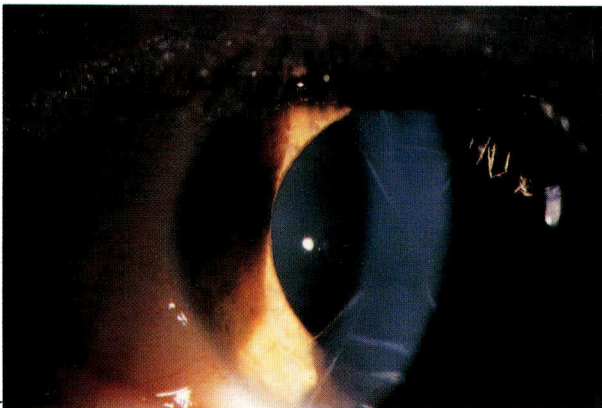

Fig. 15.67 Same case 72 hours after treatment with ciprofloxacin.

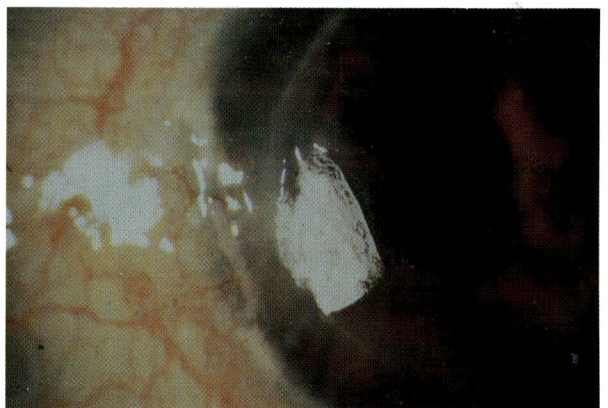

Fig. 15.70 Bacterial ulcer in a post-PKP relaxing incision.

an incision of this type is soft and offers little resistance to invasion for some years. It has been suggested that the epithelium over RK scars is somehow abnormal and perhaps more susceptible to the occurrence of infection (see Chapter 4). How this can be has never

been adequately explained, nor why these incisions should differ markedly from lacerations or PKP scars. However, there does appear to be, at least initially, disturbance of the corneal wetting mechanism post-RK [43]. While the BUT seems to return to normal in most

Table 15.5 Micro-organisms and their sensitivity to antibiotics

	Ampicillin	Bacitracin	Cefamandole	Cefazolin	Chloramphenicol	Ciprofloxacin	Clindamycin	Erythromycin	Gentamicin	Methicillin	Moxalactam	Neomycin	Norfloxacin	Penicillin G	Piperacillin	Polymyxin B	Rifampin	Sulfonamides	Tetracyclines	Tobramycin	Trimethoprim/ sulfamethoxazole	Vancomycin
Gram-positive cocci																						
Staphylococcus epidermidis	±	+	+	+	±	+	±	±	+	P	+	±	+	±	±	−	±	±	±	+	+	+
Staphylococcus aureus	−	+	+	+	±	+	±	±	+	P	+	±	+	−	−	−	±	±	±	+	+	+
Methicillin-resistant *Staph. aureus*	−	+	−	−	0	+	−	−	±	−	−	0	+	−	−	−	±	0	0	±	0	+
α-Hemolytic *Streptococcus*	+	+	+	+	+	+	+	+	−	+	+	−	0	P	+	−	−	±	±	−	+	+
β-Hemolytic *Streptococcus*	+	+	+	+	+	±	+	+	−	+	+	−	0	P	+	−	+	−	±	−	+	+
Streptococcus faecalis	P	+	−	−	0	±	−	−	P	±	−	−	+	P	+	−	0	±	±	P	±	+
Streptococcus pneumoniae	+	+	+	+	+	+	+	+	−	+	+	−	+	P	+	−	+	±	±	−	+	+
Anaerobic *Streptococcus* sp.*	±	+	+	+	+	−	+	+	−	±	+	−	0	P	+	0	0	0	±	−	0	0
Gram-positive bacilli																						
Bacillus anthracis	0	+	±	±	+	0	0	+	0	0	±	0	0	P	0	−	+	0	+	0	0	+
Bacillus sp.	0	+	0	−	+	0	0	+	P	0	0	0	0	0	±	0	−	0	0	0	P	0
Clostridium sp.	0	±	±	±	±	−	±	±	−	0	±	−	0	P	±	−	+	0	±	−	0	P
Corynebacterium sp.	±	+	+	−	0	0	0	+	0	0	0	0	0	P	0	−	+	0	0	0	0	P
Listeria monocytogenes	P	0	0	−	+	0	0	+	0	0	0	0	0	0	±	0	−	0	0	+	0	0
Gram-negative cocci																						
Neisseria gonorrhoeae	P	+	±	−	+	+	+	+	±	±	+	+	+	P	+	−	+	−	P	±	0	−
Neisseria meningitidis	+	+	±	−	+	+	+	+	±	±	0	+	0	P	+	−	+	−	+	±	0	−
Gram-negative bacilli																						
Actinobacter sp.	−	−	−	−	0	0	0	−	P	−	0	0	0	−	+	+	0	0	±	P	+	−
*Bacteroides fragilis**	−	0	−	−	P	−	P	−	−	−	±	−	0	−	±	−	0	0	−	−	−	−
Bacteroides sp.*	±	0	±	−	+	−	+	+	−	−	+	−	0	P	±	−	0	0	±	−	−	−
Bordetella pertussis	0	0	0	0	0	0	0	P	0	−	0	0	0	0	0	0	0	0	0	0	+	−
Brucella sp.	0	0	0	0	+	0	0	+	0	−	0	0	0	0	0	0	+	P	0	−	0	−
Citrobacter sp.	0	0	±	0	0	0	0	0	P	0	+	0	0	0	+	+	0	0	0	P	+	−
Enterobacter sp.	±	0	±	−	+	0	−	−	P	−	+	±	+	−	+	+	0	±	±	P	+	−
Escherichia coli	±	0	+	±	+	+	−	−	P	−	+	+	+	−	+	+	±	±	±	P	+	−
Francisella tularensis	0	0	0	0	P	0	0	0	0	−	0	0	0	0	0	0	0	0	P	0	0	−
Haemophilus influenzae	P	+	±	−	P	+	+	±	±	−	+	±	+	±	±	+	±	+	±	±	+	−
Klebsiella sp.	−	0	+	±	+	0	−	−	P	−	+	+	+	−	+	+	+	−	±	P	+	−
Moraxella sp.	+	0	±	±	0	0	0	+	±	−	+	+	0	P	+	+	0	+	0	±	+	−
Pasteurella multocida	0	0	0	−	0	+	0	0	0	−	0	0	0	P	+	+	0	0	+	0	+	−
Proteus mirabilis	±	−	±	±	±	+	−	−	P	−	+	+	+	−	+	−	+	±	−	P	+	−
Proteus sp. (indole-positive)	−	−	±	−	±	+	−	−	P	−	+	+	+	−	+	−	+	−	±	P	+	−
Pseudomonas aeruginosa	−	−	−	−	−	+	−	−	P	−	±	±	+	−	P	+	±	−	±	P	−	−
Salmonella sp.	P	−	0	−	P	0	0	−	+	−	+	0	0	±	+	+	0	−	0	+	+	−
Serratia sp.	−	0	−	−	±	+	−	−	P	−	+	+	0	−	+	−	0	−	−	P	+	−
Shigella sp.	P	−	0	−	+	0	0	−	0	−	+	0	0	±	+	+	0	−	±	0	+	−
Others																						
Actinomyces sp.*	+	+	±	±	+	0	+	0	−	0	0	−	0	P	0	0	0	±	+	−	0	+
Chlamydia trachomatis	−	0	0	0	±	+	0	P	−	−	0	−	0	−	−	0	±	P	P	−	+	−
Mycobacterium fortuitum	0	0	0	0	0	0	0	+	0	0	0	0	0	0	0	0	−	−	P	0	0	−
Mycobacterium marinum	0	0	0	0	0	0	0	0	0	0	0	0	0	0	0	0	+	−	P	0	+	−
Nocardia sp.*	+	0	0	0	0	0	0	0	0	0	0	0	0	0	0	0	0	P	+	0	+	0
Toxoplasma gondii	−	−	−	−	−	0	+	−	−	−	−	−	0	−	−	−	0	±	−	−	+	−

+, Sensitive; −, resistant; ±, variable sensitivity; 0, no information; P, drug of choice or commonly used drug; *, anaerobes.
Table compiled by R.A. Hyndiuk, and R.W. Snyder—07/13/91

cases the author has examined, it is possible that this might play a role in allowing an invading organism a foothold. It is evident that the appearance of iron lines in these corneas is somewhat higher than the general population; thus it could be that the mechanism is simply that of a sufficiently irregular surface for organisms to adhere to [44]. Whatever the mechanism might be, it is evident that these patients may be at slightly greater risk for infection and should be advised accordingly.

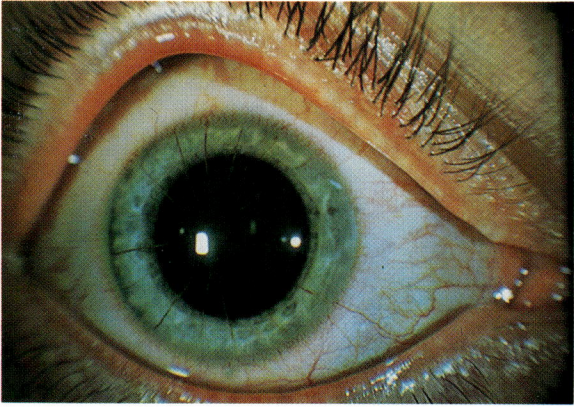

Fig. 15.71 Leaving blood in the incisions can lead to difficulty later on.

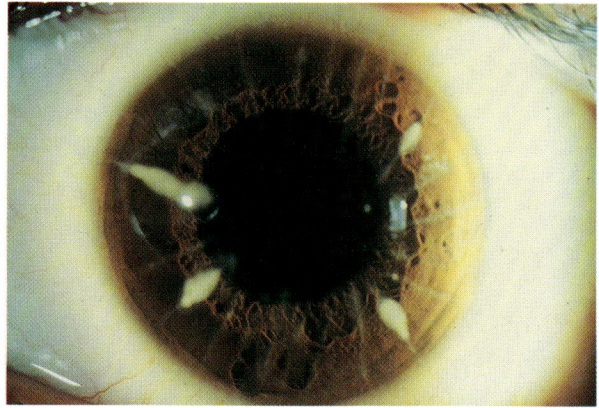

Fig. 15.72 Lipoid deposits appearing where red blood cells were not irrigated from the incisions.

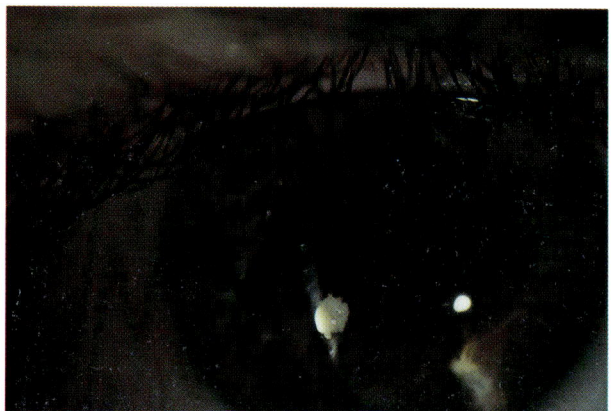

Fig. 15.73 Close-up of these lipoid deposits.

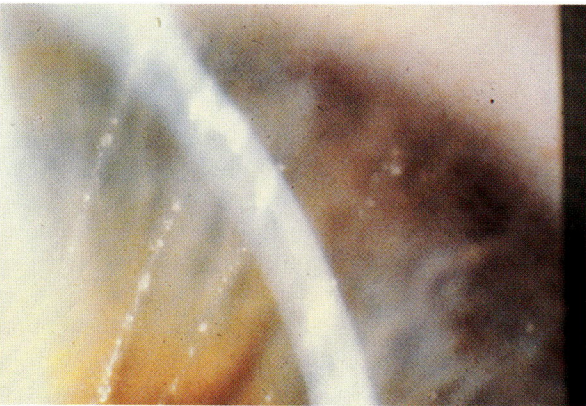

Fig. 15.74 Giant intra-incisional lipid deposit. (Courtesy of S.N. Fyodorov.)

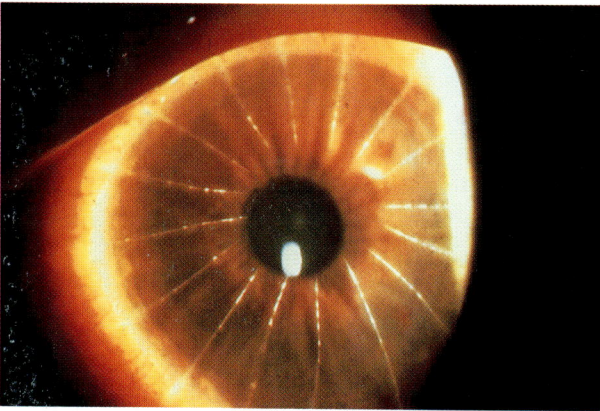

Fig. 15.75 Giant lipid deposit in an RK wound.

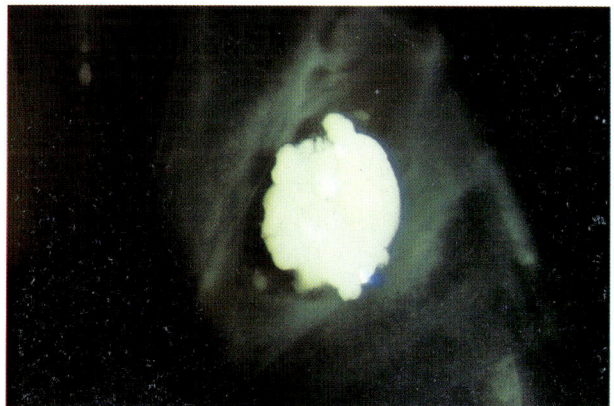

Fig. 15.76 Close-up of the lesion.

Table 15.5 is an antibiotic susceptibility table for a number of frequently encountered micro-organisms, current as of July 13th, 1991.

Intra-incisional opacities

These have been reported with decreasing frequency as more attention has been paid to post-surgical incision irrigation and the practice of keeping the cornea dry during surgery [45]. If blood is left within the incisions it is possible that the keratocytes will break it down into refractile lipid deposits. Generally these are unsightly but pose no problem. Occasionally it has been found necessary to remove these deposits with a sharp blade to reduce the glare that they can produce. Sometimes they can become quite large (Figures 15.71 through 15.77). If air is left within the

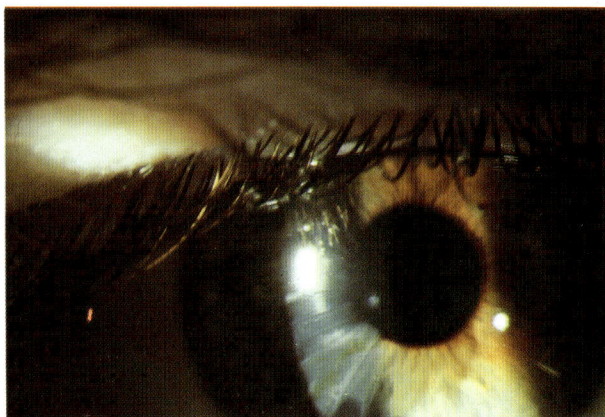

Fig. 15.77 Cornea after removal of the deposit. Note the shallow pocket remaining.

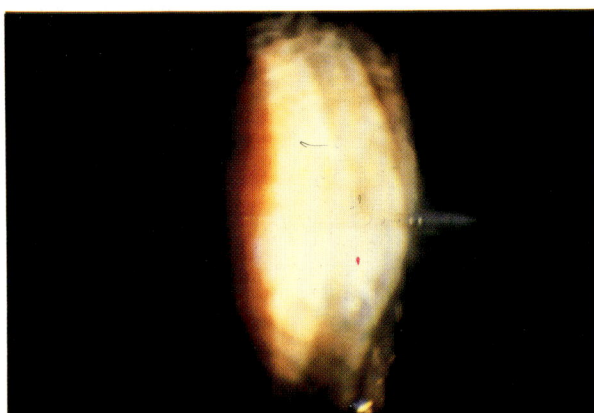

Fig. 15.78 Air-filled incisional "cyst" after RK.

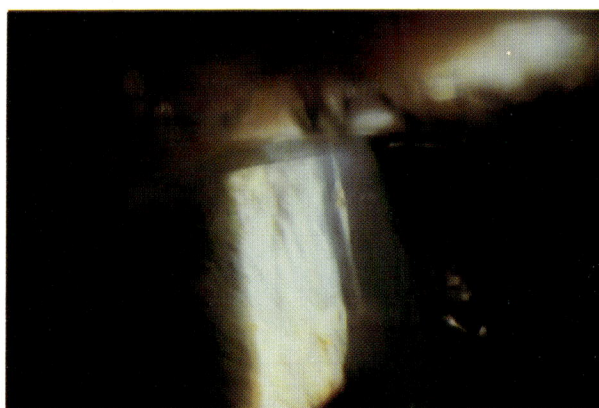

Fig. 15.79 Foreign body in an RK incision.

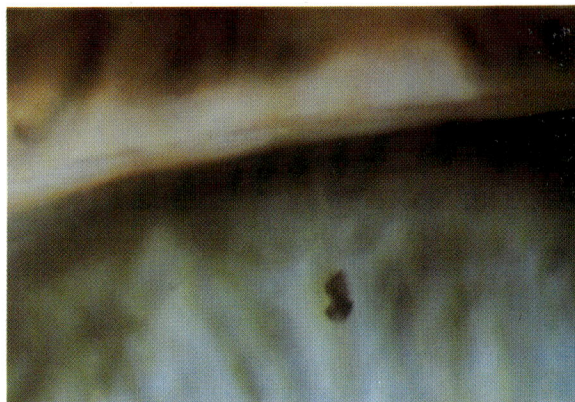

Fig. 15.80 Close-up of the intruder which turned out to be mascara.

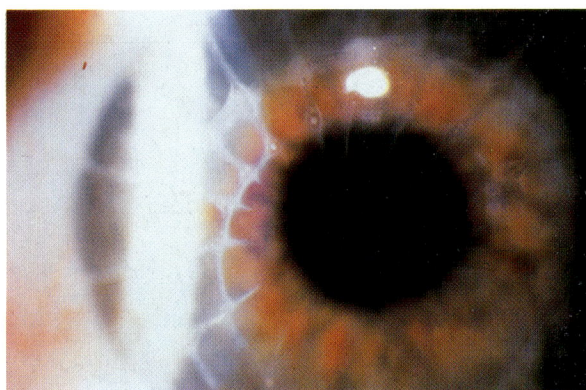

Fig. 15.81 Circular-radial keratotomy. This case resulted in marsupialization of the wounds, a "flail" cornea, and increased myopia. (Courtesy of R. Villasenor.)

Marsupialization

This very rare phenomenon has been reported only in conjunction with circular-radial keratotomy (and recently with the Mendez operation) [46]. Some numbers of these cases were performed on patients, with the result that large gaps appeared between incisions, particularly at crossing points, which then became lined with epithelium, producing small blind pockets or pouches (Figures 15.81 through 15.83). In addition, the myopia was found to have increased in all cases, along with extreme fluctuation of the vision through the day.

This is a potential problem with any incision that crosses another. The intersected area retracts, sometimes producing large gaps which then become only partially filled with the normal muco-epithelial plug. Sometimes the tips of the incision will be lost in the repair process, further increasing the gap to be filled. Retraction of this scar will, in time, induce localized flattening with the potential of creating irregular astigmatism.

wounds, encysted areas will result (Figure 15.78). These collapse in time but may need to be assisted by decompressing them with a needle tip. Rarely, meibomian secretions as well as other things can find their way into a partially open incision (Figures 15.79 and 15.80). These may have to be excised as well.

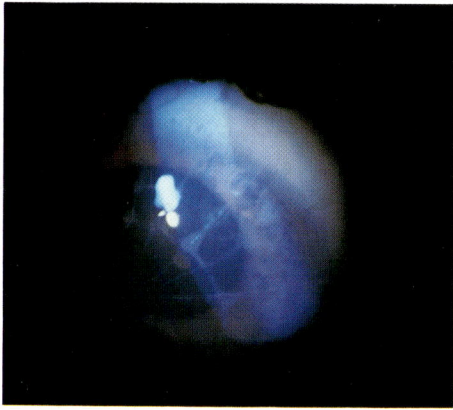

Fig. 15.82 Note the rings of dye demonstrating how tears are pumped out of the pockets with each heart beat. (Courtesy of R. Villasenor.)

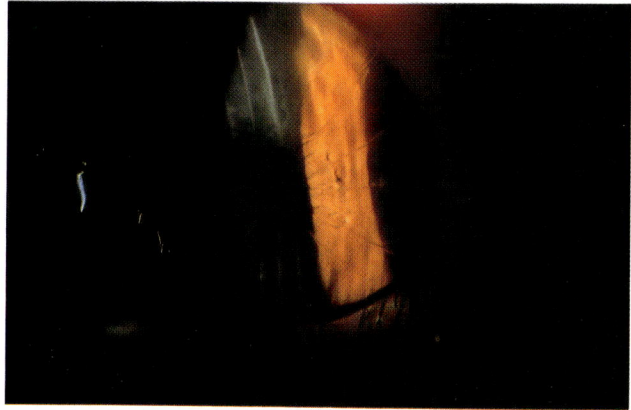

Fig. 15.85 Pseudo-bullous keratopathy. This wound communicates with the anterior chamber. The bullae are caused by aqueous under the epithelium.

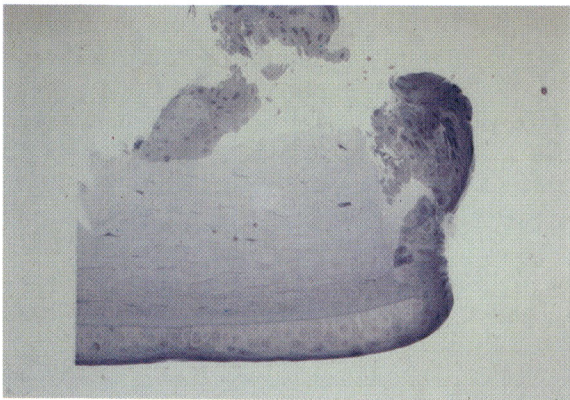

Fig. 15.83 Histologic section of one of the pockets showing marsupialization. (Courtesy of R. Villasenor.)

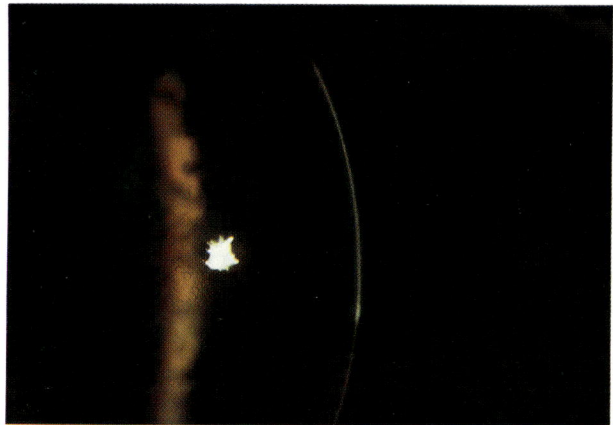

Fig. 15.86 Small area of true bullous keratopathy—the only known case following RK.

Endothelial cell loss

Recent studies have shown no significant endothelial cell loss following RK surgery—unlike that seen in the Sato operation (Figure 15.84). Earlier reports of as much as 22% cells lost were later shown to be instances clearly related to excess trauma during the performance of the surgery. Another report was later found to have been counted incorrectly. Endothelial effects demonstrated related to surgery in monkey eyes have not been duplicated in humans [2,47].

Micro-bullous keratopathy

Persistent micro-bullous keratopathy has not been reported with this surgery to date. The author has had five cases of localized microbullous keratopathy following RK surgery in older patients, however (Figures 15.85 and 15.86). In all cases the endothelial cell counts showed no significant cell loss post-RK with an initial count in the normal range for the age. In each

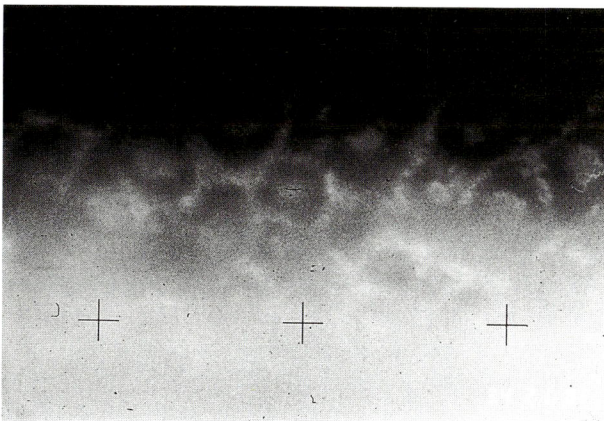

Fig. 15.84 Endothelial microscope picture of one of Sato's cases. (Courtesy of A. Momose.)

Therefore, any procedure that requires that incisions cross should be done in two stages with at least 6 months allowed to elapse between stages. In the Ruiz procedure the radial incisions should not connect with the interior ladders for the same reason.

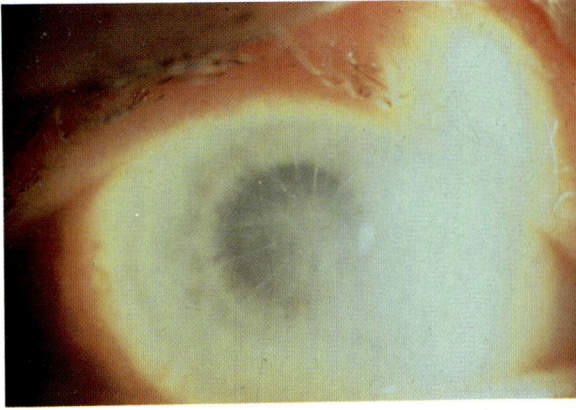

Fig. 15.87 Corneal decompensation in an eye with a history of interstitial keratitis and shallow incisions, immediately post-surgery.

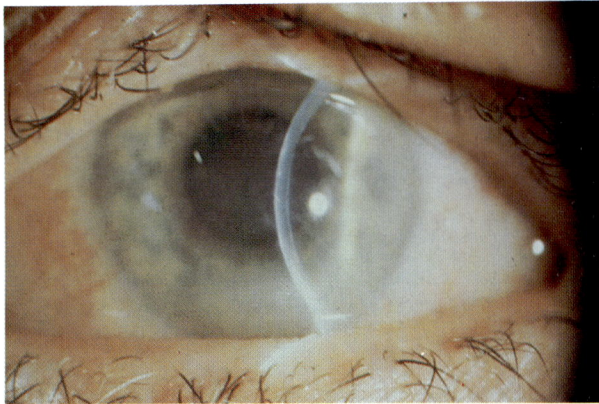

Fig. 15.88 Same eye as above, 5 months post-surgery.

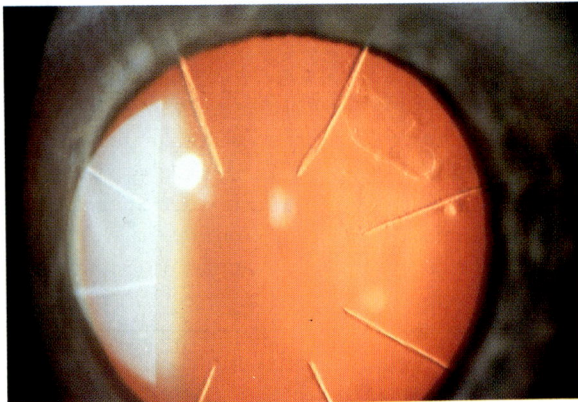

Fig. 15.89 Map-dot corneal changes supposedly not present before the RK.

case the patients had prominent arcus senilis with some increase in corneal shagreen pre-operatively but no epithelial abnormalities. All cases were high myopes requiring triple-step procedures, with three having had free-hand deepening. Two had self-sealing

micro-perforations. All cases cleared spontaneously within 2 weeks and none have shown any sequelae. One case required a second-stage procedure but did not demonstrate a recurrence of the micro-bullous keratopathy.

No cases of decompensation of the cornea as a result of this surgery have been reported to date. However, it is possible that the application of this technique to corneas that are unhealthy could precipitate such a calamity. An example of what can happen in a case having normal endothelium but abnormal epithelium and/or stroma has been demonstrated experimentally on a human volunteer (Figures 15.87 and 15.88).

Recurrent corneal erosion

Epithelial defects associated with basement membrane disease—such as recurrent corneal erosion and map-fingerprint-dot changes—have been reported following RK [28,48]. It is unclear what mechanism would account for the appearance of map-dot changes—the one case can be seen to exist between incisions (Figure 15.89). No note was made whether or not stripping of epithelium had occurred during surgery. As to the recurrent erosions, these are often associated with foreign material embedded in Bowman's layer, which probably explains why many respond to mechanical or chemical debridement. Some of the micro-wipes used in RK surgery are notorious for leaving behind particles of cellulose or other material. Perhaps such detritus is responsible for the incomplete detachment of the epithelium in these cases.

Corneal rupture

Numerous cases of severe trauma occurring to eyes at various periods post-operatively have been reported following RK [49–57]. One such case involved a direct hit from a racket ball in an eye 1 month post-surgery. The patient sustained a mild hyphema and a recession of the angle [56]. There was a transient decrease in visual acuity secondary to an associated corneal abrasion. No incisions were found to have opened and the anterior chamber remained full and deep with no evidence of leakage or secondary glaucoma.

On the other hand, a female patient 18 months post-RK was thrown through the windshield of an automobile during an accident, sustaining severe head trauma. The cornea of one eye was found to have ruptured along the 12 to 6 o'clock meridian in the incisions and ocular contents herniated anteriorly (Figure 15.90). Several of the other incisions were said to have been split as well. The eye was not lost but vision was reduced to Count Fingers. A similar case involved a male approximately 1 year post-RK. Again, the eye was not lost but vision was impaired.

Recently a case of a rupture following a blow from an elbow was reported; the eye was saved. The latest incident involved a case of the author's in which a macro-perforation had occurred during a re-operation; it required suturing. Approximately 3 months after suture removal, the patient was struck in the face by an automobile "half-axle" while repairing his car. The axle fell some 30 cm (12 in) and struck the eye directly. In this instance the previously sutured (but currently unsutured) wound opened and the chamber collapsed. The patient sought consultation after 3 days only because of persistent irritation and mild tearing (Figures 15.91 and 15.92). The unaided visual acuity was 20/60, corrected to 20/20 on the initial visit. Re-suturing of the wound with re-positioning of the iris were accomplished with minimal trauma. The anterior chamber was clear and full by the next day. The patient retains good unaided vision to this day (20/25) and is correctable to 20/20. No lens complications have occurred in this patient to date—2 years post-trauma.

Forstot and Damiano have reported eight cases of ocular trauma following RK in seven accident-prone patients in their own practice; one patient got hit with a tennis ball, twice. All patients retained the same visual acuity post-trauma that they had pre-trauma. Only two of the eight cases received direct injury which opened one incision in each case, resulting in flat chambers. Both of these were 16-incision cases and one incision opened at the site of a micro-perforation. In one of the other cases, the laceration was oblique to the RK incisions [55].

Spivack reported a case in which a woman had received severe facial trauma consequent to a plane crash in which the globes remained intact [57]. That these corneas may be vulnerable for some time is shown by the case reported by McDermott and colleagues. A woman suffered corneal rupture after trauma in an eye that had had RK 10 years previously [51].

Ocular injury accounts for a considerable number of accident cases each year. Visual loss occurs in an appalling number of these. It is obvious that RK does not necessarily predispose the patient to such a sad fate, however. Still, in both rupture cases described by Forstot and Damiano [55], each occurred in eyes that had had 16 incisions. Is this evidence that 16-incision eyes are more vulnerable than those with fewer incisions? Possibly, but both of these cases were in eyes injured within 1 year of the original surgery—one of them at 2 weeks. It is possible that while the shear strength of an eye which has had 16 incisions is less than one with eight or fewer incisions, it is also true that such eyes tend to be easily distorted, thus possibly absorbing the shock of trauma through that distortion.

At least one rupture has been reported follow-

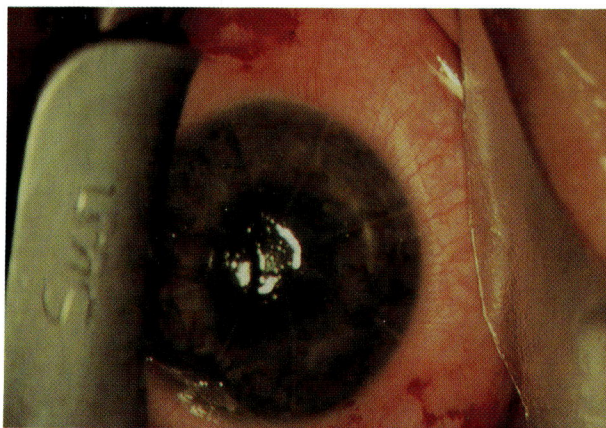

Fig. 15.90 Corneal laceration following blunt trauma (auto accident). The cornea ruptured from limbus to limbus along two RK incisions.

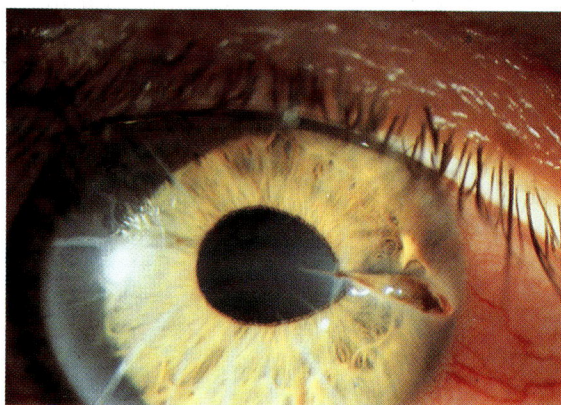

Fig. 15.91 Iris prolapse through RK incision after blunt trauma.

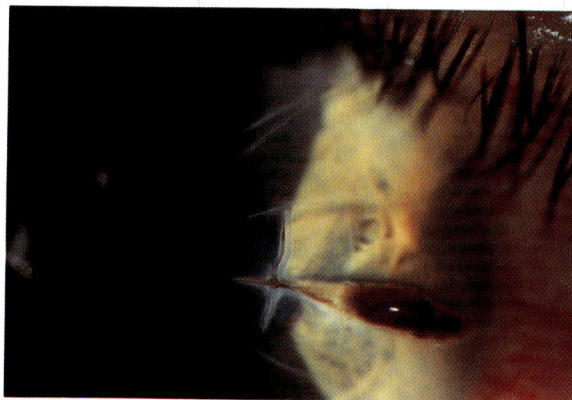

Fig. 15.92 Close-up of the same eye. Note that the chamber is formed. Vision was 20/60, uncorrected before repair.

ing blunt trauma after hexagonal keratotomy [58]. Approximately 6 months after hexagonal keratotomy the patient's left eye collided with a fist. Both nasal and temporal transverse incisions had opened. It was

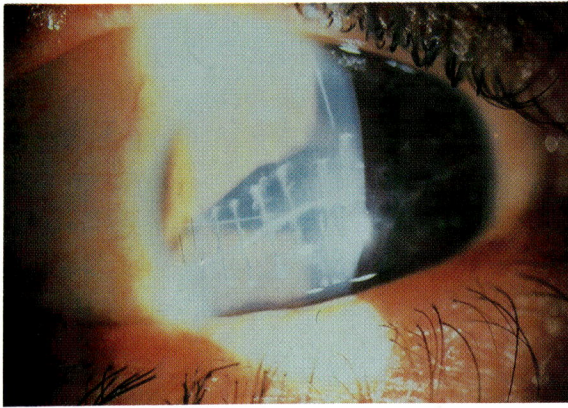

Fig. 15.93 Blunt trauma (auto accident) corneal laceration crossing an RK incision obliquely. (Courtesy of Villasenor.)

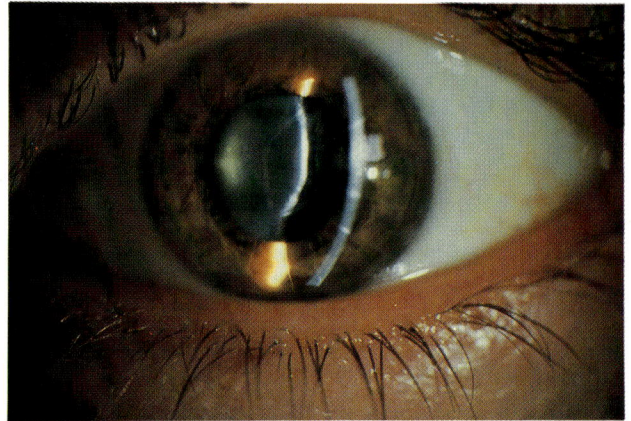

Fig. 15.94 Cataract following surgical trauma during RK. (Courtesy of B. Hewitt.)

noted that incisions at the apices were joined (some overlapped). The patient never regained useful vision in the damaged eye.

Critics of RK have pointed to the work of Larson and associates showing that eyes do not regain normal tensile strength even after 3 months and are prone to rupture along the incisions [59]. This study, while interesting, used rabbit eyes and each eye was subjected to repeated trauma until rupture occurred. Rabbits do not have a Bowman's layer in any event, which adds considerably to the integrity of the human cornea. Thus all we can conclude from this study is that rabbit eyes undergoing RK should not be exposed to repeated blunt trauma. The study of Luttrull *et al.* on the other hand, is more significant [60]. The safety of deep corneal incisions in RK was evaluated in a porcine model. All eyes were subjected to standard blunt trauma. Control eyes ruptured at the equatorial sclera. Eyes with radial incisions cut through approximately 70% of corneal thickness also ruptured at the equator. When incisions of this depth (70%) were extended across the limbus rather than stopping at the corneal–scleral junction, all ruptures occurred at the limbal portion of the incisions—which further reinforces our decision not to carry the incisions across the limbus. Eyes cut 95–100% of corneal thickness tended to rupture at the incisions, as would be expected. However, this tendency in pig eyes does not explain the oblique lacerations in Forstot and Damiano's cases, nor does it explain Figure 15.92, an RK eye which received severe blunt trauma in which the resultant laceration crosses the RK incisions—none of which opened.

Patients in whom transverse incisions cross radials may be more vulnerable to such injury none the less. Karr *et al.* reported persistent wound gape in a patient with just such an incisional pattern [61]. This patient's case was complicated by a sterile keratitis. Girard and colleagues described a patient in whom the

radials re-opened 6 months post-operatively when a circumferential incision was made in an effort to correct post-operative astigmatism [62].

All this means is that RK eyes *may* be vulnerable to trauma and patients should be cautioned. Still, how to explain the author's patient who, 1 month after bilateral RK surgery, completed a free ocean descent with scuba equipment to a depth of 130 m (435 ft)? Despite the enormous pressures to which he was subjected during the dive and the hours spent in the decompression chamber, he experienced only mild, transient blurring of vision upon surfacing. No evidence of ocular injury was found.

Hyphema (not associated with external trauma)

One case is known to have developed a small hyphema post-RK. This is believed to have been caused by one of the incisions perforating at the limbus. The blood cleared spontaneously within 24 hours—no sequelae have been reported (J. Dodick, 1984, personal communication).

Cataract formation

There have been a small number of cases of cataract formation reported to date. Five followed perforation into the anterior chamber (Figures 15.94 through 15.96). Four of these showed frank evidence of direct lens injury ([63], L.D. Bores, 1991, unpublished data). It is presumed that the fifth lens was also injured but no injury site could be unequivocally identified [64]. It is difficult to postulate how entry into the anterior chamber of the blade tip alone without trauma to the lens could produce a cataract in the immediate post-operative period. Unless withdrawal of the blade is instantaneous in the event of a micro-perforation, the chamber can deflate sufficiently to allow contact of the blade tip with the lens capsule. That this can occur

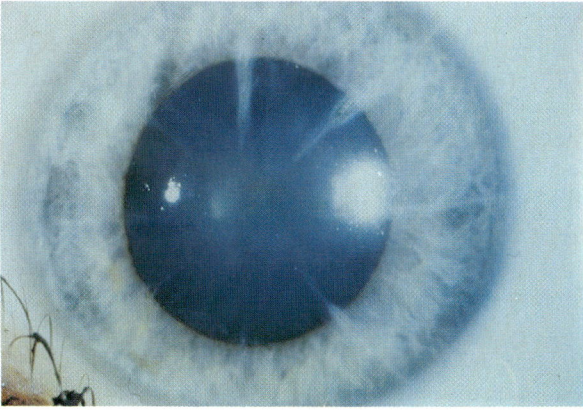

Fig. 15.95 Cataract developing in an eye following presumed intra-surgical lens trauma. (Courtesy of J.I. Barraquer.)

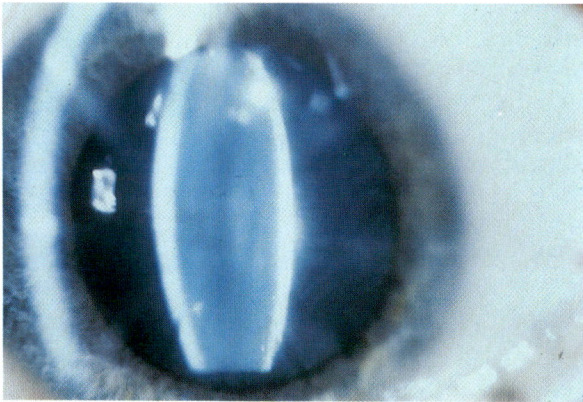

Fig. 15.96 Slit-lamp view of the same eye. (Courtesy of J.I. Barraquer.)

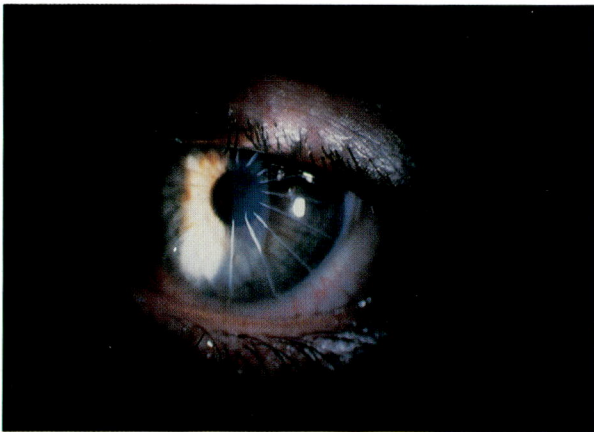

Fig. 15.97 Sixteen-incision RK case 3 months post surgery. (Courtesy of R. Nozik.)

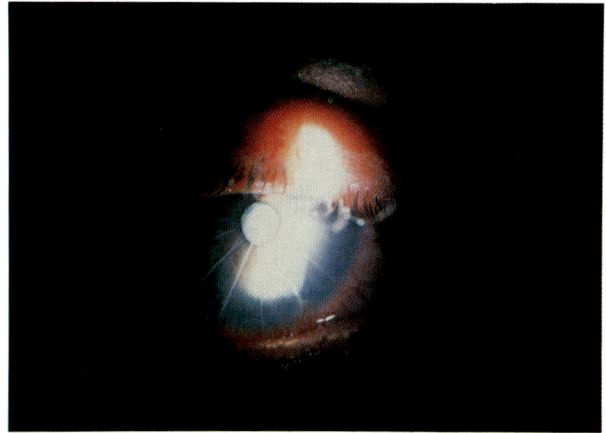

Fig. 15.98 The same eye shortly after having developed phakoanaphylaxis and cataract formation—6 months post-surgery. (Courtesy of R. Nozik.)

without notice of the physician and in the absence of evident lens trauma is borne out by the case of Nozik. In this instance, phakoanaphylaxis occurred in a female patient some considerable time after a 16-incision RK was performed. The surgeon acknowledged that a micro-perforation had occurred but that the chamber had not flattened in any way (Figures 15.97 and 15.98). Care in blade-setting, reduced blade speed, avoidance of manipulation of the incision when the chamber is shallow (free-hand deepening), and an undilated pupil should prevent the occurrence of this major complication.

Two cases of steroid-induced cataract formation have been reported. In each case the surgeon was attempting to enhance the effect of his surgery by inducing an intra-ocular pressure rise with topical steroids [41]. It has not been shown that increasing the intra-ocular pressure above normal has any permanent effect upon the outcome of the surgery; none the less some surgeons persist in this attempt. Because of the serious side-effects reported with long-term topical steroid usage, this method of treating under-correction is not recommended. Additionally, the steroid itself may interfere with the healing process and negate any possible gain. Our experience with the use of steroids at 8 weeks in which the correction was consequently reduced leads us to believe that the hazards of the long-term use of steroids far outweigh their possible benefits. Furthermore, it does not seem logical to induce a disease (glaucoma) in order to cure another (myopia).

Iron (Hudson–Stähli) lines

These areas of small brownish pigment deposits are sometimes seen in the inferior aspect of the optical zone, and are due to pooling of tears admixed with various electrolytes, especially iron (Figure 15.99 [44, 65–67]. They are less often seen with well-irrigated incisions and do not appear to degrade vision. They do not progress but may be quite large. Such lines have

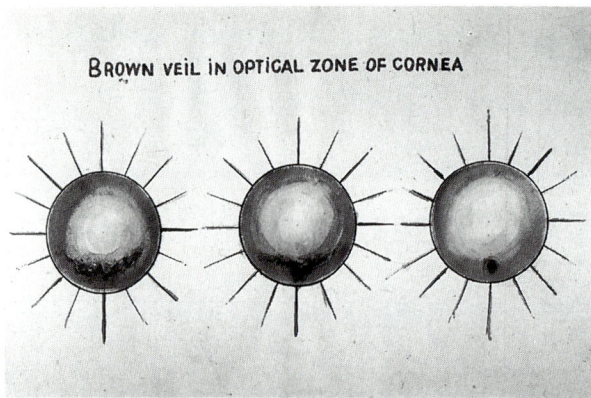

Fig. 15.99 Hudson–Stähli iron lines.

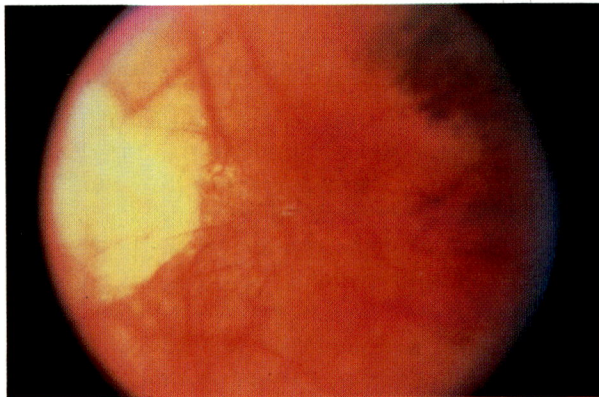

Fig. 15.100 Penetration of the globe with a retro-bulbar needle. This case had a cataract as well from direct lens trauma during surgery.

been seen after other forms of refractive surgery as well [68,69].

Retinal detachment

Only one case of this complication has been reported to date. In this case the patient had been placed on a strong miotic (phospholine iodide) post-operatively in an attempt to ameliorate an over-correction [40]. Strong miotics, particularly phospholine iodide, have been implicated in numerous instances of retinal detachment in myopic patients and their usage in these cases is decried [70–72].

Optic atrophy

The use of retro-bulbar anesthesia in this surgery has led, tragically, to acute optic atrophy in a number of cases [73]. In each instance, irretrievable visual loss has occurred. In at least three of these cases, penetration of the globe has been demonstrated (Figure 15.100) [74]. The myopic eye, being long and thin, is much more vulnerable to this hazard than the older, shorter,

cataractous eye (Figure 15.101). The use of this type of anesthesia, indiscriminately, has never been advocated in this surgery for the reason that it is fraught with known hazard and inappropriate to the situation. The fact that thousands of patients have had this surgery performed under topical anesthesia alone and under all sorts of differing conditions strengthens this viewpoint.

The author recognizes that there may be those occasions where the use of local, injectable anesthesia may be appropriate. In those rare instances, the surgeon is advised to use peri-bulbar anesthetic administration, which has been put forward as an effective and less hazardous alternative to retro-bulbar injection. The author would agree with this point of view but it is this author's strong recommendation that injectable anesthetics be avoided in these cases. In the unlikely event that such type of anesthesia *must* be used, the patient should look down toward the needle, thus swinging the posterior pole away from the tip instead of toward it, which would be the case if the patient is instructed to look up as usual (Figures 15.102 and 15.103).

Being there—a first-hand experience with radial keratotomy

We are including herewith the personal experiences of one of the author's patients—an ophthalmologist operated on almost 6 years ago. Dr Richmond has outlined his experience before [25,26]. It is our opinion that repeating it here with an update, along with the operative plan, will prove instructive to the reader. We are also including it to underscore the fact that refractive surgery is a serious undertaking with serious consequences for failure. Too many individuals have approached this surgery with a casual and cavalier attitude. This has not only damaged the eyes upon which the surgery was attempted but has undermined the credibility of refractive surgeons and ophthalmologists in general. The introduction of RK in 1978 initiated a cat-fight between town-and-gown, the ripples of which are still being felt in the profession. Its performance by surgical dilettantes has not helped heal the rift.

Dr Richmond's story is reproduced in its entirety with changes made only to conform to editorial policy and to correct minor spelling errors—nothing was left out. A discussion by the surgeon (Bores) who performed Richmond's surgery follows.

Radial keratotomy as seen through operated eyes: an ophthalmologist's view

I am a 57-year-old white male ophthalmologist who in September 1985 gambled my vision and career on the

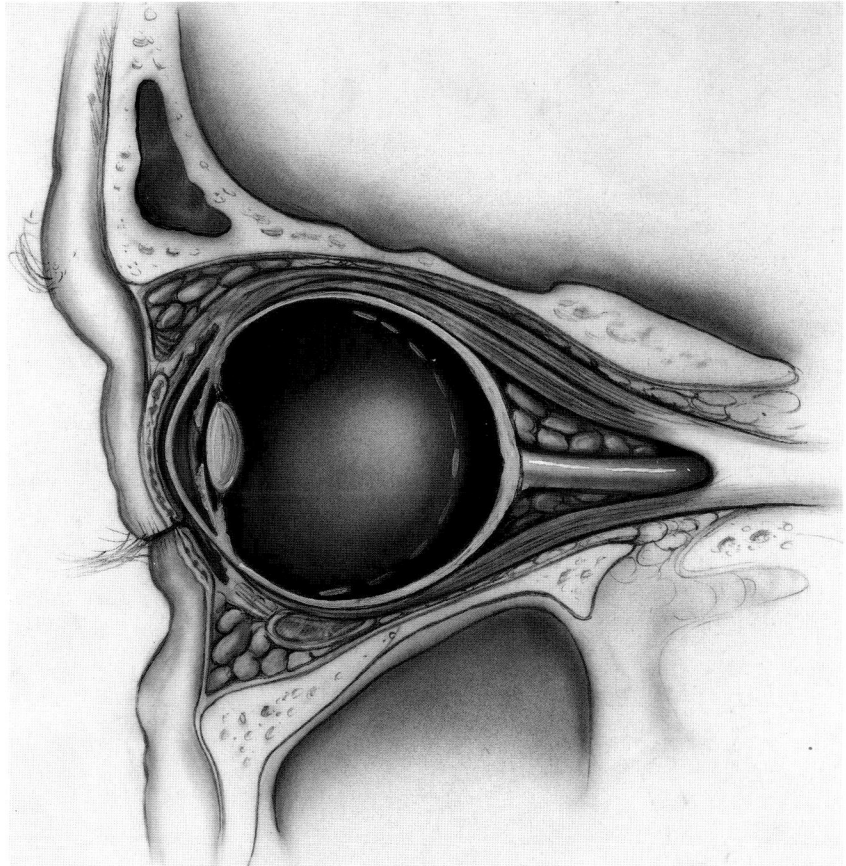

Fig. 15.101 Myopic versus emmetropic eye within the orbit.

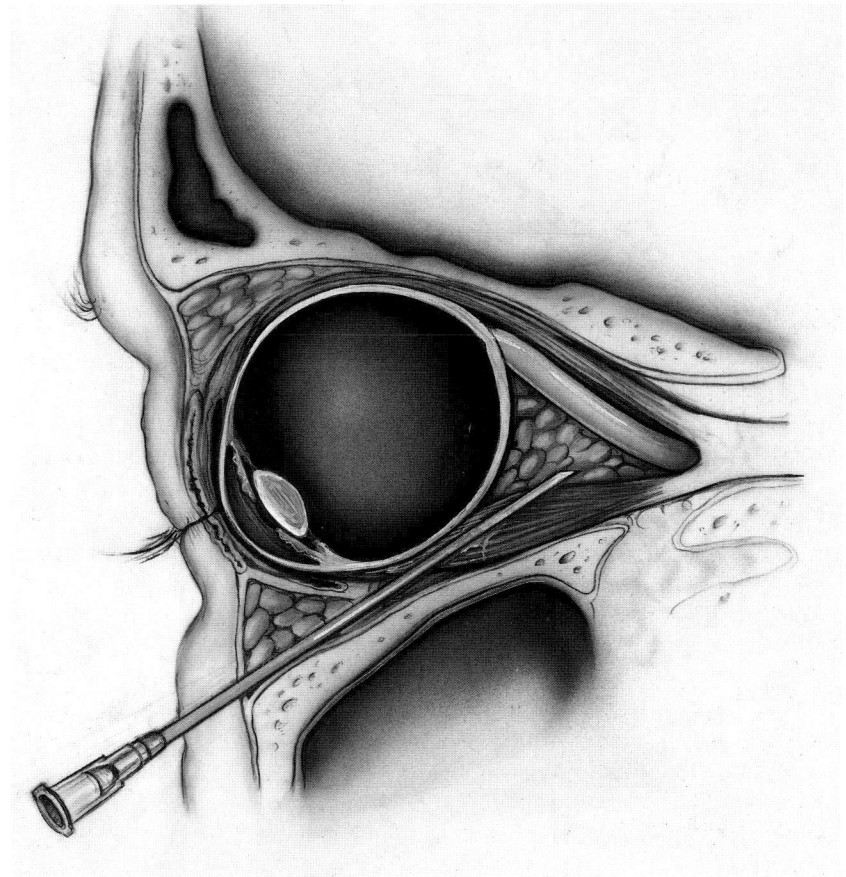

Fig. 15.102 If the patient looks down, the vulnerable posterior pole swings away from the needle tip.

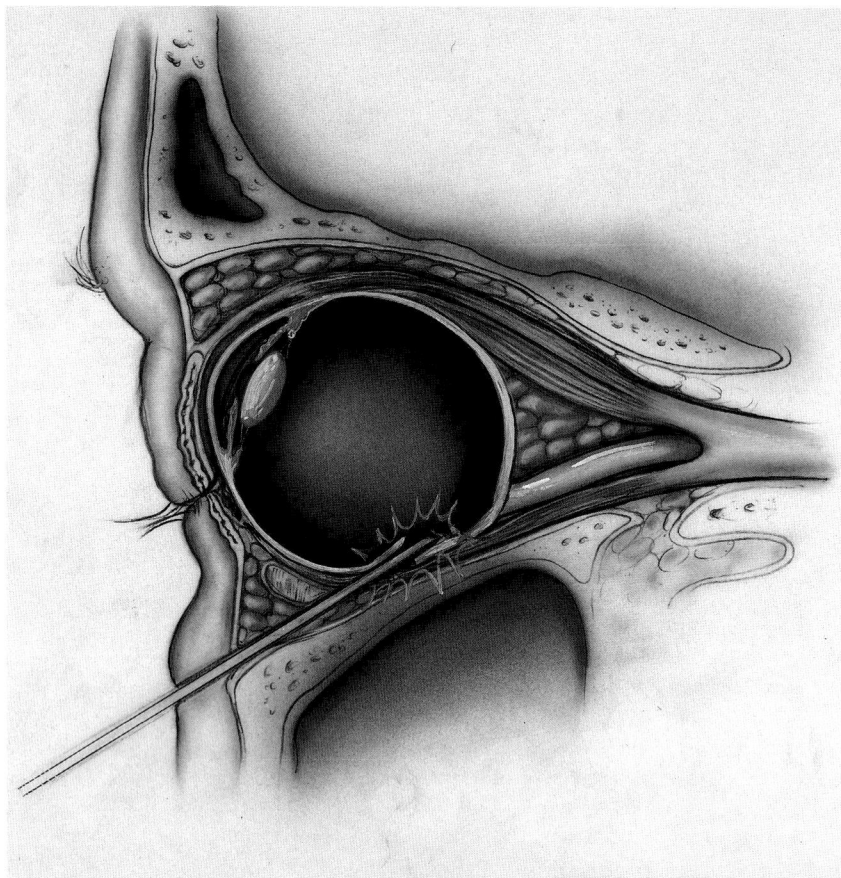

Fig. 15.103 If the patient looks up, the posterior part of the eye swings into the needle tip.

outcome of RK. I have been collecting data for an ongoing study of my post-operative course since the RKs were done. This is my story. My pre- and post-operative refractions are chronicled in Table 15.6.

To understand the motive for submitting to RK, one must understand the disdain those of us who have undergone the procedure have for glasses and contact lenses. I did not become myopic until I was a junior in high school, so I have retained vivid memories of seeing clearly without correction. From age 16 to age 45, I developed slowly progressive myopic astigmatism with no evidence of corneal pathology. If excessive near work ever caused myopia, I felt I was a candidate for such a study. In addition, I have always been athletically active and still play tennis and golf several times weekly. Glasses are a terrible nuisance for athletics, and I could never tolerate contact lenses well.

When refractive surgery re-emerged in the late 1970s, I became interested in its possibilities for me. I took two courses from the author of this book and by 1985 had decided that I would start performing RK in my practice. I did not relish the task of explaining to prospective RK patients why I was wearing moderately thick myopic glasses and yet was preparing to operate on them in order to remove their moderately thick myopic glasses. In September 1985, I had RK done on my left eye, followed 2 days later by the right eye. Despite experiencing 2 D of diurnal fluctuation of refraction, I had no significant problems resuming my practice, including performing surgery, within 10 days of my RK.

In 1985, it had not become apparent to RK surgeons that corneas could take a very long time to heal after RK. As of the date of publication of this textbook, the length required for complete corneal healing following RK is still unknown. The answer possibly is—never! In 1985, I was only expecting diurnal fluctuation of refraction to last for 6 months to 1 year. In 1991, I am still experiencing 1 D of change from morning to early afternoon with relatively stable refraction from mid-afternoon until bedtime. The dioptric change, as with most RK patients, is a minus shift that in my case is from more hyperopia to less hyperopia.

In 1985, I was expecting stabilization of final refraction by 1 year post-operation. In 1991, I am one of the 23% of RK patients experiencing one of the most disturbing long-term problems of RK, namely, continued increase in the effect of the surgery [75]. Slow healing of the corneal wounds is the suspected cause of continued effect of the surgery. Perhaps it is time for the PERK study to do a retrospective analysis of the habits of patients who are experiencing con-

Table 15.6 Summary of Richmond's post-operative progress (data courtesy Richmond, MD, Beckley, West Virginia, 1991)

Post-operative interval	Refraction				K-readings			
	OD		OS		OD		OS	
	a.m.	p.m.	a.m.	p.m.	a.m.	p.m.	a.m.	p.m.
Pre-surgery	−4.00−1.25 × 97	−4.12−1.25 × 97	−3.37−1.75 × 75	−3.50−1.75 × 75	44.62/44.25 × 97	44.62/44.25 × 97	44.50/44.00 × 75	44.50/44.00 × 75
1 year post-RK	+3.50−1.25 × 80	+2.37−1.00 × 75	+0.75−0.75 × 150	+0.25−0.50 × 150	38.50/37.50 × 80	39.75/38.37 × 81	40.00/39.62 × 80	40.75/44.25 × 85
5 months post-surgery initial suturing OD	+3.25−3.00 × 80	+1.75−2.25 × 80	+1.50−1.00 × 155	+0.50−0.75 × 155	44.50/38.75 × 75	41.00/39.50 × 75	39.25/39.50 × 81	40.12/40.00 × 76
2 weeks post-surgery additional sutures OD	+1.50−3.00 × 85	+0.25−2.25 × 92			41.00/41.12 × 61	41.25/41.00 × 61		
1 year post-surgery original suture OD; 28 months RK	+1.25−1.25 × 80	+0.75−1.25 × 80	+1.00−0.75 × 155	+0.62−0.75 × 155	40.00/38.87 × 73	40.37/39.62 × 70	39.50/39.62 × 76	40.12/40.00 × 76
$5\frac{1}{2}$ years post-surgery RK	+2.25−1.25 × 80	+0.75−0.75 × 80	+2.50−1.00 × 155	+1.50−1.00 × 150	39.62/39.12 × 70	40.00/40.12 × 64	38.75/39.12 × 73	39.87/39.87 × 70

tinued effect of the surgery. I would suspect that the frequent massaging of corneas during sports activities and close work may be of some significance in delaying healing.

My left eye had a relatively acceptable refractive error following the initial RK and despite progressive hyperopia is just now reaching a refractive error that requires more frequent use of glasses for distance vision. My right eye had a far different result and post-operative course. The initial RK resulted in significant over-correction resulting in hyperopic astigmatism.

Referring to Table 15.6, one would have expected the 11-incision [sic] RL-procedure done on my left eye to cause over-correction but instead the eight-incision R-procedure done on my right eye resulted in over-correction. [*Author's note*: Richmond is in error here: 12 incisions were performed on that eye—see the workup sheet reproduced below.]

I read of the suture technique of Lindstrom and Lindquist for correction of excessive hyperopia resulting from RK [29]. Thanks to Richard Lindstrom, my over-corrected right eye was reversed to an acceptable refractive error 2 years after the original RK. Lindstrom's original repair performed 18 months after the original RK involved blunt opening of four incisions, removal of epithelial plugs, and interrupted suture closure of the incisions using 10-0 Mersilene. When the sutures were tightened, one wound spontaneously opened and needed repairing. This asymmetric five-suture repair resulted in unwanted astigmatism. I returned 6 months later for two additional sutures. Although incisions were not opened when the two additional sutures were placed, these sutures were very effective in reducing astigmatism and residual hyperopia.

My original RK did not reduce best corrected pre-operative visual acuity. My pre-operative visual acuity was 20/15. However, the initial suture repair reduced best corrected vision in the right eye from 20/15 to 20/25. The addition of two sutures 6 months later caused no further reduction in best corrected visual acuity.

Suture correction of the right eye has left the cornea with multiple refractive surfaces. During photoptic conditions, the multiple refractive surfaces perform quite nicely. I have 20/25 distance vision uncorrected much of the day and yet retain some near vision that eliminates need for bifocals for print 20/50 and larger. Under scotopic conditions, the right eye performs less well. Under scotopic conditions, visual acuity OS without correction is in the 20/40–20/50 range at distance and no better than 20/100 at near. With correction, both distance and near acuity are approximately 20/40.

In the past year, nearly 6 years after the original RK, a dioptric change in the repaired right eye has been 0.50 D which is essentially no different from the unrepaired left cornea. Keratometric changes in the past year have been 0.87 OD and 0.25 OS.

After suture repair of the right eye, I tried another "miracle" solution. Hearing of the patient at Louisiana State University who had experienced a significant reduction of RK-induced hyperopia following hyperbaric oxygen therapy for a peripheral ulcer, I climbed into a monoplace hyperbaric oxygen chamber for four treatments in September 1988, and for two additional treatments in September 1990. Hyperbaric oxygen therapy has had no obvious benefit to me in reducing either diurnal fluctuation of refraction or for stabilizing continued effect of the surgery. The patient at Louisiana State University was unique in that contact lens wear following RK had resulted in 100% neo-vascularization of the corneal wounds. Perhaps she had exaggerated healing from hyperbaric oxygen therapy due to neo-vascularization.

It is encouraging to report that despite continuation of diurnal fluctuation of refraction and continued increase in the effect of the surgery, approximately 6 years after RK, my endothelial cell count has remained stable OU. Endothelial cell counts have been monitored by Dr George Waring and his group.

While collecting my post-operative data, I have been particularly interested in the causes of diurnal fluctuation of refractive error. I have come to the conclusion that only two factors are of major importance to explain these changes:

1 Changes of corneal stromal and epithelial hydration.
2 Some degree of mechanic corneal alteration caused by lid pressure and convergence and/or accommodation.

It is my impression that diurnal variations of intra-ocular pressure are of minimal importance when explaining diurnal fluctuation of refractive error. My corneas have never responded with a minus shift to lowering of the intra-ocular pressure. Instead, I get the opposite effect in that my corneas seem to hinge from the limbus and lowering of the intra-ocular pressure results in greater hyperopia (see comments below).

After all my trials and tribulations, would I now have RK performed if I had the advantage of 20/20 hindsight? Probably not, but I must admit that I have enjoyed being rid of glasses for a great many activities for 6 years. If the alternatives of excimer laser photo-refractive keratectomy or YAG laser stromal ablation were not promising, I might still consider RK. I would certainly follow the modern trends which dictate fewer incisions and larger optical zones as the procedure of choice for my age range. I would also favor T-incisions for astigmatism correction.

It is my personal opinion that general ophthalmologists should not be performing RK. Knowledge of all forms of refractive surgery and the ability to use them are only fair to the patients who entrust their vision to our care. Even with refinements, RK is still gross surgery in a micro-surgery arena. Four-incision RK has improved predictability, especially using "titratable" techniques of re-operation to enhance the effect, but we still do not have adequate numbers to prove that fewer incisions will reduce the threat of continued effect of the surgery [76,77].

Refractive surgery is certainly an intriguing and challenging addition to ophthalmology. Restoration of perfect uncorrected vision to an imperfect system is the goal of refractive surgery.

I have no doubt that research will continue at a rapid pace. We will learn to eliminate the bad procedures and continue those with promise. I look forward to the day when RK can be discarded for a more predictable and potentially less complicated procedure.

Discussion of the foregoing

Figures 15.104 and 15.105 are the surgical workup sheets for Dr Richmond. There is nothing unusual about this case in terms of the parameters used for the surgery nor the method employed—it was within the standard for the time performed. In fact, it appears slightly on the conservative side. Nevertheless, the patient experienced an over-correction requiring multiple suturing to reduce. In retrospect, it is obvious that a triple-step incision pattern produced the over-correction—the incisions were deeper than necessary for the patient's age. Other patients in the same age-group and with similar physical parameters have not experienced this type of complication—yet some few have. Unfortunately, we do not have, as yet, a method to gauge accurately the response of each individual patient. Therein lies the impetus for staged or incremental surgery. While the author cannot argue with the logic of individuals who choose to perform staged surgery, it is my experience that the addition of incisions in a previously operated eye is even more problematic than the primary surgery on a "virgin" eye. Besides, avoiding a perceived problem is not the way to solve it. The author's statistics do not support the PERK's findings of 23% progression of effect.

In reviewing a series of 635 consecutive, non-astigmatic, *fresh* RK cases with more than 1-year follow-up, the number of over-corrections was two—0.3%. If the same data are examined for the period prior to 1 year, the incidence is seven cases—1.1%. These cases obviously represent the state-of-the-art results and are lower than the data for earlier cases (reviewed in Chapter 8). The data for re-operations are more quixotic. Despite attempts at conservative management, 12 out of the last 123 spherical re-operations (9.8%) during the same time period resulted in over-corrections ultimately requiring intervention of one sort or another. The author works with a modified computer algorithm that predicts the outcome of the surgery at 1 year. In any series reporting over-corrections following RK, it is important to consider how many of the reported cases are unstable beyond 12 months. This is not to say that progression of effect does not occur—it obviously does. However, we still do not know exactly why this occurs but the same unknowns in corneal response to surgery exist for laser ablative procedures as well. Keep that in mind.

Richmond concludes that the variation in vision he

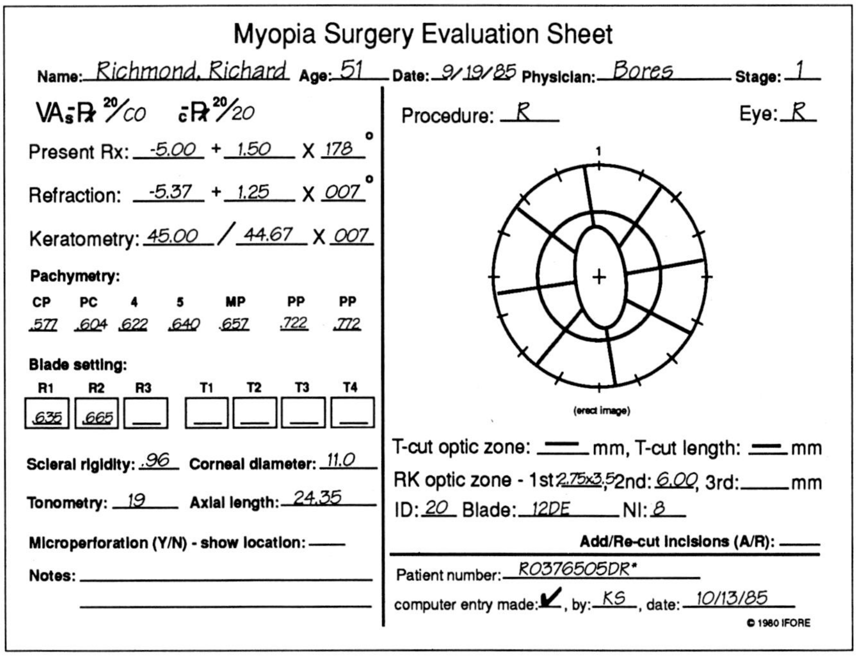
Myopia Surgery Evaluation Sheet

Name: Richmond, Richard Age: 51 Date: 9/19/85 Physician: Bores Stage: 1

VA s Rx 20/CO c Rx 20/20

Present Rx: -5.00 + 1.50 X 178°

Refraction: -5.37 + 1.25 X 007°

Keratometry: 45.00 / 44.67 X 007

Pachymetry:

CP	PC	4	5	MP	PP	PP
.577	.604	.622	.640	.657	.722	.772

Blade setting:

R1	R2	R3	T1	T2	T3	T4
.635	.665					

Scleral rigidity: .96 Corneal diameter: 11.0

Tonometry: 19 Axial length: 24.35

Microperforation (Y/N) - show location: —

Notes:

Procedure: R Eye: R

1

(erect image)

T-cut optic zone: — mm, T-cut length: — mm

RK optic zone - 1st 2.75x3.5 2nd: 6.00, 3rd: mm

ID: 20 Blade: 12DE NI: 8

Add/Re-cut Incisions (A/R): —

Patient number: R0376505DR*

computer entry made: ✓, by: KS, date: 10/13/85

© 1980 IFORE

Fig. 15.104 Surgical workup sheet for the right eye of Dr Richmond.

experiences is due to changes in stromal hydration and/or accommodation. While this may possibly be true there is good evidence that this is not the mechanism—diurnal intra-ocular pressure changes are the more likely cause [8]. Dr Richmond does not explain the mechanism whereby his intra-ocular pressure was lowered. It has been my experience that normal intra-ocular pressures are rarely affected by beta-blockers or miotics. Furthermore, the dynamics of a "thin shell" do not reflect a hinging mechanism—he has no transverse incisions to produce a hinge.

Richmond comments that four-incision RK has improved predictability. While it may be true in *his* experience, this has, unfortunately, not been supported by the literature nor by the author's personal experience with this surgery. While it may seem to make sense to do less surgery initially to decrease the possibility of an over-correction, this benefit is offset by the demonstrated fact that re-operations are notoriously unpredictable. In the author's experience, the incidence of over-corrections—immediate or late progressive—is much higher in this group than in cases having had only one surgery.

Dr Richmond's observation that RK should not be done by general ophthalmologists is "right on," however. The author would extend that admonition to include any form of refractive surgery. Our thanks go to Dr Richmond for sharing his experiences with us. It took courage to have the surgery performed in the first place, and even more to share the aftermath. The author regrets that Dr Richmond has experienced the difficulties he has had, yet we are pleased that he remains philosophic. Hopefully, we have all learned something from this recitation.

Lamellar refractive surgery

The complications of this surgery are those that can be expected of any non-penetrating surgical procedure on the cornea. Infection is usually rare, typically confined to the corneal stroma and is generally localized. It responds well to topical antibiotics but in some cases may require sub-tenon injection. Cases of severe intra-ocular infection have been reported: rare cases of endophthalmitis leading to visual loss have occurred. Induced astigmatism is by far the most common complication with this surgery and occurs in about 4% of the cases, tending to group in the higher myopia ranges.

Intra-operative problems and complications

Reference mark incorrectly placed

The reference mark may be placed either too central or too peripheral. In either case, when the corneal disk is resected, all of the mark may end up in the periphery or on the disk. When measuring the diameter of the keratectomy with the applanator, it may be clearly seen if the location of the mark is incorrect—if it is, it must be corrected.

Prophylaxis. At the beginning of the case, use a caliper set to the diameter of the section to make sure the mark straddles the edge. A 4.0 mm RK marker will work as well. Simply scribe the line from the edge of the optical zone to the limbus. Be certain to make the mark as shown in Figure 15.106.

Treatment (disk upside down). Remove disk, clean and re-suture in place correctly. Rarely, the lenticule may be irreparably damaged by collagenase secreted by the corneal epithelium and will have to be replaced by donor tissue.

Retro-bulbar injection

Hematoma

The retro-bulbar (or peri-bulbar) injection may cause a retro-bulbar hematoma which, if small, will not hinder continuation of the surgery since it is not necessary to open the eye. However, a large hematoma may produce difficulty with opening the lids and can interfere with placement of the ring and/or obtaining sufficient suction.

Prophylaxis. Use blunt needles for injection and inject a small quantity of fluid as the needle is introduced.

Anterior infiltration

If the injection is not placed within the muscle cone, it many infiltrate toward the sub-tenons or sub-conjunctival space. This will cause peri-limbal swelling which will prevent correct adaptation of the fixation ring to the globe. In this case, performing several small incisions, 5 or 6 mm from the limbus, to evacuate the fluid may be tried, or a peritomy may be done to place the ring directly over the sclera. Surgery may have to be postponed.

Prophylaxis. Only inject when certain that the muscle cone has been entered.

Perforation of the globe

This complication is vision-threatening and a real danger. The myopic globe is not only longer but thinner, consequently it is much easier to penetrate with a retro-bulbar needle than is that of a normal.

Myopia Surgery Evaluation Sheet

Name: _Richmond, Richard_ Age: _51_ Date: _9/17/85_ Physician: _Bores_ Stage: _1_

VA: s̄ Rx ²⁰/CO c̄ Rx ²⁰/20   Procedure: _RL_   Eye: _L_

Present Rx: _-4.50_ + _2.00_ X _170_ °

Refraction: _-5.25_ + _1.75_ X _165_ °

Keratometry: _44.75_ / _43.75_ X _165_

Pachymetry:

CP	PC	4	5	MP	PP	PP
.592	.605	.618	.631	.645	.700	.774

Blade setting:

R1	R2	R3	T1	T2	T3	T4
.620	.665	.740				

Scleral rigidity: _.96_ Corneal diameter: _11.0_

Tonometry: _18_ Axial length: _24.24_

Microperforation (Y/N) - show location: ——

Notes: _____

T-cut optic zone: ——— mm, T-cut length: ——— mm

RK optic zone - 1st: _3x4_, 2nd: _6.00_, 3rd: _8.00_ mm

ID: _2.5_ Blade: _12DE_ NI: _12_

Add/Re-cut Incisions (A/R): ———

Patient number: _R0377005SRL_

computer entry made: ✔, by: _KS_, date: _10/13/85_

© 1980 IFORE

Fig. 15.105 Surgical workup sheet for the left eye of Dr Richmond.

Prophylaxis. When administering the retro-bulbar, use a shorter, more flexible needle and have the patient look down. It helps to blunt the needle slightly by rubbing the tip across a sterile towel.

Pneumatic fixation ring

Insufficient lid clearance

If the inter-palpebral opening is insufficient to place the pneumatic fixation ring, due to its shape or because of proptosis due to retro-bulbar injection, a small lateral canthotomy may be performed. Remember to suture it at the end of the case. In children, use the smaller-diameter rings.

Difficulty with fixation

Scleral radius differs from that of the ring

If the scleral radius is larger than the radius of the ring, the latter makes contact only by its peripheral edge and the central edge does not contact the limbus (Figure 15.107). If the scleral radius is smaller than that of the ring, the reverse case exists (Figure 15.108). Fortunately, this occurs very rarely.

Prophylaxis. Insure that the rings at hand are the correct size for the patient. Remember that the rings for children are 110 mm in diameter, while those for the adult are 125 mm in diameter.

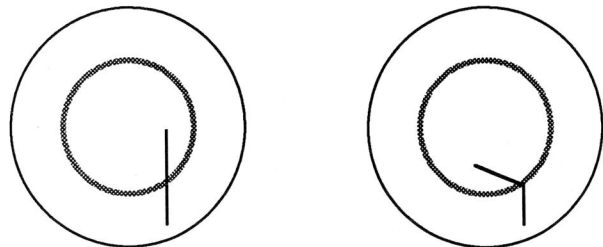

Fig. 15.106 Mismatched reference marks. The tissue has been replaced with the epithelial side down.

Lax or edematous conjunctiva blocking the suction aperture

In some cases, the conjunctiva may be so lax as to become aspirated into the ring suction aperture, thereby preventing full suction from occurring (Figure 15.109). In this case, the first step is to re-orient the ring to move the hole. If, in spite of this, the same thing happens, a small peritomy must be performed, leaving the conjunctiva of the upper area outside the pneumatic ring, and the bare sclera directly in front of the hole. Too large a peritomy may cause a tendency for the ring to decentrate. If small enough, this peritomy will not cause this problem, nor require suturing. The keratectomy must not be attempted unless the fixation provided by the ring is perfect.

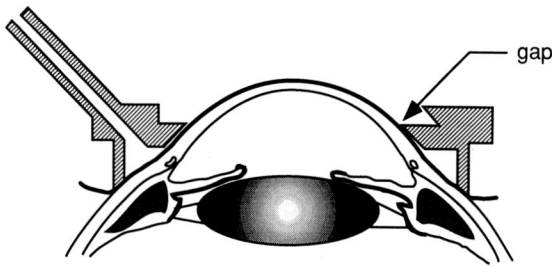

Fig. 15.107 Ring too big for eye.

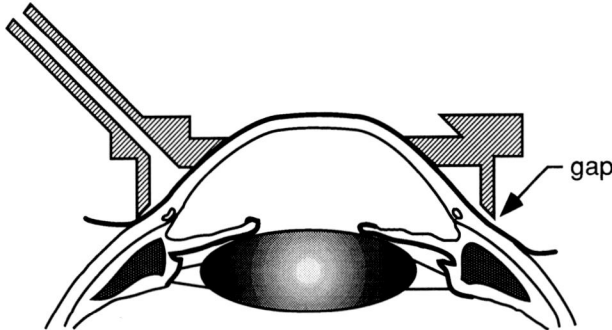

Fig. 15.108 Ring too small for eye.

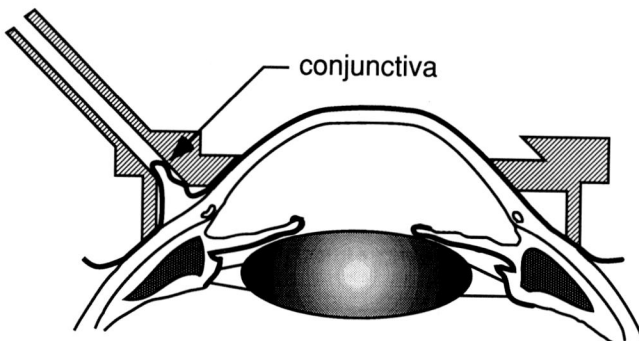

Fig. 15.109 Aspirated conjunctiva.

Insufficient pump suction on start-up

This is something that will occur upon check-out of the instrument pre-operatively. This will occur if there is a partial blockage of the vacuum path or if there is a leak in the system.

Prophylaxis. Insure proper functioning of the vacuum system before the case starts.

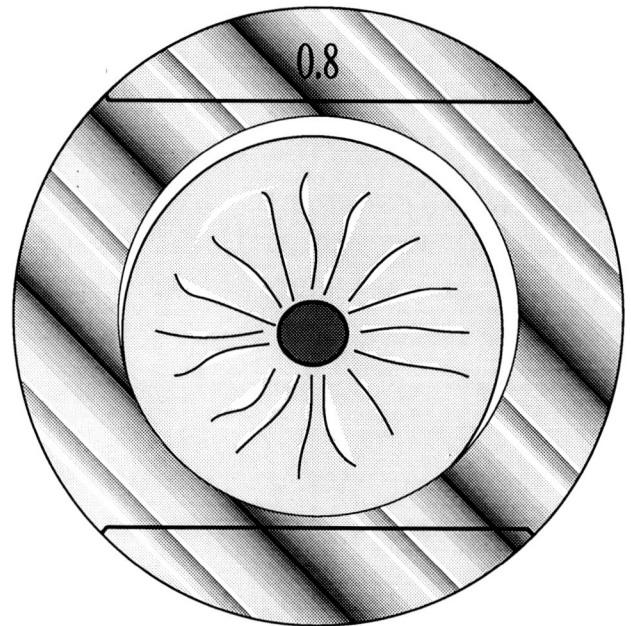

Fig. 15.110 Decentration of ring.

Difficulty with centration

In some globes with a somewhat irregular sclera, the cornea tends to be out of center in relation to the ring aperture (Figure 15.110). A small decentration of 0.50 mm toward the supero-temporal side is desirable in myopia and to the infero-nasal side in hyperopia. If the decentration is greater than this, the conjunctiva should be disinserted near the limbus on the side where the conjunctiva is showing mostly (Figure 15.111).

Section with the microkeratome

Obstacles to movement

Lid speculum problems

Care must be taken to prevent the blades of the lid speculum from extending into the path of the microkeratome. If the microkeratome strikes the speculum during its translation across the cornea, an irregularity in the section will result. Generally, an assistant can move the blades out of the way with forceps. If this cannot be done, it is better to remove the fixation ring and the lid speculum and use lid sutures—4-0 silk is adequate for this purpose. Be careful to place the sutures in the skin and away from the lid margin vascular arcade. Sometimes a problem will arise when the retro-bulbar has been excessive, or if the speculum is too small. Beware using a Guyton-Park type of speculum with lockable blades. This

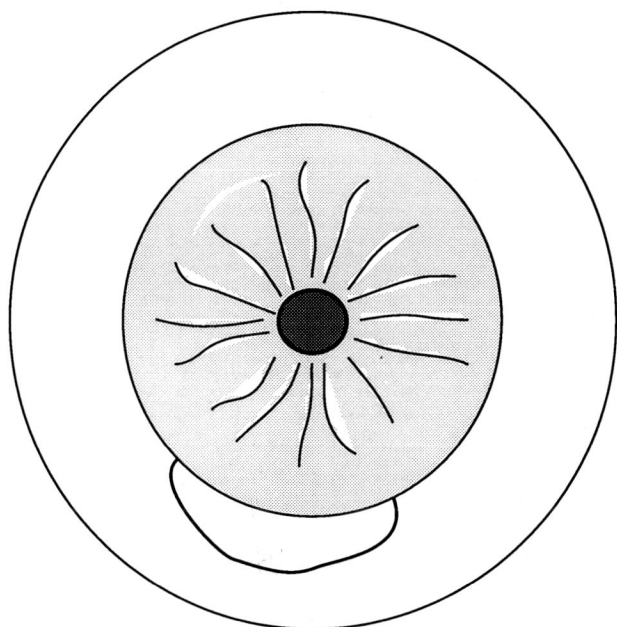

Fig. 15.111 Peritomy for decentration. The peritomy must be on the opposite side of the decentration.

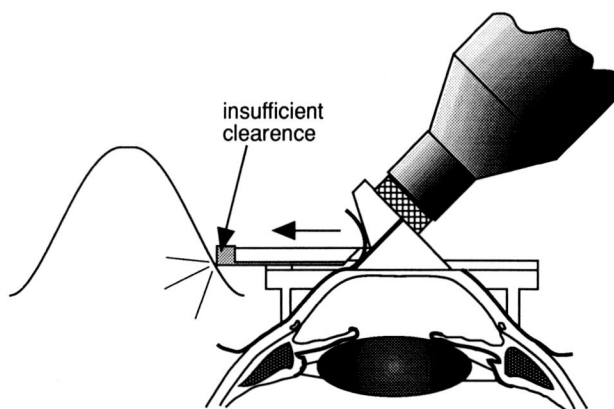

Fig. 15.112 The keratome may strike the nose, preventing complete resection of the disk.

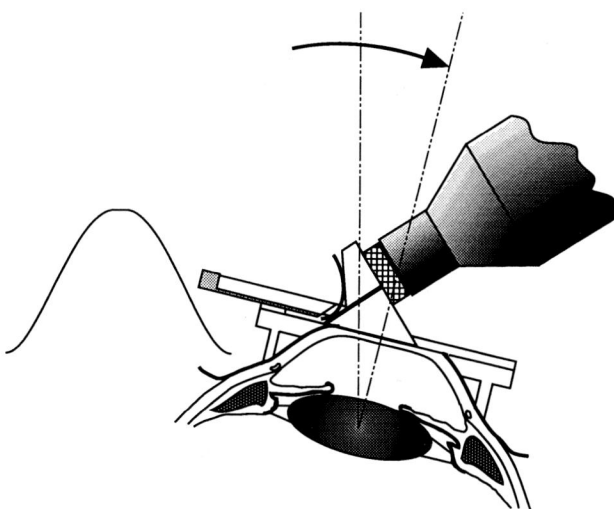

Fig. 15.113 Rotating the eye temporally will provide more clearance for the keratome.

device has been implicated in post-operative ptosis secondary to levator aponeurosis dehiscence [78].

Nose gets in the way

In cases of large noses, the head of the microkeratome may hit the nose before completing the pass (Figure 15.112). This can be prevented by taking measurements over the ring with the microkeratome off. If there is insufficient space, the globe can be abducted with the ring handle. It is recommended that, prior to moving the keratome across the eye, that eye be adducted (rotated outward) slightly with the suction ring handle (Figure 15.113).

Disk of size other than selected

Smaller disk

The cornea was wet and liquid meniscus falsified the reading, making it appear larger.

Prophylaxis. Dry the cornea before applanating. Check blades for proper dimensions. The latter cause is very unlikely today because all blades are examined and measured at the factory.

Larger disk

Inadequate seating of the applanator to the surface of the fixation ring.

Prophylaxis

Insure that the applanator seats against the ring surface.

Thicker disk

1 Higher intra-ocular pressure.
2 Wider blade (Figure 15.114a).
3 Large-diameter disk.

Thinner disk

1 Low IOP.
2 Narrower blade (Figure 15.114b).
3 Smaller-diameter disk.

(a)   (b)

>4.14 mm   <4.14 mm

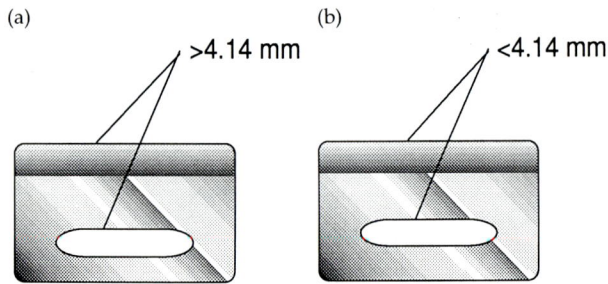

Fig. 15.114 (a) Blade too big; (b) blade too small.

Incomplete section

If the section with the microkeratome is incomplete, but the corneal disk is attached by only a small bridge of tissue, it may be sectioned with a small sharp spatula or knife. If the microkeratome stops halfway or in two-thirds of the resection, the surgery must be postponed.

Prophylaxis. Observe the disk as it exits the microkeratome. As soon as it stops emerging, the section is complete. Take care to retain pressure upon both the motor and vacuum foot-switches during the keratectomy.

Sectioning of the disk halfway or in the final third

This may occur for two reasons:
1 From having withdrawn the microkeratome from the eye too soon, with the motor running.
2 From detachment of the fixation ring during the section.

Prophylaxis. If the vacuum breaks for any reason, stop the keratome motor immediately. Insure that fixation is adequate prior to starting and don't pull up strongly on the vacuum ring. Stop the motor in any case before removing it from the ring.

Entering the anterior chamber

This can occur from a number of causes: the most obvious is setting the plate incorrectly or an error in pachymetry. Too slow translation during the keratectomy or stopping with the motor running can also cause it. The most common cause in fixed-plate microkeratomes is operating the microkeratome without a plate (Figures 15.115 and 15.116).

Irregularity in the corneal disk

Irregularity in shape. The shape of the disk may be defective because it is to a greater or lesser extent oval

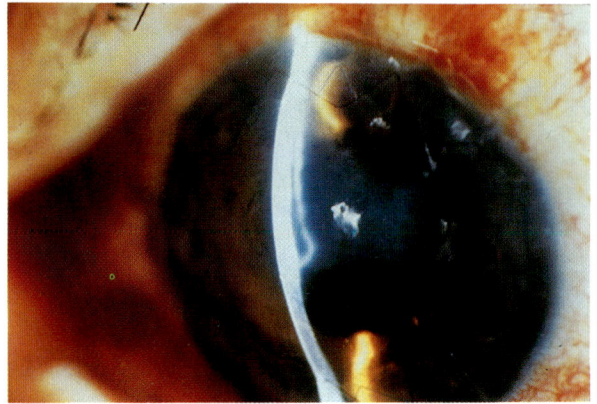

Fig. 15.115 Entry into the anterior chamber during keratectomy. (Courtesy of J.I. Barraquer.)

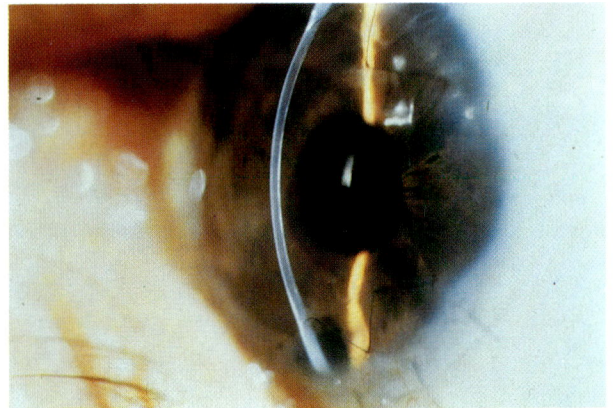

Fig. 15.116 The same eye at 1 month. (Courtesy of J.I. Barraquer.)

(Figure 15.117), pyriform (Figure 15.118), or kidney-shaped (Figure 15.119).

These accidents may be due to:
1 An irregularly shaped cornea.
2 An irregularity in the limbus (pterygium, etc.).
3 Variation in intra-ocular pressure during the resection.
4 Defective fit of the microkeratome into the ring guides.
5 Faster translation of the microkeratome at the end of the resection than at the beginning.

Prophylaxis
1 Pre-operative examination of the corneal surface and limbus.
2 Keeping the ring in a constant position, not pushing down.
3 Uniform microkeratome motion.

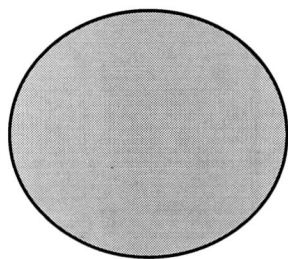

Fig. 15.117 Oval disk.

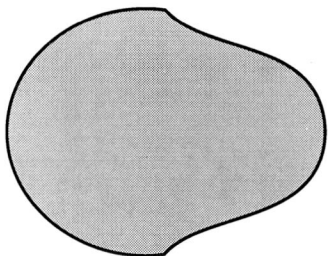

Fig. 15.118 Pyriform disk.

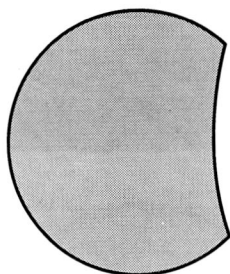

Fig. 15.119 D or kidney-shaped disk.

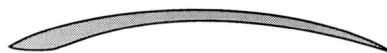

Fig. 15.120 Irregular section thickness.

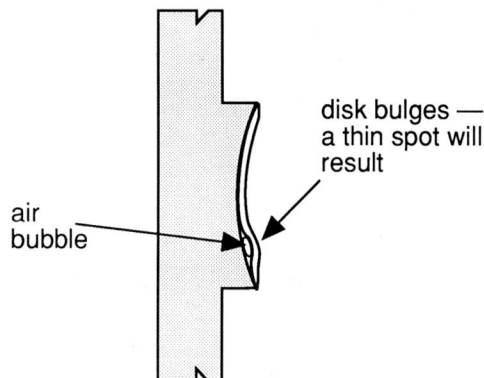

Fig. 15.121 Air under the tissue during lathing can produce an eccentric thin spot and post-operative irregular astigmatism.

Irregularity in thickness

This can occur due to insufficient or variable intra-ocular pressure during the resection (Figure 15.120). Also, if the microkeratome is moved too rapidly during the keratectomy, the tissue will be thinner. Occasionally this will occur due to a dull blade. If the corneal surface is highly irregular, the resection bed will also be irregular. If a parallel-sided disk of sufficient thickness is sutured into the bed it is possible that a smooth external surface may result. However, the center of myopic lenticules is thin and is likely to re-shape itself to the bed. In this case irregular astigmatism may result. When lathing, make sure that no air remains between the disk and the Delrin base (Figure 15.121).

Prophylaxis
1 Check blade edge.
2 Perform pre-keratectomy tonometry.
3 Keep ring stable (see above).
4 Keep the motion of microkeratome uniform (see above).

Irregularity in the section

The section looks like a Ruffles® potato chip (Figure 15.122).

Prophylaxis. Prophylaxis involves slow and uniform movement of the microkeratome. In case of a small defect, the operation can continue. Otherwise, the best solution is to replace the disk, suturing it into place and postponing the surgery.

Foreign bodies in the section interface

Interface inclusions: everything from dust to lint can find its way between the tissues, and usually will (Figure 15.123). Working without gloves; using lint-free drapes; and laminar air-flow in the operating theater can minimize this problem. The most common source for such substances is from the air (lint, hair, talcum, dust), or from small chips off the blade caused by its striking the lid speculum.

Prophylaxis. Use a laminar flow filter and avoid striking any metallic surfaces. Examine both the bed and the

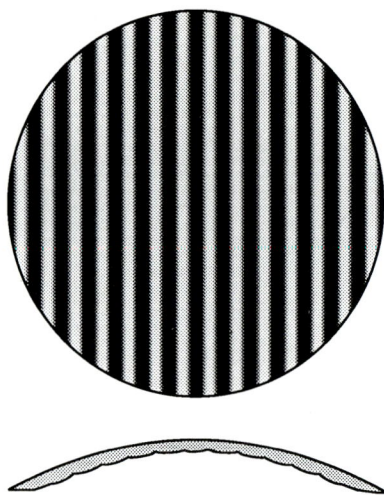

Fig. 15.122 "Ruffled" section.

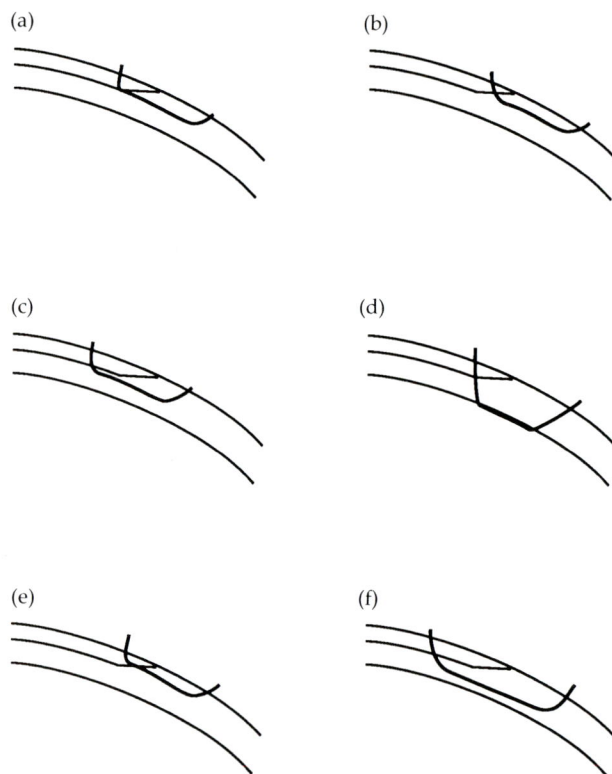

Fig. 15.124 Suturing mistakes. (a) Correct suture placement; (b) too close to lenticule edge; (c) too central and includes the resection bed; (d) too deep, enters the anterior chamber; (e) too superficial; (f) too deep and too broad.

provide easy access to the interface for the epithelium (see the section on suturing in Chapter 10).

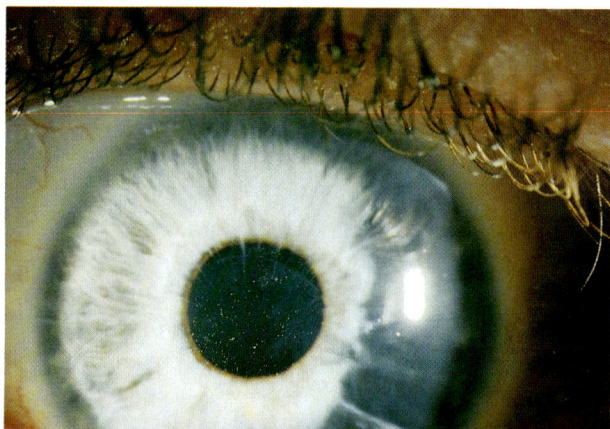

Fig. 15.123 Metallic particles and dust in the interface.

disk under the microscope with oblique lighting. Carefully scrub both surfaces with the sable brush and pick away those pieces not dislodged by the scrubbing or irrigation. Do not lay the disk on the eye to clean it. This is sure to sow epithelial cells into the interface.

Suture difficulties

When suturing the disk, the needle used must be very sharp to minimize trauma to the disk edges. Make sure that you expose the needle tip before passing it through the keratectomy edge.

Edge tearing

The bites must be placed at least 1.0 mm from the edge of the disk (Figure 15.124). If they are placed more peripherally, the tissue can be easily torn. Torn edges

Perforating or superficial suture

If a suture penetrates into the anterior chamber, it should be replaced, although the use of 10-0 nylon makes this less imperative. When the suture is superficial, there is a risk of the tissue tearing, which will result in a loose running suture and displaced disk. In addition, torn tissue impedes re-epithelialization and promotes epithelial invasion of the interface. Use of 3/8s curved needles will assist in placing the bites correctly—do not use the "fish-hook" configuration. The author uses 10-0 black nylon on an Alcon A-3 needle.

Suture breakage

If the suture breaks after the ends have been cut, prior to burying (or during) the knot, loosen the suture sufficiently so as to provide length for tying on to an additional suture. Tie the knot as shown (Figure 15.125) and pull the knot into the corneal side. Replace the suture bite (it should pass through the original hole easily) and try to tie it to the other end so that

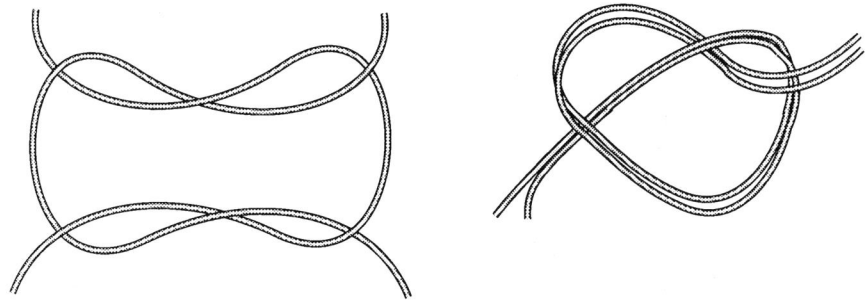

Fig. 15.125 Recommended knots to be used with broken sutures.

the new knot can be pulled into the cornea as well. Suture breakage before finishing usually occurs at the needle—the solution is obvious, if not pleasant.

Sowing epithelial cells

This can occur during cleaning (as explained above) but can also happen during suturing. If the needle is blunt or rough, it can drag cells into the interface.

Likewise, sutures placed too close to the edge of the disk could cause tearing or gaping, allowing epithelium to sneak in under the disk. Transfer of cells can occur from handling with the Colibri forceps as well. This can be minimized by not handling the disk with forceps once the first cardinal suture is in place. Keep all instruments scrupulously clean during the procedure.

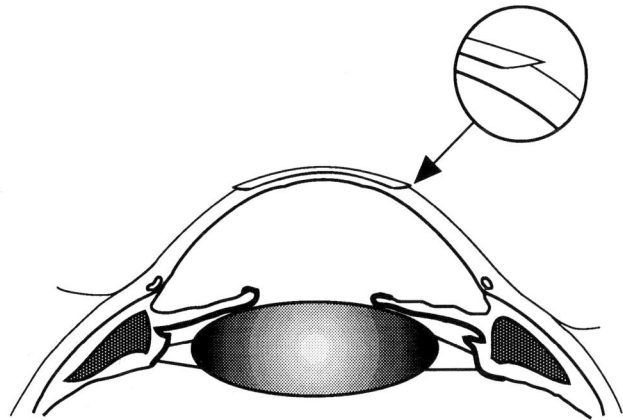

Fig. 15.126 Avoid the lenticule over-riding the resection edge.

Irregular edge gap or coaptation

In lamellar refractive surgery, the edges of the disk must not be allowed to extend beyond the edge of the resection (Figure 15.126). This can occur if the disk is too large for the bed—something that can happen in homoplastic cases—and also if care is not taken to center the tissue before completing the knotting. The epithelium will dive under the edge rather than climb over it. It is better that there be a small gap at the edge, which will not cause a problem. The suture should be adjusted before tying to insure that this gap is equal all way around. This can be facilitated by having the gap slightly larger next to the knot with the disk abutting at 180°. When the knot is tied up, there will be a small movement of the tissue toward the knot, evening the gap. Fiddling with the suture, once tied, will result in little if any movement in any direction and the risk of suture breakage is high. In homoplastic cases remember to cut the donor section 0.3 mm *smaller* in diameter.

Loose suture

Apart from providing a bad coaptation, a loose running suture will produce discomfort to the patient by accumulating mucus in the loose suture limbs and may interfere with epithelialization as well as possibly promoting neo-vascularization. To prevent this happening, before knotting it will help to "snug up" the suture with a 2-1 knot so that it will hold for the final throw. Avoid using the usual 3-2-2 throw which results in a large knot, difficult (if not impossible) to pull into the needle hole. If, after knotting the suture, it is seen to be loose, it may be tightened by placing a radial stitch in the periphery of the cornea, taking in one of the loops (limbs) of the running suture and tightening it until the running suture takes up the proper tension. More than one of these can be done (Figure 15.127).

Excessively tight suture

If the running suture is too tight, the edges of the disk can overlap the peripheral epithelium and the coaptation will be irregular and scalloped (Figure 15.128). Sub-lenticular epithelialization can occur under these circumstances as well as astigmatism from the furrowing.

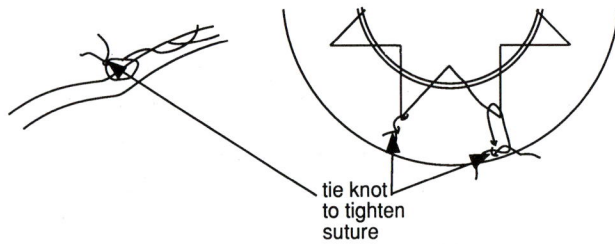

Fig. 15.127 Dealing with a loose suture.

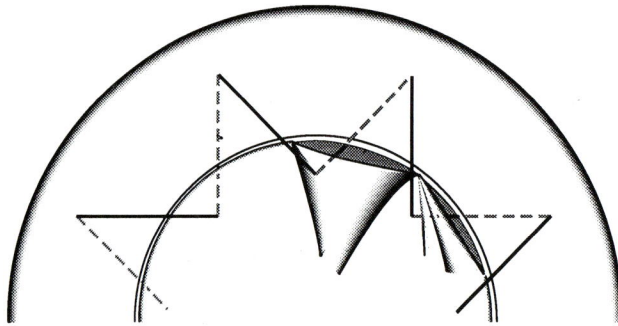

Fig. 15.128 Tight sutures produce edge-gaping.

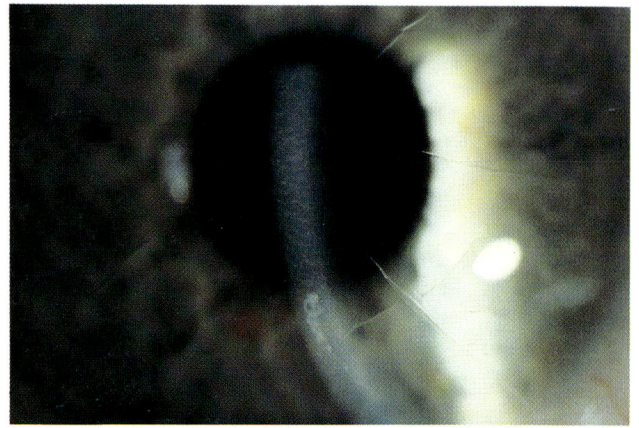

Fig. 15.129 Epithelial implantation—at lenticule edge.

Post-operative complications

The post-operative complications are generally those of any operation upon the cornea of the eye such as keratitis, ulcer, etc. Those peculiar to these procedures are induced or residual astigmatism, irregular astigmatism, sub-lenticular epithelialization, disk slough, residual refractive error, infection, and interface foreign bodies interfering with vision.

Astigmatism

Irregular astigmatism has been reported with this surgery and occurs as a result of a severely torn disk or decentration of the resection. It can also occur in keratomileusis with a disk whose thickness is not uniform. This may not always be apparent by examination at the time of surgery. The incidence of induced astigmatism is approximately 11% after keratomileusis-*in-situ*, which is about twice that of classic or freeze-lathing keratomileusis. In hyperopic lamellar keratotomy, induced astigmatism is approximately 4%, indicating that decentration of the second pass is the operative factor in the increased astigmatism seen in keratomileusis-*in-situ*.

If it occurs, it is best handled by attempting to regularize the astigmatism through the application of relaxing incisions after some months of healing. Removal and replacement of the disk are not the solution because the repeat section may also be irregular due to irregular applanation. This is unlikely to occur

in hyperopic lamellar keratotomy because nothing is removed. Irregular astigmatism may occur in keratomileusis-*in-situ* if the diameter of the second pass is less than 4.5 mm. You are advised to avoid secondary sections less than 4.5 mm—it is suggested that 5.0 mm be the minimum.

Residual or induced regular astigmatism is treated by allowing 3–4 months to elapse or until the keratometry readings stabilize. Relaxing incisions appropriate to the degree of astigmatism are then made (see Chapter 9). The same is true for residual myopia in the case of keratomileusis-*in-situ*. Relaxing incisions have been used successfully in conjunction with MKM for some time.

Epithelial ingrowth

Epithelialization of the interface is a serious complication in lamellar refractive surgery because it is progressive and usually results in loss of vision. In classic keratomileusis, it is the leading cause of lenticular loss. Rarely, epithelial cells will stop proliferating if they have been sown into the interface if they migrate in from the edge—usually they do not (Figures 15.129 through 15.134). Epithelial ingrowth is often accompanied by serous elevation and clouding of the disk (Figure 15.135).

In these cases, the disk must be totally removed from the resection bed and the epithelial cell mass carefully peeled away and removed from both surfaces. This is best accomplished by placing a single "hinge" of interrupted 10-0 nylon before removing the running suture. The epithelium must be completely removed from the coapted edge before lifting the edge of the disk. A small amount of 10% cocaine on a microsponge will loosen and destroy some of the cells.

The running suture is removed and the lenticule carefully freed from the interface. Use a gentle lifting

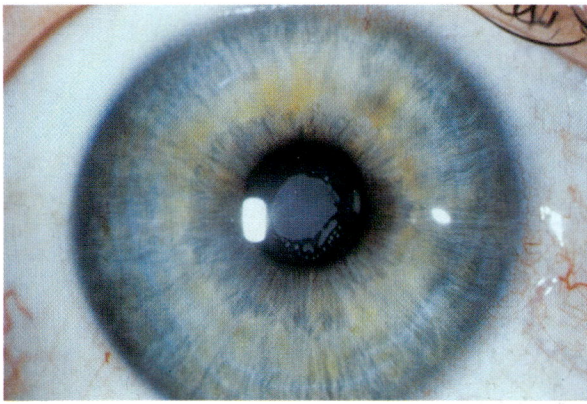

Fig. 15.130 Epithelial ingrowth—central. (Courtesy of J.I. Barraquer.)

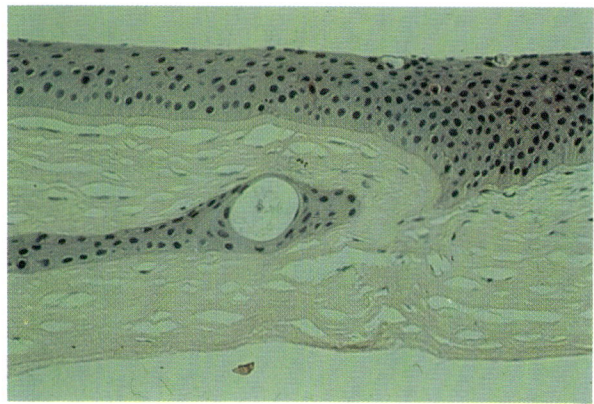

Fig. 15.133 Epithelial ingrowth—peripheral. Histologic section. (Courtesy of J.I. Barraquer.)

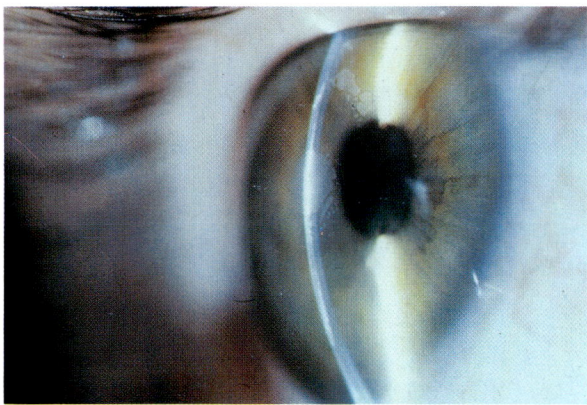

Fig. 15.131 Epithelial ingrowth—central. Slit-lamp view. (Courtesy of J.I. Barraquer.)

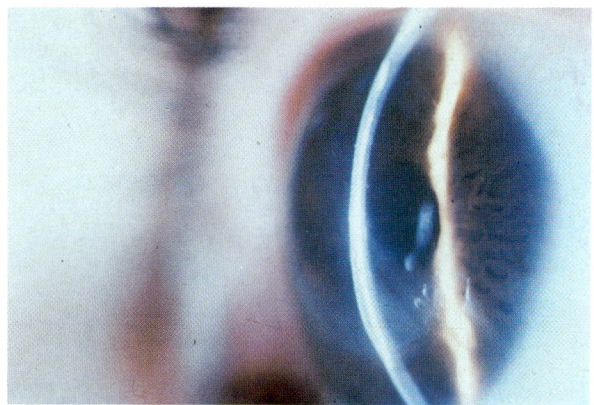

Fig. 15.134 Typical reaction to active epithelium in the interface. (Courtesy of J.I. Barraquer.)

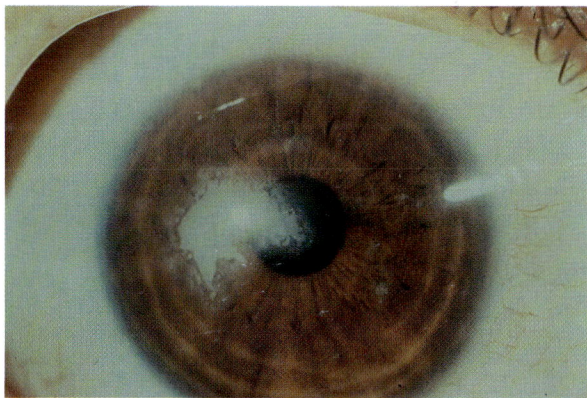

Fig. 15.132 Epithelial ingrowth—peripheral. (Courtesy of J.I. Barraquer.)

movement with a flat, blunt iris spatula such as the Katena Jaffe spatula (Figure 15.136). As the disk is lifted, the underlying ingrown epithelium will probably come up with it (Figure 15.137). At this juncture, the disk must be lifted carefully so as to leave the epithelial sheet intact, if possible. Hinge the disk over on to its top surface, Bowman's layer down. Using a dry or lightly moistened microsponge (*not* a Weck-Cel), remove the epithelium from the resection bed. Do this by making repeated one-way passes with the sponge, using a clean, new sponge each time. Repeat the process with the stromal side of the lenticule.

After the mechanic scrubbing is done, gently brush both surfaces with a Red Sable brush while irrigating with copious quantities of BSS (Jorge Krumeich suggests distilled water). Once clean, the disk can be replaced and re-sutured, taking care not to duplicate the circumstances that caused the problem in the first place (Figure 15.138).

Lenticular necrosis and sloughing

Only two cases of disk decompensation with necrosis not due to trauma have been observed in keratomileusis. The cause is still unknown but is believed to be due to contamination of the lenticule by Cidex during the surgery in one case while the other was

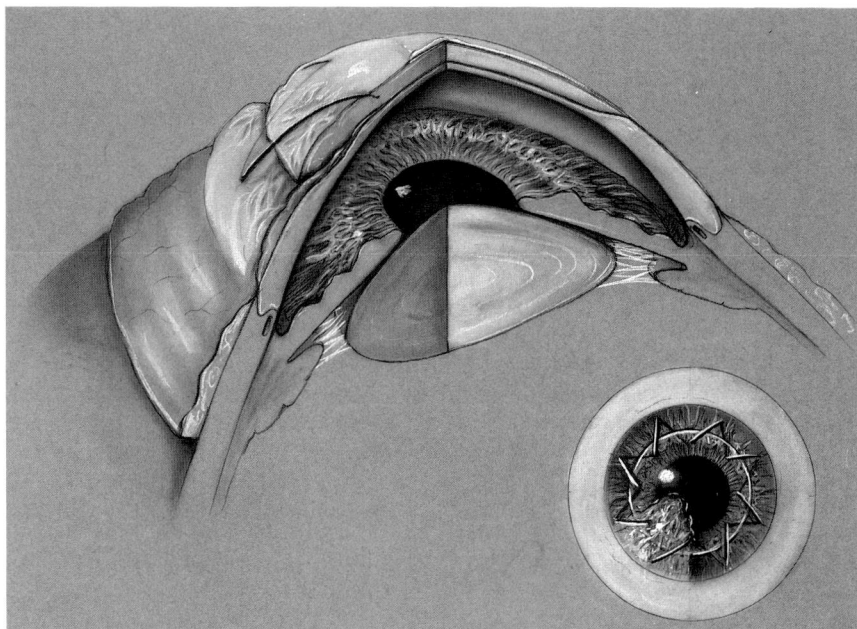

Fig. 15.135 Epithelial ingrowth.

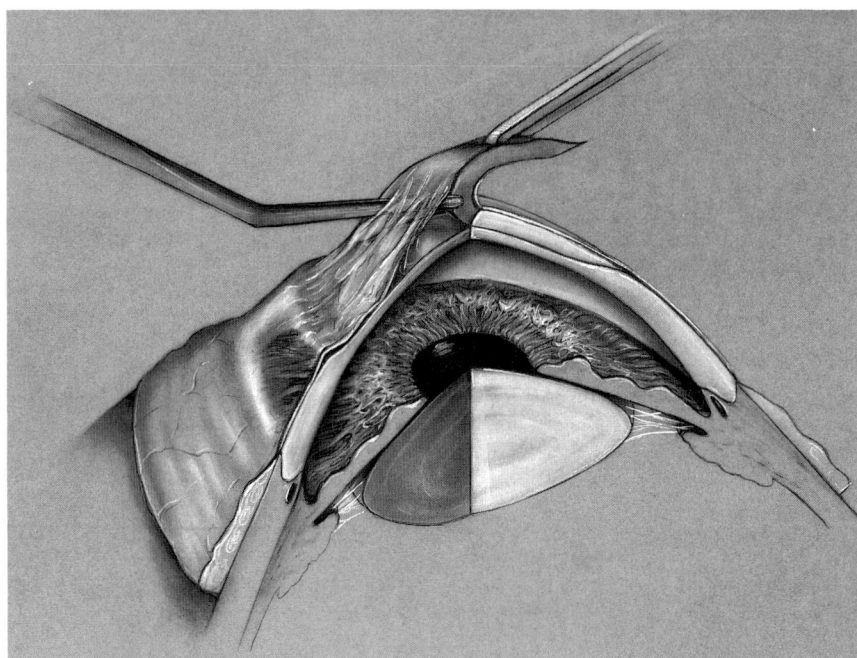

Fig. 15.136 Elevate lenticule and epithelial sheet, using spatula to separate the epithelial sheet.

associated with diabetic glycemic crisis (Figure 15.139). In the former case two subsequent lenticules failed due to poor coaptation. The problem was finally solved with a modified form of epikeratophakia. Most sloughing or displacement will occur due to direct trauma or through suture breakage. Occasionally a suture is sufficiently loose so as to allow the lid blink to tear the lenticule loose from the bed. In these cases, a replacement by donor tissue must be done as soon as possible (Figures 15.140 through 15.142).

Interface foreign bodies

Interface foreign bodies result from particulate matter entering the interface during surgery. These are most frequently lint and dust particles but may sometimes be talc and rarely metallic pieces caused by spalling. Particles not interfering with vision are best left alone. Their damage is to the surgeon's pride alone—the surgeon undertaking this surgery should possess sufficient ego to be able to cope with it. However, if these

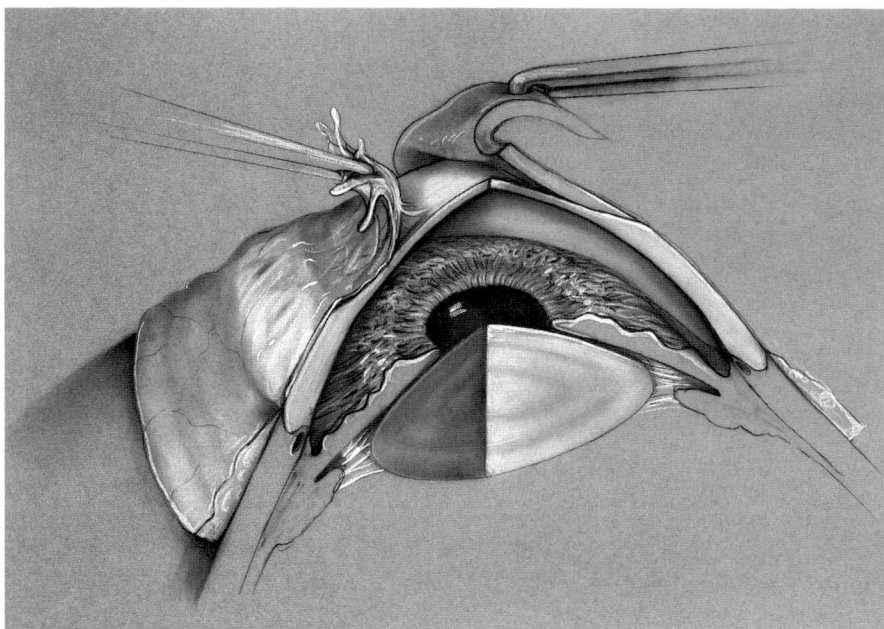

Fig. 15.137 Peel epithelium away from disk bed and lenticule.

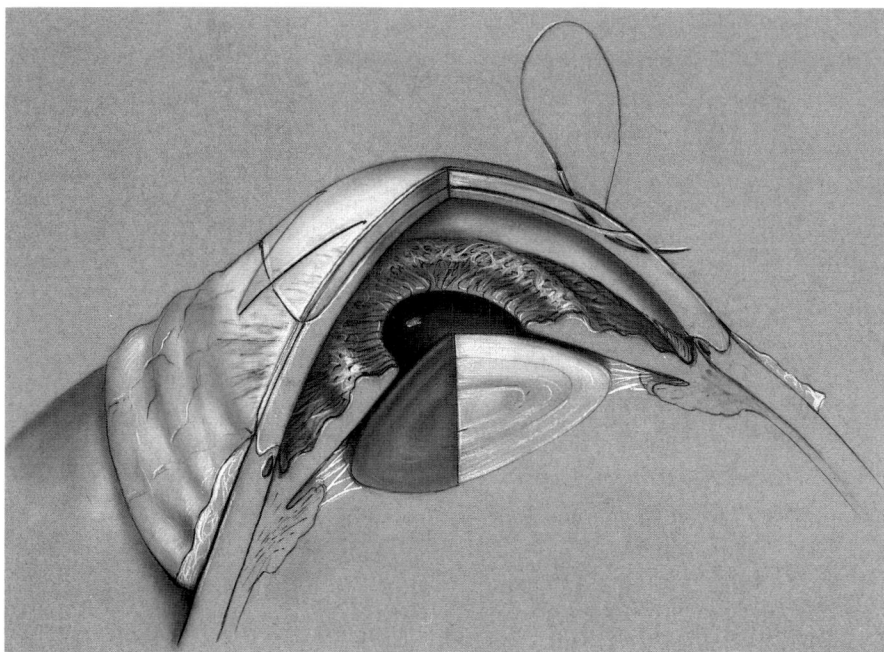

Fig. 15.138 Re-sutured lenticule.

particles are interfering with vision due to glare or obstruction, they must be removed. It may be necessary, in some cases, to separate and lift the disk from the bed over the foreign body. Begin at one edge by first removing the epithelium in the area with a cotton-tipped applicator moistened with 10% cocaine. This will swell and loosen the epithelial layer without damaging the lenticule—avoid alcohol. Gently elevate the edge of the disk with a fine spatula and tease the disk away from the bed until the foreign body can be reached (Figure 15.143). Avoid handling the tissue edge with forceps of any kind to prevent tearing or fraying. If the disk tends to bend excessively, it will have to be freed up still more. Rarely will it be necessary to remove it completely. Remove the offending material with a smooth, fine-tipped forceps. If the area of elevation is not extensive, no re-suturing will be required but is generally recommended. Patch overnight after administering antibiotic/steroids and possibly a cycloplegic/mydriatic.

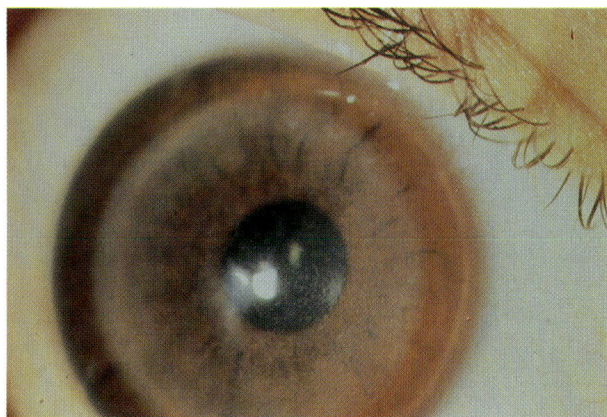

Fig. 15.139 Asceptic necrosis of MKM lenticule. (Courtesy of J.I. Barraquer.)

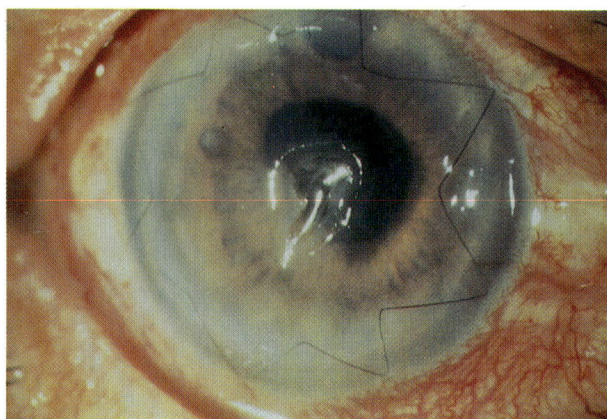

Fig. 15.140 Central necrosis of MKM lenticule following corneal abrasion. (Courtesy of J.I. Barraquer.)

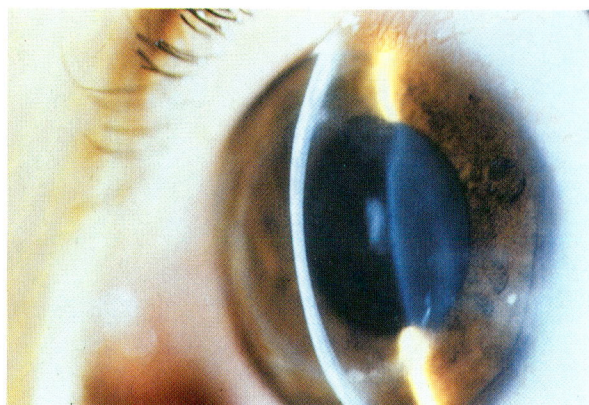

Fig. 15.141 Lenticular clouding following lathing without use of cryopreservative. (Courtesy of J.I. Barraquer.)

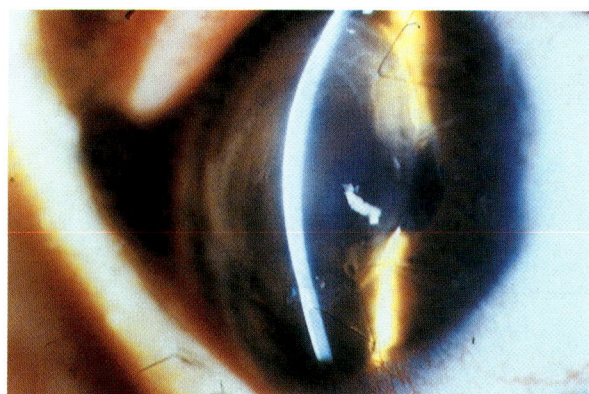

Fig. 15.142 Prolonged freezing (8 min in this case) can lead to prolonged lenticular edema and possible loss of the tissue. (Courtesy of J.I. Barraquer.)

Infection

Fortunately, infection is usually very rare in these cases and manifests—when it occurs—as a clouding within the interface. This can mimic an ingrowth of epithelium and could prove to be a diagnostic dilemma (Figures 15.144 through 15.147). Such an infection is unlikely to be present, however, within the first few days if the recommended post-operative injection of sub-tenons gentamicin has been administered. If infection is suspected, vigorous treatment with broad-spectrum topical antibiotic/steroid drops must be instituted immediately.

Over- or under-correction

The nature of surgery upon living tissue is such that accurate prediction of the outcome is not entirely possible. Therefore, occurrence of over- and under-corrections of the myopia or hyperopia is inevitable.

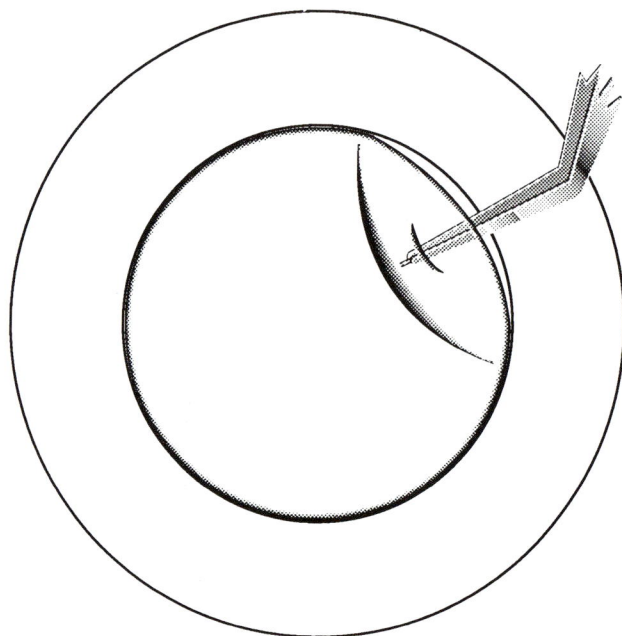

Fig. 15.143 Elevate the edge of the lenticule near the foreign body to be removed.

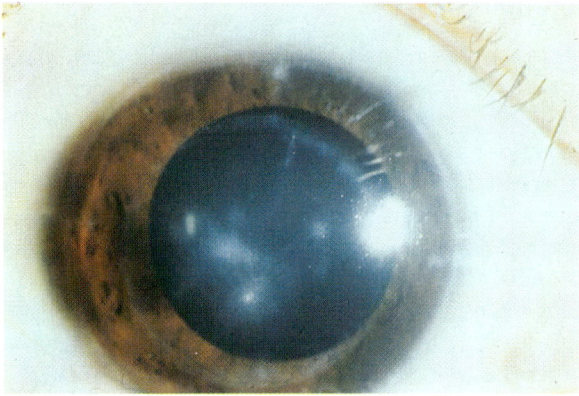

Fig. 15.144 Infection involving lenticule. In the early stages it may be difficult to distinguish from epithelium in the interface. (Courtesy of J.I. Barraquer.)

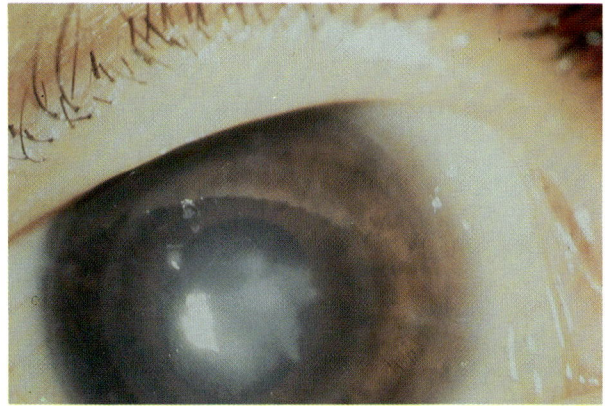

Fig. 15.146 Interface bacterial growth occurring after early contact lens use. (Courtesy of J.I. Barraquer.)

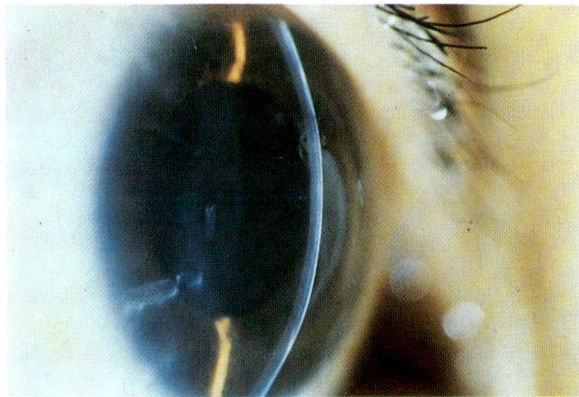

Fig. 15.145 Slit-lamp view of the same eye. (Courtesy of J.I. Barraquer.)

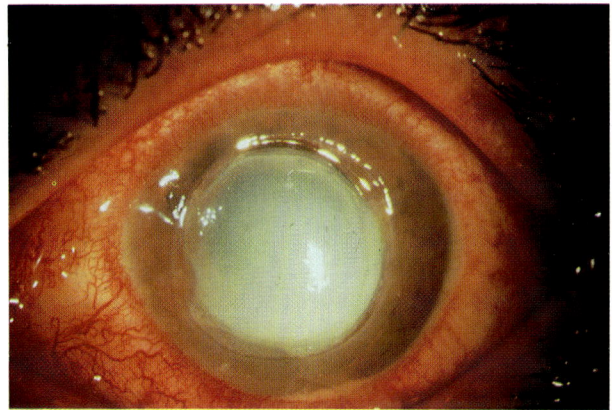

Fig. 15.147 Complete loss of epi-lenticule following infection. (Courtesy of J.I. Barraquer.)

Under-corrections

In keratomileusis. If the residual myopia is less than 5 D and greater than 1 D, RK incisions may be employed to complete the reduction of the correction toward plano. In these cases it is best to wait for at least 4 months to insure stabilization of the residual refractive error—when in doubt, wait it out. When using the calculations, input the original, pre-operative, K-readings (remember that your post-operative K-readings are meaningless). Use the sharpest blade in your armamentarium—preferably a new, double-edged one. However, be advised that incisions through the edge of the lenticule can result in a tissue response similar to that seen when T-cuts join radials (Figure 15.148).

In hyperopic lamellar keratotomy. The solution here really depends upon the degree of residual hyperopia. If it is not very great, the best solution is to do nothing surgically. If greater than 2 D, it is best to wait for at least 6 months and repeat the section at a deeper

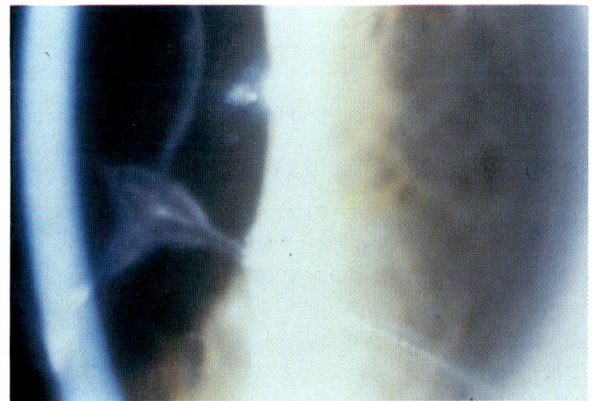

Fig. 15.148 Tissue "melting" at the intersection of RK incisions and lenticular edge. (Courtesy of J.I. Barraquer.)

setting. Be careful when selecting the depth, however, if the section is too deep—myopia of the progressive, possibly never-ending, variety can occur. Additionally, the new resection must be larger in diameter by at least 0.5 mm than the first one; do not attempt to make the new section *inside* the first one.

In epi. If the residual hyperopia is of sufficient magnitude, removal and replacement with an appropriately powered *fresh* epi-lenticule is in order.

Over-corrections

In keratomileusis. These are much more difficult to deal with than under-corrections. If the degree of induced hyperopia is creating difficulties for the patient and spectacles or contact lenses are not an option, it may seem desirable to perform hyperopic lamellar keratotomy. In these cases, at least 6 months must be allowed to elapse to insure that adequate adhesion of the lenticule to the underlying cornea has occurred. Typically, the disk diameter in hyperopic lamellar keratotomy is much smaller than that in keratomileusis and the resultant annulus remaining of the original resection may opacify or part company with the parent cornea. Most over-corrections are of a low order, however; therefore a more viable alternative would be application of a low-power hyperopic epikeratophakia lenticule. This choice is more likely to effect a reduction of the hyperopia and has the advantages that it will overlay and extend beyond the edges of the first resection. Additionally, it is replaceable in the event of difficulty. This latter alternative may not be viable for individual surgeons with no access to either a lathe or source of an appropriate lenticule, therefore it would be prudent to plan for under-correction in subsequent patients. Considering the improved communication and transportation facilities currently available, the enterprising surgeon will no doubt be able to come up with a solution to this dilemma of obtaining epi-lenticules in that event.

In hyperopic lamellar keratotomy. It may seem obvious that this problem is easily corrected with RK. *Beware!* This complication is frequently due to sections that are too deep. Here, the myopia is likely to be progressive. Sufficient time—minimum 9 months—must be allowed to elapse to make sure that progression has stopped. If it does stop, then RK may be able to reduce the myopia to acceptable levels. If the myopia continues to progress, however, the alternative is myopic epikeratophakia, preferably of the wet variety using an MKM-type, meniscus, lenticule. Avoid a PKP unless the induced keratoconus is associated with severe irregular astigmatism. Even in these cases, an epi-keratoplasty can save the day.

In epi. As in under-correction, the choice is removal and replacement of the lenticule.

Summary

While some of these problems may seem formidable, they do not occur with frequency. For example, epithelial ingrowth occurs in about 3% of cases in the author's series. Over-correction is even rarer in hyperopic lamellar keratotomy or keratomileusis. You must be aware that these problems are discussed because they have occurred to someone—they are not theoretic. Therefore, you must be prepared to face them some time in your career as a refractive surgeon. This is why the author has stated that this branch of surgery is not a "sometime thing!" You are either going to devote yourself wholly to it or you are better advised to look elsewhere for "entertainment." This surgery can be a most fulfilling and rewarding challenge. Please give it the attention and respect that it and your patients deserve.

References

1 Bourque LB, Cosand BB, Crews C, Waring GO, Lynn M, Cartwright C. Reported satisfaction, fluctuation of vision, and glare among patients one year after surgery in the Prospective Evaluation of Radial Keratotomy (PERK) study. Arch Ophthalmol 1986; 104:356–363.

2 Steel D, Jestter JV, Salz J *et al.* Modification of corneal curvature following radial keratotomy in primates. Ophthalmology 1981; 88:747–754.

3 Kuster A. Myopieprogression bei Kontaktlinsen und bei Brillentragern in 400 Fallen. [The progression of myopia in wearers of contact lenses and spectacles. 400 cases.] Klin Monatsbl Augenheilkd 1971; 159:213–219.

4 Hemenger RP, Tomlinson A, McDonnell PJ. Explanation for good visual acuity in uncorrected residual hyperopia and presbyopia after radial keratotomy. Invest Ophthalmol Visual Sci 1990; 31:1644–1646.

5 Maguire LJ, Bourne WM. Multifocal lens effect as a complication of radial keratotomy. Refract Corneal Surg 1989; 5: 394–399.

6 Bores L. *Pseudo-accommodation Following Radial Keratotomy.* Quintum Forum, Bogota, Colombia, 1987.

7 Helmholtz H. *Treatise on Physiological Optics*, vol 1, J Southall (transl). Optical Society of America, New York, 1924.

8 Feldman ST, Frucht-Pery J, Weinreb RN, Chayet A, Dreher AW, Brown SI. The effect of increased intraocular pressure on visual acuity and corneal curvature after radial keratotomy. Am J Ophthalmol 1989; 108:126–129.

9 Wyzinski P. Daily refractive changes persisting after radial keratotomy. Am J Ophthalmol 1989; 108:205–206.

10 Kiely PM, Carney LG, Smith G. Diurnal variations of corneal topography and thickness. Am J Optom Physiol Opt 1982; 59:976–982.

11 Santos CR, Waring GO, Lynn MJ *et al.* Morning-to-evening change in refraction, corneal curvature, and visual acuity 2 to 4 years after radial keratotomy in the PERK Study. Ophthalmology 1988; 95:1487–1493.

12 Schanzlin DJ, Santos CR, Waring GO. Diurnal change in refraction, corneal curvature, visual acuity, and intraocular pressure after radial keratotomy in the PERK study. Ophthalmology 1986; 93:167–175.

13 Deitz M, Sanders D, Marks R. Radial keratotomy: an over-

view of the Kansas City study. Ophthalmology 1984; 91:467–478.

14 Fyodorov SN. Surgical correction of myopia and astigmatism. Proceedings of the Keratorefractive Society Meeting 1980.

15 Bates WH. *The Bates Method for Better Eye Sight without Glasses.* Henry Holt, New York, 1943.

16 Waring GO, Lynn MJ, Strahlman ER *et al.* Stability of refraction during four years after radial keratotomy in the prospective evaluation of radial keratotomy study. Am J Ophthalmol 1991; 111:133–144.

17 Sawelson H, Marks RG. Two-year results of radial keratotomy. Arch Ophthalmol 1985; 103:505–510.

18 Rowsey JJ, Balyeat HD. Radial keratotomy: preliminary report of complications. Ophthalm Surg 1982; 13:27.

19 Salz JJ. Multiple complications following radial keratotomy in an elderly patient: a case report. Ophthalm Surg 1985; 16:579–580.

20 McDonnell PJ, Caroline PJ, Salz JJ. Irregular astigmatism after radial and astigmatic keratotomy. Am J Ophthalmol 1989; 107:42–46.

21 Salz JJ, Lee T, Jester JV *et al.* Analysis of incision depth following experimental radial keratotomy. Ophthalmology 1983; 90:655–659.

22 O'Donnell FEJ. Short incision radial keratotomy. J Cataract Refract Surg 1987; 3:102–103.

23 Bores L. Radial keratotomy. I. A safe, effective way to correct a handicap. Surv Ophthalmol 1983; 28:101–105.

24 Deitz M, Sanders D, Raanan M. Progressive hyperopia in radial keratotomy. Long-term follow-up of diamond-knife and metal-blade series. Ophthalmology 1986; 93:1284–1289.

25 Richmond RD. Radial keratotomy as seen through operated eyes: Part II. J Refract Surg 1987; 4:91–95.

26 Richmond RD. Radial keratotomy as seen through operated eyes: Part I. J Refract Surg 1987; 3:22–27.

27 Deitz M, Sanders D. Progressive hyperopia with long-term follow-up of radial keratotomy. Arch Ophthalmol 1985; 103:782–784.

28 Waring GO, Lynn MJ, Culbertson W *et al.* Three-year results of the prospective evaluation of radial keratotomy (PERK) study. Ophthalmology 1987; 94:1339–1354.

29 Lindquist TD, Rubenstein JB, Lindstrom RL. Correction of hyperopia following radial keratotomy: quantification in human cadaver eyes. Ophthalm Surg 1987; 18:432–437.

30 Grady FJ. Hexagonal keratotomy for corneal steepening. Ophthalm Surg 1988; 19:622–623.

31 Jensen RP. Experience with hexagonal keratotomy [letter]. J Cataract Refract Surg 1988; 14:580–581.

32 Schachar RA. Radial thermokeratoplasty. Int Ophthalmol Clin 1991; 31:47–57.

33 Starling JC, Hoffmann RF. A new surgical technique for the correction of hyperopia after radial keratotomy: An experimental model. J Refract Surg 1986; 2:9–14.

34 Bores LD, Myers W, Cowden J. Radial keratotomy: an analysis of the American experience. Ann Ophthalmol 1981; 13:941–948.

35 Gelender H, Flynn HWJ, Mandelbaum SH. Bacterial endophthalmitis resulting from radial keratotomy. Am J Ophthalmol 1982; 93:323–326.

36 Nirankari VS, Katzen LE, Karesh JW, Richards RD, Lakhanpal V. Ongoing prospective clinical study of radial keratotomy. Ophthalmology 1983; 90:637–641.

37 Santos CR. Herpes keratitis after radial keratotomy. Am J Ophthalmol 1982; 93:370.

38 Santos CR. Herpetic corneal ulcer following radial keratotomy. Ann Ophthalmol 1983; 15:82–85.

39 Fyodorov SN, Durnev VV. Operation of dosaged dissection of corneal circular ligament in cases of myopia of mild degree. Ann Ophthalmol 1979; 11:1885–1890.

40 Mandelbaum S, Waring GO, Forster RK, Culbertson WW, Rowsey JJ, Espinal ME. Late development of ulcerative keratitis in radial keratotomy scars. Arch Ophthalmol 1986; 104:1156–1160.

41 O'Day DM, Feman SS, Elliott JH. Visual impairment following radial keratotomy. A cluster of cases. Ophthalmology 1986; 93:319–326.

42 Shivitz IA, Arrowsmith PN. Delayed keratitis after radial keratotomy. Arch Ophthalmol 1986; 104:1153–1155.

43 Stern GA, Weitzenkorn D, Valenti J. Adherence of *Pseudomonas aeruginosa* to the mouse cornea: epithelial vs stromal adherence. Arch Ophthalmol 1982; 100:1956–1958.

44 Steinberg EB, Wilson LA, Waring GO. Stellate iron lines in the corneal epithelium after radial keratotomy. Am J Ophthalmol 1984; 98:416–421.

45 Jester JV, Villasenor RA, Miyashiro J. Epithelial inclusion cysts following radial keratotomy. Arch Ophthalmol 1983; 101:611–615.

46 Perry L, Taylor L. Worsening of myopia following a circular keratotomy. Ophthalm Surg 1982; 13:104–107.

47 Smith RS, Cutro J. Computer analysis of radial keratotomy. CLAO J 1984; 10:241–248.

48 Nelson JD, Williams P, Lindstrom RL, Doughman DJ. Map-fingerprint-dot changes in the corneal epithelial basement membrane following radial keratotomy. Ophthalmology 1985; 92:199–205.

49 McKnight SJ, Fitz J, Giangiacomo J. Corneal rupture following radial keratotomy in cats subjected to BB gun injury. Ophthalm Surg 1988; 19:165–167.

50 Pearlstein ES, Agapitos PJ, Cantrill HL, Holland EJ, Williams P, Lindstrom RL. Ruptured globe after radial keratotomy. Am J Ophthalmol 1988; 106:755–756.

51 McDermott ML, Wilkinson WS, Tukel DB, Madion MP, Cowden JW, Puklin JE. Corneoscleral rupture ten years after radial keratotomy. Am J Ophthalmol 1990; 110:575–577.

52 Bloom HR, Sands J, Schneider D. Corneal rupture from blunt trauma 22 months after radial keratotomy. Refract Corneal Surg 1990; 6:197–199.

53 Zhaboedov G, Bondareva G. Traumatic rupture of the eyeball after radial keratotomy. Vestn Oftalmol 1990; 106:64–65.

54 Binder PS, Waring GO, Arrowsmith PN, Wang C. Histopathology of traumatic corneal rupture after radial keratotomy. Arch Ophthalmol 1988; 106:1584–1590.

55 Forstot SL, Damiano RE. Trauma after radial keratotomy. Ophthalmology 1988; 95:833–835.

56 John ME, Schmitt TE. Traumatic hyphema after radial keratotomy. Ann Ophthalmol 1983; 15:930–932.

57 Spivack LE. Case report: radial keratotomy incisions remain intact despite facial trauma plane crash. J Refract Surg 1987; 3:59–60.

58 McDonnell PJ, Lean JS, Schanzlin DJ. Globe rupture from blunt trauma after hexagonal keratotomy. Am J Ophthalmol 1987; 103:241–242.

59 Larson BC, Kremer FB, Eller AW, Bernardino VBJ. Quantitated trauma following radial keratotomy in rabbits. Ophthalmol 1983; 90:660–667.

60 Luttrull JK, Jester JV, Smith RE. The effect of radial keratotomy on ocular integrity in an animal model. Arch Ophthalmol 1982; 100:319–320.

61 Karr DJ, Grutzmacher RD, Reeh MJ. Radial keratotomy complicated by sterile keratitis and corneal perforation. Histopathologic case report and review of complications. Ophthalmology 1985; 92:1244–1248.

62 Girard LJ, Rodriguez J, Nino N, Wesson M. Delayed wound

healing after radial keratotomy. Am J Ophthalmol 1985; 99: 485–486.

63 Gelender H, Gelber EC. Cataract following radial keratotomy. Arch Ophthalmol 1983; 101:1229–1231.

64 Baldone JA, Franklin RM. Cataract following radial keratotomy. Ann Ophthalmol 1983; 15:416–418.

65 Wharton KR. Corneal stellate iron lines following radial keratotomy. J Am Optom Assoc 1989; 60:362–364.

66 Steinberg EB, Waring GO, Wilson LA. Slitlamp microscopic study of corneal wound healing after radial keratotomy in the PERK study. (AMA Abstracts). Invest Ophthalmol Visual Sci 1985; 26(suppl):203.

67 Waring GO, Steinberg EB, Wilson LA. Slit lamp microscopic appearance of corneal wound healing after radial keratotomy. Am J Ophthalmol 1985; 100:218–224.

68 Koenig SB, McDonald MB, Yamaguchi T, Friedlander M, Ishii Y. Corneal iron lines after refractive keratoplasty. Arch Ophthalmol 1983; 101:1862–1865.

69 Grabner G. Eine neue zentrale, epitheliale Eisenablagerung nach Epikeratophakie bei hohergradiger Myopie. [New central, epithelial iron deposit following epikeratophakia in high-grade myopia.] Klin Monatsbl Augenheilkd 1987; 190: 424–427.

70 Casanovas J, Casanovas R. Les dangers de quelques medications ophthalmologiques recentes. [Dangers of various recent ophthalmologic drugs.] Ann Ocul (Paris) 1969; 202: 1–22.

71 Beasley H, Fraunfelder FT. Retinal detachments and topical ocular miotics. Ophthalmology 1979, 86:95–98.

72 Alpar JJ. Miotics and retinal detachment: a survey and case report. Ann Ophthalmol 1979; 11:395–401.

73 Jindra LF. Blindness following retrobulbar anesthesia for astigmatic keratotomy. Ophthalm Surg 1989; Surg 20:433–435.

74 Schneider ME, Milstein DE, Oyakawa RT, Ober RR, Campo R. Ocular perforation from a retrobulbar injection. Am J Ophthalmol 1988; 106:35–40.

75 Waring GO, Lynn MJ, Fielding B et al. Results of the prospective evaluation of radial keratotomy (PERK) study 4 years after surgery for myopia. Perk Study Group. JAMA 1990; 263:1083–1091.

76 Spigelman AV, Williams PA, Nichols BD, Lindstrom RL. Four incision radial keratotomy. J Cataract Refract Surg 1988; 14: 125–128.

77 Spigelman AV, Williams PA, Lindstrom RL. Further studies of four incision radial keratotomy. Refract Corneal Surg 1989; 5:292–295.

78 Linberg JV, McDonald MB, Safir A, Googe JM. Ptosis following radial keratotomy. Ophthalmology 1986; 93:1509–1512.

Index

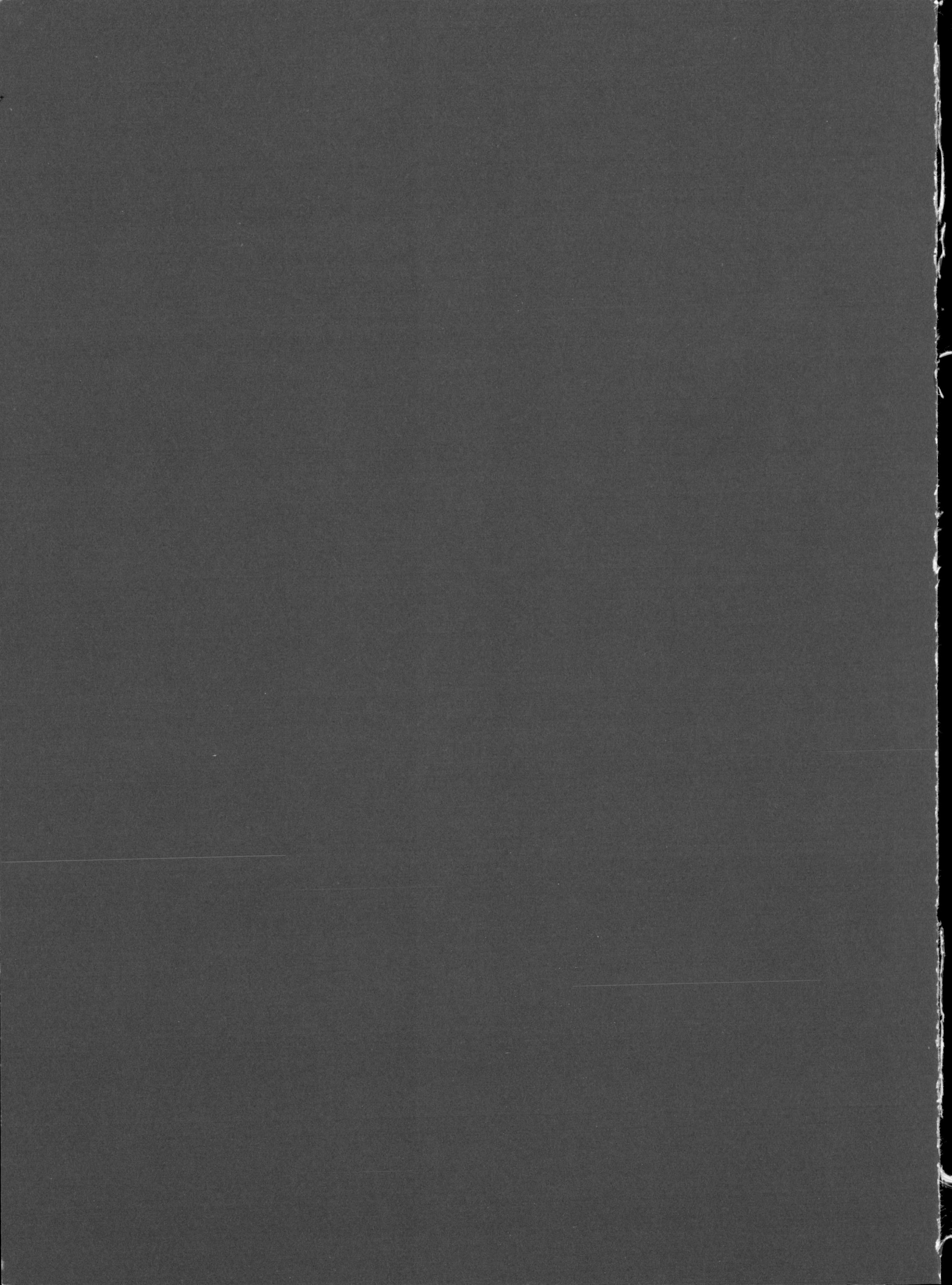